STOELTING'S

Anesthesia and Co-Existing Disease

STOELTING'S

Anesthesia and Co-Existing Disease

FIFTH EDITION

Editors

Roberta L. Hines, MD

Nicholas M. Greene Professor and Chairman,
Department of Anesthesiology,
Yale University School of Medicine,
New Haven, Connecticut

Katherine E. Marschall, MD

Assistant Professor,
Department of Anesthesiology,
Yale University School of Medicine,
New Haven, Connecticut

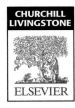

CHURCHILL
LIVINGSTONE

ELSEVIER

CHURCHILL LIVINGSTONE

1600 John F. Kennedy Boulevard
Suite 1800
Philadelphia, PA 19103-2899

STOELTING'S ANESTHESIA AND CO-EXISTING DISEASE, FIFTH EDITION
Copyright © 2008 by Churchill Livingstone, an imprint of Elsevier Inc.

ISBN: 978-1-4160-3998-3

Notice

Knowledge and best practice in this field are constantly changing. As new research and experience broaden our knowledge, changes in practice, treatment and drug therapy may become necessary or appropriate. Readers are advised to check the most current information provided (i) on procedures featured or (ii) by the manufacturer of each product to be administered, to verify the recommended dose or formula, the method and duration of administration, and contraindications. It is the responsibility of the practitioner, relying on their own experience and knowledge of the patient, to make diagnoses, to determine dosages and the best treatment for each individual patient, and to take all appropriate safety precautions. To the fullest extent of the law, neither the Publisher nor the Editors assume any liability for any injury and/or damage to persons or property arising out of or related to any use of the material contained in this book.

The Publisher

Previous editions copyright 2002, 1993, 1988, 1983.

Library of Congress Cataloging-in-Publication Data
Stoelting's anesthesia and co-existing disease. –5th ed. / editors,
Roberta L. Hines, Katherine E. Marschall.
    P. ; cm.
    Rev. ed. of: Anesthesia and co-existing disease / [edited by] Robert K. Stoelting,
Stephen F. Dierdorf. New York: Churchill Livingstone, c2002.
    Includes bibliographical references and index.
    ISBN 978-1-4160-3998-3
1. Anesthesia–Complication. 2. Therapeutics, Surgical. I. Stoelting, Robert K. II. Hines,
Roberta L. III. Marschall, Katherine E. IV. Anesthesia and co-existing disease.
V. Title: Anesthesia and co-existing disease.
    [DNLM: 1. Anesthesia–adverse effects. 2. Anesthesia–methods. 3. Anesthetics–adverse effects. 4. Intraoperative Complication. WO 245 S872 2008]
RD82.5.A53 2008
617.9'6041–dc22

2008000559

Executive Publisher: Natasha Andjelkovic
Developmental Editor: Karen Lynn Carter and Janice Gaillard
Project Manager: Mary Stermel
Design Direction: Steven Stave
Marketing Manager: Catalina Nolte

Printed in the United States of America

Last digit is the print number: 9 8 7 6 5 4 3 2

CONTRIBUTORS

Shamsuddin Akhtar, MD
Assistant Professor, Department of Anesthesiology,
Yale University School of Medicine; Attending Physician,
Yale-New Haven Hospital, New Haven, Connecticut

Michael S. Avidan, MBBCH, FCA
Associate Professor of Anesthesiology and Surgery, Washington
University of St. Louis; Division Chief, CT Anesthesiology and CT
Intensive Care, Barnes-Jewish Hospital, St. Louis, Missouri

Bruno Bissonnette, MD
Professor of Anaesthesia, University of Toronto; Director of
Neurosurgical Anaesthesia, The Hospital for Sick Children,
Toronto, Ontario, Canada

Ferne R. Braveman, MD
Professor of Anesthesiology, Vice-Chair for Clinical Affairs,
Director, Section of Obstetrical Anesthesiology, Co-Director,
Obstetrical Anesthesiology Fellowship Program, Yale University
School of Medicine; Attending Physician, Yale-New Haven
Hospital, New Haven, Connecticut

Susan Garwood, MBCHB
Associate Professor, Department of Anesthesiology,
Yale University School of Medicine; Attending Physician,
Yale-New Haven Hospital, New Haven, Connecticut

Marbelia Gonzalez, MD
Attending Anesthesiologist, Hartford Anesthesiology Associates,
Hartford Hospital, Department of Anesthesiology, Hartford,
Connecticut

Alá Sami Haddadin, MD, FCCP
Assistant Professor of Anesthesiology, Yale University School
of Medicine; Attending Physician, Yale-New Haven Hospital,
New Haven, Connecticut

Adriana Herrera, MD
Assistant Professor, Department of Anesthesiology, Yale
University School of Medicine; Attending Anesthesiologist,
Yale-New Haven Hospital, New Haven, Connecticut

Zoltan G. Hevesi, MD
Associate Professor of Anesthesiology and Surgery, University
of Wisconsin; Medical Director of Transplant Anesthesiology,
University of Wisconsin Hospital and Clinics, Madison, Wisconsin

Roberta L. Hines, MD
Nicholas M. Greene Professor and Chairman, Department of
Anesthesiology, Yale University School of Medicine, New Haven,
Connecticut

Viji Kurup, MD
Assistant Professor, Department of Anesthesiology,
Yale University School of Medicine; Attending Physician,
Yale-New Haven Hospital, New Haven,
Connecticut

William L. Lanier, Jr., MD
Professor of Anesthesiology, Mayo Clinic College of Medicine,
Rochester, Minnesota

Charles Lee, MD
Assistant Professor of Anesthesiology, Loma Linda University
School of Medicine; Director of Acute/Perioperative Pain
Service, Loma Linda University Medical Center, Loma Linda,
California

Igor Luginbuehl, MD
Assistant Professor, University of Toronto; Staff Anesthesiologist,
The Hospital for Sick Children, Toronto, Ontario, Canada

Inna Maranets, MD
Assistant Professor, Department of Anesthesiology,
Yale University School of Medicine; Attending Physician,
Yale-New Haven Hospital, New Haven, Connecticut

Katherine E. Marschall, MD
Assistant Professor, Department of Anesthesiology,
Yale University School of Medicine; Attending Physician,
Yale-New Haven Hospital, New Haven, Connecticut

Linda J. Mason, MD
Professor of Anesthesiology and Pediatrics, Loma Linda University
School of Medicine; Director of Pediatric Anesthesiology,
Loma Linda University Medical Center, Loma Linda,
California

Raj K. Modak, MS, MD
Assistant Professor of Anesthesiology, Yale University School
of Medicine; Attending Physician, Yale-New Haven Hospital,
New Haven, Connecticut

Jeffrey J. Pasternak, MS, MD
Assistant Professor of Anesthesiology, Mayo Clinic College
of Medicine, Rochester, Minnesota

Wanda M. Popescu, MD
Assistant Professor of Anesthesiology, Yale University
School of Medicine; Attending Physician, Yale-New Haven
Hospital, New Haven, Connecticut; Attending Physician,
Veterans Administration Hospital, West Haven,
Connecticut

Christine S. Rinder, MD
Associate Professor of Anesthesiology, Yale University School of Medicine; Attending Physician, Yale-New Haven Hospital, New Haven, Connecticut

Jeffrey J. Schwartz, MD
Associate Professor, Yale University School of Medicine; Attending Physician, Yale-New Haven Hospital, New Haven, Connecticut

Hossam Tantawy, MD
Assistant Professor, Department of Anesthesiology, Yale University School of Medicine; Attending Physician, Yale-New Haven Hospital, New Haven, Connecticut

Nalini Vadivelu, MD
Associate Professor, Department of Anesthesiology, Yale University School of Medicine; Attending Physician, Yale-New Haven Hospital, New Haven, Connecticut

Russell T. Wall, III, MD
Professor of Anesthesiology, Associate Dean, Georgetown University School of Medicine; Vice-Chair and Program Director, Department of Anesthesiology, Georgetown University Hopsital, Washington, DC

Matthew C. Wallace, MD
Fellow in Cardiothoracic Anesthesiology, Yale University School of Medicine, Department of Anesthesiology, New Haven, Connecticut

Kelley Teed Watson, MD
Assistant Clinical Professor, Yale University School of Medicine, New Haven, Connecticut; Cardiac Anesthesiologist, Carolina Cardiac Surgery at Self Regional Healthcare, Greenwood, South Carolina

PREFACE

In 1983, the first edition of *Anesthesia and Co-Existing Disease* was published with the stated goal "to provide a concise description of the pathophysiology of disease states and their medical management that is relevant to the care of the patient in the perioperative period." The result was a very useful basic reference text and review guide that continued through three more editions and became one of those exceptional works that is a "must have" in every anesthesiologist's personal library.

This fifth edition of *Anesthesia and Co-Existing Disease* marks a turning point and yet a continuation in the history of this book. Drs. Robert K. Stoelting and Stephen F. Dierdorf have passed the editorial "baton" to us. Together with a group of gifted medical authors, we have produced this latest edition. As with the previous editions, our goal has been to provide readers with a current and concise description of the pathophysiology of co-existing diseases, current treatment of these entities, and the impact that such diseases might have on the management of anesthesia. Common diseases receive more attention, but uncommon diseases, especially those with unique features that could be of significance in the perioperative period, are also included. References are made to the most up-to-date diagnostics, guidelines, and recommendations for medical management. There is liberal use of figures and tables to clarify the text. A consistency in writing style was sought to make this multiauthored book read as though written by only a few individuals. We are honored to have had the opportunity to carry on the tradition of this legendary work and we hope that Drs. Stoelting and Dierdorf are pleased with our efforts.

The editors wish to recognize the invaluable secretarial assistance of Gail Norup in the preparation of this manuscript.

Roberta L. Hines, MD
Katherine E. Marschall, MD

CONTENTS

Ischemic Heart Disease

Shamsuddin Akhtar

Ischemic heart disease is present in an estimated 30% of patients who undergo surgery in the United States. The aging of the population increases the likelihood that patients undergoing surgery will have co-existing ischemic heart disease. Angina pectoris, acute myocardial infarction, and sudden death are often the first manifestations of this disease. Cardiac dysrhythmias are the major cause of sudden death. The two most important risk factors for the development of coronary artery atherosclerosis are male gender and increasing age (**Table 1-1**). Additional risk factors include hypercholesterolemia, hypertension, cigarette smoking, diabetes mellitus, obesity, a sedentary lifestyle, and a family history of premature development of ischemic heart disease. Psychological factors such as type A personality and stress have also been implicated. Patients with ischemic heart disease can present with chronic stable angina or with acute coronary syndrome. The latter includes

TABLE 1-1 Risk Factors for Development of Ischemic Heart Disease

Male gender
Increasing age
Hypercholesterolemia
Hypertension
Cigarette smoking
Diabetes mellitus
Obesity
Sedentary lifestyle
Genetic factors/family history

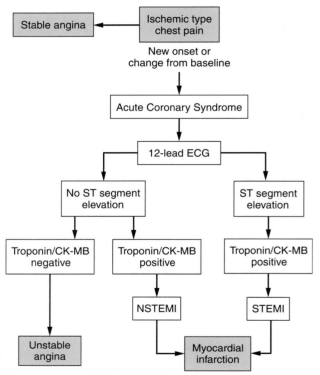

Figure 1-1 • Terminology of acute coronary syndrome. CK-MB, creatine kinase, myocardial bound isoenzyme; ECG, electrocardiogram; NSTEMI, non–ST elevation myocardial infarction; STEMI, ST elevation myocardial infarction. *(Adapted from Alpert JS, Thygesen K, Antman E, Bassand JP: Myocardial infarction redefined—a consensus document of The Joint European Society of Cardiology/American College of Cardiology Committee for the redefinition of myocardial infarction. J Am Coll Cardiol 2000;36:959–969.)*

ST elevation myocardial infarction (STEMI) on presentation and unstable angina/non–ST elevation myocardial infarction (UA/NSTEMI) (**Fig. 1-1**).

ANGINA PECTORIS

The coronary artery circulation normally supplies sufficient blood flow to meet the oxygen demands of the myocardium in response to widely varying workloads. An imbalance between

coronary blood flow (oxygen supply) and myocardial oxygen consumption (oxygen demand) can precipitate ischemia, which frequently manifests as angina pectoris. Stable angina typically develops in the setting of partial occlusion or chronic narrowing of a segment of coronary artery. When the imbalance between myocardial oxygen supply and demand becomes extreme, congestive heart failure, electrical instability with dysrhythmias, and myocardial infarction (MI) can result. Angina pectoris reflects intracardiac release of adenosine and bradykinin during ischemia. These substances stimulate cardiac chemical and mechanosensitive receptors whose afferent neurons converge with upper thoracic sympathetic fibers and other somatic nerve fibers in the spinal cord and ultimately produce thalamic and cortical stimulation that results in the typical chest pain of angina pectoris. These substances also slow atrioventricular nodal conduction and decrease contractility, thereby improving the balance between myocardial oxygen demand and supply. Atherosclerosis is the most common cause of impaired coronary blood flow resulting in angina pectoris.

Diagnosis

Angina pectoris is typically described as retrosternal chest discomfort, pain, pressure, or heaviness. The chest discomfort often radiates to the neck, left shoulder, left arm, or jaw and occasionally to the back or down both arms. Angina may also be perceived as epigastric discomfort resembling indigestion. Some patients describe angina as shortness of breath, mistaking a sense of chest constriction as dyspnea. The need to take a deep breath, rather than to breathe rapidly, often identifies shortness of breath as an anginal equivalent. Angina pectoris usually lasts several minutes and is crescendo/decrescendo in nature; a sharp pain that lasts only a few seconds or a dull ache that lasts for hours is rarely caused by myocardial ischemia. Physical exertion, emotional tension, and cold weather may induce angina; rest and/or nitroglycerin relieve it. Chronic stable angina refers to chest pain or discomfort that does not change appreciably in frequency or severity over 2 months or longer. Unstable angina by contrast is defined as angina at rest, angina of new onset, or an increase in the severity or frequency of previously stable angina. Noncardiac chest pain is often exacerbated by chest wall movement and associated with tenderness over the involved area, which is often a costochondral junction. Sharp retrosternal pain exacerbated by deep breathing, coughing, or change in body position suggests pericarditis. Esophageal spasm can produce severe substernal pressure that may be confused with angina pectoris and may be relieved by administration of nitroglycerin.

Electrocardiography

Standard Electrocardiography With myocardial ischemia, the standard 12-lead electrocardiogram (ECG) demonstrates ST segment *depression* (characteristic of subendocardial ischemia) that coincides in time with anginal chest pain. This may be accompanied by transient symmetrical T-wave inversion. Patients with chronically inverted T waves resulting from previous MI may manifest a return of the T waves to the normal upright position ("pseudonormalization") during myocardial ischemia.

Variant angina, that is, angina that results from coronary vasospasm rather than occlusive coronary artery disease, is diagnosed by ST elevation during an episode of angina pectoris.

Exercise Electrocardiography Exercise electrocardiography is useful for detecting signs of myocardial ischemia and establishing their relationship to chest pain. The appearance of a new murmur of mitral regurgitation or a *decrease* in blood pressure during exercise adds to the diagnostic value of this test. Exercise testing is not always feasible either because of the inability of a patient to exercise or the presence of conditions that interfere with interpretation of the exercise ECG (paced rhythm, left ventricular hypertrophy, digitalis administration, or preexcitation syndrome). Contraindications to exercise stress testing include severe aortic stenosis, severe hypertension, acute myocarditis, uncontrolled heart failure, and infective endocarditis.

The exercise ECG is most likely to indicate myocardial ischemia when there is at least 1 mm of horizontal or downsloping ST-segment depression during or within 4 minutes after exercise. The greater the degree of ST-segment depression is, the greater the likelihood of significant coronary artery disease. When the ST-segment abnormality is associated with angina pectoris and occurs during the early stages of exercise and persists for several minutes after exercise, significant coronary artery disease is very likely. Exercise electrocardiography is less accurate but more cost effective than imaging tests for detecting ischemic heart disease. A negative stress test does not exclude the presence of coronary artery disease, but it makes the likelihood of three-vessel or left main coronary disease extremely low.

Noninvasive Imaging Tests

Many patients who are at increased risk of coronary events cannot exercise because of peripheral vascular or musculoskeletal disease, deconditioning, or dyspnea on exertion. Noninvasive imaging tests for the detection of ischemic heart disease are usually recommended when exercise electrocardiography is not possible or interpretation of ST-segment changes would be difficult. Administration of atropine, infusion of dobutamine, or institution of artificial cardiac pacing produces a rapid heart rate to create cardiac stress. Alternatively, cardiac stress can be produced by administering a coronary vasodilator such as adenosine or dipyridamole. These drugs dilate normal coronary arteries but evoke minimal or no change in the diameter of atherosclerotic coronary arteries. After cardiac stress is induced by these interventions, either echocardiography to assess myocardial function or radionuclide tracer scanning to assess myocardial perfusion is performed.

Echocardiography Echocardiographic wall motion analysis is performed immediately after stressing the heart. An intravenous echocardiographic contrast dye can improve the accuracy of stress echocardiography. The ventricular wall motion abnormalities induced by stress correspond to the site of myocardial ischemia, thereby localizing the obstructive coronary lesion. In contrast, exercise electrocardiography can indicate the presence of ischemic heart disease but does not reliably predict the location of the obstructive coronary lesion.

Nuclear Stress Imaging Nuclear stress imaging is useful for assessing coronary perfusion. It has greater sensitivity than exercise testing for detection of ischemic heart disease. It can define vascular regions in which stress-induced coronary blood flow is limited and can estimate left ventricular systolic size and function. Tracers (e.g., thallium, technetium) can be detected over the myocardium by single-photon emission computed tomography techniques. A significant coronary obstructive lesion causes less blood flow and thus less tracer activity. Exercise increases the difference in tracer activity between normal and underperfused regions because coronary blood flow increases markedly with exercise except in those regions distal to a coronary artery obstruction. Imaging is carried out in two phases: first immediately after cessation of exercise to detect regional ischemia and then 4 hours later to detect reversible ischemia. Areas of persistently absent uptake signify old MI. The size of the perfusion abnormality is the most important indicator of the significance of the coronary artery disease detected.

Electron Beam Computed Tomography Calcium deposition occurs in atherosclerotic vessels. Coronary artery calcification can be detected by electron beam computed tomography. Although the sensitivity of electron beam computed tomography is high, it is not a very specific test and yields many false-positive results. Its routine use has not been recommended.

Coronary Angiography Coronary angiography provides the best information about the condition of the coronary arteries. It is indicated in patients who continue to have angina pectoris despite maximal medical therapy, in those who are being considered for coronary revascularization, and for the definitive diagnosis of coronary disease in individuals whose occupations could place others at risk (e.g., airline pilots). Coronary angiography is also useful for establishing the diagnosis of nonatherosclerotic coronary artery disease such as coronary artery spasm. Surgical coronary bypass is most effective when a diseased coronary artery is of reasonable size, has a high-grade proximal stenosis, and is free of significant distal plaques. The most suitable atherosclerotic lesion for coronary angioplasty is discrete, concentric, proximal, noncalcified, and less than 5 mm in length.

Coronary artery bypass surgery is likely to improve survival in patients with multivessel coronary disease and an ejection fraction of less than 40%. The presence of hypokinetic or akinetic areas of the left ventricle connote a poor prognosis. Extensive myocardial fibrosis from a previous MI is unlikely to be improved by coronary artery bypass grafting (CABG). However, some patients with ischemic heart disease have chronically impaired myocardial function ("hibernating myocardium") that demonstrates improvement in contractility following surgical revascularization.

The important prognostic determinants in patients with coronary artery disease are the anatomic extent of the atherosclerotic disease as revealed by coronary angiography, the state of left ventricular function (ejection fraction) and the stability of coronary plaque. Left main coronary artery disease is the most dangerous anatomic lesion and is associated with an unfavorable prognosis with medical therapy. Greater than 50% stenosis of the left main coronary artery is associated with a mortality rate of 15% per year. Coronary angiography cannot predict which plaques are most likely to rupture and initiate acute coronary syndromes. Vulnerable plaques, that is, those most likely to rupture and form an occlusive thrombus have a thin fibrous cap and a large lipid core containing a large number of macrophages. The presence of vulnerable plaque predicts a greater risk of MI regardless of the degree of coronary artery stenosis. Indeed, UA and acute MI most often result from rupture of a plaque that had produced less than 50% stenosis. Currently, there is no satisfactory test to measure the stability of plaques.

Treatment

Treatment of ischemic heart disease includes lifestyle modification, pharmacologic therapy, and revascularization. Treatment that prolongs life has the highest priority. So surgical revascularization (CABG) is recommended for significant left main or three-vessel coronary artery obstruction. In patients with stable angina pectoris and one- or two-vessel coronary disease, medical therapy, percutaneous transluminal coronary angioplasty (PTCA) with or without stent placement, or CABG may be used.

Lifestyle Modification

The progression of atherosclerosis may be slowed by cessation of smoking; maintenance of an ideal body weight through a low-fat, low-cholesterol diet; regular aerobic exercise; and treatment of hypertension. Lowering the low-density lipoprotein level by diet and/or drugs such as statins is associated with a substantial decrease in the risk of death due to cardiac events. Drug treatment is appropriate when the low-density lipoprotein cholesterol level exceeds 130 mg/dL. The goal of treatment is a decrease in low-density lipoprotein to less than 100 mg/dL. Patients with ischemic heart disease may benefit from further low-density lipoprotein lowering, which can be achieved by a combination of diet and statin therapy.

Hypertension increases the risk of coronary events as a result of direct vascular injury, left ventricular hypertrophy, and increased myocardial oxygen demand. Lowering the blood pressure from hypertensive levels to normal levels decreases the risk of MI, congestive heart failure, and cerebrovascular accident. In combination with lifestyle modifications, β-blockers and calcium channel blockers are especially useful for managing hypertension in patients with angina pectoris. If left ventricular dysfunction accompanies hypertension, an angiotensin-converting enzyme (ACE) inhibitor or an angiotensin receptor blocker is recommended.

Medical Treatment of Myocardial Ischemia

Antiplatelet drugs, β-blockers, calcium channel blockers, nitrates, and ACE inhibitors are used in the medical treatment of angina pectoris.

Antiplatelet Drugs Low-dose aspirin therapy (75–325 mg/day) decreases the risk of cardiac events in patients with stable or unstable angina pectoris and is recommended for all patients with ischemic heart disease. Clopidogrel (Plavix) and ticlopidine (Ticlid) effectively inhibit platelet aggregation by blocking adenosine diphosphate receptors. Clopidogrel can be used in patients who have a contraindication to or are intolerant of aspirin. Platelet glycoprotein IIb/IIIa receptor antagonists (abciximab, eptifibatide, tirofiban) inhibit platelet adhesion, activation, and aggregation. Administration of antiplatelet drugs is particularly useful after placement of an intracoronary stent.

β-Blockers β-Blockers are the principal drug treatment for patients with angina pectoris. Long-term administration of β-blockers decreases the risk of death and myocardial reinfarction in patients who have had a MI, presumably by decreasing myocardial oxygen demand. This benefit is present even in patients in whom β-blockers were traditionally thought to be contraindicated (congestive heart failure, pulmonary disease, advanced age). Drug-induced blockade of β_1-adrenergic receptors (atenolol, metoprolol, acebutolol, bisoprolol) results in heart rate slowing and decreased myocardial contractility that are greater during activity than at rest. The result is a decrease in myocardial oxygen demand with a subsequent decrease in ischemic events during exertion. The decrease in heart rate also increases the length of diastole and thereby coronary perfusion time. β_2-adrenergic blockade, (propranolol, nadolol) could increase the risk of bronchospasm in patients with reactive airway disease. Despite differences between β_1 and β_2 effects, all β-blockers seem to be equally effective in the treatment of angina pectoris. β-Blockers are contraindicated in the presence of severe bradycardia, sick sinus syndrome, severe reactive airway disease, atrioventricular heart block, and uncontrolled congestive heart failure. Diabetes mellitus is not a contraindication to β-blocker therapy, although these drugs may mask signs of hypoglycemia. The most common side effects of β-blocker therapy are fatigue and insomnia.

Calcium Channel Blockers Long-acting calcium channel blockers are comparable to β-blockers in relieving anginal pain. However, short-acting calcium channel blockers such as verapamil and diltiazem are not. Calcium channel blockers are uniquely effective in decreasing the frequency and severity of angina pectoris due to coronary artery spasm (Prinzmetal's or variant angina). They are not as effective as β-blockers in decreasing the incidence of myocardial reinfarction. The effectiveness of calcium channel blockers is due to their ability to decrease vascular smooth muscle tone, dilate coronary arteries, decrease myocardial contractility and oxygen consumption, and decrease arterial pressure. Many calcium channel blockers such as amlodipine, nicardipine, isradipine, felodipine, and long-acting nifedipine are potent vasodilators and are useful in treating both hypertension and angina. Calcium channel blockers are contraindicated in patients with severe congestive heart failure. Common side effects of calcium channel blocker therapy are hypotension, peripheral edema, and headache. They must be used cautiously in the presence of β-blockers because both classes of drugs have significant depressant effects on heart rate and myocardial contractility.

Nitrates Organic nitrates decrease the frequency, duration, and severity of angina pectoris and increase the amount of exercise needed before the onset of ST-segment depression. Nitrates dilate coronary arteries and collateral blood vessels and thereby improve coronary blood flow. Nitrates also decrease peripheral vascular resistance, which decreases left ventricular afterload and myocardial oxygen consumption. The venodilating effect of nitrates decreases venous return and hence left ventricular preload and myocardial oxygen consumption. Nitrates are contraindicated in the presence of hypertrophic obstructive cardiomyopathy and severe aortic stenosis and should not be used within 24 hours of sildenafil (Viagra), tadalafil (Cialis), or vardenafil (Levitra) because this combination may produce severe hypotension. Administration of sublingual nitroglycerin by tablet or spray produces prompt relief of angina pectoris. The most common side effect of nitrate treatment is headache. Hypotension may occur after nitrate administration in hypovolemic patients. For long-term therapy, long-acting nitrate preparations (isosorbide, nitroglycerin ointment or patches) are equally effective. The therapeutic value of organic nitrates is compromised by the development of tolerance. To avoid nitrate tolerance, a daily 8- to 12-hour interval free of nitrate exposure is recommended.

Angiotensin-Converting Enzyme Inhibitors Excessive angiotensin II plays a significant role in the pathophysiology of cardiac disorders. It can lead to development of myocardial hypertrophy, interstitial myocardial fibrosis, increased coronary vasoconstriction, and endothelial dysfunction. Angiotensin II also promotes inflammatory responses and atheroma formation. ACE inhibitors are important not only in the treatment of heart failure but also in the treatment of hypertension and in cardiovascular protection. ACE inhibitors benefit patients with evidence of vascular disease or diabetes plus one other cardiovascular risk factor even if there is no evidence of left ventricular dysfunction. Therefore, an ACE inhibitor is recommended for all patients with coronary artery disease, especially those with hypertension, left ventricular dysfunction, or diabetes. Angiotensin receptor blockers might offer similar benefits, but this has not yet been shown. Contraindications to ACE inhibitor use include documented intolerance or allergy, hyperkalemia, bilateral renal artery stenosis, and renal failure.

Revascularization Revascularization by CABG or percutaneous coronary intervention (PCI) with or without placement of intracoronary stents is indicated when optimal medical therapy fails to control angina pectoris. Revascularization is also indicated for specific anatomic lesions (left main stenosis of > 70%, combinations of two- or three-vessel disease that include a proximal left anterior descending artery stenosis of > 70%) and evidence of impaired left ventricular contractility (decreased ejection fraction). The use of coronary artery stents with PCI decreases the rate of coronary restenosis and the need for a repeat intervention.

ACUTE CORONARY SYNDROME

Acute coronary syndrome represents a hypercoagulable state. Focal disruption of an atheromatous plaque triggers the coagulation cascade with subsequent generation of thrombin and partial or complete occlusion of the coronary artery. Imbalance of myocardial oxygen supply and demand leads to ischemic chest pain. Patients who present with ischemic chest pain can be categorized based on a 12-lead ECG. Patients with ST elevation at presentation are considered to have STEMI. Patients who present with ST-segment depression or nonspecific changes on the ECG can be further categorized based on the levels of cardiac specific troponins or CK-MB. Elevation of cardiac specific biomarkers in this situation indicates NSTEMI. If cardiac specific biomarkers are normal, then UA is present (see Fig. 1-1) STEMI and UA/NSTEMI require different management and have different prognostic implications. Many more patients present with UA/NSTEMI than with STEMI.

ST Elevation Myocardial Infarction

Mortality due to acute MI remains significant, and one in 25 patients who survive hospitalization will die within 1 year. Overall early in-hospital mortality has declined significantly, undoubtedly due to early therapeutic interventions such as angioplasty, thrombolysis, aspirin, heparin, and statin therapy. Coronary angiography has documented that nearly all MIs are caused by thrombotic occlusion of a coronary artery.

Long-term prognosis of an acute MI is determined principally by the severity of left ventricular dysfunction, the presence and degree of residual ischemia, and the potential for malignant ventricular dysrhythmias. Most deaths during the first year after hospital discharge occur within the first 3 months. Ventricular function can be substantially improved during the weeks following an acute MI, particularly in patients in whom early reperfusion was achieved. Therefore, measurement of ventricular function 2 to 3 months after MI is a more accurate predictor of long-term prognosis than measurement of ventricular function during the acute phase of an infarction.

Pathophysiology

Atherosclerosis is being increasingly recognized as an inflammatory disease. The presence of inflammatory cells in atherosclerotic plaques suggests that inflammation is important in the cascade of events leading to plaque rupture. Indeed, serum markers of inflammation, such as C-reactive protein and fibrinogen, are increased in those at greatest risk of development of coronary artery disease.

STEMI occurs when coronary blood flow decreases abruptly. This decrease in blood flow is attributable to acute thrombus formation at a site when an atherosclerotic plaque fissures, ruptures, or ulcerates. This creates a local environment that favors thrombogenesis. Typically, "vulnerable" plaques, that is, those with rich lipid cores and thin fibrous caps, are most prone to rupture.

A platelet monolayer forms at the site of ruptured plaque and various chemical mediators such as collagen, adenosine diphosphate, epinephrine, and serotonin stimulate platelet aggregation. The potent vasoconstrictor thromboxane A_2 is released, further compromising coronary blood flow. Glycoprotein IIb/IIIa receptors on the platelets are activated, which enhances the ability of platelets to interact with adhesive proteins and other platelets and causes growth and stabilization of the thrombus. Further activation of coagulation leads to strengthening of the thrombus by fibrin deposition. This makes the clot more resistant to thrombolysis. It is rather paradoxical that plaques that rupture and lead to acute coronary occlusion are rarely of a size that causes significant coronary obstruction. By contrast, flow-restrictive plaques that produce angina pectoris and stimulate development of collateral circulation are less likely to rupture. Rarely, STEMI develops as a result of acute coronary spasm or coronary artery embolization.

Diagnosis

Diagnosis of acute MI requires the presence of at least two of these three criteria: (1) chest pain, (2) serial electrocardiographic changes indicative of MI, and (3) increase and decrease of serum cardiac enzymes. Almost two thirds of patients describe new-onset angina pectoris or a change in anginal pattern during the 30 days preceding an acute MI. Pain is more severe than the previous angina pectoris and does not resolve with rest. Other potential causes of severe chest pain (pulmonary embolism, aortic dissection, spontaneous pneumothorax, pericarditis, cholecystitis) should be considered. In approximately one fourth of patients, especially in the elderly and in those with diabetes, there is no or only mild pain at the time of MI.

On physical examination, patients typically appear anxious, pale, and diaphoretic. Sinus tachycardia is usually present. Hypotension caused by left or right ventricular dysfunction or cardiac dysrhythmias may be present. Rales represent congestive heart failure due to left ventricular dysfunction. A cardiac murmur may indicate ischemic mitral regurgitation.

Laboratory Studies Troponin is a cardiac-specific protein and biochemical marker for acute MI. An increase in the circulating concentration of troponin occurs early after myocardial injury. Cardiac troponins (troponin T or I) increase within 4 hours after myocardial injury and remain elevated for 7 to 10 days. When used together, elevated troponin levels and electrocardiography are powerful predictors of adverse cardiac events in patients with anginal pain. Troponin is more specific than CK-MB for determining myocardial injury.

Imaging Studies Patients with typical ECG evidence of acute MI do not require evaluation with echocardiography. However, echocardiography is useful in patients with left bundle branch block or an abnormal ECG (but without ST-segment elevation) in whom the diagnosis of acute MI is uncertain. Echocardiography will demonstrate regional wall motion abnormalities in most patients with acute MI. The time required to perform myocardial perfusion imaging with thallium and the inability to differentiate between new and old MI limits the utility of radionuclide imaging in the early diagnosis of acute MI.

Treatment

Early treatment of acute MI reduces morbidity and mortality. Initial steps include evaluation of hemodynamic stability, 12-lead ECG, and administration of oxygen to all patients suspected of acute MI. Pain relief, usually provided by intravenous morphine and/or sublingual nitroglycerin, is necessary to reduce catecholamine release and the resultant increase in myocardial oxygen requirements. Aspirin (or clopidogrel for those intolerant of aspirin) is administered to decrease further thrombus formation. The primary aim in management of STEMI is to reestablish blood flow in the obstructed coronary artery as soon as possible. This can be achieved by reperfusion therapy or coronary angioplasty with or without an intracoronary stent.

Reperfusion Therapy Thrombolytic therapy with streptokinase, tissue plasminogen activator, reteplase, or tenecteplase should be initiated within 30 to 60 minutes of hospital arrival. Thrombolytic therapy restores normal antegrade blood flow in the occluded coronary artery. Resolution of clot by thrombolytic therapy becomes much more difficult if therapy is delayed. The most feared complication of thrombolytic therapy is intracranial hemorrhage. This is most likely in elderly patients (older than 75 years of age) and those with uncontrolled hypertension. Patients with gastrointestinal bleeding and recent surgery are also at increased risk of bleeding complications. Thrombolytic therapy is *not* recommended in patients with UA/NSTEMI.

Direct Coronary Angioplasty Coronary angioplasty may be preferable to thrombolytic therapy for restoring flow to an occluded coronary artery if the resources are available. Ideally angioplasty should be performed within 90 minutes of arrival at the health care facility and within 12 hours of symptom onset. It is the modality of choice in patients with contraindication to thrombolytic therapy, severe heart failure, and/or pulmonary edema. About 5% of patients with acute MI who undergo immediate PCI require emergency cardiac surgery because of failed angioplasty or because coronary artery anatomy precluded PCI. The combined use of intracoronary stents and a platelet glycoprotein IIb/IIIa inhibitor during emergency PCI provides the maximum chance of achieving normal antegrade coronary blood flow, and this therapy decreases the need for subsequent revascularization procedures.

Coronary Artery Bypass Graft Surgery CABG can restore blood flow in an occluded coronary artery, but reperfusion can be achieved more promptly with thrombolytic therapy or coronary angioplasty. Emergency CABG is usually reserved for patients in whom angiography reveals coronary anatomy that precludes PCI, patients with a failed angioplasty and those with evidence of infarction-related ventricular septal defect or mitral regurgitation. Patients with ST-segment elevation who develop cardiogenic shock, left bundle branch block, or posterior MI within 36 hours of an acute MI are also candidates for early revascularization. Mortality from CABG is significant for the first 3 to 7 days after an acute MI.

Adjunctive Medical Therapy Intravenous heparin therapy is commonly administered for 24 to 48 hours after thrombolytic therapy to decrease thrombus regeneration. A disadvantage of unfractionated heparin use is the variability in dose response due to its binding with plasma proteins other than antithrombin. Low molecular weight heparin provides a more predictable pharmacologic profile, long plasma half-life, and a more practical means of administration (subcutaneous), without the need to monitor the activated partial thromboplastin time. Thus, low molecular weight heparin is an excellent alternative to unfractionated heparin. Direct thrombin inhibitors such as bivalirudin can be used in patients with a history of heparin-induced thrombocytopenia.

Administration of β-blockers is associated with a significant decrease in early (in-hospital) and long-term mortality and myocardial reinfarction. Early administration of β-blockers can decrease infarct size by decreasing heart rate, blood pressure, and myocardial contractility. In the absence of specific contraindications, it is recommended that *all* patients receive intravenous β-blockers as early as possible after an acute MI. β-Blocker therapy should be continued indefinitely.

All patients with a large anterior wall MI, clinical evidence of left ventricular failure, ejection fraction less than 40%, or diabetes should be treated with ACE inhibitors or an angiotensin II receptor blocker such as valsartan if they are intolerant of ACE inhibitors.

In the absence of ventricular dysrhythmias, prophylactic administration of lidocaine or other antidysrhythmic drugs is not recommended. Calcium channel blockers should not be administered routinely but should be reserved for patients with persistent myocardial ischemia despite optimal use of aspirin, β-blockers, nitrate therapy, and intravenous heparin. Glycemic control is considered part of standard care in diabetics with acute MI. Routine administration of magnesium is not recommended, but magnesium therapy is indicated in patients with torsade de pointes ventricular tachycardia. Statins have strong immune-modulating effects and should be started as soon as possible after MI, especially in patients on long-term statin therapy.

Unstable Angina/Non–ST Elevation Myocardial Infarction

UA/NSTEMI results from a reduction in myocardial oxygen supply. Typically, rupture or erosion of an atherosclerotic coronary plaque leads to thrombosis, inflammation, and vasoconstriction. Most culprit arteries have less than 50% stenosis. Embolization of platelets and clot fragments into the coronary microvasculature leads to microcirculatory ischemia and infarction and results in elevation of cardiac biomarkers. Conditions that increase myocardial oxygen demand such as thyrotoxicosis, sepsis, fever, tachycardia, anemia, and cocaine and amphetamine use may lead to UA/NSTEMI.

Diagnosis

UA/NSTEMI has three principal presentations: angina at rest (usually lasting less than 20 minutes), chronic angina pectoris that becomes more frequent and more easily provoked, and new-onset angina, which is severe, prolonged, or disabling. UA/NSTEMI can also present with hemodynamic instability or congestive heart failure. Signs of congestive heart failure (S_3 gallop, jugular venous distention, pulmonary rales, peripheral edema) or ischemia-induced papillary muscle dysfunction causing acute mitral regurgitation may be evident. Significant ST-segment depression in two or more contiguous leads and/or deep symmetrical T-wave inversions, especially in the setting of chest pain, is highly consistent with a diagnosis of myocardial ischemia and UA/NSTEMI. Elevation of cardiac biomarkers, troponins, and/or CK-MB establishes the diagnosis of acute MI (see Fig. 1-1).

Treatment

Management of UA/NSTEMI is directed at decreasing myocardial oxygen demand. Bed rest, supplemental oxygen, analgesia, and β-blocker therapy are indicated. Sublingual or intravenous nitroglycerin may improve myocardial oxygen supply. Aspirin or clopidogrel and 48 hours of intravenous heparin or subcutaneous low molecular weight heparin are strongly recommended to decrease further thrombus formation. Older age (older than 65 years of age), positive cardiac biomarkers, rales, hypotension, tachycardia, and decreased left ventricular function (ejection fraction < 40%) are associated with an increased mortality. Patients at high risk (recurrent ischemia or angina at rest, heart failure, hemodynamic instability, sustained ventricular tachycardia, PCI within the past 6 months, previous CABG, elevated troponins, angina at low-level activity) are considered for early invasive evaluation, which includes coronary angiography and revascularization by PCI or CABG, if needed. Patients at lower risk are treated medically and undergo stress testing at a later date. Cardiac angiography is usually considered for patients who demonstrate significant ischemia on stress testing.

COMPLICATIONS OF ACUTE MYOCARDIAL INFARCTION

Cardiac Dysrhythmias

Cardiac dysrhythmias, especially ventricular dysrhythmias, are a common cause of death during the early period following acute MI.

Ventricular Fibrillation

Ventricular fibrillation occurs in 3% to 5% of patients with acute MI, usually during the first 4 hours after the event.

Rapid defibrillation with 200 to 300 J of energy is necessary when ventricular fibrillation occurs. Prophylactic lidocaine is not necessary if electrical defibrillation can be promptly accomplished. Amiodarone is generally regarded as one of the most effective antidysrhythmic drugs for control of life-threatening ventricular tachyarrhythmias, especially after MI. β-Blockers may decrease the early occurrence of ventricular fibrillation. Hypokalemia is a risk factor for ventricular fibrillation. Ventricular fibrillation is often fatal when it occurs in patients with co-existing hypotension and/or congestive heart failure.

Ventricular Tachycardia

Ventricular tachycardia is common in acute MI. Short periods of nonsustained ventricular tachycardia do not appear to predispose a patient to the risk of sustained ventricular tachycardia or ventricular fibrillation. Sustained or hemodynamically significant ventricular tachycardia must be treated with prompt electrical cardioversion. Asymptomatic ventricular tachycardia can be treated with intravenous lidocaine or amiodarone.

Atrial Fibrillation

Atrial fibrillation is the most common atrial dysrhythmia seen with acute MI. It occurs in about 10% of patients. Precipitating factors include hypoxia, acidosis, heart failure, pericarditis, and sinus node ischemia. Atrial fibrillation may result from atrial ischemia or from an acute increase in left atrial pressure. The incidence of atrial fibrillation is decreased in patients receiving thrombolytic therapy. When atrial fibrillation is hemodynamically significant, cardioversion is necessary. If atrial fibrillation is well tolerated, β-blocker or calcium channel blocker therapy is indicated to control the ventricular response.

Bradydysrhythmias and Heart Block

Sinus bradycardia is common after acute MI, particularly in patients with inferior wall MI. This may reflect increased parasympathetic nervous system activity or acute ischemia of the sinus node or atrioventricular node. Treatment with atropine and/or a temporary cardiac pacemaker is needed only when there is hemodynamic compromise from the bradycardia. Second- or third-degree atrioventricular heart block occurs in approximately 20% of patients with inferior MI, and the heart block may require temporary cardiac pacing.

Pericarditis

Pericarditis is a common complication of acute MI and may cause chest pain that can be confused with continuing or recurrent angina. In contrast to the pain of myocardial ischemia, the pain of pericarditis gets worse with inspiration or lying down and may be relieved by changes in posture. A pericardial friction rub can be heard but is often transient and positional. Diffuse ST-segment and T-wave changes may be present on the ECG. In the absence of a significant pericardial effusion, treatment of pericarditis is aimed at relieving the chest pain. Aspirin or indomethacin are recommended initially. Corticosteroids can relieve symptoms dramatically but are usually reserved for refractory cases. Dressler's syndrome (postmyocardial infarction syndrome) is a delayed form of acute pericarditis developing several weeks to months after an acute MI. It is thought to be immune mediated.

Mitral Regurgitation

Mitral regurgitation due to ischemic injury to the papillary muscles and/or to the ventricular muscle to which they attach is common after acute MI. Severe mitral regurgitation is rare and usually results from partial or complete rupture of a papillary muscle. Severe mitral regurgitation is 10 times more likely to occur after an inferior wall MI than after an anterior wall MI. Severe acute mitral regurgitation typically results in pulmonary edema and cardiogenic shock. Total papillary muscle rupture usually leads to death within 24 hours. Prompt surgical therapy is required. Treatments that decrease left ventricular afterload, such as intravenous nitroprusside and an intra-aortic balloon pump, can decrease the regurgitant volume and increase forward blood flow and cardiac output and may be helpful until surgery is accomplished.

Ventricular Septal Rupture

The characteristic holosystolic murmur of ventricular septal rupture may be difficult to distinguish from the murmur of severe mitral regurgitation. Ventricular septal rupture is more likely after anterior wall rather than inferior wall MI. Emergency surgical repair is necessary when the ventricular defect is associated with hemodynamic compromise. The mortality rate associated with surgical repair of a postinfarction ventricular septal defect is about 20%. As soon as the diagnosis of ventricular septal rupture is made, intra-aortic balloon counterpulsation should be initiated and surgical repair undertaken.

Congestive Heart Failure and Cardiogenic Shock

Acute MI is often complicated by some degree of left ventricular dysfunction. This can be evident by detection of a third heart sound or decreased Pa_{O_2}. The term *cardiogenic shock* is restricted to the hypotension and oliguria that persist after the relief of chest pain, abatement of excess parasympathetic nervous system activity, correction of hypovolemia, and treatment of dysrhythmias. Cardiogenic shock is an advanced form of acute heart failure in which the cardiac output is insufficient to maintain adequate perfusion of the kidneys and other vital organs. Systolic blood pressure is low, and there may be associated pulmonary edema and arterial hypoxemia. Cardiogenic shock is usually a manifestation of infarction of more than 40% of the left ventricular myocardium.

An important aspect of the management of cardiogenic shock is the diagnosis and prompt treatment of potentially reversible mechanical complications of MI such as rupture of the left ventricular free wall, septum, or papillary muscles; cardiac tamponade; and acute, severe mitral regurgitation. Echocardiography is extremely helpful in diagnosing and quantifying these pathologies. Treatment of cardiogenic shock is dependent on blood pressure and peripheral perfusion. Norepinephrine, vasopressin, dopamine, or dobutamine may be administered in an attempt to improve blood pressure and cardiac output. In the setting of an adequate blood pressure, nitroglycerin can be used to decrease left ventricular preload and afterload. Concomitant pulmonary edema may require morphine, diuretics, or even mechanical ventilation. Restoration of some coronary blood flow to the peri-infarction zone by thrombolytic therapy, PCI, or surgical revascularization may be indicated. Circulatory assist devices can help sustain viable myocardium and support cardiac output until revascularization can be performed or the feasibility of cardiac transplantation considered. Left ventricular assist devices improve cardiac output much more than intra-aortic balloon counterpulsation, but intra-aortic balloon pumps are much more widely available. The intra-aortic balloon pump is programmed to the ECG so that it deflates just before systole and inflates during diastole. Inflation of the balloon during diastole increases diastolic blood pressure and thus improves coronary blood flow and myocardial oxygen delivery. Deflation of the balloon just before systole augments left ventricular ejection and decreases left ventricular afterload. Intravenous infusion of a combination of inotropic and vasodilator drugs may serve as a pharmacologic alternative to mechanical counterpulsation with an intra-aortic balloon pump.

Myocardial Rupture

Myocardial rupture usually causes acute cardiac tamponade and sudden death. In a very small percentage of cases, it is possible to have time for medical stabilization and emergency surgery.

Right Ventricular Infarction

Right ventricular infarction occurs in about one third of patients with acute inferior wall left ventricular MI. An isolated right ventricular infarction is very unusual. The right ventricle has a more favorable oxygen supply/demand ratio than the left ventricle because of its muscle mass and the improved oxygen delivery that results from delivery of coronary blood flow during *both* systole and diastole. The clinical triad of hypotension, increased jugular venous pressure, and clear lung fields in a patient with an inferior wall MI is virtually pathognomonic for right ventricular infarction. Kussmaul's sign (distention of the jugular vein on inspiration) is likely to be seen. Echocardiography is useful in diagnosing right ventricular infarction. Right ventricular dilation, right ventricular asynergy, and abnormal interventricular septal motion can be seen. Cardiogenic shock, although uncommon, is the most serious

complication of right ventricular infarction. About one third of patients with RV infarction develop atrial fibrillation. Heart block may occur in as many as 50% of these patients. Both of these situations may produce severe hemodynamic compromise.

Recognition of right ventricular infarction is important because pharmacologic treatments of left ventricular failure may worsen right ventricular failure. In particular, vasodilators and diuretics are very undesirable. Third-degree atrioventricular heart block should be treated promptly with temporary AV sequential pacing, recognizing the value of atrioventricular synchrony in maintaining ventricular filling in the ischemic, noncompliant right ventricle. Intravascular volume replacement is often effective in restoring cardiac output. Administration of an inotropic drug such as dopamine may occasionally be necessary if hypotension persists despite fluid infusion. Improvement in right ventricular function generally occurs over time, suggesting reversal of ischemic stunning.

Cerebrovascular Accident

Infarction of the anterior wall and apex of the left ventricle results in thrombus formation in as many as one third of patients. The risk of systemic embolization and the possibility of an ischemic cerebrovascular accident are very significant in these patients. Echocardiography is used to detect thrombus formation in the left ventricle. The presence of a left ventricular thrombus is an indication for immediate anticoagulation with heparin followed by 6 months of anticoagulation with warfarin.

Thrombolytic therapy is associated with hemorrhagic stroke in 0.3% to 1% of patients. The stroke is usually evident within the first 24 hours after treatment and is associated with a high mortality rate.

PERIOPERATIVE MYOCARDIAL INFARCTION

It is estimated that 500,000 to 900,000 perioperative MIs occur annually worldwide. The incidence of perioperative cardiac injury is a cumulative result of preoperative medical condition, the specific surgical procedure, expertise of the surgeon, the diagnostic criteria used to define MI, and the overall medical care at a particular institution. The risk of perioperative death due to cardiac causes is less than 1% for patients who do not have ischemic heart disease as evidenced by a history of angina pectoris, electrocardiographic signs of MI, or angiographically documented coronary artery disease. The incidence of perioperative MI in patients who undergo elective high-risk vascular surgery is between 5% and 15%. The risk is even higher for emergency surgery. Patients who undergo *urgent* hip surgery have an incidence of perioperative MI of 5% to 7%, whereas less than 3% of patients who undergo *elective* total knee or hip arthroplasty have a perioperative MI.

Pathophysiology

Our understanding of the mechanism of perioperative MI is evolving. Earlier observations had suggested that most postoperative MIs occurred on the third postoperative day. Newer studies report that most perioperative MIs occur in the first 24 to 48 hours after surgery. This discrepancy is likely related to the criteria used to diagnose acute perioperative MI. In older studies, postoperative MI was usually diagnosed by the development of Q waves on the ECG. It is now known that many postoperative MIs are non–Q-wave infarctions and can be diagnosed by ECG changes and/or release of cardiac biomarkers.

Postoperative ischemia occurs early in the postoperative period and is associated with perioperative MI. These MIs are preceded by tachycardia and ST depression, are often silent, and present as NSTEMI. Patients with more severe coronary artery disease are at greater risk. These observations support the hypothesis that perioperative myocardial injury develops as a consequence of increased myocardial oxygen demand (increased blood pressure and heart rate) in the context of underlying compromised myocardial oxygen supply.

Another hypothesis suggests that perioperative MI is the result of sudden development of a thrombotic process associated with vulnerable plaque rupture. This hypothesis is based on postoperative autopsy studies and angiographic evidence of thrombus present in noncritically stenosed vessels. Endothelial injury at the site of a plaque rupture triggers the cascade of platelet aggregation and release of mediators including thromboxane A_2, serotonin, adenosine diphosphate, platelet-activating factor, thrombin, and oxygen-derived free radicals. Aggregation of platelets and activation of other inflammatory and noninflammatory mediators potentiates thrombus formation and leads to dynamic vasoconstriction distal to the thrombus. The combined effects of dynamic and physical blood vessel narrowing cause ischemia and/or infarction. In the postoperative period, changes in blood viscosity, catecholamine concentrations, cortisol levels, endogenous tissue plasminogen activator concentrations, and plasminogen activator inhibitor levels create a prothrombotic state. Changes in heart rate and blood pressure as a result of the endocrine stress response can increase the propensity for plaque fissuring and endothelial damage. In combination, these factors can precipitate thrombus formation in an atherosclerotic coronary artery and lead to the development of ST-segment elevation (Q-wave) MI. Thus, two different pathophysiologic mechanisms can be responsible for perioperative MI. One could be related to acute coronary thrombosis, and the other could be the consequence of increased myocardial oxygen demand in the setting of compromised myocardial oxygen supply. These processes are not mutually exclusive. However, one process or the other can predominate in a particular patient (**Fig. 1-2**).

Diagnosis of Perioperative Myocardial Infarction

The diagnosis of acute MI traditionally requires the presence of at least two of the following three elements: (1) ischemic

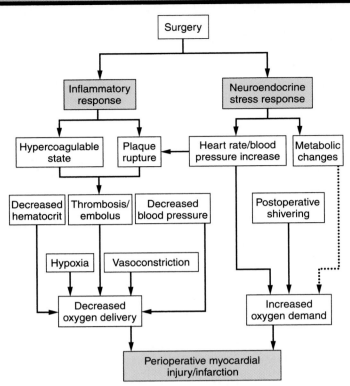

Figure 1-2 • Factors that can contribute to perioperative myocardial infarction.

chest pain, (2) evolutionary changes on the ECG, and (3) increase and decrease in cardiac biomarker levels. In the perioperative period, ischemic episodes are often silent, that is, not associated with chest pain. In addition, many postoperative ECGs are nondiagnostic. Nonspecific ECG changes, new-onset dysrhythmias, and noncardiac-related hemodynamic instability can further obscure the clinical picture of acute coronary syndrome in the perioperative period.

As in the nonoperative setting, an acute increase in troponin levels should be considered an MI in the perioperative setting. An increase in cardiac troponin is a marker of myocardial injury, and there is a good correlation between the duration of myocardial ischemia and the increase in cardiac-specific troponin. There is also a significant association between increased troponin levels and short- and long-term morbidity and mortality in surgical patients. This association exists for cardiac death, MI, myocardial ischemia, congestive heart failure, cardiac dysrhythmias, and cerebrovascular accident. Even relatively minor cardiovascular complications such as uncontrolled hypertension, palpitations, increased fatigue, or shortness of breath are correlated to increased levels of cardiac specific troponins. An increase in troponin postoperatively, even in the absence of clear cardiovascular signs and symptoms, is an important finding that requires careful attention and referral to a cardiologist for further evaluation and management.

TABLE 1–2 Clinical Predictors of Increased Perioperative Cardiovascular Risk

Major

Unstable coronary syndromes

Acute or recent MI with evidence of important ischemic risk by clinical symptoms or noninvasive study

Unstable or severe angina

Decompensated heart failure

Significant dysrhythmias

High-grade atrioventricular block

Symptomatic ventricular dysrhythmias in the presence of underlying heart disease

Supraventricular dysrhythmias with uncontrolled ventricular rate

Severe valvular heart disease

Intermediate

Mild angina pectoris

Previous MI by history or Q waves on ECG

Compensated or previous heart failure

Diabetes mellitus (particularly insulin dependent)

Renal insufficiency

Minor

Advanced age (older than 70 years)

Abnormal ECG (left ventricular hypertrophy, left bundle branch block, ST-T abnormalities)

Rhythm other than sinus

Low functional capacity

History of stroke

Uncontrolled systemic hypertension

ECG, electrocardiogram; MI, myocardial infarction.
Adapted from Fleisher LA, Beckman JA, Brown KA, et al: ACC/AHA 2006 guideline update on perioperative cardiovascular evaluation for noncardiac surgery: Focused update on perioperative beta-blocker therapy: A report of the American College of Cardiology/American Heart Association Task Force on Practice Guidelines. Circulation 2006;113: 2662–2674 with permission.

PREOPERATIVE ASSESSMENT OF PATIENTS WITH KNOWN OR SUSPECTED ISCHEMIC HEART DISEASE

History

The preoperative history is meant to elicit the severity, progression, and functional limitations imposed by ischemic heart disease. It should focus on determining the presence of major, moderate and minor clinical risk factors in a particular patient (**Table 1-2**). Myocardial ischemia, left ventricular dysfunction, and cardiac dysrhythmias are usually responsible for the signs and symptoms of ischemic heart disease. Symptoms such as angina and dyspnea may be absent at rest, emphasizing the importance of evaluating the patient's response to various physical activities such as walking or climbing stairs. Limited exercise tolerance in the absence of significant lung disease is very good evidence of decreased cardiac reserve. If a patient can climb two to three flights of stairs without symptoms, it is likely that cardiac reserve is adequate. Dyspnea after the onset of angina pectoris suggests the presence of acute left ventricular dysfunction due to myocardial ischemia. It is important to recognize the presence of incipient congestive heart failure preoperatively because the added stresses of anesthesia, surgery, fluid replacement, and postoperative pain may result in overt congestive heart failure.

Silent Myocardial Ischemia

Silent myocardial ischemia does not evoke angina pectoris and usually occurs at a heart rate and systemic blood pressure substantially lower than that present during exercise-induced ischemia. A history of ischemic heart disease or an abnormal ECG suggestive of a previous MI is associated with an increased incidence of silent myocardial ischemia. It is estimated that nearly 75% of ischemic episodes in patients with symptomatic ischemic heart disease are not associated with angina pectoris and 10% to 15% of acute MIs are silent. Treatment of silent myocardial ischemia is the same as that for classic angina pectoris. The mortality due to MI in patients with silent myocardial ischemia is similar to that in patients with classic chest pain.

Previous Myocardial Infarction

A history of MI is an important piece of information. It is common practice to delay elective surgery for some time (at least 6 weeks) following an acute myocardial infarction. Retrospective studies of large groups of adult patients have suggested that the incidence of myocardial reinfarction during the perioperative period is influenced by the time elapsed since the previous MI. Acute (1–7 days) and recent myocardial infarction (8–30 days) and UA incur the highest risk of perioperative myocardial ischemia, MI, and cardiac death.

It is important to determine whether a patient has had an angioplasty with stent placement. Stent placement (drug-eluting or bare metal stent) is routinely followed by postprocedure antiplatelet therapy to prevent acute coronary thrombosis and maintain long-term patency of the vessel. Elective noncardiac surgery should be delayed for 4 to 6 weeks after coronary angioplasty. It is prudent to delay elective noncardiac surgery for 6 weeks after PCI with bare metal stent placement and as long as 12 months in patients with drug-eluting stent placement to allow complete endothelialization of the stent and completion of antiplatelet therapy with GIIb/IIIa inhibitors such as clopidogrel.

Co-Existing Noncardiac Diseases

The history should also elicit information relevant to co-existing noncardiac disease. For example, patients with ischemic heart disease are likely to have peripheral vascular disease. A history of syncope may reflect cerebrovascular disease, a seizure disorder, or cardiac dysrhythmias. Cough is often pulmonary rather than cardiac in origin. It may be difficult to differentiate dyspnea due to cardiac dysfunction from that due to chronic lung disease, although patients with ischemic heart disease more often complain of orthopnea and paroxysmal nocturnal dyspnea. Chronic obstructive pulmonary disease is likely in patients with a long history of cigarette smoking. Diabetes mellitus often co-exists with ischemic heart disease. Renal insufficiency (creatinine > 2.0 mg/dL) increases the risk of perioperative cardiac events.

Current Medications

Medical treatment for ischemic heart disease is designed to decrease myocardial oxygen requirements, improve coronary blood flow, stabilize plaque, prevent thrombosis, and remodel the injured myocardium. These goals are achieved by the use of β-blockers, nitrates, calcium entry blockers, statins, antiplatelet drugs, and ACE inhibitors.

Effective β-blockade is suggested by a resting heart rate of 50 to 60 beats per minute. Routine physical activity is expected to increase the heart rate 10% to 20%. There is no evidence that β-blockers enhance the negative inotropic effects of volatile anesthetics. β-blocker therapy should be continued throughout the perioperative period. Atropine or glycopyrrolate can be used to treat excessive chronotropic effects of β-blockers during the perioperative period. Isoproterenol is the specific pharmacologic antagonist for excessive β-antagonist activity. The postoperative period is a time when inadvertent withdrawal of β-blocker therapy may occur and result in rebound hypertension and tachycardia.

Significant hypotension has been observed in patients treated long term with ACE inhibitors who undergo general anesthesia. Many recommend withholding ACE inhibitors for 24 hours before surgical procedures involving significant fluid shifts or blood loss. Hypotension attributable to ACE inhibitors is usually responsive to fluids or sympathomimetic drugs. If hypotension is refractory to these measures, treatment with vasopressin or one of its analogues may be required.

Antiplatelet drugs are an essential component in the pharmacotherapy of acute coronary syndrome and long-term management of ischemic heart disease. Aspirin irreversibly inhibits cyclooxygenase and prevents platelet activation. Clopidogrel (Plavix) and ticlopidine (Ticlid) bind irreversibly to adenosine diphosphate receptors on the platelets preventing transformation of platelet glycoprotein IIb/IIIa receptors and further platelet activation. The use of clopidogrel and tidopidine precludes neuroaxial anesthesia. Clopidogrel and ticlopidine can increase the risk of perioperative bleeding and necessitate platelet transfusion in urgent clinical situations.

Physical Examination

The physical examination of patients with ischemic heart disease is often normal. Nevertheless, signs of right and left ventricular dysfunction must be sought. A carotid bruit may indicate cerebrovascular disease. Orthostatic hypotension may reflect attenuated autonomic nervous system activity due to treatment with antihypertensive drugs. Jugular venous distention and peripheral edema are signs of right ventricular failure. Auscultation of the chest may reveal evidence of left ventricular dysfunction such as an S_3 gallop or rales.

Specialized Preoperative Testing

Specialized preoperative cardiac testing includes electrocardiography, echocardiography, radionuclide ventriculography, thallium scintigraphy, high-speed computed tomography, magnetic resonance imaging, and positron emission tomography scanning. Such testing is reserved for patients in whom the results are critical for guiding therapy during the perioperative period.

Electrocardiography

Preoperative evaluation that includes tests that stimulate an increase in heart rate is appealing because perioperative increases in myocardial oxygen consumption and the development of myocardial ischemia are often accompanied by tachycardia. Preoperative stress testing and/or the exercise tolerance of a patient can indicate the risk of perioperative myocardial ischemia. Preoperative exercise stress testing is usually not indicated in patients with stable coronary artery disease and acceptable exercise tolerance. Because the exercise ECG can produce a number of false-negative and false-positive results, its predictive value is limited.

Preoperative ambulatory electrocardiography in patients with coronary artery disease often reveals episodes of silent myocardial ischemia. These changes on ambulatory electrocardiography have been considered as independent predictors of adverse postoperative cardiac outcomes. However, the precise role of this test in relation to other specialized diagnostic tests remains undefined.

Echocardiography

Preoperative transthoracic or transesophageal echocardiography is useful for diagnosing left ventricular dysfunction and assessing valvular heart disease. Resting echocardiography does not contribute appreciably to the information provided by routine clinical and electrocardiographic data in predicting adverse outcomes. Echocardiographic wall motion analysis during the infusion of dipyridamole or dobutamine or atropine (pharmacologic stress testing) is a good technique for evaluating ischemic heart disease, particularly in patients with no history of MI. Dobutamine stress echocardiography provides comparable, if not better, results than myocardial perfusion scintigraphy and provides additional information about valvular function.

Radionuclide Ventriculography

Radionuclide ventriculography quantitates left and right ventricular systolic and diastolic function. The ejection fraction determined by radionuclide ventriculography does not appear to provide information that can be used to accurately predict perioperative myocardial ischemic events, but an ejection fraction less than 50% does predict an increased risk of postoperative congestive heart failure in patients undergoing abdominal aortic surgery.

Thallium Scintigraphy

Physical limitations, such as claudication or joint disease, may impair the ability of a patient to exercise. This limits the usefulness of exercise stress testing. Dipyridamole-thallium testing mimics the coronary vasodilator response associated with exercise. Like stress echocardiography, it is a useful test in patients with limited exercise capacity. Defects or "cold spots" on the nuclear scan denote areas of myocardial ischemia or infarction. The cost-effectiveness of thallium scintigraphy is best when this test is restricted to patients who cannot exercise and whose risk of perioperative cardiac complications cannot be estimated based on clinical factors.

Computed Tomography and Magnetic Resonance Imaging

High-speed computed tomography can visualize coronary artery calcification. Intravenous administration of radiographic contrast medium enhances the clarity of the images. Magnetic resonance imaging provides even greater image clarity and can delineate the proximal portions of the coronary arterial circulation. However, computed tomography and magnetic resonance imaging are more expensive and less mobile than other modalities of cardiac evaluation.

Positron Emission Tomography

Positron emission tomography is a highly sophisticated technique that demonstrates regional myocardial blood flow and metabolism. It can be used to delineate the extent of coronary artery disease and myocardial viability.

MANAGEMENT OF ANESTHESIA IN PATIENTS WITH KNOWN OR SUSPECTED ISCHEMIC HEART DISEASE UNDERGOING NONCARDIAC SURGERY

The preoperative management of patients with ischemic heart disease or risk factors for ischemic heart disease is geared toward the following goals: (1) determining the extent of ischemic heart disease and any previous interventions (CABG, PCI), (2) determining the severity and stability of the disease, and (3) reviewing medical therapy and noting any drugs that can increase the risk of surgical bleeding or contraindicate a particular anesthetic technique. The first two goals are important in risk stratification.

Risk Stratification Strategy

In stable patients undergoing elective major noncardiac surgery, six independent predictors of major cardiac complications have been described in the Lee Revised Cardiac Risk Index (**Table 1-3**). These six predictors include high risk surgery, ischemic heart disease, congestive heart failure, cerebrovascular disease, preoperative insulin-dependent diabetes mellitus. and preoperative serum creatinine greater than 2.0 mg/dL. The presence of several risk factors increases the incidence of postoperative cardiac complications such as cardiac death, cardiac arrest/ventricular fibrillation, complete heart block, acute MI, and pulmonary edema (**Fig. 1-3**). These risk factors have been incorporated into the American College of Cardiology/American Heart Association (ACC/AHA) guidelines for perioperative cardiovascular evaluation for noncardiac surgery. The principal theme of

TABLE 1-3	Cardiac Risk Factors in Patients Undergoing Elective Major Noncardiac Surgery

I. High-risk surgery
   Abdominal aortic aneurysm
   Peripheral vascular operation
   Thoracotomy
   Major abdominal operation
II. Ischemic heart disease
   History of myocardial infarction
   History of a positive exercise test
   Current complaints of angina pectoris
   Use of nitrate therapy
   Q waves on electrocardiogram
III. Congestive heart failure
   History of congestive heart failure
   History of pulmonary edema
   History of paroxysmal nocturnal dyspnea
   Physical examination showing rales or S_3 gallop
   Chest radiograph showing pulmonary vascular redistribution
IV. Cerebrovascular disease
   History of stroke
   History of transient ischemic attack
V. Insulin-dependent diabetes mellitus
VI. Preoperative serum creatinine concentration > 2 mg/dL

Adapted from Lee TH, Marcantonio ER, Mangione CM, et al: Derivation and prospective validation of a simple index for prediction of cardiac risk of major noncardiac surgery. Circulation 1999;100:1043–1049 with permission.

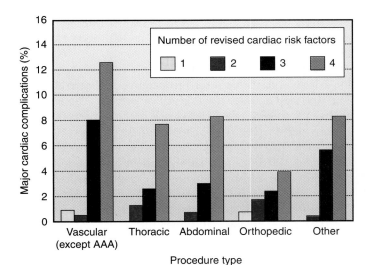

Figure 1-3 • Bars represent the rate of major cardiac complications in patients in Revised Cardiac Risk Index classes according to the type of surgery performed. Note that by definition, patients undergoing AAA (abdominal aortic aneurysm), thoracic, and abdominal procedures are excluded from class I because these operations are all considered high-risk surgery. In all subsets, there was a statistically significant trend toward greater risk with higher risk class. (*Reproduced with permission from Lee TH, Marcantonio ER, Mangione CM, et al: Derivation and prospective validation of a simple index for prediction of cardiac risk of major noncardiac surgery. Circulation 1999;100:1043–1049.*)

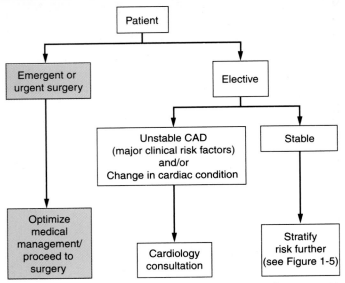

Figure 1-4 • An algorithm for preoperative assessment of patients with ischemic heart disease. Identify patients for urgent or emergent surgery and proceed to the operating room with medical management. In patients scheduled for elective surgery, the presence of major clinical risk factors or a change in medical condition may prompt further evaluation before surgery. CAD, coronary artery disease.

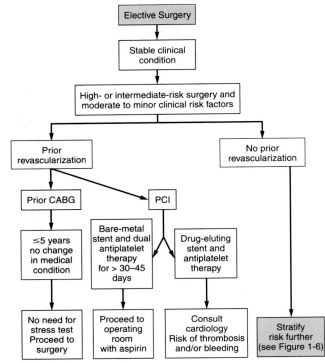

Figure 1-5 • An algorithm for preoperative assessment of patients with ischemic heart disease scheduled for elective intermediate- to high-risk surgery who are in stable clinical condition with moderate clinical risk factors. Determine previous coronary intervention and stability of cardiac condition. If no interval change in cardiac condition, proceed to surgery with medical management. For patients with intracoronary stents, determine the date of insertion and location of the stent(s), the kind of stent(s), and the status of current antiplatelet therapy. Patients on antiplatelet therapy may require consultation with the cardiologist and the surgeon. CABG, coronary artery bypass grafting; PCI, percutaneous coronary intervention.

the guidelines is that preoperative intervention is rarely necessary just to lower the risk of surgery. An intervention is indicated or not indicated irrespective of the need for surgery. Preoperative testing should be performed only if it is likely to influence perioperative management. Although no prospective, randomized study has been conducted to prove the efficacy of these guidelines, they offer a paradigm that has been widely adopted by clinicians.

The ACC/AHA guidelines provide a multistep algorithm for determining the need for preoperative cardiac evaluation. The first step assesses the urgency of surgery. The need for emergency surgery takes precedence over the need for additional work-up (**Fig. 1-4**). The second step assesses whether the patient has undergone revascularization. The third step determines whether and when the patient underwent invasive or noninvasive cardiac evaluation. If a patient has had revascularization within the past 5 years or has had an appropriate coronary evaluation in the past 2 years, with no subsequent deterioration of cardiac status, then further cardiac evaluation is not warranted (**Fig. 1-5**).

The next five steps of the ACC/AHA guidelines integrate risk stratification according to clinical risk factors, functional capacity, and surgery-specific risk factors. Clinical risk factors obtained by history, physical examination, and review of the ECG are grouped into three categories: (1) *Major clinical risk factors* (unstable coronary syndrome, decompensated heart failure, significant arrhythmias, severe valvular disease) may require delay of elective surgery and cardiology evaluation. Intensive preoperative management is necessary if surgery is urgent or emergent (see Fig. 1-4). (2) *Intermediate clinical risk factors* (stable angina pectoris, previous MI by history or pathologic Q waves, compensated or previous heart failure, insulin-dependent diabetes mellitus, renal insufficiency) are well validated markers of enhanced risk of perioperative cardiac complications. (3) *Minor clinical risk factors* (hypertension, left bundle branch block, nonspecific ST-T–wave changes, history of stroke) are recognized markers of coronary artery disease that have not been proven to independently increase perioperative cardiac risk.

Functional capacity or exercise tolerance can be expressed in metabolic equivalent of the task (MET) units. The O_2 consumption ($\dot{V}O_2$) of a 70-kg, 40-year-old man in a resting state is 3.5 mL/kg per minute or 1 MET. Perioperative cardiac risk is increased in patients with poor functional capacity, that is, who are unable to meet a 4-MET demand during normal daily activities. These people may be able to do some activities such as baking, slow ballroom dancing, golfing with a cart, walking at a speed of approximately 2 of 3 mph, but are unable to perform more strenuous activity without developing chest pain or significant shortness of breath. The ability to participate in activities requiring more than 4 METs indicates good functional capacity.

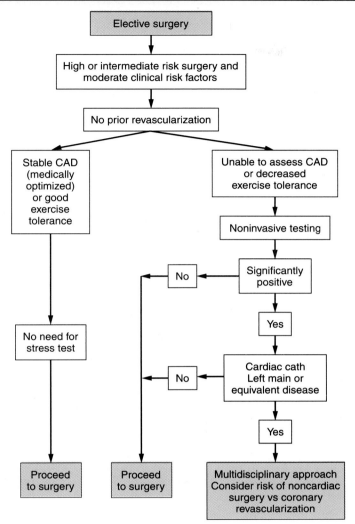

Figure 1-6 • For patients scheduled for intermediate- to high-risk surgery who have moderate clinical risk factors and poor exercise tolerance (or inability to determine exercise tolerance), consider noninvasive stress testing to determine whether significant myocardium is at risk. If significant myocardium is at risk, consider coronary angiogram. CAD, coronary artery disease.

The surgery-specific risk of noncardiac surgical procedures is graded as high, intermediate, or low. *High-risk surgery* includes emergency major surgery, aortic and other major vascular surgery, peripheral vascular surgery, and prolonged surgical procedures associated with large fluid shifts and/or blood loss. These operations are reported to have a cardiac risk greater than 5%. *Intermediate-risk surgery* includes carotid endarterectomy, head and neck surgery, intraperitoneal and intrathoracic surgery, orthopedic surgery, and prostate surgery. Such operations are reported to have a cardiac risk of less than 5%. *Low-risk procedures* such as endoscopic surgery, superficial surgery, cataract surgery, and breast surgery are reported to have a less than 1% risk of perioperative cardiac events.

According to the ACC/AHA guidelines, patients with two of the following three factors, high-risk surgery, low exercise tolerance, and moderate clinical risk factors, could be considered for further cardiac evaluation. Patients who have low functional capacity or in whom it is difficult to assess functional capacity are good candidates for further evaluation (**Fig. 1-6**). Many of these patients may not be candidates for exercise stress testing but can be referred for pharmacologic stress testing. Nuclear imaging can better detect myocardium at risk.

Preoperative coronary angiography would be most suitable in a patient with a highly positive stress test that suggests significant myocardium at risk. The aim of the angiographic study would be to identify significant coronary artery disease, that is, left main or severe multivessel coronary artery disease. Further management in such a patient would be dictated by the patient's clinical condition, the overall risk of an intervention, and available resources.

Management after Risk Stratification

The fundamental reason for risk stratification is to identify patients at increased risk so as to manage them with pharmacologic and other perioperative interventions that can lessen the risk and severity of perioperative cardiac events. Three therapeutic options are available before elective noncardiac surgery: (1) revascularization by surgery, (2) revascularization by PCI, and (3) optimal medical management.

In nonoperative settings, treatment strategies like PCI with or without stenting, CABG in selected patients, and β-blocker therapy have proven efficacy in improving long-term morbidity and mortality. Hence, patients with significant ischemic heart disease who present for noncardiac surgery are likely to be candidates for one or more of these therapies regardless of their need for surgery. Revascularization may not be necessary preoperatively. Optimal medical management can improve perioperative outcomes. Coronary intervention should be guided by the patient's cardiac condition and by the potential consequences of delaying surgery for recovery after revascularization.

Coronary Artery Bypass Grafting

For CABG surgery to be beneficial before noncardiac surgery, the institutional risk of that noncardiac surgery should be greater than the combined risk of coronary catheterization, coronary revascularization, and the reported risk of the noncardiac surgery. The indications for preoperative coronary revascularization are the same as those in the nonoperative setting. There is no value in preoperative coronary intervention in patients with stable ischemic heart disease.

Percutaneous Coronary Intervention

Angioplasty before elective noncardiac surgery could improve outcome. However, angioplasty is now often accompanied by stenting, which requires postprocedure antiplatelet therapy to prevent acute coronary thrombosis and maintain long-term patency of the vessel. Acute postoperative stent thrombosis has been reported when antiplatelet drugs were held perioperatively. Although many factors influence the chance of stent thrombosis, it is becoming clear that discontinuation of antiplatelet therapy predisposes to stent thrombosis with significant morbidity and mortality. The following precautions should be adopted: (1) determine the date, kind of stent, and any stent-related complications in patients with a history of PCI with coronary stenting; (2) consider patients with recent stent placement (< 6 weeks for bare metal stents and <1 year for drug-eluting stents) as high risk and consult an interventional cardiologist for recommendations; (3) review the timing of the proposed surgery. Discontinuing or modifying antiplatelet therapy should involve a multidisciplinary team of cardiologist, surgeon, and anesthesiologist. The procedure, especially if emergent or urgent, should ideally be performed in a center with interventional cardiology so that complications of stent thrombosis can be addressed promptly.

Pharmacologic Management

The implication in formulation of a risk stratification index is that high-risk individuals will be identified and treated to reduce their risk of perioperative cardiac complications. Few patients will require preoperative coronary revascularization. Most patients with stable ischemic heart disease or significant risk factors for ischemic heart disease will be managed pharmacologically.

Several drugs have been used to reduce perioperative cardiac injury. They were chosen because they have demonstrated efficacy in the management of coronary ischemia in the nonsurgical setting. Nitroglycerin is helpful in the management of active ischemia, but *prophylactic* administration of nitroglycerin has not been shown to be efficacious in reducing perioperative cardiac morbidity and mortality.

Perioperative use of β-blockers has been shown to be efficacious in reducing perioperative cardiac morbidity and mortality in several studies, although these had rather small numbers of patients. A large multinational, multicenter trial is under way and will help determine the true efficacy of β-blockers. Patients with three or more clinical risk factors

scheduled for vascular surgery and with significant myocardium at risk are still at appreciable risk of perioperative MI or death despite β-blocker therapy.

Questions regarding the timing of perioperative β-blocker initiation, the necessary duration of therapy, choice of drug, and target heart rate are still unresolved. Likewise, controversy exists as to the efficacy of acute perioperative β-blocker therapy versus long-term β-blocker therapy. At present, most agree that β-blockers should be administered to high-risk patients according to ACC/AHA guidelines (**Table 1-4**) and titrated to a heart rate of about 60 bpm. Abrupt perioperative withdrawal of β-blocker therapy may result in a marked increase in sympathetic nervous system activity and considerable risk of myocardial ischemia/infarction. For ease of dosing and consistency of effect, longer acting β-blockers such as atenolol or bisoprolol may be more efficacious in the perioperative period.

α_2-Agonists have analgesic, sedative, and sympatholytic effects. In patients in whom β-blockers are contraindicated, α_2-agonists can be used to help decrease perioperative cardiac injury. The role of calcium channel blockers in reducing perioperative cardiac morbidity and mortality is controversial.

It is likely that other drugs beneficial in the treatment of ischemic heart disease in the nonoperative setting, such as ACE inhibitors, statins, aspirin, and insulin may prove to be beneficial in the perioperative period as well. The beneficial cardiovascular effects of a glucose-insulin-potassium infusion have long been known. More recently, the beneficial effects of controlling hyperglycemia in patients undergoing cardiac surgery and in critically ill patients have been demonstrated. Because multiple pathophysiologic mechanisms can trigger perioperative MI, it may be that multimodal therapy with β-blockers or α_2-agonists, statins, and, possibly, insulin will be more beneficial than treatment with only a single drug (**Fig. 1-7**).

| TABLE 1-4 | Recommendations for Perioperative β-Blocker Use |

	CLINICAL RISK FACTORS				
	Already Receiving β-Blockers	Major Clinical Risk Factors or Positive Ischemia on Preoperative Stress Testing	Multiple Moderate Clinical Risk Factors	Single Moderate Clinical Risk Factor	Minor Clinical Risk Factors
Vascular surgery	++	++	+	±	*
High- or intermediate-risk surgery	++	+	+	±	*
Low-risk surgery	*	*	*	*	*

*, Insufficient data available; ++, class I recommendation, β-blockers should be used; +, class IIa recommendation, β-blockers should probably be used; ±, class IIb recommendation, β-blockers may be used.

Adapted from Fleisher LA, Beckman JA, Brown KA, et al: ACC/AHA 2006 guideline update on perioperative cardiovascular evaluation for noncardiac surgery: Focused update on perioperative beta-blocker therapy: A report of the American College of Cardiology/American Heart Association task force on practice guidelines: Circulation 2006;113:2662–2674 with permission.

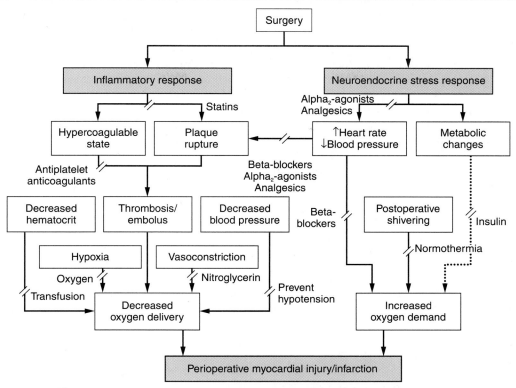

Figure 1-7 • Interventions that can modulate triggers of perioperative myocardial injury.

Anxiety reduction can be achieved by both psychological and pharmacologic means. Patients are more likely to arrive in the operating room in a relaxed state if there has been a preoperative visit during which the anesthetic was explained in detail and all questions and concerns addressed. The goal of drug-induced sedation and anxiolysis is maximum sedation and/or amnesia without significant circulatory or ventilatory depression.

Intraoperative Management

The basic challenges during induction and maintenance of anesthesia in patients with ischemic heart disease are (1) to prevent myocardial ischemia by optimizing myocardial oxygen supply and reducing myocardial oxygen demand and (2) to monitor for ischemia and to treat ischemia if it develops. Intraoperative events associated with persistent tachycardia, systolic hypertension, sympathetic nervous system stimulation, arterial hypoxemia, or hypotension can adversely affect the patient with ischemic heart disease (**Table 1-5**). Perioperative myocardial injury is closely associated with heart rate in vascular surgery patients (**Fig. 1-8**). A rapid heart rate increases myocardial oxygen requirements and decreases diastolic time for coronary blood flow and thus oxygen delivery. The increased oxygen requirements produced by hypertension are offset to some degree by improved coronary perfusion. Hyperventilation must be avoided because hypocapnia may cause coronary artery vasoconstriction.

Maintenance of the balance between myocardial oxygen supply and demand is more important than the specific anesthetic technique or drugs selected to produce anesthesia and muscle relaxation. Although isoflurane may decrease coronary

TABLE 1-5	Intraoperative Events That Influence the Balance Between Myocardial Oxygen Delivery and Myocardial Oxygen Requirements

Decreased Oxygen Delivery
Decreased coronary blood flow
Tachycardia
Diastolic hypotension
Hypocapnia (coronary artery vasoconstriction)
Coronary artery spasm
Decreased oxygen content
Anemia
Arterial hypoxemia
Shift of the oxyhemoglobin dissociation curve to the left

Increased Oxygen Requirements
Sympathetic nervous system stimulation
Tachycardia
Hypertension
Increased myocardial contractility
Increased afterload
Increased preload

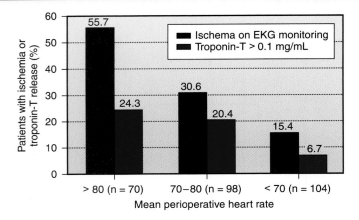

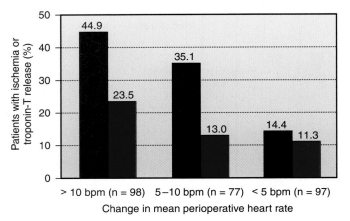

Figure 1-8 • Relationship of mean heart rate and absolute heart rate change in relation to myocardial ischemia and troponin release in patients undergoing vascular surgery. *(From Feringa HH, Bax JJ, Boersma E, et al: High-dose beta-blockers and tight heart rate control reduce myocardial ischemia and troponin T release in vascular surgery patients. Circulation 2006;114: I344–I349 with permission.)*

vascular resistance, predisposing to coronary steal syndrome, there is no evidence that this drug increases the incidence of intraoperative myocardial ischemia.

It is important to avoid persistent and excessive changes in heart rate and systemic blood pressure. A common recommendation is to keep the heart rate and blood pressure within 20% of the normal awake value. However, many episodes of intraoperative myocardial ischemia occur in the absence of hemodynamic changes. These episodes of myocardial ischemia may be due to regional decreases in myocardial perfusion and oxygenation. It is unlikely that this form of ischemia can be prevented by the anesthesiologist.

Induction of Anesthesia

Induction of anesthesia in patients with ischemic heart disease can be accomplished with an intravenous induction drug. Ketamine is not a likely choice because the associated increase in heart rate and systemic blood pressure transiently increases myocardial oxygen requirements. Tracheal intubation is facilitated by administration of succinylcholine or a nondepolarizing muscle relaxant.

Myocardial ischemia may accompany the sympathetic nervous system stimulation that results from direct laryngoscopy and tracheal intubation. Short-duration direct laryngoscopy ($\leq$15 seconds) is useful in minimizing the magnitude and duration of the circulatory changes associated with tracheal intubation. If the duration of direct laryngoscopy is not likely to be brief or if hypertension already exists, it is reasonable to consider administering drugs to minimize the pressor response. Laryngotracheal lidocaine, intravenous lidocaine, esmolol, and fentanyl have all been shown to be useful for blunting the increase in heart rate evoked by tracheal intubation.

Maintenance of Anesthesia

In patients with normal left ventricular function, tachycardia and hypertension are likely to develop in response to intense stimulation, as during direct laryngoscopy or painful surgical stimulation. Controlled myocardial depression using a volatile anesthetic may be useful in such patients to minimize the increase in sympathetic nervous system activity. The volatile anesthetic may be administered alone or in combination with nitrous oxide. Equally acceptable for maintenance of anesthesia is use of a nitrous oxide–opioid technique with the addition of a volatile anesthetic to treat any undesirable increases in blood pressure that accompany painful surgical stimulation. Overall, volatile anesthetics may be beneficial in patients with ischemic heart disease by virtue of decreasing myocardial oxygen requirements and preconditioning the myocardium to tolerate ischemic events, or they may be detrimental because of drug-induced decreases in systemic blood pressure and associated decreases in coronary perfusion pressure.

Patients with severely impaired left ventricular function may not tolerate anesthesia-induced myocardial depression. Rather than volatile anesthetics, opioids may be selected for these patients. The addition of nitrous oxide, a benzodiazepine, or a low-dose volatile anesthetic may be needed because total amnesia cannot be ensured with an opioid alone, but the addition of nitrous oxide or a volatile anesthetic may be associated with myocardial depression.

Regional anesthesia is an acceptable technique in patients with ischemic heart disease. However, the decrease in blood pressure associated with epidural or spinal anesthesia must be controlled. Prompt treatment of hypotension that exceeds 20% of the preblock blood pressure is necessary. Potential benefits of a regional anesthetic include excellent pain control, a decreased incidence of deep vein thrombosis in some patients, and the opportunity to continue the block into the postoperative period. However, the incidence of postoperative cardiac morbidity and mortality does not appear to be significantly different between general and regional anesthesia.

Hemodynamic goals for intraoperative therapy with β-blockers are unclear, and potential interactions with anesthetics that cause myocardial depression and vasodilatation must be considered. It seems prudent to maintain intraoperative heart rate at less than 80 bpm.

Choice of Muscle Relaxant

The choice of nondepolarizing muscle relaxant in patients with ischemic heart disease is influenced by the impact these drugs could have on the balance between myocardial oxygen delivery and myocardial oxygen requirements. Muscle relaxants with minimal or no effect on heart rate and systemic blood pressure (vecuronium, rocuronium, cisatracurium) are attractive choices for patients with ischemic heart disease. Histamine release and the resulting decrease in blood pressure caused by atracurium are less desirable. Myocardial ischemia has been described in patients with ischemic heart disease given pancuronium, presumably because of the modest increase in heart rate and blood pressure produced by this drug. However, these circulatory changes produced by pancuronium may be useful for offsetting the negative inotropic and chronotropic effects of some anesthetic drugs.

Reversal of neuromuscular blockade with an anticholinesterase/anticholinergic drug combination can be safely accomplished in patients with ischemic heart disease. Glycopyrrolate, which has much less chronotropic effect than atropine, is preferred in these patients.

Monitoring

Perioperative monitoring is influenced by the complexity of the operative procedure and the severity of the ischemic heart disease. An important goal when selecting monitors for patients with ischemic heart disease is to select those that allow early detection of myocardial ischemia (**Fig. 1-9**). Most myocardial ischemia occurs in the absence of hemodynamic alterations, so one should be cautious when endorsing routine use of expensive or complex monitors to detect myocardial ischemia.

Electrocardiography The simplest, most cost-effective method for detecting perioperative myocardial ischemia is electrocardiography. The diagnosis of myocardial ischemia focuses on changes in the ST segment characterized as depression or elevation of at least 1 mm. T-wave inversion and R-wave changes can also be associated with myocardial ischemia, although other factors such as electrolyte changes can also produce such changes. The degree of ST-segment depression parallels the severity of myocardial ischemia. Because visual detection of ST segments changes is unreliable, computerized ST-segment analysis has been incorporated into electrocardiography monitors. Traditionally, monitoring two leads, II and V_5, has been the standard, but it appears that monitoring three leads improves the ability to detect ischemia. Leads II, V_4, and V_5 or V_3, V_4, and V_5 are the sets of three leads recommended. There is a predictable correlation between the lead of the ECG that detects myocardial ischemia and the anatomic distribution of the diseased coronary artery (**Table 1-6**). For example, the V_5 lead (fifth intercostal space in the anterior axillary line) reflects myocardial ischemia in the portion of the left ventricle supplied by the left anterior descending coronary artery. Lead II is more likely to detect myocardial ischemia occurring in the distribution of the right coronary artery. Lead II is also very useful for analysis of cardiac rhythm disturbances.

Intraoperative monitors for ischemia

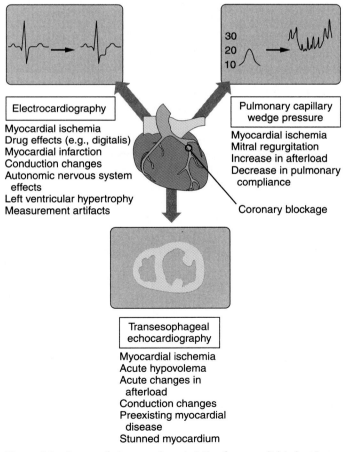

Electrocardiography

Myocardial ischemia
Drug effects (e.g., digitalis)
Myocardial infarction
Conduction changes
Autonomic nervous system
  effects
Left ventricular hypertrophy
Measurement artifacts

Pulmonary capillary
wedge pressure

Myocardial ischemia
Mitral regurgitation
Increase in afterload
Decrease in pulmonary
  compliance

Coronary blockage

Transesophageal
echocardiography

Myocardial ischemia
Acute hypovolema
Acute changes in
  afterload
Conduction changes
Preexisting myocardial
  disease
Stunned myocardium

Figure 1-9 • Causes of changes characteristic of myocardial ischemia on intraoperative monitors. *(Reproduced with permission from Fleisher LA: Real-time intraoperative monitoring of myocardial ischemia in noncardiac surgery. Anesthesiology 2000;92:1183–1188.* © *2000, Lippincott Williams & Wilkins.)*

TABLE 1-6	Relationship of Electrocardiogram Leads to Areas of Myocardial Ischemia	
ECG Lead	**Coronary Artery Responsible for Ischemia**	**Area of Myocardium That May Be Involved**
II, III, aVF	Right coronary artery	Right atrium Right ventricle Sinoatrial node Infesior aspect of left ventricle Atrioventricular node
I, aVL	Circumflex coronary artery	Lateral aspect of left ventricle
V_3–V_5	Left anterior descending coronary artery	Anterolateral aspect of left ventricle
ECG, electrocardiogram.		

Events other than myocardial ischemia that can cause ST-segment abnormalities include cardiac dysrhythmias, cardiac conduction disturbances, digitalis therapy, electrolyte abnormalities, and hypothermia. However, in patients with known or suspected coronary artery disease, it is reasonable to assume that intraoperative ST-segment changes represent myocardial ischemia. The occurrence and duration of intraoperative ST-segment changes in high-risk patients are linked to an increased incidence of perioperative MI and adverse cardiac events. The overall incidence of myocardial ischemia in the intraoperative period is lower than that in the pre- or postoperative periods.

Pulmonary Artery Catheter Intraoperative myocardial ischemia can manifest as an acute increase in pulmonary artery occlusion pressure due to changes in left ventricular compliance and systolic performance. If myocardial ischemia is global or involves the papillary muscle, V waves may appear in the pulmonary artery occlusion pressure tracing. Nonischemic causes of an increased pulmonary artery occlusion pressure include acute increases in ventricular afterload, decreases in pulmonary venous compliance, or mitral regurgitation due to nonischemic mechanisms. If only small regions of left ventricular myocardium become ischemic, overall ventricular compliance and pulmonary artery occlusion pressure will remain unchanged so the pulmonary artery catheter is a relatively insensitive monitor of myocardial ischemia. In addition, pulmonary artery occlusion pressure is measured only intermittently, and the pulmonary artery diastolic pressure is even less sensitive than the pulmonary artery occlusion pressure in detecting a change in ventricular compliance. A pulmonary artery catheter can be more useful as a guide in the treatment of myocardial dysfunction. It can be used to guide fluid replacement, to measure cardiac output, and to calculate systemic vascular resistance and thereby to evaluate the effectiveness of vasopressor, vasodilator, or inotropic therapy.

Indications for placing a pulmonary artery catheter are influenced by the information likely to be derived. Use of a pulmonary artery catheter has not beeen shown to be associated with improved outcomes. Nevertheless, the value and safety of pulmonary artery catheterization in selected patients are widely accepted. Central venous pressure and pulmonary artery occlusion pressure correlate in patients with ischemic heart disease when the ejection fraction is greater than 50%. However, if the ejection fraction is less than 50%, there is no longer a predictable correlation.

Transesophageal Echocardiography The development of new regional ventricular wall motion abnormalities is the accepted standard for the intraoperative diagnosis of myocardial ischemia. These regional wall motion abnormalities occur before ECG changes occur. However, segmental wall motion abnormalities may also occur in response to events other than myocardial ischemia. The limitations of transesophageal echocardiography include its cost, the need for extensive training in interpretation, and the fact that it cannot be inserted until after induction of anesthesia, so there is a critical period during which myocardial ischemia may develop in the absence of this monitoring.

Intraoperative Management of Myocardial Ischemia

Treatment of myocardial ischemia should be instituted when there are 1-mm ST-segment changes on the ECG. Prompt, aggressive pharmacologic treatment of changes in heart rate and/or blood pressure is indicated. A persistent increase in heart rate can be treated by intravenous administration of a β-blocker such as esmolol. Nitroglycerin is a more appropriate choice when myocardial ischemia is associated with a normal to modestly elevated blood pressure. In this situation, the nitroglycerin-induced coronary vasodilation and decrease in preload facilitate improved subendocardial blood flow but the nitroglycerin-induced decrease in afterload does not decrease systemic blood pressure to the point that coronary perfusion pressure is jeopardized.

Hypotension is treated with sympathomimetic drugs to restore coronary perfusion pressure. In addition to vasoconstrictor drugs, fluid infusion can be useful to help restore blood pressure. Regardless of the treatment, prompt restoration of blood pressure is necessary to maintain pressure-dependent flow through coronary arteries narrowed by atherosclerosis. In an unstable hemodynamic situation, circulatory support with inotropes or an intra-aortic balloon pump may be necessary. It may also be necessary to plan for early postoperative cardiac catheterization.

Postoperative Management

Although significant advances have been made in researching and refining preoperative evaluation and risk management strategies, evidence-based strategies that can specifically be adopted in the postoperative period to improve outcome have not yet been developed.

The goals of postoperative management are the same as those for intraoperative management: prevent ischemia, monitor for myocardial injury, and treat myocardial ischemia/infarction. Any situation that leads to prolonged and significant hemodynamic perturbations can stress the heart. Intraoperative hypothermia may predispose to shivering on awakening, leading to abrupt and dramatic increases in myocardial oxygen requirements. Pain, hypoxemia, hypercarbia, sepsis, and hemorrhage also lead to increased myocardial oxygen demand. The resulting oxygen supply/demand imbalance in patients with ischemic heart disease can precipitate myocardial ischemia, infarction, or death. Although most adverse cardiac events occur within the first 48 hours postoperatively, delayed cardiac events (within the first 30 days) can occur and could be the result of secondary stresses. It is imperative that patients on β-blockers continue to receive these drugs throughout the perioperative period.

Prevention of hypovolemia and hypotension is necessary postoperatively, and not only intravascular volume but also an adequate hemoglobin concentration must be maintained.

Oxygen content and oxygen delivery are significantly dependent on the concentration of hemoglobin in blood. The degree of anemia that can be safely tolerated in patients with ischemic heart disease remains to be defined.

The timing of weaning and tracheal extubation is another aspect of care that requires careful consideration. Early extubation is possible and desirable in many patients as long as they fulfill the criteria for extubation. However, patients with ischemic heart disease can become ischemic during emergence from anesthesia and/or weaning with an increased heart rate and blood pressure. These hemodynamic alterations must be managed diligently. Pharmacologic therapy with a β-blocker or combined α- and β-blockers such as labetalol can be very helpful.

Continuous ECG monitoring is useful for detecting postoperative myocardial ischemia, which is often silent. Postoperative myocardial ischemia predicts adverse in-hospital and long-term cardiac events. It should be identified, evaluated, and managed aggressively, preferably in consultation with a cardiologist.

CARDIAC TRANSPLANTATION

Heart transplantation is most often used in patients with end-stage heart failure due to a dilated cardiomyopathy or ischemic heart disease. Preoperatively, the ejection fraction is often less than 20%. Irreversible pulmonary hypertension is a contraindication to cardiac transplantation, and most centers do not consider candidates older than 65 years of age for a transplant.

Management of Anesthesia

Patients may come for cardiac transplantation with inotropic, vasodilator, or mechanical circulatory support. They should be stable hemodynamically before induction of anesthesia. Etomidate is preferred as an induction agent because it has little effect on hemodynamics. An opioid technique is often chosen for maintenance of anesthesia. Volatile anesthetics may produce undesirable degrees of myocardial depression and peripheral vasodilation. Nitrous oxide is rarely used because significant pulmonary hypertension is often present. In addition, there is concern about air embolism because large blood vessels are opened during the surgical procedure. Nondepolarizing neuromuscular blocking drugs that do not cause histamine release are usually selected. The ability of pancuronium to increase heart rate and systemic blood pressure modestly may be desirable in some patients. Many patients undergoing heart transplantation have coagulation disturbances due to passive congestion of the liver as a result of chronic congestive heart failure.

The operative technique consists of cardiopulmonary bypass and anastomosis of the aorta, pulmonary artery, and left and right atria. Immunosuppressive drugs are usually initiated during the preoperative period. Intravascular catheters are placed using strict aseptic technique. It is necessary to withdraw the central venous or pulmonary artery catheter into the superior vena cava when the heart is removed. The catheter is then repositioned into the donor heart. These catheters are often inserted into the central circulation via the left internal jugular vein so that the right internal jugular vein is available as an access site when needed to perform cardiac biopsies during the postoperative period. Transesophageal echocardiography is usually used to monitor cardiac function.

Aftzer cessation of cardiopulmonary bypass, an inotropic drug may be needed briefly to maintain myocardial contractility and heart rate. Therapy to lower pulmonary vascular resistance may be necessary and includes administration of a pulmonary vasodilator such as isoproterenol, a prostaglandin, nitric oxide, or a phosphodiesterase inhibitor. The denervated transplanted heart initially assumes an intrinsic heart rate of about 110 bpm, reflecting the absence of normal vagal tone. Stroke volume responds to an increase in preload by the Frank-Starling mechanism. These patients tolerate hypovolemia poorly. The transplanted heart does respond to direct-acting catecholamines, but drugs that act by indirect mechanisms such as ephedrine have a less intense effect. Vasopressin may be needed to treat severe hypotension unresponsive to catecholamines. The heart rate does not change in response to administration of anticholinergic or anticholinesterase drugs. About one fourth of patients develop bradycardia after transplantation that requires insertion of a permanent cardiac pacemaker.

Postoperative Complications

Early postoperative morbidity after heart transplantation surgery is usually related to sepsis and rejection. The most common early cause of death after cardiac transplantation is opportunistic infection as a result of immunosuppressive therapy. Transvenous right ventricular endomyocardial biopsies are performed to provide early warning of otherwise clinically asymptomatic allograft rejection. Congestive heart failure and development of dysrhythmias are late signs of rejection. Cyclosporine treatment is associated with drug-induced hypertension that is often resistant to antihypertensive therapy. Nephrotoxicity is another complication of cyclosporine therapy. Long-term corticosteroid use may result in skeletal demineralization and glucose intolerance.

Late complications of cardiac transplantation include development of coronary artery disease in the allograft and an increased incidence of cancer. Diffuse obliterative coronary arteriopathy affects cardiac transplant recipients over time, and the ischemic sequelae of this form of coronary artery disease are the principal limitations to long-term survival. The arterial disease is restricted to the allograft and is present in about one half of cardiac transplant recipients after 5 years. The accelerated appearance of this coronary artery disease likely reflects a chronic rejection process in the vascular endothelium. This process is not unique to cardiac allografts and is thought to be analogous to the chronic immunologically mediated changes seen in other organ allografts (chronic rejection of the kidney, bronchiolitis obliterans in the lungs, vanishing bile duct syndrome in the liver). The clinical sequelae of this obliterative coronary artery disease include myocardial ischemia, left ventricular dysfunction, cardiac dysrhythmias, and sudden death. The prognosis for transplant recipients with angiographically established coronary artery disease is poor.

Any medical regimen involving long-term immunosuppression is associated with an increased incidence of cancer, especially lymphoproliferative and cutaneous cancers. Malignancy is responsible for a significant portion of the mortality of heart transplant patients. Most posttransplantation lymphoproliferative disease is related to infection with the Epstein-Barr virus.

Anesthetic Considerations in Heart Transplant Recipients

Heart transplant patients present unique anesthetic challenges because of the hemodynamic function of the transplanted denervated heart, the side effects of immunosuppressive therapy, the risk of infection, the potential for drug interactions with complex drug regimens, and the potential for allograft rejection.

Allograft rejection results in progressive deterioration of cardiac function. The presence and degree of rejection should be noted preoperatively. The presence of infection must also be noted preoperatively because infection is a significant cause of morbidity and mortality in these patients. Invasive monitoring requires strict aseptic technique. When hepatic and renal function is normal, there is no contraindication to the use of any anesthetic drug.

Cardiac Innervation

The transplanted heart has no sympathetic, parasympathetic, or sensory innervation, and the loss of vagal tone results in a higher than normal resting heart rate. There are two P waves detectable on the ECG after heart transplantation. The native sinus node remains intact if a cuff of atrium is left to permit surgical anastomosis to the grafted heart. Because the native P wave cannot traverse the suture line, it has no influence on the chronotropic activity of the heart. Carotid sinus massage and the Valsalva maneuver have no effect on heart rate. There is no sympathetic response to direct laryngoscopy and tracheal intubation, and the denervated heart has a blunted heart rate response to light anesthesia or intense pain. The transplanted heart is unable to increase its heart rate immediately in response to hypovolemia or hypotension but responds instead with an increase in stroke volume (Frank-Starling mechanism). The needed increase in cardiac output is dependent on venous return until the heart rate increases after several minutes in response to the effect of circulating catecholamines. Because α- and β-adrenergic receptors are intact on the transplanted heart, it will eventually respond to circulating catecholamines.

Cardiac dysrhythmias may occur in heart transplant patients, perhaps reflecting a lack of vagal innervation and/or increased levels of circulating catecholamines. At rest, the heart rate reflects the intrinsic rate of depolarization of the donor sinoatrial node in the absence of any vagal tone. First-degree atrioventricular block (an increased PR interval) is common after cardiac transplantation. Some patients may require a cardiac pacemaker for treatment of bradydysrhythmias. A surgical transplantation technique that preserves the anatomic integrity of the right atrium by using anastomoses at the level of the superior and inferior vena cava rather than at the mid-atrial level results in better preservation of sinoatrial node and

tricuspid valve function. Afferent denervation renders the cardiac transplant patient incapable of experiencing angina pectoris in response to myocardial ischemia.

Responses to Drugs

Catecholamine responses are different in the transplanted heart because the intact sympathetic nerves required for normal uptake and metabolism of catecholamines are absent. The density of α and β receptors in the transplanted heart is unchanged, however, and responses to direct-acting sympathomimetic drugs are intact. Epinephrine, isoproterenol, and dobutamine have similar effects in normal and denervated hearts. Indirect-acting sympathomimetics such as ephedrine have a blunted effect on denervated hearts.

Vagolytic drugs such as atropine do not increase the heart rate. Pancuronium does not increase the heart rate and neostigmine and other anticholinesterases do not slow the heart rate of denervated hearts.

Preoperative Evaluation

Heart transplant recipients may present with ongoing rejection manifesting as myocardial dysfunction, accelerated coronary atherosclerosis, or dysrhythmias. All preoperative drug therapy must be continued, and proper functioning of a cardiac pacemaker, if in place, must be confirmed. Cyclosporine-induced hypertension may require treatment with calcium channel–blocking drugs or ACE inhibitors. Cyclosporine-induced nephrotoxicity may present as an increased creatinine concentration. Anesthetic drugs excreted mainly by renal clearance mechanisms should then be avoided. Proper hydration is important and should be confirmed preoperatively because heart transplant patients are preload dependent.

Management of Anesthesia

Experience suggests that heart transplant recipients undergoing noncardiac surgery have monitoring and anesthetic requirements similar to those of other patients undergoing the same surgery. Intravascular volume must be maintained intraoperatively because these patients are preload dependent and the denervated heart is unable to respond to sudden shifts in blood volume with an increase in heart rate. Invasive hemodynamic monitoring may be considered if the planned procedure is associated with large fluid shifts. Transesophageal echocardiography is an alternative to invasive hemodynamic monitoring in these patients. General anesthesia is usually selected because there may be an impaired response to the hypotension associated with spinal or epidural anesthesia. Anesthetic management includes avoidance of significant vasodilation and acute reductions in preload. Although volatile anesthetics may produce myocardial depression, they are usually well tolerated in heart transplant patients who do not have significant heart failure. Despite reports of cyclosporine-induced enhanced neuromuscular blockade, it does not appear that these patients require different dosing of muscle relaxants than nontransplant patients. Careful attention must be paid to appropriate aseptic technique because of the increased susceptibility to infection.

KEY POINTS

- The exercise ECG is most likely to indicate myocardial ischemia when there is at least 1 mm of horizontal or down–sloping ST-segment depression during or within 4 minutes after exercise. The greater the degree of ST-segment depression is, the greater the likelihood of significant coronary disease. When the ST-segment abnormality is associated with angina pectoris and occurs during the early stages of exercise and persists for several minutes after exercise, significant coronary artery disease is very likely.

- Noninvasive imaging tests for the detection of ischemic heart disease are used when exercise electrocardiography is not possible or interpretation of ST-segment changes would be difficult. Atropine, infusion of dobutamine, cardiac pacing, or administration of a coronary vasodilator such as adenosine and dipyridamole creates cardiac stress. After stress is induced, either echocardiography to assess myocardial function or radionuclide imaging to assess myocardial perfusion is performed.

- β–Blockers are the principal drug treatment for patients with angina pectoris. Long-term administration of β-blockers decreases the risk of death and myocardial reinfarction in patients who have had an MI, presumably by decreasing myocardial oxygen demand. This benefit is present even in patients in whom β-blockers were traditionally thought to be contraindicated (congestive heart failure, pulmonary disease, advanced age).

- Patients with acute coronary syndrome can be categorized based on a 12-lead ECG. Patients with ST elevation at presentation are considered to have ST elevation MI. Patients who present with ST-segment depression or nonspecific ECG changes can be further categorized based on the levels of cardiac-specific troponins or CK-MB. Elevation of cardiac-specific biomarkers indicates non–ST elevation MI. If cardiac-specific biomarkers are normal, then unstable angina is present

- ST elevation MI occurs when coronary blood flow decreases abruptly. This decrease in blood flow is attributable to acute thrombus formation at a site where an atherosclerotic plaque fissures, ruptures, or ulcerates, creating a local environment that favors thrombogenesis. Typically, "vulnerable" plaques, that is, those with rich lipid cores and thin fibrous caps, are most prone to rupture. Plaques that rupture are rarely of a size that causes significant coronary obstruction. By contrast, flow-restrictive plaques that produce angina pectoris and stimulate development of collateral circulation are less likely to rupture.

- The primary aim in the management of ST elevation MI is reestablishment of blood flow in the obstructed coronary artery as soon as possible. This can be achieved by reperfusion therapy or coronary angioplasty with or without an intracoronary stent.

- Administration of β-blockers is associated with a significant decrease in early (in-hospital) and long-term mortality and myocardial reinfarction. Early administration of β-blockers can decrease infarct size by decreasing heart rate, blood pressure, and myocardial contractility. In the absence of specific contraindications, it is recommended that *all* patients receive intravenous β-blockers as early as possible after acute MI.

- Non–ST elevation MI and UA result from a reduction in myocardial oxygen supply. Rupture or erosion of an atherosclerotic coronary plaque leads to thrombosis, inflammation, and vasoconstriction. Embolization of platelets and clot fragments into the coronary microvasculature leads to microcirculatory ischemia and infarction and results in elevation of cardiac biomarkers.

- Infarction of the anterior wall and/or apex of the left ventricle results in intracardiac thrombus formation in as many as one third of patients. Echocardiography can be used to detect this thrombus, and the presence of a left ventricular thrombus is an indication for immediate anticoagulation with heparin followed by 6 months of anticoagulation with warfarin. Thrombolytic therapy is associated with hemorrhagic stroke in 0.3% to 1% of patients.

- In older studies, postoperative MI was usually diagnosed by development of Q waves on the ECG. It is now known that many postoperative MIs are non–Q-wave infarctions and can be diagnosed by ECG changes and/or release of cardiac biomarkers. Two different pathophysiologic mechanisms may be responsible for perioperative MI. One is related to acute coronary thrombosis, and the other is the consequence of increased myocardial oxygen demand in the setting of compromised myocardial oxygen supply.

- Retrospective studies of large groups of patients note that the incidence of myocardial reinfarction during the perioperative period is influenced by the time elapsed since the previous MI. Acute (1–7 days) and recent (8–30 days) MI and UA incur the highest risk of perioperative myocardial ischemia, MI, and cardiac death.

- Stent placement (drug-eluting or bare metal stent) is routinely followed by postprocedure antiplatelet therapy to prevent acute coronary thrombosis and maintain long-term patency of the vessel. Elective noncardiac surgery should be delayed for 4 to 6 weeks after coronary angioplasty. It is prudent to delay elective noncardiac surgery for 30 to 45 days after a PCI with bare metal stent placement and for as long as 6 to 12 months in patients with drug-eluting stent placement

Continued

to allow complete endothelialization of the stent and completion of antiplatelet therapy.

- The simplest, most cost-effective method for detecting perioperative myocardial ischemia is electrocardiography. The diagnosis of myocardial ischemia focuses on changes in the ST segment characterized as depression or elevation of at least 1 mm. T-wave inversion can also be associated with myocardial ischemia. The degree of ST-segment depression parallels the severity of myocardial ischemia. Events other than myocardial ischemia that can cause ST-segment abnormalities include cardiac dysrhythmias, cardiac conduction disturbances, digitalis therapy, electrolyte abnormalities, and hypothermia.

- The transplanted heart has no sympathetic, parasympathetic, or sensory innervation, and the loss of vagal tone results in a higher than normal resting heart rate. Carotid sinus massage and the Valsalva maneuver have no effect on heart rate. There is no sympathetic response to direct laryngoscopy and tracheal intubation and the denervated heart has a blunted heart rate response to

light anesthesia or intense pain. The transplanted heart is unable to increase its heart rate immediately in response to hypovolemia or hypotension but responds instead with an increase in stroke volume (Frank-Starling mechanism). The needed increase in cardiac output is dependent on venous return. After several minutes, the heart rate increases in response to the effect of circulating catecholamines. Because α- and β-adrenergic receptors are intact on the transplanted heart, it eventually responds to circulating catecholamines.

- One of the late complications of cardiac transplantation is the development of coronary artery disease in the allograft. Diffuse obliterative coronary arteriopathy affects cardiac transplant recipients over time, and the ischemic sequelae of this form of coronary disease are the principal limitations to long-term survival. The arterial disease is restricted to the allograft and is present in about one half of cardiac transplant recipients after 5 years. The accelerated appearance of this coronary artery disease likely reflects a chronic rejection process in the vascular endothelium.

REFERENCES

Alpert JS, Thygesen K, Antman E, Bassand JP: Myocardial infarction redefined—a consensus document of the Joint European Society of Cardiology/American College of Cardiology Committee for the Redefinition of Myocardial Infarction. J Am Coll Cardiol 2000;36:959–969.

Antman EM, Anbe DT, Armstrong PW, et al: ACC/AHA guidelines for the management of patients with ST-elevation myocardial infarction—executive summary: A report of the American College of Cardiology/American Heart Association task force on practice guidelines (Writing Committee to Revise the 1999 Guidelines for the Management of Patients with Acute Myocardial Infarction). Circulation 2004;110: 588–636.

Braunwald E, Antman EM, Beasley JW, et al: ACC/AHA guidelines for the management of patients with unstable angina and non-ST-segment elevation myocardial infarction: Executive summary and recommendations. A report of the American College of Cardiology/American Heart Association Task Force on Practice Guidelines (Committee on the Management of Patients with Unstable Angina). Circulation 2000; 102:1193–1209.

Chobanian AV, Bakris GL, Black HR, et al: The Seventh Report of the Joint National Committee on Prevention, Detection, Evaluation and Treatment of High Blood Pressure: The JNC 7 report. JAMA 2003;289:2560–2572.

Devereaux PJ, Goldman L, Cook DJ, et al: Perioperative cardiac events in patients undergoing noncardiac surgery: A review of the magnitude of the problem, the pathophysiology of the events and methods to estimate and communicate risk. CMAJ 2005;173:627–634.

Dupuis JY, Labinaz M: Noncardiac surgery in patients with coronary artery stent: What should the anesthesiologist know? Can J Anaesth 2005;52:356–361.

Feringa HH, Bax JJ, Boersma E, et al: High-dose beta-blockers and tight heart rate control reduce myocardial ischemia and troponin T release in vascular surgery patients. Circulation 2006; 114:I344–I349.

Fleisher LA: Real-time intraoperative monitoring of myocardial ischemia in noncardiac surgery. Anesthesiology 2000;92: 1183–1188.

Fleisher LA, Beckman JA, Brown KA, et al: ACC/AHA 2007 guidelines on perioperative cardiovascular evaluation and care for noncardiac surgery: a report of the American College of Cardiology/American Heart Association Task Force on Practice Guidelines (Writing Committee to Revise the 2002 Guidelines on Perioperative Cardiovascular Evaluation for Noncardiac Surgery): developed in collaboration with the American Society of Echocardiography, American Society of Nuclear Cardiology, Heart Rhythm Society, Society of Cardiovascular Anesthesiologists, Society for Cardiovascular Angiography and Interventions, Society for Vascular Medicine and Biology, and Society for Vascular Surgery. Circulation 2007;116:e418–e499.

Gibbons RJ, Abrams J, Chatterjee K, et al: ACC/AHA 2002 guideline update for the management of patients with chronic stable angina—summary article: A report of the American College of Cardiology/American Heart Association Task Force on practice guidelines (Committee on the Management of Patients with Chronic Stable Angina). J Am Coll Cardiol 2003;41:159–168.

Kostopanagiotou G, Smyrniotis V, Arkadopoulos N, et al: Anesthetic and perioperative management of adult transplant recipients in nontransplant surgery. Anesth Analg 1999;89: 613–622.

Landesberg G, Shatz V, Akopnik I, et al: Association of cardiac troponin, CK-MB, and postoperative myocardial ischemia with long-term survival after major vascular surgery. J Am Coll Cardiol 2003;42:1547–1554.

Libby P, Theroux P: Pathophysiology of coronary artery disease. Circulation 2005;111:3481–3488.

Mangano DT, Goldman L: Preoperative assessment of patients with known or suspected coronary disease. N Engl J Med 1995;333:1750–1756.

McFalls EO, Ward HB, Moritz TE, et al: Coronary artery revascularization before elective major vascular surgery. N Engl J Med 2004;351:2795–2804.

Opie L, Poole-Wilson P: Beta-blocking agents. In Opie L, Gersh BJ (eds): Drugs for the Heart. Philadelphia, Elsevier Saunders, 2005.

Shanewise J: Cardiac transplantation. Anesthesiol Clin North Am 2004;22:753–765.

Sutton PR, Fihn SD: Chronic unstable angina. ACP Medicine. In Gibbons RJ (ed): Cardiovascular Medicine IX. WebMD Inc., 2004.

CHAPTER 2

Valvular Heart Disease

Adriana Herrera

Preoperative Evaluation
- History and Physical Examination
- Drug Therapy
- Laboratory Data
- Presence of Prosthetic Heart Valves
- Prevention of Bacterial Endocarditis

Mitral Stenosis
- Pathophysiology
- Diagnosis
- Treatment
- Management of Anesthesia

Mitral Regurgitation
- Pathophysiology
- Diagnosis
- Treatment
- Management of Anesthesia

Mitral Valve Prolapse
- Diagnosis
- Management of Anesthesia

Aortic Stenosis
- Pathophysiology
- Diagnosis
- Treatment
- Management of Anesthesia

Aortic Regurgitation
- Pathophysiology
- Diagnosis
- Treatment
- Management of Anesthesia

Tricuspid Regurgitation
- Pathophysiology
- Management of Anesthesia

Tricuspid Stenosis

Pulmonic Regurgitation

Pulmonic Stenosis

In the past 2 decades, there have been major advances in understanding the natural history of valvular heart disease and in improving cardiac function in patients with valvular heart disease. The development of better noninvasive monitors of ventricular function, improved prosthetic heart valves, better techniques for valve reconstruction, and the development of guidelines for selecting the proper timing for surgical intervention have resulted in an increased survival in this group of patients.

Valvular heart disease places a hemodynamic burden on the left and/or right ventricle that is initially tolerated as the cardiovascular system compensates for the overload. Hemodynamic overload eventually leads to cardiac muscle dysfunction, congestive heart failure (CHF), or even sudden death. Management of the patient with valvular heart disease during the perioperative period requires an understanding of the hemodynamic alterations that accompany valvular dysfunction.

The most frequently encountered cardiac valve lesions produce pressure overload (mitral stenosis, aortic stenosis) or volume overload (mitral regurgitation, aortic regurgitation) on the left atrium or left ventricle. Anesthetic management during the perioperative period is based on the likely effects of drug-induced changes in cardiac rhythm, heart rate, preload, afterload, myocardial contractility, systemic blood pressure, systemic vascular resistance, and pulmonary vascular resistance relative to the pathophysiology of the heart disease.

PREOPERATIVE EVALUATION

Preoperative evaluation of patients with valvular heart disease includes assessment of (1) the severity of the cardiac disease, (2) the degree of impaired myocardial contractility, and (3) the presence of associated major organ system disease. Recognition of compensatory mechanisms for maintaining cardiac output such as increased sympathetic nervous system activity and cardiac hypertrophy as well as consideration of current drug therapy are important. The presence of a prosthetic heart valve introduces special considerations in the preoperative evaluation, especially if noncardiac surgery is planned.

History and Physical Examination

Questions designed to define exercise tolerance are necessary to evaluate cardiac reserve in the presence of valvular heart disease and to provide a functional classification according to the criteria established by the New York Heart Association (**Table 2-1**). When myocardial contractility is impaired, patients complain of dyspnea, orthopnea, and easy fatigability. A compensatory increase in sympathetic nervous system activity may manifest as anxiety, diaphoresis, and resting tachycardia. CHF is a frequent companion of chronic valvular heart disease, and its presence is detected by noting basilar chest rales, jugular venous distention, and a third heart sound on physical examination. Typically, elective surgery is deferred until CHF can be treated and myocardial contractility optimized.

Disease of a cardiac valve rarely occurs without an accompanying murmur, reflecting turbulent blood flow across the valve. The character, location, intensity, and direction of radiation of a heart murmur provide clues to the location and severity of the valvular lesion. During systole, the aortic and pulmonic valves are open, and the mitral and tricuspid valves are closed. Therefore, a heart murmur that occurs during systole is due to stenosis of the aortic or pulmonic valves or incompetence of the mitral or tricuspid valves. During diastole, the aortic and pulmonic valves are closed, and the mitral and tricuspid valves are open. Therefore, a diastolic heart murmur is due to stenosis of the mitral or tricuspid valves or incompetence of the aortic or pulmonic valves.

Cardiac dysrhythmias are seen with all types of valvular heart disease. Atrial fibrillation is common, especially with mitral valve disease associated with left atrial enlargement. Atrial fibrillation may be paroxysmal or chronic.

Angina pectoris may occur in patients with valvular heart disease even in the absence of coronary artery disease. It usually reflects increased myocardial oxygen demand due to ventricular hypertrophy. The demands of this thickened muscle mass may exceed the ability of even normal coronary arteries to deliver adequate amounts of oxygen. Valvular heart disease and ischemic heart disease frequently co-exist. Fifty percent of patients with aortic stenosis who are older than 50 years of age have associated ischemic heart disease. The presence of coronary artery disease in patients with mitral or aortic valve disease worsens the long-term prognosis and mitral regurgitation due to ischemic heart disease is associated with an increased mortality.

Drug Therapy

Modern drug therapy for valvular heart disease may include β-blockers, calcium channel blockers, and digitalis for heart rate control, angiotensin-converting enzyme inhibitors, and vasodilators to control blood pressure and afterload and diuretics, inotropes and vasodilators as needed to control heart failure. Antidysrhythmic therapy may also be necessary. Certain cardiac lesions such as aortic and mitral stenosis require a slow heart rate to prolong the duration of diastole and improve left ventricular filling and coronary blood flow. The regurgitant valvular lesions such as aortic and mitral regurgitation require afterload reduction and a somewhat faster heart rate to shorten the time for regurgitation. Atrial fibrillation requires a controlled ventricular response so that activation of the sympathetic nervous system, as during tracheal intubation or in response to surgical stimulation, does not cause sufficient tachycardia to significantly decrease diastolic filling time and stroke volume.

Laboratory Data

The electrocardiogram (ECG) often exhibits characteristic changes due to valvular heart disease. Broad and notched P waves (P mitrale) suggest the presence of left atrial enlargement typical of mitral valve disease. Left and right ventricular hypertrophy can be diagnosed by the presence of left or right axis deviation and high voltage. Other common ECG findings include dysrhythmias, conduction abnormalities, evidence of active ischemia, or previous myocardial infarction.

TABLE 2-1	New York Heart Association Functional Classification of Patients with Heart Disease	
---	---	
Class	**Description**	
I	Asymptomatic	
II	Symptoms with ordinary activity but comfortable at rest	
III	Symptoms with minimal activity but comfortable at rest	
IV	Symptoms at rest	

TABLE 2-2 Utility of Doppler Echocardiography in Valvular Heart Disease

Determine significance of cardiac murmurs
Identify hemodynamic abnormalities associated with physical findings
Determine transvalvular pressure gradient
Determine valve area
Determine ventricular ejection fraction
Diagnose valvular regurgitation
Evaluate prosthetic valve function

The size and shape of the heart and great vessels and pulmonary vascular markings can be evaluated by chest radiography. On a posteroanterior chest radiograph, cardiomegaly can be noted if the heart size exceeds 50% of the internal width of the thoracic cage. Abnormalities of the pulmonary artery, left atrium, and left ventricle can be noted along the left heart border and right atrial and right ventricular enlargement along the right heart border. Enlargement of the left atrium can result in elevation of the left mainstem bronchus. Valvular calcifications may be identified. Vascular markings in the peripheral lung fields are sparse in the presence of significant pulmonary hypertension.

Echocardiography with Doppler color flow imaging is essential for noninvasive evaluation of valvular heart disease (**Table 2-2**). It is particularly useful in evaluating the significance of cardiac murmurs such as systolic ejection murmurs in suspected aortic stenosis and for detecting the presence of mitral stenosis. It permits determination of cardiac anatomy and function, hypertrophy, cavity dimensions, valve area, transvalvular pressure gradients, and the magnitude of valvular regurgitation.

Cardiac catheterization can provide information about the presence and severity of valvular stenosis and/or regurgitation, coronary artery disease, and intracardiac shunting and can help resolve discrepancies between clinical and echocardiographic findings. Transvalvular pressure gradients determined at the time of cardiac catheterization indicate the severity of the valvular heart disease. Mitral and aortic stenoses are considered to be severe when transvalvular pressure gradients are more than 10 mm Hg and 50 mm Hg, respectively. However, when CHF accompanies aortic stenosis, transvalvular pressure gradients may be smaller because of the inability of the dysfunctional left ventricular muscle to generate a large gradient. In patients with mitral stenosis or mitral regurgitation, measurement of pulmonary artery pressure and right ventricular filling pressure may provide evidence of pulmonary hypertension and right ventricular failure.

Presence of Prosthetic Heart Valves

Prosthetic heart valves may be mechanical or bioprosthetic. Mechanical valves are composed primarily of metal or carbon alloys and are classified according to their structure, such as caged ball, single tilting disk, or bileaflet tilting disk valves.

Bioprostheses may be heterografts, composed of porcine or bovine tissues mounted on metal supports, or homografts, which are preserved human aortic valves.

Prosthetic valves differ from one another with regard to durability, thrombogenicity, and hemodynamic profile. Mechanical valves are very durable, lasting at least 20 to 30 years, whereas bioprosthetic valves last about 10 to 15 years. Mechanical valves are highly thrombogenic and require long-term anticoagulation. Because bioprosthetic valves have a low thrombogenic potential, long-term anticoagulation is not necessary. Mechanical valves are preferred in patients who are young, have a life expectancy of more than 10 to 15 years, or require long-term anticoagulation therapy for another reason such as atrial fibrillation. Bioprosthetic valves are preferred in elderly patients and in those who cannot tolerate anticoagulation.

Assessment of Prosthetic Heart Valve Function

Prosthetic heart valve dysfunction is suggested by a change in the intensity or quality of prosthetic valve clicks, the appearance of a new murmur, or a change in the characteristics of an existing murmur. Transthoracic echocardiography can be used to assess sewing ring stability and leaflet motion of bioprosthetic valves, but mechanical valves may be difficult to evaluate because of echo reverberations from the metal. Transesophageal echocardiography may provide higher resolution images, especially of a prosthetic mitral valve. Magnetic resonance imaging can be used if prosthetic valve regurgitation or a paravalvular leak is suspected but not adequately visualized by echocardiography. Cardiac catheterization permits measurement of transvalvular pressure gradients and effective valve area of bioprosthetic valves.

Complications Associated with Prosthetic Heart Valves

Prosthetic heart valves can be associated with significant complications whose presence should be considered during the preoperative evaluation (**Table 2-3**). Because of the risk of thromboembolism, patients with mechanical prosthetic heart valves require long-term anticoagulant therapy. Subclinical intravascular hemolysis, evidenced by increased serum lactate dehydrogenase concentrations, decreased serum haptoglobin concentration, and reticulocytosis is noted in many patients with normally functioning mechanical heart valves. The incidence of pigmented gallstones is

TABLE 2-3 Complications Associated with Prosthetic Heart Valves

Valve thrombosis
Systemic embolization
Structural failure
Hemolysis
Paravalvular leak
Endocarditis

increased in patients with prosthetic heart valves, presumably as a result of chronic low-grade intravascular hemolysis. Severe hemolytic anemia is uncommon, and its presence usually indicates valvular dysfunction or endocarditis. Antibiotic prophylaxis is necessary to decrease the risk of endocarditis.

Management of Anticoagulation in Patients with Prosthetic Heart Valves

Patients may need to discontinue anticoagulation before surgery. However, this temporary discontinuation of anticoagulant therapy puts patients with mechanical heart valves or atrial fibrillation at risk of arterial or venous thromboembolism due to a rebound hypercoagulable state and to the prothrombotic effects of surgery. The risk of thromboembolism is estimated to be about 5% to 8%. Anticoagulation may be continued in patients with prosthetic heart valves who are scheduled for minor surgery in which blood loss is expected to be minimal. However, when major surgery is planned, warfarin is typically discontinued 3 to 5 days preoperatively. Intravenous unfractionated heparin or subcutaneous low molecular weight heparin is administered after discontinuation of warfarin and continued until the day before or the day of surgery. The heparin can be restarted postoperatively when the risk of bleeding has lessened and can be continued until effective anticoagulation is again achieved with oral therapy.

When possible, elective surgery should be avoided in the first month after an acute episode of arterial or venous thromboembolism.

Anticoagulant therapy is particularly important in parturients with prosthetic heart valves because the incidence of arterial embolization is greatly increased during pregnancy. However, warfarin administration during the first trimester can be associated with fetal defects and fetal death. Therefore, warfarin is discontinued during pregnancy and subcutaneous standard or low molecular weight heparin is administered until delivery. Low-dose aspirin therapy is safe for the mother and child and can be used in conjunction with the heparin therapy.

Prevention of Bacterial Endocarditis

The American Heart Association has made recommendations for prevention of infective endocarditis for the past half century. The most recent Guidelines for the Prevention of Infective Endocarditis (2007) represent a radical departure from prior recommendations and dramatically reduce the indications for antibiotic prophylaxis for endocarditis. These new guidelines are based on the best available evidence regarding this medical problem.

Current scientific data suggest that infective endocarditis is much more likely to result from frequent exposure to bacteremia associated with daily activities than from bacteremia associated with dental, GI, or GU tract procedures. For example, maintenance of good oral health and oral hygiene reduces bacteremia associated with normal daily activities (chewing, teeth brushing, flossing, use of toothpicks, etc.) and is more important than prophylactic antibiotics in reducing the risk of endocarditis. Endocarditis prophylaxis may prevent an exceedingly small number of cases of endocarditis, if any, in at-risk patients. It also appears that the risk of antibiotic-associated adverse events exceeds the benefits of endocarditis prophylaxis overall and that the common use of antibiotic prophylaxis promotes the emergence of antibiotic-resistant organisms.

Another change in thinking about endocarditis prophylaxis has resulted in these new guidelines: The AHA experts feel that infective endocarditis prophylaxis should not be directed to individuals with a high cumulative lifetime risk of getting endocarditis but rather to those individuals at highest risk of adverse outcomes if they develop endocarditis. It appears that only a very small group of patients with heart disease is likely to have the most severe forms and complications of endocarditis. The conditions associated with this high risk are listed in **Table 2-4**. The new AHA guidelines focus endocarditis prophylaxis *only on patients with these conditions*. The recommendations regarding which antibiotic to use for endocarditis prophylaxis are not dissimilar from previous recommendations and are listed in **Table 2-5**.

In summary, the major changes in the updated AHA guidelines for infective endocarditis prophylaxis are these: 1) Antibiotic prophylaxis for endocarditis prophylaxis is recommended *only* for the conditions listed in Table 2-4. It is no longer recommended for any forms of congenital heart disease except as noted in Table 2-4. 2) Antibiotic prophylaxis *is*

TABLE 2-4	Cardiac Conditions Associated with the Highest Risk of Adverse Outcomes from Endocarditis for Which Prophylaxis for Dental Procedures Is Reasonable

1. Prosthetic cardiac valve or prosthetic material used for cardiac valve repair
2. Previous infective endocarditis
3. Congenital heart disease:
   Unrepaired cyanotic congenital heart disease, including palliative shunts and conduits
   Completely repaired congenital heart defect with prosthetic material or device, whether placed by surgery or by catheter intervention, during the first 6 months after the procedure*
   Repaired congenital heart disease with residual defects at the site or adjacent to the site of a prosthetic patch or prosthetic device (which inhibit endothelialization)
4. Cardiac transplantation recipients who develop cardiac valvulopathy

Except for the conditions listed above antibiotic prophylaxis is no longer recommended for any other form of congenital heart disease.
*Prophylaxis is reasonable because endothelialization of prosthetic material occurs within 6 months after the procedure.
From Wilson W, Taubert KA, Gewitz M, et al: Prevention of infective endocarditis. Guidelines from the American Heart Association. Circulation 2007;116:1736–1754, with permission.

TABLE 2-5 Antibiotic Prophylaxis Regimens for a Dental Procedure

Situation	Agent	REGIMEN: SINGLE DOSE 30 TO 60 MIN BEFORE PROCEDURE	
		Adults	Children
Oral	Amoxicillin	2 g	50 mg/kg
Unable to take oral medication	Ampicillin OR Cefazolin or ceftriaxone	2 g IM or IV 1 g IM or IV	50 mg/kg IM or IV 50 mg/kg IM or IV
Allergic to penicillins or ampicillin—oral	Cephalexin*,† OR Clindamycin*,† OR Azithromycin or clarithromycin	2 g 600 mg 500 mg	50 mg/kg 20 mg/kg 15 mg/kg
Allergic to penicillins or ampicillin and unable to take oral medication	Cefazolin or ceftriaxone† OR Clindamycin	1 g IM or IV 600 mg IM or IV	50 mg/kg IM or IV 20 mg/kg IM or IV

*Or other first- or second-generation oral cephalosporin in equivalent adult or pediatric dosage.
†Cephalosporins should not be used in an individual with a history of anaphylaxis, angioedema, or urticaria with penicillins or ampicillin.
From Wilson W, Taubert KA, Gewitz M, et al: Prevention of infective endocarditis. Guidelines from the American Heart Association. Circulation 2007;116:1736-1754 with permission.

recommended for dental procedures that involve manipulation of gingival tissues or the periapical regions of teeth or perforation of the oral mucosa. 3) Antibiotic prophylaxis *is* recommended for invasive procedures (i.e., those that involve incision or biopsy) on the respiratory tract or infected skin, skin structures or musculoskeletal tissue. 4) Antibiotic prophylaxis *is not* recommended for GU or GI tract procedures.

It would be prudent for every anesthesiologist to familiarize him- or herself with this new document on infective endocarditis prevention.

MITRAL STENOSIS

The most common cause of mitral stenosis is rheumatic heart disease. Mitral stenosis primarily affects females. Diffuse thickening of the mitral leaflets and subvalvular apparatus, commissural fusion, and calcification of the annulus and leaflets are typically present. This process occurs slowly, and many patients do not become symptomatic for 20 to 30 years after the initial episode of rheumatic fever. Over time, the mitral valve becomes stenotic and patients may develop CHF, pulmonary hypertension, and right ventricular failure.

Much less common causes of mitral stenosis include carcinoid syndrome, left atrial myxoma, severe mitral annular calcification, thrombus formation, cor triatriatum, rheumatoid arthritis, systemic lupus erythematosus, and congenital mitral stenosis. Patients with mitral stenosis typically exhibit dyspnea on exertion, orthopnea, and paroxysmal nocturnal dyspnea as a result of high left atrial pressure. Left ventricular contractility is usually normal. Rheumatic heart disease presents as isolated mitral stenosis in about 40% of patients. If aortic and/or mitral regurgitation accompany mitral stenosis, there is often evidence of left ventricular dysfunction.

Pathophysiology

Mitral stenosis is characterized by mechanical obstruction to left ventricular diastolic filling secondary to a progressive decrease in mitral valve orifice size. This valvular obstruction produces an increase in left atrial volume and pressure. With mild mitral stenosis, left ventricular filling and stroke volume are usually maintained at rest by an increase in left atrial pressure. However, stroke volume will decrease during stress-induced tachycardia or when effective atrial contraction is lost as with atrial fibrillation.

Pulmonary venous pressure is increased in association with the increase in left atrial pressure. The result is transudation of fluid into the pulmonary interstitial space, decreased pulmonary compliance, and increased work of breathing, leading to progressive dyspnea on exertion. Overt pulmonary edema is likely when the pulmonary venous pressure exceeds the oncotic pressure of plasma proteins. If the increase in left atrial pressure is gradual, there is an increase in lymphatic drainage from the lungs and thickening of the capillary basement membrane that enables patients to tolerate increased pulmonary venous pressure without development of pulmonary edema. Episodes of pulmonary edema typically occur with atrial fibrillation, sepsis, pain, and pregnancy. Hemoptysis may occur because of pulmonary hypertension.

Diagnosis

Echocardiography is used to assess the anatomy of the mitral valve including the degree of leaflet thickening, calcification, changes in mobility, and the extent of involvement of the

TABLE 2-6 Severity of Mitral Stenosis Measured by Echocardiography

	Mild	Moderate	Severe
Mean valve gradient (mm Hg)	6	6–10	>10
Pressure half time (ms)	100	200	>300
Mitral valve area (cm^2)	1.6–2.0	1.0–1.5	<1.0

subvalvular apparatus. The severity of mitral stenosis is assessed by calculation of mitral valve area and measurement of the transvalvular pressure gradient. Echocardiography also allows evaluation of cardiac chamber dimensions, pulmonary hypertension, ventricular function, associated valvular disease, and examination of the left atrial appendage for the presence or absence of thrombus.

Patients with mitral stenosis usually become symptomatic when the size of the mitral valve orifice (normally 4–6 cm^2) has decreased at least 50%. When the mitral valve area is less than 1 cm^2, a mean atrial pressure of about 25 mm Hg is necessary to maintain adequate left ventricular filling and resting cardiac output. Pulmonary hypertension is likely if the left atrial pressure is chronically above 25 mm Hg. When the mitral transvalvular pressure gradient is higher than 10 mm Hg (normally < 5 mm Hg), it is likely that mitral stenosis is severe (**Table 2-6**). When mitral stenosis is severe, any additional stress such as fever or sepsis may precipitate pulmonary edema.

Clinically, mitral stenosis is recognized by the characteristic opening snap that occurs early in diastole and by a rumbling diastolic heart murmur best heard at the apex or in the axilla. Vibrations set in motion by the opening of the mobile but stenosed valve cause the opening snap. Calcification of the valve and greatly reduced leaflet mobility result in disappearance of the opening snap. Left atrial enlargement is often visible on chest radiography as straightening of the left heart border and elevation of the left mainstem bronchus. The double density of the enlarged left atrium, mitral calcification, and evidence of pulmonary edema or pulmonary vascular congestion may also be seen. Broad notched P waves on the ECG suggest left atrial enlargement. Atrial fibrillation is present in about one third of patients with severe mitral stenosis.

Stasis of blood in the distended left atrium predisposes patients with mitral stenosis to a higher risk of thromboembolic events. Venous thrombosis is also more likely because of the decreased physical activity of these patients.

Treatment

When symptoms of mild mitral stenosis develop, diuretics can decrease the left atrial pressure and relieve symptoms. If atrial fibrillation develops, heart rate control may be achieved with digoxin, β-blockers, calcium channel blockers, or a combination of these medications. Control of the heart rate is critical because tachycardia impairs left ventricular filling and increases left atrial pressure. Anticoagulation is required in patients with mitral stenosis and atrial fibrillation because

the risk of embolic stroke in such patients is about 7% to 15% per year. Warfarin is administered to a target international normalized ratio (INR) of 2.5 to 3.0. Surgical correction of mitral stenosis is indicated when symptoms worsen and pulmonary hypertension develops.

Mitral stenosis can sometimes be corrected by percutaneous balloon valvotomy. In the presence of heavy valvular calcification or valve deformity, surgical commissurotomy, valve reconstruction, or valve replacement is performed. In patients with concomitant severe tricuspid regurgitation (due to pulmonary hypertension), tricuspid valvuloplasty or ring annuloplasty can be performed together with the mitral valve surgery.

Management of Anesthesia

Management of anesthesia for noncardiac surgery in patients with mitral stenosis includes prevention and treatment of events that can decrease cardiac output or produce pulmonary edema (**Table 2-7**). The development of atrial fibrillation with a rapid ventricular response significantly decreases cardiac output and can produce pulmonary edema. Treatment consists of cardioversion or intravenous administration of β-blockers, calcium channel blockers, or digoxin. Excessive perioperative fluid administration, Trendelenburg position, or autotransfusion via uterine contraction increases central blood volume and can precipitate CHF.

In patients with severe mitral stenosis, a sudden decrease in systemic vascular resistance may not be tolerated because the normal response to hypotension, i.e., a reflex increase in heart rate, itself decreases cardiac output. If necessary, systemic blood pressure and systemic vascular resistance can be maintained with sympathomimetic drugs such as ephedrine and phenylephrine, the latter being preferable because it does not affect heart rate.

Pulmonary hypertension and right ventricular failure may be precipitated by numerous factors, including hypercarbia, hypoxemia, lung hyperinflation, and an increase in lung water. Right ventricular failure may require support with inotropic and pulmonary vasodilating drugs.

Preoperative Medication

Preoperative medication can be used to decrease anxiety and its associated tachycardia, but it must be appreciated that patients with mitral stenosis may be more susceptible

TABLE 2-7 Intraoperative Events That Have a Significant Impact on Mitral Stenosis

Sinus tachycardia or a rapid ventricular response during atrial fibrillation

Marked increase in central blood volume, as associated with overtransfusion or head-down positioning

Drug-induced decrease in systemic vascular resistance

Hypoxemia and hypercarbia that may exacerbate pulmonary hypertension and evoke right ventricular failure than normal patients to the ventilatory depressant effects of these drugs.

Drugs used for heart rate control should be continued until the time of surgery. Diuretic-induced hypokalemia can be detected and treated preoperatively. Orthostatic hypotension may be evidence of diuretic-induced hypovolemia. It may be acceptable to continue anticoagulant therapy for minor surgery, but major surgery associated with significant blood loss requires discontinuation of anticoagulation. The use of regional anesthesia may be obviated by the results of coagulation tests.

Induction of Anesthesia

Induction of anesthesia can be achieved with any available intravenous induction drug, with the exception of ketamine, which should be avoided because of its propensity to increase the heart rate. Tracheal intubation and muscle relaxation for the surgery is accomplished by administration of muscle relaxants that do not induce cardiovascular changes such as tachycardia and hypotension from histamine release.

Maintenance of Anesthesia

Maintenance of anesthesia is best accomplished by use of drugs with minimal effects on heart rate, myocardial contractility, and systemic and pulmonary vascular resistance. Often a nitrous/narcotic anesthetic or a balanced anesthetic that includes low concentrations of a volatile anesthetic can achieve this goal. Nitrous oxide can evoke some pulmonary vasoconstriction and increase pulmonary vascular resistance, but this is not of clinical significance unless pulmonary hypertension is present.

Muscle relaxants with minimal effects on heart rate, blood pressure, and systemic vascular resistance are best for patients with mitral stenosis. Pharmacologic reversal of nondepolarizing muscle relaxants should be accomplished slowly to help ameliorate any drug-induced tachycardia caused by the anticholinergic drug in the mixture.

Light anesthesia and surgical stimulation can result in sympathetic stimulation producing tachycardia and systemic and pulmonary hypertension. Pulmonary vasodilator administration may be necessary if pulmonary hypertension is severe. Intraoperative fluid replacement must be carefully titrated because these patients are very susceptible to volume overload and the development of pulmonary edema.

Monitoring

Use of invasive monitoring depends on the complexity of the operative procedure and the magnitude of physiologic impairment caused by the mitral stenosis. Monitoring asymptomatic patients without evidence of pulmonary congestion need be no different from monitoring patients without valvular heart disease. Conversely, transesophageal echocardiography could be useful in patients with symptomatic mitral stenosis undergoing major surgery, especially if significant blood loss is expected. Continuous monitoring of intra-arterial pressure, pulmonary artery pressure, and left atrial pressure should be considered. These monitors are helpful for confirming the adequacy of cardiac function, intravascular fluid volume, ventilation, and oxygenation. It appears that patients with significant pulmonary hypertension are at greater risk of pulmonary artery rupture from wedging the pulmonary artery catheter, so measurement of pulmonary artery occlusion pressure should be done infrequently and very carefully.

Postoperative Management

In patients with mitral stenosis, the risk of pulmonary edema and right heart failure continues into the postoperative period, so cardiovascular monitoring should continue as well. Pain and hypoventilation with subsequent respiratory acidosis and hypoxemia may be responsible for increasing heart rate and pulmonary vascular resistance. Decreased pulmonary compliance and increased work of breathing may necessitate a period of mechanical ventilation, particularly after major thoracic or abdominal surgery. Relief of postoperative pain with neuroaxial opioids can be very useful in selected patients.

MITRAL REGURGITATION

Mitral regurgitation due to rheumatic fever is usually associated with mitral stenosis. Isolated mitral regurgitation can be acute, be associated with ischemic heart disease, and result from papillary muscle dysfunction, mitral annular dilation, or rupture of chordae tendineae.

Other causes of mitral regurgitation include endocarditis, mitral valve prolapse, congenital lesions such as an endocardial cushion defect, left ventricular hypertrophy, cardiomyopathy, myxomatous degeneration, systemic lupus erythematosus, rheumatoid arthritis, ankylosing spondylitis, and carcinoid syndrome.

Pathophysiology

The basic hemodynamic derangement in mitral regurgitation is a decrease in forward left ventricular stroke volume and cardiac output. A portion of every stroke volume is regurgitated through the incompetent mitral valve back into the left atrium resulting in left atrial volume overload and pulmonary congestion. Patients with a regurgitant fraction of more than 0.6 are considered to have severe mitral regurgitation. The fraction of left ventricular stroke volume that regurgitates into the left atrium depends on (1) the size of the mitral valve orifice; (2) heart rate, which determines the duration of ventricular ejection; and (3) pressure gradients across the mitral valve. Such gradients are related to left ventricle compliance and impedance to left ventricular ejection into the aorta. Pharmacologic interventions that increase or decrease systemic vascular resistance have a major impact on the regurgitant fraction in patients with mitral regurgitation.

Patients with isolated mitral regurgitation are less dependent on properly timed left atrial contraction for left ventricular filling than are patients with co-existing mitral or aortic stenosis. Patients with rheumatic fever–induced mitral regurgitation are most likely to exhibit marked left atrial enlargement and atrial fibrillation. Myocardial ischemia as a result of mitral regurgitation is uncommon because the increased left ventricular wall tension is quickly dissipated as the stroke volume is rapidly ejected into the aorta and left atrium. When mitral regurgitation develops gradually, the volume overload produced by mitral regurgitation transforms the left ventricle into a larger, more compliant chamber that is able to deliver a larger stroke volume. This occurs through a dissolution of collagen weave, remodeling of the extracellular matrix, rearrangement of myocardial fibers, and addition of new sarcomeres with the development of ventricular hypertrophy. Development of ventricular hypertrophy and increased compliance of the left atrium permit the accommodation of the regurgitant volume without a major increase in left atrial pressure. This allows patients to maintain cardiac output and remain free of pulmonary congestion and be asymptomatic for many years. The combination of mitral regurgitation and mitral stenosis results in volume and pressure overload, resulting in a markedly increased left atrial pressure. Atrial fibrillation, pulmonary edema, and pulmonary hypertension develop much earlier in these patients than in those with isolated mitral regurgitation.

Because there has been no time for development of left atrial or left ventricular compensation, acute mitral regurgitation presents as pulmonary edema and/or cardiogenic shock.

Diagnosis

Mitral regurgitation is recognized clinically by the presence of a holosystolic apical murmur with radiation to the axilla. Left ventricular hypertrophy and cardiomegaly are also detectable on physical examination. Severe mitral regurgitation can produce left atrial and left ventricular hypertrophy detectable on an ECG and chest radiograph. Echocardiography (**Table 2-8**) confirms the presence, severity, and often the cause of the mitral regurgitation. Left atrial size and pressure, left ventricular wall thickness, cavitary dimensions, ventricular function, and pulmonary artery pressure can be measured. In addition, the left atrial appendage can be evaluated for the presence of thrombus. Many methods exist to evaluate the severity of mitral regurgitation. These include color-flow and pulsed-wave Doppler examination of the mitral valve with calculation of regurgitant volume and regurgitant fraction and measurement of the area of the regurgitant jet. The presence of a V wave in a pulmonary artery occlusion pressure waveform reflects regurgitant flow through the mitral valve, and the size of this V wave correlates with the magnitude of the mitral regurgitation.

If the severity of mitral regurgitation is in doubt or mitral valve surgery is planned, cardiac catheterization is necessary. In older patients, coronary angiography should be included in the evaluation in the catheterization laboratory.

Treatment

Unlike stenotic cardiac valve lesions, regurgitant cardiac valve lesions often progress insidiously, causing left ventricular damage and remodeling before symptoms have developed. Early surgery may be warranted to prevent muscle dysfunction from becoming severe or irreversible. Survival may be prolonged if surgery is performed before the ejection fraction is less than 60% or before the left ventricle is unable to contract to an end-systolic dimension of 45 mm (normal < 40 mm). Symptomatic patients should undergo mitral valve surgery even if they have a normal ejection fraction. Mitral valve repair is preferred to mitral valve replacement because it restores valve competence, maintains the functional aspects of the mitral valve apparatus, and avoids insertion of a prosthesis. The mitral valve apparatus is very important in sustaining left ventricular function. The absence of the subvalvular apparatus causes distortion of the left ventricular contractile geometry and impairment of left ventricular ejection. In patients in whom the valve and its apparatus cannot be preserved, valve replacement is done, but there is a postoperative decline in left ventricular ejection fraction. Patients with an ejection fraction of less than 30% or left ventricular end-systolic dimension more than 55 mm do not improve with mitral valve surgery.

Although vasodilators are useful in the medical management of acute mitral regurgitation, there is no apparent benefit to long-term use of these drugs in *asymptomatic* patients with chronic mitral regurgitation. For *symptomatic* patients, angiotensin-converting enzyme inhibitors or β-blockers (particularly carvedilol) and biventricular pacing have all been shown to decrease functional mitral regurgitation and improve symptoms and exercise tolerance.

Management of Anesthesia

Management of anesthesia for noncardiac surgery in patients with mitral regurgitation includes prevention and treatment of events that may further decrease cardiac output (**Table 2-9**),

TABLE 2-8 Grading of Mitral Regurgitation by Echocardiography			
	Mild	**Moderate**	**Severe**
Area of MR jet (cm^2)	<3	3.0-6.0	>6
MR jet area as percentage of left atrial area	20–30	30–40	>40
Regurgitant fraction (%)	20–30	30–50	>55
MR, mitral regurgitation.			

TABLE 2-9 Anesthetic Considerations in Patients with Mitral Regurgitation
Prevent bradycardia
Prevent increases in systemic vascular resistance
Minimize drug-induced myocardial depression
Monitor the magnitude of regurgitant flow with a pulmonary artery catheter (size of the V wave) and/or echocardiography

The goal is to improve forward left ventricular stroke volume and decrease the regurgitant fraction. Maintenance of a normal to slightly increased heart rate is recommended. Bradycardia may result in severe left ventricular volume overload. Increases in systemic vascular resistance can also cause decompensation of the left ventricle. Afterload reduction with a vasodilator drug such as nitroprusside with or without an inotropic drug will improve left ventricular function. In most patients, cardiac output can be maintained or improved with modest increases in heart rate and modest decreases in systemic vascular resistance. The decrease in systemic vascular resistance caused by regional anesthesia may be beneficial in some patients.

Induction of Anesthesia

Induction of anesthesia can be achieved with an intravenous induction drug. Dosing should be adjusted to prevent an increase in systemic vascular resistance or a decrease in heart rate because both of these hemodynamic changes will decrease cardiac output. Selection of a muscle relaxant should follow the same principles. Pancuronium produces a modest increase in heart rate, which can contribute to maintenance of forward left ventricular stroke volume.

Maintenance of Anesthesia

Volatile anesthetics can be administered to attenuate the undesirable increases in systemic blood pressure and systemic vascular resistance that can accompany surgical stimulation. The increase in heart rate and decrease in systemic vascular resistance plus the minimal negative inotropic effects of isoflurane, desflurane, and sevoflurane make them all acceptable choices for maintenance of anesthesia. When myocardial function is severely compromised, use of an opioid-based anesthetic is another option because of the minimal myocardial depression that opioids produce. However, potent narcotics can produce significant bradycardia, and this would be very deleterious in the presence of severe mitral regurgitation. Mechanical ventilation should be adjusted to maintain near-normal acid-base and respiratory parameters. The pattern of ventilation must provide sufficient time between breaths for venous return. Maintenance of intravascular fluid volume is very important for maintaining left ventricular volume and cardiac output in these patients.

Monitoring

Anesthesia for minor surgery in patients with asymptomatic mitral regurgitation does not require invasive monitoring. However, in the presence of severe mitral regurgitation, the use of invasive monitoring is helpful for detecting the adequacy of cardiac output and the hemodynamic response to anesthetic and vasodilator drugs and facilitating intravenous fluid replacement. Mitral regurgitation produces a V wave on the pulmonary artery occlusion waveform. Changes in V wave amplitude can assist in estimating the magnitude and direction of changes in the degree of mitral regurgitation. However, pulmonary artery occlusion pressure may be a poor measure of left ventricular end-diastolic volume in patients with *chronic* mitral regurgitation. With *acute* mitral regurgitation, the left atrium is less compliant, and pulmonary artery occlusion pressure does correlate with left atrial and left ventricular end-diastolic pressure.

MITRAL VALVE PROLAPSE

Mitral valve prolapse (MVP) is defined as the prolapse of one or both mitral leaflets into the left atrium during systole with or without mitral regurgitation; it is associated with the auscultatory findings of a midsystolic click and a late systolic murmur. MVP is the most common form of valvular heart disease, affecting 1% to 2.5% of the U.S. population. It is more common in young women. MVP can be associated with Marfan syndrome, rheumatic carditis, myocarditis, thyrotoxicosis, and systemic lupus erythematosus. Although it is usually a benign condition, MVP can have devastating complications such as cerebral embolic events, infective endocarditis, severe mitral regurgitation requiring surgery, dysrhythmias, and sudden death. Patients with abnormal mitral valve morphology appear to be the subset of patients at risk of these complications.

Diagnosis

The definitive diagnosis of MVP is based on echocardiographic findings. It has been defined as valve prolapse of 2 mm or more above the mitral annulus. MVP can occur with or without leaflet thickening and with or without mitral regurgitation. Patients with redundant and thickened leaflets have a primary (anatomic) form of MVP. This form of MVP typically occurs in patients with connective tissue diseases or in elderly men. Patients with mild bowing and normal-appearing leaflets have a normal variant (functional) form of MVP, and their risk of adverse events is probably no different than that of the general population.

Patients with MVP may experience anxiety, orthostatic symptoms, palpitations, dyspnea, fatigue, and atypical chest pain. Cardiac dysrhythmias, both supraventricular and ventricular dysrhythmias, may occur and respond well to β-blocker therapy. Cardiac conduction abnormalities are not uncommon.

Management of Anesthesia

Management of anesthesia for noncardiac surgery in patients with MVP follows the same principles outlined earlier for patients with mitral regurgitation (see Table 2-9). Management is influenced primarily by the degree of mitral regurgitation. Interestingly, the degree of MVP can be affected by left ventricular dimensions and is more dynamic than mitral valvular disease. A larger ventricle will often have less prolapse (and regurgitation) than a smaller ventricle. So events that affect how much the left ventricle fills or empties with each cardiac cycle will affect the amount of mitral regurgitation. Perioperative events that enhance left ventricular *emptying* include (1) increased sympathetic activity that increases myocardial contractility, (2) decreased systemic vascular resistance, and (3) assumption of the upright posture. Hypovolemia reduces left ventricular *filling*. Events that *decrease* left ventricular emptying and *increase* left ventricular volume may *decrease* the degree of MVP. These include hypertension/vasoconstriction, drug-induced myocardial depression, and volume resuscitation.

Preoperative Evaluation

Preoperative evaluation should focus on distinguishing patients with purely functional disease from those with significant mitral regurgitation. Functional MVP is most often present in women younger than 45 years of age. Some patients may be taking β-blockers to control dysrhythmias, and these drugs should be continued throughout the perioperative period. Patients with a history of transient neurologic events who are in sinus rhythm with no atrial thrombi are likely to be on daily aspirin (81–325 mg/day), whereas patients with atrial fibrillation and/or left atrial thrombus and previous stroke are likely to be taking warfarin. Although the ECG frequently shows premature ventricular contractions, repolarization abnormalities, and QT interval prolongation, there is no evidence that these findings predict or are associated with adverse intraoperative events. In the absence of symptoms, the finding of a systolic click and murmur does not warrant a preoperative cardiologic consultation.

Older men with an anatomic form of MVP can present with symptoms of mild to moderate CHF, including exercise intolerance, orthopnea, and dyspnea on exertion. These patients may be taking diuretics and angiotensin-converting enzyme inhibitors. Physical examination often reveals a mid-systolic to holosystolic murmur, an S_3 gallop, and signs of pulmonary congestion.

Selection of Anesthetic Technique

Most patients with MVP have normal left ventricular function and tolerate all forms of general and regional anesthesia. Volatile anesthetic-induced myocardial depression can be useful for offsetting the vasodilation that could decrease left ventricular volume and increase mitral regurgitation. There is no contraindication to the use of regional anesthesia in patients with MVP. The decrease in systemic vascular resistance should be anticipated and administration of fluids should offset any changes in left ventricular volume that could affect the degree of MVP and mitral regurgitation.

Induction of Anesthesia

When selecting an intravenous induction drug, the need to avoid a significant or prolonged decrease in systemic vascular resistance must be considered. Etomidate causes minimal myocardial depression and minimal alterations in sympathetic nervous system activity, so it is an attractive choice for induction of anesthesia in the presence of hemodynamically significant MVP. Ketamine, because of its ability to stimulate the sympathetic nervous system and enhance left ventricular emptying, may cause an increase in MVP and mitral regurgitation.

Maintenance of Anesthesia

Maintenance of anesthesia must minimize sympathetic nervous system activation due to painful intraoperative stimuli. Volatile anesthetics combined with nitrous oxide and/or opioids are useful for attenuating sympathetic nervous system activity, but their doses must be titrated to minimize an undesirable decrease in systemic vascular resistance.

Patients with hemodynamically significant MVP may not tolerate the dose-dependent myocardial depression of volatile anesthetics. However, low concentrations (about 0.5 MAC) of isoflurane, desflurane, and sevoflurane can decrease the regurgitant fraction. In patients with severe mitral regurgitation, vasodilators such as nitroprusside or nitroglycerin may be carefully titrated to maximize forward left ventricular flow and decrease left ventricular end-diastolic volume and left atrial pressure. There are no clinical data to support the use of one muscle relaxant over another in the presence of isolated MVP, but drug-induced hemodynamic alterations such as vagolysis or histamine release deserve consideration when selecting a specific drug.

Unexpected ventricular dysrhythmias can occur during anesthesia especially during operations performed in the head-up or sitting position. Presumably, in these situations, there is an increase in left ventricular emptying and accentuation of MVP. Lidocaine and β-antagonists can treat these dysrhythmias.

Maintenance of proper fluid balance blunts the decrease in venous return caused by positive pressure ventilation. Proper fluid balance also helps prevent an increase in the degree of MVP. If vasopressors are needed, an α-agonist such as phenylephrine is acceptable. An anesthetic technique that includes controlled hypotension would be unwise because the change in systemic vascular resistance would enhance the degree of MVP.

Monitoring

Routine monitoring is all that is necessary in the vast majority of patients with MVP. An intra-arterial catheter and pulmonary artery catheter are only needed in patients with significant mitral regurgitation and left ventricular dysfunction.

AORTIC STENOSIS

Aortic stenosis is a common valvular lesion in the United States, and its incidence is increasing as the U.S. population grows older. Two factors are associated with development of aortic stenosis. The first is degeneration and calcification of the aortic leaflets and subsequent stenosis. This is a process of aging. The second factor is the presence of a bicuspid rather that a tricuspid aortic valve. Aortic stenosis develops earlier in life (30–50 years of age) in individuals with a bicuspid aortic valve than in those with a tricuspid aortic valve (60–80 years of age). Aortic stenosis is associated with similar risk factors (systemic hypertension, hypercholesterolemia) as ischemic heart disease.

Pathophysiology

Obstruction to ejection of blood into the aorta due to a decrease in the aortic valve area necessitates an increase in left ventricular pressure to maintain forward stroke volume. The normal valve area is 2.5 to 3.5 cm^2. Transvalvular pressure gradients higher than 50 mm Hg and an aortic valve area less than 0.8 cm^2 characterize severe aortic stenosis. Aortic stenosis is almost always associated with some degree of aortic regurgitation.

Angina pectoris may occur in patients with aortic stenosis despite the absence of coronary disease. This is due to an increase in myocardial oxygen requirements because of concentric left ventricular hypertrophy and the increase in myocardial work necessary to offset the afterload produced by the stenotic valve. In addition, myocardial oxygen delivery is decreased because of compression of subendocardial blood vessels by the increased left ventricular pressure.

Since the initial study by Goldman and colleagues in 1977 showing that patients with aortic stenosis had an increased risk of perioperative cardiac complications, many studies have demonstrated that these patients have an increased risk of perioperative mortality and of nonfatal myocardial infarction regardless of the presence of risk factors for coronary artery disease. The perioperative risk attributable to aortic stenosis is independent of the risk attributable to coronary artery disease.

The origin of syncope in patients with aortic stenosis is controversial but may reflect an exercise-induced decrease in systemic vascular resistance that remains uncompensated because cardiac output is limited by the stenotic valve. CHF can be due to systolic and/or diastolic dysfunction.

Diagnosis

The classic clinical symptoms of critical aortic stenosis are angina pectoris, syncope, and dyspnea on exertion, a manifestation of CHF. The onset of these symptoms has been shown to correlate with an average time to death of 5, 3, and 2 years, respectively. About 75% of symptomatic patients will succumb within 3 years if they do not have a valve replacement. On physical examination, auscultation reveals a characteristic systolic murmur heard best in the aortic area. This murmur may radiate to the neck and mimic a carotid bruit. Because patients with aortic stenosis frequently have concomitant carotid artery disease, this finding deserves special attention. Because many patients with aortic stenosis are asymptomatic, it is important to listen for the systolic murmur of aortic stenosis in older patients scheduled for surgery. Chest radiography may show a prominent ascending aorta due to poststenotic aortic dilation. The ECG may demonstrate left ventricular hypertrophy.

Echocardiography with Doppler examination of the aortic valve provides a more accurate assessment of the severity of aortic stenosis (**Table 2-10**) than does clinical evaluation, and patients can be followed echocardiographically to assess the progression of their disease. Findings include identification of a trileaflet versus a bileaflet aortic valve, thickening and calcification of the aortic valve, decreased mobility of the aortic valve leaflets, left ventricular hypertrophy, and systolic or diastolic dysfunction. Aortic valve area and transvalvular pressure gradients can be measured. Cardiac catheterization and coronary angiography may be necessary when the severity of aortic stenosis cannot be determined by echocardiography.

TABLE 2-10	Severity of Aortic Stenosis Measured by Echocardiography		
	Mild	**Moderate**	**Severe**
Mean transvalvular pressure gradient (mm Hg)	<20	20 – 50	>50
Peak transvalvular pressure gradient (mm Hg)	<36	>50	>80
Aortic valve area (cm^2)	1.0–1.5	0.8–1.0	<0.8

Exercise stress testing may be an additional strategy to evaluate asymptomatic patients with moderate to severe aortic stenosis to identify those with poor exercise tolerance and/or an abnormal blood pressure response to exercise. Patients with exercise-induced symptoms might benefit from aortic valve replacement.

Treatment

In asymptomatic patients with aortic stenosis, it appears to be safe to continue medical management and to delay valve replacement surgery until symptoms develop. However, there is a small risk of sudden death or rapid progression of symptoms and then sudden death. Mortality approaches 75% within 3 years after symptoms develop unless the aortic valve is replaced. Even though most patients with aortic stenosis are elderly, the risks of surgery are acceptable unless there are also serious comorbid diseases that can worsen outcome. Aortic valve replacement relieves the symptoms of aortic stenosis dramatically, and the ejection fraction usually increases. Coronary revascularization is often done at the time of aortic valve replacement in patients with both aortic stenosis and coronary artery disease.

Percutaneous aortic balloon valvotomy has been shown to be beneficial in adolescents and young adults with congenital or rheumatic aortic stenosis. However, adults with acquired aortic stenosis experience only temporary relief of symptoms with this procedure. Balloon valvotomy may occasionally be useful for palliation of aortic stenosis in patients who are not candidates for aortic valve replacement.

Management of Anesthesia

Patients with aortic stenosis coming for noncardiac surgery are at high risk of major perioperative cardiac complications, and the risk of these complications increases with the complexity of the surgery, hence, the importance of ascertaining the severity of the aortic stenosis preoperatively. Management of anesthesia in patients with aortic stenosis includes the prevention of hypotension and any hemodynamic change that will decrease cardiac output (**Table 2-11**).

TABLE 2-11	Anesthetic Considerations in Patients with Aortic Stenosis

Maintain normal sinus rhythm
Avoid bradycardia or tachycardia
Avoid hypotension
Optimize intravascular fluid volume to maintain venous return and left ventricular filling

Normal sinus rhythm must be maintained because the left ventricle is dependent on a properly timed atrial contraction to produce an optimal left ventricular end-diastolic volume. Loss of atrial contraction, as during junctional rhythm or atrial fibrillation, may produce a dramatic decrease in stroke volume and blood pressure. The heart rate is important because it determines the time available for ventricular filling, for ejection of the stroke volume, and for coronary perfusion. A sustained increase in heart rate decreases the time for left ventricular filling and ejection and reduces cardiac output. A decrease in heart rate can cause overdistention of the left ventricle. Hypotension reduces coronary blood flow and results in myocardial ischemia and further deterioration in left ventricular function and cardiac output. Aggressive treatment of hypotension is mandatory to prevent cardiogenic shock and/or cardiac arrest. Cardiopulmonary resuscitation is unlikely to be effective in patients with aortic stenosis because it is difficult, if not impossible, to create an adequate stroke volume across a stenotic aortic valve with cardiac compression.

Induction of Anesthesia

General anesthesia is often selected in preference to epidural or spinal anesthesia because the sympathetic blockade produced by regional anesthesia can lead to significant hypotension.

Induction of anesthesia can be accomplished with an intravenous induction drug that does not decrease systemic vascular resistance. An opioid induction may be useful if left ventricular function is compromised

Maintenance of Anesthesia

Maintenance of anesthesia can be accomplished with a combination of nitrous oxide and volatile anesthetic and opioids or by opioids alone. Drugs that depress sinus node automaticity can produce junctional rhythm and loss of properly timed atrial contraction, which can cause a significant reduction in cardiac output. If left ventricular function is impaired, it is prudent to avoid any drugs that can cause additional depression of myocardial contractility. A decrease in systemic vascular resistance is also very undesirable. Maintenance of anesthesia with nitrous oxide plus opioids or with opioids alone in high doses is recommended for patients with marked left ventricular dysfunction. Neuromuscular blocking drugs with minimal hemodynamic effects are best. Intravascular fluid volume should be maintained at normal levels.

The onset of junctional rhythm or bradycardia during anesthesia and surgery requires prompt treatment with glycopyrrolate, atropine, or ephedrine. Persistent tachycardia can be treated with β-antagonists such as esmolol. Supraventricular tachycardia should be promptly terminated with electrical cardioversion. Lidocaine and a defibrillator should be kept available, as these patients have a propensity to develop ventricular dysrhythmias.

Monitoring

Intraoperative monitoring of patients with aortic stenosis must include ECG leads that reliably detect cardiac rhythm and left ventricular myocardial ischemia. The complexity of the surgery and the severity of the aortic stenosis influence the decision to use an intra-arterial catheter, a pulmonary artery catheter, or transesophageal echocardiography. Such monitors help determine whether intraoperative hypotension is due to hypovolemia or heart failure. Pulmonary artery occlusion pressure may overestimate left ventricular end-diastolic volume because of the decreased ventricular compliance.

AORTIC REGURGITATION

Aortic regurgitation results from failure of aortic leaflet coaptation caused by disease of the aortic leaflets or of the aortic root. Common causes of leaflet abnormalities include infective endocarditis, rheumatic fever, bicuspid aortic valve, and the use of anorexigenic drugs. Abnormalities of the aortic root causing aortic regurgitation include idiopathic aortic root dilation, hypertension-induced aortoannular ectasia, aortic dissection, syphilitic aortitis, Marfan syndrome, Ehlers-Danlos syndrome, rheumatoid arthritis, ankylosing spondylitis, and psoriatic arthritis. Acute aortic regurgitation is usually the result of endocarditis or aortic dissection.

Pathophysiology

The basic hemodynamic derangement in aortic regurgitation is a decrease in cardiac output because of regurgitation of a part of the ejected stroke volume from the aorta back into the left ventricle during diastole. This results in a combined pressure and volume overload on the left ventricle. The magnitude of the regurgitant volume depends on (1) the time available for the regurgitant flow to occur, which is determined by the heart rate, and (2) the pressure gradient across the aortic valve, which is dependent on the systemic vascular resistance. The magnitude of aortic regurgitation is decreased by tachycardia and peripheral vasodilation. In contrast to mitral regurgitation, with aortic regurgitation, the entire stroke volume is ejected into the aorta. Because the pulse pressure is proportional to the stroke volume and aortic elastance, the increased stroke volume increases systolic pressure and systolic hypertension increases afterload. The left ventricle compensates by developing hypertrophy and enlarging to accommodate the volume overload. Because of the increased oxygen requirements necessitated by left ventricular hypertrophy and the

TABLE 2-12 Severity of Aortic Regurgitation Graded by Echocardiography

	Mild	Moderate	Severe
Regurgitant jet width as percentage of LVOT width	25–46	47–64	>65
Regurgitant jet area as percentage of LVOT area	4–24	25–59	>60
Aortic diastolic flow reversal	None		Holodiastolic retrograde flow in the descending aorta

LVOT, left ventricular outflow tract.

decrease in aortic diastolic pressure, which decreases coronary blood flow, angina pectoris may occur in the absence of coronary artery disease.

The left ventricle can usually tolerate the chronic volume overload. However, if left ventricular failure occurs, left ventricular end-diastolic volume increases dramatically and pulmonary edema develops. A helpful indicator of left ventricular function in the presence of aortic regurgitation is the echocardiographic determination of end-systolic volume and ejection fraction, both of which remain normal until left ventricular function becomes impaired. Indeed, surgery is recommended before the ejection fraction decreases to less than 55% and left ventricular end-systolic volume increases to more than 55 mL.

Compared to patients with chronic aortic regurgitation, patients with acute aortic regurgitation experience severe volume overload in a ventricle that has had no time to compensate. This typically results in coronary ischemia, rapid deterioration in left ventricular function, and heart failure.

Diagnosis

Aortic regurgitation is recognized clinically by its characteristic diastolic murmur heard best along the left sternal border and peripheral signs of a hyperdynamic circulation including a widened pulse pressure, decreased diastolic blood pressure, and bounding pulses. In addition to the typical murmur of aortic regurgitation, there may be a low-pitched diastolic rumble (Austin-Flint murmur) that results from the regurgitant jet causing fluttering of the mitral valve. As with mitral regurgitation, symptoms of aortic regurgitation may not appear until left ventricular dysfunction is present. Symptoms at this stage are manifestations of left ventricular failure (dyspnea, orthopnea, fatigue) and coronary ischemia. With chronic aortic regurgitation, evidence of left ventricular enlargement and left ventricular hypertrophy may be seen on the chest radiograph and ECG. Echocardiography will identify any anatomic abnormalities of the aortic valve including leaflet perforation or prolapse and will identify any abnormalities in the aortic root and aortic annulus. Left ventricle size, volume, and ejection fraction can be measured, and Doppler examination can be used to identify the presence and severity of aortic regurgitation. Many methods exist to quantify aortic regurgitation. These include regurgitant jet width as a percentage of

overall left ventricular outflow tract width, pressure half-time, and diastolic flow reversal in the descending aorta (**Table 2-12**). Cardiac catheterization and cardiac magnetic resonance imaging may be useful for grading aortic regurgitation if echocardiography is insufficient.

Treatment

Surgical replacement of a diseased aortic valve is recommended before the onset of permanent left ventricular dysfunction, even if patients are asymptomatic. The operative mortality for isolated aortic valve replacement is approximately 4%. It is higher if there is concomitant aortic root replacement or coronary artery bypass grafting or if there are substantial comorbidities. The mortality rate of asymptomatic patients with normal left ventricular size and function is less than 0.2% per year.

In contrast, symptomatic patients have a mortality rate greater than 10% per year. In acute aortic regurgitation, immediate surgical intervention is necessary because the acute volume overload results in heart failure. Alternatives to aortic valve replacement with a prosthetic valve include a pulmonic valve autograft (Ross procedure) and aortic valve reconstruction.

Medical therapy of aortic regurgitation is designed to decrease systolic hypertension and ventricular wall stress and improve left ventricular function. Intravenous infusion of a vasodilator such as nitroprusside and an inotropic drug such as dobutamine may be useful for improving forward left ventricular stroke volume and reducing regurgitant volume. Long-term therapy with nifedipine or hydralazine can be beneficial and may delay the need for surgery in asymptomatic patients with good left ventricular function.

Management of Anesthesia

Management of anesthesia for noncardiac surgery in patients with aortic regurgitation is designed to maintain the forward left ventricular stroke volume (**Table 2-13**). The heart rate must be kept at more than 80 bpm because bradycardia, by increasing the duration of diastole and thereby the degree of regurgitation, produces acute left ventricular volume overload. An abrupt increase in systemic vascular resistance can also precipitate left ventricular failure. The compensations for

TABLE 2-13 | Anesthetic Considerations in Patients with Aortic Regurgitation

Avoid bradycardia
Avoid increases in systemic vascular resistance
Minimize myocardial depression

aortic regurgitation may be tenuous, and anesthetic-induced myocardial depression may upset this delicate balance. If left ventricular failure occurs, it is treated with a vasodilator for afterload reduction and an inotrope to increase contractility. Overall, modest increases in heart rate and modest decreases in systemic vascular resistance are reasonable hemodynamic goals during anesthesia. General anesthesia is the usual choice for patients with aortic regurgitation.

Induction of Anesthesia

Induction of anesthesia in the presence of aortic regurgitation can be achieved with inhalation anesthesia an intravenous induction drug. The ideal induction drug should not decrease the heart rate or increase systemic vascular resistance.

Maintenance of Anesthesia

In the absence of severe left ventricular dysfunction, maintenance of anesthesia is often provided with nitrous oxide plus a volatile anesthetic and/or opioid. The increase in heart rate, decrease in systemic vascular resistance, and minimal myocardial depression of isoflurane, desflurane, and sevoflurane make these drugs excellent choices in patients with aortic regurgitation. In patients with severe left ventricular dysfunction, high-dose opioid anesthesia may be preferred. Bradycardia and myocardial depression from concomitant use of nitrous oxide or a benzodiazepine are risks of the high-dose narcotic technique. Neuromuscular blockers with minimal or no effect on blood pressure and heart rate are typically used, although the modest increase in heart rate associated with pancuronium administration could be helpful in patients with aortic regurgitation.

Mechanical ventilation should be adjusted to maintain normal oxygenation and carbon dioxide elimination and adequate time for venous return. Intravascular fluid volume should be maintained at normal levels to provide for adequate cardiac preload. Bradycardia and junctional rhythm may require prompt treatment with intravenous atropine.

Monitoring

Minor surgery in patients with asymptomatic aortic regurgitation does not require invasive monitoring. Standard monitors should be adequate to detect any rhythm disturbances or myocardial ischemia. In the presence of severe aortic regurgitation, monitoring with a pulmonary artery catheter or transesophageal echocardiography is helpful for detection of myocardial depression, for facilitating intravascular volume replacement, and for measuring the response to administration of a vasodilating drug.

TRICUSPID REGURGITATION

Tricuspid regurgitation is usually functional, caused by tricuspid annular dilation secondary to right ventricle enlargement or pulmonary hypertension. Other causes include infective endocarditis (typically associated with intravenous drug abuse and unsterile injection), carcinoid syndrome, rheumatic heart disease, tricuspid valve prolapse, and Ebstein's anomaly. Tricuspid valve disease is often associated with mitral or aortic valve disease. Mild tricuspid regurgitation can be a normal finding at any age and is very commonly found in highly trained athletes.

Pathophysiology

The basic hemodynamic consequence of tricuspid regurgitation is right atrial volume overload. The high compliance of the right atrium and vena cava result in only a minimal increase in right atrial pressures even in the presence of a large regurgitant volume. Even surgical removal of the tricuspid valve can be well tolerated. The signs of tricuspid regurgitation include jugular venous distention, hepatomegaly, ascites, and peripheral edema. The therapy of functional tricuspid regurgitation is aimed at the cause of the lesion, that is, at improving lung function, relieving left-sided heart failure, or reducing pulmonary hypertension. Surgical intervention for isolated tricuspid valve disease is rarely done but would be considered if other cardiac surgery is planned. A tricuspid annuloplasty or valvuloplasty may be performed. Tricuspid valve replacement is rarely performed.

Management of Anesthesia

Management of anesthesia in patients with tricuspid regurgitation includes maintenance of intravascular fluid volume and central venous pressure in the high normal range to facilitate adequate right ventricular preload and left ventricular filling. Positive-pressure ventilation and vasodilating drugs may be particularly deleterious if they significantly decrease venous return. Events known to increase pulmonary artery pressure, such as hypoxemia and hypercarbia, must be avoided.

A specific anesthetic drug combination or technique cannot be recommended for management of patients with tricuspid regurgitation. Agents that produce some pulmonary vasodilation and those that maintain venous return are best. Nitrous oxide can be a weak pulmonary artery vasoconstrictor and could increase the degree of tricuspid regurgitation. Intraoperative monitoring should include measurement of right atrial pressure to guide intravenous fluid replacement and to detect changes in the amount of tricuspid regurgitation in response to administration of anesthetic drugs. With high right atrial pressures, the possibility of right-to-left intracardiac shunting through a patent foramen ovale must be considered. Meticulous de-airing of intravenous fluid systems can reduce the risk of a systemic air embolism.

TRICUSPID STENOSIS

Tricuspid stenosis is rare in the adult population. The most common cause in adults is rheumatic heart disease with co-existing tricuspid regurgitation and often mitral or aortic valve disease. Carcinoid syndrome and endomyocardial fibrosis are even rarer causes of tricuspid stenosis. Tricuspid stenosis increases right atrial pressure and increases the pressure gradient between the right atrium and right ventricle. Right atrial dimensions are increased, but the right ventricular dimensions are determined by the degree of volume overload from concomitant tricuspid regurgitation.

PULMONIC REGURGITATION

Pulmonic valve regurgitation results from pulmonary hypertension with annular dilatation of the pulmonic valve.

Other causes include connective tissue diseases, carcinoid syndrome, infective endocarditis, and rheumatic heart disease. Pulmonary regurgitation is rarely symptomatic.

PULMONIC STENOSIS

Pulmonic stenosis is usually congenital and detected and corrected in childhood. An acquired form can be due to rheumatic fever, carcinoid syndrome, or infective endocarditis. Significant obstruction can cause syncope, angina, right ventricular hypertrophy, and right ventricular failure. Surgical valvotomy can be used to relieve the obstruction.

KEY POINTS

- The most frequently encountered cardiac valve lesions produce pressure overload (mitral stenosis, aortic stenosis) or volume overload (mitral regurgitation, aortic regurgitation) on the left atrium or left ventricle.

- Angina pectoris may occur in patients with valvular heart disease even in the absence of coronary artery disease. It usually reflects increased myocardial oxygen demand due to ventricular hypertrophy. The demands of this thickened muscle mass may exceed the ability of even normal coronary arteries to deliver adequate amounts of oxygen.

- Certain cardiac lesions such as aortic and mitral stenosis require a slow heart rate to prolong the duration of diastole and improve left ventricular filling and coronary blood flow. The regurgitant valvular lesions such as aortic and mitral regurgitation require afterload reduction and a somewhat faster heart rate to shorten the time for regurgitation.

- Echocardiography with Doppler color-flow imaging is essential for noninvasive evaluation of valvular heart disease. It is particularly useful in evaluating the significance of cardiac murmurs such as systolic ejection murmurs in suspected aortic stenosis and for detecting the presence of mitral stenosis. It permits determination of cardiac anatomy and function, hypertrophy, cavity dimensions, valve area, transvalvular pressure gradients, and the magnitude of valvular regurgitation.

- Prosthetic valves differ from one another with regard to durability, thrombogenicity, and hemodynamic profile. Mechanical valves are very durable, lasting at least 20 to 30 years, whereas bioprosthetic valves last about 10 to 15 years. Mechanical valves are highly thrombogenic and require long-term anticoagulation. Because bioprosthetic valves have a low thrombogenic potential, long-term anticoagulation is not necessary.

- In 2007, there were major changes in the AHA Guidelines for Prevention of Infective Endocarditis. Antibiotic prophylaxis is now recommended *only for those patients at highest risk of adverse outcomes if they were to develop infective endocarditis.* These high-risk conditions are listed in Table 2-4. Antibiotic prophylaxis is no longer recommended for any other forms of congenital heart disease except as noted in Table 2-4. In these high-risk patients, antibiotic prophylaxis *is* recommended for dental procedures that involve manipulation of gingival tissues or the periapical regions of teeth or perforation of the oral mucosa. Antibiotic prophylaxis *is* recommended for invasive procedures (i.e., those that involve incision or biopsy) on the respiratory tract, skin, skin structures, or musculoskeletal tissues. Antibiotic prophylaxis *is not* recommended for GU or GI tract procedures.

- Management of anesthesia for noncardiac surgery in patients with mitral stenosis includes prevention and treatment of events that can decrease cardiac output or produce pulmonary edema. The development of atrial fibrillation with a rapid ventricular response significantly decreases cardiac output and can produce pulmonary edema. Excessive perioperative fluid administration, Trendelenburg position, or autotransfusion via uterine contraction increases central blood volume and can precipitate CHF. A sudden decrease in systemic vascular resistance may not be tolerated because the normal response to hypotension, that is, a reflex increase in heart rate, itself decreases cardiac output.

- The basic hemodynamic derangement in mitral regurgitation is a decrease in forward left ventricular stroke volume and cardiac output. A portion of every stroke volume is regurgitated through the incompetent mitral valve back into the left atrium resulting in left atrial volume overload and pulmonary congestion. Patients

Continued

KEY POINTS—cont'd

with a regurgitant fraction of more than 0.6 are considered to have severe mitral regurgitation. Pharmacologic interventions that increase or decrease systemic vascular resistance have a major impact on the regurgitant fraction in patients with mitral regurgitation.

- MVP is defined as the prolapse of one or both mitral leaflets into the left atrium during systole with or without mitral regurgitation; it is associated with the auscultatory findings of a midsystolic click and a late systolic murmur. MVP is the most common form of valvular heart disease, affecting 1% to 2.5% of the U.S. population. It is more common in young women. Although it is usually a benign condition, MVP can have devastating complications such as cerebral embolic events, infective endocarditis, severe mitral regurgitation requiring surgery, dysrhythmias, and sudden death. Patients with abnormal mitral valve morphology appear to be the subset of patients at risk of these complications.

- Management of anesthesia in patients with aortic stenosis includes the prevention of hypotension and any hemodynamic change that will decrease cardiac output. Normal sinus rhythm must be maintained because the left ventricle is dependent on a properly timed atrial contraction to produce an optimal left ventricular

end-diastolic volume. Loss of atrial contraction, as during junctional rhythm or atrial fibrillation, may produce a dramatic decrease in stroke volume and blood pressure. The heart rate is important because it determines the time available for ventricular filling, for ejection of the stroke volume, and for coronary perfusion. A sustained increase in heart rate decreases the time for left ventricular filling and ejection and reduces cardiac output. Hypotension reduces coronary blood flow and results in myocardial ischemia and further deterioration in left ventricular function and cardiac output. Aggressive treatment of hypotension is mandatory to prevent cardiogenic shock and/or cardiac arrest.

- The basic hemodynamic derangement in aortic regurgitation is a decrease in cardiac output because of regurgitation of a part of the ejected stroke volume from the aorta back into the left ventricle during diastole. This results in a combined pressure and volume overload on the left ventricle. The magnitude of the regurgitant volume depends on (1) the time available for the regurgitant flow to occur, which is determined by the heart rate, and (2) the pressure gradient across the aortic valve, which is dependent on the systemic vascular resistance. The magnitude of aortic regurgitation is decreased by tachycardia and peripheral vasodilation.

REFERENCES

Bekeredjian R, Grayburn PA: Valvular heart disease: Aortic regurgitation. Circulation 2005;112:125–134.

Bonow RO, Carabello BA, Kanu C: ACC/AHA 2006 guidelines for the management of patients with valvular heart disease: A report of the American College of Cardiology/American Heart Association Task Force on Practice Guidelines (writing committee to revise the 1998 guidelines for the management of patients with valvular heart disease): Developed in collaboration with the Society of Cardiovascular Anesthesiologists: Endorsed by the Society for Cardiovascular Angiography and Interventions and the Society of Thoracic Surgeons. Circulation 2006;114:e84–e231.

Carabello BA: Aortic stenosis. N Engl J Med 2002;346:677–682.

Carabello BA: Evaluation and management of patients with aortic stenosis. Circulation 2002;105:1746–1750.

Carabello BA: Is it ever too late to operate on the patient with valvular heart disease. J Am Coll Cardiol 2004;44:376–383.

Carabello BA: Modern management of mitral stenosis. Circulation 2005;112:432–437.

Carabello BA: The pathophysiology of mitral regurgitation. J Heart Valve Dis 2000;9:600–608.

Christ M, Sharkova Y, Geldner G, Maisch B: Preoperative and perioperative care for patients with suspected or established aortic stenosis facing noncardiac surgery. Chest 2005;128:2944–2953.

Kearon C, Hirsh J: Management of anticoagulation before and after elective surgery. N Engl J Med 1997;336:1506–1511.

Kertai MD, Bountioukos M, Boersma E: Aortic stenosis: An underestimated risk factor for perioperative complications in patients undergoing noncardiac surgery. Am J Med 2004;116:8–13.

Lester SJ, Heilbron B, Gin K: The natural history and rate of progression of aortic stenosis. Chest 1998;113:1109–1114.

Otto CM: Timing of surgery in mitral regurgitation. Heart 2003;89:100–105.

Perrino AC, Reeves ST: A Practical Approach to Transesophageal Echocardiography, 2nd ed. Philadelphia, Lippincott Williams & Wilkins, 2007.

Wilson W, Taubert KA, Gewitz M, et al: Prevention of infective endocarditis. Guidelines from the American Heart Association. Circulation 2007;116:1736–1754.

CHAPTER 3

Congenital Heart Disease

Inna Maranets
Roberta L. Hines

Acyanotic Congenital Heart Disease
- Atrial Septal Defect
- Ventricular Septal Defect
- Patent Ductus Arteriosus
- Aorticopulmonary Fenestration
- Aortic Stenosis
- Pulmonic Stenosis
- Coarctation of the Aorta

Cyanotic Congenital Heart Disease
- Tetralogy of Fallot
- Eisenmenger's Syndrome
- Ebstein's Anomaly

- Tricuspid Atresia
- Transposition of the Great Arteries
- Mixing of Blood between the Pulmonary and Systemic Circulations
- Truncus Arteriosus
- Partial Anomalous Pulmonary Venous Return
- Total Anomalous Pulmonary Venous Return
- Hypoplastic Left Heart Syndrome

Mechanical Obstruction of the Trachea
- Double Aortic Arch
- Aberrant Left Pulmonary Artery
- Absent Pulmonic Valve

Congenital anomalies of the heart and cardiovascular system occur in seven to 10 per 1000 live births (0.7%–1.0%). Congenital heart disease is the most common form of congenital disease and accounts for approximately 30% of the total incidence of all congenital diseases. With the decline in rheumatic heart disease, congenital heart disease has become the principal cause of heart disease with 10% to 15% of afflicted children having associated congenital anomalies of the skeletal, genitourinary, or gastrointestinal system. Nine congenital heart lesions comprise more than 80% of congenital heart disease, with a wide range of more unusual and complex lesions comprising the remainder (**Table 3-1**). The population of adults with congenital heart disease, surgically corrected or uncorrected, is estimated to exceed 1 million persons in the United States. As a result, it is not uncommon for adult patients with congenital heart disease to present for noncardiac surgery.

Transthoracic and transesophageal echocardiography has facilitated early, accurate diagnosis of congenital heart disease. Fetal cardiac ultrasonography has permitted prenatal diagnosis of congenital heart defects, allowing subsequent perinatal management. Imaging modalities, such as cardiac magnetic resonance imaging and three-dimensional echocardiography, have increased the understanding of complex cardiac malformations and allow visualization of blood flow and vascular structures. Cardiac catheterization and selective angiocardiography are the most definitive diagnostic procedures available for use in patients with congenital heart disease. As the success rate of cardiac surgery increases, more patients with complex cardiac defects will survive into adulthood and present for noncardiac surgery.

Advances in molecular biology have provided new understandings of the genetic basis of congenital heart disease.

TABLE 3-1 Classification and Incidence of Congenital Heart Disease

Disease	Incidence (%)
Acyanotic Defects	
Ventricular septal defect	35
Atrial septal defect	9
Patent ductus arteriosus	8
Pulmonary stenosis	8
Aortic stenosis	6
Coarctation of the aorta	6
Atrioventricular septal defect	3
Cyanotic Defects	
Tetralogy of Fallot	5
Transposition of the great vessels	4

TABLE 3-2 Signs and Symptoms of Congenital Heart Disease

Infants
Tachypnea
Failure to gain weight
Heart rate > 200 bpm
Heart murmur
Congestive heart failure
Cyanosis

Children
Dyspnea
Slow physical development
Decreased exercise tolerance
Heart murmur
Congestive heart failure
Cyanosis
Clubbing of digits
Squatting
Hypertension

Chromosomal abnormalities are associated with an estimated 10% of congenital cardiovascular lesions. Two thirds of these lesions occur in patients with trisomy 21; the other one third is found in patients with karyotypic abnormalities, such as trisomy 13 and trisomy 18, and in patients with Turner's syndrome. The remaining 90% of congenital cardiovascular lesions are postulated to be multifactorial in origin and occur as a result of interactions of several genes with or without external factors (rubella, ethanol abuse, lithium, maternal diabetes mellitus). A widely used acronym, CATCH-22 (*c*ardiac defects, *a*bnormal facies, *t*hymic hypoplasia, *c*left palate, *h*ypocalcemia) depicts a congenital heart disease syndrome attributed to defects in chromosome 22. An increased incidence of congenital heart disease in the offspring of affected adult patients suggests a role for single-gene defects in isolated congenital heart disease.

Signs and symptoms of congenital heart disease in infants and children often include dyspnea, slow physical development, and the presence of a cardiac murmur (**Table 3-2**). The diagnosis of congenital heart disease is apparent during the first week of life in approximately 50% of afflicted neonates and before 5 years of age in virtually all remaining patients. Echocardiography is the initial diagnostic step if congenital heart disease is suspected. Certain complications are likely to accompany the presence of congenital heart disease (**Table 3-3**). For example, infective endocarditis is a risk associated with most congenital cardiac anomalies. Cardiac dysrhythmias are not usually a prominent feature of congenital heart disease.

ACYANOTIC CONGENITAL HEART DISEASE

Acyanotic congenital heart disease is characterized by a left-to-right intracardiac shunt (**Table 3-4**). The ultimate result of this intracardiac shunt, regardless of its location, is increased pulmonary blood flow with pulmonary hypertension,

right ventricular hypertrophy, and eventually congestive heart failure. The younger the patient is at the time of correction, the greater is the likelihood that pulmonary vascular resistance will normalize. In older patients, if pulmonary vascular resistance is one third or less of the systemic vascular resistance, corrective surgery is likely to prevent or, in some cases, even cause slight regression of pulmonary vascular disease. The onset and severity of clinical symptoms vary with the site and magnitude of the vascular shunt.

Atrial Septal Defect

Atrial septal defect (ASD) accounts for about one third of the congenital heart disease detected in adults, with the frequency in females of two to three times that observed in males. Anatomically, an ASD may take the form of ostium secundum in the region of the fossa ovalis (often located near the center of the interatrial septum and varying from a single opening to a fenestrated septum), ostium primum (endocardial cushion defect characterized by a large opening in the

TABLE 3-3 Common Problems Associated with Congenital Heart Disease

Infective endocarditis
Cardiac dysrhythmias
Complete heart block
Hypertension (systemic or pulmonary)
Erythrocytosis
Thromboembolism
Coagulopathy
Brain abscess
Increased plasma uric acid concentration
Sudden death

TABLE 3–4	Congenital Heart Defects Resulting in a Left-to-Right Intracardiac Shunt or Its Equivalent

Secundum atrial septal defect
Primum atrial septal defect (endocardial cushion defect)
Ventricular septal defect
Aorticopulmonary fenestration

interatrial septum), or sinus venosus located in the upper atrial septum (**Fig. 3-1**). Secundum ASDs account for 75% of all ASDs. Additional cardiac abnormalities may occur with each type of defect and include mitral valve prolapse (ostium secundum) and mitral regurgitation due to a cleft in the anterior mitral valve leaflet (ostium primum). Most ASDs occur as a result of spontaneous genetic mutations.

The physiologic consequences of ASDs are the same regardless of the anatomic location and reflect the shunting of blood from one atrium to the other; the direction and magnitude of the shunt are determined by the size of the defect and the relative compliance of the ventricles. A small defect (< 0.5 cm in diameter) is associated with a small shunt and no hemodynamic sequelae. When the diameter of the ASD approaches 2 cm, it is likely that left atrial blood is being shunted to the right atrium (the right ventricle is more compliant than the left ventricle), resulting in increased pulmonary blood flow. A systolic ejection murmur audible in the second left intercostal space

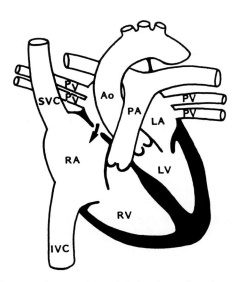

Figure 3-1 • Secundum atrial septal defect located in the center of the interatrial septum. Blood flow is along a pressure gradient from the left atrium (LA) to the right atrium (RA). The resulting left-to-right intracardiac shunt is associated with increased blood flow through the pulmonary artery (PA). A decrease in systemic vascular resistance or an increase in pulmonary vascular resistance decreases the pressure gradient across the defect, leading to a decrease in the magnitude of the shunt. Ao, aorta; IVC, inferior vena cava; LV, left ventricle; PV, pulmonary vein; RV, right ventricle; SVC, superior vena cava.

may be mistaken for an innocent flow murmur. The electrocardiogram (ECG) may reflect right axis deviation and incomplete right bundle branch block. Atrial fibrillation and supraventricular tachycardia may accompany an ASD that remains uncorrected into adulthood. The chest radiograph is likely to reveal prominent pulmonary arteries. Transesophageal echocardiography and Doppler color flow echocardiography are both useful for detecting and determining the location of ASDs.

Signs and Symptoms

Because they initially produce no symptoms or striking findings on physical examination, ASDs may remain undetected for years. A small defect with minimal right-to-left shunting (ratio of pulmonary flow to systemic flow is < 1.5) usually causes no symptoms and therefore does not require closure. When pulmonary blood flow is 1.5 times the systemic blood flow, the ASD should be surgically closed either in the cath lab or surgically to prevent right ventricular dysfunction and irreversible pulmonary hypertension. Symptoms due to large ASDs include dyspnea on exertion, supraventricular dysrhythmias, right heart failure, paradoxical embolism, and recurrent pulmonary infections. Prophylaxis against infective endocarditis is not recommended for patients with an ASD unless a concomitant valvular abnormality (mitral valve prolapse or mitral valve cleft) is present.

Management of Anesthesia

An ASD associated with a left-to-right intracardiac shunt has only minor implications for the management of anesthesia. For example, as long as the systemic blood flow remains normal, the pharmacokinetics of inhaled drugs are not significantly altered despite the increased pulmonary blood flow. Conversely, increased pulmonary blood flow could dilute drugs injected intravenously. It is unlikely, however, that this potential dilution will alter the clinical response to these drugs because the pulmonary circulation time is brief.

Any change in systemic or pulmonary vascular resistance during the perioperative period will have important implications for the patient with an ASD. For example, drugs or events that produce prolonged increases in systemic vascular resistance should be avoided because this change favors an increase in the magnitude of the left-to-right shunt at the atrial level. This is particularly true with a primum ASD defect associated with mitral regurgitation. Use of high F_{IO_2} will decrease pulmonary vascular resistance and increase pulmonary blood flow and left-to-right shunt. Conversely, decreases in systemic vascular resistance, as produced by volatile anesthetics or increases in pulmonary vascular resistance due to positive-pressure ventilation of the lungs, tend to decrease the magnitude of the left-to-right shunt.

Another consideration in the management of anesthesia in the presence of ASDs is the need to provide prophylactic antibiotics to protect against infective endocarditis when a cardiac valvular abnormality is present. In addition, meticulously avoiding the entrance of air into the circulation, as can occur through tubing used to deliver intravenous solutions, is imperative. Transient supraventricular dysrhythmias and atrioventricular conduction defects are common during the early postoperative period after surgical repair of an ASD.

Ventricular Septal Defect

Ventricular septal defect (VSD) is the most common congenital cardiac abnormality in infants and children (**Fig. 3-2**). A large number of VSDs close spontaneously by the time a child reaches 2 years of age. Anatomically, approximately 70% of these defects are located in the membranous portion of the intraventricular septum, 20% in the muscular portion of the septum, 5% just below the aortic valve causing aortic regurgitation, and 5% near the junction of the mitral and tricuspid valve (atrioventricular canal defect).

Echocardiography with Doppler flow ultrasonography confirms the presence and location of the VSD, and color-flow mapping provides information about the magnitude and direction of the intracardiac shunt. Cardiac catheterization and angiography confirm the presence and location of the VSD and determine the magnitude of the intracardiac shunting and the pulmonary vascular resistance.

Signs and Symptoms

The physiologic significance of a VSD depends on the size of the defect and the relative resistance in the systemic and pulmonary circulations. If the defect is small, there is minimal functional disturbance as pulmonary blood flow is only modestly increased. If the defect is large, the ventricular systolic

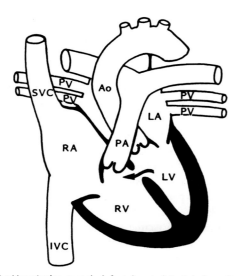

Figure 3-2 • Ventricular septal defect located just below the muscular ridge that separates the body of the right ventricle (RV) from the pulmonary artery (PA) outflow tract. Blood flow is along a pressure gradient from the left ventricle (LV) to the RV. The resulting left-to-right intracardiac shunt is associated with pulmonary blood flow that exceeds the stroke volume of the LV. A decrease in systemic vascular resistance decreases the pressure gradient across the defect and reduces the magnitude of the shunt. Ao, aorta; IVC, inferior vena cava; LA, left atrium; PV, pulmonary vein; RA, right atrium; SVC, superior vena cava.

pressures equalize and the magnitude of systemic and pulmonary blood flow is determined by the relative vascular resistances of these two circulations. Initially, systemic vascular resistance exceeds pulmonary vascular resistance, and left-to-right intracardiac shunting predominates. Over time, the pulmonary vascular resistance increases, and the magnitude of the left-to-right intracardiac shunting decreases; eventually, the shunt may become right to left with the development of arterial hypoxemia (cyanosis).

The murmur of a moderate to large VSD is holosystolic and is loudest at the lower left sternal border. The ECG and chest radiograph remain normal in the presence of a small VSD. When the VSD is large, there is evidence of left atrial and ventricular enlargement on the ECG. If pulmonary hypertension develops, the QRS axis shifts to the right, and right atrial and ventricular enlargement are noted on the ECG.

The natural history of a VSD depends on the size of the defect and the pulmonary vascular resistance. Adults with small defects and normal pulmonary arterial pressures are generally asymptomatic, and pulmonary hypertension is unlikely to develop. These patients are at risk of developing infective endocarditis even though they may not meet the criteria for surgical correction of the VSD. In the absence of surgical correction, a large VSD eventually leads to left ventricular failure or pulmonary hypertension with associated right ventricular failure. Surgical closure of the defect is recommended in these patients if the magnitude of the pulmonary hypertension is not prohibitive. Once the pulmonary/systemic vascular resistance ratio exceeds 0.7, the risk of surgical closure becomes prohibitive.

Management of Anesthesia

Antibiotic prophylaxis to protect against infective endocarditis is indicated when noncardiac surgery is planned in patients with VSDs. The pharmacokinetics of inhaled and injected drugs are not significantly altered by a VSD. As with an ASD, acute and persistent increases in systemic vascular resistance or decreases in pulmonary vascular resistance are undesirable because these changes can accentuate the magnitude of the left-to-right intracardiac shunt at the ventricular level. In this regard, volatile anesthetics (which decrease systemic vascular resistance) and positive-pressure ventilation (which increases pulmonary vascular resistance) are well tolerated. However, there may be increased delivery of depressant drugs to the heart if coronary blood flow is increased to supply the hypertrophied ventricles. Conceivably, the technique of increasing the inspired concentrations of volatile anesthetics to achieve rapid induction of anesthesia, as is often done in normal children, could result in excessive depression of the heart before central nervous system depression is achieved in children with VSD.

Right ventricular infundibular hypertrophy may be present in patients with VSDs. Normally, this is a beneficial change because it increases the resistance to right ventricular ejection, leading to a decrease in the magnitude of the left-to-right intracardiac shunt. Nevertheless, perioperative events that exaggerate this obstruction to right ventricular outflow, such as increased myocardial contractility or hypovolemia, must be minimized. Therefore, these patients are often anesthetized with volatile anesthetics. In addition, intravascular fluid volume should be maintained by prompt replacement by crystalloid or colloid (depending on the clinical scenario).

Anesthesia for placement of a pulmonary artery band is often achieved with drugs that provide minimal cardiac depression. If bradycardia or systemic hypotension develops during surgery, it may be necessary to remove the pulmonary artery band promptly. Continuous monitoring of the systemic blood pressure with an intra-arterial catheter is helpful. Administration of positive end-expiratory pressure may be useful in the presence of congestive heart failure but should be discontinued when the pulmonary artery band is in place. The high mortality rate associated with pulmonary artery banding has led to attempted complete surgical correction at an early age. Third-degree atrioventricular heart block may follow surgical closure if the cardiac conduction system is near the VSD. Premature ventricular beats may reflect the electrical instability of the ventricle due to surgical ventriculotomy. The risk of ventricular tachycardia, however, is low if postoperative ventricular filling pressures are normal.

Patent Ductus Arteriosus

A patent ductus arteriosus (PDA) is present when the ductus arteriosus (which arises just distal to the left subclavian artery and connects the descending aorta to the left pulmonary artery) fails to close spontaneously shortly after birth (**Fig. 3-3**). In the fetus, the ductus arteriosus permits pulmonary arterial blood to bypass the deflated lungs and enter the descending aorta for oxygenation in the placenta. In full-term newborns, the ductus arteriosus closes within 24 to 48 hours after delivery, but in preterm newborns, the ductus arteriosus frequently fails to close. When the ductus arteriosus fails to close spontaneously after birth, the result is continuous flow of blood from the aorta to the pulmonary artery. The pulmonary/systemic blood flow ratio depends on the pressure gradient from the aorta to the pulmonary artery, the pulmonary/systemic vascular resistance ratio, and the diameter and length of the ductus arteriosus. The PDA can usually be visualized on echocardiography, with Doppler studies confirming the continuous flow into the pulmonary circulation. Cardiac catheterization and angiography make it possible to quantify the magnitude of the shunting and the pulmonary vascular resistance and to visualize the PDA.

Signs and Symptoms

Most patients with a PDA are asymptomatic and have only modest left-to-right shunts. This cardiac defect is often detected during a routine physical examination, at which time a characteristic continuous systolic and diastolic murmur is heard. If the left-to-right shunt is large, there may be evidence of left ventricular hypertrophy on the ECG and chest radiograph. If pulmonary hypertension develops, right ventricular hypertrophy is apparent. The presence of

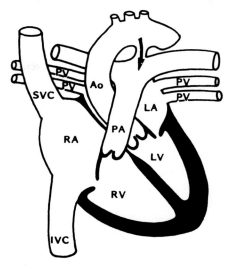

Figure 3-3 • Patent ductus arteriosus connecting the arch of the aorta (Ao) with the pulmonary artery (PA). Blood flow is from the high pressure Ao into the PA. The resulting aorta-to-pulmonary artery shunt (left-to-right shunt) leads to increased pulmonary blood flow. A decrease in systemic vascular resistance or an increase in pulmonary vascular resistance decreases the magnitude of the shunt through the ductus arteriosus. IVC, inferior vena cava; LA, left atrium; LV, left ventricle, RV, right ventricle; SVC, superior vena cava.

a PDA increases the risk of infective endocarditis. Surgical ligation of a PDA is associated with low mortality and is unlikely to require cardiopulmonary bypass. Without surgical closure, most patients remain asymptomatic until adolescence, when pulmonary hypertension and congestive heart failure may occur. Once severe pulmonary hypertension develops, surgical or percutaneous closure is contraindicated.

Treatment

It is estimated that 70% of preterm infants delivered before 28 weeks of gestation require medical or surgical closure of a PDA. Surgical ligation of a PDA can be performed in neonatal intensive care units with low morbidity and mortality rates. Nevertheless, the risks of surgical closure are significant and include intracranial hemorrhage, infections, and recurrent laryngeal nerve paralysis, especially in infants born at less than 28 weeks of gestation. Inhibition of prostaglandin synthesis with nonselective cyclooxygenase inhibitors (COX-1, COX-2) appears to be an effective medical alternative to surgery for closure of a PDA in neonates. Indomethacin, a nonselective cyclooxygenase inhibitor used for this purpose, has reduced the need for surgery by 60% and is the first-line of therapy for PDA. Adverse side effects of indomethacin include decreased mesenteric, renal, and cerebral blood flow. Ibuprofen is a nonselective cyclooxygenase inhibitor that can be used effectively to treat PDA and has less effect on organ blood flow than indomethacin.

Management of Anesthesia

Antibiotic prophylaxis for protection against infective endocarditis is recommended for patients with PDAs who are scheduled for noncardiac surgery. When surgical closure of the PDA is planned through a left thoracotomy, appropriate preparations must be taken in anticipation of the possibility of large blood loss should control of the PDA be lost during attempted ligation. The decrease in systemic vascular resistance produced by volatile anesthetics may improve systemic blood flow by decreasing the magnitude of the left-to-right shunt. Likewise, positive-pressure ventilation of the patient's lungs is well tolerated, as pulmonary vascular resistance, thereby decreasing the pressure gradient across the PDA. Conversely, increases in systemic vascular resistance or decreases in pulmonary vascular resistance should be avoided because these changes will increase the magnitude of the left-to-right shunt.

Ligation of the PDA is often associated with significant systemic hypertension during the postoperative period. This hypertension can be managed with continuous infusion of vasodilator drugs such as nitroprusside. Long-acting antihypertensive drugs can be gradually substituted for nitroprusside if systemic hypertension persists.

Aorticopulmonary Fenestration

Aorticopulmonary fenestration is characterized by a communication between the left side of the ascending aorta and the right wall of the main pulmonary artery, just anterior to the origin of the right pulmonary artery. This communication is due to failure of the aorticopulmonary septum to fuse and completely separate the aorta from the pulmonary artery. Clinical and hemodynamic manifestations of an aorticopulmonary communication are similar to those associated with a large PDA. The diagnosis is facilitated by echocardiography and angiocardiography. Treatment is surgical and requires the use of cardiopulmonary bypass. Management of anesthesia entails the same principles as described for patients with PDAs.

Aortic Stenosis

Bicuspid aortic valves occur in 2% to 3% of the U.S. population, and an estimated 20% of these patients have other cardiovascular abnormalities, such as PDA or coarctation of the aorta (see Chapter 2).[2] The deformed bicuspid aortic valve is not stenotic at birth, but with time, thickening and calcification of the leaflets (usually not apparent before 15 years of age) occur with resulting immobility. Transthoracic echocardiography with Doppler flow studies permits accurate assessment of the severity of the aortic stenosis and of left ventricular function. Cardiac catheterization is performed to determine the presence of concomitant coronary artery disease.

Aortic stenosis is associated with a systolic murmur that is audible over the aortic area (second right intercostal space) and often radiates into the neck. Most patients with congenital aortic stenosis are asymptomatic until adulthood. Infants with severe aortic stenosis, however, may present with congestive heart failure. Findings in patients with supravalvular aortic stenosis may include characteristic appearances in which the facial bones are prominent, the forehead is rounded, and the

upper lip is pursed. Strabismus, inguinal hernia, dental abnormalities, and moderate mental retardation are commonly present. The ECG in the presence of congenital aortic stenosis typically reveals left ventricular hypertrophy. Depression of the ST segment on the ECG is likely during exercise, particularly if the pressure gradient across the aortic valve is more than 50 mm Hg. Chest radiographs show left ventricular hypertrophy with or without poststenotic dilation of the aorta. Angina pectoris in the absence of coronary artery disease reflects the inability of coronary blood flow to meet increased myocardial oxygen requirements of the hypertrophied left ventricle. Syncope can occur when the pressure gradient across the aortic valve exceeds 50 mm Hg. In the presence of aortic stenosis, the myocardium must generate an intraventricular pressure that is two to three times normal, whereas pressure in the aorta remains within a physiologic range. The resulting concentric myocardial hypertrophy leads to increased myocardial oxygen requirements. Furthermore, the high velocity of blood flow through the stenotic area predisposes to the development of infective endocarditis and is associated with poststenotic dilation of the aorta. In adults with symptomatic aortic stenosis (syncope, angina pectoris, congestive heart failure), the indicated treatment is surgical valve replacement.

Pulmonic Stenosis

Pulmonic stenosis producing obstruction to right ventricular outflow is valvular in 90% of patients; in the remainder, it is supravalvular or subvalvular. Supravalvular pulmonic stenosis often co-exists with other congenital cardiac abnormalities (ASD, VSD, PDA, tetralogy of Fallot). It is a common feature of Williams syndrome, which is characterized by infantile hypercalcemia and mental retardation. Subvalvular pulmonic stenosis usually occurs in association with a VSD. Valvular pulmonic stenosis is typically an isolated abnormality, but it may occur in association with a VSD. Severe pulmonic stenosis is characterized by transvalvular pressure gradients of more than 80 mm Hg or right ventricular systolic pressures of more than 100 mm Hg. Echocardiography and Doppler flow studies can determine the site of the obstruction and the severity of the stenosis. Treatment of pulmonic stenosis is with percutaneous balloon valvuloplasty.

Signs and Symptoms

In asymptomatic patients, the presence of pulmonic stenosis is identified by the presence of a loud systolic ejection murmur, best heard at the second left intercostal space. The intensity and duration of the cardiac murmur parallel the severity of the pulmonic stenosis. Dyspnea may occur on exertion, and eventually right ventricular failure with peripheral edema and ascites develops. If the foramen ovale is patent, right-to-left intracardiac shunting of blood may occur, causing cyanosis and clubbing.

Management of Anesthesia

Management of anesthesia is designed to avoid increases in right ventricular oxygen requirements. Therefore, excessive increases in heart rate and myocardial contractility are undesirable. The impact of changes in pulmonary vascular resistance is minimized by the presence of fixed obstruction of the pulmonic valve. As a result, increases in pulmonary vascular resistance due to positive-pressure ventilation of the lungs are unlikely to produce significant increases in right ventricular afterload and oxygen requirements. These patients are extremely difficult to resuscitate if cardiac arrest occurs because external cardiac compression is not highly effective in forcing blood across a stenotic pulmonic valve. Therefore, decreases in systemic blood pressure should be promptly treated with sympathomimetic drugs. Likewise, cardiac dysrhythmias or increases in heart rate that become hemodynamically significant should be rapidly corrected.

Coarctation of the Aorta

Coarctation of the aorta typically consists of a discrete, diaphragm-like ridge extending into the aortic lumen just distal to the left subclavian artery at the site of the aortic ductal attachment (ligamentum arteriosum). This anatomic manifestation is known as postductal coarctation of the aorta and is most likely to manifest in young adults. Less commonly, the coarctation is immediately proximal to the left subclavian artery (preductal); this situation is most likely to present in infants. Coarctation of the aorta is more common in males and may occur in conjunction with a bicuspid aortic valve, PDA, mitral stenosis or regurgitation, aneurysms of the circle of Willis, and gonadal dysgenesis (Turner's syndrome).

Signs and Symptoms

Most adults with coarctation of the aorta are asymptomatic, and the problem is diagnosed during a routine physical examination when systemic hypertension is detected in the arms in association with diminished or absent femoral arterial pulses. Characteristically, systolic blood pressure is higher in the arms than in the legs, but the diastolic pressure is similar, resulting in widened pulse pressure in the arms. The femoral arterial pulses are weak and delayed. Systemic hypertension presumably reflects ejection of the left ventricular stroke volume into the fixed resistance created by the narrowed aorta. A harsh systolic ejection murmur is present along the left sternal border and in the back, particularly over the area of the coarctation. In the presence of preductal coarctation of the aorta, there is no difference in the systemic blood pressures in the arms and legs. Extensive collateral arterial circulation to the distal body through the internal thoracic, intercostal, scapular, and subclavian arteries is likely in the presence of coarctation of the aorta. In this regard, a systolic murmur may be heard in the back, reflecting this collateral blood flow.

The ECG shows signs of left ventricular hypertrophy. On the chest radiograph, increased collateral flow through the intercostal arteries causes symmetrical notching of the posterior third of the third through eighth ribs. Notching is not seen in the anterior ribs because the anterior intercostal arteries are not located in costal grooves. The coarctation may be visible as an indentation of the aorta with prestenotic or poststenotic dilation of the aorta, producing the "reversed E," or "3," sign. The coarctation may be visualized with echocardiography, and Doppler examination makes it possible to estimate the transcoarctation pressure gradient. Computed tomography, magnetic resonance imaging, and contrast aortography provide precise anatomic information regarding the location and length of the coarctation and the degree of collateral circulation.

When clinical symptoms of a previously unrecognized coarctation of the aorta manifest, they are usually characterized as headache, dizziness, epistaxis, and palpitations. Occasionally, diminished blood flow to the legs causes claudication. Women with coarctation of the aorta are at increased risk of aortic dissection during pregnancy. Complications of coarctation of the aorta include systemic hypertension, left ventricular failure, aortic dissection, premature ischemic heart disease presumably related to chronic hypertension, infective endocarditis, and cerebral vascular accidents due to rupture of intracerebral aneurysms. Patients with known coarctation of the aorta should be given prophylactic antibiotics prior to dental or surgical procedures.

Treatment

Surgical resection of the coarctation of the aorta should be considered for patients with a transcoarctation pressure gradient of more than 30 mm Hg. Although balloon dilation is a therapeutic alternative, the procedure is associated with a higher incidence of subsequent aortic aneurysm and recurrent coarctation than surgical resection.

Management of Anesthesia

Management of anesthesia for surgical resection of coarctation of the aorta must consider (1) the adequacy of perfusion to the lower portion of the body during cross-clamping of the aorta, (2) the propensity for systemic hypertension during cross-clamping of the aorta, and (3) the risk of neurologic sequelae due to ischemia of the spinal cord. Blood flow to the anterior spinal artery is augmented by radicular branches of the intercostal arteries and may be compromised during cross-clamping of the aorta for surgical resection of coarctation of the aorta. Paraplegia after surgical resection of coarctation of the aorta is a rare complication. Continuous monitoring of systemic blood pressure above and below the coarctation is achieved by placing a catheter in the right radial artery and a femoral artery. By monitoring these pressures simultaneously, it is possible to evaluate the adequacy of the collateral circulation during periods of aortic cross-clamping. Mean arterial pressures in the lower extremities should be at least 40 mm Hg to ensure adequate blood flow to the kidneys and spinal cord. If the systemic blood pressure cannot be maintained above this level, it may be necessary to use partial circulatory bypass. Somatosensory evoked potentials are useful for monitoring spinal cord function and the adequacy of its blood flow during cross-clamping of the aorta. Nevertheless, case reports of paraplegia despite normal somatosensory evoked potentials suggest that monitoring posterior (sensory) cord function does not ensure adequate blood flow to the anterior (motor) portion of the spinal cord. Excessive increases in systolic blood pressure during cross-clamping of the aorta may adversely increase the work of the heart and make surgical repair more difficult. In this situation, the use of volatile anesthetics is helpful for maintaining normal systemic blood pressures. If systemic hypertension persists, continuous intravenous infusions of nitroprusside should be considered. The disadvantages of lowering the systemic blood pressure to normal levels are excessively decreased perfusion pressure in the lower part of the body and inadequate blood flow to the kidneys and spinal cord.

Postoperative Management

Immediate postoperative complications include paradoxical hypertension, possible sequelae of a bicuspid aortic valve (infective endocarditis and aortic regurgitation), and paraplegia. Baroreceptor reflexes, activation of the renin-angiotensin-aldosterone system, and excessive release of catecholamines have been implicated as possible causes of immediate postoperative systemic hypertension. Regardless of the etiology, intravenous administration of nitroprusside with or without esmolol effectively controls the systemic blood pressure during the early postoperative period. Longer acting antihypertensive drugs may be needed if hypertension persists. Paraplegia manifesting during the immediate postoperative period is assumed to reflect ischemic damage to the spinal cord during the aortic cross-clamping required for surgical resection of the coarctation. Abdominal pain may occur during the postoperative period and is presumably due to sudden increases in blood flow to the gastrointestinal tract, leading to increased vasoactivity.

The incidence of persistent or recurrent systemic hypertension and the survival rate are influenced by the patient's age at the time of surgery. Most of the patients who undergo surgery during childhood are normotensive 5 years later, whereas those who undergo surgery after 40 years of age often manifest persistent systemic hypertension.

CYANOTIC CONGENITAL HEART DISEASE

Cyanotic congenital heart disease is characterized by a right-to-left intracardiac shunt (**Table 3-5**) with associated decreases in pulmonary blood flow and the development of arterial hypoxemia. The magnitude of shunting determines the severity of arterial hypoxemia. Erythrocytosis secondary to chronic arterial hypoxemia results in a risk of thromboembolism, especially when the hematocrit exceeds 70%. Patients with secondary erythrocytosis may exhibit coagulation defects most likely owing to deficiencies of vitamin K–dependent clotting factors in the liver and defective platelet aggregation. Development of a brain abscess is a major risk in patients

TABLE 3-5	Congenital Heart Defects Resulting in a Right-to-Left Intracardiac Shunt
Tetralogy of Fallot	
Eisenmenger's syndrome	
Ebstein's anomaly (malformation of the tricuspid valve)	
Tricuspid atresia	
Foramen ovale	

with cyanotic congenital heart disease. The onset of a brain abscess often mimics a stroke. Survival in the presence of a right-to-left intracardiac shunt requires a communication between the systemic and pulmonary circulations. Tetralogy of Fallot is the prototype of these defects. Most children with cyanotic congenital heart disease do not survive to adulthood without surgical intervention. Principles for the management of anesthesia are the same for all the cyanotic congenital cardiac defects.

Tetralogy of Fallot

Tetralogy of Fallot, the most common cyanotic congenital heart defect, is characterized by a large single VSD, an aorta that overrides the right and left ventricles, obstruction to right ventricular outflow (subvalvular, valvular, supravalvular, pulmonary arterial branches), and right ventricular hypertrophy (**Fig. 3-4**).

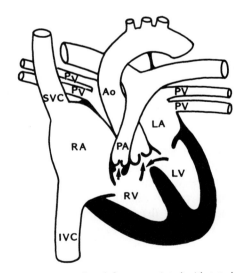

Figure 3-4 • Anatomic cardiac defects associated with tetralogy of Fallot. Defects include (1) ventricular septal defect, (2) aorta (Ao) overriding the pulmonary artery (PA) outflow tract, (3) obstruction to blood flow through a narrowed PA or stenotic pulmonic valve, and (4) right ventricular hypertrophy. Obstruction to PA outflow results in a pressure gradient that favors blood flow across the ventricular septal defect from the right ventricle (RV) to the left ventricle (LV). The resulting right-to-left intracardiac shunt combined with obstruction to ejection of the stroke volume from the RV leads to marked decreases in pulmonary blood flow and the development of arterial hypoxemia. Any event that increases pulmonary vascular resistance or decreases systemic vascular resistance increases the magnitude of the shunt and accentuates arterial hypoxemia. IVC, inferior vena cava; LA, left atrium; PV, pulmonary vein; SVC, superior vena cava.

Several abnormalities may occur in association with tetralogy of Fallot, including right aortic arch, ASD ("pentalogy of Fallot"), and coronary arterial anomalies. Right ventricular hypertrophy occurs because the VSD permits continuous exposure of the right ventricle to the high pressures present in the left ventricle. Right-to-left intracardiac shunting occurs because of increased resistance to flow in the right ventricular outflow tract, the severity of which determines the magnitude of the shunt. Because the resistance to flow across the right ventricular outflow tract is relatively fixed, changes in systemic vascular resistance (drug induced) may affect the magnitude of the shunt. Decreases in systemic vascular resistance increase right-to-left intracardiac shunting and accentuate arterial hypoxemia, whereas increases in systemic vascular resistance (squatting) decrease left-to-right intracardiac shunting with resultant increases in pulmonary blood flow.

Diagnosis

Echocardiography is used to establish the diagnosis and assess the presence of associated abnormalities, the level and severity of the obstruction to right ventricular outflow, the size of the main pulmonary artery and its branches, and the number and location of the VSDs. Right-to-left shunting through the VSD is visualized by color Doppler imaging, and the severity of the right ventricular outflow tract obstruction can be determined by spectral Doppler measurement. Cardiac catheterization further confirms the diagnosis and permits confirmation of anatomic and hemodynamic data, including the location and magnitude of the right-to-left shunt, the level and severity of the right ventricular outflow obstruction, the anatomic features of the right ventricular outflow obstruction, the anatomic features of the right ventricular outflow tract and the main pulmonary artery and its branches, and the origin and course of the coronary arteries. Magnetic resonance imaging can also provide much of this information.

Signs and Symptoms

Most patients with tetralogy of Fallot have cyanosis from birth or beginning during the first year of life. The most common auscultatory finding is an ejection murmur heard along the left sternal border resulting from blood flow across the stenotic pulmonic valve. Congestive heart failure rarely develops because the large VSD permits equilibration of intraventricular pressures and cardiac workload. Chest radiographs show evidence of decreased lung vascularity, and the heart is "boot shaped" with an upturned right ventricular apex and a concave main pulmonary arterial segment. The ECG is characterized by changes of right axis deviation and right ventricular hypertrophy. Arterial oxygen desaturation is present even when breathing 100% oxygen (Pa_{O_2} usually < 50 mm Hg). Compensatory erythropoiesis is proportional to the magnitude of the arterial hypoxemia. The Pa_{CO_2} and arterial pH are usually normal. Squatting is a common feature of children with tetralogy of Fallot. It is speculated that squatting increases the systemic vascular resistance by kinking the large arteries in the inguinal area. The resulting increase in systemic vascular resistance tends to decrease the magnitude of the right-to-left intracardiac shunt, which leads to increased pulmonary blood flow and subsequent improvement in arterial oxygenation.

Hypercyanotic Attacks Hypercyanotic attacks are characterized by sudden spells of arterial hypoxemia associated with worsening cyanosis, tachypnea, and, in some instances, loss of consciousness, seizures, cerebrovascular accidents, and even death. These attacks can occur without obvious provocation but are often associated with crying or exercise. Their mechanism is not known, but the most likely explanation is a sudden decrease in pulmonary blood flow due to spasm of the infundibular cardiac muscle or decreased systemic vascular resistance.

Treatment of hypercyanotic attacks is influenced by the cause of the pulmonary outflow obstruction. When symptoms reflect a dynamic infundibular obstruction (spasm), appropriate treatment is administration of β-adrenergic antagonists such as esmolol or propranolol. Indeed, chronic oral propranolol therapy is indicated in patients who have recurrent hypercyanotic attacks caused by spasm of the outflow tract muscle. If the cause is decreased systemic vascular resistance, treatment is intravenous administration of fluids and/or phenylephrine. Sympathomimetic drugs that display β-agonist properties are not selected because they may accentuate the spasm of the infundibular cardiac muscle. Recurrent hypercyanotic attacks indicate the need for surgical correction of the abnormalities associated with tetralogy of Fallot.

These attacks do not occur in adolescents or adults. Adults with tetralogy of Fallot manifest dyspnea and limited exercise tolerance. They may also have complications of chronic cyanosis including erythrocytosis, hyperviscosity, abnormalities of hemostasis, cerebral abscess or stroke, and infective endocarditis.

Cerebrovascular Accident Cerebrovascular accidents are common in children with severe tetralogy of Fallot. Cerebrovascular thrombosis or severe arterial hypoxemia may be the explanation for these adverse responses. Dehydration and polycythemia may contribute to thrombosis. Hemoglobin concentrations exceeding 20 g/dL are common in these patients.

Cerebral Abscess A cerebral abscess is suggested by the abrupt onset of headache, fever, and lethargy followed by persistent emesis and the appearance of seizure activity. The most likely cause is arterial seeding into areas of previous cerebral infarction.

Infective Endocarditis Infective endocarditis is a constant danger in patients with tetralogy of Fallot and is associated with a high mortality rate. Antibiotics should be administered to protect against this serious possibility whenever dental or surgical procedures are planned in these patients.

Treatment

Treatment of tetralogy of Fallot is complete surgical correction (closure of the VSD with a Dacron patch and relief of right ventricular outflow obstruction by placing a synthetic graft) when patients are extremely young. Infants with pulmonary atresia undergo Rastelli procedures. Without surgery, mortality exceeds 50% by 3 years of age. Pulmonic regurgitation due to an incompetent pulmonic valve usually results from surgical correction of the cardiac defects characteristic of tetralogy of Fallot but poses no major hazard unless the distal pulmonary arteries are hypoplastic, in which case volume overload of the right ventricle secondary to regurgitant blood flow may result. Platelet dysfunction and hypofibrinogenemia are common in these patients and may contribute to postoperative bleeding problems. Right-to-left intracardiac shunting often develops through the foramen ovale during the postoperative period. Shunting through the foramen ovale acts as a safety valve if the right ventricle is unable to function at the same efficiency as the left ventricle.

In the past, infants underwent one of three palliative procedures to increase pulmonary blood flow. All three palliative procedures involved anastomosis of a systemic artery to a pulmonary artery in an effort to increase pulmonary blood flow and improve arterial oxygenation. These palliative procedures are the Waterston procedure (side-to-side anastomosis of the ascending aorta and the right pulmonary artery), the Potts operation (side-to-side anastomosis of the descending aorta to the left pulmonary artery), and the Blalock-Taussig operation (end-to-side anastomosis of the subclavian artery to the pulmonary artery). Often, however, these procedures are associated with long-term complications such as pulmonary hypertension, left ventricular volume overload, and distortion of the pulmonary arterial branches.

Management of Anesthesia

Management of anesthesia for patients with tetralogy of Fallot requires a thorough understanding of those events and drugs that can alter the magnitude of the right-to-left intracardiac shunt. For example, when shunt magnitude is acutely increased, there are associated decreases in pulmonary blood flow and Pao_2. Furthermore, the magnitude of the right-to-left shunt may alter the pharmacokinetics of both inhaled and injected drugs.

The magnitude of a right-to-left intracardiac shunt can be increased by (1) decreased systemic vascular resistance, (2) increased pulmonary vascular resistance, and (3) increased myocardial contractility, which accentuates infundibular obstruction to ejection of blood by the right ventricle. In many respects, resistance to ejection of blood into the pulmonary artery outflow tract is relatively fixed, and hence the magnitude of the shunt is inversely proportional to the systemic vascular resistance. Pharmacologically induced responses that decrease systemic vascular resistance (volatile anesthetics, histamine release, ganglionic blockade, α-adrenergic blockade) increase the magnitude of the right-to-left shunt and accentuate arterial hypoxemia. Pulmonary blood flow can be decreased by increases in pulmonary vascular resistance that accompany such intraoperative ventilatory maneuvers as intermittent positive airway pressure or positive end-expiratory pressure. Furthermore, the loss of negative intrapleural pressure on opening the chest increases pulmonary vascular resistance and the magnitude of the shunt. Nevertheless, the advantages of controlled ventilation of the lungs during operations usually offset this potential hazard. Indeed, arterial oxygenation does not predictably deteriorate in patients with tetralogy of Fallot, either with the institution of positive pressure ventilation of the lungs or after opening of the chest.

Preoperative Preparation Preoperatively, it is important to avoid dehydration by maintaining oral feedings in extremely young patients or by providing intravenous fluids before the patient's arrival in the operating room. Crying associated with intramuscular administration of drugs used for preoperative medication can lead to hypercyanotic attacks. β-Adrenergic antagonists should be continued until the induction of anesthesia in patients receiving these drugs for prophylaxis against hypercyanotic attacks.

Induction of Anesthesia Induction of anesthesia in patients with tetralogy of Fallot is often accomplished with ketamine (3–4 mg/kg IM or 1–2 mg/kg IV). The onset of anesthesia after ketamine injection may be associated with improved arterial oxygenation, presumably reflecting increased pulmonary blood flow due to ketamine-induced increases in systemic vascular resistance, which can lead to a decrease in the magnitude of the right-to-left intracardiac shunt. Ketamine has also been alleged to increase pulmonary vascular resistance, which would be undesirable in patients with a right-to-left shunt. The efficacious response to ketamine of patients with tetralogy of Fallot, however, suggests that this concern is not clinically significant. Tracheal intubation is facilitated by administration of muscle relaxants. It should be remembered that the onset of action of drugs administered intravenously may be more rapid in the presence of right-to-left shunts because the dilutional effect in the lungs is decreased. For this reason, it may be prudent to decrease the rate of intravenous injection of depressant drugs in these patients.

Induction of anesthesia with a volatile anesthetic such as sevoflurane is acceptable but must be accomplished with caution and careful monitoring of systemic oxygenation. Although decreased pulmonary blood flow speeds the achievement of anesthetic concentrations, the hazard of decreased systemic blood pressure plus decreased systemic vascular resistance is great. Indeed, hypercyanotic attacks can occur during administration of low concentrations of volatile anesthetics. Halothane is the preferred inhalational anesthetic as it decreases contractility and maintains systemic vascular resistance.

Maintenance of Anesthesia Maintenance of anesthesia is often achieved with nitrous oxide combined with ketamine. The advantage of this combination is preservation of the systemic vascular resistance. Nitrous oxide may also increase pulmonary vascular resistance, but this potentially adverse effect is more than offset by its beneficial effects on systemic vascular resistance (no change or modest increase). The principal disadvantage of using nitrous oxide is the associated decrease in the inspired oxygen concentration. Theoretically, increased inspired oxygen concentrations could decrease pulmonary vascular resistance, leading to increased pulmonary blood flow and improved Pao_2. Therefore, it seems prudent to limit the inspired concentration of nitrous oxide to 50%. The use of an opioid or benzodiazepine may also be considered during maintenance of anesthesia, but the dose and rate of administration must be adjusted to minimize decreased systemic blood pressure and systemic vascular resistance.

Intraoperative skeletal muscle paralysis may be provided with pancuronium in view of its ability to maintain systemic blood pressure and systemic vascular resistance. An increase in heart rate associated with pancuronium is helpful for maintaining left ventricular cardiac output. Alternative nondepolarizing neuromuscular blocking drugs are often selected with consideration given to the ability of some of these drugs, when administered rapidly in high doses, to evoke the release of histamine with associated decreases in systemic vascular resistance and systemic blood pressure.

Ventilation of the patient's lungs should be controlled, but it must be appreciated that excessive positive airway pressure may adversely increase the resistance to blood flow through the lungs. Intravascular fluid volume must be maintained with intravenous fluid administration because acute hypovolemia tends to increase the magnitude of the right-to-left intracardiac shunt. In view of the predictable erythrocytosis, it is probably not necessary to consider blood replacement until approximately 20% of the patient's blood volume has been lost. It is crucial that meticulous care be taken to avoid infusion of air through the tubing used to deliver intravenous solutions because it could lead to systemic air embolization. α-Adrenergic agonist drugs such as phenylephrine must be available to treat undesirable decreases in systemic blood pressure caused by decreased systemic vascular resistance.

Patient Characteristics Following Surgical Repair of Tetralogy of Fallot

Although patients with surgically repaired tetralogy of Fallot are usually asymptomatic, their survival is often shortened because of sudden death, presumably due to cardiac causes. Ventricular cardiac dysrhythmias are common in patients following surgical correction of tetralogy of Fallot. Patients with surgically repaired tetralogy of Fallot often develop atrial fibrillation or flutter. Right bundle branch block is frequent, whereas third-degree atrioventricular heart block is uncommon. Pulmonic regurgitation may develop as a consequence of surgical repair of the right ventricular outflow tract, eventually leading to right ventricular hypertrophy and dysfunction. An aneurysm may form at the site where the right ventricular outflow tract was repaired.

Eisenmenger's Syndrome

Patients in whom a left-to-right intracardiac shunt is reversed, as a result of increased pulmonary vascular resistance, to a level that equals or exceeds the systemic vascular resistance are said to have Eisenmenger's syndrome. It is presumed that exposure of the pulmonary vasculature to increased blood flow and pressure, as may accompany a VSD or ASD, results in pulmonary obstructive disease. As obliteration of the pulmonary vascular bed progresses, the pulmonary vascular resistance increases until it equals or exceeds systemic vascular resistance and the intracardiac shunt is reversed. Shunt reversal occurs in approximately 50% of patients with an untreated VSD and approximately 10% of patients with an untreated ASD. The murmur associated with these cardiac defects disappears when Eisenmenger's syndrome develops.

Signs and Symptoms

Cyanosis and decreased exercise tolerance occur as right-to-left intracardiac shunting develops. Palpitations are common and are most often due to the onset of atrial fibrillation or atrial flutter. Arterial hypoxemia stimulates erythrocytosis, leading to increased blood viscosity and associated visual disturbances, headache, dizziness, and paresthesias. Hemoptysis may occur as a result of pulmonary infarction or rupture of dilated pulmonary arteries, arterioles, or aorticopulmonary collateral vessels. Abnormal coagulation and thrombosis often accompany arterial hypoxemia and erythrocytosis. The possibility of a cerebral vascular accident or brain abscess is increased. Syncope most likely reflects inadequate cardiac output. Sudden death is a risk in patients with Eisenmenger's syndrome. The ECG shows right ventricular hypertrophy.

Treatment

No treatment has proved effective in producing sustained decreases in pulmonary vascular resistance, although intravenous epoprostenol may be beneficial. Phlebotomy with isovolemic replacement should be undertaken in patients with moderate or severe symptoms of hyperviscosity. Pregnancy is discouraged in women with Eisenmenger's syndrome. Lung transplantation with repair of the cardiac defect or combined heart-lung transplantation is an option for selected patients with this syndrome. The presence of irreversibly increased pulmonary vascular resistance contraindicates surgical correction of the congenital heart defect that was responsible for the original left-to-right intracardiac shunt.

Management of Anesthesia

Management of anesthesia for patients with Eisenmenger's syndrome undergoing noncardiac surgery is based on maintenance of preoperative levels of systemic vascular resistance and recognizing that increases in right-to-left intracardiac shunting are likely if sudden vasodilation occurs. Continuous intravenous infusions of norepinephrine have been reported to maintain systemic vascular resistance during the perioperative period. Minimization of blood loss with the development of hypovolemia and the prevention of iatrogenic paradoxical embolization are important considerations. It may be useful to perform prophylactic phlebotomy with isovolumic replacement in patients with hematocrits higher than 65%. Preoperative administration of antiplatelet drugs is not encouraged because intraoperative blood loss may be associated with the impaired coagulation that accompanies chronic arterial hypoxemia and erythrocytosis. Opioids have been administered safely for preoperative and postoperative analgesia.

Laparoscopic procedures may pose an increased risk to these patients because insufflation of the peritoneal cavity with carbon dioxide may cause increases in the $PaCO_2$, resulting in acidosis, hypotension, and cardiac dysrhythmias. Efforts to maintain normocapnia may be accompanied by increases in airway pressures and pulmonary vascular resistance, especially as the intra-abdominal pressure increases. These events may be further exaggerated by placing the patient in the head-down position. Early tracheal extubation in these patients is preferable because of the deleterious effects of positive pressure ventilation.

Despite the potential for undesirable decreases in systemic blood pressure and systemic vascular resistance, the successful management of anesthesia using epidural anesthesia has been described in patients undergoing tubal ligation and cesarean section. If epidural anesthesia is selected, it seems prudent not to add epinephrine to the local anesthetic solution injected into the epidural space. This recommendation is based on the observation that peripheral β-agonist effects produced by the epinephrine absorbed from the epidural space into the systemic circulation could exaggerate decreases in systemic blood pressure and systemic vascular resistance associated with epidural anesthesia.

Ebstein's Anomaly

Ebstein's anomaly is an abnormality of the tricuspid valve in which the valve leaflets are malformed or displaced downward into the right ventricle. As a result, the right ventricle has a small distal effective portion and an atrialized proximal portion. The tricuspid valve is usually regurgitant but may also be stenotic. Most patients with Ebstein's anomaly have an interatrial communication (ASD, patent foramen ovale) through which there may be right-to-left shunting of blood.

Signs and Symptoms

The severity of the hemodynamic derangements in patients with Ebstein's anomaly depends on the degree of displacement and the functional status of the tricuspid valve leaflets. As a result, the clinical presentation of Ebstein's anomaly varies from congestive heart failure in neonates to the absence of symptoms in adults in whom the anomaly is discovered incidentally. Neonates often manifest cyanosis and congestive heart failure that worsens after the ductus arteriosus closes, thereby decreasing pulmonary blood flow. Older children with Ebstein's anomaly may be diagnosed because of an incidental murmur, whereas adolescents and adults are likely to present with supraventricular dysrhythmias that lead to congestive heart failure, worsening cyanosis, and occasionally syncope. Patients with Ebstein's anomaly and an interatrial communication are at risk of paradoxical embolization, brain abscess, congestive heart failure, and sudden death.

The severity of cyanosis depends on the magnitude of the right-to-left shunt. A systolic murmur caused by tricuspid regurgitation is usually present at the left lower sternal border. Hepatomegaly resulting from passive hepatic congestion due to increased right atrial pressures may be present. The ECG is characterized by tall and broad P waves (resembling right bundle branch block), and first-degree atrioventricular heart block is common. Paroxysmal supraventricular and ventricular tachydysrhythmias may occur, and as many as 20% of patients with Ebstein's anomaly have ventricular preexcitation by way of accessory electrical pathways between the atrium and ventricle (Wolff-Parkinson-White syndrome). In patients with severe disease (marked right-to-left shunting and minimal functional right ventricle) marked cardiomegaly is present that is largely due to right atrial enlargement.

Echocardiography is used to assess right atrial dilation, distortion of the tricuspid valve leaflets, and the severity of the tricuspid regurgitation or stenosis. The presence and magnitude of interatrial shunting can be determined by color Doppler imaging studies. Enlargement of the right atrium may be so massive that the apical portions of the lungs are compressed, resulting in restrictive pulmonary disease.

The hazards of pregnancy in parturients with Ebstein's anomaly include deterioration in right ventricular function due to increased blood volume and cardiac output, increased right-to-left shunting and arterial hypoxemia if an ASD is present, and cardiac dysrhythmias. Pregnancy-induced hypertension may result in the development of congestive heart failure in these women.

Treatment

Treatment of Ebstein's anomaly is based on the prevention of associated complications including antibiotic prophylaxis against infective endocarditis and administration of diuretics and digoxin for management of congestive heart failure. Patients with supraventricular dysrhythmias are treated pharmacologically or with catheter ablation if an accessory pathway is present. In severely ill neonates with Ebstein's anomaly, an arterial shunt from the systemic circulation to the pulmonary circulation is created to increase pulmonary blood flow and thus decrease cyanosis. Further staged procedures to create a univentricular heart (Glenn shunt and Fontan procedure) may also be considered in these cases. Repair or replacement of the tricuspid valve in conjunction with closure of the interatrial communication is recommended for older patients who have severe symptoms despite medical therapy. Complications of surgery to correct Ebstein's anomaly include third-degree atrioventricular heart block, persistence of supraventricular dysrhythmias, residual tricuspid regurgitation after valve repair, and prosthetic valve dysfunction when the tricuspid valve is replaced.

Management of Anesthesia

Hazards during anesthesia in patients with Ebstein's anomaly include accentuation of arterial hypoxemia due to increases in the magnitude of the right-to-left intracardiac shunt and the development of supraventricular tachydysrhythmias. Increased right atrial pressures may indicate the presence of right ventricular failure. In the presence of a probe-patent foramen ovale (present in approximately 30% of patients), an increase in right atrial pressure above the pressure in the left atrium can lead to a right-to-left intracardiac shunt through the foramen ovale. Unexplained arterial hypoxemia or paradoxical air embolism during the perioperative period may be due to shunting of blood or air through a previously closed foramen ovale. The delayed onset of pharmacologic effects after intravenous administration of drugs during anesthesia most likely reflects pooling and dilution in an enlarged right atrium. Epidural analgesia has been used safely for labor and delivery.

Tricuspid Atresia

Tricuspid atresia is characterized by arterial hypoxemia, a small right ventricle, a large left ventricle, and marked decreases in pulmonary blood flow. Poorly oxygenated blood from the right atrium passes through an ASD into the left atrium, mixes with oxygenated blood, and then enters the left ventricle, from which it is ejected into the systemic circulation. Pulmonary blood flow is via a VSD, PDA, or bronchial vessels.

Treatment

A Fontan procedure (anastomosis of the right atrial appendage to the right pulmonary artery to bypass the right ventricle and provide a direct atriopulmonary communication) is used to treat tricuspid atresia. This operation is also used to treat pulmonary artery atresia.

Management of Anesthesia

Management of anesthesia for patients undergoing Fontan procedures has been successfully achieved with opioids or volatile anesthetics. Immediately after cardiopulmonary bypass and continuing into the early postoperative period, it is important to maintain increased right atrial pressures (16–20 mm Hg) to facilitate pulmonary blood flow. An increase in pulmonary vascular resistance due to acidosis, hypothermia, peak airway pressures higher than 15 cm H_2O, or reactions to the tracheal tube may cause right-sided heart failure. Early tracheal extubation and spontaneous ventilation are desirable. Positive inotropic drugs (dopamine) with or without vasodilators (nitroprusside) are often required to optimize cardiac output and maintain low pulmonary vascular resistance. Pleural effusions, ascites, and edema of the lower extremities are not uncommon postoperatively and usually resolve within a few weeks. Right atrial pressure equal to

the pulmonary artery pressure remains elevated after this operation, averaging 15 mm Hg.

Although absence of a contractile right ventricle is compatible with long-term survival, the adaptability of the circulatory system is restricted. This decreased capacity of a single ventricle to respond to an increased workload may have a significant impact on the management of these patients for another operation. In this regard, subsequent management of anesthesia in patients who have undergone Fontan procedures is facilitated by monitoring the central venous pressure (which equals the pulmonary artery pressure in these patients) to assess the intravascular fluid volume and to detect sudden impairment of left ventricular function and increased pulmonary vascular resistance. The value of monitoring the central venous pressure reflects the absence of a contractile right ventricle and the impaired ability of a single ventricle to adapt to acute increases in afterload that may necessitate prompt administration of positive inotropic drugs. Insertion of a thermodilution pulmonary artery catheter in patients after a Fontan repair may be technically difficult secondary to the unusual anatomy. No information is available regarding the accuracy of thermodilution cardiac output measurements in such patients. Peak and mean airway pressure must be maintained as it will increase pulmonary vascular resistance and may decrease carbon dioxide significantly.

Transposition of the Great Arteries

Transposition of the great arteries results from failure of the truncus arteriosus to spiral, resulting in the aorta arising from the anterior portion of the right ventricle and the pulmonary artery arising from the left ventricle (**Fig. 3-5**). There is

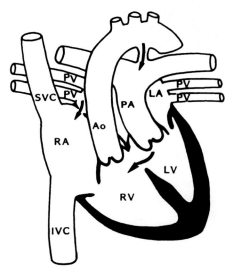

Figure 3-5 • Transposition of the great arteries. The right ventricle (RV) and left ventricle (LV) are not connected in series. Instead, the two ventricles function as parallel and independent circulations, with the aorta (Ao) arising from the RV and the pulmonary artery (PA) arising from the LV. Survival is not possible unless mixing of blood between the two circulations occurs through an atrial septal defect, ventricular septal defect, or patent ductus. IVC, inferior vena cava; LA, left atrium; PV, pulmonary vein; RA, right atrium; SVC, superior vena cava.

complete separation of the pulmonary and systemic circulations such that systemic venous blood traverses the right atrium, right ventricle, aorta, and systemic circulation; and pulmonary venous blood traverses the left atrium, left ventricle, pulmonary artery, and lungs. Survival is possible only if there is communication between the two circulations in the form of a VSD, ASD, or PDA.

Signs and Symptoms

Persistent cyanosis and tachypnea at birth may be the first clues to the presence of transposition of the great arteries. Congestive heart failure is often present, reflecting left ventricular failure due to volume overload created by the left-to-right intracardiac shunt necessary for survival. The ECG is likely to demonstrate right axis deviation and right ventricular hypertrophy because the right ventricle is the systemic ventricle. Classically, the cardiac silhouette on the chest radiograph is described as being "egg-shaped with a narrow stalk."

Treatment

The immediate management of transposition of the great arteries involves creating intracardiac mixing or increasing the degree of mixing. This goal is accomplished with infusions of prostaglandin E to maintain patency of the ductus arteriosus and/or balloon atrial septostomy (Rashkind procedure). Administration of oxygen may decrease pulmonary vascular resistance and increase pulmonary blood flow. Diuretics and digoxin are administered to treat congestive heart failure.

Two surgical switch procedures have been used to treat complete transition of the great arteries. The initial surgical procedure, known as the "atrial switch" operation (Mustard or Senning operation), involved resection of the atrial septum and its replacement with a baffle to direct the systemic venous blood into the left ventricle and pulmonary venous blood across the tricuspid valve into the right ventricle. This operation has been replaced by the "arterial switch" operation in which the pulmonary artery and ascending aorta are transected above the semilunar valves and reanastomosed with the right and left ventricles, and coronary arteries are then reimplanted, so the aorta is connected to the left ventricle and the pulmonary artery is connected to the right ventricle.

Management of Anesthesia

Management of anesthesia in the presence of transposition of the great arteries must take into account separation of the pulmonary and systemic circulations. Drugs administered intravenously are distributed with minimal dilution to organs such as the heart and brain. Therefore, doses and rates of injection of intravenously administered drugs may have to be decreased. Conversely, the onset of anesthesia produced by inhaled drugs is delayed because only small amounts of the inhaled drug reach the systemic circulation. In the final analysis, induction and maintenance of anesthesia are often accomplished with ketamine combined with muscle relaxants to facilitate tracheal intubation. Ketamine can be supplemented with opioids or benzodiazepines for maintenance of anesthesia. Nitrous oxide has limited application in these patients, as it is important to administer high inspired oxygen concentrations. The potential cardiac depressant effects of volatile anesthetics detract from the use of these drugs. Selection of muscle relaxants is influenced by the desire to avoid histamine-induced changes in systemic blood pressure. The ability of pancuronium to increase the heart rate and systemic blood pressure modestly may be useful.

Dehydration must be avoided during the perioperative period. These patients may have hematocrits in excess of 70%, which may contribute to the high incidence of cerebral venous thrombosis. This finding suggests that oral fluids should not be withheld from these patients for prolonged periods. If fluids cannot be ingested orally, an intravenous infusion should be initiated during the preoperative period. Atrial dysrhythmias and conduction disturbances may occur postoperatively.

Mixing of Blood between the Pulmonary and Systemic Circulations

Rare congenital heart defects that result in mixing of blood from the pulmonary and systemic circulations manifest as cyanosis and arterial hypoxemia of varying severity depending on the magnitude of the pulmonary blood flow. As a result of the mixing of blood from both circulations, pulmonary arterial blood has higher oxygen saturation than that of systemic venous blood, and systemic arterial blood has lower oxygen saturation than that of pulmonary venous blood.

Truncus Arteriosus

Truncus arteriosus refers to the congenital cardiac defect in which a single arterial trunk serves as the origin of the aorta and pulmonary artery (**Fig. 3-6**). This single arterial trunk overrides both ventricles, which are connected through a VSD. Mortality is high, with the median age of survival at approximately 5 to 6 weeks.

Signs and Symptoms

Presenting signs and symptoms of truncus arteriosus include cyanosis and arterial hypoxemia, failure to thrive, and congestive heart failure early in life. Peripheral pulses may be accentuated owing to the rapid diastolic runoff of blood into the pulmonary circulation. Auscultation of the chest and evaluation of the ECG do not give predictable information and are not diagnostic. Chest radiography reveals cardiomegaly and increased vascularity of the lung fields. The diagnosis is confirmed by angiocardiography performed during cardiac catheterization.

Treatment

Surgical treatment of truncus arteriosus includes banding of the right and left pulmonary arteries if pulmonary blood flow is excessive. In addition, an associated VSD can be closed so only

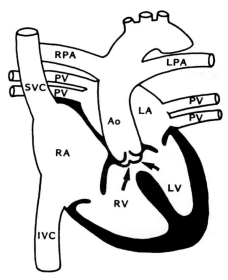

Figure 3-6 • Truncus arteriosus in which the pulmonary artery (RPA, right pulmonary artery; LPA, left pulmonary artery) and aorta (Ao) arise from a single trunk that overrides the left ventricle (LV) and right ventricle (RV). This trunk receives blood from both ventricles by virtue of a ventricular septal defect. IVC, inferior vena cava; LA, left atrium; PV, pulmonary vein; RA, right atrium; SVC, superior vena cava.

left ventricular output enters the truncus arteriosus. When this is done, a Dacron conduit with a valve is also placed between the right ventricle and pulmonary artery.

Management of Anesthesia

Management of anesthesia in the presence of truncus arteriosus is influenced by the magnitude of the pulmonary blood flow. When pulmonary blood flow in increased, the use of positive end-expiratory pressure is beneficial and may serve to decrease the symptoms of congestive heart failure. Increased pulmonary blood flow may be associated with evidence of myocardial ischemia on the ECG. When myocardial ischemia that occurs intraoperatively does not respond to (1) intravenous administration of phenylephrine or fluids or (2) the use of positive end-expiratory pressure, consideration may be given to temporary banding of the pulmonary artery to increase systemic and coronary blood flow. Patients with decreased pulmonary blood flow and arterial hypoxemia should be managed as described for tetralogy of Fallot.

Partial Anomalous Pulmonary Venous Return

Partial anomalous pulmonary venous return is characterized by the presence of left or right pulmonary veins that empty into the right side of the circulation rather than the left atrium. In approximately one half of cases, the aberrant pulmonary veins drain into the superior vena cava. In the remaining cases, pulmonary veins enter the right atrium, inferior vena cava, azygos vein, or coronary sinus. Partial anomalous pulmonary venous return may be more common than appreciated, suggested by the presence of this anomaly in approximately 0.5% of routine autopsies.

The onset and severity of symptoms produced by this abnormality depend on the amount of pulmonary blood flow routed through the right side of the heart. Fatigue and exertional dyspnea are the most frequent initial manifestations, usually appearing during early adulthood. Cyanosis and congestive heart failure are likely if more than 50% of the pulmonary venous flow enters the right side of the circulation.

Angiography is the most useful technique for confirming the diagnosis of partial anomalous pulmonary venous return. Cardiac catheterization usually demonstrates normal intracardiac pressures and increased oxygen saturations of blood in the right side of the heart. Treatment is by surgical repair.

Total Anomalous Pulmonary Venous Return

Total anomalous pulmonary venous return is characterized by drainage of all four pulmonary veins into the systemic venous system. The most common presentation of this defect, accounting for approximately one half of cases, is drainage of the four pulmonary veins into the left innominate vein in association with a left-sided superior vena cava. Oxygenated blood reaches the left atrium by way of an ASD. PDA is present in approximately one third of patients.

Signs and Symptoms

Total anomalous pulmonary venous return presents clinically as congestive heart failure in 50% of patients by 1 month of age and in 90% by 1 year. It is definitively diagnosed by angiocardiography. Mortality is approximately 80% by 1 year of age unless it is surgically corrected using cardiopulmonary bypass.

Management of Anesthesia

Management of anesthesia in the presence of total anomalous pulmonary venous return may include positive end-expiratory pressure applied to the airways in an attempt to decrease excessive pulmonary blood flow. Patients who present with pulmonary edema should undergo positive-pressure ventilation through a tube placed in the trachea before cardiac catheterization. Operative manipulation of the right atrium, which is tolerated by normal patients, may result in obstruction to flow into the right atrium in these patients, manifesting as sudden decreases in systemic blood pressure and the onset of bradycardia. Intravenous transfusions may be hazardous because any increase in right atrial pressure is transmitted directly to the pulmonary veins, leading to the possibility of pulmonary edema.

Hypoplastic Left Heart Syndrome

Hypoplastic left heart syndrome is characterized by left ventricular hypoplasia, mitral valve hypoplasia, aortic valve atresia, and hypoplasia of the ascending aorta. Extracardiac congenital anomalies do not usually accompany this syndrome. There is complete mixing of pulmonary venous and systemic venous blood in a single ventricle, which is connected in parallel to both the pulmonary and systemic circulations. Systemic blood flow is dependent on a PDA. In addition to ductal patency, infant survival depends on a balance between systemic vascular resistance and pulmonary vascular resistance because both circulations are supplied from a single ventricle in a parallel fashion. An abrupt decrease in pulmonary vascular resistance after delivery results in increased pulmonary blood flow at the expense of systemic blood flow (pulmonary steal phenomenon). When this occurs, coronary and systemic blood flow is inadequate, leading to metabolic acidosis, high-output cardiac failure, and ventricular fibrillation, despite increasingly high PaO_2 values (**Fig. 3-7**). Alternatively, any postnatal event that leads to increased pulmonary vascular resistance can decrease the pulmonary blood flow so severely that arterial hypoxemia worsens, leading to progressive metabolic acidosis and circulatory collapse (see Fig. 3-7). Because rapid changes in pulmonary vascular resistance occur during the postnatal period, the necessary fine balance between pulmonary vascular resistance and systemic vascular resistance is unstable and difficult to maintain.

Treatment

Treatment of hypoplastic left heart syndrome is surgical, beginning with a palliative procedure that eliminates the need for continued patency of the ductus arteriosus. Preoperatively,

continuous intravenous infusions of prostaglandins may be useful for preventing physiologic closure of the ductus arteriosus. In addition, administration of cardiac inotropes and sodium bicarbonate may be necessary.

The palliative procedure consists of reconstructing the ascending aorta using the proximal pulmonary artery (**Fig. 3-8**). A systemic-to-pulmonary shunt to provide pulmonary blood flow is placed between the reconstructed aorta and the distal pulmonary artery. Typically, infants are placed on cardiopulmonary bypass to permit production of whole-body hypothermia; reconstruction of the aorta is then accomplished during 40 to 60 minutes of circulatory arrest. The central shunt is placed after reinstitution of cardiopulmonary bypass and during rewarming. The completed palliative procedure leaves the single right ventricle connected in parallel to the systemic circulation and pulmonary circulation. The stage is set, however, for later correction with a Fontan procedure when pulmonary vascular resistance has decreased to adult levels (see "Tricuspid Atresia"). The Fontan procedure plus elimination of the systemic-to-pulmonary shunt separates the two circulations and facilitates development of normal arterial oxygen saturation.

Management of Anesthesia

An umbilical artery and intravenous catheter are usually placed before the arrival of these infants in the operating

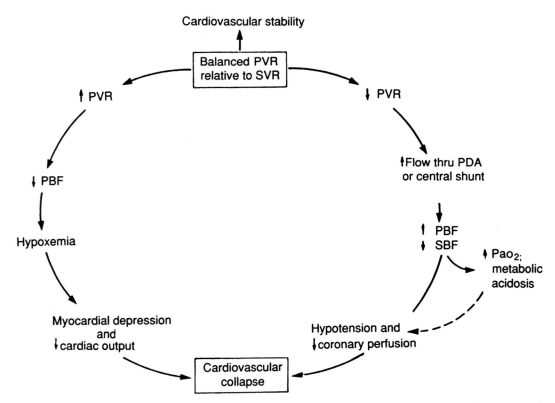

Figure 3-7 • Cardiovascular stability in the presence of hypoplastic left heart syndrome requires a balance between pulmonary vascular resistance (PVR) relative to systemic vascular resistance (SVR). An abrupt decrease in PVR after delivery can result in excessive pulmonary blood flow (PBF) relative to systemic blood flow (SBF) with cardiovascular collapse despite the absence of arterial hypoxemia. Conversely, postnatal changes that increase PVR can lead to cardiovascular collapse in the presence of arterial hypoxemia. *(From Hansen DD, Hickey PR: Anesthesia for hypoplastic left heart syndrome: Use of high-dose fentanyl in 30 neonates. Anesth Analg 1986;65:127–132, with permission.)*

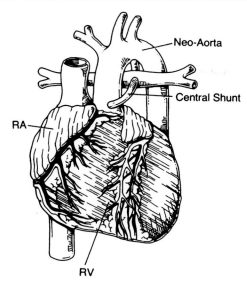

Figure 3-8 • Anatomy after the first-stage palliative procedure for hypoplastic left heart syndrome during the neonatal period. The ascending aorta has been reconstructed from the proximal pulmonary artery to form a neo-aorta. RA, right atrium; RV, right ventricle. (*From Hansen DD, Hickey PR: Anesthesia for hypoplastic left heart syndrome: Use of high-dose fentanyl in 30 neonates. Anesth Analg 1986;65:127–132, with permission.*)

room. After instituting monitoring, induction of anesthesia is often accomplished with fentanyl (50–75 µg/kg IV) administered simultaneously with pancuronium.

These infants are vulnerable to the development of ventricular fibrillation due to inadequate coronary blood flow before the palliative procedure. The danger of ventricular fibrillation and borderline cardiac status argues against the use of volatile anesthetics in these infants. A high Pa_{O_2} implies excessive pulmonary blood flow at the expense of the systemic circulation. Indeed, if the initial Pa_{O_2} is more than 100 mm Hg, maneuvers to increase pulmonary vascular resistance and decrease pulmonary blood flow are instituted. For example, a decrease in the volume of ventilation leads to increases in Pa_{CO_2} and decreases in the arterial pH, resulting in increased pulmonary vascular resistance and decreased pulmonary blood flow. If the Pa_{O_2} remains unacceptably high, institution of positive end-expiratory pressure leads to increased lung volumes and further increases in pulmonary vascular resistance. In extreme cases, temporary occlusion of one pulmonary artery serves to decrease the Pa_{O_2}.

Dopamine or isoproterenol is administered when necessary for inotropic support at the conclusion of cardiopulmonary bypass. The selection of specific inotropic drugs is influenced by pulmonary vascular resistance. The most frequent problem after cardiopulmonary bypass is too little pulmonary blood flow with associated arterial hypoxemia ($Pa_{O_2} < 20$ mm Hg). Attempts to improve the Pa_{O_2} include hyperventilation of the lungs to produce a low Pa_{CO_2} (20–25 mm Hg) and to increase the arterial pH plus infusion of isoproterenol to decrease pulmonary vascular resistance. A Pa_{O_2} higher than 50 mm Hg after cardiopulmonary bypass may indicate inadequate systemic

blood flow and the likely occurrence of progressive metabolic acidosis unless steps are taken to decrease pulmonary blood flow.

MECHANICAL OBSTRUCTION OF THE TRACHEA

The trachea can be obstructed by circulatory anomalies that produce a vascular ring or by dilation of the pulmonary artery secondary to absence of the pulmonic valve. These lesions must be considered when evaluating a child with unexplained stridor or other evidence of upper airway obstruction. The possibility of an undiagnosed vascular ring should be considered in the differential diagnosis of airway obstruction that follows placement of a nasogastric tube or an esophageal stethoscope.

Double Aortic Arch

Double aortic arch results in a vascular ring that can produce pressure on the trachea and esophagus. Compression resulting from this pressure can be manifested as inspiratory stridor, difficulty mobilizing secretions, and dysphagia. Patients with this cardiac defect usually prefer to lie with the neck extended because flexion of the neck often accentuates compression of the trachea.

Surgical transection of the smaller aortic arch is the treatment of choice for symptomatic patients. During surgery, the tracheal tube should be placed beyond the area of tracheal compression if this can be safely accomplished without producing endobronchial intubation. It must be appreciated that esophageal stethoscopes or nasogastric tubes can cause occlusion of the trachea if the tracheal tube remains above the level of vascular compression. Clinical improvement after surgical transection is often prompt. Tracheomalacia due to prolonged compression of the trachea, however, can jeopardize the patency of the trachea.

Aberrant Left Pulmonary Artery

Tracheal or bronchial obstruction can occur when the left pulmonary artery is absent and the arterial supply to the left lung is derived from a branch of the right pulmonary artery passing between the trachea and esophagus. This anatomic arrangement has been referred to as vascular sling because a complete ring is not present. The sling can cause obstruction of the right mainstem bronchus, the distal trachea, or rarely the left mainstem bronchus.

Clinical manifestations of an aberrant left pulmonary artery include stridor, wheezing, and occasionally arterial hypoxemia. In contrast to a true vascular ring, esophageal obstructions are rare, and the stridor produced by this defect is usually present during exhalation rather than inspiration. Chest radiographs may demonstrate an abnormal separation between the esophagus and the trachea. Hyperinflation or atelectasis of either lung may be present. Angiography is the most accurate approach for confirming the diagnosis.

Surgical division of the aberrant left pulmonary artery at its origin and redirection of its course anterior to the trachea, with anastomosis to the main pulmonary artery, is the treatment of choice. During the first months of life, surgical correction with deep hypothermia without cardiopulmonary bypass may be considered. Theoretically, continuous positive airway pressure or positive end-expiratory pressure should relieve the airway obstruction and associated stridor in these cases.

Absent Pulmonic Valve

Absence of the pulmonic valve results in dilation of the pulmonary artery, which can result in compression of the trachea and left mainstem bronchus. This lesion may occur as an isolated defect or in conjunction with tetralogy of Fallot. Symptoms include signs of tracheal obstruction and occasionally the development of arterial hypoxemia and congestive heart failure. Any increase in pulmonary vascular resistance, as may occur with arterial hypoxemia or hypercarbia, accentuates airway obstruction. Tracheal intubation and maintenance of 4 to 6 mm Hg of continuous positive airway pressure can be used to keep the trachea distended, reducing the magnitude of airway obstruction. Definitive treatment consists of inserting a tubular graft with an artificial pulmonic valve.

KEY POINTS

- In patients with congenital heart disease, an understanding of the relationship between systemic and pulmonary vascular resistance is essential in developing an anesthetic plan.

- New modalities for decreasing pulmonary vascular resistance have had a significant impact on the treatment of patients with intracardiac shunts

- VSDs remain the most commonly encountered congenital cardiac abnormality in infants and children.

- Transthoracic and transesophageal echocardiography facilitates early and accurate diagnosis of congenital heart disease.

- Advances in molecular biology have provided new insights into the greater bases of congenital heart disease.

- Congenital heart disease is the most common form of congenital disease and accounts for approximately 30% of the total incidence of all congenital diseases.

REFERENCES

Anand KJS, Hickey PR: Halothane-morphine compared with high-dose sufentanil for anesthesia and postoperative analgesia in neonatal cardiac surgery. N Engl J Med 1992;326:1–9.

Baum VC, Perloff JK: Anesthetic implications of adults with congenital heart disease. Anesth Analg 1993;76:1342–1358.

Brickner ME, Hillis LD, Lange RA: Congenital heart disease in adults. N Engl J Med 2000;342:256–263.

Clyman RI: Ibuprofen and patent ductus arteriosus. N Engl J Med 2000;343:728–730.

Greeley WJ, Stanley TE, Ungerleider RM, et al: Intraoperative hypoxemic spells in tetralogy of Fallot, an echocardiographic analysis of diagnosis and treatment. Anesth Analg 1989;68:815–819.

Groves ER, Groves JB: Epidural analgesia for labour in a patient with Ebstein's anomaly. Can J Anaesth 1995;42:77–79.

Hansen DD, Hickey PR: Anesthesia for hypoplastic left heart syndrome: Use of high-dose fentanyl in 30 neonates. Anesth Analg 1986;65:127–132.

Hosking MP, Beynen F: Repair of coarctation of the aorta in a child after a modified Fontan's operation: Anesthetic implications and management. Anesthesiology 1989;71:312–315.

Larson CP: Anesthesia in neonatal cardiac surgery. N Engl J Med 1992;327:124.

Mullen MP: Adult congenital heart disease. Sci Am Med 2000;1–10.

Spinnato JA, Kraynack BJ, Cooper MW: Eisenmenger's syndrome in pregnancy: Epidural anesthesia for elective cesarean section. N Engl J Med 1981;304:1215–1216.

Van Overmeire B, Smets K, Lecoutere D, et al: A comparison of ibuprofen and indomethacin for closure of patent ductus arteriosus. N Engl J Med 2000;343:674–681.

Weiss BM, Zemp L, Seifert B, et al: Outcome of pulmonary vascular disease in pregnancy: A systematic overview from 1978 through 1996. J Am Coll Cardiol 1998;31:1650–1659.

Wong RS, Baum VC, Sangivan S: Truncus arteriosus: Recognition and therapy of intraoperative cardiac ischemia. Anesthesiology 1991;74:378–380.

CHAPTER 4

Abnormalities of Cardiac Conduction and Cardiac Rhythm

Kelley Teed Watson

ANATOMY OF CARDIAC PACEMAKERS AND THE CONDUCTION SYSTEM

The conduction system of the heart is a set of very specialized cardiac cells that initiate and conduct electrical signals through the heart with precise coordination and great speed. Spontaneous depolarization is initiated in the pacemaker cells of the sinoatrial (SA) node. As the electrical impulse moves along the conduction system a wave of depolarization is propagated throughout the heart causing progressive contraction of cardiac muscle cells (**Fig. 4-1**).

The SA node is the primary site for impulse initiation, spontaneously discharging at a rate between 60 and 100 beats per minute. The SA node is located at the junction of the superior vena cava and the right atrium. It is richly innervated by sympathetic and parasympathetic nerve endings. In 60% of individuals, the arterial blood supply to the SA node comes from the right coronary artery; in the remaining 40%, the blood supply is from the left circumflex coronary artery. Impulses initiated in the SA node are rapidly conducted across the right and left atria causing them to contract.

The fibrous atrioventricular (AV) rings (annula fibrosa) of the tricuspid and mitral valves, located on either side of the AV node, electrically separate the atria from the ventricles. These rings essentially insulate the conduction tissue of the AV node and prevent electrical conduction between the atria and ventricles except via the normal conduction system. In addition to the physical separation that the fibrous rings provide, the AV node has a long refractory period to help prevent overstimulation of the ventricles by very rapid atrial impulses.

The AV node is located in the septal wall of the right atrium, anterior to the coronary sinus and above the insertion of the septal leaflet of the tricuspid valve. The blood supply to the AV node is from the right coronary artery in 85% to 90% of the population and from the left circumflex coronary artery in the remaining 10% to 15%. The AV node, like the SA node, is innervated by parasympathetic and sympathetic nerves. The AV node slows the conduction velocity of the electrical impulse, which allows time for atrial contraction, the so-called atrial kick, to contribute additional volume to the ventricle in late diastole. This volume contributes an additional 20% or so to cardiac output. After a brief slowing of the electrical impulse at the AV node, the impulse continues down the conduction tract along the bundle of His. The bundle of His quickly divides into right and the left bundles within the interventricular septum.

The right bundle branch (RBB) is a relatively thin bundle of fibers that courses down the right ventricle then branches near the right ventricular apex. Because of this late branching, the RBB is more vulnerable to interruption than the left bundle branch (LBB), which branches early and widely. This is why disruption of the more robust LBB usually indicates more extensive cardiac disease or damage.

The LBB divides into two fascicles: the left anterior superior fascicle and the left posterior inferior fascicle. The left and right bundles both receive blood supply from branches of the left anterior descending coronary artery. Infarction in the territory of the left anterior descending coronary artery can often affect the left anterior superior fascicle and the RBB, but rarely the left posterior inferior fascicle because it receives additional blood supply from the posterior descending coronary artery. The distal branches of the right and left bundles interlace into a network of Purkinje fibers.

THE ELECTROPHYSIOLOGY OF THE CONDUCTION SYSTEM

In the resting state, the inside of a cardiac cell is negative relative to the outside. Impulses are conducted through the heart by a process of progressive depolarization. Cardiac muscle cells have a resting membrane potential of -80 to -90 mV. The resting gradient is maintained by membrane bound $Na^+K^+ATPase$ that concentrates potassium intracellularly and extrudes sodium extracellularly. The membrane potential increases when the sodium and calcium channels open in response to neighboring cell membrane charge shifts. At the point at which the membrane potential reaches $+20$ mV, an action potential (or depolarization) occurs. After depolarization, cells are refractory to subsequent action potentials for a period corresponding to phase 4 of the depolarization potential (**Fig. 4-2**).

Electrocardiography

The essential monitor for diagnosis of cardiac conduction abnormalities and rhythm disturbances is the electrocardiogram (ECG). An ECG is a tracing made using electrodes on the skin that amplify cardiac electrical potentials. The normal ECG tracing is a complex composed of three waveforms: the P wave (atrial depolarization), the QRS complex (ventricular depolarization), and T wave (ventricular repolarization). The direction of the electrical signal relative to a ground electrode determines the direction of the deflection seen on the ECG. Positive signals are represented by deflections above the isoelectric line and negative signals are represented as deflections below the isoelectric line.

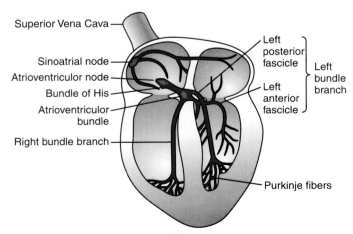

Figure 4-1 • Anatomy of the conduction system for transmission of cardiac electrical impulses.

Superior Vena Cava

Sinoatrial node

Atrioventriculor node

Bundle of His

Atrioventriculor bundle

Right bundle branch

Left posterior fascicle

Left anterior fascicle

Left bundle branch

Purkinje fibers

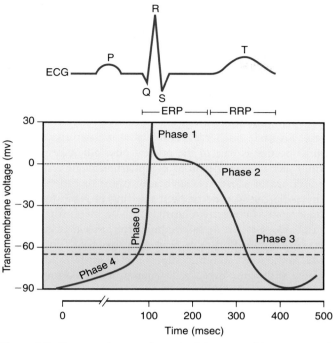

Figure 4-2 • Transmembrane action potential generated by an automatic cardiac cell and the relationship of this action potential to events depicted on the electrocardiogram. Phase 4 undergoes spontaneous depolarization from the resting membrane potential (−90 mV) until the threshold potential (*broken line*) is reached. Depolarization (phase 0) occurs when the threshold potential is reached and corresponds to the QRS complex on the electrocardiogram (ECG). Phases 1 through 3 represent repolarization, with phase 3 corresponding to the T wave on the ECG. The effective refractory period (ERP) is the time during which cardiac impulses cannot be conducted, regardless of the intensity of the stimulus. During the relative refractory period (RRP), a strong stimulus can initiate an action potential. The action potential from a contractile cardiac cell differs from an automatic cardiac cell in that phase 4 does not undergo spontaneous depolarization.

The time between atrial depolarization and the initiation of ventricular depolarization is the PR interval. The normal reference range for PR interval is 0.12 to 0.20 seconds. The QRS complex corresponds to the wave of depolarization as it emerges from the AV node and moves downward to depolarize the right and left ventricles. The QRS is normally 0.05 to 0.10 seconds in duration. Abnormal intraventricular conduction is suggested by a QRS complex that exceeds 0.12 seconds. The segment between the end of the S wave (end of ventricular contraction) and the beginning of the T wave is the ST segment. The ST segment represents the time between ventricular depolarization and the start of ventricular repolarization. It is normally isoelectric, but can be elevated to 1 mm in the absence of any cardiac abnormality. However, it is never normal for the ST segment to be depressed. The T-wave deflection should be in the same direction as the QRS complex and should not exceed 5 mm in amplitude in standard leads or 10 mm in precordial leads. Normal values for the QT interval should be corrected for the heart rate (QTc) because the QT interval varies inversely with heart rate. A normal QTc is less than 0.47 seconds. As a general rule, the QT interval is less than one half of the preceding R-R interval.

CARDIAC DYSRHYTHMIAS

Cardiac dysrhythmias are usually classified according to heart rate and the site of the abnormality. Conduction disturbances are usually classified by site and degree of blockade. The clinical significance of these abnormalities for the anesthesiologist depends on the effect they have on vital signs and the potential for deterioration into a life-threatening rhythm. In healthy adults, a wide variation in heart rate can be tolerated because normal compensatory mechanisms serve to maintain cardiac output and blood pressure. However, in the patient with cardiac disease, dysrhythmias and conduction disturbances can overwhelm normal compensatory processes and result in hemodynamic instability, cardiac and other end-organ ischemia, congestive heart failure, and even death.

MECHANISMS OF TACHYDYSRHYTHMIAS

Tachydysrhythmia can result from three mechanisms: (1) increased automaticity in normal conduction tissue or in an ectopic focus, (2) reentry of electrical potentials through abnormal pathways, and (3) triggering of abnormal cardiac potentials due to afterdepolarizations.

Automaticity

The fastest pacemaker in the heart is normally the SA node. Under abnormal conditions, other pacemakers can be accelerated and overdrive the SA node. Cardiac dysrhythmias caused by enhanced automaticity are due to repetitive firing of a focus other than the sinus node. Abnormal automaticity is not confined to secondary pacemakers within the conduction system. Almost any cell in the heart may exhibit automaticity under certain circumstances. A sustained rhythm due to accelerated firing of a pacemaker other than the SA node is called an ectopic rhythm.

The automaticity of cardiac tissue changes when the slope of phase 4 depolarization shifts or the resting membrane potential changes. Sympathetic stimulation causes an increase in heart rate by increasing the slope of phase 4 of the action potential and by decreasing the resting membrane potential. Conversely, parasympathetic stimulation results in a decrease in the slope of phase 4 depolarization and an increase in resting membrane potential to slow the heart rate.

Reentry Pathways

Dysrhythmias due to an ectopic focus often have a gradual onset and termination. This is in contrast to reentrant or triggered dysrhythmias that tend to be paroxysmal with abrupt onset and termination. Reentry requires two pathways over which cardiac impulses can be conducted at different velocities (**Fig. 4-3**). Extra electrical pathways, called accessory tracts, are embryologic remnants of tissue around the AV node that can conduct

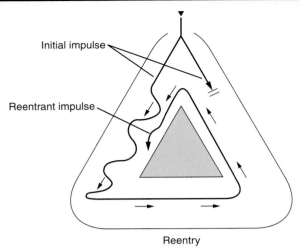

Figure 4-3 • Essential requirement for initiation of reentry excitation is a unilateral block that prevents uniform anterograde propagation of the initial cardiac impulse. Under appropriate conditions, this same cardiac impulse can traverse the area of blockade in a retrograde direction and become a reentrant cardiac impulse. *(Adapted from Akhtar M: Management of ventricular tachyarrhythmias. JAMA 1982;247:671–674. Copyright 1982 American Medical Association.)*

impulses bypassing the AV node and normal infranodal conduction tract. Normally, the conduction time through the AV node is the slowest in the heart. In a reentry circuit, there is anterograde (forward) conduction over the slower normal conduction pathway and retrograde (backward) conduction over a faster accessory pathway. Reentry pathways account for most premature beats and tachydysrhythmias. Pharmacologic or physiologic events may alter the balance between conduction velocities and refractory periods of the dual pathways, resulting in the initiation or termination of reentrant dysrhythmias.

Triggering by Afterdepolarizations

Afterdepolarizations are oscillations in membrane potential that occur during or after repolarization. Under special circumstances these afterdepolarizations can trigger a complete depolarization. Once triggered, the process may be self-sustaining and result in a triggered dysrhythmia. Triggered dysrhythmias associated with *early* afterdepolarizations are enhanced by slow heart rates and are treated by accelerating the heart rate with pacing or a positive chronotropic drug. Conversely, triggered dysrhythmias associated with *delayed* afterpotentials are enhanced by fast heart rates and can be suppressed with negative chronotropic drugs.

SUPRAVENTRICULAR DYSRHYTHMIAS

Sinus Dysrhythmia

Occasionally an ECG will show sinus rhythm that appears irregular. This is a normal variant called sinus dysrhythmia. The variation in heart rate is in response to changes in intrathoracic pressure during inspiration and expiration known as the Bainbridge reflex. Inspiration accelerates the heart rate and

expiration slows it down. Sinus dysrhythmia is common in children and young people but tends to decrease with age.

Sinus Tachycardia

Signs and Symptoms

Typically, sinus tachycardia is a nonparoxysmal elevation in heart rate. The heart rate usually speeds up and slows down gradually. Sinus tachycardia is caused by acceleration of the rate of SA node discharge secondary to sympathetic stimulation. It occurs as part of the normal physiologic response to stimuli such as fear or pain or as a pharmacologic response to medications or substances such as atropine or caffeine. Sinus tachycardia can also occur in the setting of significant heart disease such as congestive heart failure or myocardial infarction (**Table 4-1**). In these circumstances, the increased heart rate is usually an effort to increase cardiac output. Sinus tachycardia is the most common supraventricular dysrhythmia associated with acute myocardial infarction and occurs in 30% to 40% of these patients.

Diagnosis

Sinus tachycardia occurs at a heart rate of 100 to 160 bpm. The ECG during sinus tachycardia shows a normal P wave before every QRS complex. The PR interval is normal unless a co-existing conduction block exists.

Treatment

The treatment of sinus tachycardia is directed toward correcting the underlying cause of increased sympathetic

TABLE 4–1 Perioperative Causes of Sinus Tachycardia
I. Physiologic Increase in Sympathetic Tone
Pain
Anxiety/fear
Light anesthesia
Hypovolemia/anemia
Arterial hypoxemia
Hypotension
Hypoglycemia
Fever/infection
II. Pathologic Increase in Sympathetic Tone
Myocardial ischemia/infarction
Congestive heart failure
Pulmonary embolus
Hyperthyroidism
Pericarditis
Pericardial tamponade
Malignant hyperthermia
Ethanol withdrawal
III. Drug-induced Increase in Heart Rate
Atropine/glycopyrrolate
Sympathomimetic drugs
Caffeine
Nicotine
Cocaine/amphetamines

stimulation. If the patient is not hypovolemic or manifesting evidence that the heart rate is a compensation to maintain cardiac output, intravenous administration of a β-blocker may be employed to lower the heart rate and decrease myocardial oxygen demand. Caution must be exercised with the use of β-blockers in patients susceptible to bronchospasm and in patients with impaired cardiac function. Patients unable to increase their cardiac stroke volume because of cardiac damage or left ventricular dysfunction may have an abrupt and dangerous decrease in blood pressure in response to a β-blocker–induced decrease in heart rate.

Prognosis

The prognosis of patients exhibiting sinus tachycardia is related to the physiologic or pathologic process causing the acceleration of sinus node activity. Sinus tachycardia without manifestations of hemodynamic instability is not life threatening but can contribute to myocardial ischemia and congestive heart failure in susceptible patients.

Management of Anesthesia

If specific etiologies for sinus tachycardia can be determined, they should be treated. Many causes of sinus tachycardia are clinically obvious, but some of the most serious causes, such as infection, hypoxia, myocardial ischemia, and congestive heart failure, may be less obvious. Supplemental oxygen should be administered to increase oxygen supply in response to the increased oxygen demand. Avoidance of vagolytic drugs, such as pancuronium, can aid in management of sinus tachycardia intraoperatively. Sinus tachycardia is generally well tolerated in young healthy patients. However, in patients with ischemic heart disease, diastolic dysfunction, or congestive heart failure, sinus tachycardia can contribute to significant clinical deterioration.

Premature Atrial Beats

Signs and Symptoms

Premature atrial contractions (PACs) arise from ectopic foci in the atria. Typical symptoms of PACs include an awareness of a "fluttering" or a "heavy" heart beat. Precipitating factors include excessive caffeine, emotional stress, alcohol, nicotine, recreational drugs, and hyperthyroidism. Premature atrial contractions are common in patients of all ages with and without heart disease. They often occur at rest and become less frequent with exercise. They are more common in patients with chronic lung disease, ischemic heart disease, and digitalis toxicity. PACs are the second most common dysrhythmia associated with acute myocardial infarction.

Diagnosis

Atrial premature beats are recognized on the ECG by the presence of early, abnormally shaped P waves. The PR interval is variable. Most often the duration and configuration of the corresponding QRS complex are normal because activation of the ventricles occurs via the normal conduction pathway. Aberrant conduction of atrial impulses can occur, resulting in a QRS complex that is widened and may mimic a ventricular premature contraction (PVC). PACs, unlike PVCs, are *not* followed by a compensatory pause.

Treatment

Avoidance of precipitating drugs or toxins can reduce the incidence of PACs. Underlying precipitating disorders should be treated. PACs are usually hemodynamically insignificant and do not require acute therapy unless they are associated with initiation of a tachydysrhythmia. Then, treatment is directed at controlling or converting the secondary dysrhythmia.

Prognosis

PACs can occur in patients with and without heart disease. The occurrence of PACs is not a risk factor for progression to a life-threatening dysrhythmia.

Management of Anesthesia

Anesthetic management of the patient with PACs should be aimed at avoiding excessive sympathetic stimulation, and eliminating drugs that might induce PACs. Pharmacologic treatment is required only if the PACs trigger secondary dysrhythmias. The PACs can usually be suppressed with calcium channel blockers or β-blockers. The secondary dysrhythmias triggered by PACs are treated with drugs or maneuvers that improve heart rate control and/or conversion to sinus rhythm.

Supraventricular Tachycardia

Signs and Symptoms

Common symptoms during an episode of supraventricular tachycardia (SVT) include lightheadedness, dizziness, fatigue, chest discomfort, and dyspnea. Fifteen percent of patients with SVT experience overt syncope. SVT occurs most often in the absence of structural heart disease in younger individuals and occurs three times more often in women than in men. Polyuria can be associated with SVT or any other atrial tachycardia that causes AV dyssynchrony. The polyuria is caused by an increase in secretion of atrial natriuretic peptide in response to increased atrial pressures from contraction of the atria against closed AV valves during the dysrhythmia episode.

Diagnosis

SVT is any tachydysrhythmia (average heart rate of 160–180 bpm) initiated and sustained by tissue at or above the AV node. Unlike sinus tachycardia, SVT is usually paroxysmal and may begin and end very abruptly. AV nodal reentrant tachycardia (AVNRT) is the most common type of SVT and accounts for 50% of diagnosed SVTs. AVNRT is most commonly due to a reentry circuit in which there is anterograde conduction over the slower AV nodal pathway and retrograde conduction over a faster accessory pathway. Other mechanisms for SVT include enhanced automaticity of secondary pacemaker cells and triggered impulse initiation by afterdepolarizations.

Atrial fibrillation and atrial flutter are SVTs, but their electrophysiology and treatment are distinctly different from other forms of SVT so they are discussed separately.

Treatment

If hemodynamically stable, the initial treatment of SVT is often a vagal maneuver such as carotid sinus massage or a Valsalva maneuver. Termination by a vagal maneuver suggests reentry as the causative mechanism. If conservative treatment is not effective, pharmacologic treatment directed at blocking AV nodal conduction is indicated.

Adenosine, calcium channel blockers, and β-blockers may be used to terminate SVT. Adenosine's advantage over the other intravenous drugs is a rapid onset (15–30 seconds) and brief duration (10 seconds). Most AVNRT episodes are terminated by a single dose of adenosine. The effects of adenosine are potentiated by dipyridamole and carbamazepine. Patients taking theophylline may require higher doses of adenosine due to competitive inhibition with adenosine for receptor sites. Adenosine often causes cutaneous flushing. Heart transplant recipients may require a reduction in dose secondary to denervation hypersensitivity. Multifocal atrial tachycardia, atrial flutter, and atrial fibrillation do not respond to adenosine.

Intravenous administration of calcium channel-blocking drugs including verapamil and diltiazem is also useful for terminating SVT. The advantage of these drugs is a longer duration of action than adenosine. However, side effects including peripheral vasodilation and negative inotropy can contribute to an undesirable degree of hypotension. Intravenous β-blockers may also be used to control or convert SVT. Intravenous digoxin is not clinically useful in acute control of SVT because digoxin has a delayed peak effect and a narrow therapeutic index. Electrical cardioversion is indicated for SVT unresponsive to drug therapy or SVT associated with hemodynamic instability.

Prognosis

Long-term medical therapy of patients with repeated episodes of SVT includes oral verapamil, digoxin, and/or propranolol. Radiofrequency catheter ablation may also be used to treat patients with recurrent AVNRT.

Anesthetic Management

Anesthetic management in a patient with SVT should focus on avoiding factors known to produce ectopy, such as increased sympathetic tone, electrolyte imbalances, and acid-base disturbances. Because SVT is usually paroxysmal, monitoring of vital signs to detect any progression to hemodynamic instability and verbal reassurance (if the patient is awake) is all that may be needed until an episode of SVT terminates. One should evaluate and treat any potential aggravating factors and anticipate the need for antidysrhythmics and/or cardioversion.

If hemodynamically stable, a patient with SVT can be treated initially with vagal maneuvers. If conservative treatment is ineffective, pharmacologic treatment directed at blocking AV nodal conduction is indicated. Adenosine, calcium channel blockers, or β-blockers may be used.

Multifocal Atrial Tachycardia
Signs and Symptoms

Multifocal atrial tachycardia is an irregular rhythm that electrophysiologically reflects the presence of multiple ectopic atrial pacemakers.

Diagnosis

The ECG shows P waves with three or more different morphologies, and the PR intervals vary. The rhythm is frequently confused with atrial fibrillation but, unlike atrial fibrillation, the rate is not excessively rapid (**Fig. 4-4**). The atrial rhythm is usually between 100 and 180 bpm.

Treatment

Treatment of the underlying abnormality is the most successful therapy for multifocal atrial tachycardia. It is most commonly found in patients experiencing an acute exacerbation of chronic lung disease. It can also be associated with methylxanthine toxicity (theophylline and caffeine), congestive heart failure, sepsis, and metabolic or electrolyte abnormalities. The dysrhythmia tends to respond to treatment of the underlying pulmonary decompensation with bronchodilators and supplemental oxygen. Use of theophylline can aggravate or prolong the condition. Improvement in arterial oxygenation decreases ectopy.

Pharmacologic treatment of multifocal atrial tachycardia has limited success and is considered secondary. Magnesium sulfate 2 g IV over 1 hour followed by 1 to 2 g IV per hour by infusion has demonstrated some success in decreasing atrial ectopy and converting the rhythm to sinus rhythm. Verapamil 5 to 10 mg IV over 5 to 10 minutes slows the ventricular rate and will convert some patients to sinus rhythm. Likewise, β-blockers such as esmolol or metoprolol can decrease the ventricular rate but at the risk of provoking bronchospasm, which can worsen the situation. Cardioversion has *no effect* on the multiple sites of ectopy that produce this dysrhythmia.

Anesthetic Management

Patients with multifocal atrial tachycardia who must undergo urgent surgery benefit from optimization of their pulmonary status. Avoidance of medications or procedures that could worsen the pulmonary status and avoidance of hypoxemia are the mainstays of anesthetic management.

Atrial Flutter
Signs and Symptoms

Atrial flutter is characterized by an organized atrial rhythm with an atrial rate of 250 to 350 bpm with varying degrees of AV block. The majority of patients present with 2:1 AV conduction. With an atrial rate of 300 bpm, and 2:1 conduction, a patient can present with a ventricular rate of 150 bpm and significant physical symptoms and signs. Atrial flutter

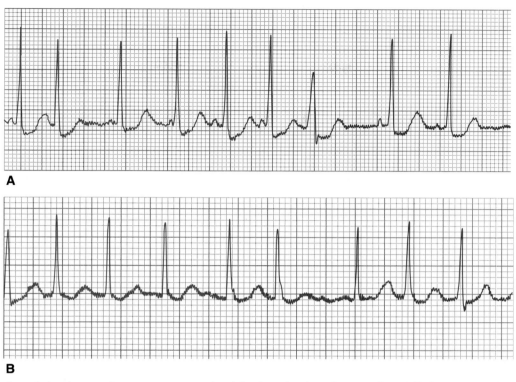

Figure 4-4 • Comparison of the electrocardiogram appearance of multifocal atrial tachycardia (**A**) and atrial fibrillation (**B**). Both rhythms are irregular. However, note several distinct P-wave morphologies and varying PR intervals with multifocal atrial tachycardia. There are no distinct P waves with atrial fibrillation.

frequently occurs in association with other dysrhythmias such as atrial fibrillation or atrial tachycardia.

Diagnosis

Atrial flutter is characterized by a regular pattern of atrial contractions called flutter waves. The rapid atrial flutter waves (F waves) result in a sawtooth appearance of the P wave on the ECG. The flutter waves are not separated by an isoelectric baseline. Most commonly, the atrial rate compared to the ventricular rate is 2:1. The ventricular rate may be regular or irregular depending on the rate of conduction. The ventricular rate is usually between 120 and 160 bpm (characteristically 150 bpm). Atrial flutter may degenerate into atrial fibrillation or, conversely, atrial fibrillation may convert to atrial flutter.

Treatment

If atrial flutter is hemodynamically significant, the treatment is cardioversion. Often less than 50 J is adequate to convert the rhythm to sinus. In the hemodynamically stable patient, overdrive pacing using transesophageal or atrial electrodes can be used for conversion to sinus rhythm. Patients with atrial flutter lasting longer than 48 hours should be anticoagulated and evaluated by transesophageal echocardiography for the presence of atrial thrombus prior to any attempt at cardioversion.

Pharmacologic control of the ventricular response and conversion to sinus rhythm can be challenging. Ventricular rate control should be the initial goal of therapy in order to avoid a potential increase in AV conduction from 2:1 to 1:1. If drug therapy slows the atrial flutter wave rate to the point that there is 1:1 conduction, hemodynamic deterioration can occur as the ventricular rate increases. Intravenous amiodarone, diltiazem, or verapamil may be used for control of the ventricular rate. If there is 1:1 conduction with a ventricular rate of 300 bpm or faster, reentry is the most likely mechanism and procainamide administration should be considered. All these drugs are helpful in controlling the ventricular rate, but none of these drugs is likely to convert atrial flutter to sinus rhythm.

Prognosis

Atrial flutter is usually associated with structural heart disease. Most patients with atrial flutter experience this dysrhythmia in conjunction with an acute exacerbation of a chronic condition, such as pulmonary disease, acute myocardial infarction, ethanol intoxication, thyrotoxicosis, or after cardiothoracic surgery. Atrial flutter occurs in approximately one third of patients with atrial fibrillation and may be associated with more intense symptoms due to a more rapid ventricular response.

Anesthetic Management

If atrial flutter occurs prior to induction of anesthesia, surgery should be postponed if possible until control of the dysrhythmia has been achieved. Management of atrial flutter occurring during anesthesia/surgery depends on the hemodynamic stability of the patient. If the atrial flutter is hemodynamically significant, treatment requires cardioversion. Synchronized cardioversion starting at 50 J is indicated. Pharmacologic control of the ventricular response with intravenous amiodarone, diltiazem, or verapamil may be attempted if vital signs are stable. The choice of pharmacologic agent depends on the co-existing medical diseases of the patient.

Atrial Fibrillation

Sign and Symptoms

Although atrial fibrillation may present as an asymptomatic finding on physical examination or the ECG, more commonly, the loss of AV synchrony and the rapid heart rate associated with this dysrhythmia result in significant symptoms. Symptoms may range from palpitations to angina pectoris, congestive heart failure, pulmonary edema, and hypotension. Atrial fibrillation is often associated with fatigue and generalized weakness. The absence of synchronized atrial contractions combined with rapid ventricular rates decreases cardiac output, sometimes to the point that heart failure occurs.

Diagnosis

Atrial fibrillation occurs when multiple areas of the atria continuously depolarize and contract in a disorganized manner. There is no uniform depolarization or contraction, only a quivering of the atrial walls. The dysrhythmia is characterized on the ECG as chaotic atrial activity with no discernible P waves (see Fig. 4-4). The rapid, disordered atrial activation and irregular electrical input to the AV node lead to sporadic ventricular contractions at a rate of approximately 180 bpm in a patient with a normal AV node. An extremely rapid ventricular response as high as 300 bpm can be seen in patients with accessory bypass tracts. When the ventricular activation occurs by an accessory tract, the QRS is often wide and can resemble ventricular tachycardia. Atrial fibrillation may be triggered by other atrial tachycardias.

Clinical Manifestations

Atrial fibrillation can be a sustained rhythm or an episodic dysrhythmia. Predisposing conditions include rheumatic heart disease (especially mitral valve disease), hypertension, thyrotoxicosis, ischemic heart disease, chronic obstructive pulmonary disease, acute alcohol intoxication, pericarditis, pulmonary embolus, and atrial septal defect. Increased left atrial size and mass are positive predictors for atrial fibrillation. Perhaps the most important clinical consequence of atrial fibrillation is a thromboembolic event causing a stroke. Loss of coordinated atrial contraction promotes stasis of blood and formation of atrial thrombi. Goals in the treatment of atrial fibrillation are control of the ventricular rate and restoration of normal sinus rhythm.

Treatment

Electrical cardioversion is the most effective method for converting atrial fibrillation to normal sinus rhythm. Cardioversion is indicated to relieve symptoms of heart failure, to improve cardiac output by restoring atrial contractility, and to reduce the risk of arterial thromboembolism. A large proportion of patients with new-onset atrial fibrillation spontaneously convert to sinus rhythm within 24 to 48 hours.

Pharmacologic cardioversion is most effective if initiated within 7 days of the onset of atrial fibrillation. Several drugs are efficacious in converting atrial fibrillation to sinus rhythm. These drugs include amiodarone, propafenone, ibutilide, and sotalol. The preferred drug for patients with significant heart disease including ischemic heart disease, left ventricular hypertrophy, left ventricular dysfunction, and heart failure is amiodarone. The efficacy of amiodarone ranges from 34% to 69% with a bolus dose (3–7 mg/kg body weight) and 55% to 95% success when the bolus is followed by a continuous drug infusion. Amiodarone also suppresses atrial ectopy and recurrence of atrial fibrillation and improves the success rate of electrical cardioversion. Adverse effects of acute amiodarone administration include bradycardia, hypotension, and phlebitis at the site of administration. Long-term therapy can be associated with visual disturbances, thyroid dysfunction, nausea, and constipation.

Control of the ventricular response in patients with atrial fibrillation is typically achieved with drugs that slow AV nodal conduction. The most commonly used drugs for this purpose are β-blockers, calcium channel blockers and digoxin. β-Blockers are useful in the prevention of recurrent atrial fibrillation and provide good heart rate control and reduce symptoms during subsequent episodes of atrial fibrillation. Potential side effects of β-blocker therapy are hypotension and bronchospasm.

Calcium channel-blocking drugs such as diltiazem and verapamil can rapidly reduce the ventricular rate during atrial fibrillation. These drugs have negative inotropic effects and must be used with caution in patients prone to heart failure.

Digoxin can be useful to control ventricular rate but is not effective for conversion of atrial fibrillation to sinus rhythm. In the acute setting of rapid atrial fibrillation, the usefulness of digoxin is limited due to the fact that the peak therapeutic effects of digoxin are delayed by several hours. Side effects associated with digitalis are dose related and most commonly include AV block and ventricular ectopy.

Prognosis

Atrial fibrillation is the most common sustained cardiac dysrhythmia in the U.S. population (0.4% incidence). The incidence of atrial fibrillation increases with age, being present in 1% of individuals younger than 60 years of age, increasing to 5% in those 70 to 75 years of age and exceeding 10% in those older than the age of 80. The most common underlying cardiovascular diseases associated with atrial fibrillation are systemic hypertension and ischemic heart disease. Valvular heart disease, congestive heart failure, and diabetes mellitus are independent risk factors for the development of atrial fibrillation. Atrial fibrillation is the most common postoperative tachydysrhythmia and frequently occurs early in the postoperative period (first 2–4 days), especially in elderly patients following cardiothoracic surgery.

Individuals with atrial fibrillation are at increased risk of stroke and are usually treated with anticoagulants. The prophylactic regimen chosen for each patient is determined by risk stratification for thromboembolism based on age and concomitant heart disease. In the acute setting, intravenous heparin is the most commonly used anticoagulant. For chronic anticoagulation, warfarin is most often used, but aspirin therapy may be sufficient for individuals considered to be at low risk of thromboembolic complications.

Anesthetic Management

If new-onset atrial fibrillation occurs prior to induction of anesthesia, surgery should be postponed if possible until control of the dysrhythmia has been achieved. Management of atrial fibrillation during anesthesia/surgery depends on the hemodynamic stability of the patient. If the atrial fibrillation is hemodynamically significant, the treatment is cardioversion. Synchronized cardioversion at 100 to 200 J is indicated. Pharmacologic control of ventricular response and conversion to sinus rhythm with intravenous amiodarone, diltiazem, or verapamil may be attempted if vital signs allow. The choice of drug depends on the co-existing medical diseases of the patient.

Patients with chronic atrial fibrillation should be maintained on their antidysrhythmic drugs perioperatively with close attention to serum magnesium and potassium levels, particularly if the patient is on digoxin. Careful coordination with the primary care team is needed to manage the transition on and off intravenous and oral anticoagulation.

VENTRICULAR RHYTHMS

Ventricular Ectopy (Premature Ventricular Beats)

Signs and Symptoms

Ventricular ectopy can occur as short episodes with spontaneous termination or as a sustained period of bigeminy or trigeminy. The occurrence of more than three consecutive PVCs is considered ventricular tachycardia. The most common symptoms that are associated with ventricular ectopy are palpitations, near syncope, and syncope. The longer the episode of ectopy is, generally, the more severe the symptoms. The volume of blood ejected by the premature beat is smaller than normal, whereas the stroke volume of the beat following the compensatory pause is larger than normal.

Diagnosis

Ventricular premature beats arise from single (unifocal) or multiple (multifocal) foci located below the AV node. Characteristic ECG findings include a premature and wide QRS complex, no preceding P wave, ST segment, and T-wave deflection opposite to the QRS deflection and a compensatory pause before the next sinus beat. The "vulnerable period," that is, the relative refractory period of the cardiac action potential, occurs at approximately the middle third of the T wave. PVCs that occur during this time may initiate repetitive beats including ventricular tachycardia or ventricular fibrillation. This clinical situation is known as the R-on-T phenomenon.

Treatment

Ventricular premature beats should be treated when they are frequent, polymorphic, occurring in runs of three or more, or taking place during the vulnerable period because these characteristics are associated with an increased incidence of ventricular tachycardia and ventricular fibrillation. The first step in the treatment of ventricular premature beats is to eliminate or correct the underlying cause (**Table 4-2**). Discontinuation of prodysrhythmic drugs or drugs that prolong the QT interval and elimination of any iatrogenic mechanical irritation of the heart such as from an intracardiac catheter can decrease the incidence of ventricular dysrhythmias. A defibrillator should be immediately available should clinical deterioration into a life-threatening dysrhythmia occur.

With the exception of β-blockers, currently available antidysrhythmic drugs have not been shown in randomized clinical trials to be effective in the primary long-term management of ventricular dysrhythmias. Many antidysrhythmic drugs have prodysrhythmic effects and/or prolong the QT interval. In fact, the prolongation of depolarization (QT length) can precipitate and increase the propensity for dysrhythmias. Amiodarone, lidocaine, and other antidysrhythmics are not

TABLE 4–2 Conditions and Factors Associated with Development of Ventricular Premature Beats
Normal heart
Arterial hypoxemia
Myocardial ischemia
Myocardial infarction
Myocarditis
Sympathetic nervous system activation
Hypokalemia
Hypomagnesemia
Digitalis toxicity
Caffeine
Cocaine
Alcohol
Mechanical irritation (central venous or pulmonary artery catheter)

indicated unless PVCs progress to ventricular tachycardia or are frequent enough to cause hemodynamic instability. Drug therapy is not at all effective in suppression of ventricular dysrhythmias due to mechanical irritation of the heart.

Prognosis

Typically, benign ventricular premature beats occur at rest and disappear with exercise. An increased frequency of PVCs with exercise may be an indication of underlying heart disease. The prognostic significance of ventricular ectopy depends on the presence and severity of co-existing structural heart disease. The incidence of PVCs in a healthy population ranges from 0.5% in those younger than 20 years old to 2.2% in those older than age 50. In the absence of structural heart disease, asymptomatic ventricular ectopy is benign with no demonstrable risk of sudden death even in the presence of ventricular tachycardia.

The occurrence of six or more PVCs per minute and repetitive or multifocal forms of ventricular ectopy, even if asymptomatic, indicates an increased risk of developing a life-threatening ventricular tachydysrhythmia. The most common pathologic conditions associated with this are myocardial ischemia, valvular heart disease, cardiomyopathy, QT interval prolongation, and the presence of electrolyte abnormalities, especially hypokalemia and hypomagnesemia.

Anesthetic Management

During an anesthetic, if a patient exhibits six or more PVCs per minute and repetitive or multifocal forms of ventricular ectopy, there is an increased risk of developing a life-threatening dysrhythmia. Treatment should include a differential diagnosis of possible causes such as acidosis, electrolyte imbalance, prodysrhythmic drugs, or mechanical stimulation by intracardiac catheters. While treatment or elimination of those factors is under way, the immediate availability of a defibrillator should be confirmed.

β-Blockers are the most successful drugs for suppressing ventricular ectopy and dysrhythmias. Amiodarone, lidocaine, and other dysrhythmics are indicated only if the PVCs progress to ventricular tachycardia or are frequent enough to cause hemodynamic instability.

Ventricular Tachycardia

Signs and Symptoms

Palpitations, presyncope, and syncope are the three most common symptoms described by patients having ventricular dysrhythmias. Ventricular tachycardia is common after an acute myocardial infarction and in the presence of inflammatory or infectious diseases of the heart. Digitalis toxicity may manifest as ventricular tachycardia.

Diagnosis

Ventricular tachycardia (also call monomorphic ventricular tachycardia) is present when three or more consecutive ventricular premature beats occur at a calculated heart rate of greater than 120 bpm (usually 150–200 bpm). It can occur as a nonsustained, paroxysmal rhythm or as a sustained rhythm. The rhythm is regular with wide QRS complexes and no discernible P waves (**Fig. 4-5**). SVT can sometimes be difficult to distinguish from ventricular tachycardia, especially if there is aberrant conduction or if the patient has a RBB block (RBBB) or LBB block (LBBB).

Torsade de pointes (TdP) (also called polymorphic ventricular tachycardia) is a distinct form of ventricular tachycardia initiated by a ventricular premature beat in the setting of abnormal ventricular repolarization (prolongation of the

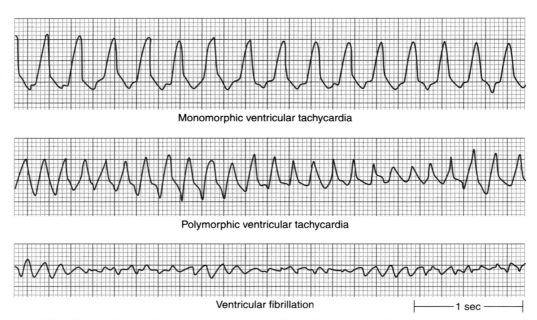

Monomorphic ventricular tachycardia

Polymorphic ventricular tachycardia

Ventricular fibrillation   ├——— 1 sec ———┤

Figure 4-5 • Comparison of the electrocardiographic appearance of monomorphic ventricular tachycardia, polymorphic ventricular tachycardia (torsade de pointes), and ventricular fibrillation.

QT interval). Drugs that prolong repolarization such as phenothiazines, tricyclic antidepressants, certain antiemetics, and most antidysrhythmics predispose to development of TdP.

Treatment On occasion, it may be impossible to differentiate ventricular tachycardia from SVT based on clinical symptoms, vital signs, or ECG findings. Patients with symptomatic or unstable ventricular tachycardia or SVT should be cardioverted immediately. If vital signs are stable and the ventricular tachycardia is persistent or recurrent after cardioversion, amiodarone 150 mg over 10 minutes is recommended. This may be repeated as needed to a maximum total dose of 2.2 g in 24 hours. Recommended alternative drugs include procainamide, sotalol, and lidocaine. Pulseless ventricular tachycardia requires immediate cardioversion/defibrillation and cardiopulmonary resuscitation (CPR).

Prognosis

Ventricular dysrhythmias, often asymptomatic, can be found in 70% to 80% of persons older than the age of 60. The prognosis depends on the presence or absence of structural heart disease. In the perioperative environment, mechanical ventilation, drug therapy, insertion of central catheters, and other interventions can be iatrogenic causes of ventricular dysrhythmias. The risk of sudden death in patients with structurally normal hearts experiencing ventricular dysrhythmias is low. However, treatment with a β-blocker or calcium channel blocker can suppress the dysrhythmia and alleviate symptoms. Catheter ablation or implantation of a cardioverter/defibrillator are options for treatment of drug-refractory ventricular tachycardia.

Anesthetic Management

The occurrence of paroxysmal nonsustained ventricular tachycardia during anesthesia necessitates an investigation into possible causes since this dysrhythmia can become sustained and/or deteriorate into ventricular fibrillation. The occurrence of sustained ventricular tachycardia with or without a pulse demands immediate action. In addition to electrical therapy and drug treatment of ventricular tachycardia, endotracheal intubation and evaluation and correction of acid-base and electrolyte disturbances may be required.

Ventricular Fibrillation

Signs and Symptoms

Ventricular fibrillation is an irregular ventricular rhythm incompatible with life because there is no associated stroke volume or cardiac output. A pulse or blood pressure *never* accompanies ventricular fibrillation. If a patient with presumed ventricular fibrillation is awake or responsive, the ECG must be reevaluated before treatment decisions are made.

Diagnosis

Ventricular fibrillation is a rapid, grossly irregular ventricular rhythm with marked variability in QRS cycle length, morphology, and amplitude (see Fig. 4-5).

Treatment

Electrical defibrillation is the only effective method to convert ventricular fibrillation to a rhythm capable of generating a cardiac output. Defibrillation involves delivery of an electrical current through the heart to depolarize all myocardial cells at once. Ideally, a single pacemaker focus will then restore myocardial synchrony. This treatment should be instituted as soon as possible because cardiac output, coronary blood flow, and cerebral blood flow are extremely low, even with vigorous external cardiac compression. Survival is highest if defibrillation occurs within 3 to 5 minutes of cardiac arrest.

When ventricular fibrillation is refractory to electrical treatment, administration of epinephrine 1 mg IV or vasopressin 40 units IV may improve the response to electrical defibrillation. After three defibrillation attempts with epinephrine or vasopressin therapy, administration of amiodarone, lidocaine, or, in the case of TdP, magnesium is indicated.

In any pulseless arrest, contributing factors should be sought and treated. The differential diagnosis includes hypoxia, hypovolemia, acidosis, hypokalemia, hyperkalemia, hypoglycemia, hypothermia, drug or environmental toxins, cardiac tamponade, tension pneumothorax, coronary ischemia, pulmonary embolus, and hemorrhage.

Prognosis

Ventricular fibrillation is the most common cause of sudden cardiac death. Most victims have underlying ischemic heart disease. Ventricular tachycardia often precedes the onset of ventricular fibrillation. Long-term treatment of recurrent episodic ventricular tachycardia or fibrillation may be managed successfully with a permanent automatic implanted cardioverter/defibrillator (ICD).

Anesthetic Management

Ventricular fibrillation during anesthesia is a critical event. CPR must be initiated immediately. The single most important factor that increases survival in patients experiencing ventricular fibrillation is time to defibrillation. Survival is best if defibrillation occurs within 3 to 5 minutes of cardiac arrest. Standardized Advanced Cardiac Life Support algorithms should be followed for electrical, pharmacologic, and adjunctive therapy. The cause of the ventricular fibrillation must be found and corrected to maximize resuscitative efforts.

VENTRICULAR PRE-EXCITATION SYNDROMES

The normal conduction system of the heart from atrium to ventricle is a single conduction pathway through the AV node and His-Purkinje system. There can be alternate (accessory) pathways that function as electrically active muscle bridges that bypass the normal conduction pathway and create the potential for reentrant tachycardias. These accessory pathways are congenital and most likely represent remnants of fetal atrioventricular muscular connections left by incomplete development of the annulus fibrosus.

Wolff-Parkinson-White Syndrome

Signs and Symptoms

Symptomatic tachydysrhythmias associated with the Wolff-Parkinson-White (WPW) syndrome typically begin during early adulthood. Paroxysmal palpitations with or without dizziness, syncope, dyspnea, or angina pectoris are common during the tachydysrhythmias associated with this syndrome. Pregnancy may be associated with the initial manifestation of WPW syndrome in some women, and some patients may first manifest WPW syndrome during the perioperative period. WPW syndrome is associated with an increased incidence of sudden death, but it is very unusual for sudden death to be the first manifestation of WPW syndrome.

Diagnosis

The diagnosis of WPW syndrome is reserved for patients who have both preexcitation and tachydysrhythmia. Ventricular preexcitation causes an earlier than normal deflection of the QRS complex called a delta wave. Delta waves can mimic the Q waves of a myocardial infarction.

AVNRT is the most common tachydysrhythmia in WPW syndrome patients. It accounts for 95% of the dysrhythmias seen with this syndrome. This tachydysrhythmia is usually triggered by a PAC or a PVC. AVNRT is classified as either orthodromic (narrow QRS complex) or antidromic (wide QRS complex). Orthodromic AVNRT is much more common (90%–95% of patients) and has a narrow QRS complex because the cardiac impulse is conducted from the atrium through the normal AV node–His-Purkinje system. These impulses return from the ventricle to the atrium using the accessory pathway.

In the less common antidromic form of AVNRT, the cardiac impulse is conducted from the atrium to the ventricle through the accessory pathway and returns from the ventricles to the atria via the normal AV node. The wide QRS complex seen in antidromic AVNRT makes it difficult to distinguish this dysrhythmia from ventricular tachycardia on the ECG.

Atrial fibrillation and atrial flutter are uncommon in WPW syndrome but are potentially more serious because they can result in very rapid ventricular response rates and even ventricular fibrillation.

Treatment

Orthodromic Atrioventricular Nodal Reentrant Tachycardia Treatment of orthodromic AVNRT (narrow complex) in stable conscious patients should begin with vagal maneuvers (carotid sinus massage or Valsalva maneuver). If vagal maneuvers are unsuccessful, adenosine, verapamil, β-blockers, or amiodarone may be successful.

Antidromic Atrioventricular Nodal Reentrant Tachycardia Treatment of antidromic AVNRT (wide complex) is intended to block conduction of the cardiac impulses along the accessory pathway. Drugs that slow AV nodal conduction, such as adenosine, verapamil, β-blockers, and digoxin, will not be effective in the treatment of wide-complex AVNRT.

These drugs slow AV nodal conduction but may increase conduction along the accessory pathway. As a result, they may produce a marked increase in ventricular rate.

Treatment of antidromic AVNRT with stable vital signs includes intravenous administration of procainamide 10 mg/kg IV infused at a rate not to exceed 50 mg/min. Procainamide slows conduction of cardiac impulses along the accessory pathway and may slow the ventricular response rate and terminate the wide-complex tachydysrhythmia. Electrical cardioversion is indicated if the ventricular response cannot be controlled by drug therapy.

Special Considerations for Atrial Fibrillation in Wolff-Parkinson-White Syndrome Atrial fibrillation in the setting of WPW syndrome can be associated with anterograde conduction via the accessory pathway and the risk of extreme ventricular response rates and/or ventricular fibrillation. It can be treated with intravenous procainamide. Verapamil and digoxin are *contraindicated* in this situation because they may accelerate conduction through the accessory pathway. Electrical cardioversion is used in the presence of hemodynamic instability. Long-term management of tachydysrhythmia in patients with WPW syndrome may include antidysrhythmic drugs or radiofrequency catheter ablation of the accessory pathway.

Prognosis

Since WPW syndrome was first described in 1930, the understanding of WPW syndrome and reentrant tachycardias has improved enormously. Preexcitation occurs in the general population at a rate of 1.5 per 1000. Of these, 50% to 60% will become symptomatic. There is a bimodal age distribution in initial symptoms, first in early childhood, then in young adulthood. There is a strong association of Ebstein's anomaly of the tricuspid valve with preexcitation. The incidence of sudden cardiac death in WPW syndrome patients is 0.15% to 0.39% per patient year. It is very unusual for sudden death to be the initial manifestation of WPW syndrome. Although antidysrhythmics can provide therapeutic management of the dysrhythmias associated with WPW syndrome, catheter ablation is considered the best treatment for symptomatic WPW syndrome. It is curative in 95% of patients and has a low complication rate.

Anesthetic Management

Patients with known WPW syndrome presenting for surgery should continue to receive their antidysrhythmic drugs. The goal during management of anesthesia is to avoid any event (for example, increased sympathetic nervous system activity due to pain, anxiety, or hypovolemia) or drug (digoxin, verapamil) that could enhance anterograde conduction of cardiac impulses through an accessory pathway. Drugs known to be effective in the management of the tachydysrhythmia associated with the WPW syndrome must be immediately available. The equipment for electrical cardioversion must also be available.

PROLONGED QT SYNDROME

Signs and Symptoms

There are two types of prolonged (long) QT syndromes (LQTS): congenital and acquired. Syncope is the hallmark of the inherited forms of prolonged QT syndrome. These events are commonly associated with stress, emotion, exercise, or other situations associated with sympathetic stimulation. A rare autosomal recessive form of prolonged QT syndrome, called Jervell Lange-Nielsen syndrome, is associated with congenital deafness. Acquired iatrogenic prolonged QT syndrome is far more common than inherited forms of LQTS.

Diagnosis

There are several genetically determined syndromes that manifest a long QT interval. The more common are the Romano-Ward and Timothy syndromes. These are inherited as autosomal dominant disorders and usually present as syncope in late childhood. Manifestations can occur as early as the first year of life or as late as the sixth decade. The prolongation of repolarization in LQTS results in a dispersion of refractory periods throughout the myocardium. This abnormality in repolarization allows afterdepolarizations to trigger PVCs. Under certain circumstances, the triggered PVCs initiate a ventricular reentry rhythm manifesting as polymorphic ventricular tachycardia (TdP).

By definition, LQTS demonstrates a prolongation of the QTc exceeding 460 to 480 milliseconds. During a syncopal episode, the most common finding on the ECG is polymorphic ventricular tachycardia (TdP). TdP is ventricular tachycardia in a patient with a history of long QTc and is electrocardiographically characterized by a "twisting of the peaks" or rotation about the baseline of the ECG. This description refers to the constantly changing cycle length, axis, and morphology of the QRS complexes around the isoelectric baseline during TdP (see Fig. 4-5). This dysrhythmia may be repetitive, episodic, or sustained and may degenerate into ventricular fibrillation.

Treatment

Treatment of LQTS includes correction of electrolyte abnormalities, particularly those of magnesium or potassium. Any drugs associated with QT prolongation should be discontinued. Additional treatment options include β-blocker therapy, cardiac pacing, and ICD implantation.

β-Blockers are effective in prevention of ventricular dysrhythmias in LQTS. Studies have shown a considerable reduction in cardiac events and mortality in congenital LQTS patients treated with β-blocker therapy (from 50% to < 5% over a 10-year period). Cardiac pacing is a treatment option in LQTS because TdP is often preceded by bradycardia. Programming a pacemaker to pace at a higher "backup" rate than usual will prevent bradycardia that can herald TdP. Pacing is usually employed in combination with β-blocker therapy. In recent years, ICDs with pacing capability have emerged as the life-saving therapy in patients with recurrent symptoms and recalcitrant TdP despite β-blocker therapy.

Prognosis

Typically, women have longer QT intervals than men. This difference is more pronounced at slower heart rates. The incidence of congenital and acquired prolonged QT syndrome is higher in women. Not surprisingly, the incidence of TdP is also higher in women. The strongest predictor of the risk of syncope or sudden death in patients with congenital prolonged QT syndrome is a QTc exceeding 500 milliseconds.

Acquired LQTS may be caused by many prescription medications such as antibiotics, antidysrhythmics, antidepressants, and antiemetics. Data suggest that TdP occurs in 1% to 10% of patients receiving QT-prolonging antidysrhythmic drugs. However, the incidence of TdP is much less in patients receiving noncardiovascular QT-prolonging drugs. LQTS can be associated with hypokalemia, hypomagnesemia, severe malnutrition, and intracranial catastrophes such as subarachnoid hemorrhage.

Anesthetic Management

A preoperative ECG to rule out LQTS is useful in the presence of a family history of sudden death or a history of unexplained syncope. If patients present with a prolonged QTc, the choice of anesthetic drugs deserves special attention. Isoflurane and sevoflurane have been shown to prolong the QTc in otherwise healthy children and adults. However, currently there is insufficient information to favor one volatile anesthetic over another. Droperidol and other antiemetic drugs also increase the QT interval.

Events known to prolong the QT interval should be avoided, such as abrupt increases in sympathetic stimulation associated with preoperative anxiety and noxious stimulation intraoperatively, acute hypokalemia due to iatrogenic hyperventilation, and administration of drugs known to prolong the QTc. Consideration may be given to establishing β-blockade prior to induction in patients believed to be at particular risk. A defibrillator should be available because the likelihood of perioperative ventricular fibrillation is increased.

MECHANISMS OF BRADYDYSRHYTHMIAS

Bradycardia is a heart rate less than 60 bpm. Trained athletes often exhibit resting bradycardia as may normal individuals during sleep. However, an inability to increase the heart rate adequately during exercise, bradycardia associated with symptoms (such as syncope, dizziness, and chest pain), or a heart rate less than 40 bpm in the absence of physical conditioning or sleep is considered abnormal. Bradydysrhythmias are most commonly caused by SA node dysfunction or a conduction block. With significant sinus bradycardia, secondary pacemakers in the conduction system may provide electrical stimuli to support the heart rate.

Sinus Bradycardia

Signs and Symptoms

Sinus bradycardia is due to a decrease in the normal discharge rate of the SA node (**Table 4-3**). In some, it presents without symptoms, whereas in others it will show signs and symptoms of decreased cardiac output and poor tissue perfusion. Altered mental status, dizziness, seizures, angina, heart failure, syncope, hypotension, end-organ failure, and other manifestations of cardiogenic shock may accompany severe sinus bradycardia.

Diagnosis

Sinus bradycardia occurs at a heart rate of less than 60 bpm. On the ECG, there is a regular rhythm with a normal-appearing P wave before each QRS complex.

Treatment

In asymptomatic patients with sinus bradycardia, no treatment is required. However, these patients should be monitored for evidence of further electrophysiologic or hemodynamic deterioration.

In mildly symptomatic patients, any potential contributing factors such as excess vagal tone or drugs should be eliminated. In severely symptomatic patients, that is, those with chest pain or syncope, immediate transcutaneous or transvenous pacing is indicated. Atropine 0.5 mg IV every 3 to 5 minutes (to a maximum of 3 mg) may be given but should not delay initiation of pacing. It should be noted that small doses of atropine (< 0.5 mg IV) can cause a further *slowing* of the heart rate.

An epinephrine or dopamine infusion may be titrated to response while awaiting cardiac pacing. Glucagon may be useful in some patients with bradycardia due to β-blocker or calcium channel blocker overdose that is unresponsive to atropine. The dose of glucagon is 3 mg IV as a bolus followed by a continuous infusion at 3 mg/hr.

Prognosis

Under normal conditions, the SA node overdrives other potential pacemakers in the heart. If the SA node does not fire, other slower pacemaker cells will usually take over pacemaker function. These secondary pacemakers are slower than the SA node. If the SA node does not fire, there is normally a pause in electrical activity before a secondary pacemaker begins to fire. Each group of potential pacemaker cells has an intrinsic rate. The SA node usually fires between 60 and 100 times per minute Cells near the AV node, the so-called junctional pacemaker, fire at 40 to 60 bpm. Ventricular pacemaker cells fire at 30 to 45 bpm. Even ventricular muscle cells can initiate electrical impulses and act as ectopic pacemakers.

Anesthetic Management

Sinus bradycardia in asymptomatic patients requires no treatment. However, these patients should be monitored for any evidence of worsening bradycardia or clinical deterioration. In mildly symptomatic patients with sinus bradycardia, elimination or treatment of the cause of the bradydysrhythmia is prudent. If severely symptomatic, immediate transcutaneous or transvenous pacing is indicated, with or without the pharmacologic support noted previously.

Bradycardia Associated with Spinal and Epidural Anesthesia

Bradycardia during neuraxial blockade can occur in patients of any age and any American Society of Anesthesiologists physical class, whether or not they are sedated. The incidence of profound bradycardia and cardiac arrest during neuraxial anesthesia is approximately 1.5 per 10,000 cases. By contrast, cardiac arrest during general anesthesia occurs at a rate of 5.5 per 10,000 cases. Bradycardia or asystole may develop suddenly (within seconds or minutes) in a patient with a previously normal or even increased heart rate, or the heart rate slowing may be progressive. Bradycardia can occur at any time during neuraxial blockade but most often occurs approximately an hour after the anesthetic is initiated. The risk of bradycardia and asystole may persist into the postoperative period even after the sensory and motor blockade has diminished.

Oxygen saturation is usually normal prior to the onset of bradycardia. Approximately half of patients who arrest during neuraxial anesthesia complain of shortness of breath, nausea, restlessness, light-headedness, or tingling fingers and manifest a deterioration in mental status prior to arrest.

The underlying mechanism responsible for bradycardia and asystole during spinal and epidural anesthesia is not known. Proposed theories include reflex-induced bradycardia resulting from decreased venous return and activation of vagal reflex arcs mediated by baroreceptors and stretch receptors in the sinus node resulting in a paradoxical Bezold-Jarisch response. Another possible mechanism is the unopposed

---

TABLE 4–3 Perioperative Causes of Sinus Bradycardia
I. Vagal Stimulation
Oculocardiac reflex: traction on eye muscles
Celiac plexus stimulation: traction on the mesentery
Laryngoscopy
Abdominal insufflation
Nausea
Pain
Electroconvulsive therapy
II. Drugs
β-Agonists
Calcium channel blockers
Opioids (fentanyl/sufentanyl)
III. Succinylcholine
IV. Hypothermia
V. Hypothyroidism
VI. Athletic heart syndrome
VII. Sinoatrial nodal disease or ischemia

parasympathetic nervous system activity that results from the anesthetic-induced sympathectomy. Blockade of cardiac accelerator fibers originating from thoracic sympathetic ganglia (T1-4) may alter the balance of autonomic nervous system input to the heart resulting in the emergence of relatively unopposed parasympathetic influences on the SA node and AV node. Secondary factors such as hypovolemia, opioid administration, sedation, hypercarbia, concurrent medical illnesses, and long-term use of medications that slow the heart rate could also contribute to development of bradycardia.

Bradydysrhythmias associated with spinal or epidural anesthesia should be treated aggressively. Bradycardia can occur despite prophylactic therapy with atropine and/or intravenous fluids. Recalcitrant bradycardia necessitates transcutaneous or transvenous pacing. In the clinical scenario of severe bradycardia, preparation should be made for management of asystole. Asystole is treated with CPR. Pharmacologic management should follow Advanced Cardiac Life Support protocols and include therapy with atropine, epinephrine, and/or vasopressin.

Bradycardia Associated with Sinus Node Dysfunction

Dysfunction of the SA node, also referred to as sick sinus syndrome, is a common cause of bradycardia. Sick sinus syndrome with symptomatic bradycardia accounts for more than 50% of the indications for placement of a permanent cardiac pacemaker. The prevalence of sinus node dysfunction may be as high as one in 600 patients older than 65 years of age.

Many patients with sick sinus syndrome are asymptomatic. Others may have syncope or palpitations. Episodes of SVT may punctuate periods of bradycardia accounting for another common name for sinus node dysfunction, that is, tachycardia-bradycardia syndrome. In patients with ischemic heart disease, periods of bradycardia may contribute to development of congestive heart failure and periods of tachycardia can precipitate angina pectoris.

Junctional Rhythm
Signs and Symptoms

Junctional (nodal) rhythm is due to activity of a cardiac pacemaker in the tissues surrounding the AV node. Junctional pacemakers usually have an intrinsic rate of 40 to 60 bpm. If the junctional rhythm has an accelerated rate, it is called a junctional tachycardia. Junctional rhythms often result in atrioventricular dyssynchrony. The loss of atrial kick can result in fatigue, generalized weakness, angina pectoris, congestive heart failure, pulmonary edema, and hypotension. The absence of synchronized atrial contraction and rapid ventricular rates during a junctional tachycardia can severely impair cardiac output.

Diagnosis

The impulse initiated by a junctional pacemaker travels to the ventricles along the normal conduction pathway but can also be conducted retrograde into the atria. The site of the junctional pacemaker determines whether the P wave precedes the QRS complex (with a shortened PR interval), follows the QRS complex, or is buried within the QRS complex and not visible. A junctional rhythm may respond normally to exercise and the diagnosis of junctional rhythm may be an incidental finding on the ECG. However, junctional rhythm can be suspected if the jugular venous pulsation shows cannon *a* waves. Junctional tachycardia is a narrow-complex tachycardia at a rate usually less than 120 bpm.

Treatment

Junctional rhythm that occurs in association with myocarditis, myocardial ischemia, or digitalis toxicity should be managed by treating the underlying disorder. Junctional rhythms are not uncommon during general anesthesia especially if volatile anesthetics such as halothane and enflurane are administered. Transient junctional rhythm during an anesthetic requires no treatment. Atropine can be used to accelerate the heart rate if a junctional rhythm becomes hemodynamically significant.

Prognosis

Junctional rhythm can occur in association with many different disorders. It is often an escape rhythm because of depressed sinus node function, SA block, or delayed conduction in the AV node. Junctional tachycardia can result from increased automaticity of junctional tissues with digitalis toxicity or ischemia. Junctional rhythms are usually considered benign and require no treatment even in the setting of acute myocardial infarction. However, if myocardial ischemia precipitated a junctional rhythm, that ischemia may also cause ventricular dysrhythmias and deterioration in overall cardiac function.

Anesthetic Management

Junctional rhythms are not infrequent during general anesthesia with halogenated anesthetics. Transient junctional rhythm requires no treatment. The loss of atrioventricular synchrony during a junctional rhythm can, however, result in myocardial ischemia, heart failure, or hypotension. Atropine at a dose of 0.5 mg can be used to treat hemodynamically significant junctional rhythms.

CONDUCTION DISTURBANCES

An intact cardiac conduction system normally ensures conduction of each sinus impulse from the atria to the ventricles. Abnormalities of the conduction system can disrupt this process and lead to heart block (**Table 4-4**). The site of the conduction abnormality, the risk of progression to complete heart block, and the likelihood that a secondary pacemaker beyond the site of conduction blockade will generate an adequate heart rate are all issues of significance in treating patients with heart block.

A variety of acute and chronic conditions can cause or contribute to heart block. These include acute myocardial infarction (especially in the distribution of the right coronary

TABLE 4–4 Classification of Heart Block
First-degree atrioventricular heart block
Second-degree atrioventricular heart block
Mobitz type 1 (Wenckebach)
Mobitz type 2
Unifascicular heart block
Left anterior hemiblock
Left posterior hemiblock
Right bundle branch block
Left bundle branch block
Bifascicular heart block
Right bundle branch block plus left anterior hemiblock
Right bundle branch block plus left posterior hemiblock
Third-degree heart block (trifascicular, complete)
Nodal
Infranodal

artery), digitalis toxicity, excess β-blockade or calcium channel blockade, myocarditis, rheumatic fever, mononucleosis, Lyme disease, and infiltrative diseases such as sarcoidosis and amyloidosis.

First-Degree Atrioventricular Heart Block

Signs and Symptoms

First-degree AV heart block demonstrates a prolonged PR interval, indicating a delay in passage of the cardiac impulse through the AV node. A prolonged PR interval is often a result of the normal degeneration of the cardiac conduction system that accompanies aging. Other causes include myocardial ischemia (involving the blood supply to the AV node), drugs affecting AV node conduction (digitalis and amiodarone), and processes that enhance parasympathetic nervous system activity and vagal tone. First-degree AV block is usually asymptomatic.

Diagnosis

First-degree AV block is defined as a PR interval greater than 0.2 seconds. Each P wave is conducted and has a corresponding QRS complex of normal duration. The site of conduction block is the AV node.

Treatment

First-degree AV block is usually asymptomatic and rarely requires treatment. In some patients, elimination of drugs that slow AV conduction or clinical factors that enhance vagal tone can reverse first-degree block. Other patients may require correction of ischemia to the AV node. Atropine administration can speed conduction of cardiac impulses through the AV node. However, in patients with significant heart disease, the increase in oxygen consumption due to the increase in heart rate produced by atropine may contribute to myocardial ischemia.

Prognosis

First-degree AV block can be found in patients without structural heart disease and in those with increased vagal

tone, digitalis toxicity, inferior wall myocardial infarction, and myocarditis. Patients with first-degree AV block appear to have no significant increase in mortality compared to matched controls.

Anesthetic Management

Anesthetic management of the patient with first-degree heart block should be aimed at avoiding any clinical situation or drug that increases vagal tone or slows AV conduction. Patients with risk factors such as coronary ischemia and systemic infection should have these clinical conditions treated and medically optimized prior to surgery. Digoxin levels should be checked prior to surgery, and serum potassium should be maintained at normal levels in patients receiving digoxin.

Second-Degree Atrioventricular Heart Block

Signs and Symptoms

Mobitz type 1 block (Wenckebach) demonstrates progressive prolongation of the PR interval until a beat is dropped. It is thought to occur because each successive depolarization produces a prolongation of the refractory period of the AV node. This process continues until an atrial impulse reaches the AV node during its absolute refractory period and conduction of that impulse is blocked completely. A pause allows the AV node to recover and then the process resumes.

Mobitz type 1 block is caused by delayed conduction of cardiac impulses through the AV node. This type of block is often transient and *asymptomatic*. It can be a result of myocardial ischemia or infarction, myocardial fibrosis or calcification, or infiltrative or inflammatory diseases of the myocardium or can occur after cardiothoracic surgery. It can also be associated with certain drugs such as calcium channel blockers, β-blockers, digoxin, and sympatholytic drugs.

Mobitz type 2 block is a complete interruption in the conduction of a cardiac impulse, usually at a point below the AV node in the bundle of His or in a bundle branch. Mobitz type 2 block is usually *symptomatic*, with palpitations and near syncope being common complaints. It has a much higher potential to progress to third-degree AV block than does Mobitz type 1 block.

Diagnosis

Second-degree AV block can be suspected when a P wave is present without a corresponding QRS complex. Second-degree AV heart block can be categorized as Mobitz type 1 block (Wenckebach) or Mobitz type 2 block. Mobitz type 1 block shows progressive prolongation of the PR interval until a beat is entirely blocked (dropped beat) followed by a repeat of this sequence. In contrast, Mobitz type 2 block is characterized by sudden and complete interruption of conduction without PR prolongation. Mobitz type 2 block is usually associated with permanent damage to the conduction system and may progress to third-degree block, especially in the setting of acute myocardial infarction.

Treatment

Mobitz type 1 block does not usually require treatment unless the decreased ventricular rate results in signs of hypoperfusion. Symptomatic patients may be treated with atropine as needed. If atropine is unsuccessful, pacing may be indicated.

Treatment for Mobitz type 2 block includes transcutaneous or transvenous cardiac pacing. Atropine is unlikely to improve the bradycardia due to Mobitz type 2 block.

Prognosis

The prognosis for Mobitz type 1 block is good since reliable secondary pacemakers in the AV node can usually take over pacing duties and maintain adequate cardiac output. Mobitz type 2 block has a more serious prognosis because it frequently progresses to third-degree heart block. Reliable secondary pacemakers are not usually present in Mobitz type 2 block or in third-degree heart block because these disorders are associated with serious disease involving the infranodal conduction system.

Anesthetic Management

Therapeutic decisions for patients presenting with second-degree heart block depend on the ventricular response and the symptoms of the patient. The heart rate with Mobitz type 1 block is usually good, and rarely does Mobitz type 1 block progress to third-degree heart block. In the presence of an acceptable ventricular rate and an adequate cardiac output, no other treatment is needed. However, continued vigilance is needed to detect any clinical deterioration.

In Mobitz type 2 block, conduction can fail suddenly and unexpectedly without a change in PR interval. Because this disorder is generally due to disease within the His-Purkinje system, the QRS is often widened. Mobitz type 2 block has a high rate of progression to third-degree heart block and can manifest as a slow escape rhythm insufficient to sustain an acceptable cardiac output. A cardiac pacemaker is mandatory in this circumstance.

BUNDLE BRANCH BLOCKS

Conduction disturbances that occur at various levels of the branches of the His-Purkinje system are described as bundle branch blocks or intraventricular conduction defects. A complete bundle branch block has a QRS duration of 120 milliseconds or more. In patients with isolated chronic RBBB, the progression to complete AV block is rare. Patients with bifascicular block (RBBB and left anterior or posterior fascicular block) or LBBB have a 6% incidence of progression to complete heart block. In the setting of acute myocardial infarction, the development of new bifascicular block plus first-degree AV block is associated with a very high risk (40%) of progression to complete heart block. These patients should undergo prophylactic temporary cardiac pacing. Alternating bundle branch blocks, even if asymptomatic, are a sign of advanced conduction system disease and are an indication for permanent pacing.

Intraventricular conduction disturbances are usually associated with significant structural heart disease, especially dilated cardiomyopathies. They are a marker of poor prognosis, both in terms of heart failure and increased mortality.

Right Bundle Branch Block

Signs and Symptoms

In patients without structural heart disease, RBBB is more common than LBBB. However, RBBB can be associated with structural heart disease such as atrial septal defect, valvular disease, and ischemic heart disease. The intraventricular conduction delay resulting from a RBBB is seldom symptomatic. Bifascicular heart block is present when RBBB exists in combination with block of one of the fascicles of the LBB. RBBB plus left anterior hemiblock is more common than RBBB plus left posterior hemiblock.

Diagnosis

RBBB is due a disruption of the cardiac impulse as it travels over the RBB. It is recognized on the ECG by a widened QRS complex (> 0.1 second in duration) and an rSR′ QRS complex in leads V_1-V_2. There is also a deep S wave in leads I and V_6.

Bifascicular heart block is present when RBBB is associated with block of one of the fascicles of the LBB. RBBB plus left anterior hemiblock is the more frequent combination, present on approximately 1% of all ECGs in adults. Each year approximately 1% to 2% of these patients progress to third-degree heart block. The combination of RBBB and left posterior hemiblock is infrequent, but it often progresses to third-degree AV block.

Treatment

Acute treatment of RBBB or RBBB with left anterior hemiblock consists of observation and elimination of drugs or clinical factors known to contribute to conduction disturbances. Pacing capability should be available in the event of progression of the block to complete heart block.

Prognosis

RBBB is present in approximately 1% of hospitalized adult patients. It does not always imply cardiac disease and is often of no clinical significance. Patients with isolated RBBB rarely progress to advanced AV block.

Anesthetic Management

A theoretical concern in patients with bifascicular heart block is that perioperative events (changes in blood pressure, arterial oxygenation, serum electrolyte concentrations) might compromise the conduction of cardiac impulses in the one remaining intact fascicle, leading to the onset of third-degree heart block. There is no evidence, however, that surgery performed with general or regional anesthesia predisposes patients with pre-existing bifascicular heart block to the development of third-degree heart block. Prophylactic placement of a cardiac pacemaker is, therefore, not needed.

Left Bundle Branch Block

Signs and Symptoms

Bundle branch blocks can be chronic or intermittent. LBBB is often a marker of serious heart disease, such as hypertension, coronary artery disease, aortic valve disease, and cardiomyopathy. Isolated LBBB is often asymptomatic.

Diagnosis

LBBB is recognized on the ECG as a QRS complex of more than 0.12 second in duration and the absence of Q waves in leads 1 and V_6. Abnormal conduction of impulses through the fascicles of the LBB can be characterized as unifascicular (hemiblock) or as bifascicular (complete). Block of the left anterior fascicle is the most common hemiblock. Left posterior hemiblock is uncommon because the posterior fascicle of the LBB is larger and better perfused than the anterior fascicle. Although hemiblock is a form of intraventricular heart block, the duration of the QRS complex is normal or only minimally prolonged.

Treatment

Some patients have an LBBB only after a critical heart rate is reached. In others, LBBB is associated with ischemic heart disease, left ventricular hypertrophy, or cardiomyopathy. Treatment of these contributing disorders can decrease the incidence of LBBB in susceptible patients.

Prognosis

LBBB, in contrast to RBBB, has more ominous clinical implications. LBBB is often associated with ischemic heart disease, left ventricular hypertrophy accompanying chronic systemic hypertension, or cardiac valve disease. Patients with isolated LBBB rarely progress to advanced AV block. The appearance of LBBB has been observed during anesthesia, particularly during hypertensive or tachycardic episodes and may be a sign of myocardial ischemia. It is very difficult to diagnose a myocardial infarction by ECG in the presence of LBBB because ST-segment and T-wave changes (repolarization abnormalities) are already present as part of the bundle branch block. An SVT can be mistaken for ventricular tachycardia in the patient with LBBB because the QRS complexes are wide.

Management of Anesthesia

The presence of a LBBB has special implications if insertion of a pulmonary artery catheter is planned. Third-degree heart block can occur if the central catheter induces RBBB in the patient with pre-existing LBBB. RBBB (usually transient) occurs during insertion of a pulmonary artery catheter in approximately 2% to 5% of patients.

Third-Degree Atrioventricular Heart Block

Signs and Symptoms

Third-degree heart block is complete interruption of AV conduction. It can be transient or permanent. Third-degree heart block develops in approximately 8% of patients with acute inferior wall myocardial infarction. In this situation, the heart block is usually transient, although it may last for several days.

The onset of third-degree AV block may be signaled by an episode of vertigo or syncope. Other symptoms include weakness and dyspnea. A syncopal episode caused by third-degree heart block is called a Stokes-Adams attack. Congestive heart failure can occur from the decreased cardiac output produced by the bradycardia that accompanies third-degree AV block.

Diagnosis

Third-degree heart block (complete heart block) is characterized by the complete absence of conduction of cardiac impulses from the atria to the ventricles. Continued activity of the ventricles is due to impulses from an ectopic pacemaker distal to the site of the conduction block. If the conduction block is near the AV node, the heart rate is usually 45 to 55 bpm and the QRS complex appears normal. When the conduction block is below the AV node (infranodal), the heart rate is usually 30 to 40 bpm and the QRS complex is wide.

Treatment

Treatment of third-degree AV block consists of transcutaneous or transvenous cardiac pacing. If the block persists, placement of a permanent cardiac pacemaker is indicated.

Prognosis

The most common cause of third-degree AV block in adults is fibrotic degeneration of the distal cardiac conduction system. This condition is associated with aging and is called Lenègre's disease. Degenerative and calcific changes in more proximal conduction tissue adjacent to the mitral valve annulus can also interrupt cardiac conduction and is called Lev's disease.

Management of Anesthesia

Previous placement of a transvenous pacemaker or availability of transcutaneous cardiac pacing is necessary before an anesthetic is administered for insertion of a permanent cardiac pacemaker. Isoproterenol may be needed to maintain an acceptable heart rate and act as a "chemical pacemaker" until the artificial cardiac pacemaker is functional. Caution must be exercised when administering antidysrhythmic drugs to patients with third-degree AV block because these drugs may suppress the ectopic ventricular pacemakers that are responsible for maintaining the heart rate.

TREATMENT OF CARDIAC DYSRHYTHMIAS

Abnormal physiologic parameters should be corrected before initiating antidysrhythmic drug therapy or inserting an artificial cardiac pacemaker. Establishing physiologic acid-base values, normalization of serum electrolyte concentrations, and stabilization of autonomic nervous system activity are important and maximize the possibility of re-establishing normal sinus rhythm.

Antidysrhythmic Drugs

Antidysrhythmic drugs are administered when the correction of identifiable precipitating events is not sufficient to suppress dysrhythmias. These drugs act by altering various electrophysiologic characteristics of myocardial cells. The majority of antidysrhythmia drugs work by one of three mechanisms: (1) suppressing automaticity in pacemaker cells by decreasing the slope of phase 4 depolarization, (2) prolonging the effective refractory period in order to eliminate reentry circuits, and (3) facilitating impulse conduction along normal conduction pathways in order to prevent conduction over a reentrant pathway. Antidysrhythmia drugs can produce changes on the ECG such as an increased PR interval or a prolonged QRS duration.

Adenosine

Adenosine is formed by serial dephosphorylation of adenosine triphosphate. It is an α-agonist and the drug of choice for pharmacologic termination of hemodynamically stable AV nodal reentrant tachycardia. Sixty percent of patients will terminate this dysrhythmia at a dose of 6 mg, and an additional 32% of patients will respond at a dose of 12 mg adenosine. The pharmacologic actions of adenosine are rapidly terminated by active transport of the drug into red blood cells and endothelial cells where it is metabolized. Adenosine has a half-life of approximately 10 seconds. To be effective, it should be rapidly injected and flushed quickly through the intravenous tubing with saline.

Common side effects of adenosine include facial flushing, dyspnea, and chest pressure. Generally, these effects are transient, lasting less than 60 seconds. Less common side effects include nausea, lightheadedness, headache, sweating, palpitations, hypotension, and blurred vision. Dipyridamole pretreatment increases the potency of adenosine and carbamazepine potentiates the action of adenosine. Caffeine and theophylline antagonize the actions of adenosine. Patients with a heart transplant require only one third to one fifth the usual dose of adenosine because the transplanted heart is denervated. Adenosine is contraindicated in patients with sick sinus syndrome and second- or third-degree heart block unless the patient has a functioning cardiac pacemaker.

Amiodarone

Amiodarone is an antidysrhythmic that has a structural similarity to thyroxine and procainamide. It acts on sodium, potassium, and calcium channels to produce α- and β-blocking effects that result in prolongation of the refractory period of myocardial cells. Amiodarone is an indicated treatment for ventricular fibrillation and pulseless ventricular tachycardia unresponsive to defibrillation, CPR, and vasopressors. In this situation, amiodarone improves the likelihood of defibrillation in patients with ventricular fibrillation or unstable ventricular tachycardia.

Amiodarone is metabolized in the liver and slows the metabolism and increases the blood levels of other drugs metabolized by the liver such as warfarin, quinidine, procainamide, disopyramide, mexiletine, and propafenone. It also increases the blood levels of digoxin.

β-Adrenergic Blockers

β-Blockers ameliorate the effects of circulating catecholamines and decrease heart rate and blood pressure. These cardioprotective effects are particularly important in patients with acute coronary syndromes. β-Blockers are indicated in patients with preserved left ventricular function who require ventricular rate control in atrial fibrillation, atrial flutter, and narrow-complex tachycardias originating at or above the AV node.

Side effects of β-blockade include bradycardia, AV conduction delays, and hypotension. Contraindications to β-blocker therapy include second- or third-degree heart block, hypotension, severe congestive heart failure, and reactive airway disease (asthma or chronic obstructive pulmonary disease). β-Blockers are *not* useful in the treatment of atrial fibrillation or atrial flutter associated with WPW syndrome. Indeed, they may contribute to clinical deterioration in this situation.

Calcium Channel Blockers

Verapamil and diltiazem are calcium channel blockers. Verapamil inhibits the influx of extracellular calcium across myocardial and vascular smooth muscle cell membranes. This inhibits the contractile process of myocardial muscle and dilates coronary and systemic arteries. Verapamil slows conduction and increases refractoriness of the AV node so reentrant dysrhythmias can be terminated and the ventricular rate in patients with atrial tachydysrhythmias can be slowed. Verapamil is indicated for treatment of narrow-complex tachycardia (SVT) in patients who have failed vagal maneuvers and adenosine therapy. It is also indicated for ventricular rate control with atrial flutter or atrial fibrillation. In patients with an accessory bypass tract, such as those with WPW syndrome, verapamil can cause acceleration of conduction through the accessory tract and increase the ventricular rate so it is contraindicated in this situation. Calcium channel blockers have negative inotropic properties and should be avoided in patients with left ventricular dysfunction or heart failure. Verapamil is not effective in treating tachycardias originating below the AV node. Verapamil therapy can prolong the PR interval. If given to patients already receiving β-blockers, second- or third-degree heart block can result. The initial dose of verapamil is typically 2.5 to 5 mg IV over 2 minutes. This can be repeated if needed to a maximum total dose of 0.15 mg/kg. Hemodynamic effects peak in 5 minutes and persist for 20 to 30 minutes

Diltiazem has a similar mechanism of action as verapamil and is indicated for treatment of the same dysrhythmias as verapamil. However, diltiazem has a less negative inotropic effect and causes less peripheral vasodilation than verapamil. The degree of AV node inhibition is similar for both drugs. The recommended dose for diltiazem is 0.25 mg/kg IV over 2 minutes. This can be repeated if needed. Successful dysrhythmia treatment can be followed by a maintenance infusion of diltiazem at 5 to 15 mg/hr.

Digoxin

Digoxin is a cardiac glycoside that was approved for use by the U.S. Food and Drug Administration in 1952 and has been used since that time for the treatment of congestive heart failure and atrial fibrillation. Digoxin inhibits the myocardial cell $Na^+K^+ATPase$ membrane pump. The inotropic effects of digoxin are due to an increase in intracellular calcium that allows for greater activation of contractile proteins.

In addition to its inotropic effects, digoxin also increases phase 4 depolarization and shortens the action potential. This decreases conduction velocity through the AV node and prolongs the AV nodal refractory period. Digoxin is effective in controlling ventricular rate in atrial fibrillation, although it does not convert atrial fibrillation to sinus rhythm. Onset of therapeutic effects following intravenous administration of digoxin is 5 to 30 minutes, with the peak effect in 2 to 6 hours. Digoxin has a narrow toxic to therapeutic ratio (therapeutic index), especially in the presence of hypokalemia. High serum digoxin levels can cause a variety of symptoms and signs including life-threatening dysrhythmias. A digoxin-specific antibody is available for treatment of digitalis toxicity.

Lidocaine

Lidocaine is an antidysrhythmic drug with few immediate side effects. It produces its clinical effects by blocking sodium channels. Lidocaine is recommended as a treatment for ventricular ectopy and short bursts of ventricular tachycardia. It is also an alternative treatment to amiodarone in cardiac arrest associated with ventricular fibrillation or pulseless ventricular tachycardia. The recommended dose is 1.0 to 1.5 mg/kg IV. Half this dose can be repeated at 5- to 10-minute intervals to a maximum total dose of 3 mg/kg. Lidocaine is rapidly redistributed out of the plasma and myocardium so multiple loading doses may be needed to achieve therapeutic blood levels. To sustain therapeutic effect, lidocaine must be administered by a continuous infusion. Therapeutic doses of lidocaine have minimal negative inotropic effects.

During lidocaine therapy, monitoring of mental status is desirable because the first signs of lidocaine toxicity are usually central nervous symptoms such as tinnitus, drowsiness, dysarthria, confusion, and seizures. When administered in combination with other antidysrhythmic drugs, lidocaine can cause some myocardial depression or sinus node dysfunction.

Lidocaine undergoes extensive first-pass hepatic metabolism so clinical conditions that result in decreased hepatic blood flow, such as general anesthesia, can result in higher than normal blood levels of lidocaine. Cimetidine therapy can also increase the plasma concentration of lidocaine.

Magnesium

There are a few observational studies supporting the use of magnesium in the termination of TdP ventricular tachycardia associated with QT prolongation. However, there is no evidence that magnesium is likely to be effective in ventricular tachycardia associated with a normal QT interval.

In ventricular fibrillation or pulseless ventricular tachycardia associated with TdP, magnesium can be given in a dose of 1 to 2 g over 5 minutes. If a pulse is present with the torsade, then the same dose can be administered but more slowly, over 30 to 60 minutes.

Procainamide

Procainamide is a class 1 antidysrhythmic drug that slows conduction, decreases automaticity, and increases refractoriness of myocardial cells. It can be used in patients with preserved ventricular function in the following situations: ventricular tachycardia with a pulse, atrial flutter or fibrillation, atrial fibrillation in WPW syndrome, and SVT resistant to adenosine and vagal maneuvers.

Procainamide can be administered at a rate of 50 mg/min IV until the dysrhythmia is suppressed, significant hypotension occurs, or the QRS complex is prolonged by 50%. Procainamide must be used with caution in patients with pre-existing QT prolongation and in combination with other drugs that prolong the QT interval. To maintain therapeutic effect, procainamide can be given as a maintenance infusion at a rate of 1 to 4 mg/min. Doses should be reduced in renal failure.

Sotalol

Sotalol prolongs the duration of the action potential and increases the refractoriness of cardiac cells. It also has β-blocking properties. It can be used to treat ventricular tachycardia or atrial fibrillation/atrial flutter in patients with WPW syndrome. Sotalol is not a first-line antidysrhythmic drug.

Epinephrine

Epinephrine is a vasopressor with α- and β-adrenergic effects that is commonly used during CPR. The α effects of epinephrine can be beneficial during CPR to increase coronary and cerebral perfusion. Although it has been used for many years during CPR, there are few objective studies to show definitive proof that epinephrine improves survival. The suggested dose is 1 mg IV every 3 to 5 minutes. Occasionally, larger doses may be needed to treat cardiac arrest due to β-blocker or calcium channel blocker overdose. In addition to the intravenous route, epinephrine can be administered via the intratracheal route if intravenous access has not yet been established.

Vasopressin

Vasopressin is a potent peripheral vasoconstrictor that does not work by α- or β-adrenergic mechanisms. Currently, epinephrine and vasopressin are recommended interchangeably to treat cardiac arrest. If vasopressin is chosen, the dose is 40 units IV. Vasopressin may replace the first or second dose of epinephrine in the treatment of cardiac arrest.

Atropine

Atropine sulfate is a vagolytic drug that is used to increase heart rate, blood pressure, and systemic vascular resistance. In the situation of asystole or pulseless electrical activity, atropine may improve survival. The recommended dose is 1 mg IV every 3 to 5 minutes as needed to a maximum total dose of 3 mg.

Isoproterenol

Isoproterenol is a potent bronchodilator and sympathomimetic structurally similar to epinephrine. It has potent β_1 and β_2-agonist actions with no α-adrenergic properties. The actions of isoproterenol are mediated intracellularly by cyclic adenosine monophosphate. Isoproterenol stimulates β_1 receptors, which results in an increase in inotropy and chronotropy. The systolic blood pressure may increase, but the diastolic blood pressure is usually decreased secondary to drug-induced peripheral vasodilation. Isoproterenol does dilate the coronary vasculature, but the increased oxygen demand resulting from its β_1 effects outweighs the benefit of the increased myocardial blood flow. Isoproterenol increases myocardial excitability and automaticity, resulting in an increased heart rate, an increased propensity for dysrhythmias, and, possibly, myocardial ischemia.

Isoproterenol may be used to treat symptomatic bradycardia in heart transplant recipients. An initial intravenous dose of 1 µg/min is titrated slowly upward until the desired effect is achieved.

Dopamine

Dopamine is a catecholamine with dose-related effects. At low doses (3–5 µg/kg per minute), dopamine increases renal, mesenteric, coronary, and cerebral blood flow via activation of dopaminergic receptors. At moderate doses (5–7 µg/kg per minute), β effects predominate, and at high doses (> 10 µg/kg per minute), the α receptor stimulation causes peripheral vasoconstriction and a reduction in renal blood flow. Dopamine can be used to treat symptomatic bradycardia unresponsive to atropine.

Electrical Cardioversion

Electrical *cardioversion* entails delivery of an electrical discharge via two chest electrodes, one placed anteriorly and one placed posteriorly. Delivery of the current is synchronized to the R wave of the ECG so that the current is delivered during the QRS complex. If the shock were delivered during the relative refractory period of the ventricle, that is, during the T wave, the electrical stimulus could evoke ventricular tachycardia or ventricular fibrillation. In contrast, during electrical *defibrillation*, it is not possible to synchronize the electrical current to the ECG because there are neither defined QRS complexes nor effective cardiac contractions. Cardioversion can begin at an output of 50 to 100 J and increase in increments of 50 to 100 J as necessary. Defibrillation attempts start with an output of 150 to 200 J.

Synchronized cardioversion is used to treat acute unstable supraventricular tachycardias (such as SVT, atrial flutter, and atrial fibrillation) and to convert chronic stable rate-controlled atrial flutter or atrial fibrillation to sinus rhythm.

Cardioversion can also be used to treat ventricular tachycardia with a pulse. Digitalis-induced dysrhythmias are refractory to cardioversion, and attempts at cardioversion in this situation could trigger more serious ventricular dysrhythmias.

Cardioversion of patients with atrial fibrillation carries the risk of systemic embolization. Therefore, it is recommended that elective cardioversion be preceded by anticoagulation if the dysrhythmia has been present for more than 48 hours. Before elective cardioversion, patients are fasted for at least 6 hours and electrolyte imbalances are corrected. Normally, elective cardioversion is performed under conditions of intravenous sedation/amnesia or very brief general anesthesia with standard anesthetic monitoring. Propofol and short-acting benzodiazepines are commonly used for this procedure. Antidysrhythmic drugs, advanced airway equipment, and emergency cardiac pacing devices should be immediately available. Ventricular ectopy or bradycardia, secondary to related sinus node dysfunction, can occur post-cardioversion.

Defibrillation

Modern defibrillators are classified according to the type of waveform delivered as either monophasic and biphasic. Monophasic devices were the original defibrillators. Most modern defibrillators are biphasic devices. Neither type of defibrillator has been shown to be consistently more successful in termination of pulseless rhythms or improving early survival. The optimal energy dose for a biphasic defibrillator has not been determined, and the manufacturer of each device has dose suggestions specific to its equipment.

Maximizing the success of defibrillation involves not just defibrillator output but thoracic impedance, electrode position, electrode size, and the logistics of defibrillation in the presence of implanted pacemakers or ICDs. When transthoracic impedance is too high, an energy shock will not achieve defibrillation. To reduce impedance, conductive gels should always be used with defibrillation paddles. Self-adhesive defibrillation pads have an integrated conductive surface. In excessively hairy patients, electrode contact with the skin can be suboptimal, resulting in air pockets between the defibrillator paddles and the skin from poor adhesion. This causes increased impedance and can be very dangerous because the air pocket can ignite in an oxygen-rich environment. Routine use of self-adhesive defibrillation pads or gel pads with paddles can minimize the risk of current arcing and fire. At times, the pad area may need to be shaved to achieve good electrode contact. In addition to the impedance caused by the chest wall, the electrical current is impeded by passage through air. The defibrillator current should, therefore, be delivered during expiration.

Standard electrodes come in several sizes. As a rule of thumb, it is best to use the largest pads available that can fit on the chest and not overlap.

Defibrillation/cardioversion electrodes should not be placed directly over pulse generators or ICDs. Delivery of a high current near a pacemaker or ICD can cause the device to malfunction and delivery of current to the area over the generator can block or divert the current path and result in suboptimal current delivery to the myocardium. All permanently implanted devices should be evaluated after defibrillation or cardioversion to ensure proper function.

Radiofrequency Catheter Ablation

Radiofrequency catheter ablation uses an intracardiac electrode catheter inserted percutaneously under local anesthesia into a large vein (femoral, subclavian, internal jugular, or brachial) to produce small, well-demarcated areas of thermal injury that destroy the myocardial tissue responsible for initiation or maintenance of dysrhythmias. Cardiac dysrhythmias amenable to radiofrequency catheter ablation include reentrant supraventricular dysrhythmias and some ventricular dysrhythmias. The procedure is usually performed under conscious sedation.

Artificial Cardiac Pacemakers

Transcutaneous Cardiac Pacing

Patient with symptomatic bradycardia or severe conduction block require immediate pacing. Transcutaneous pacing is a recommended treatment for symptomatic bradydysrhythmias with a pulse.

The cutaneous chest and back electrodes should be placed over areas of lesser skeletal muscle mass, and low-density constant-current impulses should be delivered. This improves the likelihood of effective cardiac stimulation and minimizes painful skeletal muscle or cutaneous stimulation. Transcutaneous pacing should be considered a temporizing measure until transvenous cardiac pacing can be instituted.

Permanently Implanted Cardiac Pacemakers

Permanent cardiac pacing was originally designed for the management of Stokes-Adams (syncopal) attacks in patients with complete heart block. Currently, the most common indication for permanent pacemaker insertion is sinus node dysfunction (sick sinus syndrome). Cardiac pacing is the only long-term treatment for symptomatic bradycardia regardless of cause. Technical advances in cardiac pacing have included the creation of dual-chamber devices, rate response algorithms, and implantable cardioverter/defibrillators. These advances have expanded the indications for cardiac pacing beyond symptomatic bradycardia to include neurogenic syncope, hypertrophic obstructive cardiomyopathy, and cardiac resynchronization therapy for congestive heart failure.

An artificial cardiac pacemaker system consists of a device that generates electrical impulses (pulse generator) and sensing and pacing electrodes and is powered by a lithium-iodide battery. Electrical impulses originating in the pulse generator are transmitted through the specialized leads to excite endocardial cells and produce a propagating wave of depolarization in the myocardium. Electronic circuitry can modulate the frequency and amount of current flow and, in addition, sense spontaneous electrical activity in the heart. Common programmable features of cardiac pacemakers include pacing mode, output, sensitivity, rate, refractory period, and rate adaptation.

An artificial cardiac pacemaker can be inserted intravenously (endocardial lead) or via a subcostal approach (epicardial or myocardial lead). Electrical impulses are formed in the pulse generator and transmitted to the endocardial or myocardial surface of the heart, resulting in myocardial contraction.

Pacing Modes

A five-letter generic code is used to describe the various characteristics of cardiac pacemakers. The first letter denotes the cardiac chamber(s) being paced (A, atrial; V, ventricular; D, dual chamber). The second letter denotes the cardiac chamber(s) that detects (senses) electrical signals (A, atrial; V, ventricular; D, dual). The third letter indicates the response to sensed signals (I, inhibition; T, triggering; D, dual: inhibition and triggering). The fourth letter, "R," denotes activation of rate response features, and the fifth position denotes the chamber(s) in which multisite pacing is delivered. The most common pacing modes are AAI, VVI, and DDD.

DDD Pacing

In most dual-chamber pacing modes, the atrial pacemaker output is inhibited if an intrinsic atrial signal is sensed, and, if no intrinsic ventricular activity is sensed by the end of a programmable AV interval, ventricular output is activated. If intrinsic ventricular activity is sensed, however, the ventricular output is inhibited. Dual-chamber pacemakers provide the important benefits of maintaining AV synchrony. Atrial events either sensed and paced initiate or trigger the AV interval so AV synchrony is maintained over a wide range of heart rates. The DDD pacing mode permits the pacemaker to respond to increases in sinus node discharge rate, such as during exercise. Maintenance of AV synchrony in patients with sick sinus syndrome may contribute to a lower incidence of atrial fibrillation and thromboembolic events.

DDD pacing also minimizes the incidence of pacemaker syndrome. *Pacemaker syndrome* is a constellation of symptoms that can be associated with ventricular pacing including syncope, weakness, orthopnea, paroxysmal nocturnal dyspnea, hypotension, and pulmonary edema. The symptoms of pacemaker syndrome are due to loss of AV synchrony and the resultant decrease in cardiac output. Loss of AV synchrony reduces resting cardiac output by approximately 20% to 30%. Additionally, increases in atrial pressure that result from contraction of the atrium against closed mitral and tricuspid valves (a result of asynchrony) activate baroreceptors that induce reflex peripheral vasodilation. Symptoms of the pacemaker syndrome are eliminated by pacing in a mode that restores AV synchrony.

DDI Pacing

In the DDI pacing mode, there is sensing in both the atrium and ventricle, but the only response to a sensed event is inhibition (inhibited pacing of the atrium and ventricle). DDI pacing is useful when there are frequent atrial tachydysrhythmias that might be inappropriately tracked by a DDD pacemaker and result in rapid ventricular rates.

Rate-Adaptive Pacemakers

A rate-adaptive pacemaker is considered for patients who do not have an appropriate heart rate response to exercise ("chronotropic incompetence"). This syndrome may be due to drug treatment with negative chronotropic drugs such as β-blockers or calcium channel blockers or due to pathologic processes such as sick sinus syndrome. Normally, AV synchrony contributes more to cardiac output at rest and at low levels of exercise, whereas rate adaptation (i.e., a higher heart rate) is more important at higher levels of exercise. Rate-responsive pacing uses sensors to detect physical or physiologic indices of exercise and mimics the rate response of a normal sinus node. The indices used to modulate rate response include activity (body movement), minute ventilation, QT interval, and stroke volume.

Choice of Pacing Mode

The choice of pacing mode depends on the primary indication for the artificial pacemaker. If the patient has SA node disease and no evidence of disease of the AV node or bundle of His, an atrial pacemaker (AAI) could be placed. However, the rate of progression to second- or third-degree AV heart block in patients with sick sinus syndrome is approximately 1% to 5% per year. Accompanying disease of the AV node or His bundle or the need for drug treatment to slow AV nodal conduction requires a dual-chamber (DDD or DDI) system. Patients with sinus node disease, AV node disease, or lower conduction system disease whose heart rates do not respond to an increase in metabolic demands should be considered for placement of a rate-adaptive pacing system.

Individuals experiencing episodes of symptomatic bradycardia due to SA node or AV node disease may benefit from placement of a single-chamber ventricular (VVI) pacemaker. Neurocardiogenic syncope (due to carotid sinus hypersensitivity), vasovagal syncope, and hypertrophic cardiomyopathy can be treated with dual-chamber pacemakers. Cardiac resynchronization therapy using biatrial or biventricular pacing is being employed in patients with electromechanical asynchrony and intraventricular conduction block. The criteria for cardiac resynchronization therapy include drug refractory heart failure (symptoms at rest or with minimal exertion), left ventricular ejection fraction less than 35%, left ventricular dilation, and prolongation of the QRS complex more than 130 milliseconds.

Complications of Permanent Cardiac Pacing

The incidence of complications surrounding pacemaker insertion is approximately 5%. The incidence of late complications is 2% to 7%. Early complications can be associated with venous access and include pneumothorax, hemothorax, and air embolism. Pneumothoraces are often small and asymptomatic. However, tension pneumothorax should always be considered if hypotension or pulseless electrical activity develops during or immediately after pacemaker placement. Hemothorax can result from trauma to the great vessels secondary to inadvertent arterial puncture. Arterial cannulation must be immediately recognized and treated with manual compression or arterial repair. Arterial damage can be minimized by placing a small guidewire under fluoroscopic guidance prior to placement of the much larger introducer sheath. Variable amounts of air can be introduced into the low-pressure venous system during the procedure. Small amounts are generally well tolerated, but entrainment of larger amounts of air can result in respiratory distress, oxygen desaturation, hypotension, and cardiac arrest.

Early pacemaker failure is usually due to electrode displacement or breakage. Pacemaker failure that occurs more than 6 months after implantation is usually due to premature battery depletion. The lithium-iodide batteries used in pulse generators are not rechargeable, and battery depletion requires surgical replacement of the entire generator. Modern pulse generators have an expected longevity of 5 to 9 years. Improved shielding of pacemakers has eliminated most problems related to external electrical fields (microwaves, electrocautery, magnetic resonance imaging) that produced inhibition of ventricular pacing. Many artificial cardiac pacemakers are designed to convert to an asynchronous mode rather than be completely inhibited when an external electrical field is encountered. Most pacemakers can be manually converted to an asynchronous mode by placing an external magnet over the pulse generator. Many functions of an artificial cardiac pacemaker can be adjusted using a magnetically activated potentiometer held externally near the pulse generator.

Implanted Cardioverter-Defibrillator Therapy

The single most important factor determining survival from cardiac arrest due to ventricular fibrillation is the time between arrest and the first defibrillation attempt. In witnessed cardiac arrest due to ventricular fibrillation, patients who are defibrillated within the first 3 minutes have a survival rate of 74%. ICDs were approved for use by the U.S. Food and Drug Administration in 1985. By the year 2000, more than 80,000 ICDs had been implanted worldwide. An ICD responds to a dysrhythmia by delivering an internal electrical shock within 15 seconds of the onset of the dysrhythmia. This provides a time interval for spontaneous dysrhythmia reversal, which, in fact, is a very common event.

The ICD system consists of a pulse generator and leads for dysrhythmia detection and current delivery. In addition to internal defibrillation, an ICD can produce antitachycardia and antibradycardia pacing and synchronized cardioversion. Detailed diagnostic data concerning intracardiac electrograms and event markers are stored in the memory of the device and can be retrieved for analysis. The pulse generator is a small computer powered by a lithium battery that is sealed within a titanium case. The lead system consists of pacing electrodes and a large surface area defibrillation coil. The defibrillation circuit is completed by the titanium case of the pulse generator, which acts as a defibrillation electrode. The pulse generator is usually implanted into a subcutaneous pocket. The position of the pulse generator is important because the position affects the defibrillation wave front.

The left pectoral region is the ideal location for the pulse generator. Right-sided implantation can result in a significantly higher defibrillation threshold. The transvenous leads consist of pacing and sensing electrodes and one or two defibrillation coils. Dual-chamber ICDs require another electrode, a coronary sinus lead, for resynchronization therapy in patients with severe heart failure.

ICDs employ electrical defibrillation as the sole therapy for the treatment of ventricular fibrillation. The ICD senses ventricular depolarization and amplifies, filters, and rectifies the signal. The signal is compared to the programmed sensing thresholds and to the R-R intervals in algorithms. If the device detects ventricular fibrillation, the capacitor charges, and, prior to shock delivery, a confirmatory algorithm is fulfilled by signal analysis. This process prevents inappropriate shocks for self-terminating events or spurious signals. The process takes approximately 10 to 15 seconds from dysrhythmia detection to shock delivery. During this time, the patient may experience presyncope or syncope.

Approximately half of patients with ICDs will have an adverse event related to the device within the first year after implantation. Lead-related problems, such as failure to sense or pace, inappropriate therapy, and dislodgment remain the most common problems. One of the most devastating complications is ICD infection. The estimated infection rate is approximately 0.6%, which is similar to the infection rate associated with pacemaker implantation. Device infection requires explantation of the entire ICD system.

Surgery in Patients with Cardiac Devices

The presence of an artificial cardiac pacemaker or ICD in a patient scheduled for surgery unrelated to the device introduces special considerations for preoperative evaluation and subsequent management of anesthesia.

Preoperative Evaluation

Preoperative evaluation of the patient with an artificial cardiac pacemaker or ICD includes determining the reason for device placement and assessment of its current function. Especially in a patient with an ICD, preoperative evaluation and perioperative planning should be coordinated with a cardiologist and the pacemaker representative for that specific device. ICDs are often switched off preoperatively and therapy reinstituted postoperatively. However, with many more ICDs implanted as part of pacing and resynchronization therapy, management decisions are now more complex. Early involvement of consultants is desirable.

A preoperative history of vertigo, presyncope, or syncope in a patient with a pacemaker could reflect pacemaker dysfunction. The rate of discharge of an atrial or ventricular *asynchronous* (fixed rate) cardiac pacemaker (usually 70–72 bpm) is a useful indicator of pulse generator function. A 10% decrease in heart rate from the initial heart rate setting may reflect battery depletion. An irregular heart rate could indicate competition of the pulse generator with the patient's intrinsic heart rate or failure of the pulse generator to sense R waves.

The ECG is not a diagnostic aid if the intrinsic heart rate is greater than the preset pacemaker rate. In such cases, proper function of a ventricular synchronous or sequential artificial cardiac pacemaker is best confirmed by electronic evaluation. A chest radiograph can be useful to evaluate the external condition of pacemaker electrodes.

Management of Anesthesia

Management of anesthesia in patients with artificial cardiac pacemakers includes (1) monitoring the ECG to confirm proper functioning of the pulse generator and (2) ensuring the availability of equipment and drugs to maintain an acceptable intrinsic heart rate should the artificial cardiac pacemaker unexpectedly fail. Insertion of a pulmonary artery catheter does not disturb epicardial electrodes but might become entangled in, or dislodge, a recently placed transvenous (endocardial) electrode. The danger of lead dislodgment is minimal 4 weeks after implantation. The choice of drugs to produce anesthesia is not altered by the presence of a properly functioning artificial cardiac pacemaker.

Improved shielding of cardiac pacemakers has reduced the problems associated with electromagnetic interference from electrocautery. The electrical artifact produced by electrocautery can be sensed by a pacemaker as either interference or an intrinsic R wave. If the pacemaker senses interference and is not certain whether an R wave is being produced, the unit will go into asynchronous (fixed rate) mode to guarantee delivery of a paced beat. Alternatively, the electrical artifact from electrocautery could be sensed as an R wave resulting in inhibition of the pulse generator. This would be a critical event if there is no underlying intrinsic cardiac rhythm. Examination of the pulse oximeter waveform, palpation of a pulse, or auscultation of heart sounds can confirm continued cardiac activity. An external magnet may be used to convert the pacemaker to the asynchronous mode. However, asynchronous pacing carries the risk of the R-on-T phenomenon.

The grounding electrode for electrocautery should be as far as possible from the pulse generator to minimize detection of the cautery current by the pulse generator. It is also useful to keep the electrocautery current as low as possible and to apply electrocautery in short bursts, especially if current is being applied in close proximity to the pulse generator. The presence of a *temporary* transvenous cardiac pacemaker creates a situation in which there is a direct connection between an external electrical source and the endocardium. There is a risk of ventricular fibrillation due to microshock currents.

Ventricular fibrillation in a patient with a permanent cardiac pacemaker or ICD (that is turned off) is managed in the conventional manner. However, care must be taken that the defibrillator paddles are not placed directly over the pulse generator. An acute increase in stimulation threshold may follow external defibrillation causing loss of capture. If this occurs, transcutaneous cardiac pacing or temporary transvenous pacing may be required.

There is no evidence that anesthetic drugs alter the stimulation threshold of artificial cardiac pacemakers. Nevertheless,

TABLE 4–5	Factors That Can Alter the Threshold of Cardiac Pacemakers

Hyperkalemia
Hypokalemia
Arterial hypoxemia
Myocardial ischemia/infarction
Catecholamines

it is prudent to avoid events such as hyperventilation that can acutely change the serum potassium concentration (**Table 4-5**). Conceivably, succinylcholine could increase the stimulation threshold because of an acute increase in serum potassium concentration. Succinylcholine could also inhibit a normally functioning cardiac pacemaker by causing contraction of skeletal muscle groups (myopotentials) that the pulse generator interprets as intrinsic R waves. Clinical experience suggests that succinylcholine is usually a safe drug in the patient with an artificial cardiac pacemaker, and if myopotential inhibition does occur, it is generally transient.

Anesthesia for Cardiac Pacemaker Insertion

Most pacemakers are inserted using conscious sedation in the cardiac catheterization laboratory or monitored anesthesia care in the operating room. Routine anesthetic monitoring is employed. A functioning cardiac pacemaker should be in place or transcutaneous cardiac pacing available before administration of anesthetic drugs. Drugs such as atropine or isoproterenol should be available should a decrease in heart rate compromise hemodynamics before the new pacemaker is functional.

KEY POINTS

- Cardiac dysrhythmias are classified according to heart rate and the site of the abnormality. Conduction disturbances are classified by site and degree of blockade. The clinical significance of these abnormalities depends on the effect that they have on vital signs (hemodynamic instability, cardiac and end-organ ischemia, congestive heart failure) and/or the potential for deterioration into a life-threatening rhythm.

- Tachydysrhythmias can result from three mechanisms: (1) increased automaticity in normal conduction tissue or in an ectopic focus, (2) reentry of electrical potentials through abnormal pathways, and (3) triggering of abnormal cardiac potentials due to afterdepolarizations.

- Typically, benign ventricular premature beats occur at rest and disappear with exercise. An increase in premature ventricular contractions with exercise may be an indication of underlying cardiac disease. The prognostic significance of ventricular ectopy depends on the presence and severity of coexisting structural heart disease. In the absence of structural heart disease, asymptomatic ventricular ectopy is benign with no demonstrable risk of sudden death.

- The normal conduction system of the heart from atrium to ventricle is a single conduction pathway through the AV node and His-Purkinje system. There can be alternate (accessory) pathways that function as electrically active muscle bridges that bypass the normal conduction pathway and create the potential for reentrant tachycardias.

- Torsade de pointes is ventricular tachycardia in a patient with a long QTc and is electrocardiographically characterized by a "twisting of the peaks." This description refers to the constantly changing cycle length, axis, and morphology of the QRS complexes around the isoelectric baseline.

- Antidysrhythmic drugs work by one of three mechanisms: (1) suppressing automaticity in cardiac pacemaker cells by decreasing the slope of phase 4 depolarization, (2) prolonging the effective refractory period in order to eliminate reentry circuits, and (3) facilitating impulse conduction along the normal conduction pathway in order to prevent conduction over a reentrant pathway.

- Mobitz type 1 block (Wenckebach) demonstrates progressive prolongation of the PR interval until a beat is dropped. A pause allows the AV node to recover and then the process resumes. In contrast, Mobitz type 2 block is characterized by sudden and complete interruption of conduction without PR prolongation. Mobitz type 2 block is usually associated with permanent damage to the conduction system and may progress to third-degree block.

- Third-degree heart block (complete heart block) is characterized by complete absence of conduction of cardiac impulses from the atria to the ventricles. Continued activity of the ventricles is due to impulses from an ectopic focus distal to the site of block. If the conduction block is near the AV node, the heart rate is usually 45 to 55 bpm and the QRS complex has a normal width. If the conduction block is below the AV node (infranodal), the heart rate is usually 30 to 40 bpm and the QRS complex is wide.

- Improved shielding of permanent cardiac pacemakers has eliminated most problems related to external electrical fields (microwaves, electrocautery, magnetic resonance imaging) that produced inhibition of ventricular pacing. Many pacemakers are designed to convert to an asynchronous mode rather than be completely inhibited when an external electrical field is encountered. Most pacemakers can be manually converted to asynchronous mode by placing an external magnet over the pulse generator.

Continued

KEY POINTS—cont'd

- An ICD senses ventricular depolarization, amplifies and filters the signal, and then compares the signal to sensing thresholds and R-R intervals in an algorithm. If the device detects ventricular fibrillation, the capacitor charges, and, prior to shock delivery, a confirmatory algorithm is fulfilled by signal analysis. This process prevents inappropriate shocks for self-terminating events or spurious signals. The process takes approximately 10 to 15 seconds from dysrhythmia detection to shock delivery.

REFERENCES

Blomstrom-Lundqvist C, Scheinman MM, Aliot EM, et al: ACC/AHA/ESC guidelines for the management of patients with supraventricular arrhythmias—executive summary. A report of the American College of Cardiology/American Heart Association Task Force on Practice Guidelines and the European Society of Cardiology Committee for Practice Guidelines. Developed in collaboration with NASPE-Heart Rhythm Society. J Am Coll Cardiol 2003;42:1493–1531.

Erb TO, Kanter RJ, Hall JM, et al: Comparison of electrophysiologic effects of propofol and isoflurane-based anesthetics in children undergoing radiofrequency catheter ablation for supraventricular tachycardia. Anesthesiology 2002;96:1386–1394.

Fuster A, Ryden LE, Cannom DS, et al: ACC/AHA/ESC 2006 guidelines for the management of patients with atrial fibrillation: A report of the American College of Cardiology/American Heart Association Task Force on Practice Guidelines and the European Society of Cardiology Committee for Practice Guidelines. Developed in collaboration with the European Heart Rhythm Association and the Heart Rhythm Society. Circulation 2006;114:e257–e354.

Kopp SL, Horlocker TT, Warner ME, et al: Cardiac arrest during neuraxial anesthesia: Frequency and predisposing factors associated with survival. Anesth Analg 2005;100:855–865.

Latini S, Pedata FJ: Adenosine in the central nervous system: Release mechanisms and extracellular concentrations. J Neurochem 2001;79:463–484.

Trohman RG, Kim MH, Pinski SL: Cardiac pacing: State of the art. Lancet 2004;364:1701–1716.

2005 American Heart Association Guidelines for cardiopulmonary resuscitation and emergency cardiovascular care, part 7.2: Management of cardiac arrest. Circulation 2005;112(Suppl IV):IV-67–IV-78.

Zipes DP, Camm AJ, Borggrefe M, et al: ACC/AHA/ESC 2006 guidelines for management of patients with ventricular arrhythmias and the prevention of sudden cardiac death: A report of the American College of Cardiology/American Heart Association Task Force and the European Society of Cardiology Committee for Practice Guidelines. Circulation 2006;114:e385–e484.

CHAPTER 5

Systemic and Pulmonary Arterial Hypertension

Matthew C. Wallace
Alá Sami Haddadin

Systemic Hypertension
- Pathophysiology
- Treatment of Essential Hypertension
- Treatment of Secondary Hypertension
- Hypertensive Crises
- Management of Anesthesia in Patients with Essential Hypertension

Pulmonary Arterial Hypertension
- Definition
- Clinical Presentation and Evaluation
- Physiology and Pathophysiology
- Treatment of Pulmonary Hypertension
- Anesthetic Management
- Perioperative Preparation and Induction

SYSTEMIC HYPERTENSION

An adult is considered to be hypertensive when the systemic blood pressure is 140/90 mm Hg or more on at least two occasions measured at least 1 to 2 weeks apart (**Table 5-1**). Prehypertension is said to exist when systolic blood pressure is 120 to 139 or diastolic blood pressure is 80 to 89. Based on this definition, systemic hypertension is the most common circulatory derangement in the United States, affecting approximately 25% of adults. The incidence of systemic hypertension increases progressively with age and is higher in the African American population (**Fig. 5-1**). Hypertension is a significant risk factor for the development of ischemic heart disease (**Fig. 5-2**) and a major cause of congestive heart failure (**Fig. 5-3**), cerebral vascular accident (stroke), arterial aneurysm, and end-stage renal disease. It is estimated that less than one third of patients with hypertension in the United States are aware of their condition and are adequately treated.

Pathophysiology
Systemic hypertension is characterized as essential or primary hypertension when a cause for the increased blood pressure cannot be identified. It is termed secondary hypertension when an identifiable cause is present.

Essential Hypertension
Essential hypertension, which accounts for more than 95% of all cases of hypertension, is characterized by a familial incidence and inherited biochemical abnormalities. Pathophysiologic factors implicated in the genesis of essential hypertension include increased sympathetic nervous system activity in response to stress, overproduction of

TABLE 5–1	Classification of Systemic Blood Pressure for Adults	
Category	Systolic Blood Pressure (mm Hg)	Diastolic Blood Pressure (mm Hg)
Normal	<120	<80
Prehypertension	120–139	80–89
Stage 1 hypertension	140–159	90–99
Stage 2 hypertension	≥160	≥100

Reprinted with permission from Chobanian AV, et al: Seventh Report of the Joint National Committee on Prevention, Detection, Evaluation and Treatment of High Blood Pressure. Hypertension 2003;42:1206–1252.

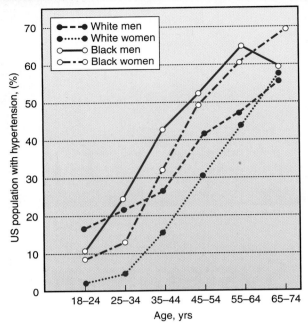

Figure 5-1 • Prevalence of hypertension (>160/90 mm Hg) among the adult population in the United States. (*Reprinted with permission from Tjoa HI, Kaplan NM: Treatment of hypertension in the elderly. JAMA 1990;264:1015–1018.*)

sodium-retaining hormones and vasoconstrictors, high sodium intake, inadequate dietary intake of potassium and calcium, increased renin secretion, deficiencies of endogenous vasodilators such as prostaglandins and nitric oxide (NO), and the presence of medical diseases such as diabetes mellitus and obesity. The final common pathway in the pathophysiology of essential hypertension is salt and water retention. Hypertension, insulin resistance, dyslipidemia, and obesity often occur concomitantly, and an estimated 40% of persons with hypertension also manifest hypercholesterolemia. Alcohol and tobacco use is associated with essential hypertension. Obstructive sleep apnea, which is present in a substantial proportion of the adult population, causes temporary increases in blood pressure in association with hypoxemia, arousal, and activation of the sympathetic nervous system. There is evidence that obstructive sleep apnea leads to sustained

hypertension independent of known confounding factors such as obesity. Indeed, an estimated 30% of hypertensive patients manifest obstructive sleep apnea.

A history of ischemic heart disease, angina pectoris, left ventricular hypertrophy, congestive heart failure, cerebrovascular disease, stroke, peripheral vascular disease, or renal insufficiency

Figure 5-2 • Ischemic heart disease (IHD) mortality rate in each decade of age versus usual blood pressure at the start of that decade. Mortality rates are termed "floating" because multiplication by a constant appropriate for a particular population would allow prediction of the absolute rate in that population. (*Reprinted with permission from Lewington S, et al: Age-specific relevance of usual blood pressure to vascular mortality: A meta-analysis of individual data for one million adults in 61 prospective studies. Lancet 2002;360:1903–1913. Copyright 2002.*)

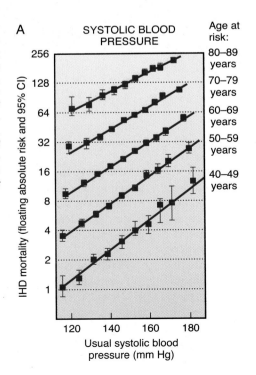

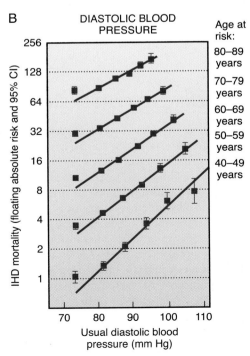

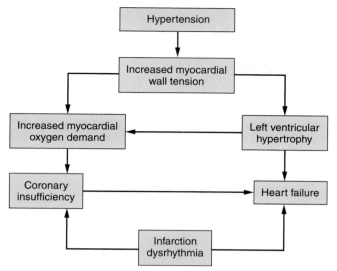

Figure 5-3 • Chronic increases in systemic blood pressure initiate a series of pathophysiologic changes that may culminate in congestive heart failure.

suggests end-organ disease due to chronic, poorly controlled essential hypertension. Laboratory evaluation is intended to document target organ damage and includes blood urea nitrogen and serum creatinine assays to quantify renal function. Hypokalemia in the presence of essential hypertension suggests primary aldosteronism. Fasting blood glucose concentrations should be evaluated because 50% of hypertensive patients manifest glucose intolerance. An ECG is useful for detecting evidence of ischemic heart disease or left ventricular hypertrophy.

Secondary Hypertension

Secondary hypertension has a demonstrable cause but accounts for less than 5% of all cases of systemic hypertension. Renovascular hypertension due to renal artery stenosis is the most common cause of secondary hypertension. This and other more common causes of secondary hypertension with their notable signs and symptoms are listed in **Table 5-2**. A more comprehensive list of causes of secondary hypertension is seen in **Table 5-3**.

TABLE 5–2 Common Causes of Secondary Hypertension		
Causes	**Clinical Findings**	**Laboratory Evaluation**
Renovascular disease	Epigastric or abdominal bruit Severe hypertension in young patient	MRI angiography Aortography Duplex ultrasonography CT angiography
Hyperaldosteronism	Fatigue Weakness Headache Paresthesia Nocturnal polyuria and polydypsia	Urinary potassium Serum potassium Plasma renin Plasma aldosterone
Aortic coarctation	Elevated blood pressure in upper limbs relative to lower limbs Weak femoral pulses Systolic bruit	Aortography Echocardiography MRI or CT
Pheochromocytoma	Episodic headache, palpitations, and diaphoresis Paroxysmal hypertension	Plasma metanephrines Urinary catecholamines Spot urine metanephrines Adrenal CT/MRI scan
Cushing's syndrome	Truncal obesity Proximal muscle weakness Purple striae "Moon facies" Hirsutism	Dexamethasone suppression test Urinary cortisol Adrenal CT scan Glucose tolerance test
Renal parenchymal disease	Nocturia Edema	Urinary glucose, protein and casts Serum creatinine Renal ultrasonography Renal biopsy
Pregnancy-induced hypertension	Peripheral and pulmonary edema Headache Seizures Right upper quadrant pain	Urinary protein Uric acid Cardiac output Platelet count

CT, computed tomography; MRI, magnetic resonance imaging.

TABLE 5-3 Other Causes of Secondary Hypertension

Systolic and Diastolic Hypertension
Renal
  Renal transplantation
  Renin-secreting tumors
Endocrine
  Acromegaly
  Hyperparathyroidism
Obstructive sleep apnea
Postoperative hypertension
Neurologic disorders
  Increased intracranial pressure
  Spinal cord injury
  Guillain-Barre syndrome
  Dysautonomia
Drugs
  Glucocorticoids
  Mineralocorticoids
  Cyclosporine
  Sympathomimetics
  Tyramine and monoamine oxidase inhibitors
  Nasal decongestants
Sudden withdrawal from antihypertensive drug therapy
  (central acting and β-adrenergic antagonists)

Isolated Systolic Hypertension
Aging with associated aortic rigidity
Increased cardiac output
  Thyrotoxicosis
  Anemia
  Aortic regurgitation
Decreased peripheral vascular resistance
  Arteriovenous shunts
  Paget's disease

Treatment of Essential Hypertension

Decreasing blood pressure by lifestyle modification and pharmacologic therapy is intended to decrease morbidity and mortality. The standard goal of therapy is to decrease systemic blood pressure to lower than 140/90 mm Hg, but in the presence of diabetes mellitus or renal disease, the goal is lower than 130/80 mm Hg. Treatment resulting in normalization of blood pressure has been particularly successful in decreasing the incidence of cerebrovascular accidents. Decreasing blood pressure decreases the morbidity and mortality associated with ischemic heart disease (**Fig. 5-4**). It slows or prevents progression to a more severe stage of hypertension and decreases the risk of congestive heart failure and renal failure. The benefits of antihypertensive drug therapy appear to be greater in elderly patients than in younger patients.

Patients with concomitant risk factors (hypercholesterolemia, diabetes mellitus, tobacco abuse, family history, age older than 60 years) and evidence of target organ damage (angina pectoris, prior myocardial infarction, left ventricular hypertrophy, cerebrovascular disease, nephropathy, retinopathy, peripheral vascular disease) are most likely to benefit from pharmacologic antihypertensive therapy. Patients who do not manifest clinical evidence of cardiovascular disease or target organ damage may benefit from a trial of lifestyle modification and subsequent reevaluation before initiation of pharmacologic therapy.

Lifestyle Modification

Lifestyle modifications of proven value for lowering blood pressure include weight reduction or prevention of weight gain, moderation of alcohol intake, increased physical activity, maintenance of recommended levels of dietary calcium and

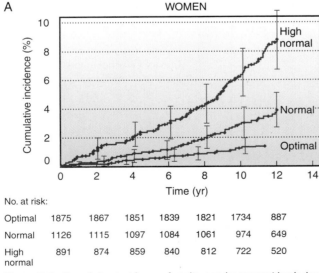

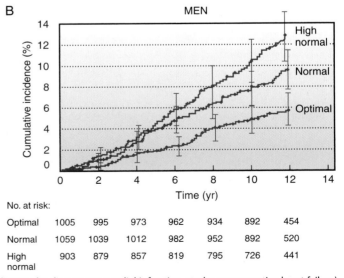

A WOMEN						
No. at risk:						
Optimal	1875	1867	1851	1839	1821	1734	887
Normal	1126	1115	1097	1084	1061	974	649
High normal	891	874	859	840	812	722	520

B MEN						
No. at risk:						
Optimal	1005	995	973	962	934	892	454
Normal	1059	1039	1012	982	952	892	520
High normal	903	879	857	819	795	726	441

Figure 5-4 • Cumulative incidence of cardiovascular events (death due to cardiovascular disease, myocardial infarction, stroke, or congestive heart failure) in women (**A**) and men (**B**) without hypertension according to blood pressure category at the baseline examination. Optimal blood pressure: <120/80, normal blood pressure: <130/85, high-normal blood pressure: <140/90. (*Adapted from Vasan RS, et al: Impact of high-normal blood pressure on the risk of cardiovascular disease. N Engl J Med 2001;345:1291–1297. Copyright © 2001, Massachusetts Medical Society. All rights reserved.*)

potassium, and moderation in dietary salt intake. Smoking cessation is critical because smoking is an independent risk factor for cardiovascular disease.

Weight loss may be the most efficacious of all nonpharmacologic interventions in the treatment of hypertension. Weight loss also enhances the efficacy of antihypertensive drug therapy. Alcohol consumption is associated with an increase in blood pressure, and excessive use of alcohol may cause resistance to antihypertensive drugs. However, moderate alcohol ingestion has been shown to decrease overall cardiovascular risk in the general population. At least 30 minutes of moderate intensity physical activity, such as brisk walking or bicycling, can lower blood pressure in both normotensive and hypertensive individuals.

There is an inverse relationship between dietary potassium and calcium intake and blood pressure in the general population. The antihypertensive efficacy of dietary salt restriction (such as the Dietary Approaches to Stop Hypertension eating plan) shows small but consistent decreases in systemic blood pressure (**Fig. 5-5**). It is possible that the role of sodium restriction in lowering blood pressure is most beneficial in a subset of patients with low renin activity such as the elderly and African Americans. Sodium restriction can minimize diuretic-induced hypokalemia and may enhance the ease of blood pressure control with diuretic therapy. Additional benefits of salt restriction include protection from osteoporosis and fractures by decreasing urinary calcium excretion and favorable effects on left ventricular hypertrophy. Salt substitutes in which sodium is replaced with potassium are useful for hypertensive patients who do not have renal dysfunction.

Pharmacologic Therapy

Initiation of drug therapy should occur in tandem with lifestyle modification. After drug therapy is started, patients are seen every 1 to 4 weeks to titrate the antihypertensive drug dose and then every 3 to 4 months once the desired degree of blood pressure control has been achieved. Use of long-acting drugs is preferable because patient compliance and consistency of blood pressure control are superior with once-daily dosing. In the Seventh Report of the Joint National Committee on Prevention, Detection, Evaluation, and Treatment of High Blood Pressure, thiazide diuretics are recommended as initial therapy for uncomplicated hypertension (**Fig. 5-6**). Thiazide diuretics can also increase the efficacy of multidrug regimens. The hypertensive patient may have comorbid conditions that present compelling indications for antihypertensive therapy with drugs of a particular class (**Table 5-4**). For example, hypertension in patients with heart failure is typically treated with an angiotensin-converting enzyme (ACE) inhibitor. These compelling indications are based on the results of multiple outcome studies. If monotherapy is unsuccessful, a second drug, usually of a different class, is added. A large variety of antihypertensive drugs are available, and many of these drugs present unique and potentially significant advantages and side effects (**Table 5-5**).

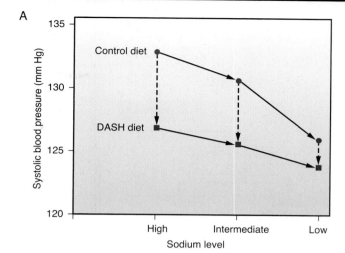

A

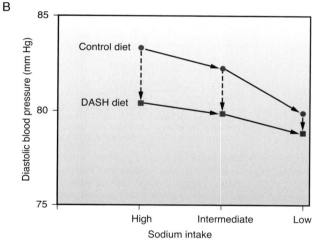

B

Figure 5-5 • The effect on systolic blood pressure (**A**) and diastolic blood pressure (**B**) of reduced sodium intake and the Dietary Approaches to Stop Hypertension (DASH) diet. (*Reprinted with permission from Sacks FM, et al: Effects on blood pressure of reduced dietary sodium and the Dietary Approaches to Stop Hypertension (DASH) Diet. N Engl J Med 2001;344:3–10. Copyright © 2001, Massachusetts Medical Society. All rights reserved.*)

Treatment of Secondary Hypertension

Treatment of secondary hypertension is often surgical. Pharmacologic therapy is reserved for patients in whom surgery is not possible. Certain disease entities, such as pheochromocytoma, may require a combined approach for optimal outcome.

Surgical Therapy

Surgical therapy is reserved for identifiable causes of secondary hypertension, and includes correction of renal artery stenosis via angioplasty or direct repair and adrenalectomy for adrenal adenoma or pheochromocytoma.

Pharmacologic Therapy

For patients in whom renal artery revascularization is not possible, blood pressure control may be accomplished with

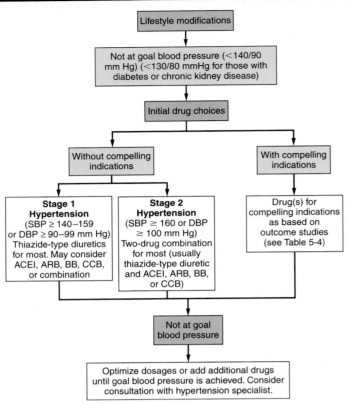

Figure 5-6 • Algorithm for treatment of hypertension. ACEI, angiotensin-converting enzyme inhibitor; ARB, angiotensin receptor blocker; BB, β-blocker; CCB, calcium channel blocker; DBP, diastolic blood pressure; SBP, systolic blood pressure. *(Reprinted with permission from Chobanian AV, et al: Seventh Report of the Joint National Committee on Prevention, Detection, Evaluation, and Treatment of High Blood Pressure. Hypertension 2003;42:1206–1252.)*

TABLE 5–4 Compelling Indications for Specific Classes of Antihypertensive Drugs	
Comorbid Condition	**Class of Antihypertensive Drugs**
Postmyocardial infarction	ACE inhibitor Aldosterone antagonist β-Blocker
Heart failure	ACE inhibitor Aldosterone antagonist ARB β-Blocker Diuretic
High risk of coronary artery disease	ACE inhibitor β-Blocker Calcium channel blocker Diuretic
Diabetes	ACE inhibitor ARB β-Blocker Calcium channel blocker Diuretic
Chronic kidney disease	ACE inhibitor ARB
Recurrent stroke prevention	ACE inhibitor Diuretic
ACE, angiotensin-converting enzyme; ARB, angiotensin receptor blocker.	

ACE inhibitors alone or in combination with diuretics. Renal function and serum potassium concentration must be carefully monitored when ACE inhibitor therapy is initiated in these patients. Primary aldosteronism in women is treated with an aldosterone antagonist such as spironolactone, but amiloride is used in men for this purpose because spironolactone may cause gynecomastia.

Hypertensive Crises

Definition

Hypertensive crises typically present with a blood pressure of higher than 180/120 and can be categorized as either a hypertensive urgency or a hypertensive emergency, based on the presence or absence of impending or progressive target organ damage. Patients with chronic systemic hypertension can tolerate a higher systemic blood pressure than previously normotensive individuals and are more likely to present with urgencies rather than emergencies.

Hypertensive Emergency

Patients with evidence of acute or ongoing target organ damage (encephalopathy, intracerebral hemorrhage, acute left ventricular failure with pulmonary edema, unstable angina, dissecting aortic aneurysm, acute myocardial infarction, eclampsia, microangiopathic hemolytic anemia, or renal insufficiency) require prompt pharmacologic intervention to lower the systemic blood pressure. Encephalopathy rarely develops in patients with chronic hypertension until the diastolic blood pressure exceeds 150 mm Hg, whereas parturients with pregnancy-induced hypertension may develop signs of encephalopathy with diastolic blood pressures less than 100 mm Hg. Even in the absence of symptoms, a parturient with a diastolic blood pressure higher than 109 mm Hg is considered a hypertensive emergency and requires immediate management. The goal of treatment in hypertensive emergencies is to decrease the diastolic blood pressure promptly but gradually. A precipitous decrease in blood pressure to normotensive levels may provoke coronary or cerebral ischemia. Typically, mean arterial pressure is reduced by about 20% within the first 60 minutes and then more gradually. Thereafter, the blood pressure can be reduced to 160/110 over the next 2 to 6 hours as tolerated by the absence of symptomatic hypoperfusion of target organs.

Hypertensive Urgency

Hypertensive urgencies are situations in which BP is severely elevated, but the patient is not exhibiting evidence of target organ damage. These patients can present with headache, epistaxis, or anxiety. Selected patients may benefit from oral antihypertensive therapy because noncompliance with or

TABLE 5-5 Commonly Used Antihypertensive Drugs

Class	Subclass	Generic Name	Trade Name
Diuretics	Thiazides	Chlorothiazide	Diuril
		Hydrochlorothiazide	Hydrodiuril, Microzide
		Indapamide	Lozol
		Metolazone	Zaroxolyn, Mykrox
	Loop	Bumetanide	Bumex
		Furosemide	Lasix
		Torsemide	Demadex
	Potassium-sparing	Ameloride	Midamor
		Spironolactone	Aldactone
		Triamterene	Dyrenium
Adrenergic antagonists	β-Blockers	Atenolol	Tenormin
		Bisoprolol	Zebeta
		Metoprolol	Lopressor
		Nadolol	Corgard
		Propranolol	Inderal
		Timolol	Blocadren
	α_1-blockers	Doxazosin	Cardura
		Prazosin	Minipress
		Terazosin	Hytrin
	Combined α- and β-blockers	Carvedilol	Coreg
		Labetalol	Normodyne, Trandate
	Centrally acting	Clonidine	Catapress
		Methyldopa	Aldomet
Vasodilators		Hydralazine	Apresoline
ACE inhibitors		Benazepril	Lotensin
		Captopril	Capoten
		Enalapril	Vasotec
		Fosinopril	Monopril
		Lisinopril	Prinivil, Zestril
		Moexipril	Univasc
		Quinipril	Accupril
		Ramipril	Altace
		Trandolapril	Mavik
Angiotensin receptor blockers		Candesartan	Atacand
		Eprosartan	Teveten
		Irbesartan	Avapro
		Losartan	Cozaar
		Olmesartan	Benicar
		Telmisartan	Micardis
		Valsartan	Diovan
Calcium channel blockers	Dihydroperidine	Amlodipine	Norvasc
		Felodipine	Plendil
		Israpidine	Dynacirc
		Nicardipine	Cardene
		Nifedipine	Adalat, Procardia
		Nisoldipine	Sular
	Nondihydroperidine	Diltiazem	Cardiazem, Dilacor, Tiazac
		Verapamil	Calan, Isoptin, Coer, Covera

ACE, angiotensin-converting enzyme.

TABLE 5-6 Treatment of Hypertensive Emergencies

Etiology/Manifestation	Primary Agents	Cautions	Comments
Encephalopathy and intracranial hypertension	Nitroprusside, labetalol, fenoldopam, nicardipine	Cerebral ischemia may result from lower blood pressure due to altered autoregulation Risk of cyanide toxicity Nitroprusside increases intracranial pressure	Lower blood pressure may lessen bleeding in intracerebral hemorrhage Elevated BP often resolves spontaneously
Myocardial ischemia	Nitroglycerin	Avoid β-blockers in acute congestive heart failure	Include morphine and oxygen therapy
Acute pulmonary edema	Nitroglycerin, nitroprusside, fenoldopam	Avoid β-blockers in acute congestive heart failure	Include morphine, loop diuretic, and oxygen therapy
Aortic dissection	Esmolol, vasodilators Trimethaphan	Vasodilators may cause reflex tachycardia	Goal: lessening of pulsatile force of left ventricular contraction
Renal insufficiency	Fenoldopam, nicardipine	Tachyphylaxis occurs with fenoldopam	May require emergent hemodialysis Avoid ACE inhibitors and ARBs
Preeclampsia and eclampsia	Methyldopa, hydralazine Magnesium sulfate Labetalol, nicardipine	Lupus-like syndrome with hydralazine Risk of flash pulmonary edema Calcium channel blockers may reduce uterine blood flow and inhibit labor	Definitive therapy is delivery ACE inhibitors and ARBs are contraindicated during pregnancy due to teratogenicity
Pheochromocytoma	Phentolamine, phenoxybenzamine, propranolol	Unopposed α-adrenergic stimulation following β-blockade worsens hypertension	
Cocaine intoxication	Nitroglycerin, nitroprusside, phentolamine	Unopposed α-adrenergic stimulation following β-blockade worsens hypertension	

unavailability of prescribed medications is often the factor responsible for this problem.

Pharmacologic Therapy

The initial choice of pharmacologic therapy for a hypertensive emergency lies in an analysis of the patient's comorbidities and the symptoms and signs at presentation (**Table 5-6**). An intra-arterial catheter to continuously monitor systemic blood pressure is recommended during treatment with potent vasoactive substances. For most types of hypertensive emergencies, sodium nitroprusside 0.5 to 10.0 μg/kg/min intravenously is a drug of choice. The immediate onset and short duration of action allow effective minute-by-minute titration, but sodium nitroprusside use can be complicated by lactic acidosis and cyanide toxicity. Nicardipine infusion is another option and may improve both cardiac and cerebral ischemia. The dopamine (DA_1-specific) agonist fenoldopam increases renal blood flow and inhibits sodium reabsorption, making it an excellent drug in patients with renal insufficiency. Esmolol infusion can be effective alone or in combination with other drugs. Labetalol, an α- and β-blocker, can also be very effective in the acute treatment of hypertension.

Management of Anesthesia in Patients with Essential Hypertension

Despite earlier suggestions that antihypertensive medications be discontinued preoperatively, it is now accepted that most drugs that effectively control systemic blood pressure should be continued throughout the perioperative period to ensure optimum control of blood pressure. A summary of the anesthetic management of patients with hypertension is shown in **Table 5-7**.

Preoperative Evaluation

Preoperative evaluation of patients with essential hypertension should determine the adequacy of blood pressure control, and antihypertensive drug therapy that has rendered patients normotensive should be continued throughout the perioperative period. It seems reasonable to support the concept that

TABLE 5-7 Management of Anesthesia for Hypertensive Patients

Preoperative Evaluation
Determine adequacy of blood pressure control
Review pharmacology of drugs being administered to control blood pressure
Evaluate for evidence of end-organ damage
Continue drugs used for control of blood pressure

Induction and Maintenance of Anesthesia
Anticipate exaggerated blood pressure response to anesthetic drugs
Limit duration of direct laryngoscopy
Administer a balanced anesthetic to blunt hypertensive responses
Consider placement of invasive hemodynamic monitors
Monitor for myocardial ischemia

Postoperative Management
Anticipate periods of systemic hypertension
Maintain monitoring of end-organ function

It is not uncommon for the blood pressure on admission to the hospital to be increased (white coat syndrome), reflecting patient anxiety. Subsequent blood pressures are typically lower. However, this subset of patients who manifest anxiety-related hypertension are likely to have exaggerated pressor responses to direct laryngoscopy and are more likely than others to develop perioperative myocardial ischemia or to require antihypertensive therapy during the perioperative period.

End-organ damage (angina pectoris, left ventricular hypertrophy, congestive heart failure, cerebrovascular disease, stroke, peripheral vascular disease, renal insufficiency) should be evaluated preoperatively. Patients with essential hypertension are presumed to have ischemic heart disease until proven otherwise. Renal insufficiency secondary to chronic hypertension is a marker of a widespread hypertensive disease process.

It is useful to review the pharmacology and potential side effects of the drugs being used for antihypertensive therapy (see Table 5-5). Many of these drugs interfere with autonomic nervous system function. Preoperatively, this may manifest as orthostatic hypotension. During anesthesia, exaggerated decreases in blood pressure seen with blood loss, positive pressure ventilation, or sudden changes in body position could reflect impaired vascular compensation due to these autonomic inhibitory effects. Administration of vasopressors, such as phenylephrine and ephedrine, results in predictable and appropriate blood pressure responses in these patients.

Another compelling reason to continue antihypertensive therapy throughout the perioperative period is the risk of rebound hypertension should certain drugs, especially β-adrenergic antagonists and clonidine, be abruptly discontinued. Antihypertensive agents that act independent of the autonomic nervous system such as ACE inhibitors are not associated with rebound hypertension.

Bradycardia may be a manifestation of a selective alteration in sympathetic nervous system activity. There is no evidence, however, that heart rate responses to surgical stimulation or surgical blood loss are absent in patients treated with antihypertensive drugs and clinical experience does not support the theoretical possibility that exaggerated decreases in heart rate could occur when drugs that normally increase

hypertensive patients should be made normotensive prior to elective surgery. The incidence of hypotension and evidence of myocardial ischemia during maintenance of anesthesia is increased in patients who are hypertensive prior to induction of anesthesia. Also the magnitude of blood pressure decreases during anesthesia is greater in hypertensive than in normotensive patients. However, intraoperative *increases* in blood pressure commonly occur in patients with a history of hypertension, whether or not the blood pressure is controlled preoperatively (**Table 5-8**).

There is no evidence that the incidence of postoperative complications is increased when hypertensive patients (diastolic blood pressure as high as 110 mm Hg) undergo elective surgery (see Table 5-8). However, co-existing hypertension may increase the incidence of postoperative myocardial reinfarction in patients with a history of myocardial infarction and the incidence of neurologic complications in patients undergoing carotid endarterectomy. In hypertensive patients who exhibit signs of target organ damage, postponement of an elective procedure is justified if that end-organ damage can be improved or if further evaluation of that damage could alter the anesthetic plan.

TABLE 5-8 Risk of General Anesthesia and Elective Surgery in Hypertensive Patients

Preoperative Systemic Blood Pressure Status	Incidence of Perioperative Hypertensive Episodes (%)	Incidence of Postoperative Cardiac Complications (%)
Normotensive	8*	11
Treated and rendered normotensive	27	24
Treated but remain hypertensive	25	7
Untreated and hypertensive	20	12

*$P < .05$ compared with other groups in the same column.
Reprinted with permission from Goldman L, Caldera DL: Risk of general anesthesia and elective operation in the hypertensive patient. Anesthesiology 1979;50:285–292.

parasympathetic nervous system activity, such as anticholines-terase drugs, are administered. Decreased anesthetic requirements parallel the sedative effects produced by clonidine. Hypokalemia (<3.5 mEq/L) despite potassium supplementation is a common preoperative finding in patients being treated with diuretics, but this drug-induced hypokalemia does not increase the incidence of cardiac dysrhythmias. Hyperkalemia can be seen patients being treated with ACE inhibitors who are also receiving potassium supplementation or have renal dysfunction.

Angiotensin-Converting Enzyme Inhibitors There is a risk that hemodynamic instability and hypotension will occur during anesthesia in patients receiving ACE inhibitors. Three systems exist to maintain normal blood pressure. Following blunting of autonomic responses by induction of anesthesia and blunting of the renin-angiotensin-aldosterone system by an ACE inhibitor, the only remaining system to support blood pressure is the vasopressin system, and so blood pressure is likely to be volume dependent (**Fig. 5-7**). ACE inhibitors may also decrease cardiac output by attenuating the venoconstrictor effect of angiotensin on capacitance vessels. This will result in a decrease in venous return. Maintenance of intravascular fluid volume is crucial during surgery in patients on long-term treatment with these drugs. Surgical procedures involving major fluid shifts have been associated with hypotension in patients being treated with ACE inhibitors. This hypotension has been responsive to fluid infusion and administration of sympathomimetic drugs. Hypotension resistant to such measures may require administration of vasopressin or a vasopressin agonist. Careful titration of anesthetic drugs may prevent or limit the hypotension attributable to ACE inhibitors.

It may be prudent to discontinue ACE inhibitors 24 to 48 hours preoperatively in patients at high risk of intraoperative hypovolemia and hypotension. The major disadvantage of

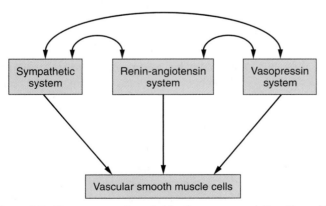

Figure 5-7 • Vasopressor systems in blood pressure regulation. Three different vasopressor systems are involved in blood pressure regulation. Each acts on the same target, i.e., the vascular smooth muscle cell, by inducing an increase in free cytosolic calcium followed by cell contraction. Each system is related to the others and may act as a compensatory mechanism. (*Reprinted with permission from Colson P, Ryckwaert F, Coriat P: Renin angiotensin system antagonists and anesthesia. Anesth Analg 1999; 89:1143–1155.*)

drug discontinuation is the potential loss of blood pressure control.

Angiotensin Receptor Blockers Angiotensin receptor blockers (ARBs) effectively treat hypertension by preventing angiotensin II from binding to its receptor. As with ACE inhibitors, blockade of the renin-angiotensin-aldosterone system by ARBs increases the potential for hypotension during anesthesia. Hypotension requiring vasoconstrictor treatment occurs more often after induction of anesthesia in patients continuing ARB treatment than in those in whom treatment had been discontinued on the day before surgery. In addition, the hypotensive episodes experienced by patients treated with ARBs may be refractory to conventional vasoconstrictors such as ephedrine and phenylephrine, necessitating use of vasopressin or one of its analogues. For these reasons, it is recommended that ARBs be discontinued on the day before surgery.

Induction of Anesthesia

Induction of anesthesia with rapidly acting intravenous drugs may produce an exaggerated decrease in blood pressure due to peripheral vasodilation in the presence of a decreased intravascular fluid volume, as is likely in the presence of diastolic hypertension. Hypotension during induction is more noticeable in patients continuing ACE inhibitor or ARB therapy up until the time of surgery.

Direct laryngoscopy and tracheal intubation can produce significant hypertension in patients with essential hypertension, even if these patients have been rendered normotensive preoperatively. Evidence of myocardial ischemia is likely to occur in association with the hypertension and tachycardia that accompany laryngoscopy and intubation. Intravenous induction drugs do not predictably suppress the circulatory responses evoked by tracheal intubation. Patients at high risk for developing myocardial ischemia may benefit from maneuvers that suppress tracheal reflexes and blunt the autonomic responses to tracheal manipulation such as deep inhalation anesthesia or injection of an opioid, lidocaine, β-blocker, or vasodilator. In addition, the duration of laryngoscopy is important in limiting the pressor response to this painful stimulus. Direct laryngoscopy that does not exceed 15 seconds in duration helps minimize blood pressure changes.

Maintenance of Anesthesia

The hemodynamic goal during maintenance of anesthesia is to minimize wide fluctuations in blood pressure. Management of intraoperative blood pressure lability is as important as preoperative control of hypertension in these patients.

Regional anesthesia can certainly be used in hypertensive patients. However, a high sensory level of anesthesia with its associated sympathetic denervation can unmask unsuspected hypovolemia.

Intraoperative Hypertension The most likely intraoperative blood pressure change is hypertension produced by painful stimulation, i.e., light anesthesia. Indeed, the incidence of perioperative hypertensive episodes is increased in patients diagnosed with essential hypertension, even if the blood pressure was controlled preoperatively (see Table 5-8). Volatile anesthetics are useful in attenuating sympathetic nervous system activity responsible for pressor responses. Volatile anesthetics produce dose-dependent decreases in blood pressure, reflecting decreases in systemic vascular resistance and myocardial depression. There is no evidence that one volatile anesthetic drug is preferable to another to control intraoperative hypertension.

A nitrous oxide–opioid technique can be used for maintenance of anesthesia, although it is likely that a volatile agent will be needed at times to control hypertension, for example, during periods of abrupt change in surgical stimulation. Antihypertensive medication by bolus or by continuous infusion is an alternative to the use of a volatile anesthetic for blood pressure control intraoperatively. There is no evidence that a specific neuromuscular blocker is best for patients with hypertension. Pancuronium can modestly increase blood pressure, but there is no evidence that this pressor response is exaggerated in the presence of essential hypertension.

Intraoperative Hypotension Hypotension during maintenance of anesthesia may be treated by decreasing the depth of anesthesia and/or by increasing fluid infusion rates. Sympathomimetic drugs such as ephedrine or phenylephrine may be necessary to restore vital organ perfusion pressures until the underlying cause of hypotension can be ascertained and corrected. Despite the suppressant effect of many antihypertensive drugs on the autonomic nervous system, extensive clinical experience has confirmed that the response to sympathomimetic drugs is both appropriate and predictable. Intraoperative hypotension in patients being treated with ACE inhibitors or ARBs is responsive to administration of intravenous fluids, sympathomimetic drugs, and/or vasopressin. Cardiac rhythm disturbances that result in loss of sequential atrioventricular contraction such as junctional rhythm and atrial fibrillation can also create hypotension and must be treated promptly.

Monitoring Monitoring in patients with essential hypertension is influenced by the complexity of the surgery. Electrocardiography is particularly useful in recognizing the occurrence of myocardial ischemia during periods of intense painful stimulation such as laryngoscopy and tracheal intubation. Invasive monitoring with an intra-arterial catheter and a central venous or pulmonary artery catheter may be useful if extensive surgery is planned and there is evidence of left ventricular dysfunction or other significant end-organ damage. Transesophageal echocardiography is an excellent monitor of left ventricular function and adequacy of intravascular volume replacement, but it requires specially trained personnel and equipment and may not be universally available.

Postoperative Management

Postoperative hypertension is common in patients with essential hypertension. This hypertension requires prompt assessment and treatment to decrease the risk of myocardial ischemia, cardiac dysrhythmias, congestive heart failure, stroke, and bleeding. Hypertension that persists despite adequate treatment of postoperative pain may necessitate administration of an intravenous antihypertensive medication such as labetalol. Gradually, conversion can be made to the patient's usual regimen of oral antihypertensive medication.

PULMONARY ARTERIAL HYPERTENSION

This section deals with idiopathic pulmonary arterial hypertension. (See Chapter 6 for a discussion of pulmonary hypertension associated with heart or lung disease.) Primary pulmonary hypertension (PAH) is a rare disease with an incidence of one to two cases per million people in the general population. While the majority of cases of pulmonary hypertension not associated with other medical conditions are sporadic, familial autosomal dominant inheritance accounts for 10% of these cases. The median period of survival after a diagnosis of idiopathic PAH is 2.8 years, with most patients succumbing to progressive right ventricular (RV) failure. Patients with idiopathic PAH are at risk of perioperative RV failure, hypoxemia, and coronary ischemia. Their risk may be as high as 28% for respiratory failure, 12% for cardiac dysrhythmias, 11% for congestive heart failure, and 7% for overall perioperative mortality for noncardiac surgery.

Definition

The pulmonary arteries normally have a systolic pressure of 18 to 25 mm Hg, a diastolic pressure of 6 to 10 mm Hg, and a mean pressure of 12 to 16 mm Hg. Pulmonary arterial hypertension is defined as a mean pulmonary artery pressure higher than 25 mm Hg at rest or higher than 30 mm Hg with exercise. Idiopathic PAH, previously called primary pulmonary hypertension, is that which occurs in the absence of left-sided heart disease, myocardial disease, congenital heart disease, and any clinically significant respiratory, connective tissue, or chronic thromboembolic disease. With idiopathic PAH, pulmonary artery occlusion pressure is no more than 15 mm Hg, and pulmonary vascular resistance (PVR) is higher than 3 Wood units (mm Hg/L/min) (**Table 5-9**). The 2003 Third World Symposium on Pulmonary Arterial Hypertension produced a document describing a new classification of pulmonary hypertension in Venice, Italy, as illustrated in **Table 5-10**.

TABLE 5-9	Calculation of Pulmonary Vascular Resistance
$\dfrac{(\overline{PAP} - PAOP) \times 80}{CO}$	PVR is expressed in dynes/sec/cm^{-5}, with normal PVR = 50–150 dynes/sec/cm^{-5}
$\dfrac{(\overline{PAP} - PAOP)}{CO}$	PVR is expressed in Wood units (mm Hg/L/min), with normal PVR = 1 Wood unit
CO, cardiac output (L/min); PAOP, pulmonary artery occlusion pressure (mm Hg); $\overline{PAP}$, mean pulmonary artery pressure (mm Hg);	

TABLE 5–10 Diagnostic Classification of Pulmonary Hypertension

1. Pulmonary arterial hypertension
   1.1 Idiopathic
   1.2 Familial
   1.3 Associated with . . .
      1.3.1 Collagen vascular disease
      1.3.2 Congenital systemic-to-pulmonary shunts
      1.3.3 Portal hypertension
      1.3.4 HIV infection
      1.3.5 Drugs and toxins
      1.3.6 Other (thyroid disorders, glycogen storage disease, Gaucher's disease, hereditary hemorrhagic telangiectasia, hemoglobinopathies, myeloproliferative disorders, splenectomy)
   1.4 Associated with significant venous or capillary involvement
      1.4.1 Pulmonary veno-occlusive disease
      1.4.2 Pulmonary capillary hemangiomatosis
   1.5 Persistent pulmonary hypertension of the newborn
2. Pulmonary hypertension with left heart disease
   2.1 Left-sided atrial or ventricular heart disease
   2.2 Left-sided valvular disease
3. Pulmonary hypertension associated with lung diseases and/or hypoxemia
   3.1 Chronic obstructive pulmonary disease
   3.2 Intersitital lung disease
   3.3 Sleep-disordered breathing
   3.4 Alveolar hypoventilation disorders
   3.5 Chronic exposure to high altitude
   3.6 Developmental abnormalities
4. Pulmonary hypertension due to chronic thrombotic and/or embolic disease
   4.1 Thromboembolic obstruction of proximal pulmonary arteries
   4.2 Thromboembolic obstruction of distal pulmonary arteries
   4.3 Nonthrombotic pulmonary embolism (tumor, parasites, foreign material)
5. Miscellaneous (sarcoidosis, histiocytosis X, lymphangiomatosis, compression of pulmonary vessels [adenopathy, tumor, fibrosing mediastinitis])

HIV, human immunodeficiency virus.
Reprinted with permission from Simonneau G, Galiè N, Rubin L J, et al: Clinical classification of pulmonary hypertension. J Am Coll Cardiol 2004;43(12 Suppl):5S–12S. Copyright 2004, the American College of Cardiology Foundation.

distention, peripheral edema, hepatomegaly, and ascites. The laboratory evaluation and diagnostic studies used in the workup of pulmonary hypertension of any cause are listed in **Table 5-11**. A 6-minute walk test can be administered to assess functional status and noninvasively follow the progress of therapy. Right heart catheterization provides a definitive means to determine disease severity and to ascertain which patients can respond to vasodilator therapy. A potent vasodilator such as prostacyclin, NO, adenosine,

TABLE 5–11 Clinical Findings in Pulmonary Hypertension

Diagnostic Modality	Key Findings
Chest radiograph	Prominent pulmonary arteries Right atrial and right ventricular enlargement Parenchymal lung disease
Electrocardiography	P pulmonale Right axis deviation Right ventricular strain or hypertrophy Complete or incomplete right bundle branch block
Two-dimensional echocardiography	Right atrial enlargement Right ventricular hypertrophy, dilation, or volume overload Tricuspid regurgitation Elevated estimated pulmonary artery pressures Congenital heart disease
Pulmonary function tests	Obstructive or restrictive pattern Low diffusing capacity
V/Q scan	Ventilation/perfusion mismatching
Pulmonary angiography	Vascular filling defects
Chest CT scan	Main pulmonary artery size > 30 mm Vascular filling defects Mosaic perfusion defects
Abdominal ultrasound or CT scan	Cirrhosis Portal hypertension
Blood tests	Antinuclear antibody Rheumatoid factor Complete blood count Coagulation profile HIV titers Thyroid-stimulating hormone
Sleep study	High respiratory disturbance index

CT, computed tomography; HIV, human immunodeficiency virus; V/Q, ventilation/perfusion.
Reprinted with permission from Dincer HE, Presberg KW: Current management of pulmonary hypertension. Clin Pulm Med 2004;11:40–53.

Clinical Presentation and Evaluation

PAH often presents with vague symptoms including breathlessness, weakness, fatigue, and abdominal distention. Syncope and angina pectoris are indicative of severe limitations of cardiac output and possible myocardial ischemia. On physical examination, the patient may exhibit a parasternal lift, murmurs of pulmonic insufficiency (Graham-Steell murmur) and/or tricuspid regurgitation, a pronounced pulmonic component of S2, an S3 gallop, jugular venous or prostaglandin E_1 is administered. The vasodilator test is considered positive, i.e., the patient is a responder, if PVR and mean pulmonary arterial pressure both decrease acutely by 20% or more. Only about one fourth of patients will have a favorable response to the vasodilator test.

Physiology and Pathophysiology

The normal pulmonary circulation can accommodate flow rates ranging from 6 to 25 L/min with minimal changes in pulmonary artery pressure. As a result of pulmonary vasoconstriction, vascular wall remodeling and thrombosis in situ, PAH develops. RV wall stress increases in response to the increase in afterload produced by pulmonary hypertension. Both RV stroke volume and the volume available for left ventricular filling are reduced, leading to low cardiac output and systemic hypotension. RV dilation in response to the increased wall stress results in annular dilation of right-sided heart valves producing tricuspid regurgitation and/or pulmonic insufficiency. The right ventricle receives coronary blood flow during both systole and diastole. RV myocardial perfusion

can be dramatically limited as RV wall stress increases and RV systolic pressure approaches systemic systolic pressure.

Patients with PAH are at risk of hypoxemia by three mechanisms: (1) as right-sided pressures increase, right-to-left shunting can occur through a patent foramen ovale; (2) in the presence of a relatively fixed cardiac output, the increased oxygen extraction associated with exertion will produce hypoxemia; and (3) V/Q mismatch can result in perfusion of poorly ventilated alveoli. If hypoxic pulmonary vasoconstriction occurs, overall pulmonary hypertension will be worsened.

Treatment of Pulmonary Hypertension

A sample treatment algorithm is summarized in **Figure 5-8**.

Oxygen, Anticoagulation, and Diuretics

Oxygen therapy can be helpful in reducing the magnitude of hypoxic pulmonary vasoconstriction. It has been studied primarily in patients with chronic obstructive pulmonary disease, and in this situation, it clearly improves survival and reduces progression of pulmonary hypertension.

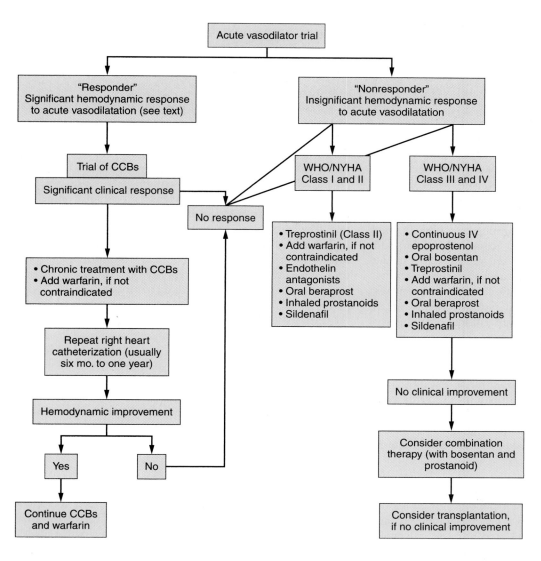

Figure 5-8 • Outpatient treatment of pulmonary arterial hypertension. CCBs, calcium channel blockers; NYHA, New York Heart Association; WHO, World Health Organization. *(Reprinted with permission from Dincer HE, Presberg KW: Current management of pulmonary hypertension. Clin Pulm Med 2004;11:40–53.)*

Anticoagulation may be recommended because of the increased risk of thrombosis and thromboembolism due to sluggish pulmonary blood flow, dilation of the right heart, venous stasis, and the limitation in physical activity imposed by this disease. Diuretics can be used to decrease preload in patients with right heart failure, especially when hepatic congestion, ascites, and severe peripheral edema are present.

Calcium Channel Blockers

The first class of drugs to provide dramatic long-term benefit in patients with PAH was calcium channel blockers. Calcium channel blockers are administered to patients who exhibit a positive response to a vasodilator trial in the cardiac catheterization laboratory. Nifedipine, diltiazem, and amlodipine are the most commonly used calcium channel blockers for this purpose and have been shown to improve 5-year survival.

Phosphodiesterase Inhibitors

Phosphodiesterase inhibitors produce pulmonary vasodilation and improve cardiac output. Sildenafil (Viagra) administration has been associated with improved exercise capacity and reduction in RV mass, although long-term mortality benefits have not yet been proven. Phosphodiesterase inhibitors inhibit the hydrolysis of cyclic guanosine monophosphate, reducing intracellular calcium concentration and effecting smooth muscle relaxation. They are effective when given alone and can augment the efficacy of inhaled NO.

Inhaled Nitric Oxide

Inhaled NO in concentrations of 20 to 40 ppm can be used to treat PAH. When inhaled, NO diffuses into vascular smooth muscle where it activates guanylate cyclase, increasing intracellular cyclic guanosine monophosphate, which reduces intracellular calcium concentration, resulting in smooth muscle relaxation. After diffusing into the intravascular space, NO binds to hemoglobin, forming nitrosylmethemoglobin, which is rapidly metabolized to methemoglobin and excreted by the kidneys. All NO is rendered inactive in the pulmonary circulation, thereby minimizing systemic effects. Because it is administered via inhalation, NO is preferentially distributed to well-ventilated alveoli, causing vasodilation in these areas. This improves ventilation/perfusion matching and improves oxygenation. NO has been shown to improve oxygenation and lower pulmonary arterial pressure in acute respiratory distress syndrome and in other conditions associated with severe pulmonary hypertension, but it has not been shown to reduce mortality in these situations. Problems associated with NO administration include rebound pulmonary hypertension, platelet inhibition, methemoglobinemia, formation of toxic nitrate metabolites, and the technical requirements for its application.

Prostacyclins

Prostacyclins are systemic and pulmonary vasodilators that also have antiplatelet activity. The prostacyclins reduce PVR and improve cardiac output and exercise tolerance. However, complications such as worsened intrapulmonary shunting, rebound pulmonary hypertension, and problems associated with the route of administration, such as systemic hypotension, infection, and bronchospasm, can occur. Prostacyclins can be administered by continuous infusion in the short term and the long term (by a pump attached to a permanent indwelling central venous catheter), by inhalation, and by intermittent subcutaneous injection. All prostacyclins demonstrate significant improvements in cardiopulmonary hemodynamics, at least in the short term, but have not yet provided evidence of sustained improvement or a decrease in mortality. Currently used prostacyclins include epoprostenol (Flolan), treprostinil (Remodulin), and iloprost (Ventalis).

Endothelin Receptor Antagonists

Endothelin interacts with two receptors: endothelin A and endothelin B. The endothelin A receptors cause pulmonary vasoconstriction and smooth muscle proliferation, whereas the endothelin B receptors produce vasodilation via enhanced endothelin clearance and increased production of NO and prostacyclin. Endothelin receptor antagonists have been shown to lower PA pressure and PVR and to improve RV function, exercise tolerance, quality of life, and mortality. The only endothelin receptor antagonist currently available for general use in the United States is bosentan (Tracleer).

Surgical Treatment

RV assist devices can be used in severe pulmonary hypertension and right heart failure. Balloon atrial septostomy is an investigational procedure that creates an atrial septal defect and allows right-to-left shunting of blood to decompress the right heart. At the expense of an expected and generally well-tolerated decrease in arterial oxygen saturation, it has been shown to improve exercise tolerance. Currently, this procedure is reserved for treatment of terminal right heart failure and as a bridge to cardiac transplantation. The benefits of extracorporeal membrane oxygenation are well established in children, but this modality has not found widespread use in the adult population. Lung transplantation is the only curative therapy for many types of PAH. Long-term survival is similar with single or bilateral lung transplantation.

Anesthetic Management

The risk of right heart failure is significantly increased in patients with PAH during the perioperative period. Mechanisms for this include increased RV afterload, hypoxemia, hypotension, and inadequate RV preload. Medications for PAH should be continued throughout the perioperative period. Continuous infusions of pulmonary vasodilators should be maintained at their usual doses to prevent rebound pulmonary hypertension. Diuretics may be needed to control edema, but excessive diuresis may dangerously reduce RV preload. Reduction in systemic vascular resistance by inhalational anesthetics or sedatives may be dangerous because of the relatively fixed cardiac output. Hypoxia, hypercarbia, and acidosis must be aggressively controlled because these conditions increase PVR. Maintenance of sinus rhythm is crucial. The atrial "kick" is necessary for adequate right and left ventricular filling.

Preoperative Preparation and Induction

In a patient with newly diagnosed PAH who is not yet on long-term therapy, administration of sildenafil or L-arginine preoperatively may be helpful. Patients on long-term pulmonary vasodilator therapy must have that therapy continued. Systems for inhalation of NO or prostacyclin should be immediately available. Sedatives should be used with caution because respiratory acidosis may increase PVR. Opioids, propofol, thiopental, and depolarizing or nondepolarizing neuromuscular blockers may all be used safely. Ketamine and etomidate may suppress some mechanisms of pulmonary vasorelaxation and should be avoided. Epidural anesthesia has been used for cesarean delivery and other suitable surgical procedures, but close attention must be paid to intravascular volume and systemic vascular resistance. It is also important to remember that prostacyclins and NO can inhibit platelet function. The level of regional anesthesia should be induced slowly and with invasive hemodynamic monitoring so that adjustment in cardiac variables can be made promptly.

Monitoring

Central venous catheterization is recommended, although care must be taken in the placement of central venous and pulmonary artery catheters because disruption of sinus rhythm by the catheter or wire can be a critical event. Intra-arterial blood pressure monitoring is recommended.

Maintenance

Inhalational anesthetics, neuromuscular blockers and opioids, except those associated with histamine release, can be used for maintenance of anesthesia. Hypotension can be corrected with norepinephrine, phenylephrine, or fluids. A potent pulmonary vasodilator such as milrinone, nitroglycerin, NO, or prostacyclin should be available to treat severe pulmonary hypertension should it develop. During mechanical ventilation, fluid balance and ventilator adjustments must be set to prevent a decrease in venous return.

Postoperative Period

Patients with PAH are at risk of sudden death in the early postoperative period due to worsening PAH, pulmonary thromboembolism, dysrhythmias, and fluid shifts. These patients must be monitored intensively in the postoperative period to help maintain hemodynamic variables and oxygenation at acceptable levels. Optimal pain control is an essential component of the postoperative care of these patients.

Obstetric Population

Forceps delivery to decrease patient effort is recommended. Nitroglycerin should be immediately available at the time of uterine involution because the return of uterine blood to the central circulation may be poorly tolerated in the parturient with PAH.

KEY POINTS

- The goal of pharmacologic therapy of hypertension is to decrease the systemic blood pressure to less than 140/90 mm Hg. However, in the presence of diabetes mellitus or renal disease, the goal is set at < 130/80 mm Hg.

- Preoperative evaluation of a patient with essential hypertension should determine the adequacy of blood pressure control, the antihypertensive drug therapy that has rendered the patient normotensive, and evaluation of possible target organ damage.

- Despite the desire to render patients normotensive before elective surgery, there is no evidence that the incidence of postoperative complications is increased when hypertensive patients (diastolic blood pressure as high as 110 mm Hg) undergo elective surgery.

- Hypotension requiring vasoconstrictor treatment occurs more often after induction of anesthesia in patients on long-term treatment with ACE inhibitors and ARBs than in those in whom such treatment has been discontinued on the day before surgery.

- Direct laryngoscopy and tracheal intubation may result in a significant increase in blood pressure in patients with essential hypertension, even if these patients have been treated with antihypertensive drugs and are rendered normotensive preoperatively.

- PAH is defined as a mean pulmonary artery pressure of > 25 mm Hg at rest or > 30 mm Hg with exercise.

- Smooth muscle hyperplasia, intimal fibrosis, medial hypertrophy, obliteration of smallblood vessels, and neoplastic forms of endothelial cell growth called plexiform lesions are all part of the pathophysiology of pulmonary hypertension. In addition, platelet function is enhanced, and in situ thrombosis is a common finding.

- NO diffuses into the vascular smooth muscle where it activates guanylate cyclase, increasing intracellular cyclic guanosine monophosphate, which reduces the intracellular calcium concentration resulting in smooth muscle relaxation.

- Calcium channel blockers, prostacyclins, NO, endothelin receptor blockers, and phosphodiesterase inhibitors are pulmonary vasodilators useful in the treatment of patients with PAH. All long-term pulmonary vasodilator therapy must be continued throughout the perioperative period.

- In the perioperative period, the risk of right heart failure or sudden death is significantly increased in patients with PAH. This may be due to increased RV afterload, inadequate RV preload, hypoxemia, hypotension, dysrhythmias, or pulmonary thromboembolism.

REFERENCES

Aggarwal M, Kahn I: Hypertensive crisis: Hypertensive emergencies and urgencies. Cardiol Clin 2006;24:135–146.

Bedford RF, Feinstein B: Hospital admission blood pressure: A predictor for hypertension following endotracheal intubation. Anesth Analg 1980;59:367–370.

Behina R, Molteni A, Igic R: Angiotensin-converting enzyme inhibitors: Mechanisms of action and implications in anesthesia practice. Curr Pharm Design 2003;9:763–776.

Bertrand M, Godet G, Meersschaert K, et al: Should the angiotensin II antagonists be discontinued before surgery? Anesth Analg 2001;92:26–30.

Blaise G, Langleben D, Hubert B: Pulmonary arterial hypertension: Pathophysiology and anesthetic approach. Anesthesiology 2003;99:1415–1432.

Brabant SM, Bertrand M, Eyraud D, et al: The hemodynamic effects of anesthetic induction in vascular surgical patients chronically treated with angiotensin II receptor antagonists. Anesth Analg 1999;88:1388–1392.

Colson P, Ryckwaert F, Coriat P: Renin angiotensin system antagonists and anesthesia. Anesth Analg 1999;89:1143–1155.

Dincer HE, Presberg KW: Current management of pulmonary hypertension. Clin Pulm Med 2004;11:40–53.

Galié N, Manes A, Branzi A: Evaluation of pulmonary arterial hypertension. Curr Opin Cardiol 2004;19:575–581.

Goldman L, Caldera DL: Risks of general anesthesia and elective operation in the hypertensive patient. Anesthesiology 1979;50:285–292.

Haj RM, Cinco JE, Mazer CD, et al: Treatment of pulmonary hypertension with selective pulmonary vasodilators. Curr Opin Anaesth 2006;19:88–95.

Hanada S, Kawakami H, Goto T, Morita S: Hypertension and anesthesia. Curr Opin Anesth 2006;19:315–319.

Howell SJ, Sear JW, Foëx P: Hypertension, hypertensive heart disease and perioperative cardiac risk. Br J Anaesth 2004;92:570–583.

Howell ST, Sear YM, Yates D, et al: Hypertension, admission blood pressure and perioperative cardiovascular risk. Anaesthesia 1996;51:1000–1004.

Licker M, Schweizer A, Hohn L, et al: Cardiovascular responses to anesthetic induction in patients chronically treated with angiotensin-converting enzyme inhibitors. Can J Anaesth 2000;47:433–440.

Moser M, Setaro JF: Resistant or difficult-to-control hypertension. JAMA 2006;355:385–392.

Peppard PE, Young T, Palta M, et al: Prospective study of the association between sleep-disordered breathing and hypertension. N Engl J Med 2000;342:1378–1384.

Prys-Roberts C: Anaesthesia and hypertension. Br J Anaesth 1984;56:711–724.

Ramakrishna G, Sprung J, Ravi BS, et al: Impact of pulmonary hypertension on the outcomes of noncardiac surgery: Predictors of perioperative morbidity and mortality. J Am Coll Cardiol 2005;45:1691–1699.

The Seventh Report of the Joint National Committee on Prevention, Detection, Evaluation, and Treatment of High Blood Pressure (JNC VII): NIH Publication No. 03-5233, December 2003. Also Hypertension 2003;42:1206–1252.

Steen PA, Tinker JH, Tarhan S: Myocardial reinfarction after anesthesia and surgery: An update: Incidence, mortality and predisposing factors. JAMA 1978;239:2566–2570.

Stone JG, Foex P, Sear JW, et al: Risk of myocardial ischaemia during anaesthesia in treated and untreated hypertensive patients. Br J Anaesth 1988;61:675–679.

Weksler N, Klein M, Szendro G, et al: The dilemma of preoperative hypertension: To treat and operate, or to postpone surgery? J Clin Anesth 2003;15:179–183.

CHAPTER 6

Heart Failure and Cardiomyopathies

Wanda M. Popescu

Peripartum Cardiomyopathy
- Signs and Symptoms
- Diagnosis
- Treatment
- Prognosis
- Management of Anesthesia

Secondary Cardiomyopathies with Restrictive Physiology
- Signs and Symptoms
- Diagnosis
- Treatment
- Prognosis
- Management of Anesthesia

Cor Pulmonale
- Pathophysiology
- Signs and Symptoms
- Diagnosis
- Treatment
- Prognosis

Management of Anesthesia
- Preoperative Management
- Intraoperative Management
- Postoperative Management

HEART FAILURE

Definition

Heart failure is a complex pathophysiologic state described by the inability of the heart to fill with or eject blood at a rate appropriate to meet tissue requirements. The clinical syndrome is characterized by symptoms of dyspnea and fatigue and signs of circulatory congestion or hypoperfusion.

Epidemiology and Costs

Heart failure is a major health problem in the United States, affecting about 5 million adults. Each year an additional 550,000 patients are diagnosed with heart failure. Heart failure is mainly a disease of the elderly so aging of the population contributes to its increased incidence. The incidence of heart failure approaches 10 per 1000 in the population age 65 or older. Systolic heart failure (SHF) is more common among middle-aged men due to the high incidence of coronary artery disease (CAD). Diastolic heart failure (DHF) is usually seen in elderly women due to the increased incidence of hypertension, obesity, and diabetes after menopause.

Heart failure is the most common Medicare hospital discharge diagnosis. More Medicare dollars are spent on the diagnosis and treatment of heart failure than on any other disease. It is estimated that yearly the total direct and indirect cost of heart failure in the United States is 38 billion dollars.

Etiology

Heart failure is a clinical syndrome arising from diverse causes. The principal pathophysiology of heart failure is the inability of the heart to fill or empty the ventricle. Heart failure is most often due to (1) impaired myocardial contractility secondary to ischemic heart disease or cardiomyopathy; (2) cardiac valve abnormalities; (3) systemic hypertension; (4) diseases of the pericardium; or (5) pulmonary hypertension (cor pulmonale). The most common cause of right ventricular failure is left ventricular (LV) failure.

FORMS OF VENTRICULAR DYSFUNCTION

Heart failure may be described in various ways: systolic or diastolic, acute or chronic, left sided or right sided, high output or low output. Early in the course of heart failure, the various categories may have different clinical and therapeutic implications. Ultimately, however, all forms of heart failure develop high ventricular end-diastolic pressure due to altered ventricular function and neurohormonal regulation.

SYSTOLIC AND DIASTOLIC HEART FAILURE

Decreased ventricular systolic wall motion reflects systolic dysfunction, whereas diastolic dysfunction is characterized by abnormal ventricular relaxation and reduced compliance. There are differences in both myocardial architecture and function in SHF and DHF. Clinical signs and symptoms do not reliably differentiate systolic dysfunction from diastolic dysfunction.

Systolic Heart Failure

Causes of SHF include CAD, dilated cardiomyopathy (DCM), chronic pressure overload (aortic stenosis and chronic hypertension), and chronic volume overload (regurgitant valvular lesions and high output cardiac failure). CAD typically results in regional defects in ventricular contraction, which may become global over time, whereas all other causes of SHF produce global ventricular dysfunction. Ventricular dysrhythmias are common in patients with LV dysfunction. Patients with left bundle branch block and SHF are at high risk of sudden death.

A decreased ejection fraction, the hallmark of chronic LV systolic dysfunction, is closely related to the increase in the diastolic volume of the left ventricle (**Fig. 6-1**). Measuring the LV ejection fraction via echocardiography, radionuclide imaging or ventriculography provides the quantification necessary to document the severity of ventricular systolic dysfunction.

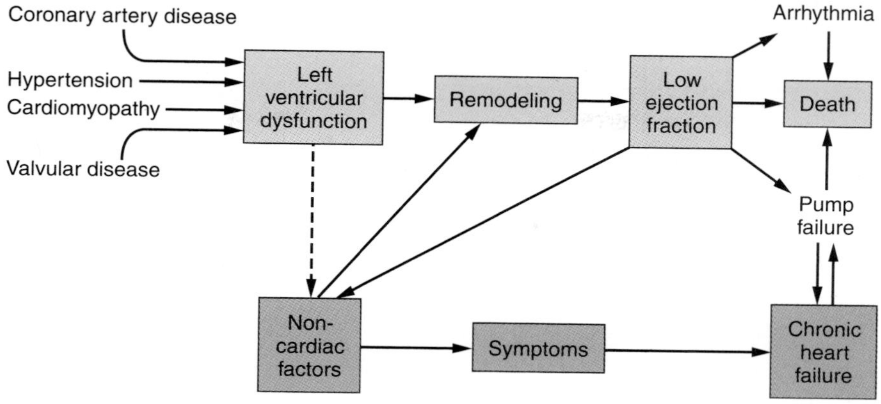

Figure 6-1 • Left ventricular dysfunction regardless of cause, results in progressive remodeling of the ventricular chamber leading to dilation and a low ejection fraction. Cardiac dysrhythmias, progressive cardiac failure, and premature death are likely. Noncardiac factors such as neurohormonal stimulation, vasoconstriction, and renal sodium retention may be stimulated by left ventricular dysfunction and ultimately contribute to remodeling of the left ventricle and to the symptoms (dyspnea, fatigue, edema) considered characteristic of the clinical syndrome of congestive heart failure. *(Adapted from Cohn JN: The management of chronic heart failure. N Engl J Med 1996;335:490–498. Copyright 1996 Massachusetts Medical Society.)*

Diastolic Heart Failure

Symptomatic heart failure in patients with normal or near-normal LV systolic function is most likely due to diastolic dysfunction. However, DHF may co-exist in patients with SHF. The prevalence of DHF is age dependent, increasing from less than 15% in patients younger than 45 years of age to 35% in those between the ages of 50 and 70 years to more than 50% in patients older than 70 years. DHF can be classified into four stages. Class I DHF is characterized by an abnormal LV relaxation pattern with normal left atrial pressure. Classes II, III, and IV are characterized by abnormal relaxation as well as reduced LV compliance resulting in an increase in LV end-diastolic pressure (LVEDP). As a compensatory mechanism, the pressure in the left atrium increases so that LV filling can occur despite the increase in LVEDP. Factors that predispose to decreased ventricular distensibility include myocardial edema, fibrosis, hypertrophy, aging, and pressure overload. Ischemic heart disease, long-standing essential hypertension, and progressive aortic stenosis are the most common causes of DHF. In contrast to SHF, DHF affects women more than men. Hospitalization and mortality rates are similar in patients with SHF and DHF. The major differences between SHF and DHF are presented in **Table 6-1**.

ACUTE AND CHRONIC HEART FAILURE

Acute heart failure is defined as a change in the signs and symptoms of heart failure requiring emergency therapy. Chronic heart failure is present in patients with long-standing cardiac disease. Typically, chronic heart failure is accompanied by venous congestion, but blood pressure is maintained. In acute heart failure due to a sudden decrease in cardiac output, systemic hypotension is typically present without signs of peripheral edema. Acute heart failure encompasses three clinical entities: (1) worsening chronic heart failure; (2) new-onset heart failure such as with cardiac valve rupture, large myocardial infarction, or severe hypertensive crisis; and (3) terminal heart failure, which is refractory to therapy.

LEFT-SIDED AND RIGHT-SIDED HEART FAILURE

The clinical signs and symptoms of heart failure are produced by increased ventricular pressures and subsequent fluid accumulation upstream from the affected ventricle. In left-sided heart failure, high LVEDP promotes pulmonary venous congestion. The patient complains of dyspnea, orthopnea, and paroxysmal nocturnal dyspnea, which can evolve to pulmonary edema. Right-sided heart failure causes systemic venous congestion. Peripheral edema and congestive hepatomegaly are the most prominent clinical manifestations. Right-sided heart failure may be caused by pulmonary hypertension or right ventricular myocardial infarction, but the most common cause is left-sided heart failure.

LOW-OUTPUT AND HIGH-OUTPUT HEART FAILURE

The normal cardiac index varies between 2.2 and 3.5 L/min/m². It may be difficult to diagnose low-output heart failure because a patient may have a cardiac index that is nearly normal in the resting state but does not respond adequately to stress or exercise. The most common causes of low-output heart failure are CAD, cardiomyopathy, hypertension, valvular disease, and pericardial disease.

Causes of high cardiac output include anemia, pregnancy, arteriovenous fistulas, severe hyperthyroidism, beriberi, and Paget's disease. The ventricle fails not only because of the increased hemodynamic burden placed on it but also because of direct myocardial toxicity as caused by thyrotoxicosis and beriberi and myocardial anoxia caused by severe and prolonged anemia.

TABLE 6-1 Characteristics of Patients with Diastolic Heart Failure and Patients with Systolic Heart Failure

Characteristic	Diastolic Heart Failure	Systolic Heart Failure
Age	Frequently elderly	Typically 50–70 years old
Sex	Frequently female	More often male
Left ventricular ejection fraction	Preserved, ≥40%	Depressed, ≤40%
Left ventricular cavity size	Usually normal, often with concentric left ventricular hypertrophy	Usually dilated
Chest radiography	Congestion ± cardiomegaly	Congestion and cardiomegaly
Gallop rhythm present	Fourth heart sound	Third heart sound
Hypertension	+++	++
Diabetes mellitus	+++	++
Previous myocardial infarction	+	+++
Obesity	+++	+
Chronic lung disease	++	0
Sleep apnea	++	++
Dialysis	++	0
Atrial fibrillation	+ Usually paroxysmal	+ Usually persistent

+, occasionally associated with; ++, often associated with; +++, usually associated with; 0, no association.

PATHOPHYSIOLOGY OF HEART FAILURE

Heart failure is a complex phenomenon at both the clinical and cellular levels. Our understanding of the pathophysiology of heart failure is in constant evolution. The initiating mechanisms of heart failure are pressure overload (aortic stenosis, essential hypertension), volume overload (mitral or aortic regurgitation), myocardial ischemia/infarction, myocardial inflammatory disease, and restricted diastolic filling (constrictive pericarditis, restrictive myocarditis). In the failing ventricle, various adaptive mechanisms are initiated to help maintain a normal cardiac output. These include (1) the Frank-Starling relationship; (2) activation of the sympathetic nervous system (SNS); (3) alterations in the inotropic state, heart rate, and afterload; and (4) humoral-mediated responses. In more advanced stages of heart failure, these mechanisms become maladaptive and ultimately lead to myocardial remodeling, which is the key pathophysiologic change responsible for the development and progression of heart failure.

Frank-Starling Relationship

The Frank-Starling relationship describes the increase in stroke volume that accompanies an increase in LV end-diastolic volume and pressure (**Fig. 6-2**). Stroke volume increases because the tension developed by contracting muscle is greater when the resting length of that muscle is increased. The magnitude of the increase in stroke volume produced by changing the tension of ventricular muscle fibers depends on myocardial contractility. For example, when myocardial contractility is decreased, as in the presence of heart failure, a lesser increase in stroke volume is achieved

relative to any given increase in LV end-diastolic pressure (see **Fig. 6-2**). Constriction of venous capacitance vessel shifts blood centrally, increases preload, and helps maintain cardiac output by the Frank-Starling relationship.

Activation of Sympathetic Nervous System

Activation of the SNS promotes arteriolar and venous constriction. Arteriolar constriction serves to maintain systemic blood pressure despite a decrease in cardiac output. Increased venous tone shifts blood from peripheral sites to the central circulation, thereby enhancing venous return and maintaining cardiac output by the Frank-Starling relationship. Furthermore, arteriolar constriction causes redistribution of blood

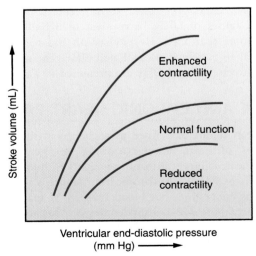

Figure 6-2 • Frank-Starling relationship states that stroke volume is directly related to the ventricular end-diastolic pressure.

from the kidneys, splanchnic organs, skeletal muscles, and skin to maintain coronary and cerebral blood flow despite overall decreases in cardiac output. The decrease in renal blood flow activates the renin-angiotensin-aldosterone system (RAAS), which increases renal tubular reabsorption of sodium and water, resulting in an increase in blood volume and ultimately cardiac output by the Frank-Starling relationship. These compensatory responses may be effective in the short term, but they contribute to the deterioration of heart failure in the long term. For example, fluid retention, increased venous return, and increased afterload can impose more work on the failing myocardium, increase myocardial energy expenditure, and further reduce cardiac output and tissue perfusion. Interruption of this vicious circle is the purpose of the current therapeutic strategies for heart failure.

Although heart failure is associated with SNS activation, a down-regulation of β-adrenergic receptors is observed. Plasma and urinary concentrations of catecholamines are increased in patients in heart failure and correlate with worse clinical outcomes. High plasma levels of norepinephrine are directly cardiotoxic and promote myocyte necrosis and cell death, which lead to ventricular remodeling. Therapy with β-blockers attempts to decreases these deleterious effects of catecholamines on the heart.

Alterations in the Inotropic State, Heart Rate, and Afterload

The inotropic state describes myocardial contractility as reflected by the velocity of contraction developed by cardiac muscle. The maximum velocity of contraction is referred to as V_{max}. When the inotropic state of the heart is increased, as in the presence of catecholamines, V_{max} is increased. Conversely, V_{max} is decreased when myocardial contractility is impaired as in heart failure.

Afterload is the tension the ventricular muscle must develop to open the aortic or pulmonic valve. The afterload presented to the left ventricle is increased in the presence of systemic arteriolar constriction and hypertension. The forward LV stroke volume in patients with heart failure can be increased by administering vasodilating drugs.

In the presence of SHF and low cardiac output, the stroke volume is relatively fixed with any increase in CO being dependent on an increase in heart rate. Tachycardia is an expected finding in the presence of SHF with a low ejection fraction and reflects activation of the sympathetic nervous system. However, in the presence of DHF, tachycardia can produce a decrease in CO due to inadequate ventricular filling time. Therefore, heart rate control is a target for therapy of DHF.

Humoral-Mediated Responses and Biochemical Pathways

As heart failure progresses, various neurohumoral pathways are activated in order to maintain adequate cardiac output during exercise and ultimately even at rest. Generalized

vasoconstriction is initiated via several mechanisms including increased activity of the SNS and RAAS, parasympathetic withdrawal, high levels of circulating vasopressin, endothelial dysfunction, and release of inflammatory mediators.

In an attempt to counterbalance these mechanisms, the heart evolves into "an endocrine organ." This concept emerged more than 20 years ago when Bold and colleagues reported the presence of a potent diuretic and vasodilator in the atria of rats. Atrial natriuretic peptide is stored in atrial muscle and released in response to increases in atrial pressures, such as produced by tachycardia or hypervolemia. More recently, B-type natriuretic peptide (BNP) was discovered. It is secreted by both the atrial and ventricular myocardium. In the failing heart, the ventricle becomes the principal site for BNP production. The natriuretic peptides promote blood pressure control and protect the cardiovascular system from the effects of volume and pressure overload. Physiologic effects of the natriuretic peptides include diuresis, natriuresis, vasodilation, antihypertrophy, anti-inflammation, and inhibition of the RAAS and SNS. The responsiveness to elevated levels of endogenous natriuretic peptides is blunted over time in heart failure. However, exogenous administration of BNP can be useful in the treatment of acute heart failure.

Myocardial Remodeling

Myocardial remodeling is the result of the various endogenous mechanisms that the body uses to maintain cardiac output. It is the process by which mechanical, neurohormonal, and genetic factors change the LV size, shape, and function. The process includes myocardial hypertrophy, myocardial dilation and wall thinning, increased interstitial collagen deposition, myocardial fibrosis, and scar formation due to myocyte death. Myocardial hypertrophy represents the compensatory mechanism to chronic pressure overload. This mechanism is limited because hypertrophied cardiac muscle functions at a lower inotropic state than normal cardiac muscle. Cardiac dilation occurs in response to volume overload and increases the CO by the Frank-Starling relationship. However, increased cardiac wall tension produced by the enlarged ventricular radius is also associated with increased myocardial oxygen requirements and decreased cardiac efficiency. The most common cause of myocardial remodeling is ischemic injury, and it encompasses both hypertrophy and dilation of the left ventricle. Angiotensin-converting enzyme inhibitors (ACEIs) have been proven to promote a "reverse-remodeling" process. Therefore, they are first-line therapy for heart failure.

SIGNS AND SYMPTOMS OF HEART FAILURE

The hemodynamic consequences of heart failure are decreased cardiac output, increased LVEDP, peripheral vasoconstriction, retention of sodium and water, and decreased oxygen delivery to the tissues with a widened arterial-venous oxygen difference. LV failure results in signs and symptoms of pulmonary edema, whereas right ventricular failure results in systemic venous hypertension and peripheral edema. Patient fatigue and organ system dysfunction are related to inadequate CO.

Symptoms of Heart Failure

Dyspnea reflects increased work of breathing due to stiffness of the lungs produced by interstitial pulmonary edema. It is one of the earliest subjective findings of LV failure. Initially, this symptom occurs only with exertion. It can be quantified by asking the patient how many flights of stairs can be climbed or the distance that can be walked at a normal pace before dyspnea occurs. Patients experiencing angina pectoris may interpret substernal discomfort as breathlessness. Dyspnea can be caused by many other diseases such as asthma, chronic obstructive pulmonary disease (COPD), airway obstruction, anxiety, and neuromuscular weakness. Dyspnea related to heart failure will be linked to other supporting evidence such as a history of orthopnea, paroxysmal nocturnal dyspnea, a third heart sound, rales on physical examination, and elevated BNP levels.

Orthopnea reflects the inability of the failing left ventricle to handle the increased venous return associated with the recumbent position. Clinically, this will be manifested as a dry, nonproductive cough that develops when in the supine position and that is relieved by sitting up. The orthopneic cough differs from the productive morning cough characteristic of patients with chronic bronchitis and must be differentiated from the cough produced by ACEIs. Paroxysmal nocturnal dyspnea is shortness of breath that awakens a patient from sleep. This symptom must be differentiated from anxiety-provoked hyperventilation or wheezing due to accumulation of secretions in patients with chronic bronchitis. Paroxysmal nocturnal dyspnea and wheezing caused by pulmonary congestion ("cardiac asthma") are accompanied by radiographic evidence of pulmonary congestion.

A hallmark of decreased cardiac reserve and low cardiac output is fatigue and weakness at rest or with minimal exertion. During exercise, the failing ventricle is unable to increase its output in order to deliver adequate amounts of oxygen to the muscles. These findings, although nonspecific, are very common in patients with heart failure.

Heart failure patients may complain of anorexia, nausea, or abdominal pain related to increased liver congestion and prerenal azotemia. Decreases in cerebral blood flow may produce confusion, difficulty concentrating, insomnia, anxiety, or memory deficits. Nocturia may contribute to insomnia.

Physical Examination

The classic physical findings in patients with LV failure are tachypnea and the presence of moist rales. These rales may be confined to the lung bases in patients with a mild degree of LV failure, or they may be diffuse in those with acute pulmonary edema. Other findings in heart failure include resting tachycardia and a third heart sound (S_3 gallop or ventricular diastolic gallop). This heart sound is produced by blood entering and distending a relatively noncompliant left ventricle. Despite peripheral vasoconstriction, severe heart failure

may manifest as systemic hypotension with cool and pale extremities. Lip and nail bed cyanosis may be present. A narrow pulse pressure with a high diastolic pressure reflects a decreased stroke volume. Marked weight loss, also known as cardiac cachexia, is a sign of severe chronic heart failure. Weight loss is caused by a combination of factors including an increase in the metabolic rate, anorexia and nausea, decreased intestinal absorption of food caused by splanchnic venous congestion, and the presence of high levels of circulating cytokines.

In the presence of right heart or biventricular failure, jugular venous distention may be present or inducible by pressing on the liver (hepatojugular reflux). The liver is typically the first organ to become engorged with blood in the presence of right or biventricular failure. The hepatic engorgement may be associated with right upper quadrant pain and tenderness or even jaundice in severe cases. Pleural effusions (usually right sided) may be present. Bilateral pitting pretibial leg edema is typically present with right ventricular failure and reflects both venous congestion and sodium and water retention.

DIAGNOSIS OF HEART FAILURE

The diagnosis of heart failure is based on the history, physical examination, and interpretation of laboratory and diagnostic tests. The signs and symptoms of heart failure have already been noted.

Laboratory Diagnosis

The differential diagnosis of dyspnea can be difficult. The use of serum BNP as a biomarker for heart failure has helped physicians establish the etiology of dyspnea. Plasma BNP levels below 100 pg/mL indicate that heart failure is unlikely (90% negative predictive value); BNP in the range of 100 to 500 pg/mL suggests an intermediate probability for heart failure; levels above 500 pg/mL are consistent with the diagnosis of heart failure (90% positive predictive value). Plasma levels of BNP may be affected by other factors such as sex, advanced age, renal clearance, obesity, pulmonary embolism, atrial fibrillation, and/or other cardiac tachydysrhythmias. Therefore, these factors have an impact on the interpretation of BNP levels.

A complete metabolic profile is indicated in the evaluation of patients with heart failure. Decreases in renal blood flow may lead to prerenal azotemia characterized by a disproportionate increase in blood urea nitrogen concentration relative to the serum creatinine concentration. When moderate liver congestion is present, liver function tests may be mildly elevated, and when liver engorgement is severe, the prothrombin time may be prolonged. Hyponatremia, hypomagnesemia, and hypokalemia may be present.

Electrocardiography

Patients with heart failure usually have an abnormal 12-lead electrocardiogram (ECG). Therefore, this test has a low predictive value for the diagnosis of heart failure. The ECG may show evidence of a previous myocardial infarction, LV hypertrophy, conduction abnormalities (left bundle branch block, widened QRS), or various cardiac dysrhythmias, especially atrial fibrillation and ventricular dysrhythmias.

Chest Radiography

Chest radiography (posteroanterior and lateral) may be useful in the evaluation of a heart failure patient by detecting the presence of pulmonary disease, cardiomegaly, pulmonary venous congestion, and interstitial or alveolar pulmonary edema. An early radiographic sign of LV failure and associated pulmonary venous hypertension is distention of the pulmonary veins in the upper lobes of the lungs. Perivascular edema appears as hilar or perihilar haze. The hilus appears large with ill-defined margins. Kerley lines, reflecting edematous interlobular septae in the upper lung fields (Kerley A lines), lower lung fields (Kerley B lines), or basilar regions of the lungs producing a honeycomb pattern (Kerley C lines) may also be present. Alveolar edema produces homogeneous densities in the lung fields, typically in a butterfly pattern. Pleural effusion and pericardial effusion may be observed. Radiographic evidence of pulmonary edema may lag behind the clinical evidence of pulmonary edema by up to 12 hours. Likewise, radiographic patterns of pulmonary congestion may persist for several days after normalization of cardiac filling pressures and resolution of symptoms.

Echocardiography

Echocardiography is the most useful test in the diagnosis of heart failure. A comprehensive two-dimensional echocardiogram coupled with Doppler flow examination can assess whether any abnormalities of the myocardium, cardiac valves, or pericardium are present. This examination addresses the following topics: ejection fraction, LV structure and functionality, the presence of other structural abnormalities such as valvular and pericardial disease and the presence of diastolic dysfunction and right ventricular function. This information can be presented as numerical estimates of ejection fraction, LV size and wall thickness, left atrial size, and pulmonary artery pressure. Assessment of diastolic function provides information about LV filling and left atrial pressure. A preoperative echocardiographic evaluation can serve as a baseline for comparison with perioperative echocardiography if a patient's condition deteriorates.

CLASSIFICATION OF HEART FAILURE

Heart failure has been classified in various ways. The most commonly used classification is that of the New York Heart Association and is based on the functional status of the patient at a particular time. Functional status may worsen or improve. These patients have structural heart disease and symptoms of heart failure. There are four functional classes:

Class I: Ordinary physical activity does not cause symptoms
Class II: Symptoms occur with ordinary exertion
Class III: Symptoms occur with less than ordinary exertion
Class IV: Symptoms occur at rest

This classification is useful because the severity of the symptoms has an excellent correlation with survival and quality of life. However, the American College of Cardiology and the American Heart Association published the 2005 Guideline Update for the Diagnosis and Management of Chronic Heart Failure and introduced a new classification based on the progression of the disease. This classification has four stages:

Stage A: Patients at high risk of heart failure but without structural heart disease or symptoms of heart failure
Stage B: Patients with structural heart disease but without symptoms of heart failure
Stage C: Patients with structural heart disease with previous or current symptoms of heart failure
Stage D: Patients with refractory heart failure requiring specialized interventions

This classification is meant to be complementary to the New York Heart Association classification and to be used in guiding therapy.

MANAGEMENT OF HEART FAILURE

Current therapeutic strategies are aimed at reversing the pathophysiologic alterations present in heart failure and at interrupting the vicious circle of maladaptive mechanisms (**Fig. 6-3**). Short-term therapeutic goals in patients with heart failure include relieving symptoms of circulatory congestion, increasing tissue perfusion, and improving the quality of life. However, management of heart failure involves more than the treatment of symptoms. The processes that contributed to the LV dysfunction may progress independently of the development of symptoms. Therefore, the long-term therapeutic goal is to prolong life by slowing or reversing the progression of ventricular remodeling.

Management of Chronic Heart Failure

The current recommended therapy of chronic heart failure is based on results of large, adequately powered, randomized trials and on the American College of Cardiology/American Heart Association and European Society of Cardiology guidelines for the diagnosis and treatment of chronic heart failure. According to these guidelines, treatment options include lifestyle modification, patient and family education, medical therapy, corrective surgery, implantable devices, and cardiac transplantation (**Fig. 6-4**).

Lifestyle modifications are aimed at decreasing the risk of heart disease and include smoking cessation, a healthy diet with moderate sodium restriction, weight control, exercise, moderate alcohol consumption, and adequate glycemic control.

Management of Systolic Heart Failure

The major classes of drugs used for medical management of SHF include inhibitors of RAAS, β-adrenergic blockers, diuretics, digoxin, vasodilators, and statins. Most heart

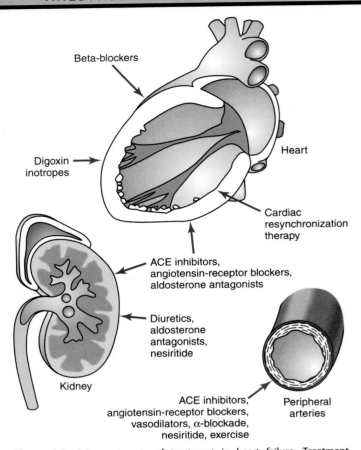

Beta-blockers

Digoxin
inotropes

Heart

Cardiac
resynchronization
therapy

ACE inhibitors,
angiotensin-receptor blockers,
aldosterone antagonists

Diuretics,
aldosterone
antagonists,
nesiritide

Kidney

ACE inhibitors,
angiotensin-receptor blockers,
vasodilators, α-blockade,
nesiritide, exercise

Peripheral
arteries

Figure 6-3 • Primary targets of treatment in heart failure. Treatment options for patients with heart failure affect the pathophysiologic mechanisms that are stimulated in heart failure. Angiotensin-converting enzyme inhibitors (ACEIs) and angiotensin II receptor blockers decrease afterload by interfering with the renin-angiotensin-aldosterone system, resulting in peripheral vasodilation. They also affect left ventricular hypertrophy, remodeling, and renal blood flow. Aldosterone production by the adrenal glands is increased in heart failure. It stimulates renal sodium retention and potassium excretion and promotes ventricular and vascular hypertrophy. Aldosterone antagonists counteract the many effects of aldosterone. Diuretics decrease preload by stimulating natriuresis in the kidneys. Digoxin affects the $Na^+K^+ATPase$ pump in the myocardial cell, increasing contractility. Inotropes such as dobutamine and milrinone increase myocardial contractility. β-Blockers inhibit the sympathetic nervous system and adrenergic receptors. They slow the heart rate, decrease blood pressure, and have a direct beneficial effect on the myocardium by enhancing reverse remodeling. Selected agents that also block α-adrenergic receptors can cause vasodilation. Vasodilator therapy such as combination therapy with hydralazine and isosorbide dinitrate decreases afterload by counteracting peripheral vasoconstriction. Cardiac resynchronization therapy with biventricular pacing improves left ventricular function and favors reverse remodeling. Nesiritide (brain natriuretic peptide) decreases preload by stimulating diuresis and decreases afterload by vasodilation. Exercise improves peripheral blood flow by eventually counteracting peripheral vasoconstriction. It also improves skeletal-muscle physiology. *(Reproduced with permission from Jessup M, Brozena S: Heart failure. N Engl J Med 2003;348:2007–2018. Copyright © 2003 Massachusetts Medical Society. All rights reserved.)*

failure patients are managed on a combination of drugs. Therapy with ACEIs and β-blockers favorably influences long-term outcome.

Inhibitors of the Renin-Angiotensin-Aldosterone System

Inhibition of the RAAS can be performed at several levels: by inhibiting the enzyme that converts angiotensin I to angiotensin II, by blocking the angiotensin II receptor, or by blocking the aldosterone receptor.

Angiotensin-Converting Enzyme Inhibitors

ACEIs block the conversion of angiotensin I to angiotensin II. This decreases the activation of the RAAS and decreases the degradation of bradykinin. Beneficial effects include promoting vasodilation, reducing water and sodium reabsorption, and supporting potassium conservation. This class of drugs has been proven to decrease ventricular remodeling and even to potentiate the "reverse-remodeling" phenomenon. In large clinical trials, ACEIs have consistently been shown to reduce morbidity and mortality of patients in any stage of heart failure. For this reason, they are considered the first line of treatment in heart failure. It appears, however, that the African American population does not derive as much clinical benefit from ACEI therapy as the white population. Side effects of ACEIs include hypotension, syncope, renal dysfunction, hyperkalemia, and development of a nonproductive cough and angioedema. Treatment with ACEIs should be started at low doses to avoid significant hypotension. Then the dose can be gradually increased until the target dose defined by clinical trials is reached.

Angiotensin II Receptor Blockers

As their name implies, angiotensin receptor blockers block angiotensin II receptors. These drugs have similar but not superior efficacy compared to ACEIs. Currently, angiotensin receptor blockers are only recommended for patients who cannot tolerate ACEIs. In some patients treated with ACEIs, angiotensin levels may return to normal due to alternative pathways of angiotensin production. Such patients may benefit from the addition of an angiotensin receptor blocker to the medical therapy.

Aldosterone Antagonists

In advanced stages of heart failure, there are high circulating levels of aldosterone. Aldosterone stimulates sodium and water retention, hypokalemia, and ventricular remodeling. Spironolactone, an aldosterone antagonist, may reverse all these effects. There is strong clinical evidence showing reduced mortality and hospitalization rates with the use of a low dose of aldosterone antagonist in New York Heart Association class III and IV patients. During therapy with spironolactone, patients should have renal function and potassium levels monitored and the dose of spironolactone adjusted accordingly.

β-Blockers

β-Blockers are used to reverse the harmful effects of SNS activation in heart failure. Recent clinical trials have

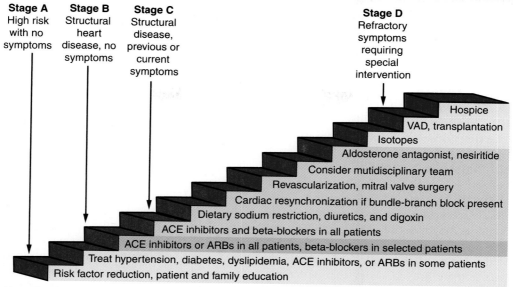

Figure 6-4 • Stages of heart failure and treatment options for systolic heart failure. Patients with stage A heart failure are at high risk of heart failure but do not yet have structural heart disease or symptoms of heart failure. This group includes patients with hypertension, diabetes, coronary artery disease, previous exposure to cardiotoxic drugs, or a family history of cardiomyopathy. Patients with stage B heart failure have structural heart disease but no symptoms of heart failure. This group includes patients with left ventricular hypertrophy, previous myocardial infarction, left ventricular systolic dysfunction, or valvular heart disease, all of whom would be considered to have New York Heart Association (NYHA) class I symptoms. Patients with stage C heart failure have known structural heart disease and current or previous symptoms of heart failure. Their current symptoms may be classified as NYHA class I, II, III, or IV. Patients with stage D heart failure have refractory symptoms of heart failure at rest despite maximal medical therapy, are hospitalized, and require specialized interventions or hospice care. All such patients would be considered to have NYHA class IV symptoms. ACE, angiotensin-converting enzyme; ARB, angiotensin receptor blocker; VAD, ventricular assist device. *(Reproduced with permission from Jessup M, Brozena S: Heart failure. N Engl J Med 2003;348:2007–2018. Copyright © 2003 Massachusetts Medical Society. All rights reserved.)*

consistently shown that these drugs reduce morbidity and the number of hospitalizations and improve both quality of life and survival. β-Blockers improve the ejection fraction and decrease ventricular remodeling. American College of Cardiology and the American Heart Association guidelines recommend β-blockers as an integral part of the therapy for heart failure. Caution should be used when administering β-blockers to patients with reactive airway disease, diabetics with frequent hypoglycemic episodes, and patients with bradydysrhythmias or heart block.

Diuretics

Diuretics can relieve circulatory congestion and the accompanying pulmonary and peripheral edema more rapidly than any other drugs. Symptomatic improvement can be noted within hours. Diuretic-induced decreases in ventricular diastolic pressure will decrease diastolic ventricular wall stress and prevent the persistent cardiac distention that interferes with subendocardial perfusion and negatively affects myocardial metabolism and function. Thiazide and/or loop diuretics are recommended as an essential part of the therapy of heart failure. Potassium and magnesium supplementation may be needed in patients chronically treated with diuretics in order to prevent cardiac dysrhythmias. Excessive doses of diuretics may cause hypovolemia, prerenal azotemia, or an undesirably low cardiac output and are associated with worse clinical outcomes.

Digitalis

Digitalis enhances the inotropy of cardiac muscle and decreases activation of the SNS and the RAAS. These latter effects are related to the ability of digitalis to restore the inhibitory effects of cardiac baroreceptors on central SNS outflow. It is unclear whether digitalis treatment improves survival, but digoxin may impede the worsening of heart failure and result in fewer hospitalizations. Digitalis can be added to standard therapy when patients are still symptomatic despite treatments with diuretics, ACEIs, and β-blockers. Patients with the combination of atrial fibrillation and heart failure present another subgroup that may benefit from digoxin therapy. Caution should be used when administering this drug to elderly patients or to those with impaired renal function since they are particularly prone to development of digitalis toxicity. Manifestations of digitalis toxicity include anorexia, nausea, blurred vision, and cardiac dysrhythmias. Treatment of toxicity may include reversing hypokalemia, treating cardiac dysrhythmias, administering antidigoxin antibodies, and/or placing a temporary cardiac pacemaker.

Vasodilators

Vasodilator therapy relaxes vascular smooth muscle, decreases resistance to LV ejection, and increases venous capacitance. In patients with dilated left ventricles, administration of vasodilators results in increased stroke volume and decreased ventricular filling pressures. African Americans seem to respond very well to vasodilator therapy and show improved clinical outcomes when treated with a combination of hydralazine and nitrates.

Statins

By their anti-inflammatory and lipid-lowering effects, statins have been proven to decrease morbidity and mortality in patients with SHF. Promising studies suggest that DHF patients could derive similar benefits from statin therapy.

Management of Diastolic Heart Failure

The management of SHF is based on the results of large-scale randomized trials, but the therapy of DHF remains mostly empirical. It is generally accepted that the best treatment strategy for DHF is prevention. American College of Cardiology and the American Heart Association guidelines recommend that patients at risk of developing DHF should be preemptively treated. Unfortunately, there are no drugs that selectively improve diastolic distensibility. Current treatment options include a low-sodium diet, cautious use of diuretics to relieve pulmonary congestion without an excessive decrease in preload, maintenance of normal sinus rhythm at a heart rate that optimizes ventricular filling, and correction of precipitating factors such as acute myocardial ischemia and systemic hypertension. Long-acting nitrates and diuretics may alleviate the symptoms of DHF but do not alter the natural history of the disease. Statin therapy early in the course of the disease may play an important role in decreasing ventricular remodeling and reducing disease progression. The general concepts of managing patients with DHF are outlined in **Table 6-2**.

Surgical Management of Heart Failure

Part of the overall management of heart failure includes trying to eliminate the cause of the disease. LV ischemia may be treated with percutaneous coronary interventions or coronary artery bypass surgery. Increasingly severe symptoms in the presence of correctable cardiac valve lesions may be alleviated surgically. Ventricular aneurysmectomy may be useful in patients with large ventricular scars after myocardial infarction. The definitive treatment for heart failure is heart transplantation. However, the limited supply of donors renders this treatment unattainable in most patients.

Ventricular assist devices include extracorporeal membrane oxygenators and implantable pulsatile devices. These mechanical pumps take over function of the damaged ventricle and facilitate restoration of normal hemodynamics and tissue blood flow. These devices may be useful in patients who require ventricular assistance to allow the heart to rest and recover its function and in those who are awaiting cardiac transplantation.

Cardiac resynchronization therapy (CRT) is aimed at patients with advanced stages of heart failure who have a ventricular conduction delay (QRS prolongation on the ECG). Such a conduction delay creates a mechanical dyssynchrony that impairs ventricular function and worsens prognosis. CRT, also known as biventricular pacing, consists of the placement of a dual-chamber cardiac pacemaker but with an additional lead introduced into the coronary sinus/coronary vein until it reaches the dyssynchronous LV wall. With this lead in place, the heart contracts more efficiently and ejects a larger cardiac output. CRT is recommended for New York Heart Association Class II/IV patients with an LV ejection fraction less than 35% and a QRS duration between 120 and 150 milliseconds. Patients undergoing CRT may have fewer symptoms, better exercise tolerance, and improved ventricular function compared to similar patients on pharmacologic therapy alone. The reverse remodeling induced by CRT may also improve survival in these patients. Unfortunately, approximately one third of patients do not respond to this form of therapy.

Implanted cardioverter/defibrillators (ICDs) are used for prevention of sudden death in patients with advanced heart failure. Approximately one half of deaths in heart failure patients are sudden and due to cardiac dysrhythmias. Current recommendations for ICDs in patients at risk of sudden death are listed in **Table 6-3**.

Management of Acute Heart Failure

Patients may experience acute heart failure as a result of decompensated chronic heart failure or de novo. Anesthesiologists deal with acute heart failure when caring for patients in overt heart failure who present for emergency surgery or

TABLE 6-2 Management Strategies for Diastolic Heart Failure	
Goals	**Management Strategies**
Prevent development of diastolic heart failure by decreasing risk factors	Treat coronary artery disease Treat hypertension Control weight gain Treat diabetes mellitus
Allow adequate filling time of left ventricle by decreasing heart rate	β-Blockers, calcium channel blockers, digoxin
Control volume overload	Diuretics, long-acting nitrates, low-sodium diet
Restore and maintain sinus rhythm	Cardioversion, amiodarone, digoxin
Decrease ventricular remodeling	Angiotensin-converting enzyme inhibitors, statins
Correct precipitating factors	Aortic valve replacement Coronary revascularization

TABLE 6–3 Indications for Implantable Cardioverter Defibrillator Placement for Prevention of Sudden Death	
Cause of Heart Failure	**Condition**
Coronary artery disease	Ejection fraction < 30%
	Ejection fraction < 40% if electrophysiologic study demonstrates inducible ventricular dysrhythmias
All other causes	After first episode of syncope or aborted ventricular tachycardia/ventricular fibrillation

patients who decompensate intraoperatively. Acute heart failure therapy has three phases: the emergency phase, the in-hospital management phase, and the predischarge phase. For the anesthesiologist, the emergency phase is of most interest and is the phase that is addressed here. The hemodynamic profile of acute heart failure is characterized by high ventricular filling pressures, low cardiac output, and hyper- or hypotension. Traditional therapy includes diuretics, vasodilators, inotropic drugs, mechanical assisted devices (intra-aortic balloon pump, ventricular assist device), and emergency cardiac surgery. Newer therapy includes calcium sensitizers, exogenous BNP, and nitric oxide synthase inhibitors.

Diuretics and Vasodilators

Loop diuretics can improve symptoms rapidly, but in high doses, they may have deleterious effects on clinical outcomes. It may be more desirable to use a combination of a low dose of loop diuretic with an intravenous vasodilator. Nitroglycerin and nitroprusside reduce LV filling pressure and systemic vascular resistance and increase stroke volume. However, nitroprusside may have a negative impact on clinical outcome in patients with acute myocardial infarction.

Inotropic Support

Positive inotropic drugs have been the mainstay of treatment for patients in cardiogenic shock. Their positive inotropic effect is produced via an increase in cyclic adenosine monophosphate, which promotes an increase in intracellular calcium levels and, thereby, an improvement in excitation-contraction coupling. Catecholamines (epinephrine, norepinephrine, dopamine, and dobutamine) do so by direct β-receptor stimulation, whereas phosphodiesterase inhibitors (amrinone, milrinone) block the degradation of cyclic adenosine monophosphate. Side effects of inotropic drugs include tachycardia, increased myocardial energy demand and oxygen consumption, dysrhythmias, worsening of DHF, and downregulation of β-receptors. Long-term use of these drugs may result in cardiotoxicity and accelerate myocardial cell death.

Calcium Sensitizers

Myofilament calcium sensitizers are a new class of positive inotropic drugs that increase contractility without increasing intracellular levels of calcium. Therefore, there is no significant increase in myocardial oxygen consumption or heart rate and no propensity for dysrhythmias. The most widely used medication in this class is levosemindan. It is an inodilator increasing myocardial contractile strength and promoting dilation of systemic, pulmonary, and coronary arteries. It does not

worsen diastolic function. Studies have shown that levosemindan may be particularly useful in the setting of myocardial ischemia. Levosemindan is included in the European guidelines for treatment of acute heart failure, but it is not yet available for use in the United States.

Exogenous B-Type Natriuretic Peptide

Nesiritide (Natrecor) is recombinant BNP that binds to both the A- and B-type natriuretic receptors. It promotes arterial, venous, and coronary vasodilation, thereby decreasing LVEDP and improving dyspnea. Nesiritide induces diuresis and natriuresis. It has many effects similar to nitroglycerin but generally produces less hypotension and more diuresis than nitroglycerin.

Nitric Oxide Synthase Inhibitors

The inflammatory cascade stimulated by heart failure results in production of a large amount of nitric oxide in the heart and vascular endothelium. These high levels of nitric oxide have a negative inotropic and profound vasodilatory effect leading to cardiogenic shock and vascular collapse. Inhibition of nitric oxide synthase should decrease these harmful effects. L-NAME (*N*-nitro-L-arginine methyl ester) is the principal drug in this class under investigation.

Mechanical Devices

If the etiology of acute heart failure is a large myocardial infarction, the insertion of an intra-aortic balloon pump should be considered. The intra-aortic balloon pump is a mechanical device inserted via the femoral artery and positioned just below the left subclavian artery. Its balloon inflates in diastole increasing aortic diastolic blood pressure and coronary perfusion pressure. The balloon deflates in systole creating a "suction" effect that enhances LV ejection. Complications of intra-aortic balloon pump placement include femoral artery or aortic dissection, bleeding, thrombosis, and infection.

In severe cardiogenic shock, emergency insertion of LV and/or right ventricular assist devices may be necessary for survival.

Prognosis

Despite advances in therapy, the number of heart failure deaths continues to increase steadily. The mortality rate during the first 4 years following the diagnosis of heart failure approaches 40%. Certain factors have been associated with a poor prognosis and include increased urea and creatinine levels, hyponatremia, hypokalemia, severely depressed ejection fraction, high levels of endogenous BNP, very limited exercise tolerance, and the presence of multifocal premature ventricular contractions. The prognosis in heart failure patients depends on the underlying heart disease and on the presence or absence of a specific precipitating factor. If a correctable cause of heart failure can be effectively eliminated, prognosis improves.

MANAGEMENT OF ANESTHESIA

Preoperative Evaluation and Management

The presence of heart failure has been described as the single most important risk factor for predicting perioperative cardiac morbidity and mortality. In the preoperative period, all precipitating factors for heart failure should be sought and aggressively treated before proceeding with elective surgery.

Patients treated for heart failure are usually on several medications that may affect anesthetic management. It is generally accepted that diuretics may be discontinued on the day of surgery. Maintaining β-blocker therapy is essential since many studies have shown that β-blockers reduce perioperative morbidity and mortality. Due to inhibition of the RAAS, ACEIs may put patients at increased risk of intraoperative hypotension. This hypotension can be treated with a sympathomimetic drug such as ephedrine, an α-agonist such as phenylephrine, or vasopressin or one of its analogues. If ACEIs are being used to prevent ventricular remodeling in heart failure patients and kidney dysfunction in diabetic patients, then stopping the medication for 1 day will not significantly alter these effects. However, if ACEIs are used to treat hypertension, then discontinuing therapy the day of or the day before surgery may result in significant hypertension. Angiotensin receptor blockers produce profound RAAS blockade and should be discontinued the day before surgery. Digoxin therapy can be continued until the day of surgery.

Results of recent electrolyte, renal function, and liver function tests and the most recent ECG and echocardiogram should be evaluated.

Intraoperative Management

All types of general anesthetics have been successfully used in patients with heart failure. However, drug doses may need to be adjusted. Opioids seem to have a particularly beneficial effect in heart failure patients because of their effect on the δ-receptor, which inhibits adrenergic activation. Positive pressure ventilation and positive end-expiratory pressure may be beneficial in decreasing pulmonary congestion and improving arterial oxygenation.

Monitoring is adjusted to the complexity of the operation. Intra-arterial pressure monitoring is justified when a major operation is required in a patient with heart failure. Monitoring of ventricular filling and fluid status is a more challenging task. Fluid overload during the perioperative period may contribute to the development or worsening of heart failure. Intraoperative use of a pulmonary artery catheter may help in evaluation of optimal fluid loading, but in patients with DHF and poor ventricular compliance, accurate assessment of LV end-diastolic volume may be quite difficult. Transesophageal echocardiography may be a better alternative, allowing not only monitoring of ventricular filling but also ventricular wall motion and valvular function. However, transesophageal echocardiography requires trained personnel to perform and interpret the study and may not be readily available in all circumstances.

Regional anesthesia is acceptable for suitable operations in heart failure patients. In fact, the modest decrease in systemic vascular resistance secondary to peripheral SNS blockade may increase cardiac output. However, the decreased systemic vascular resistance produced by epidural or spinal anesthesia is not always predictable or easy to control. The pros and cons of regional anesthesia must be carefully weighed in heart failure patients.

Special consideration must be given to patients who have undergone cardiac transplantation and now require other surgeries. These patients are on long-term immunosuppressive therapy and are at high risk of infection. Strict aseptic technique is necessary when performing any invasive procedure such as central line placement or neuraxial block. The transplanted heart is denervated. Therefore, an increase in heart rate can only be achieved by administering direct acting β-adrenergic agonists such as isoproterenol and epinephrine. An increase in heart rate will *not* occur with administration of atropine or pancuronium. A blunted response to α-adrenergic agonists may also be observed. The transplanted heart increases cardiac output by increasing stroke volume. Therefore, these patients are preload dependent and require adequate intravascular volume.

Postoperative Management

Patients who have evidence of acute heart failure during surgery should be transferred to an intensive care unit where invasive monitoring can be continued postoperatively. Pain should be aggressively treated since its presence and hemodynamic consequences may worsen heart failure. Patients should have their usual medications restarted as soon as possible.

CARDIOMYOPATHIES

The definition of cardiomyopathies used by the American Heart Association expert consensus panel in its 2006 document entitled "Contemporary Definition and Classification of the Cardiomyopathies" states:

Cardiomyopathies are a heterogeneous group of diseases of the myocardium associated with mechanical and/or electrical dysfunction that usually (but not invariably) exhibit inappropriate ventricular hypertrophy or dilation and are due to a variety of causes that frequently are genetic. Cardiomyopathies either are confined to the heart or are part of generalized systemic disorders, often leading to cardiovascular death or progressive heart failure-related disability.

TABLE 6–4 Classification of Primary Cardiomyopathies

Genetic	Hypertrophic cardiomyopathy
	Arrhythmogenic right ventricular cardiomyopathy
	Left ventricular noncompaction
	Glycogen storage disease
	Conduction system disease (Lenègre's disease)
	Ion channelopathies: long QT syndrome, Brugada syndrome, short QT syndrome,
Mixed	Dilated cardiomyopathy
	Primary restrictive nonhypertrophied cardiomyopathy
Aquired	Myocarditis (inflammatory cardiomyopathy): viral, bacterial, rickettsial, fungal, parasitic (Chagas disease)
	Stress cardiomyopathy
	Peripartum cardiomyopathy

According to the new American Heart Association classification, cardiomyopathies are divided into two major groups: primary cardiomyopathies and secondary cardiomyopathies. Primary cardiomyopathies are those exclusively (or predominantly) confined to the heart muscle. Primary cardiomyopathies can be genetic, acquired, or of mixed origin. Secondary cardiomyopathies demonstrate pathophysiologic involvement of the heart in the context of a multiorgan disorder. **Tables 6-4** and **6-5** list the most common cardiomyopathies classified according to the new guidelines. It is important to emphasize that the previously used terms *ischemic cardiomyopathy*, *restrictive cardiomyopathy*, and *obliterative cardiomyopathy* no longer exist in the new American Heart Association classification.

This section addresses the cardiomyopathies most often seen in the operating room: hypertrophic cardiomyopathy (HCM), DCM, peripartum cardiomyopathy, and secondary cardiomyopathies with restrictive physiology.

HYPERTROPHIC CARDIOMYOPATHY

Hypertrophic cardiomyopathy (HCM) is a complex cardiac disease with unique pathophysiologic characteristics and a great diversity of morphologic, functional, and clinical features. The disease can affect patients of all ages and has a prevalence in the general population approaching 1 in 500. It is the most common genetic cardiovascular disease and is

TABLE 6-5 Classification of Secondary Cardiomyopathies

Infiltrative	Amyloidosis
	Gaucher's disease
	Hunter's syndrome
Storage	Hemochromatosis
	Glycogen storage disease
	Niemann-Pick disease
Toxic	Drugs: cocaine, alcohol
	Chemotherapy drugs: doxorubicin, daunarubicin, cyclophosphamide
	Heavy metals: lead, mercury
	Radiation therapy
Inflammatory	Sarcoidosis
Endomyocardial	Hypereosinophilic (Löffler's) syndrome
	Endomyocardial fibrosis
Endocrine	Diabetes mellitus
	Hyper- or hypothyroidism
	Pheochromocytoma
	Acromegaly
Neuromuscular	Duchenne-Becker dystrophy
	Neurofibromatosis
	Tuberous sclerosis
Autoimmune	Lupus erythematosus
	Rheumatoid arthritis
	Scleroderma
	Dermatomyositis
	Polyarteritis nodosa

transmitted as an autosomal dominant trait with variable penetrance. The disease is characterized by LV hypertrophy in the absence of any other cardiac disease capable of inducing ventricular hypertrophy such as hypertension or aortic stenosis. The most common form of HCM presents as hypertrophy of the septal and anterolateral free wall. Histologic features of this disease include hypertrophied myocardial cells and areas of patchy myocardial scarring.

The pathophysiology of HCM is related to the following issues: myocardial hypertrophy, dynamic LV outflow tract (LVOT) obstruction, systolic anterior movement of the mitral valve and mitral regurgitation, diastolic dysfunction, myocardial ischemia, and dysrhythmias. During systole, vigorous contraction of the hypertrophied septum accelerates blood flow through the narrow LVOT creating a Venturi effect on the anterior leaflet of the mitral valve and inducing systolic anterior movement. The presence of systolic anterior movement further induces dynamic LVOT obstruction as well as significant mitral regurgitation (**Fig. 6-5**). LVOT obstruction can be present at rest or induced with a Valsalva maneuver. Situations that worsen LVOT obstruction are presented in **Table 6-6**. With HCM, diastolic dysfunction is seen more commonly than LVOT obstruction. The hypertrophied myocardium exhibits a prolonged relaxation time and a decreased compliance. Myocardial ischemia is present in patients with HCM, whether or not they have CAD. Myocardial ischemia is caused by several factors including abnormal coronary arteries, a mismatch between ventricular mass and coronary artery size, increased LVEDP compromising coronary perfusion, decreased diastolic filling time, increased oxygen consumption due to hypertrophy, and the presence of a metabolic derangement in the use of oxygen at the cellular

TABLE 6-6	Factors Influencing Left Ventricular Outflow Tract Obstruction in Patients with Hypertrophic Cardiomyopathy

Events That Increase Outflow Obstruction
Increased myocardial contractility
  β-Adrenergic stimulation (catecholamines)
  Digitalis
Decreased preload
  Hypovolemia
  Vasodilators
  Tachycardia
  Positive pressure ventilation
Decreased afterload
  Hypotension
  Vasodilators

Events That Decrease Outflow Obstruction
Decreased myocardial contractility
  β-Adrenergic blockade
  Volatile anesthetics
  Calcium entry blockers
Increased preload
  Hypervolemia
  Bradycardia
Increased afterload
  Hypertension
  α-Adrenergic stimulation

level. Dysrhythmias in patients with HCM result from the disorganized cellular architecture, myocardial scarring, and expanded interstitial matrix. Dysrhythmias are the cause of sudden death in young adults with HCM.

Signs and Symptoms

The clinical course of HCM varies widely, with most patients remaining asymptomatic throughout life. Some, however, have symptoms of severe heart failure and others die suddenly. The principal symptoms of HCM are angina pectoris, fatigue or syncope (may represent aborted sudden death), tachydysrhythmias, and heart failure. Interestingly, the angina pectoris of HCM is often relieved by lying down. Presumably, the change in LV size that accompanies this positional change decreases LV outflow obstruction.

Cardiac physical examination may reveal a double apical impulse, gallop rhythm, and cardiac murmurs and thrills. The murmurs can result from LV outflow obstruction or mitral regurgitation and can be confused with aortic or mitral valve disease. The intensity of these murmurs can change markedly with certain maneuvers. For example, the Valsalva maneuver, which increases LV outflow obstruction, will enhance the systolic murmur along the left sternal border. The murmur of mitral regurgitation intensifies as well with a Valsalva maneuver. Nitroglycerin and standing (versus lying down) also increase the loudness of these murmurs.

Sudden death is a recognized complication of HCM. The severity of ventricular hypertrophy is directly related to the risk of sudden death. Young individuals with massive hypertrophy,

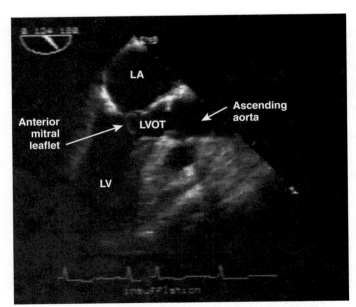

Figure 6-5 • Two-dimensional echocardiographic image showing the anterior leaflet of the mitral valve abutting the hypertrophied interventricular septum and obstructing the left ventricular outflow tract (LVOT) during systole in a patient with hypertrophic cardiomyopathy. LA, left atrium; LV, left ventricle.

even with few or no symptoms, deserve consideration for an intervention to prevent sudden death. Sudden death is especially likely to occur in patients between the ages of 10 and 30 years. For this reason, there is general agreement that young HCM patients should not participate in competitive sports. Most patients with mild hypertrophy are at low risk of sudden death.

Diagnosis

The ECG typically depicts LV hypertrophy. In asymptomatic patients, unexplained LV hypertrophy may be the only sign of the disease. The 12-lead ECG is abnormal in 75% to 90% of patients with HCM. ECG abnormalities include high QRS voltage due to hypertrophy, ST-segment and T-wave alterations, abnormal Q waves resembling those seen with myocardial infarction, and left atrial enlargement. The diagnosis of HCM should be considered in any young patient whose ECG is consistent with previous myocardial infarction because not all patients with HCM have evidence of LV hypertrophy on the ECG.

Echocardiography can demonstrate the presence of myocardial hypertrophy. Ejection fraction is usually more than 80%, reflecting the hypercontractile condition of the heart. Echocardiography can also assess the mitral valve apparatus and the presence of systolic anterior movement. Color flow Doppler can reveal the presence of LVOT obstruction by demonstrating turbulent flow as well as mitral regurgitation. Pressure gradients across the LVOT can be measured. Echocardiography is also useful in evaluating diastolic function.

Cardiac catheterization allows direct measurement of the increased LV end-diastolic pressure and the pressure gradients between the left ventricle and the aorta. Provocative maneuvers may be required to evoke evidence of LVOT obstruction. Ventriculography characteristically shows cavity obliteration.

The definitive diagnosis of HCM is made by endomyocardial biopsy and DNA analysis, but these diagnostic modalities are usually reserved for patients in whom the diagnosis cannot be otherwise established.

Treatment

The diverse clinical and genetic features of HCM make it impossible to define precise guidelines for management (**Fig. 6-6**). However, it is recognized that some patients are at high risk of sudden death and must be treated aggressively. Pharmacologic therapy to improve diastolic filling, reduce LV outflow obstruction, and possibly decrease myocardial ischemia is the primary means of relieving the signs and symptoms of HCM. Surgery to remove the area of hypertrophy causing outflow tract obstruction is considered in only approximately 5% of patients who have both marked outflow obstruction and severe symptoms unresponsive to medical therapy.

Medical Therapy

β-Blockers and calcium channel blockers have been used extensively to treat HCM. The beneficial effects of β-blockers on dyspnea, angina pectoris, and exercise tolerance are likely due to the decreased heart rate with consequent prolongation

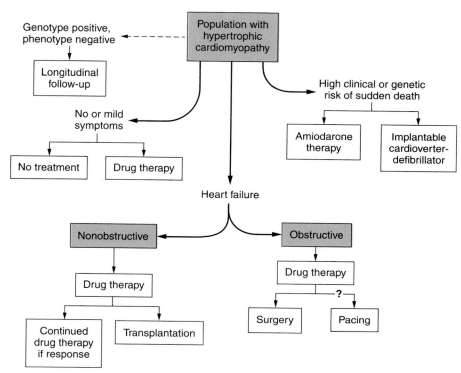

Figure 6-6 • Clinical presentations of hypertrophic cardiomyopathy and corresponding treatment strategies. Size of the *arrows* indicates the approximate proportion of patients in each subgroup. *Dashed arrow* indicates uncertainties as to the size of this subgroup. (*Adapted from Spirito P, Seidman CE, McKenna WJ, et al: The management of HCM. N Engl J Med 1997;336:775–785. Copyright 1997 Massachusetts Medical Society.*)

of diastole and a lengthening of the time for passive ventricular filling. β-Blockers can lessen myocardial oxygen requirements and decrease the dynamic outflow tract obstruction during exercise by blunting SNS activity. Similarly, calcium channel blockers, such as verapamil and diltiazem, have beneficial effects on the symptoms of HCM because they improve ventricular filling and decrease myocardial ischemia. Patients who develop congestive heart failure despite treatment with β-blockers or calcium channel blockers may improve with the addition of a diuretic. However, because of the presence of diastolic dysfunction and the requirement for relatively high ventricular filling pressures to achieve adequate cardiac output, diuretic administration must be done very cautiously. Patients at high risk of sudden death may require amiodarone therapy or placement of an internal cardioverter/defibrillator.

Atrial fibrillation often develops in patients with HCM and is associated with an increased risk of thromboembolism, congestive heart failure, and sudden death. Amiodarone is the most effective antidysrhythmic drug for prevention of paroxysms of atrial fibrillation in these patients. β-Blockers and calcium channel blockers can control the heart rate. Long-term anticoagulation is indicated in those with recurrent or chronic atrial fibrillation.

Surgical Therapy

The small subgroup of patients with HCM who have both large outflow tract gradients (≥50 mm Hg) and severe symptoms of congestive heart failure despite medical therapy are candidates for surgery. Surgical reduction of the outflow gradient is usually achieved by removing a small amount of cardiac muscle from the ventricular septum (septal myomectomy). Surgery abolishes or greatly reduces the LVOT gradient in most patients. Intraventricular systolic and end-diastolic pressures are markedly reduced, and these changes favorably influence LV filling and myocardial oxygen requirements.

Prognosis

The overall annual mortality of HCM is approximately 1%. However, the subset of patients at high risk of sudden death (family history of sudden death or history of malignant ventricular dysrhythmias) have a mortality rate of 5% per year. Only approximately one fourth of patients diagnosed with HCM will develop signs of LVOT obstruction.

Management of Anesthesia

Management of anesthesia in patients with HCM is directed toward minimizing LVOT obstruction. Any drug or event that decreases myocardial contractility or increases preload or afterload reduces LVOT obstruction. Conversely, sympathetic stimulation, hypovolemia, and vasodilation worsen LVOT obstruction (see **Table 6-6**). Intraoperatively, HCM patients may develop severe hypotension, myocardial ischemia, acute heart failure, and supraventricular or ventricular tachydysrhythmias. Previously unrecognized HCM may become

manifest intraoperatively as unexplained hypotension or development of a systolic murmur in association with acute hemorrhage or drug-induced vasodilation.

Preoperative Evaluation and Management

Given the prevalence of HCM in the general population, patients with this disorder will present to the operating room with a fair frequency. Patients already diagnosed with this disease should have an updated cardiac evaluation prior to elective surgery. Such evaluation should include a 12-lead ECG and an echocardiographic examination. Patients taking β-blockers or calcium channel blockers should continue these medications throughout the perioperative period. Patients with an ICD should have the unit turned off in the immediate preoperative period and have an external defibrillator immediately available in the operating room.

A more challenging task is the preoperative evaluation of patients with HCM in whom the diagnosis has not yet been made. These patients are often young and appear healthy. Every patient should be asked preoperatively about any possible cardiac symptoms or a family history of cardiac disease or sudden death. The presence of a systolic murmur should raise suspicion of a possible HCM diagnosis. If the ECG is found to be abnormal in this context, cardiologic evaluation is prudent.

In HCM patients, preoperative medication to allay anxiety and the associated activation of the sympathetic nervous system may be advisable. Expansion of intravascular volume during the preoperative period may also be useful in preventing LVOT obstruction and minimizing the adverse effects of positive-pressure ventilation on the central blood volume.

Intraoperative Management

Regional or general anesthesia can be selected for patients with HCM as long as the anesthesiologist is aware of the main pathophysiologic mechanisms that trigger LVOT obstruction and develops an anesthetic plan tailored to these specific needs.

Induction of anesthesia with an intravenous drug is acceptable, remembering the importance of avoiding sudden decreases in systemic vascular resistance and increases in heart rate and contractility. A modest degree of direct myocardial depression is acceptable. Administration of a volatile anesthetic or β-adrenergic antagonist before direct laryngoscopy can blunt the SNS response typically evoked by tracheal intubation. Positive-pressure ventilation can significantly decrease preload and predispose a hypovolemic patient to dynamic LVOT obstruction. To help avoid this, smaller tidal volumes and higher respiratory rates should be used and positive end-expiratory pressure should be avoided. Preload reduction and severe hypotension due to LVOT obstruction can also be encountered when abdominal insufflation is performed for laparoscopic surgery. The surgeon should be advised about this possibility, and the abdomen should be insufflated slowly and at pressures not exceeding 15 mm Hg.

Nondepolarizing muscle relaxants that have only minimal effects on the systemic circulation should be used for skeletal muscle relaxation in HCM patients. The increased heart rate that may accompany administration of pancuronium or the histamine release of other neuromuscular blockers should be avoided.

Anesthesia should be maintained with drugs that produce mild depression of myocardial contractility and have minimal effects on preload and afterload. A volatile anesthetic in a moderate dose is often used for this purpose.

Invasive monitoring of blood pressure may be helpful. Transesophageal echocardiography is particularly useful in HCM patients during surgery and anesthesia because of the unique pathophysiology of this disorder. Neither central venous pressure monitoring nor pulmonary artery pressure monitoring can diagnose LVOT obstruction or systolic anterior movement nor do these monitors give an accurate assessment of LV filling.

Hypotension that occurs in response to a decrease in preload or afterload should be treated with an α-adrenergic agonist such as phenylephrine. Drugs with β-adrenergic agonist activity, such as ephedrine, dopamine, and dobutamine, are contraindicated in treating hypotension in these patients because the drug-induced increase in myocardial contractility and heart rate increases LVOT obstruction. Prompt replacement of blood loss and titration of intravenous fluids is important for maintaining preload and blood pressure. However, because of the diastolic dysfunction, aggressive fluid replacement may result in pulmonary edema. Vasodilators should not be used to lower blood pressure because the decrease in systemic vascular resistance will accentuate LVOT obstruction (see **Table 6-6**).

Maintenance of normal sinus rhythm is very important because adequate ventricular filling is dependent on left atrial contraction. Patients who develop intraoperative supraventricular tachydysrhythmias should undergo immediate pharmacologic or electrical cardioversion. A cardioverter/defibrillator must be readily available in the operating room. β-Blockers such as metoprolol and esmolol are indicated to slow persistently elevated heart rates.

Parturients

Pregnancy is usually well tolerated in patients with HCM despite the pregnancy-induced decrease in systemic vascular resistance and the risk of impaired venous return due to aortocaval compression. Parturients with HCM may present major anesthetic challenges because events such as labor pain producing catecholamine release and "bearing down" (Valsalva maneuver) may increase LVOT obstruction. There is no evidence that regional anesthesia increases complication rates in parturients with HCM undergoing vaginal delivery. Epidural anesthesia has been successfully administered to these patients. Maintenance of euvolemia or slight hypervolemia is helpful. Should hypotension unresponsive to fluid administration occur following institution of regional anesthesia, phenylephrine should be used to increase afterload. Oxytocin must be administered carefully because of its vasodilating properties and compensatory tachycardia and

because of the abrupt inflow of large amounts of blood into the central circulation as a consequence of uterine contraction.

Pulmonary edema has been observed in parturients with HCM after delivery, emphasizing the delicate fluid requirements of these patients. Treatment of pulmonary edema in the presence of HCM may include phenylephrine if hypotension is present and esmolol to slow the heart rate, prolong diastolic filling time, and decrease myocardial contractility, all of which will decrease LVOT obstruction. Diuretics, digoxin, and nitrates *cannot* be used to treat pulmonary edema in this situation. They worsen the situation by provoking further LVOT obstruction.

Postoperative Management

Patients with HCM must be vigilantly monitored in the recovery room or intensive care unit in the immediate postoperative period. All factors that stimulate sympathetic activity such as pain, shivering, anxiety, hypoxia, and hypercarbia should be eliminated. As in the operating room, maintenance of euvolemia and prompt treatment of hypotension are crucial.

DILATED CARDIOMYOPATHY

DCM is a primary myocardial disease characterized by LV or biventricular dilation, systolic dysfunction, and normal LV wall thickness. The etiology of DCM is usually unknown but may be genetic or associated with infection such as viral coxsackie B infection. There is a familial transmission pattern in approximately 30% of cases, usually autosomal dominant. Many types of secondary cardiomyopathies have the features of DCM. These include the cardiomyopathies associated with alcohol, cocaine, the peripartum state, pheochromocytoma, infectious diseases (human immunodeficiency virus), uncontrolled tachycardia, Duchenne's muscular dystrophy, thyroid disease, chemotherapeutic drugs, radiation therapy, hypertension, CAD, and valvular disease. African American men have an increased risk of developing DCM. DCM is the most common type of cardiomyopathy, the third most common cause of heart failure, and the most common indication for cardiac transplantation.

Signs and Symptoms

The initial manifestation of DCM is usually with signs and symptoms of heart failure. Chest pain on exertion that mimics angina pectoris occurs in some patients. Ventricular dilation may be so marked that functional mitral and/or tricuspid regurgitation occurs. Supraventricular and ventricular dysrhythmias, conduction system abnormalities, and sudden death are common. Systemic embolization is also common as a result of the formation of mural thrombi in dilated and hypokinetic cardiac chambers.

Diagnosis

The electrocardiogram often shows ST segment and T-wave abnormalities and left bundle branch block. Cardiac dysrhythmias are common and include ventricular premature beats and atrial fibrillation. Chest radiography may show enlargement of all four cardiac chambers, but LV dilatation is the principal morphologic feature of DCM.

Echocardiography typically reveals dilation of all four chambers but especially the left ventricle. There is global hypokinesis. Regional wall motion abnormalities may be seen in DCM and do not necessarily imply the presence of CAD. Mural thrombi can be detected and valvular regurgitation secondary to annular dilation is a common finding.

Laboratory testing should be performed to eliminate other causes of cardiac dilation such as hyperthyroidism. Coronary arteriography is usually normal in patients with DCM. Right heart catheterization reveals a high pulmonary capillary wedge pressure, high systemic vascular resistance, and a low cardiac output. Endomyocardial biopsy is not recommended.

Treatment

Treatment of DCM includes general supportive measures such as adequate rest, weight control, low-sodium diet, fluid restriction, abstinence from tobacco and alcohol, and decreased physical activity during periods of cardiac decompensation. Cardiac rehabilitation, if possible, will improve general conditioning.

The medical management of DCM is similar to the medical management of chronic heart failure. Patients with DCM are at risk of systemic and pulmonary embolization because blood stasis in the hypocontractile ventricle leads to activation of the coagulation cascade. The risk of cardiac embolization is greatest in patients with severe LV dysfunction, atrial fibrillation, a history of thromboembolism, or echocardiographic evidence of intracardiac thrombus. Anticoagulation with warfarin is often instituted in patients with idiopathic DCM and symptomatic heart failure.

Although asymptomatic, nonsustained ventricular tachycardia is common in patients with DCM. However, suppression of this dysrhythmia with drug therapy does not improve survival. An ICD can decrease the risk of sudden death in patients with heart failure who have survived a previous cardiac arrest (see Table 6-3).

DCM remains the principal indication for cardiac transplantation in adults and children. Patients most likely to benefit from a heart transplant are those formerly vigorous persons younger than 60 years of age with intractable symptoms of heart failure despite optimal medical therapy.

Prognosis

Symptomatic patients with DCM referred to tertiary care medical centers have a 5-year mortality rate of 50%. If the cardiomyopathy involves both the left and right ventricles, the prognosis is worse. Hemodynamic abnormalities that predict a poor prognosis include an ejection fraction less than 25%, pulmonary capillary wedge pressure higher than 20 mm Hg, cardiac index less than 2.5 L/min/m^2, systemic hypotension, pulmonary hypertension, and increased central venous pressure. Alcoholic cardiomyopathy is largely reversible if complete abstinence from alcohol is maintained.

Management of Anesthesia

Since DCM is a cause of heart failure, the anesthetic management of these patients is the same as described in the heart failure section of this chapter.

Regional anesthesia may be an alternative to general anesthesia in selected patients with DCM. However, anticoagulant therapy may limit this option.

PERIPARTUM CARDIOMYOPATHY

Peripartum cardiomyopathy is a rare, dilated form of cardiomyopathy of unknown cause that occurs during the peripartum period, that is, the third trimester of pregnancy until 5 months after delivery. It occurs in women with no history of heart disease. The estimated incidence of peripartum cardiomyopathy is 1:3000 to 1:4000 live births. Risk factors include obesity, multiparity, advanced maternal age (older than 30 years of age), multifetal pregnancy, preeclampsia, and being African American. Possible etiologies of this cardiomyopathy include viral myocarditis, an abnormal immune response to pregnancy, or maladaptive responses to the hemodynamic stresses of pregnancy.

Signs and Symptoms

The signs and symptoms of peripartum cardiomyopathy are those of heart failure: dyspnea, fatigue, and peripheral edema. However, these signs and symptoms are common in the final trimester of pregnancy, and there are no specific criteria for differentiating subtle symptoms of heart failure from normal late pregnancy. Clinical conditions that may mimic heart failure, such as amniotic fluid or pulmonary embolism, should be excluded when considering the diagnosis of peripartum cardiomyopathy.

Diagnosis

The diagnosis of peripartum cardiomyopathy is based on the onset of unexplained LV dysfunction and echocardiographic documentation of a new finding of dilated cardiac chambers with LV systolic dysfunction during the period surrounding parturition.

Treatment

The goal of treatment is to alleviate the symptoms of heart failure. Diuretics, vasodilators, and digoxin can be used. ACEIs are teratogenic but can be useful following delivery. During pregnancy, vasodilation is accomplished with hydralazine and nitrates. Intravenous immunoglobulin may have a beneficial effect. Thromboembolic complications are not uncommon, and anticoagulation is often recommended. Heart transplantation may be considered in patients who do not improve over time.

Prognosis

The mortality rate of peripartum cardiomyopathy ranges from 25% to 50%, with most deaths occurring within 3 months after delivery. Death is usually a result of progression of congestive heart failure or sudden death associated with cardiac dysrhythmias or thromboembolic events. The prognosis appears to depend on the degree of normalization of LV size and function within 6 months of delivery.

Management of Anesthesia

The management of anesthesia in parturients with peripartum cardiomyopathy requires assessment of cardiac status and careful planning of the analgesia and/or anesthesia required for delivery. Regional anesthesia may provide a desirable decrease in afterload.

SECONDARY CARDIOMYOPATHIES WITH RESTRICTIVE PHYSIOLOGY

Secondary cardiomyopathies with restrictive physiology are due to systemic diseases that produce myocardial infiltration and severe diastolic dysfunction. The most common of these cardiomyopathies is caused by amyloidosis. Other systemic diseases such as hemochromatosis, sarcoidosis, and carcinoid may produce a similar type of cardiomyopathy. The diagnosis should be considered in patients presenting with heart failure but no evidence of cardiomegaly or systolic dysfunction. The condition results from increased stiffness of the myocardium due to the deposition of these abnormal substances. Although there is impaired diastolic function and reduced ventricular compliance, systolic function is usually normal. Cardiomyopathies with restrictive physiology must be differentiated from constrictive pericarditis that has a similar physiology. A clinical history of pericarditis makes the diagnosis of constrictive pericarditis more likely.

Signs and Symptoms

Because cardiomyopathies with restrictive physiology can affect both ventricles, symptoms and signs of LV and/or right ventricular failure may be present. In advanced stages of this cardiomyopathy, all the signs and symptoms of heart failure can be present, but there is no cardiomegaly. Amyloidosis cardiomyopathy often presents with thromboembolic complications. Atrial fibrillation is also common. Cardiac conduction disturbances are particularly common in amyloidosis and sarcoidosis. Over time, this involvement of the conduction system can lead to heart block or ventricular dysrhythmias resulting in sudden death.

Diagnosis

The ECG may demonstrate conduction abnormalities. The chest radiograph may show signs of pulmonary congestion and/or pleural effusion, but cardiomegaly is absent. Chemical laboratory tests should be employed as needed to diagnose the systemic disease responsible for the cardiac infiltration.

Echocardiography will demonstrate significant diastolic dysfunction and normal systolic function. The atria are enlarged due to the high atrial pressures, but the ventricles are normal in size. In cardiac amyloidosis, the ventricular mass appears speckled, a characteristic sign of amyloid deposition. Various echocardiographic criteria can differentiate secondary cardiomyopathies with restrictive physiology from constrictive pericarditis. Endomyocardial biopsy can elucidate the exact etiology of the infiltrative cardiomyopathy.

Treatment

Symptomatic treatment is similar to that for DHF. It includes administration of diuretics to treat pulmonary and systemic congestion. Excessive diuresis may decrease ventricular filling pressures and cardiac output and result in hypotension and hypoperfusion. Digoxin must be used with great caution because it is potentially dysrhythmogenic in patients with amyloidosis. The development of atrial fibrillation with loss of the atrial contribution to ventricular filling may substantially worsen diastolic dysfunction, and a rapid ventricular response may further compromise cardiac output. Maintenance of normal sinus rhythm is extremely important. Because stroke volume tends to be fixed in the presence of cardiomyopathy with restrictive physiology, the onset of bradycardia may precipitate acute heart failure, so significant bradycardia or severe conduction system disease may require implantation of a cardiac pacemaker. With cardiac sarcoidosis, malignant ventricular dysrhythmias are common and may necessitate insertion of an ICD. Anticoagulation may be needed in patients with atrial fibrillation and/or low cardiac output. Cardiac transplantation is *not* a treatment option because myocardial infiltration will recur in the transplanted heart.

Prognosis

The prognosis of secondary cardiomyopathy with restrictive physiology is very poor.

Management of Anesthesia

Management of anesthesia for patients with restrictive cardiomyopathy uses the same principles as for patients with cardiac tamponade (see Chapter 7). Because stroke volume is relatively fixed, it is important to maintain normal sinus rhythm and to avoid any significant decrease in the heart rate. Maintenance of venous return and intravascular fluid volume is also necessary to maintain an acceptable cardiac output. Anticoagulant therapy will negatively influence the decision to select regional anesthesia.

COR PULMONALE

Cor pulmonale is right ventricular enlargement (hypertrophy and/or dilation) that may progress to right heart failure. It is caused by diseases that induce pulmonary hypertension. Cor pulmonale can be caused by several types of lung disease including COPD, restrictive lung disease, and respiratory insufficiency of central origin (obesity-hypoventilation syndrome). It can also result from idiopathic pulmonary artery hypertension, that is, the pulmonary hypertension that occurs in the absence of left-sided heart disease, myocardial disease, congenital heart disease, or any other clinically significant respiratory, connective tissue, or chronic thromboembolic disease. The most common cause of cor pulmonale is COPD.

This disorder usually presents in persons older than 50 years of age because of its association with COPD. Men are afflicted five times more often than women.

Pathophysiology

The main pathophysiologic determinant of cor pulmonale is pulmonary hypertension. By various mechanisms, chronic lung disease induces an increase in pulmonary vascular resistance. Chronic alveolar hypoxia ($Pao_2 < 55$ mm Hg) is the most important factor in this process. Acute hypoxia, such as seen in exacerbations of COPD or during sleep in patients with obesity-hypoventilation syndrome, causes pulmonary vasoconstriction. Long-standing chronic hypoxia promotes pulmonary vasculature remodeling and an increase in pulmonary vascular resistance. Even mild hypoxemia may result in vascular remodeling, so it appears that other factors are also involved in the development of cor pulmonale.

Due to pulmonary hypertension, the right ventricle has an increased workload and right ventricular hypertrophy develops. Over time, right ventricular dysfunction occurs and eventually right ventricular failure is present.

Signs and Symptoms

Clinical manifestations of cor pulmonale may be obscured by co-existing lung disease. Clinical signs occur late in the course of the disease, and the most prominent of these is peripheral edema. As right ventricular function deteriorates, dyspnea increases and effort-related syncope can occur. Accentuation of the pulmonic component of the second heart sound, a diastolic murmur due to incompetence of the pulmonic valve, and a systolic murmur due to tricuspid regurgitation connote severe pulmonary hypertension. Evidence of overt right ventricular failure consists of increased jugular venous pressure and hepatosplenomegaly.

Diagnosis

The ECG may show signs of right atrial and right ventricular hypertrophy. Right atrial hypertrophy is suggested by peaked P waves in leads II, III, and aVF ("p" pulmonale). Right axis deviation and a partial or complete right bundle branch block are often seen with right ventricular hypertrophy. A normal ECG, however, does not exclude the presence of pulmonary hypertension.

Radiographic signs of cor pulmonale include an increase in width of the right pulmonary artery and a decrease in pulmonary vascular markings in the lung periphery. On the lateral projection of a chest radiograph, right ventricular enlargement is reflected by a decrease in the retrosternal space. However, this is a late sign.

Echocardiography can be a very useful diagnostic tool. It can provide numeric estimates of pulmonary artery pressure, assessment of the size and function of the right atrium and ventricle, and evaluation of the presence and severity of tricuspid or pulmonic regurgitation. Transthoracic echocardiography is often difficult to perform in patients with COPD because the hyperinflated lungs impair transmission of the ultrasound waves.

Treatment

Treatment of cor pulmonale is geared to reducing the workload of the right ventricle by decreasing pulmonary vascular resistance and pulmonary artery pressure. If the pulmonary artery vasoconstriction has a reversible component, as is likely during an acute exacerbation of COPD, this goal can be achieved by returning the Pao_2, $Paco_2$, and arterial pH to normal.

Supplemental oxygen to maintain the Pao_2 above 60 mm Hg ($Spo_2 > 90\%$) is useful in both the acute and long-term treatment of right heart failure. Long-term oxygen therapy decreases the mortality of cor pulmonale and improves cognitive function and quality of life.

Diuretics and digitalis may be used to treat right heart failure that does not respond to correction of arterial blood gases. Diuretics must be administered very carefully because diuretic-induced metabolic alkalosis, which encourages CO_2 retention, may aggravate ventilatory insufficiency by depressing the effectiveness of carbon dioxide as a stimulus to breathing. Diuresis can also increase blood viscosity and myocardial work. Digitalis can be used for treatment of atrial fibrillation, but it must be used very cautiously because the risk of digitalis toxicity is increased in the presence of hypoxemia, acidosis, and electrolyte imbalances

When cor pulmonale is progressive despite maximum medical therapy, transplantation of one or both lungs or a heart-lung transplant will provide dramatic relief of cardiorespiratory failure.

Prognosis

The prognosis of patients with cor pulmonale is dependent on the disease responsible for initiating pulmonary hypertension. Patients with COPD in whom arterial oxygenation can be maintained at near-normal levels and whose pulmonary hypertension is mild have a favorable prognosis. Prognosis is poor in patients with severe, irreversible pulmonary hypertension.

MANAGEMENT OF ANESTHESIA

Preoperative Management

Preoperative preparation of patients with cor pulmonale due to chronic lung disease is directed toward (1) eliminating and controlling acute and chronic pulmonary infection, (2) reversing bronchospasm, (3) improving clearance of airway secretions, (4) expanding collapsed or poorly ventilated alveoli, (5) hydration, and (6) correcting any electrolyte imbalances. Preoperative measurement of arterial blood gases will provide guidelines for perioperative management. Antibiotic endocarditis prophylaxis should be considered for patients with valvular disease (tricuspid or pulmonic insufficiency).

Intraoperative Management

Induction of general anesthesia can be accomplished using any available method or drug. Adequate depth of anesthesia should be present before tracheal intubation because this stimulus can elicit reflex bronchospasm in lightly anesthetized patients.

Anesthesia is typically maintained with a volatile anesthetic combined with other drugs. Volatile anesthetics are effective bronchodilators. Large doses of opioids should be avoided because they can contribute to prolonged ventilatory depression in the postoperative period. Muscle relaxants associated with histamine release should also be avoided because of the adverse effect of histamine on airway resistance and pulmonary vascular resistance.

Positive-pressure ventilation improves oxygenation, presumably due to better ventilation-to-perfusion matching. Humidification of inhaled gases helps maintain hydration, liquefaction of secretions, and mucociliary function.

Intraoperative monitoring of patients with cor pulmonale is influenced by the invasiveness of the operation. An intra-arterial catheter permits frequent determination of arterial blood gases and subsequent adjustments in the inspired concentration of oxygen. Central venous catheters or pulmonary artery catheters may be useful depending on the complexity of the surgery. A trend value of right atrial pressure can provide some information about right ventricular function. Direct measurement of pulmonary artery pressure helps determine the time to treat pulmonary hypertension and the response to treatment. Transesophageal echocardiography is an alternative method for monitoring right ventricular function and fluid status. However, as noted previously, the need for trained personnel and expensive equipment prevents this monitoring modality from being universally available.

Regional anesthetic techniques can be used in appropriate situations in patients with cor pulmonale, but regional anesthesia is best avoided for operations that require high sensory and motor levels of anesthesia. Loss of function of the accessory muscles of respiration may be very deleterious in patients with pulmonary disease. In addition, any decrease in systemic vascular resistance in the presence of fixed pulmonary hypertension can produce a very significant degree of systemic hypotension.

Postoperative Management

The respiratory and cardiovascular status of a patient with cor pulmonale must be vigilantly monitored in the postoperative period and any factors that exacerbate pulmonary hypertension, such as hypoxia and hypercarbia, must be avoided. Oxygen therapy should be maintained as needed.

KEY POINTS

- Heart failure is a complex pathophysiologic state described by the inability of the heart to fill with or eject blood at a rate appropriate to tissue requirements. Heart failure is characterized by specific symptoms (dyspnea and fatigue) and signs of circulatory congestion (rales, peripheral edema) or hypoperfusion.

- Heart failure has a high prevalence in the United States (5 million people) and imposes a great financial burden on the society. Efforts must be made to prevent or arrest the progression of this disease.

- The principal pathophysiologic derangement in heart failure development and progression is ventricular remodeling. The main treatment goals in heart failure patients are avoiding or decreasing ventricular remodeling and promoting reverse remodeling. Therapies proven to decrease morbidity and mortality and to induce the reverse remodeling phenomenon include ACEIs, β-blockers, and cardiac resynchronization therapy.

- The management of acute heart failure in the operating room includes the use of low-dose loop diuretics in combination with vasodilators, positive inotropic drugs, exogenous BNP, and/or mechanical devices.

- Hypertrophic cardiomyopathy is the most common genetic cardiac disorder. Its pathophysiology is related to the development of LVOT obstruction and ventricular dysrhythmias that can cause sudden death.

- Factors that induce LVOT obstruction in HCM include hypovolemia, tachycardia, an increase in myocardial contractility, and a decrease in afterload. LVOT obstruction is managed by hydration, increasing afterload (phenylephrine), and decreasing heart rate and myocardial contractility (β-blockers and calcium channel blockers).

- DCM is the most common form of cardiomyopathy and the second most common cause of heart failure. The treatment and anesthetic implications are similar to those of patients with chronic heart failure.

- Cor pulmonale is right ventricular enlargement (hypertrophy and/or dilation) that may progress to right heart failure. It is caused by diseases that promote development of pulmonary hypertension.

- The most important pathophysiologic determinant of development of pulmonary hypertension and cor pulmonale in patients with chronic lung disease is alveolar hypoxia. The best available treatment to improve the prognosis in these patients is long-term oxygen therapy.

REFERENCES

Gheorghiade M, Zannad F, Sopko G, et al: International Working Group on Acute Heart Failure Syndromes: Acute heart failure syndromes: Current state and framework for future research. Circulation 2005;112:3958–3968.

Groban L, Butterworth J: Perioperative management of chronic heart failure. Anesth Analg 2006;103:57–75.

Hunt SA, Abraham WT, Chin MH, et al: ACC/AHA 2005 Guideline Update for the Diagnosis and Management of Chronic Heart Failure in the Adult: A report of the American College of Cardiology/American Heart Association Task Force on Practice Guidelines (Writing Committee to Update the 2001 Guidelines for the Evaluation and Management of Heart Failure): Developed in collaboration with the American College of Chest Physicians and the International Society for Heart and Lung Transplantation: Endorsed by the Heart Rhythm Society. Circulation 2005;112:154–235.

Jessup M, Brozena S: Heart failure. N Engl J Med 2003;348:2007–2018.

Maron BJ, Towbin JA, Thiene G, et al: Contemporary definition and classification of the cardiomyopathies: An American Heart Association Scientific Statement from the Council on Clinical Cardiology, Heart Failure and Transplantation Committee; Quality of Care and Outcomes Research and Functional Genomics and Transplantational Biology Interdisciplinary Working Groups; and Council on Epidemiology and Prevention. Circulation 2006;113:1807–1816.

Poliac LC, Barron ME, Maron BJ: Hypertrophic cardiomyopathy. Anesthesiology 2006;104:183–192.

Rauch H, Motsch J, Böttiger BW: Newer approaches to the pharmacologic management of heart failure. Curr Opin Anesthesiol 2006;19:75–81.

Swedberg K, Cleland J, Dargie H, et al: Guidelines for the diagnosis and treatment of chronic heart failure: Executive summary (update 2005): The Task Force for the Diagnosis and Treatment of Chronic Heart Failure of the European Society of Cardiology. Eur Heart J 2005;26:1115–1140.

Weitzenblum E: Chronic cor pulmonale. Heart 2003;89:225–230.

Yan AT, Yan RT, Liu PP: Narrative review: Pharmacotherapy for chronic heart failure: Evidence from recent clinical trials. Ann Intern Med 2005;142:132–145.

CHAPTER 7

Pericardial Diseases and Cardiac Trauma

Raj K. Modak

Acute Pericarditis
- Diagnosis
- Treatment
- Relapsing Pericarditis
- Pericarditis after Cardiac Surgery

Pericardial Effusion and Cardiac Tamponade
- Signs and Symptoms
- Diagnosis
- Treatment
- Management of Anesthesia

Constrictive Pericarditis
- Signs and Symptoms
- Diagnosis
- Treatment
- Management of Anesthesia

Pericardial and Cardic Trauma
- Pericardial Trauma
- Myocardial Contusion

Pericardial diseases may have diverse causes but result in responses that are clinically and pathologically similar. The three most frequent responses to pericardial injury are characterized as acute pericarditis, pericardial effusion, and constrictive pericarditis. Cardiac tamponade is a possibility whenever pericardial fluid accumulates under pressure. Management of anesthesia in patients with pericardial disease is facilitated by an understanding of the alterations in cardiovascular function produced by pericardial disease.

ACUTE PERICARDITIS

Viral infection is often presumed to be the cause of acute pericarditis that occurs as a primary illness (**Table 7-1**). Most cases of acute pericarditis follow a transient and uncomplicated clinical course and so the syndrome is often termed *acute benign pericarditis*. Acute benign pericarditis is unaccompanied by either a substantial pericardial effusion or cardiac tamponade and rarely progresses to constrictive pericarditis.

Pericarditis can occur after myocardial infarction. It most commonly occurs 1 to 3 days following a transmural myocardial infarction as a result of the interaction between the healing necrotic myocardium and the pericardium. Dressler's syndrome is a delayed form of acute pericarditis that may follow acute myocardial infarction. It occurs weeks to months after a myocardial infarction. It is thought that Dressler's syndrome is the result of an autoimmune process that is initiated by the entry of necrotic myocardium into the circulation where it acts as an antigen.

Diagnosis

The clinical diagnosis of acute pericarditis is based on the presence of chest pain, pericardial friction rub, and changes on

TABLE 7-1 Causes of Acute Pericarditis and Pericardial Effusion

Infectious
　Viral
　Bacterial
　Fungal
　Tuberculous
Postmyocardial infarction (Dressler's syndrome)
Posttraumatic/postcardiotomy
Metastatic disease
Drug induced
Mediastinal radiation
Systemic disease
　Rheumatoid arthritis
　Systemic lupus erythematosus
　Scleroderma

the electrocardiogram (ECG). Chest pain associated with acute pericarditis typically has an acute onset and is described as a severe pain located over the anterior chest. This pain typically worsens with inspiration, which helps to distinguish it from pain due to myocardial ischemia. Patients often report relief by changing from the supine position to sitting forward. Low-grade fever and sinus tachycardia are also present. Auscultation of the chest often reveals a friction rub, especially when the symptoms are acute. These high-pitched scratchy sounds occur when volumes in the heart are undergoing the most dramatic changes as during early ventricular filling and ventricular ejection. Pericardial friction rubs are present throughout the cardiac cycle, making it possible to differentiate these from pleural rubs whose sounds are related to inspiration.

Inflammation of the superficial myocardium is the most likely explanation for the diffuse changes seen on the ECG. Classically, the ECG changes associated with acute pericarditis evolve through four stages: stage I, diffuse ST segment elevation and PR segment depression; stage II, normalization of the ST and PR segments; stage III, widespread T-wave inversions; and stage IV, normalization of the T waves. The ST elevation seen early is usually present in all leads, but in postmyocardial infarction pericarditis, the changes may be more localized. The diffuse distribution and the absence of reciprocal ST segment depression distinguish these changes from the ECG changes of myocardial infarction. Depression of the PR segment seen on the ECG reflects superficial injury of the atrial myocardium and may be the earliest sign of acute pericarditis on the ECG. Patients with uremic pericarditis frequently do not have the typical ECG abnormalities of pericarditis. Acute pericarditis in the absence of an associated pericardial effusion does not alter cardiac function.

Treatment

Salicylates or nonsteroidal anti-inflammatory drugs may be useful in decreasing pericardial inflammation. Aspirin is most commonly prescribed, and ketorolac has also been used successfully. Symptomatic relief of the pain of acute pericarditis can also be provided by oral analgesics such as codeine. In some settings, relief may be achieved with the use of colchicine. Corticosteroids such as prednisone can also relieve the symptoms of acute pericarditis. However, their use early in the course of acute pericarditis is associated with an increased incidence of relapse after drug discontinuation. Therefore, the use of steroid therapy is usually reserved for patients who do not respond to conventional therapy.

Relapsing Pericarditis

Acute pericarditis due to any cause may follow a recurrent or chronic relapsing course. Relapsing pericarditis has two clinical presentations: incessant and intermittent. *Incessant pericarditis* applies to patients in whom discontinuation or attempts to wean from anti-inflammatory drugs nearly always results in a relapse within a period of 6 weeks or less. *Intermittent pericarditis* refers to patients with symptom-free intervals longer than 6 weeks without drug treatment. In many patients, the symptoms of relapsing pericarditis include weakness, fatigue, and headache and are associated with chest discomfort. Although relapsing pericarditis is uncomfortable, it is rarely life-threatening. Treatment may include standard treatments for acute pericarditis and/or corticosteroids (prednisone) or immunosuppressive drugs such as azathioprine.

Pericarditis after Cardiac Surgery

The postcardiotomy syndrome presents primarily as acute pericarditis. The cause of this syndrome may be infective or autoimmune. It may follow blunt or penetrating trauma, hemopericardium, or epicardial pacemaker implantation. Most commonly, it is seen in cardiac surgical patients in whom pericardiotomy was performed. The incidence of postcardiotomy syndrome associated with cardiac surgery is between 10% and 40%. It is more common in pediatric patients. Patients after cardiac transplantation are at lower risk, presumably due to their immunosuppressed state. Cardiac tamponade is a rare complication of postcardiotomy syndrome with an incidence ranging from 0.1% to 6%. The treatment of postcardiotomy syndrome is similar to that of other forms of acute pericarditis.

PERICARDIAL EFFUSION AND CARDIAC TAMPONADE

Pericardial fluid may accumulate in the pericardial cavity with virtually any form of pericardial disease. The pathophysiologic effects of a pericardial effusion depend on whether the fluid is under increased pressure. Cardiac tamponade occurs when the pressure of the fluid in the pericardial space impairs cardiac filling. Common causes of atraumatic and traumatic pericardial effusions are listed in Table 7-1. The etiology of as many as 20% of pericardial effusions is idiopathic. Neoplastic pericardial effusion is a common cause of cardiac tamponade in nonsurgical patients.

Pericardial fluid may be classified as transudative or exudative. Serosanguineous (exudative) fluid is typically seen when the pericardial disease is due to cancer, tuberculosis, or radiation exposure. Serosanguineous pericardial effusion also occurs in patients with end-stage renal disease who are on dialysis. Traumatic injury usually presents as hemopericardium. Perforation of the heart and subsequent cardiac tamponade may also result from the insertion of central venous catheters or pacemaker wires.

Signs and Symptoms

The signs and symptoms of a pericardial effusion depend on its size and duration (acute versus chronic). The pericardial space normally holds 15 to 50 mL of pericardial fluid. This fluid is an ultrafiltrate of plasma that comes from the visceral pericardium. Native pericardial fluid lubricates the heart and facilitates normal cardiac motion within the pericardial sac. Acute changes in pericardial volume as small as 100 mL may result in increased intrapericardial pressure and development of cardiac tamponade. Conversely, large volumes can be accommodated if the pericardial effusion develops gradually. In this situation, the pressure-volume relationship is altered and cardiac tamponade may not develop because the pericardium stretches to accommodate the volume of the effusion (**Fig. 7-1**). The development of a chronic pericardial effusion in this setting can result in effusion volumes in excess of 2 L. If the pressure in the pericardium remains low, large effusions can be tolerated without significant signs and symptoms. However, as pericardial pressure increases, right atrial pressure increases in parallel, such that right atrial pressure becomes an accurate reflection of intrapericardial pressure. At this point, patients may have signs and symptoms of cardiac tamponade.

Cardiac Tamponade

Cardiac tamponade presents as a spectrum of hemodynamic abnormalities of varying severity rather than as an all-or-none phenomenon. Symptoms of large pericardial effusions reflect compression of adjacent anatomic structures, specifically the esophagus, trachea, and lung. In this situation, common symptoms are anorexia, dyspnea, cough, and chest pain. Symptoms such as dysphagia, hiccups, and hoarseness may indicate higher pressure on these same adjacent tissues.

Two important physical signs of cardiac tamponade and constrictive pericarditis were described by Dr. Adolf Kussmaul in 1873. *Kussmaul's sign* is distention of the jugular veins during inspiration. *Pulsus paradoxus* was described by Kussmaul as "a pulse simultaneously slight and irregular, disappearing during inspiration and returning on expiration." The modern definition of pulsus paradoxus is a decrease in systolic blood pressure > 10 mm Hg during inspiration (**Fig. 7-2**). This hemodynamic change reflects selective impairment of diastolic filling of the left ventricle. Pulsus paradoxus is seen in about 75% of patients with acute cardiac tamponade but in only about 30% of patients with chronic pericardial effusion. Kussmaul's sign and pulsus paradoxus both represent dyssynchrony or opposing responses of the right and left ventricles to filling during the respiratory cycle. Another term for this is *ventricular discordance*.

Beck's triad consists of quiet heart sounds, increased jugular venous pressure, and hypotension. It is present in

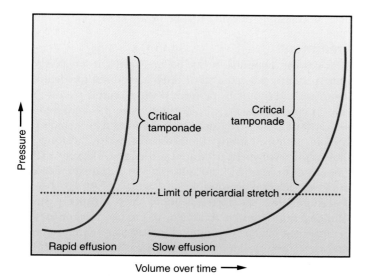

Figure 7-1 • Pericardial pressure-volume curves are shown in which the intrapericardial volume increases slowly or rapidly over time. On the left, rapidly increasing pericardial fluid quickly exceeds the limit of pericardial stretch, causing a steep increase in pericardial pressure. On the right, a slower rate of pericardial filling takes longer to exceed the limit of pericardial stretch because there is more time for the pericardium to stretch and for compensatory mechanisms to become activated. *(From Spodick DH: Acute cardiac tamponade. N Engl J Med 2003;349:684–690. Copyright 2003 Massachusetts Medical Society, with permission.)*

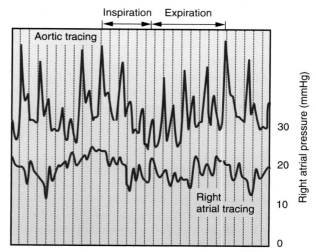

Figure 7-2 • In the presence of cardiac tamponade, the arterial blood pressure decreases more than 10 mm Hg during inspiration as a reflection of a concomitant decrease in left ventricular stroke volume. This contrasts with the opposite response observed during inspiration in the absence of cardiac tamponade, accounting for its designation as a paradoxical pulse (pulsus paradoxus).

one third of patients with acute cardiac tamponade. Another triad (quiet heart sounds, increased central venous pressure, and ascites) has been described with chronic pericardial effusion. More commonly, symptomatic patients with chronic pericardial effusion exhibit sinus tachycardia, jugular venous distention, hepatomegaly, and peripheral edema. The Ewart sign is an uncommon sign of pericardial effusion. It is an area of bronchial breath sounds and dullness to percussion caused by compression of the left lower lobe by the pericardial effusion. It is noted at the inferior angle of the left scapula.

Depending on the severity of cardiac tamponade, systemic blood pressure may be decreased or maintained in the normal range. Central venous pressure is almost always increased. Activation of the sympathetic nervous system is an attempt to maintain cardiac output and blood pressure by tachycardia and peripheral vasoconstriction. Cardiac output is maintained as long as central venous pressure exceeds right ventricular end-diastolic pressure. A progressive increase in intrapericardial pressure, however, eventually results in equalization of right atrial pressure and right ventricular end-diastolic pressure. Ultimately, the increased intrapericardial pressure leads to impaired diastolic filling of the heart, decreased stroke volume, and hypotension.

Cardiac tamponade may be the cause of low cardiac output syndrome during the early postoperative period after cardiac surgery. Cardiac tamponade may occur as a complication of various invasive procedures in the cardiac catheterization laboratory and intensive care unit. Acute cardiac tamponade may also be due to hemopericardium caused by aortic dissection, penetrating cardiac trauma, or acute myocardial infarction.

Loculated Pericardial Effusions

Loculated pericardial effusion may selectively compress one or more cardiac chambers producing localized cardiac tamponade. This is most frequently seen following cardiac surgery when blood accumulates behind the sternum and selectively compresses the right ventricle and right atrium. A similar response may be seen following anterior chest wall trauma. Transesophageal echocardiography is superior to transthoracic echocardiography for demonstrating a localized pericardial effusion.

Diagnosis

Echocardiography is the most accurate and practical method for diagnosing pericardial effusion and cardiac tamponade. Echocardiography can detect pericardial effusions as small as 20 mL. The measurement of the echo-free space between the heart and pericardium allows easy assessment of effusion size and may provide information about the cause of the effusion. Computed tomography and magnetic resonance imaging are also useful in detecting both pericardial effusion and pericardial thickening. The ECG may show low voltage in the presence of a large effusion. Chest radiography often shows a characteristic "water bottle heart," but this sign is not

TABLE 7-2 Signs and Symptoms of Cardiac Tamponade
Increased central venous pressure
Pulsus paradoxus
Equalization of cardiac filling pressures
Hypotension
Decreased voltage on the electrocardiogram
Activation of the sympathetic nervous system

specific for pericardial effusion. Pericardiocentesis may be useful for diagnosing metastatic disease or infection.

Echocardiography, although definitive for diagnosing pericardial effusion, cannot always confirm the presence of cardiac tamponade (**Table 7-2**). However, the presence of early diastolic inward wall motion of the right atrium or right ventricle ("collapse"), reflecting the similarity of intracavitary and intrapericardial pressure, is suggestive of the presence of cardiac tamponade. Echocardiography can also demonstrate ventricular discordance. Pulsed-wave Doppler examination of peak mitral and tricuspid inflow velocities will show a decrease in mitral flow and an increase in tricuspid flow during inspiration if tamponade is present. Ventricular septal deviation toward the left can also be seen during inspiration. Eventually with cardiac tamponade there will be equilibration of pressures within the cardiac chambers. Clinically, this can be confirmed by right heart catheterization. Pulmonary artery occlusion pressure and pulmonary artery diastolic pressure (both estimates of left atrial pressure and left ventricular end-diastolic pressure), right atrial pressure, and right ventricular end-diastolic pressure will be nearly equal.

Treatment

Mild cardiac tamponade can be managed conservatively in some patients, but removal of fluid is required for definitive treatment and should be performed when central venous pressure is increased. Pericardial fluid may be removed by pericardiocentesis or by surgical techniques that include subxiphoid pericardiostomy, thoracoscopic pericardiostomy, or thoractomy with pericardiostomy. Removal of even a small amount of pericardial fluid can result in a dramatic decrease in intrapericardial pressure.

Temporizing measures likely to help maintain stroke volume until definitive treatment of cardiac tamponade can be instituted include expanding intravascular volume, administering catecholamines to increase myocardial contractility, and correcting metabolic acidosis. Expansion of intravascular fluid volume can be achieved by intravenous infusion of either colloid or crystalloid solution. However, improvement in hemodynamic function may be limited and pericardiocentesis should not be delayed.

Continuous intravenous infusion of a catecholamine such as isoproterenol may be an effective temporizing measure for increasing myocardial contractility and heart rate. Atropine may be necessary to treat the bradycardia that results from vagal reflexes evoked by increased intrapericardial pressure. Dopamine infusion, which increases systemic vascular resistance, could also be employed to treat cardiac tamponade. As with intravascular fluid replacement, pericardiocentesis should never be delayed in preference to drug therapy.

Correction of metabolic acidosis is essential when considering management of cardiac tamponade. Metabolic acidosis due to low cardiac output should be treated to correct the myocardial depression seen with severe acidosis and to improve the inotropic effects of catecholamines.

Management of Anesthesia

General anesthesia and positive-pressure ventilation in the presence of hemodynamically significant cardiac tamponade can result in life-threatening *hypotension*. This hypotension can be due to anesthesia-induced peripheral vasodilation, direct myocardial depression, or decreased venous return from the increased intrathoracic pressure associated with positive-pressure ventilation. Pericardiocentesis under local anesthesia is often preferred for the initial management of hypotensive patients with cardiac tamponade. After the hemodynamic status has been improved by percutaneous pericardiocentesis, general anesthesia and positive-pressure ventilation can be instituted to permit surgical exploration and more definitive treatment of the cardiac tamponade. Induction and maintenance of anesthesia with ketamine or a benzodiazepine in combination with nitrous oxide are often selected. The circulatory effects of pancuronium are particularly useful for producing skeletal muscle relaxation in these patients. Intraoperative monitoring usually includes intra-arterial and central venous pressure monitoring.

If it is not possible to relieve cardiac tamponade before induction of anesthesia, the principal goals of anesthetic induction are to maintain adequate cardiac output and blood pressure. Anesthesia-induced decreases in myocardial contractility, systemic vascular resistance, and heart rate must be avoided. Increased intrathoracic pressure caused by straining or coughing during induction or by mechanical ventilation may further decrease venous return. Some advocate prepping and draping for incision prior to induction of anesthesia and endotracheal intubation. This would allow the shortest possible time from an adverse hemodynamic consequence of anesthesia/mechanical ventilation until relief of the tamponade. Ketamine is useful for induction and maintenance of anesthesia because it increases myocardial contractility, systemic vascular resistance, and heart rate. Induction of anesthesia with a benzodiazepine followed by maintenance with nitrous oxide plus fentanyl (or another synthetic narcotic) combined with pancuronium for skeletal muscle relaxation has also been used successfully. Continuous monitoring of blood pressure and central venous pressure should be initiated prior to induction of anesthesia. Administration of intravenous fluids and/or continuous infusion of a catecholamine may be useful for maintaining cardiac output until the cardiac tamponade is relieved by surgical drainage. After release of a severe tamponade, there is often a significant swing in blood pressure from hypotension to *hypertension*. This change should be anticipated and appropriate treatment should be immediate, especially if the etiology of the tamponade is an aortic hematoma, dissection, or aneurysm.

CONSTRICTIVE PERICARDITIS

Constrictive pericarditis is most often idiopathic or a result of previous cardiac surgery or exposure to radiotherapy. Tuberculosis may also cause constrictive pericarditis. *Chronic constrictive pericarditis* is characterized by fibrous scarring and adhesions that obliterate the pericardial cavity creating a "rigid shell" around the heart. Calcification may develop in long-standing cases. *Subacute constrictive pericarditis* is more common than chronic calcific pericarditis, and the resulting constriction in this situation is fibroelastic.

Signs and Symptoms

Pericardial constriction typically presents with symptoms and signs due to a combination of increased central venous pressure and low cardiac output. Symptoms of pericardial constriction include decreased exercise tolerance and fatigue. Jugular venous distention, hepatic congestion, ascites, and peripheral edema are signs of pericardial constriction that mimic right ventricular failure. Pulmonary congestion is usually lacking. Increased and eventual equalization of right atrial pressure, right ventricular artery end-diastolic pressure, and pulmonary artery occlusion pressure are features that occur in the presence of both constrictive pericarditis and cardiac tamponade. As pericardial pressure increases, right atrial pressure increases in parallel, and, therefore, the central venous pressure is an accurate reflection of intrapericardial pressure. Atrial dysrhythmias (atrial fibrillation or flutter) are often seen in patients with chronic constrictive pericarditis, presumably reflecting involvement of the sinoatrial node by the disease process.

Constrictive pericarditis is similar to cardiac tamponade in that both conditions impede diastolic filling of the heart and result in increased central venous pressure and ultimately in a decreased cardiac output. Diagnostic signs, however, differ in the two conditions. Pulsus paradoxus is a regular feature of cardiac tamponade but is not often seen with constrictive pericarditis. Kussmaul's sign (increased central venous pressure during inspiration) occurs more often in patients with constrictive pericarditis than in those with cardiac tamponade. An early diastolic sound ("pericardial knock") is often heard in patients with constrictive pericarditis but does not occur in cardiac tamponade. A prominent y-descent of the jugular venous pressure (Friedreich's sign) reflects the predominance of right ventricular filling in early diastole that is seen with constrictive pericarditis. This rapid early diastolic filling is also detected by a dip in early diastolic pressure. The ventricle is completely filled by the end of the rapid filling phase and diastasis, that is, a constant ventricular volume, persists for the remainder of diastole. Corresponding to this prolonged diastasis, ventricular diastolic pressure remains

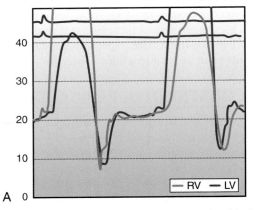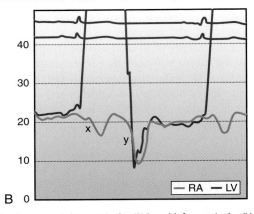

Figure 7-3 • Pressure recordings in a patient with constrictive pericarditis. **A**, Simultaneous right ventricular (RV) and left ventricular (LV) pressure tracings with equalization of diastolic pressure as well as "dip and plateau" morphology. **B**, Simultaneous right atrial (RA) and LV pressure with equalization of RA and LV diastolic pressure. Note the prominent y descent. *(From Vaitkus PT, Cooper KA, Shuman WP, Hardin NJ: Images in cardiovascular medicine: Constrictive pericarditis. Circulation 1996;93:834–835, with permission.)*

unchanged for the latter two thirds of diastole. This pattern of ventricular diastolic pressure in constrictive pericarditis is referred to as the "square root sign" or "dip and plateau" morphology (**Fig. 7-3A**).

Diagnosis

Constrictive pericarditis is difficult to diagnose and its signs and symptoms are therefore often erroneously attributed to liver disease or idiopathic pericardial effusion. The clinical diagnosis of constrictive pericarditis depends on the confirmation of an increased central venous pressure without other signs or symptoms of heart disease. Heart size and lung fields appear normal on chest radiography, but pericardial calcification can be seen in 30% to 50% of cases. The ECG may show only minor, nonspecific abnormalities. Echocardiography can be quite helpful in many instances by demonstrating abnormal septal motion and pericardial thickening that suggest the presence of constrictive pericarditis. Transesophageal echocardiography, computed tomography of the chest, and magnetic resonance imaging are superior to transthoracic echocardiography for demonstrating pericardial thickening. As with cardiac tamponade, ventricular discordance is a feature of constrictive pericarditis. Pulsed-wave Doppler studies often show exaggerated respiratory variation in mitral and tricuspid diastolic flow velocities. Cardiac catheterization demonstrates characteristic abnormalities, including increased central venous pressure, nondilated and normally contracting right and left ventricles, near-equilibration of right- and left-sided cardiac filling pressures, and a dip-plateau waveform in the right ventricle (see Figs. 7-3A and B). Many features considered characteristic of constrictive pericarditis may also be present in patients with restrictive cardiomyopathy, but several features help to distinguish these two entities (**Table 7-3**). Ventricular discordance is a feature of constrictive pericarditis but not of restrictive cardiomyopathy. Kussmaul's sign and pulsus paradoxus are present in constrictive pericarditis but lacking in restrictive cardiomyopathy. Two echocardiographic techniques can also

help in this evaluation. Pulsed-wave Doppler ultrasonography will demonstrate ventricular discordance in constrictive pericarditis. Tissue Doppler ultrasonography can be used to interrogate the motion of the mitral valve annulus. In restrictive cardiomyopathy, motion of the mitral annulus is restricted. In constrictive pericarditis, the motion of the mitral annulus is normal. Cardiac catheterization can demonstrate ventricular discordance by observing simultaneously recorded right and left ventricular systolic pressures. If discordance is present, right ventricular peak systolic pressure increases on inspiration while left ventricular peak pressure decreases. This observation of ventricular discordance indicates the presence of constrictive pericarditis rather than restrictive cardiomyopathy.

Treatment

Constrictive pericarditis that develops as a complication of acute pericarditis will occasionally resolve spontaneously. In nearly all patients, however, the definitive treatment of constrictive pericarditis consists of surgical stripping and removal of the adherent constricting pericardium. This procedure may result in considerable bleeding from the epicardial surface of the heart. Cardiopulmonary bypass may occasionally be used to facilitate pericardial stripping, especially if hemorrhage is difficult to control. Unlike cardiac tamponade in which hemodynamic improvement occurs immediately, surgical removal of constricting pericardium is not followed by an immediate improvement in cardiac output or a reduction in right atrial pressure. Typically, right atrial pressure returns to normal within 3 months of surgery. The absence of immediate hemodynamic improvement may reflect disuse atrophy of myocardial muscle fibers or persistent constrictive effects from sclerotic epicardium that is not removed with the pericardium. Inadequate long-term relief following surgical removal of constricting pericardium may reflect associated myocardial disease, especially in patients with radiation-induced pericardial disease.

TABLE 7-3 Features Useful for Differentiating Constrictive Pericarditis from Restrictive Cardiomyopathy

Feature	Constrictive Pericarditis	Restrictive Cardiomyopathy
Medical history	Previous pericarditis, cardiac surgery, trauma, radiotherapy, connective tissue disease	No such history
Mitral or tricuspid regurgitation	Usually absent	Often present
Ventricular septal movement with respiration	Movement toward left ventricle on inspiration	Little movement toward left ventricle
Respiratory variation in mitral and tricuspid flow velocity	Greater than 25% in most cases	Less than 15% in most cases
Equilibration of diastolic pressures in all cardiac chambers	Within 5 mm Hg in nearly all cases	In only a small proportion of cases
Respiratory variation of ventricular peak systolic pressures	Right and left ventricular peak systolic pressures are out of phase (discordant)	Right and left ventricular peak systolic pressures are in-phase
MRI/CT	Show pericardial thickening in most cases	Rarely shows pericardial thickening
Endomyocardial biopsy	Normal or nonspecific	Shows amyloid in some cases

Adapted from Hancock EW: Differential diagnosis of restrictive cardiomyopathy and constrictive pericarditis. Heart 2001;86:343–349.

Management of Anesthesia

Anesthetic drugs and techniques that minimize changes in heart rate, systemic vascular resistance, venous return, and myocardial contractility are selected. Combinations of opioids, benzodiazepines, and nitrous oxide with or without low doses of volatile anesthetics are acceptable for maintenance of anesthesia. Muscle relaxants with minimal circulatory effects are the best choices, although a modest increase in heart rate as seen with administration of pancuronium is also acceptable. Preoperative optimization of intravascular volume is essential. When hemodynamic compromise (hypotension) due to increased intrapericardial pressure is present prior to surgery, management of anesthesia is as described for cardiac tamponade.

Invasive monitoring of arterial and central venous pressure is helpful because removal of adherent pericardium may be a tedious and long operation often associated with significant fluid/blood losses. Cardiac dysrhythmias are common, presumably reflecting direct mechanical stimulation of the heart. Intravenous fluids and blood products will be necessary to treat the significant fluid/blood losses associated with pericardiectomy.

Postoperative ventilatory insufficiency may necessitate continued mechanical ventilation. Cardiac dysrhythmias and low cardiac output may require treatment during the postoperative period.

PERICARDIAL AND CARDIAC TRAUMA

Blunt injuries to the chest can result in cardiovascular injury. The severity of this injury can be as mild as bruising or as severe as death within minutes. There may be serious cardiovascular injury despite the lack of obvious external signs of trauma. Trauma, especially in motor vehicle crashes, is the primary cause of blunt chest injury. In automobile accidents, rapid deceleration of the chest as it impacts the steering wheel serves as the main mechanism of injury. Sudden deceleration from speeds as low as 20 miles per hour can result in serious injury. Soft mobile tissues can be crushed by their impact on the sternum and ribs. Shear forces on internal thoracic structures can result in tears in fragile tissues. Injuries to the aorta include aortic hematoma, dissection, and rupture. The pericardium can be lacerated or ruptured, and the heart can herniate through the pericardial defect. The heart itself can be contused or ruptured or suffer damage to its internal structures (valves) or to its blood supply. Because of its immediate substernal location, the right ventricle is more likely than the left ventricle to be seriously injured. Blood from aortic or cardiac injury can fill the pericardial space causing cardiac tamponade. Pulmonary contusion may also result from blunt chest trauma and can manifest as hypoxemia, consolidation on chest radiograph, or pleural effusion. Hemorrhage into the tracheobronchial tree may accompany pulmonary contusion.

Pericardial Trauma

Autopsy studies indicate that pericardial lacerations are common in persons sustaining severe chest wall injuries due to rapid deceleration. Lacerations can be limited to the pericardium or can involve adjacent structures such as the pleura and diaphragm. Pericardial-pleural tears can result in cardiac herniation and strangulation. The diaphragmatic portion of the pericardium can rupture when the diaphragm is injured and can result in bowel herniating into the pericardial sac or the heart herniating into the abdomen.

A retrospective study of blunt cardiac and pericardial injury found that in patients with pericardial rupture, 18% also had diaphragmatic tears, 9% had right-sided pleural tears, and 9% had mediastinal tears. Nearly 30% of these patients had cardiac herniation, and this was associated with a survival rate of only 33%.

Small herniations may manifest as impaired cardiac filling or ischemia if coronary blood flow becomes impaired. Larger herniations can result in strangulation of the heart by impairing ventricular filling and ejection

Diagnosis

The nonspecific signs and symptoms of pericardial rupture and cardiac herniation make the diagnosis difficult. Suspicion of pericardial trauma/pericardial rupture could be raised when unexplained alterations in pulse and blood pressure occur after initial resuscitation, especially if a sternal fracture and/or multiple rib fractures are present. Palpation and auscultation can reveal an abnormal location for the heart. Mediastinal air on a chest radiograph should be investigated further to rule out pneumopericardium, which would indicate the presence of a pericardial laceration. Rarely, chest radiography or computed tomography shows evidence of cardiac herniation.

Treatment

Minor injury or a small laceration of the pericardium can often go unnoticed. These patients may develop an "idiopathic" pericarditis with or without pericardial effusion. Severe lacerations associated with hemodynamic instability and cardiac herniation require emergency thoracotomy. However, institution of mechanical ventilation may precipitate hemodynamic collapse. Cardiac output should be maintained by fluids and/or inotropic drugs as needed until the herniation is released.

Myocardial Contusion
Signs and Symptoms

The symptoms of myocardial contusion typically include chest pain and palpitations. The chest pain can resemble angina pectoris but is not relieved by nitroglycerin. Dysrhythmias frequently complicate myocardial contusion, but cardiac failure is uncommon.

Diagnosis

The presence of chest pain and ECG changes, especially in young patients, should prompt questions about recent chest trauma that might have seemed trivial at the time of its occurrence. Electrocardiographic changes include ST-T wave abnormalities, supraventricular and ventricular dysrhythmias, and atrioventricular nodal dysfunction. However, diffuse nonspecific ST-T wave abnormalities are commonly noted in trauma patients, even in the absence of myocardial contusion.

Cardiac contusion can be recognized by transthoracic or transesophageal echocardiography, which can demonstrate impaired ventricular wall motion, valvular regurgitation, or pericardial effusion. Wall motion abnormalities usually resolve within a few days.

Serum concentrations of creatine kinase and its MB fraction increase but are often difficult to interpret because of the release of creatine kinase from injured skeletal muscles. However, the cardiac biomarkers troponin I and T can provide specific information about myocardial injury.

Treatment

The treatment of myocardial contusion is directed toward improving the symptoms and anticipating possible complications. Life-threatening dysrhythmias can occur within the first 24 to 48 hours after injury. Severely contused hearts may also require hemodynamic support. Patients with severe myocardial contusion may have other injuries that require emergent surgical intervention. Invasive hemodynamic monitoring together with electrocardiographic monitoring is prudent in this situation. Anesthetic drugs that depress myocardial function should be avoided. A cardioverter/defibrillator and drugs for dysrhythmia treatment should be immediately available.

KEY POINTS

- Most cases of acute pericarditis are due to viral infection and follow a transient and uncomplicated clinical course. Therefore, this syndrome is often termed acute benign pericarditis.

- The postcardiotomy syndrome presents primarily as acute pericarditis. It may follow blunt or penetrating trauma, hemopericardium, or epicardial pacemaker implantation. Most commonly, however, it is seen after cardiac surgery in which pericardiotomy was performed.

- The pathophysiologic effects of a pericardial effusion depend on whether the fluid is under increased pressure or not. Cardiac tamponade occurs when the pressure of the fluid in the pericardial space impairs cardiac filling.

- Pulsus paradoxus is defined as a decrease in systolic blood pressure greater than 10 mm Hg during inspiration. This hemodynamic change reflects selective impairment of diastolic filling of the left ventricle. Pulsus paradoxus represents dyssynchrony or opposing responses of the right and left ventricles to filling during the respiratory cycle. Another term for this is ventricular discordance.

- Cardiac output is maintained during cardiac tamponade as long as central venous pressure exceeds right ventricular end-diastolic pressure, but a progressive increase in intrapericardial pressure will eventually result in equalization of right atrial pressure and right ventricular end-diastolic pressure. Ultimately, the increased intrapericardial

KEY POINTS—cont'd

pressure leads to impaired diastolic filling of the heart, decreased stroke volume, and hypotension.

- Temporizing measures likely to help maintain stroke volume until definitive treatment of cardiac tamponade is undertaken include expanding intravascular volume, administering catecholamines to increase myocardial contractility, and correcting metabolic acidosis.

- Removal of pericardial fluid is the definitive treatment of cardiac tamponade and should be performed when central venous pressure is increased. Pericardial fluid may be removed by percutaneous pericardiocentesis or by surgical techniques. Removal of even a small amount of pericardial fluid can result in a dramatic decrease in intrapericardial pressure.

- Pericardiocentesis under local anesthesia is often preferred for the initial management of hypotensive patients with cardiac tamponade. After the hemodynamic status has been improved by percutaneous pericardiocentesis, general anesthesia and positive-pressure ventilation can be instituted to permit surgical exploration and more definitive treatment of the tamponade.

- Many features considered characteristic of constrictive pericarditis may also be present in patients with restrictive cardiomyopathy, but several features help to distinguish between these two entities. Kussmaul's sign and pulsus paradoxus are present with constrictive pericarditis but lacking with restrictive cardiomyopathy. Ventricular discordance is a feature of constrictive pericarditis but not of restrictive cardiomyopathy.

- Trauma, especially motor vehicle trauma, is the primary cause of blunt chest injury. Rapid deceleration of the chest as it impacts the steering wheel serves as the main mechanism of cardiovascular injury. Injuries to the aorta include aortic hematoma, dissection, and rupture. The pericardium can be lacerated or ruptured, and the heart can herniate through the pericardial defect. The heart itself can be contused or ruptured or suffer damage to its internal structures (valves) or to its blood supply. Because of its immediate substernal location, the right ventricle is more likely than the left ventricle to be seriously injured.

REFERENCES

Alpert MA, Ravenscraft MD: Pericardial involvement in end-stage renal disease. Am J Med Sci 2003;325:228–236.

Asher CR, Klein AL: Diastolic heart failure: Restrictive cardiomyopathy, constrictive pericarditis, and cardiac tamponade: Clinical and echocardiographic evaluation. Cardiol Rev 2002;10:218–229.

Goyle KK, Walling AD: Diagnosing pericarditis. American Family Physician 2002;66:1695–1702.

Hancock EW: Differential diagnosis of restrictive cardiomyopathy and constrictive pericarditis. Heart 2001;86:343–349.

Karam N, Patel P, deFilippi C: Diagnosis and management of chronic pericardial effusions. Am J Med Sci 2001;322:79–87.

Little WC, Freeman GL: Pericardial disease. Circulation 2006;113: 1622–1632.

Shabetai R: Recurrent pericarditis: Recent advances and remaining questions. Circulation 2005;112:1921–1923.

Soler-Soler J, Sagrista-Sauleda J, Permanyer-Miralda G: Management of pericardial effusion. Heart 2001;86:235–240.

Soler-Soler J, Sagrista-Sauleda J, Permanyer-Miralda G: Relapsing pericarditis. Heart 2004;90:1364–1368.

Spodick DH: Acute pericarditis: Current concepts and practice. JAMA 2003;289:1150–1153.

Sybrandy KC, Cramer MJ, Burgersdijk C: Diagnosing cardiac contusion: Old wisdom and new insights. Heart 2003;89:485–489.

Wall MJ Jr, Mattox KL, Wolf DA: The cardiac pendulum: Blunt rupture of the pericardium with strangulation of the heart. J Trauma 2005;59:136–141.

CHAPTER 8

Vascular Disease

Marbelia Gonzalez

Diseases of the Thoracic and Abdominal Aorta

Aneurysms and Dissection of the Thoracic Aorta
- Etiology
- Classification
- Signs and Symptoms
- Diagnosis
- Preoperative Evaluation
- Indications for Surgery
- Management of Anesthesia
- Postoperative Management

Aneurysms of the Abdominal Aorta
- Diagnosis
- Treatment
- Preoperative Evaluation
- Rupture of an Abdominal Aortic Aneurysm
- Management of Anesthesia
- Postoperative Management
- Endovascular Aortic Aneurysm Repair

Peripheral Vascular Disease
- Risk Factors
- Signs and Symptoms
- Diagnostic Tests
- Treatment
- Management of Anesthesia
- Postoperative Management
- Subclavian Steal Syndrome
- Coronary-Subclavian Steal Syndrome

Acute Arterial Occlusion
- Signs and Symptoms
- Diagnosis

- Treatment
- Management of Anesthesia

Systemic Vasculitis
- Takayasu's Arteritis
- Thromboangiitis Obliterans (Buerger's Disease)
- Wegener's Granulomatosis
- Temporal Arteritis
- Polyarteritis Nodosa
- Kawasaki Disease

Raynaud's Phenomenon
- Classification
- Etiology
- Diagnosis
- Treatment
- Management of Anesthesia

Carotid Artery Disease
- Cerebrovascular Anatomy

Carotid Endarterectomy
- Preoperative Evaluation
- Management of Anesthesia
- Postoperative Management and Complications
- Endovascular Treatment of Carotid Disease

Peripheral Venous Disease
- Prevention of Venous Thromboembolism

Cardiac complications are the leading cause of perioperative morbidity and mortality in patients undergoing noncardiac surgery. Compared to the general surgical population, the incidence of these complications is higher in patients undergoing vascular surgery.

Vascular surgery patients have a higher incidence of coronary artery disease and are at a particularly high risk of perioperative myocardial infarction. However, the risk of perioperative cardiac complications differs based on the type of vascular surgery performed. For example, peripheral vascular procedures actually have a higher rate of cardiovascular complications than central vascular procedures such as aortic aneurysm repair. The recent trend toward endovascular management of aortic and peripheral vascular disease may change cardiovascular risk substantially.

DISEASES OF THE THORACIC AND ABDOMINAL AORTA

Diseases of the aorta are most often aneurysmal. Occlusive disease is more likely to occur in peripheral arteries. The aorta and its major branches are affected by two entities that may be present simultaneously or occur at different stages of the same disease process. An *aneurysm* is a dilatation of all three layers of an artery. The most common definition is a 50% increase in diameter compared to normal. Arterial diameter depends on age, gender, and body habitus. Aneurysms may occasionally produce symptoms because of compression of surrounding structures, but rupture with exsanguination is the most dreaded complication. Aneurysms of the aorta may involve the ascending or descending portions of the thoracic aorta or the abdominal aorta.

Dissection of an artery occurs when blood enters the media layer. The media of large arteries is made up of organized lamellar units that decrease in number in relation to the distance from the heart. The initiating event of an aortic dissection is a tear in the intima. Blood surges through the intimal tear into an extraluminal channel called the *false lumen*. Blood in the false lumen can reenter the true lumen anywhere along the course of the dissection. The origins of aortic branch arteries arising from the area involved in the dissection may be compromised and the aortic valve rendered incompetent. This sequence of events occurs over minutes to hours. A delay in diagnosis or treatment can be fatal.

ANEURYSMS AND DISSECTION OF THE THORACIC AORTA

Dissection of the aorta can originate anywhere along the length of the aorta, but the most common points of origin are in the thorax, in the ascending aorta just above the aortic valve and just distal to the origin of the left subclavian artery near the insertion of the ligamentum arteriosum. Aneurysm is the most common condition of the thoracic aorta requiring surgical treatment.

Etiology

Systemic hypertension is the most important risk factor for thoracic aortic dissection. Predisposition to aortic dissection can also be a result of several nonhereditary and hereditary factors. Nonhereditary conditions include those related to manipulation of or surgery on the aorta and blunt trauma. Deceleration injury, as from an automobile accident, is an important cause of blunt trauma–related thoracic aortic dissection. The dissection typically involves the descending thoracic aorta and begins at the point of fixation of the aorta to the thorax, that is, the ligamentum arteriosum just distal to the origin of the left subclavian artery. Iatrogenic aortic dissection may occur as a complication of aortic cannulation, aortic cross-clamping, or at points at which the aorta was incised for aortic valve replacement or proximal anastomosis of a bypass graft. Aortic dissection predominates in men, but there is also an association with pregnancy. Approximately half of all aortic dissections in women younger than 40 years of age occur during pregnancy, usually during the third trimester.

Thoracic aortic aneurysms and dissections associated with known genetic syndromes are well described. These inherited diseases of blood vessels include conditions affecting both large arteries such as the aorta and those involving the microvasculature. Four major inherited disorders are known to affect major arteries. These include Marfan syndrome (MS), Ehlers-Danlos syndrome, bicuspid aortic valve, and nonsyndromic familial aortic dissection. Important recent observations have changed the thinking about the pathophysiology of aortic disease associated with these entities. It was once believed that mutant connective tissue proteins corrupted proteins from the normal allele (dominant negative effect). When this was combined with the normal wear and tear to which the aorta is subjected, dilatation and dissection resulted. It is now known that matrix proteins in addition to their mechanical properties have important roles in the homeostasis of the smooth muscle cells that produce them. Matrix proteins exert a key metabolic function by their ability to sequester, store, and participate in the precisely controlled activation and release of bioactive molecules. In the inherited disorders associated with aortic dissection, this loss of function (biochemical rather than mechanical) is thought to alter smooth muscle cell homeostasis. The end result is a change in matrix metabolism that causes structural weakness in the aorta.

Although the genetics of thoracic aortic aneurysm disease in patients with MS are well documented, less is known about familial patterns of aneurysm occurrence not associated with any particular collagen or vascular disease. Up to 19% of people with thoracic aortic aneurysm and dissection do not have syndromes traditionally considered to predispose them to aortic disease. However, these individuals often have several relatives with thoracic aortic aneurysm disease, suggesting a strong genetic predisposition.

MS is one of the most prevalent hereditary connective tissue disorders. Its inheritance pattern is autosomal dominant. MS is caused by mutations in the fibrillin 1 gene. Fibrillin is an important connective tissue protein in the capsule of the ocular lens, arteries, lung, skin, and dura mater. Fibrillin mutations can result in disease manifestations in each of these tissues. Because fibrillin is an integral part of elastin, the recognition of the mutations in fibrillin led to the assumption that the clinical manifestations of MS in the aorta were secondary to an inherent weakness of the aortic wall exacerbated by aging. However, histologic studies of the aortas of MS patients also demonstrate abnormalities in matrix metabolism that can result in matrix destruction.

Ehlers-Danlos syndrome represents a group of connective tissue disorders associated with skin fragility, easy bruisability, and osteoarthritis. There are several forms of the syndrome, but an increased risk of premature death occurs only in Ehlers-Danlos syndrome type IV. This vascular form of Ehlers-Danlos syndrome is caused by mutations in the type III procollagen gene. Type III collagen is abundant in the intestine and arterial walls. The alteration in type III collagen associated with Ehlers-Danlos syndrome type IV accounts for the most common clinical presentation of these patients, that is, arterial dissection or intestinal rupture.

Bicuspid aortic valve is the most common congenital anomaly resulting in aortic dilatation/dissection. It occurs in 1% of the general population. Histologic studies show elastin degradation in the aorta just above the aortic valve. Echocardiography shows that aortic root dilatation is common even in younger patients with bicuspid aortic valve. Bicuspid aortic valve clusters in families and is found in approximately 9% of first-degree relatives of affected individuals.

Nonsyndromic familial aortic dissection and aneurysm is found in approximately 20% of patients referred for repair of thoracic aneurysm or dissection. These families do not meet the clinical criteria for MS and do not have biochemical abnormalities in type III collagen. In most of these families, the inheritance pattern appears dominant with variable penetrance. At least three chromosomal regions have so far been mapped in families with nonsyndromic thoracic aortic aneurysm disease. The specific biochemical abnormalities predisposing to thoracic aortic aneurysm disease remain to be identified.

Classification

Aortic aneurysms can be classified morphologically as either fusiform or saccular. A fusiform aneurysm is a uniform dilation involving the entire circumference of the aortic wall, whereas a saccular aneurysm is an eccentric dilation of the aorta that communicates with the main lumen by a variably sized neck. Aneurysms can also be classified based on the pathology found in the aortic wall (e.g., such as due to atherosclerosis or cystic medial necrosis).

Arteriosclerosis is the primary lesion associated with aneurysms in the infrarenal abdominal aorta, thoracoabdominal aorta, and descending thoracic aorta. Aneurysms affecting the ascending aorta are primarily the result of lesions that cause degeneration of the aortic media, a pathologic process termed cystic medial necrosis.

Aneurysms of the thoracoabdominal aorta may also be classified according to their anatomic location. Two classifications widely used for aortic dissection (**Fig. 8-1**) are the DeBakey and Stanford classifications. The DeBakey classification includes types I to III. In type I, the intimal tear originates

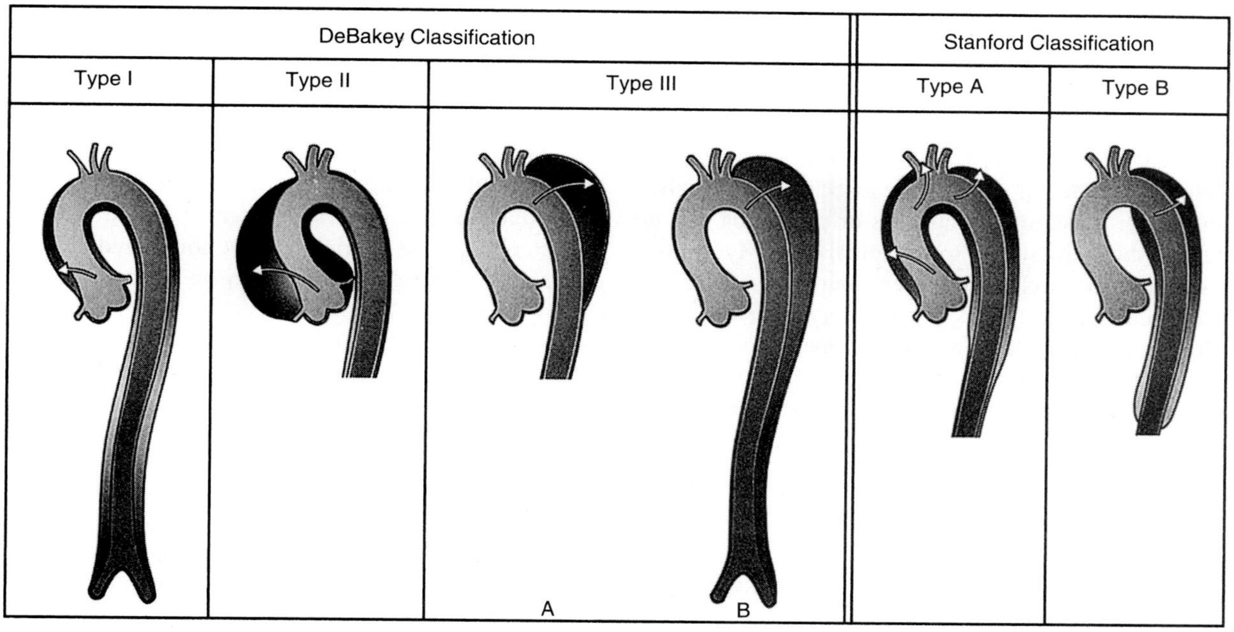

DeBakey Classification			Stanford Classification	
Type I	Type II	Type III	Type A	Type B

Figure 8-1 • The two most widely used classifications of aortic dissection. The DeBakey classification includes three types: type I, the intimal tear usually originates in the proximal ascending aorta and the dissection involves the ascending aorta and variable lengths of the aortic arch and descending and abdominal aorta; type II, the dissection is confined to the ascending aorta; type III, the dissection is confined to the descending thoracic aorta (type IIIa) or extends into the abdominal aorta and iliac arteries (type IIIb). The Stanford classification has two types: type A, all cases in which the ascending aorta is involved by the dissection, with or without involvement of the arch or the descending aorta; type B, cases in which the ascending aorta is not involved. *(From Kouchoukos NT, Dougenis D: Surgery of the thoracic aorta. N Engl J Med 1997;336:1876–1888. Copyright 1997 Massachusetts Medical Society with permission.)*

in the ascending aorta and the dissection involves the ascending aorta, arch, and variable lengths of the descending thoracic and abdominal aorta. In DeBakey type II, the dissection is confined to the ascending aorta. In type III, the dissection is confined to the descending thoracic aorta (type IIIa) or extends into the abdominal aorta and iliac arteries (type IIIb). The Stanford classification describes thoracic aneurysms as type A or B. Type A includes all cases in which the ascending aorta is involved by the dissection, with or without involvement of the arch or descending aorta. Type B includes all cases in which the ascending aorta is not involved.

Signs and Symptoms

Many patients with thoracic aortic aneurysm are asymptomatic at the time of presentation with the aneurysm being detected during testing for other disorders. Symptoms due to thoracic aneurysm typically reflect impingement of the aneurysm on adjacent structures. Hoarseness results from stretching of the left recurrent laryngeal nerve. Stridor is due to compression of the trachea. Dysphagia is due to compression of the esophagus. Dyspnea results from compression of the lungs. Plethora and edema result from compression of the superior vena cava. Patients with ascending aortic aneurysms associated with dilation of the aortic valve annulus may present with signs of aortic regurgitation and congestive heart failure.

Acute, severe, sharp pain in the anterior chest, the neck, or between the shoulder blades is the typical presenting symptom of thoracic aortic dissection. The pain may migrate as the dissection advances along the aorta. Patients with aortic dissection often appear as if they are in shock (vasoconstricted), yet the systemic blood pressure may be quite elevated. Other symptoms and signs of acute aortic dissection reflect occlusion of branches of the aorta such as diminution or absence of peripheral pulses. Neurologic complications of aortic dissection may include stroke caused by occlusion of a carotid artery, ischemic peripheral neuropathy associated with ischemia of an arm or a leg, and paraparesis or paraplegia due to impairment of the blood supply to the spinal cord. Myocardial infarction may reflect occlusion of a coronary artery. Gastrointestinal ischemia may occur. Renal artery obstruction is manifested by an increase in serum creatinine concentration. Retrograde dissection into the sinus of Valsalva with rupture into the pericardial space leading to cardiac tamponade is a major cause of death. Approximately 90% of patients with acute dissection of the ascending aorta who are not treated surgically die within 3 months.

Diagnosis

Widening of the mediastinum on chest radiograph may be diagnostic of a thoracic aortic aneurysm. However, enlargement of the ascending aorta may be confined to the retrosternal area so the aortic silhouette can appear normal. Computed tomography (CT) and magnetic resonance imaging can be used to diagnose thoracic aortic disease, but in acute aortic dissection, the diagnosis is most rapidly and safely made using transesophageal echocardiography with color Doppler imaging. Angiography of the aorta may be required for patients undergoing elective surgery on the thoracic aorta so that the complete extent of the dissection and the location of all compromised aortic branches can be defined.

Preoperative Evaluation

Because myocardial ischemia/infarction, respiratory failure, renal failure, and stroke are the principal causes of morbidity and mortality associated with surgery on the thoracic aorta, preoperative assessment of the function of these organ systems is needed. Assessment for the presence of myocardial ischemia, previous myocardial infarction, valvular dysfunction, and heart failure is important in risk stratification and in planning maneuvers for risk reduction. A preoperative percutaneous coronary intervention or coronary artery bypass grafting may be indicated in some patients with ischemic heart disease. Adjustment of drugs for manipulation of preload and afterload may be very advantageous in those with heart failure or significant aortic regurgitation.

Cigarette smoking and the presence of chronic obstructive pulmonary disease are important predictors of respiratory failure after thoracic aorta surgery. Spirometric tests of lung function and arterial blood gas analysis may better define this risk. Reversible airway obstruction and pulmonary infection should be treated with bronchodilators, antibiotics, and chest physiotherapy. Smoking cessation is very desirable.

The presence of preoperative renal dysfunction is the single most important predictor of the development of acute renal failure after surgery on the thoracic aorta. Preoperative hydration and avoidance of hypovolemia, hypotension, low cardiac output, and nephrotoxic drugs during the perioperative period are important in decreasing the likelihood of postoperative renal failure.

Duplex imaging of the carotid arteries or angiography of the brachiocephalic and intracranial arteries may be performed preoperatively in patients with a history of stroke or transient ischemic attacks. Patients with severe stenosis of one or both common or internal carotid arteries could be considered for carotid endarterectomy before elective surgery on the thoracic aorta.

Indications for Surgery

Thoracic aortic aneurysm repair is an elective procedure considered when aneurysm size exceeds a diameter of 5 cm. Some liberalization of this size limit may be given to patients with a significant family history or a previous diagnosis of any of the hereditable diseases that affect blood vessels. A number of important technical advances have decreased the risk of surgery on the thoracic aorta. These advances include the use of adjuncts such as distal aortic perfusion, profound hypothermia with circulatory arrest, monitoring of evoked potentials in the brain and spinal cord, and cerebrospinal fluid drainage.

Ascending and aortic arch dissection requires emergent or urgent surgery. Descending thoracic aortic dissection is generally associated with better survival compared to a dissection involving the ascending aorta and is rarely treated with urgent surgery.

Type A Dissection

The International Registry of Acute Aortic Dissection represents 21 large referral centers from around the world. This registry has shown that the in-hospital mortality rate of ascending aortic dissection is approximately 27% in patients subjected to timely and successful surgery. This is in contrast to an in-hospital mortality rate of 56% in those treated medically. Other independent predictors of in-hospital death include age, visceral ischemia, hypotension, renal failure, cardiac tamponade, coma, and pulse deficits.

Long-term survival rate, i.e., survival at 1 to 3 years after hospital discharge is 90% to 96% in the surgically treated group and 69% to 89% in those treated medically who survive the initial hospitalization. Thus, aggressive medical treatment and imaging surveillance of patients who, for various reasons, are unable to undergo surgery appears prudent.

Ascending Aorta

All patients with acute dissection involving the ascending aorta should be considered candidates for surgery. The most commonly performed procedures are replacement of the ascending aorta and aortic valve with a composite graft (a Dacron graft containing a prosthetic valve) or replacement of the ascending aorta and resuspension of the aortic valve.

Aortic Arch

In patients with acute aortic arch dissection, resection of the aortic arch (that is, the segment of aorta that extends from the origin of the innominate artery to the origin of the left subclavian artery) is indicated. Surgery on the aortic arch requires cardiopulmonary bypass, profound hypothermia, and a period of circulatory arrest. With current techniques, a period of circulatory arrest of 30 to 40 minutes at a body temperature of 15° to 18°C can be tolerated by most patients. Focal and diffuse neurologic deficits are the major complications associated with resection of the aortic arch. These occur in 3% to 18% of patients.

Descending Thoracic Aorta

For patients with degenerative or chronic aneurysms, elective resection is advisable if the aneurysm exceeds 5 to 6 cm in diameter or if symptoms are present.

Patients with an acute type B aortic dissection that is uncomplicated, that is, presents with normal hemodynamics, no periaortic hematoma, and no branch vessel involvement can be treated with medical therapy. Such therapy consists of (1) intra-arterial monitoring of systemic blood pressure and urinary output and (2) administration of drugs to control blood pressure and the force of left ventricular contraction. β-Blockers and nitroprusside are commonly used for this purpose. This patient population has a mortality rate of 10% to 12%.

Surgery is indicated for patients with type B aortic dissection who have signs of impending rupture (persistent pain, hypotension, left-sided hemothorax); ischemia of the legs, abdominal viscera, or spinal cord; and/or renal failure.

Surgical treatment of distal aortic dissection is associated with 29% in-hospital mortality.

Endovascular Repair Endovascular placement of intraluminal stent grafts to treat patients with aneurysms of the descending thoracic aorta may be particularly useful in the elderly and in those with co-existing medical conditions, such as hypertension, chronic obstructive pulmonary disease, and renal insufficiency, that would significantly increase the risk of conventional operative treatment. Endovascular treatment of aortic aneurysms is achieved by transluminal placement of one or more stent-graft devices across the longitudinal extent of the lesion. The prosthesis bridges the aneurysmal sac to exclude it from high-pressure aortic blood flow, thereby allowing for sac thrombosis around the stent and possible remodeling of the aortic wall.

Currently, endovascular aneurysm repair of the intrathoracic aorta has been focused on the descending thoracic aorta, that is, the portion distal to the left subclavian artery. The thoracic aorta poses several unique challenges to endovascular repair compared to endovascular repair of the abdominal aorta. First, the hemodynamic forces are significantly more severe and place greater mechanical demands on thoracic endografts. The potential for device migration, kinking, and late structural failure is an important concern. Second, greater flexibility is required of thoracic devices to conform to the natural curvature of the proximal descending aorta and to lesions with tortuous morphology. Third, because larger devices are necessary to accommodate the diameter of the thoracic aorta, arterial access is more problematic. Fourth, as with conventional open thoracic aneurysm repair, paraplegia remains a potential complication of the endovascular approach despite the absence of aortic cross-clamping.

Three endograft devices are currently undergoing clinical trials for use in thoracic aortic aneurysm repair. Although each device has unique features, all employ the same basic structural design. The endovascular devices are composed of a stent (nitinol or stainless steel) covered with fabric (polyester or polytetrafluoroethylene).

The literature on thoracic stent grafting consists mostly of small- to medium-sized case series with short- to medium-term follow-up. All these studies illustrate a common pattern of outcomes. Overall, successful device deployment is achieved in 85% to 100% of cases and perioperative mortality ranges from 0% to 14%, falling within or below elective surgery mortality rates of 5% to 20%. Outcomes have improved over time with accumulated technical expertise, technologic advances in the devices, and improved patient selection criteria. Current reported experience with thoracic stent grafting demonstrates successful deployment in 87% of cases, 30-day mortality of 2% to 5% for elective cases, and paraplegia and endoleak rates of 4% to 9%.

Endoleaks are the most prevalent stent-graft treatment complications. Endoleaks occur more commonly at the proximal or distal stent attachment sites (type I endoleak). Type I endoleaks are serious and require expeditious intervention since they represent a direct communication between the aneurysm sac and aortic blood flow. Treatment options include transcatheter coil

139

or glue embolization, balloon angioplasty, placement of endovascular graft extensions, and open surgical repair.

Unique Risks of Surgery Surgical resection of thoracic aortic aneurysms can be associated with a number of serious, even life-threatening complications. There is the risk of spinal cord ischemia (anterior spinal artery syndrome) with resulting paraparesis or paraplegia. Cross-clamping and unclamping the aorta introduces the potential for adverse hemodynamic responses such as myocardial ischemia and heart failure. Hypothermia, an important neuroprotective maneuver, can be responsible for the development of coagulopathy. Renal insufficiency/renal failure occurs in up to 30% of patients. Approximately 6% of patients will require hemodialysis. Pulmonary complications are common. The incidence of respiratory failure approaches 50%. Cardiac complications are the leading cause of mortality.

Anterior Spinal Artery Syndrome

Cross-clamping the thoracic aorta can result in ischemic damage to the spinal cord (**Fig. 8-2**). The frequency of spinal cord injury ranges from 0.2% after elective infrarenal abdominal aortic aneurysm repair to 8% in elective thoracic aortic aneurysm repair up to 40% in the setting of acute aortic dissection or rupture involving the descending thoracic aorta. Manifestations of anterior spinal artery syndrome include flaccid paralysis of the lower extremities and bowel and bladder dysfunction. Sensation and proprioception are spared.

Spinal Cord Blood Supply

The spinal cord is supplied by one anterior spinal artery and two posterior spinal arteries. The anterior spinal artery begins at the fusion of branches of both vertebral arteries and

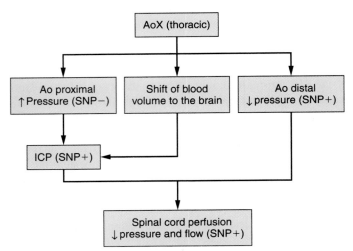

Figure 8-2 • Spinal cord blood flow and perfusion pressure during thoracic aortic occlusion, with or without sodium nitroprusside (SNP) infusion. The *arrows* represent the response to aortic cross-clamping per se. AoX, aortic cross-clamping; ICP, intracranial pressure; SNP+, the effects enhanced by SNP infusion; SNP−, the effects counteracted by SNP infusion. *(Adapted from Gelman S. The pathophysiology of aortic cross-clamping and unclamping. Anesthesiology 1995;82:1026-60. © 1995, Lippincott Williams & Wilkins).*

relies on reinforcement of its blood supply by six to eight radicular arteries, the largest and most important of which is the great radicular artery of Adamkiewicz. Multiple levels of the spinal cord do not receive feeding radicular branches, thus leaving watershed areas that are particularly susceptible to ischemic injury. These areas are in jeopardy during aortic occlusion or hypotension. Damage can also result from surgical resection of the artery of Adamkiewicz (because the origin is unknown) or exclusion of the origin of the artery by the cross-clamp. In this situation, not only is the anterior spinal artery blood flow reduced directly, but the potential for collateral blood flow to the spinal cord is also reduced because aortic pressure distal to the cross-clamp is very low.

Risk Factors The risk of paraplegia during thoracic aortic surgery is determined by the interaction of four factors: (1) the decrease in spinal cord blood flow, (2) the rate of neuronal metabolism, (3) postischemia reperfusion, and (4) postreperfusion blood flow. The duration of aortic cross-clamping is critical in determining the risk of paraplegia. A brief period of thoracic aortic cross-clamping (< 30 minutes) is usually tolerated. If cross-clamp time is more than 30 minutes, the risk of spinal cord ischemia is significant and techniques for spinal cord protection are indicated. These include partial circulatory assistance (left atrium-to-femoral artery shunt), reimplantation of critical intercostal arteries when possible, cerebrospinal fluid drainage, maintenance of proximal hypertension during cross-clamping, reduction of spinal cord metabolism by moderate hypothermia (30° to 32°C), avoidance of hyperglycemia, and the use of mannitol, corticosteroids, and/or calcium channel blockers.

Hemodynamic Responses to Aortic Cross-clamping

Thoracic aortic cross-clamping and unclamping are associated with severe hemodynamic and homeostatic disturbances in virtually all organ systems because of the decrease in blood flow distal to the aortic clamp and substantial increase in blood flow above the level of aortic occlusion. There is a substantial increase in systemic blood pressure and systemic vascular resistance with no significant change in heart rate. A reduction in cardiac output usually accompanies these changes. Systemic hypertension is attributed to increased impedance to aortic outflow (increased afterload). In addition, there is blood volume redistribution caused by collapse and constriction of the venous vasculature distal to the aortic cross-clamp. An increase in preload results. Evidence of this blood volume redistribution can be seen as an increase in filling pressures (central venous pressure, pulmonary capillary occlusion pressure, left ventricular end-diastolic pressure). Substantial differences in the hemodynamic response to aortic cross-clamping can be seen at different levels of clamping: thoracic, supraceliac, and infrarenal cross-clamping. Changes in mean arterial pressure, end-diastolic and end-systolic left ventricular area and ejection fraction, and wall motion abnormalities as assessed by transesophageal echocardiography are minimal during infrarenal aortic cross-clamping but dramatic during intrathoracic aortic cross-clamping. Some of these differences result in part from different patterns of blood volume redistribution. Preload may not increase if the aorta is clamped distal to the celiac artery because the blood volume from the distal venous vasculature may be redistributed into the splanchnic circulation. To tolerate the increase in afterload and preload, an increase in myocardial contractility and an autoregulatory increase in coronary blood flow are required. If coronary blood flow and myocardial contractility cannot increase, left ventricular dysfunction is likely. Indeed, echocardiography often indicates abnormal wall motion of the left ventricle during aortic cross-clamping suggesting the presence of myocardial ischemia. Hemodynamic responses to aortic cross-clamping are blunted in patients with aortoiliac occlusive disease.

Pharmacologic interventions intended to offset the hemodynamic effects of aortic cross-clamping, especially clamping of the thoracic aorta, are related to the effects of the administered drug on arterial and/or venous capacitance. For example, vasodilators such as nitroprusside and nitroglycerin often reduce the clamp-induced decrease in cardiac output and ejection fraction. The most plausible explanation for this effect is a drug-induced decrease in systemic vascular resistance and afterload and increased venous capacitance.

However, it is important to recognize that perfusion pressures distal to the aortic cross-clamp are decreased and are directly dependent on proximal aortic pressure, i.e., the pressure above the level of aortic clamping. Blood flow to tissues distal to aortic occlusion (kidneys, liver, spinal cord) occurs through collateral vessels or through a shunt. It decreases dramatically during aortic clamping. Blood flow to vital organs distal to the aortic clamp depends on perfusion pressure and not on cardiac output or intravascular volume.

Clinically, drugs and volume replacement must be adjusted to maintain distal aortic perfusion pressure even if that results in an increase in blood pressure proximal to the clamp. Strategies for myocardial preservation during and after aortic cross-clamping include decreasing afterload and normalizing preload, coronary blood flow, and contractility. Modalities such as temporary shunts, reimplantation of arteries supplying distal tissues (spinal cord), and hypothermia may influence the choice of drugs and endpoints of treatment.

Cross-clamping the thoracic aorta just distal to the left subclavian artery is associated with severe decreases (approximately 90%) in spinal cord blood flow and renal blood flow, glomerular filtration rate, and urinary output. Infrarenal aortic cross-clamping is associated with a large increase in renal vascular resistance and a decrease in renal blood flow (approximately 30%). Renal dysfunction results from renal hypoperfusion. Renal failure following aortic surgery almost always results from acute tubular necrosis. Ischemia-reperfusion insults to the kidneys play a central role in the pathogenesis of this renal failure.

Cross-clamping the thoracic aorta is associated not only with a decrease in distal aortic-anterior spinal artery pressure but also with an increase in cerebrospinal fluid pressure. Presumably, intracranial hypertension due to systemic hypertension above the clamp produces redistribution of blood volume and engorgement of the intracranial compartment (intracranial hypervolemia). This results in redistribution of cerebrospinal fluid into the spinal fluid space and a decrease in the compliance of the spinal fluid space. Cerebrospinal fluid drainage might increase spinal cord blood flow, and decrease the incidence of neurologic complications.

Pulmonary damage associated with aortic cross-clamping and unclamping is reflected by an increase in pulmonary vascular resistance (particularly with unclamping of the aorta), an increase in pulmonary capillary membrane permeability, and development of pulmonary edema. The mechanisms involved may include pulmonary hypervolemia and the effects of various vasoactive mediators.

Aortic cross-clamping is associated with formation and release of hormonal factors (activation of the sympathetic nervous system and the renin-angiotensin-aldosterone system) and other mediators (prostaglandins, oxygen free radicals, complement cascade). These mediators may aggravate or blunt the harmful effects of aortic cross-clamping and unclamping. Overall, injury to the spinal cord, lungs, kidneys, and abdominal viscera is principally due to ischemia and subsequent reperfusion injury due to the aortic cross-clamp (local effects) and/or to release of mediators from ischemic and reperfused tissues (distant effects).

Hemodynamic Responses to Aortic Unclamping

Unclamping the thoracic aorta is associated with substantial decreases in systemic vascular resistance and systemic blood pressure. Cardiac output may increase, decrease, or remain unchanged. Left ventricular end-diastolic pressure decreases and myocardial blood flow increases. Gradual release of the aortic clamp is recommended to allow time for volume replacement and to slow the washout of the vasoactive and cardiodepressant mediators from ischemic tissues.

The principal causes of declamping hypotension include (1) central hypovolemia caused by pooling of blood in reperfused tissues, (2) hypoxia-mediated vasodilation causing an increase in vascular capacitance in the tissues below the level of aortic clamping, and (3) accumulation of vasoactive and myocardial depressant metabolites in these tissues. Vasodilation and hypotension may be further aggravated by the transient increase in carbon dioxide release and oxygen consumption in these tissues following unclamping. Correction of metabolic acidosis does not significantly influence the degree of hypotension following aortic declamping

Management of Anesthesia

Management of anesthesia in patients undergoing thoracic aortic aneurysm resection requires consideration of monitoring systemic blood pressure, neurologic function, and intravascular volume and planning the pharmacologic interventions and hemodynamic management that will be needed to control hypertension during the period of aortic cross-clamping. Proper monitoring is more important than the selection of anesthetic drugs in these patients.

Monitoring Blood Pressure

Surgical repair of a thoracic aortic aneurysm requires aortic cross-clamping just distal to the left subclavian artery or between the left subclavian artery and the left common carotid artery. Therefore, blood pressure monitoring must be via an artery in the right arm since occlusion of the aorta can prevent measurement of blood pressure in the left arm. Monitoring blood pressure both above (right radial artery) and below (femoral artery), less commonly done, the aneurysm may be useful. This approach permits assessment of cerebral, renal, and spinal cord perfusion pressure during cross-clamping.

Blood flow to tissues below the aortic cross-clamp is dependent on perfusion pressure rather than on preload and cardiac output. Therefore, during cross-clamping of the thoracic aorta, proximal aortic pressures should be maintained as high as the heart can safely withstand unless other modalities (such as temporary shunts or hypothermia) are implemented. Sympathomimetic or vasodilator drugs may be needed to adjust perfusion pressure above and below the level of the aortic cross-clamp. Esmolol can be used to provide blood pressure control comparable to that seen with nitroprusside but without the reflex tachycardia and decrease in PaO_2 that may accompany administration of nitroprusside. A common recommendation is to maintain mean arterial pressure near 100 mm Hg above the cross-clamp and above 50 mm Hg in the areas distal to the cross-clamp.

The use of vasodilators to treat hypertension above the level of the aortic cross-clamp must be balanced against the likelihood of a decrease in perfusion pressure in the tissues below the clamp. Indeed, nitroprusside may decrease spinal cord perfusion pressure both by decreasing distal aortic pressure and by increasing cerebrospinal fluid pressure as a result of cerebral vasodilation (see Fig. 8-2). It is prudent to limit the use of drugs that decrease proximal aortic pressure and cause cerebral vasodilation. Use of temporary shunts to bypass the occluded thoracic aorta (proximal aorta–to–femoral artery or left atrium–to–femoral artery shunts) may be considered when attempting to maintain renal and spinal cord perfusion. Partial cardiopulmonary bypass is another option to maintain distal aortic perfusion.

Monitoring Neurologic Function

Somatosensory evoked potentials and electroencephalography are monitoring methods for evaluating central nervous system viability during the period of aortic cross-clamping. Unfortunately, intraoperative monitoring of somatosensory evoked potentials is not completely reliable for detecting spinal cord ischemia during aortic surgery because somatosensory evoked potential monitoring reflects dorsal column (sensory tracts) function. Ischemic changes of anterior spinal cord function (motor tracts) are not detected. Monitoring motor evoked potentials would reflect anterior spinal cord function but is impractical since it prohibits use of neuromuscular blocking drugs.

Monitoring Cardiac Function

During operations on the thoracic aorta, transesophageal echocardiography can provide valuable information about the presence of atherosclerosis in the thoracic aorta, the competence of cardiac valves, ventricular function, the adequacy of myocardial perfusion, and the intravascular volume status. A pulmonary artery catheter provides data that can complement the information obtained from transesophageal echocardiography.

Monitoring Intravascular Volume and Renal Function

Optimization of systemic hemodynamics including circulating blood volume represents the most effective measure for protecting the kidneys from the ischemic effects produced by aortic cross-clamping. Use of diuretics such as mannitol prior to aortic clamping may also be useful. Mannitol improves renal cortical blood flow and glomerular filtration rate. Endothelial swelling is decreased and an osmotic diuresis occurs.

In the future, specific antagonists of hormonal and humoral factors that are formed and released from ischemic tissues during and after the period of aortic cross-clamping may become available to prevent or ameliorate vital organ ischemia.

Induction and Maintenance of Anesthesia

Induction of anesthesia and tracheal intubation must minimize undesirable increases in systemic blood pressure, which could exacerbate an aortic dissection or rupture an aneurysm. Use of a double-lumen endobronchial tube permits collapse of the left lung and facilitates surgical exposure during resection of a thoracic aneurysm.

General anesthesia can be maintained with volatile anesthetics and/or opioids. General anesthesia may cause some reduction in cerebral metabolic rate that may be particularly desirable during this surgery. The choice of neuromuscular blocking drug may be influenced by the dependence of a particular drug on renal clearance.

Postoperative Management

Posterolateral thoracotomy is among the most painful of surgical incisions because major muscles are transected and ribs are removed. Additionally, chest tube insertion sites can be very painful. Amelioration of pain is essential for patient comfort and to facilitate coughing and maneuvers designed to prevent atelectasis. Pain relief is commonly provided by neuroaxial opioids and/or local anesthetics. Intrathecal or epidural catheters providing intermittent or continuous infusion of analgesic medications can be adapted to provide an element of patient-controlled analgesia as well. Inclusion of local anesthetic drugs in these solutions may produce sensory and motor anesthesia and delay recognition of anterior spinal artery syndrome. Moreover, when a neurologic deficit is recognized, the epidural may be implicated as the cause of the paraplegia. If neuraxial analgesia is used during the immediate postoperative period, opioids are preferred over local anesthetics to prevent masking of anterior spinal artery syndrome.

Patients recovering from thoracic aortic aneurysm resection are at risk of developing cardiac, pulmonary, and renal failure during the immediate postoperative period. Cerebrovascular accidents may result from air or thrombotic emboli that occur during surgical resection of the diseased aorta. Patients with co-existing cerebrovascular disease may be more vulnerable to the development of new central nervous system complications. Spinal cord injury may manifest during the immediate postoperative period as paraparesis or flaccid paralysis. Delayed appearance of paraplegia (12 hours to 21 days postoperatively) has been associated with postoperative hypotension in patients with severe atherosclerotic disease in whom marginally adequate collateral circulation to the spinal cord is present.

Systemic hypertension is not uncommon and may jeopardize the integrity of the surgical repair and/or predispose to myocardial ischemia. The role of pain in the etiology of hypertension must be considered. Institution of antihypertensive therapy with drugs such as nitroglycerin, nitroprusside, hydralazine, and labetalol may be appropriate. Some patients benefit from concomitant administration of β-blockers to attenuate manifestations of a hyperdynamic circulation.

ANEURYSMS OF THE ABDOMINAL AORTA

Abdominal aortic aneurysms have traditionally been viewed as resulting from atherosclerosis. This atherosclerosis involves several highly interrelated processes, including lipid disturbances, platelet activation, thrombosis, endothelial dysfunction, inflammation, oxidative stress, vascular smooth muscle cell activation, altered matrix metabolism, remodeling, and genetic factors. Atherosclerosis represents a response to vessel wall injury caused by factors including infection, inflammation, increased protease activity within the arterial wall, genetically regulated defects in collagen and fibrillin, and mechanical factors. The primary event in the development of an abdominal aortic aneurysm is proteolytic degradation of the extracellular matrix proteins elastin and collagen. Various proteolytic enzymes including matrix metalloproteinases are critical during degradation and remodeling of the aortic wall. Oxidative stress, lymphocytic and monocytic infiltration with immunoglobulin deposition in the aortic wall, and biomechanical wall stress also contribute to the formation and rupture of aneurysms. In addition, 12% to 19% of first-degree relatives (usually men) of a patient with an abdominal aortic aneurysm will develop an aneurysm. Specific genetic markers and biochemical changes that produce this pathology remain to be elucidated.

Diagnosis

Abdominal aortic aneurysms are usually detected as asymptomatic, pulsatile abdominal masses. Abdominal ultrasonography is a very sensitive test for the detection of abdominal aortic aneurysms. CT is also very sensitive and is more accurate than ultrasonography in estimating aneurysm size.

Improvements in CT technology, such as the advent of helical CT and CT angiography, have increased the role of CT imaging in the evaluation and treatment of abdominal aortic aneurysms. Helical CT provides excellent three-dimensional anatomic detail and is particularly useful for evaluating the feasibility of endovascular stent-graft repair of the aneurysm.

Magnetic resonance imaging is useful for accurate measurement of aneurysm size and evaluation of relevant vascular anatomy without the need for ionizing radiation or contrast medium.

Treatment

Surgery is usually recommended for abdominal aortic aneurysms larger than 5 cm in diameter. This recommendation is based on clinical studies indicating that the risk of rupture within a 5-year period is 25% to 41% in aneurysms larger than 5 cm. Smaller aneurysms are less likely to rupture. Patients with aneurysms less than 5.0 cm in diameter should be followed-up with serial ultrasonography. These recommendations are only guidelines. Each patient must be evaluated for the presence of risk factors for accelerated aneurysm growth and rupture such as tobacco use and family history. If the abdominal aortic aneurysm expands by more than 0.6 to 0.8 cm per year, repair is usually recommended. Surgical risk and overall health are also part of the evaluation for the timing of aneurysm repair. Endovascular aneurysm repair is an alternative to surgical repair.

Preoperative Evaluation

Co-existing medical conditions, especially coronary artery disease, chronic obstructive pulmonary disease, and renal dysfunction are important to identify preoperatively in an attempt to minimize postoperative complications. Myocardial ischemia/infarction is responsible for most postoperative deaths following elective abdominal aortic aneurysm resection. Other postoperative cardiac events include cardiac dysrhythmias and congestive heart failure. Preoperative evaluation of cardiac function might include exercise or pharmacologic stress testing with or without echocardiography or radionuclide imaging. Severe reductions in vital capacity and forced expiratory volume in 1 second and abnormal renal function may mitigate against AAA resection or significantly increase the risk of elective aneurysm repair.

Rupture of an Abdominal Aortic Aneurysm

The classic triad (hypotension, back pain, and a pulsatile abdominal mass) is present in only approximately half of patients who have a ruptured abdominal aortic aneurysm. Renal colic, diverticulitis, and gastrointestinal hemorrhage may be confused with a ruptured abdominal aortic aneurysm.

Most abdominal aortic aneurysms rupture into the left retroperitoneum. Although hypovolemic shock may be present, exsanguination may be prevented by clotting and the tamponade effect of the retroperitoneum. Euvolemic resuscitation may be deferred until the aortic rupture is surgically controlled in the operating room because euvolemic resuscitation and the resultant increase in blood pressure without surgical control of bleeding may lead to loss of retroperitoneal tamponade, further bleeding, hypotension, and death.

Unstable patients with a suspected ruptured abdominal aortic aneurysm require immediate operation and control of the proximal aorta without preoperative confirmatory testing or optimal volume resuscitation.

Management of Anesthesia

Management of anesthesia for resection of an abdominal aortic aneurysm requires consideration of commonly associated medical conditions in this patient group: ischemic heart disease, hypertension, chronic obstructive pulmonary disease, diabetes mellitus, and renal dysfunction. Monitoring intravascular volume and cardiac, pulmonary, and renal function is essential during the perioperative period. Systemic blood pressure is monitored continuously by an intra-arterial catheter. Pulmonary artery catheterization is indicated in most patients because it is not always possible to predict whether central venous pressure will parallel left ventricular filling pressure, particularly in patients with previous myocardial infarction, angina pectoris, or congestive heart failure. If appropriate personnel and equipment are available, echocardiography can be very useful for evaluating the cardiac response to aortic cross-clamping and unclamping, assessment of left ventricular filling volume, and regional and global myocardial function. Urine output is monitored continuously.

No single anesthetic drug or technique is ideal for all patients undergoing elective abdominal aortic aneurysm repair. Combinations of volatile anesthetics and/or opioids are commonly used with or without nitrous oxide. Continuous epidural anesthesia combined with general anesthesia may offer advantages related to decreasing overall anesthetic drug requirements, attenuation of the increased systemic vascular resistance associated with aortic cross-clamping, and facilitation of postoperative pain management. Nevertheless, there is no evidence that the combination of epidural anesthesia and general anesthesia decreases postoperative cardiac or pulmonary morbidity compared to high-risk patients who undergo the same aortic surgery with general anesthesia alone. However, postoperative epidural analgesia may favorably influence the postoperative course. Anticoagulation during abdominal aortic surgery introduces the controversy regarding placement of an epidural catheter and the remote risk of epidural hematoma formation.

Patients undergoing abdominal aortic aneurysm repair usually experience significant fluid and blood losses. A combination of balanced salt and colloid solutions (and blood if needed) guided by appropriate monitoring of cardiac and renal function facilitates maintenance of adequate intravascular volume, cardiac output, and urine formation. Balanced salt and/or colloid solutions should be infused during aortic cross-clamping to build up an intravascular volume reserve and thereby minimize declamping hypotension. If urinary output is decreased despite adequate fluid and blood replacement, diuretic therapy with mannitol or furosemide might be considered. The efficacy of low-dose dopamine in preserving renal function during abdominal aortic aneurysm surgery is unproven.

Infrarenal aortic cross-clamping and declamping are significant events during abdominal aortic surgery. The anticipated consequences of abdominal aortic cross-clamping include increased systemic vascular resistance (afterload) and decreased venous return (see "Hemodynamic Responses to Aortic Cross-clamping"). Often myocardial performance and circulatory variables remain acceptable after the aorta is clamped at an infrarenal level. An alteration in anesthetic depth or infusion of vasodilators may be necessary in some patients to maintain myocardial performance at acceptable levels.

Hypotension may occur when the aortic cross-clamp is removed (see "Hemodynamic Responses to Aortic Unclamping"). Prevention of declamping hypotension and maintenance of a stable cardiac output can often be achieved by volume loading to pulmonary capillary occlusion pressures higher than normal before the cross-clamp is removed. Likewise, gradual opening of the aortic cross-clamp may minimize the decrease in systemic blood pressure by allowing some pooled venous blood to return to the central circulation. The role of washout of acid metabolites from ischemic areas below the cross-clamp when the clamp is released is much less important than central hypovolemia in producing declamping hypotension, and sodium bicarbonate pretreatment does not reliably blunt declamping hypotension. If hypotension persists more than a few minutes after removing the cross-clamp, the presence of unrecognized bleeding or inadequate volume replacement must be considered. Echocardiography at this time may be particularly helpful in determining the adequacy of volume replacement and cardiac function.

Postoperative Management

Patients recovering from abdominal aortic aneurysm repair are at risk of developing cardiac, pulmonary, and renal dysfunction during the postoperative period. Assessment of graft patency and lower extremity blood flow is important. Adequate analgesia either with neuraxial opioids or patient-controlled analgesia is very important in facilitating early tracheal extubation.

Systemic hypertension is common during the postoperative period and may be more likely in patients with preoperative hypertension. Overzealous intraoperative hydration and/or postoperative hypothermia with compensatory vasoconstriction may exacerbate postoperative hypertension. Postoperative hypertension should be treated by either eliminating any specific cause or by institution of antihypertensive therapy. Preoperative administration of clonidine may attenuate hypertension during the postoperative period.

Endovascular Aortic Aneurysm Repair

Over the past decade, many endovascular devices to repair abdominal aortic aneurysms have been developed. Endovascular repair involves gaining access to the lumen of the abdominal aorta, usually via small incisions over the femoral vessels. General or regional anesthesia is acceptable for this procedure. Monitoring consists of at least intravascular blood pressure and urine output monitoring. The potential for conversion to an open aneurysm repair must be considered.

The U.S. Food and Drug Administration approved endografts for abdominal aortic aneurysm repair in 1999, and now 5-year outcome data are becoming available. It appears that in-hospital and 30-day mortality rates are lower for endovascular repair than for open repair. However, at 5 years, there is no significant difference in all-cause mortality between the endovascular and open repair groups. The incidence of conversion to an open repair is approximately 3%.

PERIPHERAL VASCULAR DISEASE

Peripheral arterial disease results in compromised blood flow to the extremities. Chronic impairment of blood flow to the extremities is most often due to atherosclerosis, whereas arterial embolism is most likely to be responsible for acute arterial occlusion (**Table 8-1**). Vasculitis may also be responsible for compromised peripheral blood flow.

The most widely accepted definition of peripheral arterial disease is an ankle-brachial index of less than 0.90, that is, the ratio of the systolic blood pressure at the ankle (as measured by Doppler ultrasonography) to the systolic blood pressure in the brachial artery is less than 0.9. An ankle-brachial index of less than 0.90 correlates extremely well with angiogram-positive disease.

Peripheral atherosclerosis resembles atherosclerosis seen in the aorta, coronary arteries, and extracranial cerebral arteries. The prevalence of peripheral atherosclerosis increases with age, exceeding 70% in individuals older than 75 years of age.

TABLE 8-1 Peripheral Vascular Diseases
Chronic peripheral arterial occlusive disease (atherosclerosis)
Distal abdominal aorta or iliac arteries
Femoral arteries
Subclavian steal syndrome
Coronary-subclavian steal syndrome
Acute peripheral arterial occlusive disease (embolism)
Systemic vasculitis
Takayasu's arteritis
Thromboangiitis obliterans
Wegener's granulomatosis
Temporal arteritis
Polyarteritis nodosa
Other vascular syndromes
Raynaud's phenomenon
Kawasaki disease

Peripheral arterial disease has been estimated to reduce quality of life in approximately 2 million symptomatic Americans, and millions more without claudication are likely to suffer peripheral arterial disease–associated impairment. Among patients who present with claudication, 80% have femoropopliteal stenosis, 40% have tibioperoneal stenosis, and 30% have lesions in the aorta or iliac arteries.

Atherosclerosis is a systemic disease. Consequently, patients with PAD have a three to five times overall greater risk of cardiovascular ischemic events, such as myocardial infarction, ischemic stroke, and death than those without this disease. Critical limb ischemia is associated with a very high intermediate-term morbidity and mortality due mostly to cardiovascular events.

Risk Factors

Risk factors associated with development of peripheral atherosclerosis are similar to those that cause ischemic heart disease: diabetes mellitus, hypertension, tobacco use, dyslipidemia, hyperhomocysteinemia, and a family history of premature atherosclerosis. The risk of significant PAD and claudication is doubled in smokers compared to nonsmokers and continued cigarette smoking increases the risk of progression from stable claudication to severe limb ischemia and amputation.

The prognosis of patients with lower extremity peripheral arterial disease is related to an increased risk of cardiovascular ischemic events due to concomitant coronary artery disease and cerebrovascular disease. These cardiovascular ischemic events are much more frequent than actual ischemic limb events.

Signs and Symptoms

Intermittent claudication and rest pain are the principal symptoms of peripheral arterial disease. Intermittent claudication occurs when the metabolic requirements of exercising skeletal muscles exceed oxygen delivery. Rest pain occurs when the arterial blood supply does not meet even the minimal nutritional requirements of the affected extremity. Even minor trauma to an ischemic foot may produce a nonhealing skin lesion.

Decreased or absent arterial pulses are the most reliable physical findings associated with peripheral arterial disease. Bruits auscultated in the abdomen, pelvis, or inguinal area and decreased femoral, popliteal, posterior tibial, or dorsalis pedis pulses may indicate the anatomic site of arterial stenosis. Signs of chronic leg ischemia include subcutaneous atrophy, hair loss, coolness, pallor, cyanosis, and dependent rubor.

Diagnostic Tests

Doppler ultrasonography and the resulting pulse volume waveform are used to identify arterial vessels with stenotic lesions. In the presence of severe ischemia, the arterial waveform may be entirely absent. The ankle-brachial index is a quantitative means to assess the presence and severity of peripheral arterial stenosis. The ratio is less than 0.9 with claudication, less than 0.4 with rest pain, and less than 0.25 with ischemic ulceration or impending gangrene. Duplex ultrasonography can identify areas of plaque formation and calcification as well as blood flow abnormalities caused by arterial stenoses. Transcutaneous oximetry can be used to assess the severity of skin ischemia in patients with peripheral arterial disease. The normal transcutaneous oxygen tension of a resting foot is approximately 60 mm Hg. It may be less than 40 mm Hg in patients with skin ischemia. Results from noninvasive tests and clinical evaluation are usually sufficient for the diagnosis of peripheral arterial disease. Magnetic resonance imaging and contrast angiography are used as a prelude to endovascular intervention or surgical reconstruction.

Treatment

Medical therapy of peripheral arterial disease includes exercise programs and identification and treatment or modification of risk factors for atherosclerosis. Supervised exercise training programs can improve the walking capacity of patients with peripheral arterial disease even though no improvement in blood flow to the extremity can be demonstrated. Presumably improvement in exercise capacity is due to changes in the efficiency of skeletal muscle metabolism. Patients who stop smoking have a more favorable prognosis than those who continue to smoke. Aggressive lipid-lowering therapy slows the progression of peripheral atherosclerosis as does treatment of diabetes mellitus. Treatment of hypertension results in cardiovascular risk reduction. Antihypertensive drug therapy often does not include β-adrenergic antagonists because these drugs may evoke peripheral cutaneous vasoconstriction that may be particularly harmful in patients with critical limb ischemia. However, β-blockers do not adversely affect claudication. Antihypertensive vasodilator drugs do not alleviate the symptoms of claudication or decrease the complications of critical limb ischemia.

Revascularization procedures are indicated in patients with disabling claudication, ischemic rest pain, or impending limb loss. The prognosis of the limb is determined by the extent of arterial disease, the acuity of limb ischemia, and the feasibility and rapidity of restoring arterial circulation. In patients with chronic arterial occlusive disease and continuous progression of symptoms, that is, development of new wounds, rest pain, or gangrene, the prognosis is very poor unless revascularization can be accomplished. In patients with acute occlusive events due to arterial embolism in an extremity with little underlying arterial disease, the long-term prognosis of the limb is related to the rapidity and completeness of revascularization before the onset of irreversible ischemic tissue or nerve damage.

Revascularization can be achieved by endovascular interventions or surgical reconstruction. Percutaneous transluminal angioplasty of iliac arteries has a high initial success rate that may be further improved by stent placement. Femoral and popliteal artery percutaneous transluminal angioplasty has a lower success rate than iliac artery percutaneous

transluminal angioplasty. However, with the introduction of the nitinol self-expanding SMART stent, the patency rate of the superficial femoral artery 12 months after the procedure is approximately 80%, which is a substantial improvement over previous patency rates. Despite improvement in long-term outcome after percutaneous transluminal angioplasty and stenting of peripheral vessels, restenosis remains a significant problem, particularly in long lesions, small-diameter vessels, and restenotic lesions. Current therapeutic approaches are focusing on mechanical devices, stents, stent grafts, vascular irradiation, and drugs, although none of these approaches has yet been successful in solving this problem.

The potential to grow new arteries both in the coronary and in the peripheral circulation generates much excitement. Preliminary results with the use of vascular endothelial growth factor to induce angiogenesis in animals and humans have been encouraging, but much more research needs to be done before this can become a common therapeutic tool in the treatment of peripheral arterial disease.

The operative procedures used for vascular reconstruction depend on the location and severity of the peripheral arterial stenosis. Aortobifemoral bypass is the standard surgical procedure used to treat aortoiliac disease. Intra-abdominal aortoiliac reconstructive surgery may not be feasible in patients with severe comorbid conditions. However, in these patients, axillobifemoral bypass can circumvent the abdominal aorta and achieve revascularization of both legs. Femoral-femoral bypass can be performed in patients with unilateral iliac artery obstruction. Infrainguinal bypass procedures using saphenous vein grafts or synthetic grafts include femoropopliteal and tibioperoneal reconstruction. Lumbar sympathectomy is rarely used to treat critical limb ischemia. It appears that ischemic blood vessels in these limbs are already maximally vasodilated. Amputation is necessary for patients with advanced limb ischemia in whom revascularization is not possible or has failed.

The operative risk of reconstructive peripheral arterial surgery, as for abdominal aortic aneurysm resection, is primarily related to the presence of associated atherosclerotic vascular disease, particularly ischemic heart disease and cerebrovascular disease. The increased incidence of perioperative myocardial infarction and cardiac death in peripheral arterial disease patients is due to the high prevalence of coronary artery disease in this patient population. Mortality following revascularization surgery is usually a result of myocardial infarction in patients with preoperative evidence of ischemic heart disease, a history of coronary artery bypass grafting, or congestive heart failure. In patients with severe or *unstable* ischemic heart disease and claudication, treatment of the ischemic heart disease by percutaneous coronary intervention or coronary artery bypass grafting might be considered before performing revascularization surgery. However, in patients with anatomically significant but *stable* coronary artery disease, elective vascular surgery can be accomplished with mortality and morbidity outcomes similar to those of patients who undergo coronary artery revascularization prior to elective vascular surgery.

Management of Anesthesia

Management of anesthesia for surgical revascularization of the lower extremities incorporates principles similar to those described for the management of patients for abdominal aortic aneurysm repair. For example, the principal risk during reconstructive peripheral vascular surgery is ischemic heart disease. Because patients with claudication are usually unable to perform an exercise stress test, pharmacologic stress testing with or without echocardiography or nuclear imaging is helpful to detect the presence and severity of ischemic heart disease preoperatively.

The American College of Cardiology/American Heart Association guidelines on perioperative β-blocker therapy identify the following groups of patients as candidates for perioperative β-blockade: (1) patients undergoing vascular surgery with or without evidence of preoperative ischemia and with or without high or intermediate risk factors, (2) patients receiving long-term β-blocker therapy, and (3) patients undergoing vascular surgery even if they have only low risk factors.

The choice of anesthesia technique must be individualized for each patient. Regional anesthesia and general anesthesia offer specific advantages and disadvantages. Patient preference, technical factors such as obesity or previous spine surgery, and use of antiplatelet/anticoagulant drugs may preclude the use of a regional technique. Regional anesthesia may also be poorly tolerated in patients with severe chronic obstructive pulmonary disease, orthopnea, or dementia. Epidural or spinal anesthesia offers the advantages of increased graft blood flow, postoperative analgesia, less activation of the coagulation system, and fewer postoperative respiratory complications. Placement of an epidural catheter at least 1 hour before intraoperative heparinization is not associated with an increased incidence of untoward neurologic events. Epidural analgesia may also attenuate postoperative stress-induced hypercoagulability.

General anesthesia may be necessary when in situ and/or repeat procedures may require long operative hours or if vein harvesting from the upper extremities is needed. There is no strong evidence suggesting an advantage of one particular type of general anesthesia over another.

During aortoiliac or aortofemoral surgery in patients with peripheral vascular occlusive disease but adequate collateral circulation, infrarenal aortic cross-clamping is associated with fewer hemodynamic derangements than occur in patients undergoing resection of an abdominal aortic aneurysm. Likewise, the hemodynamic changes associated with unclamping the abdominal aorta are less in these patients. Because major hemodynamic alterations are not likely to be seen, some will use a central venous pressure catheter in lieu of a pulmonary artery catheter, especially in the absence of symptomatic left ventricular dysfunction. Monitoring left ventricular function and intravascular volume may also be facilitated by use of transesophageal echocardiography.

Heparin is commonly administered before application of a vascular cross-clamp to decrease the risk of thromboembolic complications. However, distal embolization may still occur. Even embolization to the kidneys can occur as a result of atheroembolic debris being dislodged by the aortic cross-clamp. Care when manipulating and clamping an atherosclerotic artery is as important in minimizing the likelihood of distal embolization as administration of heparin. Spinal cord damage associated with surgical revascularization of the legs is extremely unlikely, and special monitoring for this complication is not necessary.

Postoperative Management

Postoperative management includes provision of analgesia, treatment of fluid and electrolyte derangements, and control of heart rate and blood pressure to reduce the incidence of myocardial ischemia/infarction. Dexmedetomidine, an α_2-agonist, can attenuate the increase in heart rate and plasma catecholamine concentrations during emergence from anesthesia in vascular surgery patients. In addition, dexmedetomidine can produce analgesia and sedation without cardiac or respiratory depression. Thus, it is an alternative to more traditional methods of postoperative analgesia and hemodynamic management in these patients.

Subclavian Steal Syndrome

Occlusion of the subclavian or innominate artery proximal to the origin of the vertebral artery may result in reversal of flow through the ipsilateral vertebral artery into the distal subclavian artery (**Fig. 8-3**). This reversal of flow diverts blood flow from the brain to supply the arm (subclavian steal syndrome). Symptoms of central nervous system ischemia (syncope, vertigo, ataxia, hemiplegia) and/or arm ischemia are usually present. Exercise of the ipsilateral arm accentuates these hemodynamic changes and may cause neurologic symptoms. There is often an absent or diminished pulse in the ipsilateral arm, and systolic blood pressure is likely to be at least 20 mm Hg lower in that arm. A bruit may be heard over the subclavian artery. Stenosis of the left subclavian artery is responsible for this syndrome in most patients. Subclavian endarterectomy may be curative.

Coronary-Subclavian Steal Syndrome

A rare complication of using the internal mammary artery for coronary revascularization is the coronary-subclavian steal syndrome. This syndrome occurs when proximal stenosis in the left subclavian artery produces reversal of blood flow through the patent internal mammary artery graft (**Fig. 8-4**). This steal syndrome is characterized by angina pectoris, signs of central nervous system ischemia, and a 20-mm Hg or more decrease in systolic blood pressure in the ipsilateral arm. Angina pectoris associated with coronary-subclavian steal syndrome requires surgical bypass grafting.

ACUTE ARTERIAL OCCLUSION

Acute arterial occlusion differs from the gradual development of arterial occlusion caused by atherosclerosis and is usually a

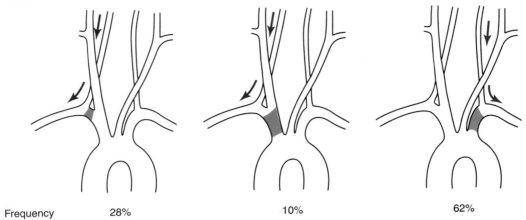

Frequency   28%   10%   62%

Figure 8-3 • Comparison of the frequency of occurrence of left, right, and bilateral subclavian steal syndrome *(Adapted from Heidrich H, Bayer O: Symptomatology of the subclavian steal syndrome. Angiology 1969;20:406–413.)*

result of cardiogenic embolism. Systemic emboli may arise from a mural thrombus in the left ventricle that develops due to myocardial infarction or dilated cardiomyopathy. Other cardiac sources of systemic emboli are valvular heart disease, prosthetic heart valves, infective endocarditis, and left atrial myxoma. Atrial fibrillation either due to valvular heart disease or occurring in the absence of valvular heart disease is a very important predisposing factor in systemic embolization. Noncardiac causes of acute arterial occlusion include atheroemboli from the aorta or iliac or femoral arteries.

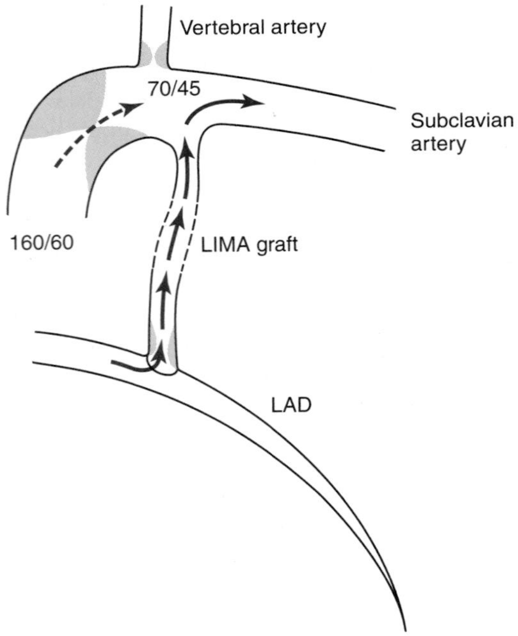

Figure 8-4 • Coronary-subclavian steal syndrome. Development of subtotal stenosis of the left subclavian artery may produce reversal of flow through a patent internal mammary graft (LIMA), thereby diverting flow destined for the left anterior descending (LAD) coronary artery. *(Adapted from Martin JL, Rock P: Coronary-subclavian steal syndrome: Anesthetic implications and management in the perioperative period. Anesthesiology 1988;68:933–936.)*

Aortic dissection and trauma can acutely occlude an artery by disrupting the integrity of the vessel lumen.

Signs and Symptoms

Acute arterial occlusion in an extremity presents with signs of limb ischemia: intense pain, paresthesias, and motor weakness distal to the site of arterial occlusion. There is loss of a palpable peripheral pulse, cool skin, and sharply demarcated skin color changes (pallor or cyanosis) distal to the arterial occlusion. Large embolic fragments often lodge at an arterial bifurcation such as the aortic bifurcation or the femoral artery bifurcation.

Diagnosis

Noninvasive tests can provide additional evidence of peripheral arterial occlusion and reveal the severity of the ischemia, but such testing should not delay definitive treatment. Arteriography may be used to define the site of acute arterial occlusion and the appropriateness of revascularization surgery.

Treatment

Surgical embolectomy is used to treat acute systemic embolism, typically thromboembolism, to a large peripheral artery. Embolectomy is rarely feasible for atheromatous embolism because the atheromatous material usually fragments into very small pieces. However, the primary source of atheroembolism may be resectable, especially if it is distal to the renal artery. Once the diagnosis of acute arterial embolism is confirmed, anticoagulation with heparin is initiated to prevent propagation of the thrombus. Intra-arterial thrombolysis with urokinase or recombinant tissue plasminogen activator may restore vascular patency in acutely occluded arteries and synthetic bypass grafts. The clinical outcome is highly dependent on the severity of the associated heart disease. Amputation is necessary in some patients.

Management of Anesthesia

Management of anesthesia for surgical treatment of acute arterial occlusion due to a systemic embolism is similar to that for patients with chronic peripheral arterial disease.

SYSTEMIC VASCULITIS

Peripheral vascular disease may manifest as part of a systemic vasculitis or inflammation of blood vessel walls due to a connective tissue disease, sepsis, or malignancy. The diagnosis of vasospastic disorders due to systemic vasculitis is facilitated by biopsy of an involved organ and detection of autoantibodies directed against cytoplasmic (extranuclear) components of neutrophils. An immune mechanism is the most likely cause of systemic vasculitis.

Takayasu's Arteritis

Takayasu's arteritis is a rare, idiopathic, chronic, progressive occlusive vasculitis that causes narrowing, thrombosis, or aneurysms of systemic and pulmonary arteries. Inflammatory changes are seen preferentially in large blood vessels such as the aorta and its branches. It has alternative names such as pulseless disease, occlusive thromboaortopathy, and aortic arch syndrome. The disease occurs most often in young Asian women. Takayasu's arteritis is diagnosed definitively based on contrast angiography.

Signs and Symptoms

Clinical signs and symptoms of Takayasu's arteritis occur as a consequence of progressive obliteration of the lumen of the aorta and its main branches (**Table 8-2**). Decreased perfusion to the brain because of involvement of the carotid arteries may manifest as vertigo, visual disturbances, seizures, or a stroke with hemiparesis or hemiplegia. Hyperextension of the head may decrease carotid blood flow further in these patients. Indeed, these patients often hold their heads in flexed ("drooping") positions to prevent syncope. Involvement of the subclavian arteries can lead to loss of arm pulses. Bruits are often audible over a stenosed carotid or subclavian artery.

TABLE 8–2 Signs and Symptoms of Takayasu's Arteritis
Central Nervous System
Vertigo
Visual disturbances
Syncope
Seizures
Cerebral ischemia or infarction
Cardiovascular System
Multiple occlusions of peripheral arteries
Ischemic heart disease
Cardiac valve dysfunction
Cardiac conduction defects
Lungs
Pulmonary hypertension
Ventilation-perfusion mismatch
Kidneys
Renal artery stenosis
Musculoskeletal System
Ankylosing spondylitis
Rheumatoid arthritis

Vasculitis of the pulmonary arteries occurs in approximately 50% of patients and can manifest as pulmonary hypertension. Ventilation-perfusion abnormalities owing to occlusion of small pulmonary arteries may contribute to hypoxemia. Myocardial ischemia may reflect inflammation of the coronary arteries. Cardiac valves and the cardiac conduction system may also be involved. Renal artery stenosis can lead to both decreased renal function and development of renovascular hypertension. Ankylosing spondylitis and rheumatoid arthritis may accompany this syndrome.

Treatment

Takayasu's arteritis is treated with corticosteroids. Anticoagulants or antiplatelet drugs may be administered to select patients. Hypertension may respond well to treatment with calcium channel blockers or angiotensin-converting enzyme inhibitors. Life-threatening or incapacitating arterial occlusions are sometimes amenable to surgical intervention.

Management of Anesthesia

Takayasu's arteritis may be encountered incidentally in patients presenting for surgery or obstetric care or in patients presenting for vascular surgery, such as carotid endarterectomy. Management of anesthesia must consider the drug therapy of this syndrome as well as the multiple organ system involvement by this vasculitis. For example, long-term corticosteroid therapy likely results in suppression of adrenocortical function and suggests the need for supplemental corticosteroid administration during the perioperative period. During the preoperative evaluation, it is useful to establish the effect of changes in head position on cerebral function. In this regard, hyperextension of the head during direct laryngoscopy and tracheal intubation could compromise blood flow through the carotid arteries.

Choice of Anesthesia

Regional anesthesia may be difficult in the presence of Takayasu's arteritis. Certainly, anticoagulation precludes use of this technique. Associated musculoskeletal changes can make performance of lumbar epidural or spinal anesthesia difficult. Hypotension produced by regional anesthesia could jeopardize perfusion pressure to vital organs, especially the brain, but regional anesthesia in an awake patient can be a useful method for monitoring cerebral function when cerebrovascular disease is prominent. Both epidural anesthesia and spinal anesthesia have been used successfully for cesarean delivery in patients with Takayasu's arteritis.

General anesthesia prevents the sympathectomy caused by regional anesthesia and may help support the blood pressure. Selection of short-acting anesthetic drugs that allow for prompt awakening and evaluation of mental status may be particularly useful in these patients.

Regardless of the technique or drugs selected to produce anesthesia, adequate arterial perfusion pressure must be maintained during the perioperative period. Decreases in systemic blood pressure caused either by decreased cardiac output or systemic vascular resistance must be recognized promptly and treated as needed. Excessive hyperventilation must be avoided because of its effect on cerebral blood flow.

Monitoring It may be difficult to measure blood pressure noninvasively in the upper extremities due to narrowing of the subclavian and brachial arterial lumens. It is unclear whether intra-arterial cannulation of arteries that might be involved in this inflammatory process is safe and/or whether the data so obtained are meaningful. Some will cannulate the radial artery for blood pressure monitoring, and others prefer to monitor systemic blood pressure via a femoral intra-arterial catheter. Monitoring systemic blood pressure in both the radial and femoral arteries may be a consideration in some patients.

Electrocardiographic monitoring and urine output measurement provide some data as to the adequacy of coronary and renal blood flow. A pulmonary artery catheter or transesophageal echocardiography might be required for certain major operations. In patients with significant compromise of carotid artery blood flow, intraoperative electroencephalographic monitoring may be useful for detecting cerebral ischemia.

Thromboangiitis Obliterans (Buerger's Disease)

Thromboangiitis obliterans is an inflammatory vasculitis leading to occlusion of small- and medium-sized arteries and veins in the extremities. The disease is most prevalent in men, and the onset is typically before age 45. The most important predisposing factor is tobacco use. The disorder has been identified as an autoimmune response triggered when nicotine is present. The traditional diagnosis of Buerger's disease is based on five criteria: smoking history, onset before age 50, infrapopliteal arterial occlusive disease, upper limb involvement or phlebitis migrans, and the absence of risk factors for atherosclerosis other than smoking. The diagnosis of thromboangiitis obliterans is confirmed by biopsy of active vascular lesions.

Signs and Symptoms

Involvement of extremity arteries causes forearm, calf, or foot claudication. Severe ischemia of the hands and feet can cause rest pain, ulcerations, and skin necrosis. Raynaud's phenomenon is commonly associated with thromboangiitis obliterans, and cold exacerbates the symptomatology. Periods of vasospasm may alternate with periods of quiescence. Migratory superficial vein thrombosis develops in approximately 40% of patients.

Treatment

The most effective treatment for patients with thromboangiitis obliterans is smoking cessation. Surgical revascularization is not usually feasible because of the involvement of small distal blood vessels. There is no proven effective drug therapy, and the efficacy of platelet inhibitors, anticoagulants, and thrombolytic therapy is not established. Recently, gene therapy with vascular endothelial growth factor was found to be helpful in healing ischemic ulcerations and relieving rest pain. Cyclophosphamide therapy has been tried because of the autoimmune nature of the disease.

Management of Anesthesia

Management of anesthesia in the presence of thromboangiitis obliterans requires avoidance of events that might damage already ischemic extremities. Positioning and padding of pressure points must be meticulous. The operating room ambient temperature should be warm and inspired gases should be warmed and humidified to maintain normal body temperature. Systemic blood pressure should be measured noninvasively rather than by intraarterial means. Co-existing pulmonary disease and elevated carboxyhemoglobin concentrations are considerations in these cigarette smokers.

Regional or general anesthesia can be administered to these patients. If regional anesthetic techniques are selected, it may be prudent to omit epinephrine from the local anesthetic solution to avoid any possibility of accentuating vasospasm.

Wegener's Granulomatosis

Wegener's granulomatosis is characterized by formation of necrotizing granulomas in inflamed blood vessels in the central nervous system, airways, lungs, cardiovascular system, and kidneys (**Table 8-3**). Patients may present with sinusitis, pneumonia, or renal failure. The laryngeal mucosa may be replaced by granulation tissue resulting in narrowing of the glottic opening or subglottic area. Vasculitis may result in occlusion of pulmonary vessels. There may be a random interstitial distribution of pulmonary granulomas with surrounding infection and hemorrhage. Progressive renal failure is the most frequent cause of death in patients with Wegener's granulomatosis. Tests for antineutrophil cytoplasmic antibodies have a high degree of specificity for Wegener's granulomatosis, suggesting a role for immune dysfunction and hypersensitivity to unidentified antigens in the etiology of this vasculitis. Treatment of Wegener's granulomatosis

TABLE 8-3 Signs and Symptoms of Wegener's Granulomatosis
Central Nervous System
Cerebral aneurysms
Peripheral neuropathy
Respiratory Tract and Lungs
Sinusitis
Laryngeal stenosis
Epiglottic destruction
Ventilation-perfusion mismatch
Pneumonia
Hemoptysis
Bronchial destruction
Cardiovascular System
Cardiac valve destruction
Disturbances of cardiac conduction
Myocardial ischemia
Kidneys
Hematuria
Azotemia
Renal failure

with cyclophosphamide can produce dramatic remissions. Approximately 90% of patients achieve remission with treatment, but more than half experience a relapse at periods ranging from 3 months to 16 years. At the time of relapse, the same or different organs can be involved compared to the initial presentation.

Management of anesthesia in patients with Wegener's granulomatosis requires an appreciation of the widespread organ system involvement of this disease. The potential depressant effects of cyclophosphamide on the immune system and the association of hemolytic anemia and leukopenia with administration of this drug should be considered. Cyclophosphamide may also decrease plasma cholinesterase activity, but prolonged skeletal muscle paralysis after administration of succinylcholine has not been described.

Avoidance of trauma during direct laryngoscopy is important since bleeding from granulomas and dislodgment of friable ulcerated tissue can occur. A smaller than expected endotracheal tube may be required if the glottic opening is narrowed by granulomatous changes. Suctioning the airway may be required to remove necrotic debris. The likely presence of pulmonary disease emphasizes the need for supplemental oxygen during the perioperative period. Arteritis that involves peripheral vessels may obviate placement of an indwelling arterial catheter to monitor blood pressure or limit the frequency of arterial punctures to obtain samples for blood gas analysis.

A careful neurologic examination should be performed before the decision is made to recommend regional anesthesia to a patient with Wegener's granulomatosis. The choice and doses of neuromuscular blocking drugs may be influenced by the magnitude of renal dysfunction. Succinylcholine administration may not be prudent in the presence of skeletal muscle atrophy owing to neuritis. Volatile anesthetics could be associated with exaggerated myocardial depression if the disease process involves the myocardium and heart valves. Electrocardiography will detect cardiac conduction abnormalities.

Temporal Arteritis

Temporal arteritis is inflammation of the arteries of the head and neck, manifesting most often as headache, scalp tenderness, or jaw claudication. This diagnosis is suspected in any patient older than age 50 complaining of a unilateral headache. Superficial branches of the temporal arteries are often tender and enlarged. Arteritis of branches of the ophthalmic artery may lead to ischemic optic neuritis and unilateral blindness. Indeed, prompt initiation of treatment with corticosteroids is indicated in patients with visual symptoms to prevent blindness. Evidence of arteritis on a biopsy specimen of the temporal artery is present in approximately 90% of patients.

Polyarteritis Nodosa

Polyarteritis nodosa is a vasculitis that most often occurs in women and often in association with hepatitis B antigenemia and allergic reactions to drugs. Small- and medium-sized arteries are involved with inflammatory changes resulting in glomerulitis, myocardial ischemia, peripheral neuropathy,

and seizures. Hypertension is common, presumably reflecting renal disease. Renal failure is the most common cause of death. A polyarteritis-like vasculitis may accompany acquired immunodeficiency syndrome.

The diagnosis of polyarteritis nodosa depends on histologic evidence of vasculitis on biopsy and demonstration of characteristic aneurysms on arteriography. Treatment is empirical and usually includes corticosteroids and cyclophosphamide, removal of offending drugs, and treatment of underlying diseases such as cancer.

Management of anesthesia in patients with polyarteritis nodosa should take into consideration the likelihood of co-existing renal disease, cardiac disease, and systemic hypertension. Supplemental corticosteroids are appropriate in patients who have been receiving these drugs as treatment for this disease.

Kawasaki Disease

Kawasaki disease (mucocutaneous lymph node syndrome) occurs primarily in children and manifests as fever, conjunctivitis, inflammation of the mucous membranes, swollen erythematous hands and feet, truncal rash, and cervical lymphadenopathy. Vasculitis appears early in the disease. Subsequently, coronary arteries and other medium-sized muscular arteries show evidence of focal segmental destruction. Coronary artery aneurysms or ectasia develops in approximately 25% of affected children. Complications of this syndrome include pericarditis, myocarditis, angina pectoris, myocardial infarction, and cerebral hemorrhage. This syndrome might be caused by a retrovirus. Treatment consists of γ globulin and aspirin.

Management of anesthesia in these children must consider the possibility of intraoperative myocardial ischemia. Peripheral nerve block to provide a sympathectomy to inflamed peripheral arteries may be a consideration when viability of the digits is threatened.

RAYNAUD'S PHENOMENON

Raynaud's phenomenon is episodic vasospastic ischemia of the digits. It affects women more often than men. Raynaud's phenomenon is characterized by digital blanching, cyanosis, and rubor after cold exposure and rewarming. Blanching represents the ischemic phase of the phenomenon caused by digital vasospasm. Cyanosis results when deoxygenated blood is present in the capillaries and veins. Rubor manifests with rewarming and represents a hyperemic phase as the digital vasospasm wanes. Burning and throbbing pain typically follow an ischemic episode.

Classification

Raynaud's phenomenon is categorized as primary (also called Raynaud's disease) or secondary when it is associated with other diseases. These other diseases are immunologic disorders, most often scleroderma or systemic lupus erythematosus (**Table 8-4**). Raynaud's disease is typically bilateral and occurs most frequently as a mild condition in many young adult women. Secondary Raynaud's phenomenon tends to be

TABLE 8–4 Secondary Causes of Raynaud's Phenomenon

Connective Tissue Diseases
Scleroderma
Systemic lupus erythematosus
Rheumatoid arthritis
Dermatomyositis

Peripheral Arterial Occlusive Disease
Atherosclerosis
Thromboangiitis obliterans
Thromboembolism
Thoracic outlet syndrome

Neurologic Syndromes
Carpal tunnel syndrome
Reflex sympathetic dystrophy
Cerebral vascular accident
Intervertebral disc herniation

Trauma
Cold thermal injury (frostbite)
Percussive injury (vibrating tools)

Drugs
β-Adrenergic antagonists
Tricyclic antidepressants
Antimetabolites
Ergot alkaloids
Amphetamines

unilateral and may be the first symptom in patients who develop scleroderma, although the systemic disease may not become apparent until years later.

Etiology

Several mechanisms have been postulated as to the cause of Raynaud's phenomenon. These include increased sympathetic nervous system activity, digital vascular hyperreactivity to vasoconstrictive stimuli, circulating vasoactive hormones, and decreased intravascular pressure. The role of increased sympathetic nervous system activity is unclear, and sympathectomy does not predictably produce beneficial effects. Patients with Raynaud's disease do have increased numbers of α_2-adrenergic receptors in the digital arteries, and many patients have low systemic blood pressure. Decreased digital vascular pressure caused by proximal arterial occlusive disease or by digital vascular obstruction could increase the likelihood of digital vasospasm when vasoconstrictive stimuli occur.

Diagnosis

Noninvasive tests that can be used to evaluate patients with Raynaud's phenomenon include digital pulse volume recording and measurement of digital systolic blood pressure and digital blood flow. Measurement of the erythrocyte sedimentation rate and titers of antinuclear antibodies, rheumatoid factor, cryoglobulins, and cold agglutinins can be useful to define specific secondary causes of Raynaud's phenomenon. Angiography is not necessary to diagnose this disorder but

may be useful if digital ischemia is due to atherosclerosis or thrombosis and revascularization is being considered.

Raynaud's phenomenon is the initial complaint in most patients who present with a limited form of scleroderma called CREST syndrome. CREST is an acronym for subcutaneous calcinosis, Raynaud's phenomenon, esophageal dysmotility, sclerodactyly (scleroderma limited to the fingers), and telangiectasia. Raynaud's phenomenon should be distinguished from acrocyanosis, which is characterized by persistent bluish discoloration of the hands or feet that intensifies during cold exposure. Acrocyanosis affects men and women equally, and the prognosis is good, with loss of digital tissue being very unlikely.

Treatment

Primary and secondary Raynaud's phenomenon can often be managed conservatively by protecting the hands and feet from exposure to cold. In addition to the hands and feet, the trunk and head should be kept warm to reduce the risk of reflex vasoconstriction. Pharmacologic intervention is indicated in patients who do not respond satisfactorily to conservative measures. Calcium channel blockers such as nifedipine and sympathetic nervous system antagonists such as prazosin can be used to treat Raynaud's phenomenon. In rare instances, surgical sympathectomy might be considered for treatment of persistent, severe digital ischemia.

Management of Anesthesia

There are no specific recommendations as to the choice of drugs to produce general anesthesia in patients with Raynaud's phenomenon. Increasing the ambient temperature of the operating room and maintaining normothermia are basic considerations. Systemic blood pressure is usually monitored via a noninvasive technique. In some instances, the risk/benefit ratio of radial arterial cannulation for major surgery must be considered. In patients with CREST syndrome, cannulation of a larger artery (such as the femoral artery) should be considered if direct intra-arterial blood pressure monitoring is needed.

Regional anesthesia is acceptable for peripheral operations in patients with Raynaud's phenomenon. If a regional anesthetic technique is selected, it may be prudent not to include epinephrine in the anesthetic solution as the catecholamine could provoke undesirable vasoconstriction.

CAROTID ARTERY DISEASE

Cerebrovascular accidents (strokes) are characterized by sudden neurologic deficits due to ischemic, hemorrhagic, or thrombotic events. Ischemic stroke is described by the area of the brain affected and the etiologic mechanism. Hemorrhagic stroke is classified as intracerebral or subarachnoid. A transient ischemic attack is a sudden vascular-related focal neurologic deficit that resolves within 24 hours. Transient ischemic attacks are not separate disease entities but rather evidence of an impending ischemic stroke.

Stroke is the leading cause of disability and the third leading cause of death in the United States. The pathogenesis of stroke differs somewhat among ethnic groups. Extracranial carotid artery disease and cardiogenic embolism more commonly cause ischemic strokes in non-Hispanic whites, whereas intracranial thromboembolic disease is more common in African Americans. Women have lower stroke rates than men until they reach 75 years of age. Then stroke rates are at their highest.

Cerebrovascular Anatomy

The blood supply to the brain (20% of cardiac output) is brought via two pairs of blood vessels: the internal carotid arteries and the vertebral arteries (**Fig. 8-5**). These vessels join to form the major intracranial blood vessels (anterior cerebral arteries, middle cerebral arteries, posterior cerebral arteries) and the circle of Willis. Occlusion of a specific major intracranial artery results in a constellation of predictable clinical neurologic deficits. Isolated infarction of the anterior cerebral artery is uncommon. Neurologic deficits following middle cerebral artery occlusion are extensive, reflecting the large areas of brain supplied by this artery and its branches.

The major branches of the vertebral arteries are the arteries to the spinal cord and the posteroinferior cerebellar arteries that supply the inferior cerebellum and lateral medulla. The two vertebral arteries then unite to form the basilar artery. Occlusion of the vertebral arteries or basilar artery results in signs and symptoms that depend on the level of the infarction. The basilar artery terminates by dividing into two posterior cerebral arteries, which supply the medial temporal lobe, occipital lobe, and parts of the thalamus.

Conventional angiography can demonstrate acute vascular occlusion or an embolus lodged at a vascular bifurcation. The vasculature can also be visualized noninvasively by CT angiography and magnetic resonance angiography. Transcranial Doppler ultrasonography can provide indirect evidence of major vascular occlusion and offers the advantage of real-time bedside monitoring in patients undergoing thrombolytic therapy.

Acute Ischemic Stroke

Acute ischemic stroke most likely reflects cardioembolism, large-vessel atherothromboembolism (such as from disease at the carotid bifurcation) or small-vessel occlusive disease (lacunar infarction). Patients with long-standing diabetes mellitus or systemic hypertension are most likely to experience acute ischemic stroke due to small-vessel occlusive disease. Echocardiography is very useful in evaluating the source of cardioembolism.

Risk Factors Systemic hypertension is the most significant risk factor for acute ischemic stroke. Adequate treatment of systolic or diastolic hypertension dramatically reduces the risk of first stroke. Cigarette smoking substantially increases the risk of acute ischemic stroke. Hyperlipidemia appears to be a risk factor for the occurrence of acute ischemic stroke, and treatment of patients with statin drugs is associated with a decreased risk of stroke. Diabetes mellitus is another common risk factor for stroke. Excessive alcohol consumption (more than six drinks daily) seems to increase the risk of stroke, whereas moderate alcohol consumption (one or two drinks daily) may be protective. An increased homocysteine level is an independent risk factor for the development of stroke.

CAROTID ENDARTERECTOMY

Surgical treatment of symptomatic carotid artery stenosis greatly decreases the risk of stroke, especially in men with severe carotid stenosis. Two large randomized trials, The North American Symptomatic Carotid Endarterectomy Trial and the European Carotid Surgery Trial, both reported favorable results for symptomatic patients with high-grade stenosis (70%–90%) compared to medically managed patients. Data from transcranial Doppler and duplex ultrasonography studies suggest that carotid artery stenosis with a residual luminal diameter of 1.5 mm (70%–75% stenosis) represents the point at which a pressure drop occurs across the stenosis, that is, the stenosis becomes hemodynamically significant. Therefore, if collateral cerebral blood flow is not adequate, transient ischemic attacks and ischemic infarction can occur.

Surgical treatment for asymptomatic disease is still controversial. It appears that the absolute risk reduction is small (approximately 1% per year for the first few years) but is higher with longer follow-up. Thus, the stroke prevention results in this patient group can be durable, but any benefit of surgical correction of asymptomatic carotid stenosis is negated by a high perioperative complication rate. Only those centers

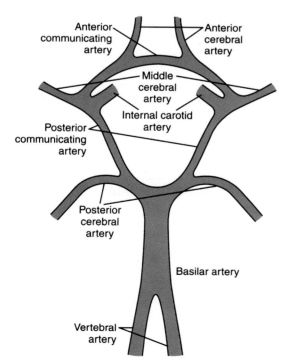

Figure 8-5 • Cerebral circulation and the circle of Willis. The cerebral blood supply comes from the vertebral arteries (arising from the subclavian arteries) and the internal carotid arteries (arising from the common carotid arteries).

153

with complication rates of 3% or less should contemplate performing carotid endarterectomy in asymptomatic patients.

Carotid angioplasty and stenting may become alternatives to carotid endarterectomy.

Preoperative Evaluation

In addition to the neurologic evaluation, patients scheduled for carotid endarterectomy should be examined for co-existing cardiovascular and renal disease. Predictably, patients with cerebrovascular occlusive disease have occlusive disease in other arteries. Ischemic heart disease is a major cause of morbidity and mortality following carotid endarterectomy. The reported incidence of perioperative myocardial infarction ranges from 0% to 4%. Patients with severe coronary artery disease and severe carotid occlusive disease present a dilemma. A staged approach with carotid endarterectomy first could result in significant morbidity/mortality from cardiac causes. On the other hand, coronary revascularization first may result in a higher incidence of stroke. No randomized studies have been performed to determine the benefit of combined versus staged procedures. The management of such a patient must be individualized.

Chronic essential hypertension is a common finding in patients with cerebrovascular disease. It is useful to establish the usual range of blood pressure for each patient preoperatively to provide a guide for acceptable perfusion pressures during anesthesia and surgery. The effect of a change in head position on cerebral function should also be ascertained. Extreme head rotation, flexion, or extension in patients with co-existing vertebral artery disease could lead to angulation or compression of that artery. Recognition of this response preoperatively allows hazardous head positions (especially hyperextension) to be avoided while patients are unconscious during general anesthesia

Management of Anesthesia

Anesthetic management for carotid endarterectomy must include protection of the heart and brain from ischemic events. Control of heart rate, blood pressure, pain, and stress responses are necessary. In addition, at the conclusion of surgery, the patient must be sufficiently awake to undergo neurologic examination.

Carotid endarterectomy can be performed under regional (cervical plexus block) or general anesthesia. Regional anesthesia allows a patient to remain awake to facilitate neurologic assessment during carotid artery cross-clamping. This technique requires patient cooperation. Blood pressure lability may be greater in patients undergoing carotid endarterectomy under general anesthesia. However, the anesthetic-induced decrease in cerebral metabolic oxygen consumption may provide some degree of cerebral protection. No particular anesthetic drug(s) can be recommended for induction and maintenance of general anesthesia. However, two goals must be met: maintenance of hemodynamic stability and prompt emergence allowing immediate assessment of neurologic status in the operating room.

Maintenance of an adequate blood pressure is important during carotid endarterectomy because autoregulation may be abnormal in these patients. Vasopressors or vasodilators may be needed to maintain an appropriate perfusion pressure during carotid cross-clamping. Surgical manipulation of the carotid sinus may cause marked alterations in heart rate and blood pressure. It is generally accepted that changes in regional cerebral blood flow associated with changes in $Paco_2$ are unpredictable in these patients. Therefore, maintenance of normocarbia is recommended.

Monitoring usually includes an intra-arterial catheter. Patients with poor left ventricular function and/or severe coronary artery disease might require a central venous or pulmonary artery catheter or transesophageal echocardiography, but this is not often necessary. The hemodynamic goals for cerebral and coronary perfusion are similar, and achievement of these goals benefits both organ systems. Particular care must be taken during central venous access attempts to prevent inadvertent carotid puncture that could cause a hematoma that compromises collateral blood flow during carotid cross-clamping.

When carotid endarterectomy is performed under general anesthesia, monitoring for cerebral ischemia, hypoperfusion, and cerebral emboli can be considered. The principal reason to monitor cerebral function in these patients is to select which patients would benefit from use of a carotid artery shunt during carotid cross-clamping. The standard electroencephalogram is a sensitive indicator of inadequate cerebral perfusion during carotid cross-clamping, and intraoperative neurologic complications correlate with the electroencephalographic changes of cerebral ischemia. However, the utility of electroencephalographic monitoring during carotid endarterectomy is limited by several factors: (1) electroencephalography may not detect subcortical or small cortical infarcts, (2) false-negative results are not uncommon (patients with previous strokes or transient ischemic attacks have a high incidence of false-negative test results), and (3) the electroencephalogram can be affected not only by cerebral ischemia but also by changes in temperature, blood pressure, and depth of anesthesia. Somatosensory evoked potential monitoring can detect specific changes produced by decreased regional cerebral blood flow, but it can be difficult to determine whether these changes are due to anesthesia, hypothermia, changes in blood pressure, or cerebral ischemia. Stump pressure (internal carotid artery back pressure) is a poor indicator of the adequacy of cerebral perfusion. Transcranial Doppler ultrasonography allows continuous monitoring of blood flow velocity and the presence of microembolic events. It could be used to determine the need for shunt placement, to recognize shunt malfunction, and to manage postoperative hyperperfusion. Overall, awake neurologic assessment is the simplest, most cost-effective, and most reliable method of cerebral function monitoring during carotid endarterectomy.

Postoperative Management and Complications

In the immediate postoperative period after carotid endarterectomy, patients must be observed for cardiac, airway, and neurologic complications. These include hyper- or hypotension, myocardial ischemia/infarction, development of significant soft-tissue edema or a hematoma in the neck, and the onset of neurologic signs and symptoms that signal a new stroke or acute thrombosis at the endarterectomy site.

Hypertension is frequently observed during the immediate postoperative period, often in patients with co-existing essential hypertension. The increase in blood pressure often reaches a maximum 2 to 3 hours after surgery and may persist for 24 hours. Hypertension should be treated to avoid the hazards of cerebral edema and myocardial ischemia. The incidence of new neurologic deficits is increased threefold in patients who are hypertensive postoperatively. Continuous infusion of nitroprusside or nitroglycerin and the use of longer acting drugs such as hydralazine or labetalol are options for blood pressure control. The mechanism of this postoperative hypertension may be related to altered activity of the carotid sinus or loss of carotid sinus function due to denervation during surgery.

Hypotension is also commonly observed during the immediate postoperative period. This hypotension can be explained based on carotid sinus hypersensitivity. The carotid sinus previously "shielded" by atheromatous plaque is now able to perceive blood pressure oscillations more clearly and goes through a period of hyperresponsiveness to these stimuli. Hypotension due to carotid sinus hypersensitivity is usually treated with vasopressors such as phenylephrine. It typically resolves within 12 to 24 hours.

Cranial nerve dysfunction is possible after carotid endarterectomy with most injuries being transient. Patients should be examined for evidence of hypoglossal, recurrent laryngeal, or superior laryngeal nerve injury. Such injury may produce difficulty swallowing or protecting the airway and could result in aspiration.

Carotid body denervation can also occur after carotid artery surgery and impair the cardiac and ventilatory responses to hypoxemia. This can be clinically significant after bilateral carotid endarterectomy or with administration of narcotics.

Endovascular Treatment of Carotid Disease

The technique of carotid artery stenting is under development for the treatment of carotid artery disease. It may become the leading alternative to carotid endarterectomy. The major complication of carotid stenting is microembolization of atherosclerotic material into the cerebral circulation during the procedure. Embolic protection devices for use during carotid stenting have been developed to prevent or decrease the risk of embolization of this material and therefore to decrease the risk of stroke. The Stenting and Angioplasty with Protection in Patients at High Risk for Endarterectomy (SAPPHIRE) study is the first randomized multicenter trial comparing the safety and efficacy of carotid stenting with embolic protection to carotid endarterectomy in high-risk patients. The main finding of this trial was that the results of carotid artery stenting with the use of an emboli protection device were similar to the results of carotid endarterectomy in the prevention of stroke, death, or myocardial infarction among patients for whom surgery poses an increased risk.

The Carotid Revascularization Endarterectomy vs. Stenting Trial (CREST) and Stent-Supported Percutaneous Angioplasty of the Carotid Artery vs. Endarterectomy Trial, when completed, will provide more data regarding clinical outcomes in low- to medium-risk patient populations and help establish guidelines for the use of endovascular techniques in the treatment of carotid artery occlusive disease.

PERIPHERAL VENOUS DISEASE

Deep vein thrombosis (usually involving a leg vein) and subsequent pulmonary embolism are a leading cause of postoperative morbidity and mortality. Formation of a clot inside a blood vessel is designated a thrombus to distinguish it from normal extravascular clotting of blood. An embolus is a fragment of the thrombus that breaks off and travels in the blood until it lodges at a site of vascular narrowing. An embolus originating in a vein commonly lodges in the pulmonary vasculature, whereas an embolus originating in an artery usually occludes a more distal, smaller artery

Factors that predispose to thromboembolism are multiple and include events associated with anesthesia and surgery (**Table 8-5**). For example, venous stasis associated with postoperative immobility or pregnancy results in failure to dilute or promptly clear activated clotting factors thereby predisposing to thrombus formation. Any condition that causes a roughened endothelial vessel wall such as infection, trauma, and drug-induced irritation also predisposes to thrombus formation.

Deep Vein Thrombosis

Deep vein thrombosis is detectable in a substantial number of patients older than age 40 after prostatectomy or hip surgery.

TABLE 8–5 Factors Predisposing to Thromboembolism
Venous stasis
Recent surgery
Trauma
Lack of ambulation
Pregnancy
Low cardiac output (congestive heart failure, myocardial infarction)
Stroke
Abnormality of the venous wall
Varicose veins
Drug-induced irritation
Hypercoagulable state
Surgery
Estrogen therapy (oral contraceptives)
Cancer
Deficiencies of endogenous anticoagulants (antithrombin III, protein C, protein S)
Stress response associated with surgery
Inflammatory bowel disease
History of previous thromboembolism
Morbid obesity
Advanced age

Most of these thromboses are subclinical and resolve completely when mobility is restored. A few travel to the lungs and produce pulmonary embolism. Venous stasis, endothelial damage, and hypercoagulability predispose to venous thrombosis. Thrombi formed in veins below the knees or in the arms rarely give rise to significant pulmonary emboli, whereas thrombi that extend into the iliofemoral venous system can produce a life-threatening pulmonary embolism. Likewise, thrombi formed in the right atrium as a result of atrial fibrillation are common sources of pulmonary embolism.

Diagnosis

Superficial thrombophlebitis is rarely associated with pulmonary embolism. The intense inflammation that accompanies superficial thrombophlebitis rapidly leads to total vein occlusion. Typically, the vein can be palpated as a cordlike structure surrounded by an area of erythema, warmth, and edema. The presence of fever suggests bacterial infection. Treatment of superficial vein thrombosis is usually conservative, consisting of elevation, application of heat, and administration of antibiotics if infection is suspected.

The diagnosis of deep vein thrombosis by clinical signs is unreliable. B-mode ultrasonography with vein compression is highly sensitive for detecting proximal vein thrombosis (popliteal or femoral vein) but less sensitive for detecting calf vein thrombosis (**Fig. 8-6**). This method is preferred for evaluation of patients with suspected deep vein thrombosis because it is less invasive than venography and more accurate than impedance plethysmography. Venous thrombosis can be diagnosed with a sensitivity and specificity of more than 95%.

Most postoperative venous thrombi arise in the lower legs, especially in soleal sinuses and in large veins draining the gastrocnemius muscle. However, in approximately 20% of patients, thrombi originate in more proximal veins. Left untreated, deep vein thrombosis can extend into larger and more proximal veins, and such extension may be responsible for subsequent fatal pulmonary emboli.

Thrombophilia refers to a hereditary tendency to experience recurrent thrombosis. Laboratory abnormalities associated with initial and recurrent venous thrombosis/embolism include congenital deficiencies of antithrombin III, protein C, protein S, or plasminogen. Congenital resistance to activated protein C and increased levels of antiphospholipid antibodies are also associated with venous thromboembolism. A family history of unexplained venous thrombosis may be present.

Treatment

Anticoagulation is the first-line treatment for all patients with a diagnosis of deep vein thrombosis. Therapy is initiated with heparin (unfractionated or low molecular weight heparin) because this drug produces an immediate anticoagulant effect. Heparin can be administered by continuous intravenous infusion or subcutaneous injection. Heparin has a narrow therapeutic window, and the response of individual patients can vary considerably. Advantages of low molecular weight heparin over unfractionated heparin include a longer half-life, a more predictable dose response, and less risk of bleeding complications.

An oral vitamin K antagonist (warfarin) is initiated within 24 hours of heparin therapy and adjusted to achieve a prothrombin time with an international normalized ratio between

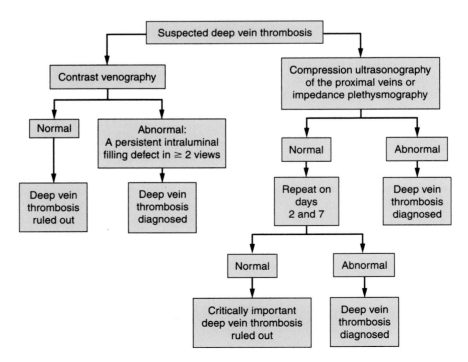

Figure 8-6 • Steps in the diagnosis of deep vein thrombosis. (*Adapted from Ginsberg JS: Management of venous thromboembolism. N Engl J Med 1996; 335:1816–1828. Copyright 1996 Massachusetts Medical Society.*)

2.0 and 3.0. Heparin is discontinued when warfarin has achieved its therapeutic effect. Oral anticoagulants may be continued for 3 to 6 months or longer.

Inferior vena cava filters may be inserted into patients with recurrent pulmonary embolism despite adequate anticoagulant therapy or in whom anticoagulation is contraindicated.

Complications of Anticoagulation

Approximately 5% of patients treated with unfractionated heparin develop significant bleeding. Fewer episodes of bleeding seem to occur with the use of low molecular weight heparin. Approximately 3% of patients receiving unfractionated heparin develop immune-mediated thrombocytopenia (heparin-induced thrombocytopenia) with platelet counts less than 100,000 cells/mm^3. Paradoxically, heparin-induced thrombocytopenia can be complicated by further extension of venous thromboses or development of new arterial thromboses. Treatment of heparin-induced thrombocytopenia is empirical and includes discontinuation of heparin (**Fig. 8-7**).

Prevention of Venous Thromboembolism
Clinical Risk Factors

Clinical risk factors identify patients who can benefit from prophylactic measures aimed at reducing the risk of development of deep vein thrombosis (**Table 8-6**). Patients at low risk require only minimal prophylactic measures, such as early postoperative ambulation and the use of compression stockings,

which augment propulsion of blood from the ankles to the knees. The risk of deep vein thrombosis may be much higher in patients older than age 40 who are undergoing operations lasting more than 1 hour, especially orthopedic surgery on the lower extremities, pelvic or abdominal surgery, and surgery that requires a prolonged convalescence period with bed rest or limited mobility. The presence of cancer also increases the risk of thrombotic complications.

Subcutaneous heparin in doses of 5000 units twice daily prevents deep vein thrombosis in patients at moderate risk following abdominal and orthopedic surgery. Intermittent external pneumatic compression of the legs is protective in patients at moderate risk of deep vein thrombosis (see Table 8-6).

Regional Anesthesia

The incidence of postoperative deep vein thrombosis and pulmonary embolism in patients having total knee or total hip replacement can be substantially decreased (20%–40%) by administration of epidural or spinal anesthesia compared to general anesthesia. Postoperative epidural analgesia does not augment this benefit but may allow earlier ambulation, which can reduce the risk of deep vein thrombosis.

Presumably, the beneficial effects of regional anesthesia compared to general anesthesia are due to (1) vasodilation, which maximizes venous blood flow and (2) the ability to provide excellent postoperative analgesia and early ambulation.

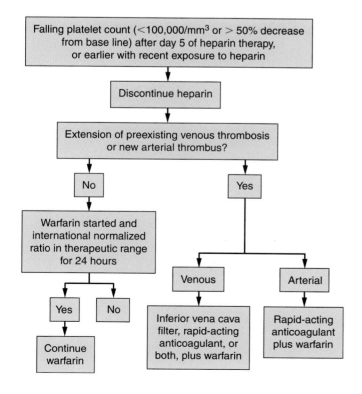

Figure 8-7 • Steps in the management of patients with venous thromboembolism and heparin-induced thrombocytopenia. (Adapted from Ginsberg JS: Management of venous thromboembolism. N Engl J Med 1996;335:1816–1828. Copyright 1996 Massachusetts Medical Society.)

TABLE 8-6 Risk and Predisposing Factors for the Development of Deep Vein Thrombosis after Surgery or Trauma

Event	Low Risk	Moderate Risk	High Risk
General surgery	<40 years old Operation < 60 minutes	>40 years old Operation > 60 minutes	>40 years old Operation > 60 minutes Previous deep vein thrombosis Previous pulmonary embolism Extensive trauma Major fractures
Orthopedic surgery			Knee or hip replacement
Trauma			Extensive soft-tissue injury Major fractures Multiple trauma sites
Medical conditions	Pregnancy	Postpartum period Myocardial infarction Congestive heart failure	Stroke
Incidence of deep vein thrombosis without prophylaxis	2%	10%–40%	40%–80%
Symptomatic pulmonary embolism	0.2%	1%–8%	5%–10%
Fatal pulmonary embolism	0.002%	0.1%–0.4%	1%–5%
Recommended steps to minimize deep vein thrombosis	Graduated compression stockings Early ambulation	External pneumatic compression Subcutaneous heparin Intravenous dextran	External pneumatic compression Subcutaneous heparin Intravenous dextran Vena caval filter Warfarin

Adapted from Weinmann EE, Salzman EW: Deep-vein thrombosis. N Engl J Med 1994;331:1630–1642.

KEY POINTS

- Atherosclerosis is a systemic disease. Patients with peripheral arterial disease have a three to five times greater risk of cardiovascular ischemic events such as myocardial infarction, ischemic stroke, and death than those without this disease. Critical limb ischemia is associated with a very high intermediate-term morbidity and mortality due to cardiovascular events.

- Development of atherosclerosis involves several highly interrelated processes including lipid disturbances, platelet activation, thrombosis, endothelial dysfunction, inflammation, oxidative stress, vascular smooth muscle cell activation, altered matrix metabolism, remodeling, and genetic factors.

- Aortic cross-clamping and unclamping are associated with significant hemodynamic disturbances because of the decrease in blood flow distal to the aortic clamp and the increase in blood flow proximal to the level of aortic occlusion. There is a substantial increase in systemic blood pressure. This hypertension is attributed to increased impedance to aortic outflow (increased afterload). The hemodynamic response to aortic cross-clamping differs based on the level of clamping: thoracic, supraceliac, or infrarenal cross-clamping.

- Perfusion pressures distal to the aortic cross-clamp are decreased and are directly dependent on the pressure above the level of aortic clamping to aid in blood flow through collateral vessels or through a shunt. Blood flow to vital organs distal to the aortic clamp depends on perfusion pressure and not on cardiac output or intravascular volume.

- Aortic cross-clamping is associated with formation and release of hormonal factors (activation of the sympathetic nervous system and the renin-angiotensin-aldosterone system) and other mediators (prostaglandins, oxygen free radicals, complement cascade). These mediators may aggravate or blunt the harmful effects of aortic cross-clamping and unclamping. Overall, injury to the spinal cord, lungs, kidneys, and abdominal viscera is principally due to ischemia and subsequent reperfusion injury due to the aortic cross-clamp (local effects) and/or to release of mediators from ischemic and reperfused tissues (distant effects).

KEY POINTS—cont'd

- The principal causes of declamping hypotension include (1) central hypovolemia caused by pooling of blood in reperfused tissues, (2) hypoxia-mediated vasodilation causing an increase in vascular capacitance in the tissues below the level of aortic clamping, and (3) accumulation of vasoactive and myocardial depressant metabolites in these tissues.

- Aortic, carotid, and peripheral arterial endovascular procedures have emerged as alternative less invasive methods of arterial repair. In-hospital and 30-day mortality rates are lower for endovascular repair of an abdominal aortic aneurysm than for open repair. However, at 5 years, there is no significant difference in all-cause mortality between endovascular and open repair groups. The incidence of conversion to an open repair is approximately 3%.

- Acute arterial occlusion is typically caused by cardiogenic embolism. Systemic emboli may arise from a mural thrombus in the left ventricle that develops due to myocardial infarction or dilated cardiomyopathy. Other cardiac sources of systemic emboli are valvular heart disease, prosthetic heart valves, infective endocarditis, and left atrial myxoma. Atrial fibrillation is a very important predisposing factor in systemic embolization. Noncardiac causes of acute arterial occlusion include atheroemboli from the aorta and iliac or femoral arteries.

- Thromboangiitis obliterans is an inflammatory vasculitis leading to occlusion of small- and medium-sized arteries and veins in the extremities. The disease is most prevalent in men, and the onset is typically before age 45. The most important predisposing factor is tobacco use. The disorder apparently involves an autoimmune response triggered when nicotine is present.

- Data from transcranial Doppler and carotid duplex ultrasonography studies suggest that a carotid artery stenosis with a residual luminal diameter of 1.5 mm (70%–75% stenosis) represents the point at which a pressure drop occurs across the stenosis, that is, the stenosis becomes hemodynamically significant. Therefore, if collateral cerebral blood flow is not adequate, transient ischemic attacks and ischemic infarction can occur.

- Hypertension is frequently observed during the immediate postoperative period after carotid endarterectomy. Hypertension at this time may be related to co-existing essential hypertension or to altered activity of the carotid sinus or loss of carotid sinus function due to denervation during the surgery. Hypertension should be treated to avoid the hazards of cerebral edema and myocardial ischemia.

- Hypotension may be observed during the immediate postoperative period after carotid endarterectomy. This hypotension can be related to carotid sinus hypersensitivity. The carotid sinus previously shielded by atheromatous plaque is now able to perceive blood pressure oscillations more clearly and goes through a period of hyperresponsiveness to these stimuli.

- Patients at low risk for deep vein thrombosis require only minimal prophylactic measures, such as early postoperative ambulation and use of compression stockings. The risk of deep vein thrombosis may be much higher in patients older than age 40 who are undergoing operations lasting more than 1 hour, especially orthopedic surgery on the lower extremities, pelvic or abdominal surgery, and surgery that requires a prolonged convalescence with bed rest or limited mobility. The presence of cancer also increases the risk of thrombotic complications. Subcutaneous heparin (minidose heparin) and intermittent external pneumatic compression of the legs help prevent deep vein thrombosis in patients at moderate risk following abdominal and orthopedic surgery.

REFERENCES

Asymptomatic Carotid Surgery Trial (ACST) Collaborative Group: Prevention of disabling and fatal strokes by successful carotid endarterectomy in patients without recent neurological symptoms: Randomised controlled trial. Lancet 2004;363:1491–1502.

Chaturvedi S, Bruno A, Feasby T, et al: Carotid endarterectomy—an evidence-based review: Report of the therapeutics and technology assessment subcommittee of the American Academy of Neurology. Neurology 2005;65:794–801.

Cremonesi A, Setacci C, Angelo Bignamini A, et al: Carotid artery stenting: First consensus document of the ICCS-SPREAD Joint Committee. Stroke 2006;37:2400–2409.

European Carotid Surgery Trialists' Collaborative Group: MRC European Carotid Surgery Trial: Interim results for symptomatic patients with severe (70–99%) or with mild (0–29%) carotid stenosis. Lancet 1991;337:1235–1243.

EVAR Trial Participants: Endovascular aneurysm repair versus open repair in patients with abdominal aortic aneurysm (EVAR trial 1): Randomised controlled trial. Lancet 2005;365:2179–2186.

EVAR Trial Participants: Endovascular aneurysm repair and outcome in patients unfit for open repair of abdominal aortic aneurysm (EVAR trial 2): Randomised controlled trial. Lancet 2005;365:2187–2192.

Freeman A, Shulman S: Kawasaki disease: Summary of the American Heart Association guidelines. Am Fam Physician 2006;74:1441–1448.

Geerts WH, Heit JA, Clagett GP, et al: Prevention of venous thromboembolism. Chest 2001;119:132S–175S.

Gelman S: The pathophysiology of aortic cross-clamping and unclamping. Anesthesiology 1995;82:1026–1060.

Hirsch AT, Haskal ZJ, Hertzer NR, et al: ACC/AHA 2005 practice guidelines for the management of patients with peripheral arterial disease (lower extremity, renal, mesenteric, and abdominal aortic): A collaborative report from the American Association for Vascular Surgery/Society for Vascular Surgery, Society for Cardiovascular Angiography and Interventions, Society for Vascular Medicine and Biology, Society of Interventional Radiology, and the ACC/AHA Task Force on Practice Guidelines (writing committee to develop guidelines for the management of patients with peripheral arterial disease): Endorsed by the American Association of Cardiovascular and Pulmonary Rehabilitation; National Heart, Lung, and Blood Institute; Society for Vascular Nursing; TransAtlantic Inter-Society Consensus; and Vascular Disease Foundation. Circulation 2006;113:e463–e654.

Katzen BT, Dake MD, MacLean AA, Wang DS: Endovascular repair of abdominal and thoracic aortic aneurysms. Circulation 2005;112:1663–1675.

Kouchoukos NT, Dougenis D: Surgery of the thoracic aorta. N Engl J Med 1997;336:1876–1888.

McFalls EO, Ward HB, Moritz TE, et al: Coronary artery revascularization before elective major vascular surgery. N Engl J Med 2004;351:2795–2804.

Norris EJ, Beattie C, Perler BA, et al: Double masked randomized trial comparing alternate combinations of intraoperative anesthesia and postoperative analgesia in abdominal aortic surgery. Anesthesiology 2001;95:1054–1067.

North American Symptomatic Carotid Endarterectomy Trial Collaborators: Beneficial effect of carotid endarterectomy in symptomatic patients with high-grade carotid stenosis. N Engl J Med 1991;325:445–453.

Sharrock NE, Ranawat CS, Urquhart B, et al: Factors influencing deep vein thrombosis after total hip arthroplasty under epidural anesthesia. Anesth Analg 1993;76:765–771.

Trimarchi S, Nienaber CA, Rampoldi V, et al: Role and results of surgery in acute type B aortic dissection: Insights from the International Registry of Acute Aortic Dissection (IRAD). Circulation 2006;114:357–364.

Tsai TT, Evangelista A, Nienaber CA, et al: Long-term survival in patients presenting with type A acute aortic dissection. Insights from the International Registry of Acute Aortic Dissection (IRAD). Circulation 2006;114(Suppl I):I-350–I-356.

Yadav JS, Wholey MH, Kuntz RE, et al: Protected carotid-artery stenting versus endarterectomy in high-risk patients. N Engl J Med 2004;351:1493–1501.

CHAPTER 9

Respiratory Diseases

Viji Kurup

Patients with preoperative respiratory diseases are at increased risk of perioperative respiratory complications. There is increasing awareness of the importance of postoperative pulmonary complications in contributing to morbidity, mortality, and increased hospital length of stay. Pulmonary complications also play an important part in determining long-term mortality after surgery. Modification of disease severity and patient optimization preoperatively significantly decreases the incidence of these complications.

Respiratory diseases can be divided into the following groups for discussion of their influence on anesthetic management: acute upper respiratory tract infection (URI), asthma, chronic obstructive pulmonary disease (COPD), acute respiratory failure, restrictive lung disease, pulmonary embolism, and lung transplantation.

ACUTE UPPER RESPIRATORY TRACT INFECTION

Every year approximately 25 million patients visit their doctor with uncomplicated URI. The common cold syndrome results in about 20 million days of absence from work and 22 million days of absence from school. It is likely then that there will be a population of patients scheduled for elective surgery who have an active URI.

Infectious (viral or bacterial) nasopharyngitis accounts for approximately 95% of all URIs with the most common viruses being rhinovirus, coronavirus, influenzavirus, parainfluenza virus, and respiratory syncytial virus. Noninfectious nasopharyngitis is allergic and vasomotor in origin.

Signs and Symptoms .
Patients with a URI present with a broad spectrum of signs and symptoms. Sneezing, runny nose, and a history of allergies point to an allergic etiology. When associated with infection, there is usually a history of fever, purulent nasal discharge, productive cough, fever, and malaise. On examination, the patient may be tachypneic or wheezing or appear toxic.

Diagnosis
The diagnosis of a URI is usually based on clinical signs and symptoms. Although viral cultures and laboratory tests are available to confirm the diagnosis of a URI, they lack sensitivity and are impractical in a busy clinical setting.

Management of Anesthesia
Preoperative
Most studies regarding the effects of URI on postoperative complications have been done in pediatric patients. There is evidence to show an increased incidence of respiratory complications in patients with a history of copious secretions, endotracheal intubation, prematurity, parental smoking, nasal congestion, and reactive airway disease and in those having airway surgery. Those with clear systemic signs of infection such as fever, purulent rhinitis, productive cough, and rhonchi who are undergoing elective surgery, particularly airway surgery, are at considerable risk of perioperative adverse events. Consultation with the surgeon regarding the urgency of the case must be undertaken. Patients who have had a URI for days or weeks and are stable or improving can be safely managed without postponing surgery. Delaying surgery does not reduce the incidence of adverse respiratory events if anesthesia is administered within 4 weeks of the URI. Airway hyperreactivity may require 6 weeks or more to heal. The economic and practical aspects of canceling surgery should be taken into consideration before a decision is made to postpone surgery.

Viral infections, particularly during the infectious phase, can cause morphologic and functional changes in the respiratory epithelium. The relationship between epithelial damage, viral infection, airway reactivity, and anesthesia remains unclear. Tracheal mucociliary flow and pulmonary bactericidal activity can be decreased by general anesthesia. It is possible that positive pressure ventilation may help in spreading infection from the upper to the lower respiratory tract. The immune response of the body is altered by surgery and anesthesia. A reduction in B-lymphocyte numbers, T-lymphocyte responsiveness, and antibody production may be associated with anesthesia, but the clinical significance of this remains to be elucidated.

Intraoperative
The anesthetic management of patients with a URI should include adequate hydration, focus on reducing secretions, and limit manipulation of a potentially sensitive airway. The laryngeal mask airway may be a good alternative to endotracheal intubation to reduce the risk of bronchospasm from airway manipulation. The role of prophylactic bronchodilators to reduce the incidence of perioperative bronchospasm has not been clearly established.

Postoperative
Reported adverse respiratory events in patients with a URI include bronchospasm, laryngospasm, airway obstruction, postintubation croup, desaturation, and atelectasis. Long-term complications from anesthetizing patients with a URI have not been demonstrated. Intraoperative and immediate postoperative hypoxemia is common and amenable to treatment with supplemental oxygen.

ASTHMA

Asthma is a disease characterized by chronic airway inflammation, reversible expiratory airflow obstruction in response to various stimuli, and bronchial hyperreactivity. It is estimated that asthma affects 4% to 5% of the U.S. population. Data from the National Center for Health Statistics indicate that 30.8 million people had a diagnosis of asthma in 2002. Adults missed 11.8 million workdays due to asthma. Bronchial asthma can occur at any age but typically appears early in life. Approximately one half of cases develop before age 10 and another third occur before age 40. In childhood, there is 2:1 male/female preponderance, but the sex ratio equalizes by age 30.

Signs and Symptoms

Asthma is an episodic disease with acute exacerbations interspersed with symptom-free periods. Most attacks are short-lived, lasting minutes to hours, and clinically the patient seems to recover completely after an attack. However, there can be a phase in which the patient experiences some degree of airway obstruction daily. This phase can be mild, with or without superimposed severe episodes, or much more serious, with significant obstruction persisting for days or weeks. Status asthmaticus is defined as life-threatening bronchospasm that persists despite treatment.

Clinical manifestations of asthma include wheezing, productive or nonproductive cough, dyspnea, chest discomfort or tightness that may lead to "air hunger," and eosinophilia.

Pathogenesis

Asthma is a heterogeneous disease and genetic (atopic) and environmental factors such as viruses, occupational exposure, and allergens contribute to its initiation and continuance. Stimuli inciting an episode of asthma are summarized in **Table 9-1**.

Factors that support the allergen-induced immunologic model of the etiology of asthma include the following: (1) Atopy is the single greatest risk factor for the development of asthma. (2) A personal and/or family history of allergic

TABLE 9-1 Stimuli Inciting Symptoms of Asthma
1. Allergens
2. Pharmacologic agents: aspirin, β-antagonists, some nonsteroidal anti-inflammatory drugs, sulfiting agents
3. Infections: respiratory viruses
4. Exercise: the attacks typically follow exertion rather than occur during it
5. Emotional stress: endorphins and vagal mediation

diseases such as rhinitis, urticaria, and eczema is often present. (3) There is usually a positive wheal-and-flare skin reaction to intradermal injection of extracts of airborne antigens. (4) Serum immunoglobulin E levels are increased and/or there is a positive response to provocative tests involving the inhalation of specific antigens. (5) Evidence of genetic linkage of high total serum IgE levels and atopy has been observed.

An alternative explanation for the characteristic features of asthma is abnormal autonomic nervous system regulation of neural function, specifically an imbalance between excitatory (bronchoconstrictor), and inhibitory (bronchodilator) neural input. It is likely that chemical mediators released from mast cells interact with the autonomic nervous system. Some chemical mediators can stimulate airway receptors to trigger reflex bronchoconstriction, while other mediators sensitize bronchial smooth muscle to the effects of acetylcholine. In addition, stimulation of muscarinic receptors can facilitate mediator release from mast cells providing a positive feedback loop for sustained inflammation and bronchoconstriction.

Diagnosis

Forced expiratory volume in 1 second (FEV_1) and maximum mid-expiratory flow rate are direct measures of the severity of expiratory airflow obstruction (**Fig. 9-1** and **Table 9-2**). These measurements provide objective data that can be used to assess the severity and monitor the course of an exacerbation of asthma. The typical asthmatic patient who presents to the hospital for treatment has an FEV_1 less than 35% of normal and a maximum mid-expiratory flow rate that is 20% or less

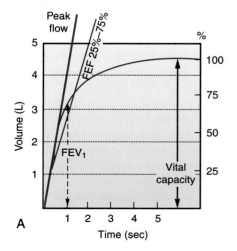

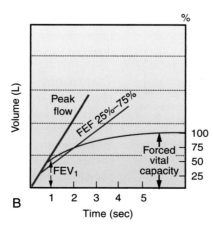

Figure 9-1 • Spirographic changes of a normal subject (**A**) and a patient in bronchospasm (**B**). The forced exhaled volume in 1 second (FEV_1) is typically less than 80% of the vital capacity in the presence of obstructive airway disease. Peak flow and maximum mid-expiratory flow rate ($FEF_{25\%-75\%}$) are also decreased in these patients (**B**). (*Adapted from Kingston HGG, Hirshman CA: Perioperative management of the patient with asthma. Anesth Analg 1984;63:844–855.*)

TABLE 9–2 Classification of Asthma Based on Severity of Expiratory Airflow Obstruction

Severity	FEV$_1$ (% Predicted)	FEF$_{25\%-75\%}$ (% Predicted)	Pao$_2$ (mm Hg)	Paco$_2$ (mm Hg)
Mild (asymptomatic)	65–80	60–75	>60	<40
Moderate	50–64	45–59	>60	<45
Marked	35–49	30–44	<60	>50
Severe (status asthmaticus)	<35	<30	<60	>50

FEF$_{25\%-75\%}$, forced exhaled flow at 25% to 75% of forced vital capacity; FEV$_1$, forced exhaled volume in 1 second.
Adapted from Kingston HGG, Hirschman CA: Perioperative management of the patient with asthma. Anesth Analg 1984;63:844–855.

of normal. Flow-volume loops show characteristic downward scooping of the expiratory limb of the loop. Flow-volume loops in which the inhaled or exhaled portion of the loop is flat help distinguish wheezing caused by airway obstruction (foreign body, tracheal stenosis, mediastinal tumor) from asthma (**Figs. 9-2** and **9-3**). During moderate to severe asthmatic attacks, the functional residual capacity (FRC) may increase substantially but total lung capacity usually remains within the normal range. Diffusing capacity for carbon monoxide is not changed. Bronchodilator responsiveness can provide supporting evidence when asthma is suspected on clinical grounds. In patients with expiratory airflow obstruction, an increase in airflow after inhalation of a bronchodilator suggests asthma. Abnormalities in pulmonary function tests may persist for several days after an acute asthmatic attack despite the absence of symptoms. Since asthma is an episodic illness, its diagnosis may be suspected even when pulmonary function tests are normal.

Mild asthma is usually accompanied by a normal Pao$_2$ and Paco$_2$. Tachypnea and hyperventilation observed during an acute asthmatic attack do not reflect arterial hypoxemia but rather neural reflexes in the lungs. Hypocarbia and respiratory alkalosis are the most common arterial blood gas findings in the presence of asthma. As the severity of expiratory airflow obstruction increases, the associated ventilation-to-perfusion mismatching may result in a Pao$_2$ less than 60 mm Hg while breathing room air. The Paco$_2$ is likely to increase when the FEV$_1$ is less than 25% of the predicted value. Fatigue of the skeletal muscles necessary for breathing may contribute to the development of hypercarbia.

Chest radiographs may demonstrate hyperinflation of the lungs. They can also be useful in diagnosing pneumonia or congestive heart failure, which may be confused with asthma. The electrocardiogram may show evidence of acute right heart failure and ventricular irritability during an asthmatic attack.

The differential diagnosis of asthma includes viral tracheobronchitis, sarcoidosis, rheumatoid arthritis with bronchiolitis, and extrinsic compression (thoracic aneurysm, mediastinal neoplasm) or intrinsic compression (epiglottitis, croup) of the upper airway. Upper airway obstruction produces a characteristic flow-volume loop (see Fig. 9-3). A history of recent trauma, surgery, or tracheal intubation may be present in patients with upper airway obstruction mimicking asthma. Congestive heart failure and pulmonary embolism may cause dyspnea and wheezing. Wheezing in association with pulmonary edema has been characterized as "cardiac asthma." Improvement after inhaled bronchodilator administration does not exclude cardiac asthma as a cause of wheezing.

Treatment

Historically, treatment of asthma has been directed at preventing and controlling bronchospasm with bronchodilator drugs. However, recognition of the consistent presence of airway inflammation in patients with asthma has resulted in a change in pharmacologic therapy. The emphasis now is on preventing and controlling bronchial inflammation. Bronchodilator therapy does not influence inflammatory changes in the airways and could mask underlying inflammation by relieving symptoms and allowing continued exposure to

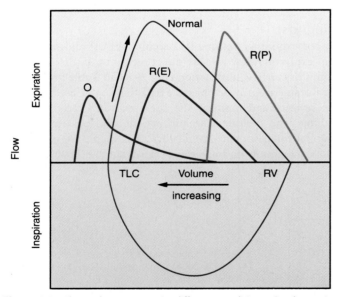

Figure 9-2 • Flow-volume curves in different conditions: O, obstructive disease; R(E), extraparenchymal restrictive disease with limitation in inspiration and expiration; R(P), parenchymal restrictive disease. Forced expiration is plotted in all conditions; forced inspiration is shown only for the normal curve. RV, residual volume; TLC, total lung capacity. By convention, lung volume increases to the left on the abscissa. The *arrow* alongside the normal curve indicates the direction of expiration from TLC to RV. *(Adapted from Weinberger SE: Disturbances of respiratory function. In Fauci B, Braunwald E, Isselbacher KJ, et al [eds]: Harrison's Principles of Internal Medicine, 14th ed. New York, McGraw-Hill, 1998.)*

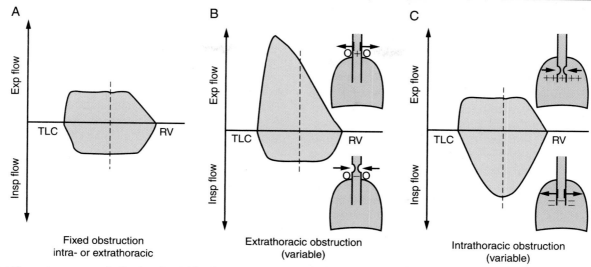

Figure 9-3 • Flow-volume curves in fixed and variable obstruction. **A**, Fixed obstruction, intra- or extrathoracic. **B**, Extrathoracic obstruction (variable). **C**, Intrathoracic obstruction (variable). Exp, expiratory; Insp, inspiratory; RV, residual volume; TLC, total lung capacity. *(Adapted from Benumof J [ed]: Anesthesia for Thoracic Surgery, 2nd ed. Philadelphia, WB Saunders, 1995.)*

allergens. The various drugs used to treat asthma are listed in **Table 9-3**.

Asthma treatment has two components. The first is the use of "controller" treatments, which modify the airway environment such that acute airway narrowing occurs less frequently. Controller treatments include inhaled and systemic corticosteroids, theophylline, and antileukotrienes. The other component of asthma treatment is the use of "reliever" or rescue agents for acute bronchospasm. Reliever treatments include β-adrenergic agonists and anticholinergic drugs.

Serial determination of pulmonary function tests is useful for monitoring the response to treatment. When the FEV_1 returns to approximately 50% of normal, patients usually have minimal or no symptoms. The adequacy of long-term asthma therapy can also be assessed by periodic testing of the degree of airway hyperresponsiveness to exogenous stimuli such as methacholine or histamine, by sputum eosinophil counts, and by the amount of nitric oxide in exhaled air.

Status Asthmaticus

Status asthmaticus is defined as unresolving bronchospasm that, despite treatment, is considered life threatening. Emergency treatment of status asthmaticus consists of repeated administration of $β_2$-agonists by inhalation using a

TABLE 9-3	Pharmacologic Agents Used in the Treatment of Asthma		
Class	**Drug**	**Actions**	**Adverse Effects**
Anti-inflammatory drugs	Corticosteroids: beclomethasone, triamcinolone, flunisolide, fluticasone, budesonide	Decrease airway inflammation, reduce airway hyperresponsiveness	Dysphonia, myopathy of laryngeal muscles, oropharyngeal candidiasis
	Cromolyn	Inhibit mediator release from mast cells, membrane stabilization	
	Leukotriene modifiers: zafirlukast (Accolate), pranlukast (Ultair), montelukast (Singulair), zileuton (Zyflo)	Reduce synthesis of leukotrienes by inhibiting 5-lipoxygenase enzyme	Increased hepatic enzyme levels
Bronchodilators	β-adrenergic agonists: albuterol, metaproterenol, salmeterol	Stimulate $β_2$-receptors of tracheobronchial tree	Tachycardia, tremors, dysrhythmias, hypokalemia
	Anticholinergics: ipratropium, atropine, glycopyrrolate	Decrease vagal tone by blocking muscarinic receptors in airway smooth muscle	
Methylxanthines	Theophylline	Increase cAMP by inhibiting phosphodiesterase, block adenosine receptors, release endogenous catecholamines	Disrupted sleep cycle, nervousness, nausea, vomiting, anorexia, headache, dysrhythmias
cAMP, cyclic adenosine monophosphate.			

metered-dose inhaler or a nebulizer. β_2-Agonists can be administered every 15 to 20 minutes for several doses without significant adverse hemodynamic effects, although patients may experience unpleasant sensations resulting from adrenergic overstimulation. Intravenous corticosteroids are administered early in the treatment because it takes several hours for their effect to appear. The corticosteroids most commonly selected are (1) cortisol (Solu-Cortef) 2 mg/kg IV followed by 0.5 mg/kg per hour by infusion and (2) methylprednisolone (Solu-Medrol) 60 to 125 mg IV every 6 hours. Supplemental oxygen is administered to help maintain arterial oxygen saturation above 90%. Empirical broad-spectrum antibiotic therapy is often initiated. Traditional treatments such as vigorous hydration, inhaled saline mist, mucolytic therapy, and chest physiotherapy have limited benefit.

Measurements of lung function can be very helpful in assessing the severity of status asthmaticus and the response to treatment. Patients whose FEV_1 or peak expiratory flow rate is decreased to 25% of normal or less are at risk of the development of hypercarbia and respiratory failure. The presence of hypercarbia ($Pa_{CO_2} > 50$ mm Hg) despite aggressive anti-inflammatory and bronchodilator therapy is a sign of respiratory fatigue that requires tracheal intubation and mechanical ventilation. The pattern of mechanical ventilation is very important in the patient with status asthmaticus. Because of the bronchoconstriction, high peak airway pressures may be required to deliver acceptable tidal volumes. High gas flows allow for a shorter inspiratory time and a greater time for exhalation. The expiratory phase must be prolonged to allow for complete exhalation and to prevent auto peak end-expiratory pressure (PEEP). To prevent barotrauma, some recommend a degree of permissive hypercarbia. When the FEV_1 or peak expiratory flow rates reach 50% of normal or more, patients usually have minimal or no symptoms. At this point, the frequency and intensity of bronchodilator therapy can be decreased and weaning from mechanical ventilation can ensue.

When patients are resistant to therapy, it is likely that expiratory airflow obstruction is caused predominantly by airway edema and intraluminal secretions. Indeed, patients with status asthmaticus are at risk of asphyxia due to the presence of mucus-plugged airways. In rare circumstances, when life-threatening status asthmaticus persists despite aggressive pharmacologic therapy, it may be necessary to consider general anesthesia to produce bronchodilation. Halothane, enflurane, isoflurane, and sevoflurane have all been described as effective bronchodilators in this situation.

Management of Anesthesia

Advances in understanding the pathogenesis and management of bronchospasm have made anesthesia and the perioperative period much safer for patients with asthma.

Preoperative

Preoperative evaluation of patients with asthma requires an assessment of disease severity and the effectiveness of current pharmacologic management and the potential need for additional therapy prior to surgery. The goal of preoperative evaluation is to formulate an anesthetic plan that prevents or blunts expiratory airflow obstruction.

Preoperative evaluation begins with a clinical history to elicit the severity and characteristics of the patient's asthma (**Table 9-4**). On physical examination, the general appearance of the patient and use of accessory muscles of respiration should be noted. Auscultation of the chest to detect wheezing or crepitations is important. Blood eosinophil counts often parallel the degree of airway inflammation, and airway hyperreactivity provides an indirect assessment of the current status of the disease. Pulmonary function tests (especially FEV_1) before and after bronchodilator therapy may be indicated in patients scheduled for major elective surgery. Chest physiotherapy, antibiotic therapy, and bronchodilator therapy during the preoperative period can often improve reversible components of asthma. Measurement of arterial blood gases is indicated if there is any question about the adequacy of ventilation or oxygenation.

The use of anticholinergic drugs should be individualized, remembering that these drugs can increase the viscosity of airway secretions, making them more difficult to remove from the airway. Furthermore, achievement of a decrease in airway resistance by inhibition of postganglionic cholinergic receptors is unlikely with intramuscular doses of anticholinergic drugs are used for preanesthetic medication.

Anti-inflammatory and bronchodilator therapy should be continued until the time of anesthesia induction. Supplementation with "stress dose" corticosteroids may be indicated before major surgery if hypothalamic-pituitary-adrenal suppression by drugs used to treat asthma is a possibility. However, hypothalamic-pituitary-adrenal suppression is very unlikely with inhaled corticosteroids. In selected patients, a preoperative course of oral corticosteroids may be useful.

Patients should be free of wheezing and have a peak expiratory flow greater than 80% of predicted or at the level of the patient's personal best value prior to surgery.

TABLE 9-4 Characteristics of Asthma to Be Evaluated Preoperatively
Age at onset
Triggering events
Hospitalization for asthma
Frequency of emergency department visits
Need for intubation and mechanical ventilation
Allergies
Cough
Sputum characteristics
Current medications
Anesthetic history

Intraoperative

During induction and maintenance of anesthesia in asthmatic patients, it is necessary to suppress airway reflexes to avoid bronchoconstriction in response to mechanical stimulation of these hyperreactive airways. Stimuli that do not ordinarily evoke airway responses can precipitate life-threatening bronchoconstriction in patients with asthma.

By avoiding instrumentation of the airway and tracheal intubation, regional anesthesia is an attractive option when the operative site is suitable for this. Concerns about high sensory levels of anesthesia leading to sympathetic blockade and consequent bronchospasm are unfounded.

When general anesthesia is selected, induction of anesthesia is most often accomplished with an intravenous induction drug. The incidence of wheezing is higher in asthmatic patients receiving thiopental for induction than in those given propofol. Thiopental itself does not cause bronchospasm, but it may inadequately suppress upper airway reflexes so airway instrumentation may trigger bronchospasm. The mechanism of propofol's relative bronchodilating effect is unknown. Ketamine may produce smooth muscle relaxation and contribute to decreased airway resistance, especially in patients who are actively wheezing.

After unconsciousness is produced, the lungs are often ventilated for a time with a gas mixture containing a volatile anesthetic. The goal is to establish a depth of anesthesia that depresses hyperreactive airway reflexes sufficiently to permit tracheal intubation without precipitating bronchospasm. The lesser pungency of halothane and sevoflurane (compared with isoflurane and desflurane) may make coughing, which can trigger bronchospasm, less likely. An alternative method to suppress airway reflexes prior to intubation is the intravenous or intratracheal injection of lidocaine 1 to 3 minutes before tracheal intubation.

After endotracheal intubation, it may be difficult to differentiate light anesthesia from bronchospasm as the cause of a decrease in pulmonary compliance. Administration of neuromuscular-blocking drugs relieves the difficulty of ventilation due to light anesthesia but has no effect on bronchospasm.

Skeletal muscle relaxation is usually provided with nondepolarizing muscle relaxants. Drugs with limited ability to evoke the release of histamine should be selected. Although histamine release has been attributed to succinylcholine, there is no evidence that this drug is associated with the appearance of increased airway resistance in asthmatic patients.

Theoretically, antagonism of neuromuscular blockade with anticholinesterase drugs could precipitate bronchospasm secondary to stimulation of postganglionic cholinergic receptors in airway smooth muscle. Such bronchospasm does not predictably occur after administration of anticholinesterase drugs, probably because of the protective bronchodilating effects provided by the simultaneous administration of anticholinergic drugs.

Intraoperatively, the desirable level of arterial oxygenation and ventilation are best provided by mechanical ventilation. In asthmatic patients, a slow inspiratory flow rate provides optimal distribution of ventilation relative to perfusion. Sufficient time for exhalation is necessary to prevent air trapping. Humidification and warming of inspired gases may be especially useful in patients with exercise-induced asthma, in whom bronchospasm is presumably due to transmucosal loss of heat. Liberal administration of fluids during the perioperative period is important for maintaining adequate hydration and ensuring the presence of less viscous airway secretions that can be removed more easily.

At the conclusion of surgery, it is prudent to remove the endotracheal tube while anesthesia is still sufficient to suppress hyperreactive airway reflexes. When it is deemed unwise to extubate the trachea before the patient is fully awake, suppressing airway reflexes and/or the risk of bronchospasm by administration of intravenous lidocaine or pretreatment with inhaled bronchodilators should be considered.

Intraoperative Bronchospasm

Intraoperatively, bronchospasm is often due to factors other than asthma (**Table 9-5**). Treatment with bronchodilator drugs should not be instituted until causes of wheezing such as mechanical obstruction to the breathing circuit, the airway, or the endotracheal tube are considered. Bronchospasm due to asthma may respond to deepening the anesthetic with a volatile agent. If bronchospasm persists, then institution of β-agonist therapy should be considered.

If bronchospasm persists despite β$_2$-agonist therapy and deep general anesthesia, corticosteroid administration may be necessary. It must be recognized that several hours may pass before the therapeutic effect of corticosteroids becomes apparent.

Emergency surgery in the asthmatic patient introduces a conflict between protection of the airway in someone at risk of aspiration and the risk of triggering bronchospasm. In addition, there may be insufficient time to optimize bronchodilator therapy prior to surgery. Regional anesthesia may be preferable if the site of surgery is suitable.

TABLE 9–5 Differential Diagnosis of Intraoperative Bronchospasm and Wheezing

Mechanical obstruction of endotracheal tube
  Kinking
  Secretions
  Overinflation of the tracheal tube cuff
Inadequate depth of anesthesia
  Active expiratory efforts
  Decreased functional residual capacity
Endobronchial intubation
Pulmonary aspiration
Pulmonary edema
Pulmonary embolus
Pneumothorax
Acute asthmatic attack

CHRONIC OBSTRUCTIVE PULMONARY DISEASE

COPD is a common condition, mainly related to smoking. The burden of the disease is increasing, and it is projected that by 2020, COPD will rank fifth as the worldwide burden of disease. COPD is characterized by the progressive development of airflow limitation that is not fully reversible. It includes chronic bronchitis with obstruction of small airways and emphysema with enlargement of air sacs, destruction of lung parenchyma, loss of elasticity, and closure of small airways.

The risk factors for development of COPD are (1) cigarette smoking; (2) respiratory infection; (3) occupational exposure to dust especially in coal mining, gold mining, and the textile industry; and (4) genetic factors such as α_1-antitrypsin deficiency.

Signs and Symptoms

Physical findings vary with the severity of COPD, and during the early stages of the disease, the physical examination may be normal. As expiratory airflow obstruction increases in severity, tachypnea and a prolonged expiratory phase are evident. Breath sounds are likely to be decreased and expiratory wheezes are common.

Diagnosis

A chronic productive cough and progressive exercise limitation are the hallmarks of the persistent expiratory airflow obstruction characteristic of COPD (**Tables 9-6** and **9-7**). Although these symptoms are nonspecific, a diagnosis of COPD is likely if the patient is a long-term cigarette smoker. Patients with predominant chronic bronchitis present with a chronic productive cough, whereas patients with predominant emphysema complain of dyspnea. Patients with emphysema experience dyspnea during the activities of daily living when the FEV_1 is less than 40% of normal. Orthopnea is often present in patients with advanced COPD, especially if there are substantial airway secretions. The orthopnea of COPD may be difficult to differentiate from that due to congestive heart failure. Transient periods of sputum discoloration occur in association with respiratory tract infection. Wheezing is common with mucus accumulation in the airways and may mimic asthma. The combination of chronic bronchitis and reversible bronchospasm is referred to as asthmatic bronchitis.

Pulmonary Function Tests

Pulmonary function tests reveal decreases in the FEV_1/forced vital capacity (FVC) ratio and even greater decreases in the forced expiratory flow between 25% and 75% of vital capacity ($FEF_{25\%-75\%}$). Measurement of lung volumes reveals an increased residual volume and normal to increased FRC and TLC (**Fig. 9-4**). Slowing of expiratory airflow and gas trapping behind prematurely closed airways are responsible for the increase in residual volume. The pathophysiologic "advantage" of an increased residual volume and FRC in patients with COPD is an enlarged airway diameter and increased elastic recoil for exhalation. The cost is the greater work of breathing at the higher lung volumes.

Chest Radiography

Radiographic abnormalities may be minimal, even in the presence of severe COPD. Hyperlucency due to arterial vascular deficiency in the lung periphery and hyperinflation (flattening of the diaphragm with loss of its normal domed appearance and a very vertical cardiac silhouette) suggest the diagnosis of emphysema. If bullae are present, the diagnosis of emphysema is certain. However, only a small percentage of patients with emphysema have bullae. Computed tomography of the chest can also be useful for diagnosing emphysema. Chronic bronchitis is rarely diagnosed by chest radiography.

Arterial Blood Gases

Arterial blood gases can be used to categorize patients with COPD as "pink puffers" (Pao_2 usually higher than 60 mm Hg and $Paco_2$ normal) or "blue bloaters" (Pao_2 usually less than 60 mm Hg and $Paco_2$ chronically increased to more than 45 mm Hg). Individuals characterized as pink puffers are

TABLE 9–6 Comparative Features of Chronic Obstructive Pulmonary Disease		
Feature	**Chronic Bronchitis**	**Pulmonary Emphysema**
Mechanism of airway obstruction	Decreased airway lumen due to mucus and inflammation	Loss of elastic recoil
Dyspnea	Moderate	Severe
FEV_1	Decreased	Decreased
Pao_2	Marked decrease ("blue bloater")	Modest decrease ("pink puffer")
$Paco_2$	Increased	Normal to decreased
Diffusing capacity	Normal	Decreased
Hematocrit	Increased	Normal
Cor pulmonale	Marked	Mild
Prognosis	Poor	Good
FEV_1, forced expiratory volume in 1 second.		

TABLE 9-7 Spirometric Classification of the Severity of COPD Based on Postbronchodilator FEV$_1$ Measurements.

Stage	Characteristics
0: At risk	Normal spirometry Chronic symptoms (cough, sputum production)
I: Mild COPD	FEV$_1$/FVC < 70% FEV$_1$ ≥ 80% predicted, with or without chronic symptoms (cough, sputum production)
II: Moderate COPD	FEV$_1$/FVC < 70% 50% ≤ FEV$_1$, <80% predicted, with or without chronic symptoms (cough, sputum production)
III: Severe COPD	FEV$_1$/FVC < 70% 30% ≤ FEV$_1$, <50% predicted, with or without chronic symptoms (cough, sputum production)
IV: Very severe COPD	FEV$_1$/FVC < 70% FEV$_1$ < 30% predicted or FEV$_1$ < 50% predicted plus chronic respiratory failure, i.e., Pa$_{O_2}$ < 60 mm Hg and/or Pc$_{O_2}$ > 50 mm Hg

COPD, chronic obstructive pulmonary disease; FEV$_1$, forced expiratory volume in 1 second; FVC, forced vital capacity.
Adapted from the Global Initiative for Chronic Obstructive Lung Disease: Global strategy for the diagnosis, management and prevention of COPD: Update 2005. At www.goldcopd.com

typically thin and free of signs of right heart failure and have severe emphysema. Blue bloaters typically exhibit cough and sputum production, frequent respiratory tract infection, and recurrent episodes of cor pulmonale. These patients may have some pathologic changes consistent with emphysema but more often meet the criteria for chronic bronchitis.

The consequences of these two arterial blood gas patterns on the cardiovascular system differ. Blue bloaters develop pulmonary hypertension because arterial hypoxemia and respiratory acidosis evoke pulmonary vascular vasoconstriction. They also develop secondary erythrocytosis due to the hypoxemia. Chronic pulmonary hypertension may produce right ventricular hypertrophy and cor pulmonale. Right ventricular failure results in systemic venous congestion, jugular venous distention, peripheral edema, hepatic congestion, and, occasionally, ascites.

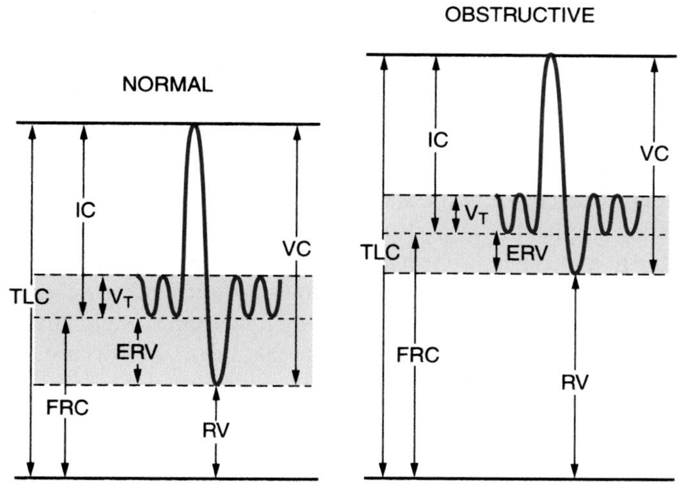

Pink puffers have emphysematous lung destruction with loss of pulmonary capillaries and destroyed alveolar walls. This loss of the pulmonary capillary vascular bed can be measured as a decreased diffusing capacity. Pa$_{O_2}$ is typically only mildly depressed, so pulmonary vasoconstriction is minimal and secondary erythrocytosis does not occur.

Treatment

Treatment of COPD is designed to relieve existing symptoms and slow the progression of the disease.

Cessation of Smoking and Supplemental Oxygen Administration

Smoking cessation and chronic oxygen administration are the only two therapeutic interventions that favorably alter the natural progression of COPD. Smoking cessation causes the symptoms of chronic bronchitis to diminish or entirely disappear, and it eliminates the accelerated loss of lung function observed in those who continue to smoke. Chronic oxygen administration (home oxygen therapy) is recommended if the Pa$_{O_2}$ is less than 55 mm Hg, the hematocrit is more than 55%, or there is evidence of cor pulmonale. The goal of supplemental oxygen administration is to achieve a Pa$_{O_2}$ between 60 and 80 mm Hg. This goal can usually be accomplished by delivering oxygen through a nasal cannula at 2 L/min. Ultimately, the flow rate for oxygen is titrated as needed according to arterial blood gas measurements. Relief of arterial hypoxemia with supplemental oxygen administration is more effective than any known drug therapy in decreasing pulmonary vascular resistance and preventing excessive erythrocytosis.

Drug Therapy

Bronchodilators are the mainstay of current drug therapy for COPD. Bronchodilators cause only a small increase in FEV$_1$ but may alleviate symptoms by decreasing hyperinflation

Figure 9-4 • Lung volumes in chronic obstructive pulmonary disease compared with normal values. In the presence of obstructive lung disease, the vital capacity (VC) is normal to decreased, the residual volume (RV) and functional residual capacity (FRC) are increased, the TLC (total lung capacity) is normal to increased, and the RV/TLC ratio is increased. ERV, expiratory reserve volume; IC, inspiratory capacity; V$_T$, tidal volume.

and dyspnea. They may thus improve exercise tolerance, despite the fact that there is little improvement in spirometric measurements. An additional benefit of β_2-agonists may be fewer infections since these drugs decrease the adhesion of bacteria such as *Haemophilus influenzae* to airway epithelial cells. COPD is often more effectively treated by anticholinergic drugs than by β_2-agonists. This is in contrast to asthma in which β_2-agonists are usually more effective. Inhaled corticosteroids are widely prescribed for COPD. Intermittent broad-spectrum antibiotic (ampicillin, cephalosporins, erythromycin) administration is indicated for acute episodes of increased dyspnea associated with excessive or purulent sputum production. Annual vaccination against influenza is beneficial. Pneumococcal vaccine is also recommended. Exacerbations of COPD may be due to viral infection of the upper respiratory tract or may be noninfective so antibiotic treatment is not always warranted. Diuretic therapy may be considered for patients with cor pulmonale and right ventricular failure with peripheral edema. Diuretic-induced chloride depletion may produce a hypochloremic metabolic alkalosis that depresses the ventilatory drive and may aggravate chronic carbon dioxide retention. Physical training programs can increase the exercise capacity of patients with COPD despite the absence of detectable effects on the FEV_1. However, prompt deconditioning occurs when the exercise program is abandoned.

Lung Volume Reduction Surgery

Lung volume reduction surgery may be considered in selected patients with emphysema who have regions of overdistended, poorly functioning lung tissue. Surgical removal of these overdistended areas allows more normal areas of the lung to expand and improves not only lung function but quality of life.

Management of anesthesia for lung volume reduction surgery includes use of a double-lumen endobronchial tube to permit lung separation, avoidance of nitrous oxide, and avoidance of excessive positive airway pressure. Monitoring central venous pressure as a guide to fluid management in this situation is not likely to be reliable.

Management of Anesthesia
Preoperative

The history and physical examination of patients with COPD provide a more accurate assessment of the likelihood of postoperative pulmonary complications than pulmonary function tests or measurement of arterial blood gases. A history of poor exercise tolerance, chronic cough, or unexplained dyspnea combined with diminished breath sounds, wheezing, and a prolonged expiratory phase predict an increased risk of postoperative pulmonary complications. Preoperative preparation of patients with COPD includes smoking cessation, treatment of bronchospasm, and eradication of bacterial infection.

Preoperative Pulmonary Function Testing The value of routine preoperative pulmonary function testing remains controversial. The results of pulmonary function tests and arterial blood gases can be useful for predicting pulmonary function following lung resection, but they do not reliably predict the likelihood of postoperative pulmonary complications after nonthoracic surgery. Clinical findings (smoking, diffuse wheezing, productive cough) are more predictive of pulmonary complications than spirometric results. Patients with mild pulmonary disease undergoing peripheral surgery do not require pulmonary function tests. If in doubt, simple spirometry with measurement of FEV_1 is sufficient.

Even patients defined as high risk by spirometry ($FEV_1 < 70\%$ of predicted, FEV_1/FVC ratio $< 65\%$) or arterial blood gases ($PaCO_2 > 45$ mm Hg) can undergo surgery including lung resection with an acceptable risk of postoperative pulmonary complications. These pulmonary function tests should be viewed as a management tool to optimize preoperative pulmonary function but not as a means to predict risk. Indications for a preoperative pulmonary evaluation (which may include consultation with a pulmonologist and/or pulmonary function tests) typically include (1) hypoxemia on room air or the need for home oxygen therapy without a known etiology, (2) bicarbonate more than 33 mEq/L or PCO_2 more than 50 mm Hg in a patient whose pulmonary disease has not been previously evaluated, (3) a history of respiratory failure due to a problem that still exists, (4) severe shortness of breath attributed to respiratory disease, (5) planned pneumonectomy, (6) difficulty assessing pulmonary function by clinical signs, (7) distinguishing among potential etiologies of significant respiratory compromise, (8) determining the response to bronchodilators, and (9) suspected pulmonary hypertension.

Right ventricular function should be carefully assessed by clinical examination and echocardiography in patients with advanced pulmonary disease.

Flow Volume Loops Ventilatory function is measured under static conditions for measurement of lung volumes and under dynamic conditions for measurement of flow rates. In assessing lung function, expiratory flow rates can be plotted against lung volumes to produce flow-volume curves. When flow rates during inspiration are added to these curves, flow-volume loops are obtained. The flow rate is zero at total lung capacity before the start of expiration. Once forced expiration begins, the peak flow rate is achieved rapidly and then falls in a linear fashion as the lung volume decreases to residual volume. During maximal inspiration from residual volume to total lung capacity, the inspiratory flow is most rapid at the midpoint of inspiration, making the inspiratory curve U shaped.

In patients with COPD, there is a decrease in the expiratory flow rate at any given lung volume. The expiratory curve is concave upward due to uniform emptying of the airways. The residual volume is increased due to air trapping. In patients with restrictive lung disease, there is a decrease in all lung volumes (see Fig. 9-2).

Fixed lesions of the upper airway, which include tracheal stenosis and goiters, produce plateaus in both the inspiratory

TABLE 9–8 Risk-Reduction Strategies to Decrease the Incidence of Postoperative Pulmonary Complications

Preoperative
Encourage cessation of smoking for at least 6 weeks
Treat evidence of expiratory airflow obstruction
Treat respiratory infection with antibiotics
Initiate patient education regarding lung volume expansion maneuvers

Intraoperative
Use minimally invasive surgery (endoscopic) techniques when possible
Consider use of regional anesthesia
Avoid surgical procedures likely to require more than 3 hours

Postoperative
Institute lung volume expansion maneuvers (voluntary deep breathing, incentive spirometry, continuous positive airway pressure)
Maximize analgesia (neuraxial opioids, intercostal nerve blocks, patient-controlled analgesia)

Adapted from Smetana GW: Preoperative pulmonary evaluation. N Engl J Med 1999;340:937–944, copyright 1999 Massachusetts Medical Society.

and expiratory cycles of the flow-volume loop (see Fig. 9-3A). Variable extrathoracic obstruction is typically a result of vocal cord paralysis and causes a plateau in the inspiratory limb (see Fig. 9-3B). Variable intrathoracic obstruction caused by endobronchial tumors causes a plateau in the expiratory limb of the flow volume loop (see Fig. 9-3C).

Risk Reduction Strategies

Strategies to decrease the incidence of postoperative pulmonary complications include preoperative, intraoperative, and postoperative interventions (**Table 9-8**).

Smoking Cessation and Pulmonary Complications Approximately 20% of American adults smoke. Cigarette smoking is the single most important risk factor for development of COPD and death due to lung disease. The effects of smoking on different organ systems are shown in **Table 9-9**. Smoking cessation is strongly encouraged by the U.S. Public Health Service (http://www.surgeongeneral.gov/tobacco). They recommend systematically identifying all tobacco users who come in contact with the health care system to urge and help them to quit smoking.

Among smokers, predictive factors for the development of pulmonary complications are a lower DLCO than predicted and a smoking history of more than 60 pack-years. Those who have smoked more than 60 pack-years have double the risk of

any pulmonary complication and triple the risk of pneumonia compared to those who have smoked less than 60 pack-years. Smoking cessation causes the symptoms of chronic bronchitis to diminish or disappear and eliminates the accelerated loss of lung function observed in those who continue to smoke.

Acute Effects of Smoking Cessation The adverse effects of carbon monoxide on oxygen-carrying capacity and of nicotine on the cardiovascular system are short-lived. The elimination half-life of carbon monoxide is approximately 4 to 6 hours when breathing room air. Within 12 hours after cessation of smoking the Pao_2 at which hemoglobin is 50% saturated with oxygen (P_{50}) increases from 22.9 to 26.4 mm Hg, and the plasma levels of carboxyhemoglobin decrease from 6.5% to approximately 1%. Carbon monoxide may have negative inotropic effects. Despite the favorable effects on plasma carboxyhemoglobin concentration, short-term abstinence from cigarettes has not been proven to decrease the incidence of postoperative pulmonary complications. The sympathomimetic effects of nicotine on the heart are transient, lasting only 20 to 30 minutes.

Cigarette smoking causes mucus hypersecretion, impairment of mucociliary transport, and narrowing of small airways. In contrast to the favorable effect of short-term abstinence from smoking on carboxyhemoglobin concentrations, improved ciliary and small airway function and decreased sputum

TABLE 9–9 Effects of Smoking on Different Organ Systems

Cardiac Effects of Smoking
1. Smoking is a risk factor for development of cardiovascular disease
2. Carbon monoxide decreases oxygen delivery and increases myocardial work
3. Smoking releases catecholamines and causes coronary vasoconstriction
4. Smoking decreases exercise capacity

Respiratory Effects of Smoking
1. Smoking is the major risk factor for development of chronic pulmonary disease
2. Smoking decreases mucociliary activity
3. Smoking results in hyperreactive airways
4. Smoking decreases pulmonary immune function

Other Organ System Effects
1. Smoking impairs wound healing

production occur slowly over a period of weeks after smoking cessation. Cigarette smoking may interfere with normal immune responses and could interfere with the ability of smokers to respond to pulmonary infection following anesthesia and surgery. Return of normal immune function requires at least 6 weeks of abstinence from smoking. Some components of cigarette smoke stimulate hepatic enzymes. As with immune responses, it likely takes 6 weeks for hepatic enzyme activity to return to normal following cessation of smoking.

Despite the clear advantages of long-term smoking cessation, there can be disadvantages to smoking cessation in the immediate preoperative period. These include an increase in sputum production, a fear of inability to handle stress by the patient, nicotine withdrawal symptoms including irritability, restlessness, sleep disturbances, and depression.

Countless methods have been devised to aid in smoking cessation. Most involve some form of counseling and pharmacotherapy. Nicotine replacement therapy with various delivery systems including patches, inhalers, nasal sprays, lozenges, and gum is generally well tolerated. The major side effect is local irritation at the site of drug delivery. The atypical antidepressant bupropion (Wellbutrin) in a sustained-release formulation can also aid in smoking cessation. The drug is typically started 1 to 2 weeks before smoking is stopped.

Smoking cessation prior to surgery is widely encouraged. A decrease in postoperative pulmonary complications due to smoking cessation is thought to be related to physiologic improvement in ciliary action, macrophage activity, and small airway function, as well as a decrease in sputum production. However, these changes take weeks to months to occur.

Intraoperative

Regional anesthesia is suitable for operations that do not invade the peritoneum and for surgical procedures performed on the extremities. Lower intraabdominal surgery can also be performed using a regional technique. General anesthesia is the usual choice for upper abdominal and intrathoracic surgery. The choice of anesthetic technique or specific anesthetic drugs does not seem to alter the incidence of postoperative pulmonary complications. Studies in patients with COPD suggest that there is a higher incidence of postoperative respiratory failure in patients who have general anesthesia, but whether this reflects the nature or complexity of the surgery and/or the operative site or the selection of anesthetic drugs or technique is unclear. Whether there is a relationship between the duration of anesthesia and the incidence of postoperative pulmonary complications is controversial. Some suggest that operations lasting longer than 3 hours are more likely to be associated with postoperative pulmonary complications.

COPD patients are susceptible to development of acute respiratory failure during the postoperative period. Continued tracheal intubation and mechanical ventilation may be necessary, particularly after upper abdominal or intrathoracic surgery. Alternatively, postoperative analgesia with neuraxial opioids that permits pain-free breathing may permit earlier tracheal extubation.

Regional Anesthesia Regional anesthesia via peripheral nerve block such as an axillary block carries a lower risk of pulmonary complications than either spinal or general anesthesia. Regional anesthesia is a useful choice in patients with COPD only if large doses of sedative and anxiolytic drugs will not be needed. It must be appreciated that COPD patients can be extremely sensitive to the ventilatory depressant effects of sedative drugs. Elderly patients may be especially susceptible to this depression of ventilation. Often small doses of a benzodiazepine, such as midazolam, in increments of 1 to 2 mg IV, can be administered without producing undesirable degrees of ventilatory depression. Regional anesthetic techniques that produce sensory anesthesia above T6 are not recommended because such high blocks can impair the ventilatory functions requiring active exhalation such as expiratory reserve volume, peak expiratory flow, and maximum minute ventilation. Clinically, this is manifested as a cough that is inadequate to clear airway secretions.

General Anesthesia General anesthesia is often provided with volatile anesthetics. Volatile anesthetics are useful because of the ability of these drugs (especially desflurane and sevoflurane) to be rapidly eliminated through the lungs. Residual ventilatory depression during the early postoperative period is thereby minimized. Furthermore, volatile anesthetics produce bronchodilation.

Nitrous oxide is frequently administered in combination with a volatile anesthetic. When using nitrous oxide, there is the potential for passage of this gas into pulmonary bullae. This could lead to enlargement or even rupture of the bullae resulting in development of a tension pneumothorax. Another potential disadvantage of nitrous oxide is the limitation on the inspired oxygen concentration that it imposes. It is important to remember that inhaled anesthetics may attenuate regional hypoxic pulmonary vasoconstriction and produce more intrapulmonary shunting. Increasing F_{IO_2} may be necessary to offset this loss of hypoxic pulmonary vasoconstriction.

Opioids may be less useful than inhaled anesthetics for maintenance of anesthesia in patients with COPD because they can be associated with prolonged ventilatory depression as a result of their slow rate of metabolism or elimination. Even the duration of ventilatory depression produced by drugs such as thiopental and midazolam may be prolonged in patients with COPD compared to normal individuals. A high inspired concentration of nitrous oxide may be necessary to ensure amnesia when opioids are used for maintenance of anesthesia. This may be difficult to achieve if a high F_{IO_2} is also needed.

An endotracheal tube bypasses nearly the entire natural airway humidification system so humidification of inspired gases and use of low gas flows will be needed to keep airway secretions moist.

Controlled mechanical ventilation is useful for optimizing oxygenation in patients with COPD who are undergoing operations requiring general anesthesia. Large tidal volumes (10–15 mL/kg) combined with slow inspiratory flow rates minimize the likelihood of turbulent airflow and help maintain optimal ventilation-to-perfusion matching. Slow respiratory rates (6 to 10 breaths per minute) provide sufficient time for complete exhalation to occur, which is particularly important if air trapping is to be minimized. They also allow sufficient time for venous return and are less likely to be associated with undesirable degrees of hyperventilation. The hazard of pulmonary barotrauma in the presence of bullae should be appreciated, particularly when high positive airway pressures are required to provide adequate ventilation. The intraoperative use of large tidal volumes and slow respiratory rates can be as efficacious as PEEP in maintaining arterial oxygenation. The detrimental cardiovascular effects of PEEP and the detrimental effects of PEEP on expiratory airflow can thereby be avoided.

If spontaneous breathing is permitted during anesthesia in patients with COPD, it should be appreciated that the ventilatory depression produced by volatile anesthetics may be greater in these patients than in normal individuals.

Postoperative

Prophylaxis against the development of postoperative pulmonary complications is based on maintaining adequate lung volumes especially FRC and facilitating an effective cough. Identification of the FRC as the most important lung volume during the postoperative period provides a specific goal for therapy.

Lung Expansion Maneuvers Lung expansion maneuvers (deep breathing exercises, incentive spirometry, chest physiotherapy, positive-pressure breathing techniques) are of proven benefit for preventing postoperative pulmonary complications in high-risk patients. These techniques decrease the risk of atelectasis by increasing lung volumes. All regimens seem to be efficacious in decreasing the frequency of postoperative pulmonary complications (approximately twofold compared to no therapy). Incentive spirometry is simple and inexpensive and provides objective goals for and monitoring of patient performance. Patients are given a particular inspired volume as a goal to achieve and hold. This provides sustained lung inflation, which is important for reexpanding collapsed alveoli. The major disadvantage of incentive spirometry is the need for patient cooperation to accomplish the treatment. Preoperative education in lung expansion maneuvers decreases the incidence of pulmonary complications to a greater degree than if education begins after surgery, but there is no evidence that instituting lung expansion maneuvers preoperatively is of value.

Intermittent positive-pressure breathing can decrease the incidence of postoperative pulmonary complications, but its cost and complexity have resulted in a decline in its use. Continuous positive airway pressure is reserved for the prevention of postoperative pulmonary complications in patients who are not able to perform deep-breathing exercises or incentive spirometry. Nasal positive airway pressure can minimize the expected decrease in lung volumes after surgery but less costly lung expansion maneuvers are available.

Postoperative neuraxial analgesia with opioids may permit early tracheal extubation. The sympathetic blockade, muscle weakness, and loss of proprioception that are produced by local anesthetics are not produced by neuraxial opioids. Therefore, early ambulation is possible. Ambulation serves to increase FRC and improve oxygenation, presumably by improving ventilation-to-perfusion matching. Neuraxial opioids may be especially useful after intrathoracic and upper abdominal surgery. Breakthrough pain may require treatment with systemic opioids administered by bolus or via patient-controlled analgesia. Sedation may accompany neuraxial opioid administration and delayed respiratory depression can be seen, especially when poorly lipid-soluble opioids such as morphine have been used.

The quality of neuraxial analgesia (epidural or spinal) may be superior to that provided by parenteral administration of opioids, but it has not been possible to document that neuraxial analgesia decreases the incidence of clinically significant postoperative pulmonary complications or is superior to parenteral opioids in this regard. Postoperative neuraxial analgesia is recommended after high-risk thoracic, abdominal, and major vascular surgery. Intermittent or continuous intercostal nerve blocks may be an alternative if neuraxial analgesia is ineffective or technically difficult.

Mechanical Ventilation Continued mechanical ventilation during the immediate postoperative period may be necessary in patients with severe COPD who have undergone major abdominal or intrathoracic surgery. Patients with preoperative FEV_1/FVC ratios less than 0.5 or with a preoperative Pa_{CO_2} of more than 50 mm Hg are likely to need some postoperative mechanical ventilation. If the Pa_{CO_2} has been chronically increased, it is important not to correct the hypercarbia too quickly because this will result in a metabolic alkalosis that can be associated with cardiac dysrhythmias and central nervous system irritability and even seizures.

When continued mechanical ventilation is necessary, F_{IO_2} and ventilator settings should be adjusted to maintain the Pa_{O_2} between 60 and 100 mm Hg and the Pa_{CO_2} in a range that maintains the pHa at 7.35 to 7.45. The decision to discontinue mechanical support of ventilation and to perform tracheal extubation is based on the patient's clinical status and indices of pulmonary function.

Chest Physiotherapy A combination of chest physiotherapy and postural drainage plus deep-breathing exercises taught during the preoperative period may decrease the incidence of postoperative pulmonary complications. Presumably, vibrations produced on the chest wall by physiotherapy result in dislodgment of mucus plugs from peripheral airways. Appropriate positioning facilitates elimination of loosened mucus.

CHRONIC OBSTRUCTIVE PULMONARY DISEASE AND ACUTE RESPIRATORY FAILURE

Patients with severe COPD often adapt to some degree of arterial hypoxemia and hypercarbia. Acute deterioration in lung function is most often triggered by events such as pneumonia, congestive heart failure, and increased metabolic production of carbon dioxide as produced by febrile states. The increasing hypoxemia and hypercarbia that accompany these exacerbations of COPD lead to increasing dyspnea and alterations in consciousness that may be associated with retention of secretions and a further deterioration in gas exchange. The vicious cycle can be interrupted by treating the event that initiated the acute deterioration and providing support to improve gas exchange until the underlying precipitating event has resolved.

Treatment

Analysis of arterial blood gases is crucial for proper treatment of acute exacerbations of COPD. Supplemental oxygen is administered to maintain the Pao_2 above 60 mm Hg. Mild hypercarbia is common when oxygen is administered to patients with COPD and is acceptable as long as the pHa does not decrease below 7.2. Bronchopulmonary drainage is stimulated by encouragement to cough, administration of inhaled bronchodilators and systemic corticosteroids, and treatment of underlying infection with antibiotics. Acute exacerbations of COPD are often accompanied by persistent respiratory acidosis and excessive work of breathing.

Mechanical support of ventilation is necessary when hypercarbia is severe enough to decrease the pHa below 7.2 and when patients show signs of mental status deterioration or respiratory muscle fatigue. Tracheal intubation must be performed when there is hemodynamic instability or somnolence or secretions cannot be cleared. For patients who remain alert despite hypercarbia, delivery of positive-pressure ventilation via a tight-fitting face mask (noninvasive ventilation) is an alternative to tracheal intubation. The most common method of noninvasive ventilation delivers a specified amount of inspiratory pressure (15–20 cm H_2O) combined with a low level of expiratory pressure (3–5 cm H_2O) to decrease the effort required to trigger the ventilator.

Advantages of noninvasive ventilation include a lower risk of nosocomial infection, shorter length of intensive care unit stay, decreased need for sedation, and decreased mortality. A complication of noninvasive ventilation with a face mask is skin necrosis over the bridge of the nose.

When tracheal intubation is required to treat acute exacerbations of COPD, the initial ventilator settings should include a large tidal volume and slow breathing rate. Patients with chronic hypercarbia should not have their $Paco_2$ decreased abruptly to normal because this can result in respiratory alkalosis and cardiac dysrhythmias. The ventilator should be adjusted to return the $Paco_2$ to the previous baseline level to avoid development of severe hyperinflation and significant auto-PEEP, which increases the risk of barotrauma, leads to erroneous interpretation of measurements from central venous and pulmonary artery catheters, increases the work of breathing, and interferes with venous return.

Risk Factors for Postoperative Pulmonary Complications

The major risk factors for the development of postoperative pulmonary complications are shown in **Table 9-10**. Obesity and mild to moderate asthma have not been shown to be independent risk factors. An algorithm for reducing pulmonary complications in patients undergoing noncardiothoracic surgery is shown in **Figure 9-5**.

LESS COMMON CAUSES OF EXPIRATORY AIRFLOW OBSTRUCTION

Causes of expiratory airflow obstruction occurring less often than chronic bronchitis and emphysema include bronchiectasis, cystic fibrosis, bronchiolitis obliterans, and tracheal stenosis.

TABLE 9–10	Major Risk Factors Associated with Postoperative Pulmonary Complications

Patient Related
1. Age > 60 years
2. ASA class > II
3. Congestive heart failure
4. Preexisting pulmonary disease (COPD)
5. Functionally dependent
6. Cigarette smoking

Procedure Related
1. Emergency surgery
2. Abdominal, thoracic surgery, head and neck surgery, neurosurgery, vascular/aortic aneurysm surgery
3. Prolonged duration of anesthesia (>2.5 hours)
4. General anesthesia

Test Predictors
1. Albumin level < 3.5 g/dL

ASA, American Society of Anesthesiologists; COPD, chronic obstructive pulmonary disease.
Adapted from Smetana GW, Lawrence VA, Cornell JE: Preoperative pulmonary risk stratification for noncardiothoracic surgery. A systematic review for the American College of Physicians. Ann Intern Med 2006;144:581–595.

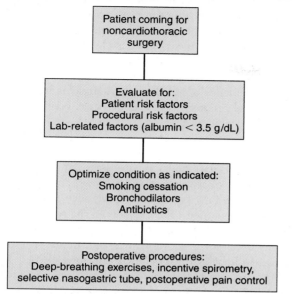

Figure 9-5 • Algorithm for decreasing pulmonary complications in patients undergoing noncardiothoracic surgery. *(Adapted from Qaseem A, Snow V, Fitterman N, et al: Risk assessment for and strategies to reduce perioperative pulmonary complications for patients undergoing noncardiothoracic surgery: A guideline from the American College of Physicians. Ann Intern Med 2006;144:575–580.)*

Bronchiectasis

Bronchiectasis is a chronic suppurative disease of the airways that, if sufficiently widespread, may cause expiratory airflow obstruction similar to that seen with COPD. Despite the availability of antibiotics, bronchiectasis is an important cause of chronic productive cough with purulent sputum and accounts for a significant number of patients who develop massive hemoptysis.

Pathophysiology

Bronchiectasis is characterized by a localized, irreversible dilation of a bronchus caused by destructive inflammatory processes involving the bronchial wall. Bacterial or mycobacterial infections are presumed to be responsible for most cases of bronchiectasis. The most important consequence of bronchiectatic destruction of airways is an increased susceptibility to recurrent or persistent bacterial infection, reflecting impaired mucociliary activity and pooling of mucus in dilated airways. Once bacterial superinfection is established, it is nearly impossible to eradicate and daily expectoration of purulent sputum persists.

Diagnosis

The history of a chronic cough productive of purulent sputum is highly suggestive of bronchiectasis. Digital clubbing occurs in most patients with significant bronchiectasis and is a valuable diagnostic clue, especially since this change is not characteristic of COPD. Pulmonary function changes vary considerably and range from no change to alterations characteristic of COPD or restrictive lung disease. Computed tomography provides excellent images of bronchiectatic airways and can be used to confirm the presence and extent of the disease.

Treatment

Bronchiectasis is treated by administration of antibiotics and postural drainage. Periodic sputum culture guides antibiotic selection. Pseudomonas is the most common organism cultured. Hemoptysis can be controlled with appropriate antibiotic therapy. However, massive hemoptysis (>200 mL over a 24-hour period) may require surgical resection of the involved lung or selective bronchial arterial embolization. Postural drainage is useful to assist in expectoration of secretions that pool distal to the diseased airways. Chest physiotherapy with chest percussion and vibration is another aid for bronchopulmonary drainage. Surgical resection has played a declining role in the management of bronchiectasis during the modern antibiotic era and is only considered in the rare instance when severe symptoms persist or recurrent complications occur.

Management of Anesthesia

Prior to elective surgery, the pulmonary status of patients with bronchiectasis is optimized by antibiotic therapy and postural drainage. Airway management might include use of a double-lumen endobronchial tube to prevent spillage of purulent sputum into normal areas of the lungs. Instrumentation of the nares should be avoided because of the high incidence of chronic sinusitis in these patients.

Cystic Fibrosis

Cystic fibrosis is the most common life-shortening autosomal recessive disorder. It affects an estimated 30,000 persons in the United States.

Pathophysiology

The cause of cystic fibrosis is a mutation in a single gene on chromosome 7 that encodes the cystic fibrosis transmembrane conductance regulator. The result of this mutation is defective chloride ion transport in epithelial cells in the lungs, pancreas, liver, gastrointestinal tract, and reproductive organs. Decreased chloride transport is accompanied by decreased transport of sodium and water, resulting in dehydrated, viscous secretions that are associated with luminal obstruction as well as destruction and scarring of various exocrine glands. Pancreatic insufficiency, meconium ileus at birth, diabetes mellitus, obstructive hepatobiliary tract disease, and azoospermia are often present but the primary cause of morbidity and mortality in patients with cystic fibrosis is chronic pulmonary infection.

Diagnosis

The presence of a sweat chloride concentration higher than 80 mEq/L plus the characteristic clinical manifestations (cough, chronic purulent sputum production, exertional dyspnea) or a family history of the disease confirm the diagnosis of cystic

175

fibrosis. Chronic pansinusitis is almost universal. The presence of normal sinuses on radiographic examination is strong evidence that cystic fibrosis is not present. Malabsorption with a response to pancreatic enzyme treatment is evidence of the exocrine insufficiency associated with cystic fibrosis. Obstructive azoospermia confirmed by testicular biopsy is also strong evidence of cystic fibrosis. Bronchoalveolar lavage typically shows a high percentage of neutrophils, a sign of airway inflammation. COPD is present in virtually all adult patients with cystic fibrosis and follows a relentless course.

Treatment

Treatment of cystic fibrosis is similar to that for bronchiectasis and is directed toward alleviation of symptoms (mobilization and clearance of lower airway secretions and treatment of pulmonary infection) and correction of organ dysfunction (pancreatic enzyme replacement).

Clearance of Airway Secretions The abnormal viscoelastic properties of the sputum in patients with cystic fibrosis lead to sputum retention, resulting in airway obstruction. The principal nonpharmacologic approach to enhancing clearance of pulmonary secretions is chest physiotherapy with postural drainage. High-frequency chest compression with an inflatable vest and airway oscillation with a flutter valve may provide alternative methods to physiotherapy that are less time-consuming and do not require trained personnel.

Bronchodilator Therapy Bronchial reactivity to histamine and other provocative stimuli is greater in patients with cystic fibrosis than in normal subjects. Bronchodilator therapy is considered if patients have an increase of 10% or more in FEV_1 in response to an inhaled bronchodilator.

Reduction in Viscoelasticity of Sputum The abnormal viscosity of airway secretions is primarily due to the presence of neutrophils and their degradation products. DNA released from neutrophils forms long fibrils that contribute to the viscosity of the sputum. Recombinant human deoxyribonuclease I can cleave this DNA and increase the clearance of sputum in these patients.

Antibiotic Therapy Patients with cystic fibrosis have periodic exacerbations of pulmonary infection that are identified primarily based on an increase in symptoms and in sputum production. Antibiotic therapy is based on identification and susceptibility testing of bacteria isolated from the sputum. In patients in whom cultures yield no pathogens, bronchoscopy to remove lower airway secretions may be indicated. Many patients with cystic fibrosis are given long-term maintenance antibiotic therapy in the hope of suppressing chronic infection and the development of bronchiectasis.

Management of Anesthesia Management of anesthesia in patients with cystic fibrosis invokes the same principles as outlined for patients with COPD and bronchiectasis. Elective surgical procedures should be delayed until optimal pulmonary function can be ensured by controlling bronchial infection and facilitating removal of airway secretions. Vitamin K treatment may be necessary if hepatic function is poor or if absorption of fat-soluble vitamins from the gastrointestinal

tract is impaired. Maintenance of anesthesia with volatile anesthetics permits the use of high inspired concentrations of oxygen, decreases airway resistance by decreasing bronchial smooth muscle tone, and decreases the responsiveness of hyperreactive airways. Humidification of inspired gases, hydration, and avoidance of anticholinergic drugs is important for maintaining secretions in a less viscous state. Frequent tracheal suctioning may be necessary.

Primary Ciliary Dyskinesia

Primary ciliary dyskinesia is characterized by congenital impairment of ciliary activity in respiratory tract epithelial cells and sperm tails (spermatozoa are alive but immobile). As a result of impaired ciliary activity in the respiratory tract, chronic sinusitis, recurrent respiratory infections, and bronchiectasis develop. In addition to male infertility, fertility is decreased in females since oviducts also have ciliated epithelium. The triad of chronic sinusitis, bronchiectasis and situs inversus is known as Kartagener's syndrome. It is speculated that the normal asymmetrical positioning of body organs is dependent on normal ciliary function of the embryonic epithelium. In the absence of normal ciliary function, placement of organs to the left or the right is random. As expected, approximately one half of patients with congenitally nonfunctioning cilia manifest situs inversus. Isolated dextrocardia is almost always associated with congenital heart disease.

Preoperative preparation is directed at treating active pulmonary infection and determining the presence of any significant organ inversion. In the presence of dextrocardia, it is necessary to reverse the electrocardiogram leads to permit accurate interpretation. Inversion of the great vessels is a reason to select the left internal jugular vein for central venous cannulation. Uterine displacement in parturients is logically to the right in these patients. Should a double-lumen endobronchial tube be considered, it is necessary to appreciate the altered anatomy introduced by pulmonary inversion. In view of the high incidence of sinusitis, nasopharyngeal airways should be avoided.

Bronchiolitis Obliterans

Bronchiolitis is a disease of childhood and is most often the result of infection with respiratory syncytial virus. Bronchiolitis obliterans is a rare cause of COPD in adults. The process may accompany viral pneumonia, collagen vascular disease (especially rheumatoid arthritis), and inhalation of nitrogen dioxide ("silo filler's disease"), or it may be a sequela of graft-versus-host disease after bone marrow transplantation. Bronchiolitis obliterans organizing pneumonia is a clinical entity that shares certain features of interstitial lung disease and bronchiolitis obliterans. Treatment of bronchiolitis obliterans is usually ineffective, although corticosteroids may be administered in an attempt to suppress inflammation involving the bronchioles. Bronchiolitis obliterans organizing pneumonia, however, does respond well to corticosteroid therapy. Symptomatic improvement may accompany the use of bronchodilators.

Tracheal Stenosis

Tracheal stenosis typically develops after prolonged endotracheal intubation. Tracheal mucosal ischemia that may progress to destruction of cartilaginous rings and subsequent circumferential constricting scar formation is minimized by the use of high-volume cuffs on tracheal tubes. Infection and hypotension may also contribute to events that culminate in tracheal stenosis.

Diagnosis

Tracheal stenosis becomes symptomatic when the lumen of the adult trachea is decreased to less than 5 mm. Symptoms may not develop until several weeks after tracheal extubation. Dyspnea is prominent even at rest. These patients must use accessory muscles of respiration during all phases of the breathing cycle and must breathe slowly. Peak expiratory flow rates are decreased. Stridor is usually audible. Flow-volume loops display flattened inspiratory and expiratory curves (see Fig. 9-3A). Tomograms of the trachea demonstrate tracheal narrowing.

Management of Anesthesia

Tracheal dilation is useful in some patients, but surgical resection of the stenotic tracheal segment with primary anastomosis is often required. Translaryngeal endotracheal intubation is accomplished. After surgical exposure, the distal normal trachea is opened and a sterile cuffed tube inserted and attached to the anesthetic circuit. Maintenance of anesthesia with volatile anesthetics is useful for ensuring maximum inspired concentrations of oxygen. High-frequency ventilation is useful in selected patients. Anesthesia for tracheal resection may be facilitated by the addition of helium to the inspired gases. This decreases the density of these gases and may improve flow through the area of tracheal narrowing.

Restrictive Lung Disease

Restrictive pulmonary diseases include both acute and chronic intrinsic pulmonary disorders as well as extrinsic (extrapulmonary) disorders involving the pleura, chest wall, diaphragm, and neuromuscular function. Restrictive lung disease is characterized by decreases in all lung volumes, decreased lung compliance, and preservation of expiratory flow rates (**Fig. 9-6**).

Acute Intrinsic Restrictive Lung Disease

Pulmonary edema is due to leakage of intravascular fluid into the interstitium of the lungs and into the alveoli. Acute pulmonary edema can be caused by increased capillary pressure (hydrostatic or cardiogenic pulmonary edema) or by increased capillary permeability. Pulmonary edema typically manifests as bilateral symmetrical opacities on chest radiography. A perihilar distribution ("butterfly pattern") of the lung opacity is common. However, this pattern of lung opacity is more commonly seen with increased capillary pressure than with increased capillary permeability. The presence of air bronchograms on chest radiograph suggests permeability pulmonary edema. Cardiogenic pulmonary edema is characterized by extreme dyspnea, tachypnea, and signs of sympathetic nervous system activation (hypertension, tachycardia, diaphoresis) that may be more pronounced than in patients with capillary permeability pulmonary edema. Pulmonary edema caused by increased capillary permeability is characterized by a high concentration of protein and secretory products in the edema fluid. Diffuse alveolar damage is typically present with the increased permeability pulmonary edema associated with acute respiratory distress syndrome (ARDS).

Aspiration Pneumonitis

Aspirated acidic gastric fluid is rapidly distributed throughout the lung and produces destruction of surfactant-producing cells and damage to the pulmonary capillary endothelium. As a result, there is atelectasis and leakage of intravascular fluid into the lungs producing capillary permeability pulmonary edema. The clinical picture is similar to that of ARDS. Arterial hypoxemia is typically present. In addition, there may be tachypnea, bronchospasm, and acute pulmonary hypertension.

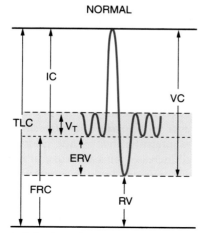
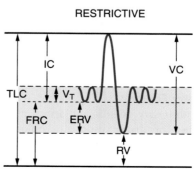

Figure 9-6 • Lung volumes in restrictive lung disease compared to normal values. ERV, expiratory reserve volume; IC, inspiratory capacity; RV, residual volume; TLC, total lung capacity; VC, vital capacity; V_T, tidal volume.

Chest radiographs may not demonstrate evidence of aspiration pneumonitis for 6 to 12 hours after the event. Evidence of aspiration, when it does appear, is most likely to be in the right lower lobe if the patient aspirated while in the supine position.

Measurement of gastric fluid pH is useful as it reflects the pH of the aspirated fluid. Measurement of tracheal aspirate pH is of no value because the aspirated gastric fluid is rapidly diluted by airway secretions. The aspirated gastric fluid is also rapidly distributed to peripheral lung regions so lung lavage is not useful unless there has been aspiration of particulate material.

Aspiration pneumonitis is best treated by delivery of supplemental oxygen and PEEP. Bronchodilation may be needed to relieve bronchospasm. There is no evidence that prophylactic antibiotics decrease the incidence of pulmonary infection or alter outcome. Corticosteroid treatment of aspiration pneumonitis is controversial. Despite the absence of confirmatory evidence that corticosteroids are beneficial, some will treat aspiration pneumonitis with very large doses of methylprednisolone or dexamethasone.

Neurogenic Pulmonary Edema

Neurogenic pulmonary edema develops in a small proportion of patients experiencing acute brain injury. Typically, this form of pulmonary edema occurs minutes to hours after central nervous system injury and may manifest during the perioperative period. There is a massive outpouring of sympathetic impulses from the injured central nervous system, resulting in generalized vasoconstriction and a shift of blood volume into the pulmonary circulation. Presumably, increased pulmonary capillary pressure leads to transudation of fluid into the interstitium and alveoli. Pulmonary hypertension and hypervolemia can also injure blood vessels in the lungs.

The association of pulmonary edema with a recent central nervous system injury should suggest the diagnosis of neurogenic pulmonary edema. The principal entity in the differential diagnosis is aspiration pneumonitis. Unlike neurogenic pulmonary edema, chemical pneumonitis resulting from aspiration frequently persists longer and is often complicated by secondary bacterial infection.

Treatment of neurogenic pulmonary edema is directed at the cause of the central nervous system injury, at decreasing intracranial pressure, and at support of oxygenation and ventilation. Diuretics should not be used unless there is hypervolemia because development of hypovolemic hypotension could aggravate the central nervous system injury.

Drug-Induced Pulmonary Edema

Acute noncardiogenic pulmonary edema can occur after administration of a number of drugs, especially opioids (heroin) and cocaine. High permeability pulmonary edema is suggested by high protein concentrations in the pulmonary edema fluid. Cocaine can also cause pulmonary vasoconstriction, acute myocardial ischemia, and myocardial infarction.

There is no evidence that naloxone speeds resolution of opioid-induced pulmonary edema. Treatment of patients who develop drug-induced pulmonary edema is supportive and may include tracheal intubation for airway protection and mechanical ventilation.

High-Altitude Pulmonary Edema

High-altitude pulmonary edema may occur at heights ranging from 2500 to 5000 meters and is influenced by the rate of ascent to that altitude. The onset of symptoms is often gradual but typically occurs within 48 to 72 hours at high altitude. Fulminant pulmonary edema may be preceded by the less severe symptoms of acute mountain sickness. The etiology of this high permeability pulmonary edema is presumed to be hypoxic pulmonary vasoconstriction, which increases pulmonary vascular pressures. Treatment includes administration of oxygen and prompt descent from the high altitude. Inhalation of nitric oxide may improve oxygenation.

Reexpansion of Collapsed Lung

Rapid expansion of a collapsed lung may lead to pulmonary edema in that lung. The risk of reexpansion pulmonary edema after relieving a pneumothorax or pleural effusion is related to the amount of air or liquid that was present in the pleural space (>1 L increases the risk), the duration of collapse (>24 hours), and the rapidity of reexpansion. High protein concentrations in the edema fluid suggest that enhanced capillary membrane permeability is important in the development of this form of pulmonary edema. Treatment of reexpansion pulmonary edema is supportive.

Negative-Pressure Pulmonary Edema

Negative-pressure pulmonary edema may follow relief of acute upper airway obstruction (postobstructive pulmonary edema) caused by postextubation laryngospasm, epiglottitis, tumors, obesity, hiccups, or obstructive sleep apnea in spontaneously breathing patients. The time at onset of pulmonary edema after relief of airway obstruction ranges from a few minutes to as long as 2 to 3 hours. Tachypnea, cough, and failure to maintain oxygen saturation above 95% are common presenting signs and may be confused with pulmonary aspiration or pulmonary embolism. It is possible that many cases of postoperative oxygen desaturation are due to unrecognized negative-pressure pulmonary edema.

The pathogenesis of negative-pressure pulmonary edema is related to the development of high negative intrapleural pressure by vigorous inspiratory efforts against an obstructed upper airway. High negative intrapleural pressure decreases the interstitial hydrostatic pressure, increases venous return, and increases left ventricular afterload. In addition, such negative pressure leads to intense sympathetic nervous system activation, hypertension, and central displacement of blood volume. Together these factors produce acute pulmonary edema by increasing the transcapillary pressure gradient.

Maintenance of a patent upper airway and administration of supplemental oxygen are sufficient treatment because this form of pulmonary edema is typically transient and self-limited. Mechanical ventilation may occasionally be needed for a brief period of time. Hemodynamic monitoring reveals normal right and left ventricular function. Central venous pressure and pulmonary artery occlusion pressure are normal. Radiographic evidence of pulmonary edema resolves within 12 to 24 hours.

Management of Anesthesia

Preoperative Elective surgery should be delayed in patients with acute restrictive pulmonary disease, and every effort must be made to optimize cardiorespiratory function. Large pleural effusions may need to be drained. Persistent hypoxemia may require mechanical ventilation and PEEP. Hemodynamic monitoring may be useful in both the assessment and treatment of pulmonary edema.

Intraoperative These patients are critically ill. Intraoperative management should be a continuation of critical care management and include a plan for intraoperative ventilator management. The best way to ventilate patients with acute respiratory failure and restrictive lung disease has not been determined by clinical trials. However, because the pathophysiology is similar to that of acute lung injury and because there is the risk of hemodynamic compromise and barotrauma with the use of large tidal volumes and high airway pressures, it is reasonable to ventilate with low tidal volumes (e.g., 6 mL/kg) with a compensatory increase in ventilatory rate (14–18 breaths per minute) attempting to keep the end-inspiratory plateau pressure less than 30 cm H_2O. Typical anesthesia ventilators may not be adequate for patients with severe ARDS and more sophisticated intensive care unit ventilators may be needed in occasional patients. Patients with restrictive lung disease typically breathe rapidly and shallowly, so tachypnea is likely during the weaning process and should not be used as the sole reason for delaying extubation if gas exchange and other assessments are satisfactory.

CHRONIC INTRINSIC RESTRICTIVE LUNG DISEASE

Chronic intrinsic restrictive lung disease is characterized by changes in the intrinsic properties of the lungs, most often due to pulmonary fibrosis. Pulmonary hypertension and cor pulmonale develop as progressive pulmonary fibrosis results in the loss of pulmonary vasculature. Dyspnea is prominent and breathing is rapid and shallow.

Sarcoidosis

Sarcoidosis is a systemic granulomatous disorder that involves many tissues but has a predilection for intrathoracic lymph nodes and the lungs. As many as two thirds of patients have no symptoms at the time of presentation, and the disease is identified because of an abnormal chest radiograph. Patients may present with respiratory symptoms such as dyspnea and cough. Ocular sarcoidosis may produce uveitis; myocardial sarcoidosis may produce conduction defects and dysrhythmias. The most common form of neurologic involvement in sarcoidosis is unilateral facial nerve palsy. Endobronchial sarcoid is common. Laryngeal sarcoidosis occurs in up to 5% of patients and may interfere with the passage of adult-size tracheal tubes. Cor pulmonale may develop. Hypercalcemia occurs in less than 10% of patients but is a classic manifestation of sarcoidosis.

Mediastinoscopy may be necessary to provide lymph node tissue for the diagnosis of sarcoidosis. Angiotensin-converting enzyme activity is increased in patients with sarcoidosis presumably due to production of this enzyme by cells within the granuloma. However, this increase in angiotensin-converting enzyme activity does not have useful diagnostic or prognostic significance. Corticosteroids are administered to suppress the manifestation of sarcoidosis and to treat the hypercalcemia.

Hypersensitivity Pneumonitis

Hypersensitivity pneumonitis is characterized by diffuse interstitial granulomatous reactions in the lungs after inhalation of dust containing fungi, spores, animal, or plant material. Signs and symptoms of hypersensitivity pneumonitis include the onset of dyspnea and cough 4 to 6 hours after inhaling the antigens. This is followed by leukocytosis, eosinophilia, and often arterial hypoxemia. Chest radiographs show multiple pulmonary infiltrates. Repeated episodes of hypersensitivity pneumonitis lead to pulmonary fibrosis.

Eosinophilic Granuloma

Pulmonary fibrosis accompanies the disease process known as eosinophilic granuloma (histiocytosis X). No treatment has been clearly shown to be beneficial in this disease.

Pulmonary Alveolar Proteinosis

Pulmonary alveolar proteinosis is a disease of unknown etiology characterized by the deposition of lipid-rich proteinaceous material in the alveoli. Dyspnea and arterial hypoxemia are the typical clinical manifestations. This process may occur independently or in association with chemotherapy, acquired immunodeficiency syndrome, or inhalation of mineral dusts. Although spontaneous remission may occur, treatment of severe cases requires whole-lung lavage to remove alveolar material and improve macrophage function. Lung lavage in patients with hypoxemia may further decrease the level of oxygenation. Airway management during anesthesia for lung lavage includes placement of a double-lumen endobronchial tube to facilitate lavage of each lung and optimize oxygenation during lavage.

Lymphangioleiomyomatosis

Lymphangioleiomyomatosis is the proliferation of smooth muscle in airways, lymphatics, and blood vessels that occurs in females of reproductive age. Pulmonary function tests show restrictive and obstructive lung disease with decreases in diffusing capacity. Lymphangioleiomyomatosis presents clinically as progressive dyspnea, hemoptysis, recurrent pneumothorax, and pleural effusions.

Nearly all lymphangioleiomyomatosis cells express progesterone receptors. Progesterone or tamoxifen can be used for treatment, but there is progressive deterioration in pulmonary function, and most patients die within 10 years of the onset of symptoms.

Management of Anesthesia

Preoperative Patients usually present with dyspnea and nonproductive cough. Cor pulmonale may be present. Coarse breath sounds with crepitations are heard on auscultation. A chest radiograph may show a ground glass or nodular pattern. Arterial blood gases reveal hypoxemia with normocarbia. Pulmonary function tests show restrictive ventilatory defects and CO diffusing capacity is decreased. A vital capacity of less than 15 mL/kg indicates severe pulmonary dysfunction. Infection should be treated, secretions cleared, and smoking stopped preoperatively.

Intraoperative Patients with restrictive lung disease tolerate apneic periods very poorly due to their small FRC and low oxygen stores. General anesthesia, the supine position, and controlled ventilation all contribute to further decreases in FRC. Alterations in FRC and the risk of hypoxia continue into the postoperative period. Uptake of inhaled anesthetics is faster in these patients because of the small FRC. Peak airway pressures should be kept as low as possible to minimize the risk of barotrauma.

CHRONIC EXTRINSIC RESTRICTIVE LUNG DISEASE

Chronic extrinsic restrictive lung disease is most often due to disorders of the thoracic cage (chest wall) that interfere with lung expansion (**Table 9-11**). The lungs are compressed and lung volumes are reduced. The work of breathing is increased due to the abnormal mechanical properties of the chest and the increased airway resistance that results from decreased lung volumes. Any thoracic deformity may cause compression of pulmonary vasculature and lead to right ventricular dysfunction. Recurrent pulmonary infection resulting from poor cough dynamics may lead to development of COPD.

Obesity

Obesity imposes a restrictive load on the thoracic cage directly by the weight that has been added to the rib cage and indirectly by the large abdominal panniculus, which impedes movement of the diaphragm when these individuals assume the supine position. FRC is decreased and the likelihood of ventilation-to-perfusion mismatching and hypoxemia is increased. Obese patients may experience significant dyspnea during exercise because of the increased work required to move the weight of the chest and abdomen. The rapid shallow breathing pattern during exercise reflects the combined effects of mass loading and diminished compliance of the respiratory system. Daytime hypercapnia may develop

TABLE 9-11 Causes of Restrictive Lung Disease
Acute Intrinsic Restrictive Lung Disease (Pulmonary Edema)
Acute respiratory distress syndrome
Aspiration
Neurogenic problems
Opioid overdose
High altitude
Re-expansion of collapsed lung
Upper airway obstruction (negative pressure)
Congestive heart failure
Chronic Intrinsic Restrictive Lung Disease
Sarcoidosis
Hypersensitivity pneumonitis
Eosinophilic granuloma
Alveolar proteinosis
Lymphangioleiomyomatosis
Drug-induced pulmonary fibrosis
Chronic Extrinsic Restrictive Lung Disease
Obesity
Ascites
Pregnancy
Deformities of the costovertebral skeletal structures
Kyphoscoliosis
Ankylosing spondylitis
Deformities of the sternum
Flail chest
Neuromuscular disorders
Spinal cord transaction
Guillain-Barré syndrome
Myasthenia gravis
Eaton-Lambert syndrome
Muscular dystrophies
Disorders of the Pleura and Mediastinum
Pleural effusion
Pneumothorax
Mediastinal mass
Pneumomediastinum

in morbidly obese patients, especially in the presence of obstructive sleep apnea.

Deformities of the Costovertebral Skeletal Structures

The two basic types of costovertebral skeletal deformity are scoliosis (lateral curvature with rotation of the vertebral column) and kyphosis (anterior flexion of the vertebral column), which are most commonly present in combination as kyphoscoliosis. Idiopathic kyphoscoliosis (accounts for 80% of cases) commonly begins during late childhood or early adolescence and may progress in severity during the years of rapid skeletal growth. Mild to moderate kyphoscoliosis (scoliotic angle < 60 degrees) is associated with minimal to mildly restrictive ventilatory defects. Dyspnea may occur during exercise, but, as the skeletal deformity worsens, the vital capacity declines and dyspnea becomes a common complaint with even moderate exertion. Severe deformities (scoliotic angle > 100 degrees) may lead to chronic alveolar hypoventilation, hypoxemia, secondary erythrocytosis, pulmonary hypertension, and cor pulmonale. Respiratory failure is most likely in patients with kyphoscoliosis associated with a vital capacity less than 45% of the predicted value and a scoliotic angle of more than 110 degrees. Compression of underlying lung tissue results in an increased alveolar-to-arterial oxygen difference. Patients with severe kyphoscoliosis are at increased risk of developing pneumonia and hypoventilation induced by central nervous system depressant drugs. Supplemental oxygen therapy augmented by nocturnal ventilatory support may be useful.

Deformities of the Sternum

Deformities of the sternum and costochondral articulations are characterized by pectus excavatum (inward concavity of the lower sternum) and pectus carinatum (outward protuberance of the upper, middle, or lower sternum). In most patients with pectus excavatum, there are no significant functional limitations. Lung volumes and cardiovascular function are preserved. Surgical correction is indicated when the sternal deformity is accompanied by evidence of pulmonary restriction or cardiovascular dysfunction.

Flail Chest

Multiple rib fractures, especially when they occur in a parallel vertical orientation, can produce a flail chest characterized by paradoxical inward movement of the unstable portion of the thoracic cage while the remainder of the thoracic cage moves outward during inspiration. The same portion of the chest then moves outward with exhalation. The pathophysiology of a flail chest can also result from dehiscence of a median sternotomy, such as following cardiac surgery. Tidal volumes are diminished because the region of the lung associated with the chest wall abnormality paradoxically increases its volume during exhalation and deflates during inspiration. The result is progressive hypoxemia and alveolar hypoventilation. Treatment of flail chest is positive-pressure ventilation until definitive stabilization procedures can be accomplished or rib fractures stabilize.

Neuromuscular Disorders

Neuromuscular disorders that interfere with the transfer of central nervous system input to skeletal muscles necessary for inspiration and exhalation can result in restrictive lung disease. Abnormalities of the spinal cord, peripheral nerves, neuromuscular junction, or skeletal muscles may result in restrictive pulmonary defects characterized by an inability to generate normal respiratory pressures. In contrast to the mechanical disorders of the thoracic cage, in which an effective cough is typically preserved, expiratory muscle weakness characteristic of neuromuscular disorders prevents generation of sufficient expiratory airflow velocity to provide a forceful cough. The extreme example is cervical spinal cord injury in which paralysis of abdominal and intercostal muscles severely decreases the ability to cough. Acute respiratory failure is likely when atelectasis associated with pneumonia (caused by retained secretions due to an ineffective cough) occurs or depressant drugs are administered.

Patients with neuromuscular disorders are somewhat dependent on the state of wakefulness to maintain adequate ventilation. During sleep, hypoxemia and hypercapnia may develop and contribute to the development of cor pulmonale. Vital capacity is an important indicator of the total impact of a neuromuscular disorder on ventilation.

Diaphragmatic Paralysis

In the absence of respiratory complications, neuromuscular disorders rarely progress to the point of hypercapnic respiratory failure unless diaphragmatic weakness or paralysis is present. Thus, quadriplegic patients who have preserved phrenic nerve and diaphragmatic function are unlikely to develop respiratory failure in the absence of pneumonia or administration of central nervous system depressant drugs. In the supine position, patients with diaphragmatic paralysis may develop a ventilatory pattern similar to that seen with a flail chest (abdominal contents push the diaphragm into the chest). In the upright posture these patients experience a significant increase in vital capacity and improved oxygenation and ventilation. Most cases of unilateral diaphragmatic paralysis are the result of neoplastic invasion of the phrenic nerve. In the absence of associated pleuropulmonary disease, most adult patients with unilateral diaphragmatic paralysis remain asymptomatic with the defect being detected as an incidental finding on chest radiography. In contrast, infants are more dependent on bilateral diaphragmatic function for adequate respiratory pump function. In these patients and symptomatic adults, plication of the hemidiaphragm may be necessary to prevent flail motion of the thoracic cage.

Transient diaphragmatic dysfunction may occur after abdominal surgery. Lung volumes are decreased, the alveolar-to-arterial oxygen difference increases, and respiratory frequency increases. These changes may be caused by irritation of the diaphragm, which causes reflex inhibition of phrenic nerve activity. As a result of postoperative diaphragmatic dysfunction, atelectasis and arterial hypoxemia may occur. Incentive spirometry may alleviate these abnormalities.

Spinal Cord Transection

Breathing is maintained solely or predominantly by the diaphragm in quadriplegic patients (transection must be at or below C4 or the diaphragm is paralyzed). Because the diaphragm is active only during inspiration, cough, which requires activity by expiratory muscles, including those of the abdominal wall, is almost totally absent. Intercostal muscles are required to stabilize the upper rib cage against inward collapse when negative intrathoracic pressure is produced by descent of the diaphragm. With diaphragmatic breathing, there is a paradoxical inward motion of the upper thorax during inspiration. The result is a diminished tidal volume. When quadriplegic patients are placed in the upright position, the weight of the abdominal contents pulls on the diaphragm and the absence of abdominal muscle tone results in less efficient function of the diaphragm. Abdominal binders serve to replace lost abdominal muscle tone and may be useful whenever tidal volume decreases in the upright posture. Quadriplegic patients have mild degrees of bronchial constriction caused by the parasympathetic tone that is unopposed by sympathetic activity from the spinal cord. Use of anticholinergic bronchodilating drugs can reverse this abnormality. Respiratory failure almost never occurs in quadriplegic patients in the absence of complications such as pneumonia.

Guillain-Barré Syndrome

Respiratory insufficiency that requires mechanical ventilation occurs in 20% to 25% of patients with Guillain-Barré syndrome. Ventilatory support is needed, on average, for 2 months. A small number of patients have persistent skeletal muscle weakness and are susceptible to recurring episodes of respiratory failure in association with pulmonary infection.

Disorders of Neuromuscular Transmission

Myasthenia gravis is the most common of the disorders affecting neuromuscular transmission that may result in respiratory failure. The myasthenic syndrome (Eaton-Lambert syndrome) may be confused with myasthenia gravis. Prolonged skeletal muscle paralysis or weakness may occur following administration of nondepolarizing neuromuscular blocking drugs.

Muscular Dystrophy

Patients with pseudohypertrophic (Duchenne's) muscular dystrophy, myotonic dystrophy, and other forms of muscular dystrophy are predisposed to pulmonary complications and respiratory failure. Chronic alveolar hypoventilation caused by inspiratory muscle weakness may develop. Expiratory muscle weakness impairs cough and accompanying weakness of the swallowing muscles may lead to pulmonary aspiration of gastric contents. As with all neuromuscular syndromes, central nervous system depressant drugs should be avoided or administered in minimal doses when necessary. Nocturnal ventilation with noninvasive techniques such as nasal intermittent positive-pressure or external negative-pressure ventilation may be useful.

Disorders of the Pleura and Mediastinum

Disorders of the pleura and mediastinum may contribute to mechanical changes that interfere with optimal lung expansion.

Pleural Fibrosis

Pleural fibrosis may follow hemothorax, empyema, or surgical pleurodesis for the treatment of recurrent pneumothoraces. Despite obliteration of the pleural space, functional restrictive lung abnormalities can remain but are usually minor. Surgical decortication to remove thick fibrous pleura is technically difficult and is considered only if the restrictive lung disease is symptomatic.

Pleural Effusion

Pleural effusion is most often confirmed by chest radiography when blunting of the sharp costophrenic angle is seen with as little as 25 to 50 mL of pleural fluid. Larger amounts of fluid produce a characteristic homogeneous opacity that forms a concave meniscus with the chest wall. Ultrasonography and computed tomography are also useful in evaluating a pleural effusion. In patients with congestive heart failure, pleural fluid may collect in the interlobular fissure as an interlobular effusion. Various types of fluid may accumulate in the pleural space, including blood (hemothorax), pus (empyema), lipids (chylothorax), and serous liquid (hydrothorax). All these conditions present with an identical radiographic appearance.

The diagnosis and treatment of pleural effusion are by thoracentesis. The pleural fluid can be either transudative or exudative and the distinction points to potential diagnoses and the need for further evaluation. Bloody pleural effusion is common in patients with malignant disease, trauma, or pulmonary infarction.

Pneumothorax

Pneumothorax is the presence of gas in the pleural space owing either to disruption of the parietal pleura (external penetrating injury) or visceral pleura (tear or rupture in the lung parenchyma). When gas originates in the lung, the rupture may occur in the absence of known lung disease (simple pneumothorax) or as a result of parenchymal disease (secondary pneumothorax). Idiopathic spontaneous pneumothorax occurs most often in tall, thin males 20 to 40 years of age and is due to rupture of apical subpleural blebs. Smoking cigarettes increases the risk of primary spontaneous pneumothorax by 20-fold. Most episodes of spontaneous pneumothorax occur while patients are at rest. Exercise or airline travel does not increase the likelihood of spontaneous pneumothorax.

Signs and Symptoms Dyspnea is always present with a pneumothorax. Most patients also have ipsilateral chest pain and cough. Arterial hypoxemia, hypotension, and hypercarbia may occur. Physical findings are often subtle, emphasizing the importance of considering this diagnosis whenever dyspnea and chest pain occur acutely. Tachycardia is the most common physical finding. In patients with a large pneumothorax, the findings on physical examination of the affected side may include decreased chest wall movement, hyperresonance to percussion, and decreased or absent breath sounds.

Treatment Treatment of a symptomatic pneumothorax is by evacuation of air from the pleural space by aspiration through a small-bore plastic catheter or placement of a chest tube. Aspiration of a pneumothorax followed by catheter removal is successful in 70% of patients with a small- to moderate-sized primary spontaneous pneumothorax. When the pneumothorax is small (< 15% of the volume of the hemithorax) and symptoms are absent, observation may suffice. Supplemental oxygen accelerates the reabsorption of air by the pleura. Continued air leak from the lung requires chest tube placement. Most air leaks resolve within 7 days. Complications of chest tube drainage include pain, pleural infection, hemorrhage, and pulmonary edema related to lung reexpansion. Recurrent pneumothoraces may require surgical intervention or chemical pleurodesis.

Tension Pneumothorax

Tension pneumothorax develops when gas enters the pleural space during inspiration and is prevented from escaping during exhalation. The result is a progressive increase in the amount of air trapped under increasing pressure (tension). Tension pneumothorax occurs in less than 2% of patients experiencing an idiopathic spontaneous pneumothorax, but it is a common manifestation of rib fractures, insertion of central lines, and barotrauma in patients receiving mechanical ventilation. Dyspnea, hypoxemia, and hypotension may be severe. Immediate evacuation of gas through a needle or a small-bore catheter placed into the second anterior intercostal space may be lifesaving.

Mediastinal Tumors

In the evaluation of mediastinal widening, contrast-enhanced computed tomography can distinguish between vascular structures, soft tissues, and calcifications Lymphoma, thymoma, teratoma, and retrosternal goiter are common causes of an anterior mediastinal mass. Large mediastinal tumors may be associated with progressive airway obstruction, loss of lung volumes, pulmonary artery or cardiac compression, and superior vena cava obstruction.

Superior vena cava syndrome is a constellation of signs that develops in patients with a mediastinal tumor that obstructs venous drainage in the upper thorax. Increased venous pressure leads to (1) dilation of collateral veins in the thorax and neck; (2) edema and cyanosis of the face, neck, and upper chest; (3) edema of the conjunctiva; and (4) evidence of increased intracranial pressure including headache and altered mental status. Dyspnea is common. Cancer accounts for nearly all cases of superior vena cava syndrome.

Mediastinitis

Acute mediastinitis usually results from bacterial contamination after esophageal perforation. Symptoms include chest pain and fever. It is treated with broad-spectrum antibiotics and surgical drainage.

Pneumomediastinum

Pneumomediastinum may follow a tear in the esophagus or tracheobronchial tree or alveolar rupture, although it most often occurs independent of known causes. Spontaneous pneumomediastinum has been observed after recreational cocaine use. Symptoms of retrosternal chest pain and dyspnea are typically abrupt in onset and usually follow exaggerated breathing efforts (cough, emesis, Valsalva maneuver). Subcutaneous emphysema may be extensive in the neck, arms, abdomen, and scrotum. Gas in the mediastinum may decompress into the pleural space leading to pneumothorax, usually on the left. The diagnosis of pneumomediastinum is established by chest radiography. Spontaneous pneumomediastinum resolves without specific therapy. When pneumomediastinum is a result of organ rupture, surgical drainage and repair may be necessary.

Bronchogenic Cysts

Bronchogenic cysts are fluid- or air-filled cysts arising from the primitive foregut that are lined with respiratory epithelium. They are usually located in the mediastinum or in the lung parenchyma. These cysts may be asymptomatic, the focus of recurrent pulmonary infection, or the cause of life-threatening airway obstruction. Cysts located in the mediastinum are more likely to be filled with fluid than air and are usually not in direct communication with the airways. These masses cause symptoms of airway compression as they grow. Surgical excision may be necessary.

Theoretical concerns in patients with bronchogenic cysts include the hazards of nitrous oxide and use of positive-pressure ventilation. Nitrous oxide can diffuse into air-filled bronchogenic cysts and cause their expansion with associated life-threatening respiratory or cardiovascular compromise. Institution of positive-pressure ventilation may have a ball-valve effect, particularly in cysts that extrinsically compress the tracheobronchial tree, resulting in air trapping. Despite these concerns, clinical experience confirms that nitrous oxide and positive-pressure ventilation may often be safely used in patients with bronchogenic cysts.

Management of Anesthesia
Preoperative

Preoperative evaluation of patients with mediastinal tumors includes chest radiography, a flow-volume loop, chest imaging studies, and clinical evaluation for evidence of tracheobronchial compression. The size of the mediastinal mass and the degree of tracheal compression can be established by computed tomography, and this study is a useful predictor of whether airway difficulties during anesthesia are to be expected. Flexible fiberoptic bronchoscopy under topical anesthesia may also be useful for evaluating airway obstruction. Interestingly, the severity of preoperative pulmonary symptoms bears no relationship to the degree of respiratory compromise that can be encountered during anesthesia. Indeed, a number of asymptomatic patients have developed unexpected airway obstruction during anesthesia. Preoperative radiation therapy should be considered whenever possible. In symptomatic patients requiring a diagnostic tissue biopsy, a local anesthetic technique, if feasible, is best. Patients with mediastinal tumors may be asymptomatic while awake yet develop airway obstruction during anesthesia in the supine position. During anesthesia, the tumor may increase in size due to venous engorgement and its position may shift somewhat. As a result, it may compress the airway, the vena cava, the pulmonary artery, or the atria and create life-threatening hypoxemia, hypotension, or even cardiac arrest.

Intraoperative

Restrictive lung disease does not influence the choice of drugs used for induction or maintenance of anesthesia.

Drugs with prolonged respiratory depressant effects that may persist into the postoperative period should be avoided. A high index of suspicion for the presence of a pneumothorax and the need to avoid or discontinue nitrous oxide must be maintained. Regional anesthesia can be considered for peripheral operations, but it must be appreciated that sensory levels above T10 can be associated with impairment of the respiratory muscle activity needed by patients with restrictive lung disease to maintain acceptable ventilation. Mechanical ventilation during the intraoperative period facilitates optimal oxygenation and ventilation. Since the lungs are poorly compliant, increased inspiratory airway pressures may be necessary. Postoperative mechanical ventilation is often required in patients with significantly impaired pulmonary function. Restrictive lung disease contributes to the risk of postoperative pulmonary complications.

The method of induction of anesthesia and tracheal intubation in the presence of mediastinal tumors depends on the preoperative assessment of the airway. External edema associated with superior vena cava syndrome may be accompanied by similar edema inside the mouth and hypopharynx. If edema due to caval obstruction is severe, it may be necessary to establish intravenous access in the legs rather than in the arms. A central venous or pulmonary artery catheter can be inserted through the femoral vein. Invasive blood pressure monitoring should be considered. Symptomatic patients may need to be in the sitting position to breathe adequately. If so, anesthetic induction in this position may proceed after the airway has been secured. Topical anesthesia of the airway with or without sedation can be used to facilitate fiberoptic laryngoscopy. In very young patients, an inhalation induction with maintenance of spontaneous ventilation may be necessary. If severe airway obstruction occurs, it can be alleviated by placing the patient in the lateral or prone position. Spontaneous ventilation throughout surgery is recommended whenever possible. Worsening of superior vena cava syndrome may occur as a result of generous intraoperative fluid replacement. Diuretics may decrease the tumor volume, but the reduction in preload in these patients with already compromised venous return may result in significant hypotension. Surgical bleeding is often increased due to increased central venous pressure.

Postoperative

Postoperatively, tumor swelling as a result of partial resection or biopsy may increase airway obstruction and require reintubation of the trachea.

DIAGNOSTIC PROCEDURES IN PATIENTS WITH LUNG DISEASE

Fiberoptic bronchoscopy has generally replaced rigid bronchoscopy for visualizing the airways and obtaining samples for culture, cytology, and biopsy. Pneumothorax occurs in 5% to 10% of patients after transbronchial lung biopsy and in 10% to 20% of patients after percutaneous needle biopsy of peripheral lung lesions. The principal contraindication to pleural biopsy is a coagulopathy.

Mediastinoscopy is performed under general anesthesia through a small transverse incision just above the suprasternal notch. Blunt dissection along the pretracheal fascia is performed, permitting biopsy of paratracheal lymph nodes to the level of the carina. Complications include pneumothorax, mediastinal hemorrhage, venous air embolism, and injury to the recurrent laryngeal nerve leading to hoarseness and vocal cord paralysis. The mediastinoscope can also exert pressure against the right innominate artery, causing loss of pulses in the right arm and compromise of right carotid artery blood flow.

Acute Respiratory Failure

Respiratory failure is the inability to provide adequate arterial oxygenation and/or elimination of carbon dioxide.

Diagnosis

Acute respiratory failure is considered to be present when the Pao_2 is less than 60 mm Hg despite supplemental oxygen and in the absence of a right-to-left intracardiac shunt. In the presence of acute respiratory failure, $Paco_2$ can be increased, unchanged, or decreased depending on the relationship of alveolar ventilation to metabolic production of carbon dioxide. A $Paco_2$ higher than 50 mm Hg in the absence of respiratory compensation for metabolic alkalosis is consistent with the diagnosis of acute respiratory failure.

Acute respiratory failure is distinguished from chronic respiratory failure based on the relationship of $Paco_2$ to arterial pH (pHa). Acute respiratory failure is typically accompanied by abrupt increases in $Paco_2$ and by corresponding decreases in pHa. In the presence of chronic respiratory failure, pHa is usually between 7.35 and 7.45 despite an increased $Paco_2$. This normal pHa reflects renal compensation for the respiratory acidosis via renal tubular reabsorption of bicarbonate.

Respiratory failure is often accompanied by a decrease in FRC and lung compliance. Increased pulmonary vascular resistance and pulmonary hypertension are likely to develop if respiratory failure persists.

Acute/Adult Respiratory Distress Syndrome

Adult ARDS is caused by an inflammatory injury to the lung and is manifested clinically as acute hypoxemic respiratory failure.

Epidemiology and Pathogenesis

Clinical disorders and risk factors associated with the development of ARDS include events associated with direct lung injury and those that cause indirect injury to the lungs in the setting of a systemic process (**Table 9-12**). Overall, sepsis is associated with the highest risk of progression of acute lung injury to ARDS. The acute phase of ARDS manifests as the rapid onset of respiratory failure accompanied by arterial hypoxemia refractory to treatment and radiographic findings

TABLE 9–12 Treatment of Acute Respiratory Failure

Supplemental oxygen
Tracheal intubation
Mechanical ventilation
Positive end-expiratory pressure
Optimize intravascular fluid volume
Diuretic therapy
Inotropic support
Glucocorticoids (?)
Removal of secretions
Control of infection
Nutritional support
Inhaled β-adrenergic agonists

?, questionable efficacy.

characterized by gradual resolution of the hypoxemia and improved lung compliance. Typically, the radiographic abnormalities resolve completely.

Signs and Symptoms

Arterial hypoxemia resistant to treatment with supplemental oxygen is usually the first sign. Radiographic signs may appear before symptoms develop. Patients usually have a normal pulmonary capillary wedge pressure. Pulmonary hypertension can occur due to pulmonary artery vasoconstriction and obliteration of portions of the pulmonary capillary bed and, when severe, can cause right heart failure. Death from ARDS is most often a result of sepsis or multiple organ failure rather than respiratory failure, although some deaths can be directly related to lung injury.

Diagnosis

Diagnosis of ARDS is dependent on the presentation of acute, refractory hypoxemia, diffuse infiltrates on chest radiography consistent with pulmonary edema, and a pulmonary capillary wedge pressure less than 18 mm Hg. The $Pa_{O_2}/F_{I_{O_2}}$ ratio is typically less than 200 mm Hg. A less severe form of ARDS is acute lung injury with similar presentation but the $Pa_{O_2}/F_{I_{O_2}}$ ratio is less than 300 mm Hg. An algorithm for clinical differentiation between cardiogenic and noncardiogenic pulmonary edema is shown in **Figure 9-7**.

indistinguishable from those of cardiogenic pulmonary edema. There is an influx of protein-rich edema fluid into the alveoli as a result of increased alveolar capillary membrane permeability. There is evidence of neutrophil-mediated lung injury. Proinflammatory cytokines may be produced locally in the lungs. This acute phase usually resolves completely, but in some patients, it may progress to fibrosing alveolitis with persistent arterial hypoxemia and decreased pulmonary compliance. The recovery or resolution phase of ARDS is

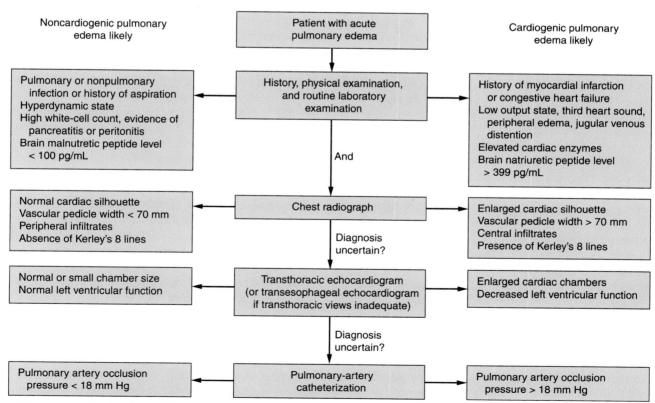

Figure 9-7 • Algorithm for the clinical differentiation between cardiogenic and noncardiogenic pulmonary edema. (*Adapted from Ware LB, Matthay MA: Acute pulmonary edema. N Engl J Med 2005;353:2788–2796. Copyright Massachusetts Medical Society, 2005.*)

TABLE 9–13	Clinical Disorders Associated with Acute Lung Injury and Acute Respiratory Distress Syndrome

Direct Lung Injury
Pneumonia
Aspiration of gastric contents
Pulmonary contusion
Fat emboli
Near-drowning
Inhalational injury
Indirect Lung Injury
Sepsis
Trauma associated with shock
Multiple blood transfusions
Cardiopulmonary bypass
Drug overdose
Acute pancreatitis

Treatment

Treatment of acute respiratory failure is directed at initiating specific therapies that support oxygenation and ventilation. The three principal goals in the management of acute respiratory failure are (1) correction of hypoxemia, (2) removal of excess carbon dioxide, and (3) provision of a patent upper airway.

Improved supportive care of patients with acute lung injury and ARDS may contribute to improved survival rates (**Table 9-13**). There should be a thorough search for the underlying cause of ARDS, with particular attention paid to the possibility of a treatable infection such as sepsis and pneumonia. Prevention or early treatment of nosocomial infection is critical. Adequate nutrition should be provided preferably through the use of enteral feedings. Prevention of gastrointestinal bleeding and thromboembolism is important. At the present time, routine use of surfactant therapy or inhaled nitric oxide is not recommended. However, in the future, strategies that hasten the resolution phase of ARDS, including the ability to remove alveolar fluid and sustain improvements in oxygenation, may become as important as traditional ventilatory management. Inhaled β-agonists may be of value in removal of pulmonary edema fluid, stimulating the secretion of surfactant, and even exerting antiinflammatory effects that may help restore the proper vascular permeability to the lungs.

Tracheal Intubation and Mechanical Ventilation The initial steps in the treatment of patients with acute respiratory failure and ARDS who cannot be adequately oxygenated are tracheal intubation and mechanical ventilation. Inspired oxygen concentrations are adjusted to maintain the PaO_2 between 60 and 80 mm Hg. The higher tidal volumes (12–15 mL/kg) used in the past for treatment of ARDS may be associated with decreased pulmonary compliance and can result in alveolar overdistention and barotraumas. The risk of barotrauma can be lessened by adjustment of tidal volumes such that increases in peak airway pressure do not exceed 35 to 40 cm H_2O. Ideal tidal volume is determined by assessing lung mechanics rather than by measuring arterial blood gases.

Application of PEEP is one of the most effective ways to improve oxygenation in patients with ARDS. PEEP helps prevent alveolar collapse at end-expiration and thereby increases lung volumes (especially FRC), improves ventilation-to-perfusion matching, and decreases the magnitude of right-to-left intrapulmonary shunting. PEEP does not decrease the amount of extravascular lung water or prevent the formation of pulmonary edema fluid. However, edema fluid is likely to be redistributed to the interstitial lung regions, causing previously flooded alveoli to become ventilated.

Application of PEEP is indicated when high concentrations of inspired oxygen ($FiO_2 > 0.5$) are needed for prolonged periods to maintain an acceptable PaO_2 and may introduce the risk of oxygen toxicity. It is possible that PEEP may decrease the shear stress associated with the opening and closing of alveoli in ARDS. The lowest level of PEEP necessary to achieve acceptable oxygenation at nontoxic oxygen concentrations should be employed. High levels of PEEP decrease cardiac output and increase the incidence of barotrauma. The level of PEEP that results in optimal pulmonary compliance is usually similar to the level associated with optimal oxygenation. PEEP is typically added in 2.5- to 5.0-cm H_2O increments until the PaO_2 is at least 60 mm Hg with an FiO_2 less than 0.5. Most patients show maximal improvement in oxygen transport and pulmonary compliance with levels of PEEP below 15 cm H_2O. Excessive levels of PEEP can decrease the PaO_2 by overdistending alveoli and thereby compressing the capillaries surrounding these alveoli and shunting more blood to less ventilated areas.

An important adverse effect of PEEP is decreased cardiac output due to interference with venous return and leftward displacement of the interventricular septum, which restricts left ventricular filling. The decrease in cardiac output caused by PEEP is exaggerated in the presence of hypovolemia. Replacement of intravascular fluid volume and administration of inotropic drugs may offset the effects of PEEP on venous return and improve myocardial contractility. A pulmonary artery catheter is useful for monitoring the adequacy of intravascular fluid replacement, myocardial contractility, and tissue oxygenation in patients being treated with PEEP. Measurement of pulmonary artery occlusion pressures may be complicated by transmission of PEEP (intra-alveolar pressure) to the pulmonary capillaries, causing an erroneous interpretation of pulmonary artery occlusion pressure.

Inverse-Ratio Ventilation Inverse-ratio ventilation is characterized by an inspiratory time that exceeds the expiratory time, i.e., the inspiratory/expiratory ratio is greater than 1. This is accomplished by adding an end-inspiratory pause to maintain the alveolar pressure briefly at the plateau level. Arterial oxygenation may be improved without increasing minute ventilation or PEEP. Risks of inverse-ratio ventilation include barotrauma and hypotension due to development of auto-PEEP as a result of the shortened expiratory time. Although inverse-ratio ventilation may improve oxygenation in some patients with ARDS, prospective studies have not confirmed a specific benefit in most patients.

Fluid and Hemodynamic Management The rationale for restricting fluids in patients with acute lung injury and ARDS is to decrease the magnitude of the pulmonary edema. Pulmonary artery occlusion pressures below 15 mm Hg may reflect inadequate intravascular fluid volume. Urine outputs of 0.5 to 1.0 mL/kg per hour are consistent with an adequate cardiac output and intravascular fluid volume. Diuresis using furosemide may be effective in reversing some effects of excessive fluid administration as evidenced by improved oxygenation and resolution of pulmonary infiltrates. Measurement of central venous pressure is not a reliable guide for monitoring intravascular fluid volume in patients with ARDS.

A reasonable goal of fluid therapy is to maintain the intravascular fluid volume at the lowest level consistent with adequate organ perfusion as assessed by metabolic acid-base balance and renal function. If organ perfusion cannot be maintained after restoration of intravascular fluid volume, as in patients with septic shock, treatment with vasopressors may be necessary to improve organ perfusion pressures and normalize tissue oxygen delivery.

Corticosteroids Despite the recognized role of inflammation in acute lung injury and ARDS, the value of corticosteroid administration early in the course of the disease remains unproven. Corticosteroids may have value in the treatment of the later fibrosing-alveolitis phase of ARDS or as rescue therapy in patients with severe ARDS that is not resolving.

Removal of Secretions Optimal removal of airway secretions is facilitated by adequate systemic hydration and humidification of inspired gases. Tracheal suctioning, chest physiotherapy and postural drainage may also enhance secretion removal. Fiberoptic bronchoscopy may be indicated to remove thicker accumulated secretions that are contributing to atelectasis.

Control of Infection Control of infection using specific antibiotic therapy based on sputum culture and sensitivity is a valuable adjunct to the management of ARDS. However, the use of prophylactic antibiotics is not recommended because this practice leads to overgrowth with resistant organisms. Not uncommonly, the earliest evidence of infection in patients with ARDS is further deterioration in pulmonary function.

Nutritional Support Nutritional support is important to prevent skeletal muscle weakness. Hypophosphatemia may contribute to skeletal muscle weakness and to the poor contractility of the diaphragm that may accompany acute respiratory failure and ARDS. Increased caloric intake, especially that associated with hyperalimentation, increases the respiratory quotient and thereby increases the production of carbon dioxide, necessitating greater alveolar ventilation. In the severely compromised patient, this need for greater ventilation might not be possible without mechanical support of ventilation.

Mechanical Support of Ventilation

Supplemental oxygen can be provided to spontaneously breathing patients using a nasal cannula, Venturi mask, nonrebreathing mask, or T piece. These devices seldom provide inspired oxygen concentrations higher than 50% and therefore are only of value in correcting the hypoxemia resulting from mild to moderate ventilation-to-perfusion mismatching. When these methods of oxygen delivery fail to maintain the Pa_{O_2} above 60 mm Hg, continuous positive airway pressure by face mask can be tried. Continuous positive airway pressure may increase lung volumes by opening collapsed alveoli and decreasing right-to-left intrapulmonary shunting. A disadvantage of continuous positive airway pressure by face mask is that the tight mask fit required may increase the risk of aspiration should the patient vomit. Maintenance of the Pa_{O_2} above approximately 80 mm Hg is of no benefit because hemoglobin saturation with oxygen is nearly 100% at this level. In some patients, it is necessary to perform tracheal intubation and institute mechanical ventilation to maintain acceptable oxygenation and ventilation. Typical devices that provide positive-pressure ventilation include volume-cycled and pressure-cycled ventilators.

Volume-Cycled Ventilation Volume-cycled ventilation provides a fixed tidal volume, and inflation pressure is the dependent variable. A pressure limit can be set and when inflation pressure exceeds this value, a pressure relief valve prevents further gas flow. This valve prevents the development of dangerously high peak airway and alveolar pressures and warns that a change in pulmonary compliance has occurred. Large increases in peak airway pressure may reflect worsening pulmonary edema, development of a pneumothorax, kinking of the tracheal tube, or the presence of mucus plugs in the tracheal tube or large airways. Tidal volume is maintained despite smaller changes in peak airway pressure. This is in contrast to pressure-cycled ventilators. A disadvantage of volume-cycled ventilation is the inability of these devices to compensate for leaks in the delivery system. The primary modalities of ventilation using volume-cycled ventilation are assist-control ventilation and synchronized intermittent mandatory ventilation (**Fig. 9-8**).

Assist-Control Ventilation In the control mode, a preset respiratory rate ensures that a patient receives a predetermined number of mechanically delivered breaths even if there are no inspiratory efforts. However, in the assist mode, if the patient can create a small negative airway pressure, a breath at the preset tidal volume will be delivered.

Synchronized Intermittent Mandatory Ventilation The synchronized intermittent mandatory ventilation technique allows patients to breathe spontaneously at any rate and tidal volume while a certain minute ventilation is provided by the ventilator. The gas delivery circuit is modified to provide sufficient gas flow for spontaneous breathing and to permit periodic mandatory breaths that are synchronous with the patient's inspiratory efforts. Theoretical advantages of synchronized intermittent mandatory ventilation compared to assist-control ventilation include continued use of respiratory muscles, lower mean airway and mean intrathoracic pressure, prevention of respiratory alkalosis, and improved patient-ventilator coordination.

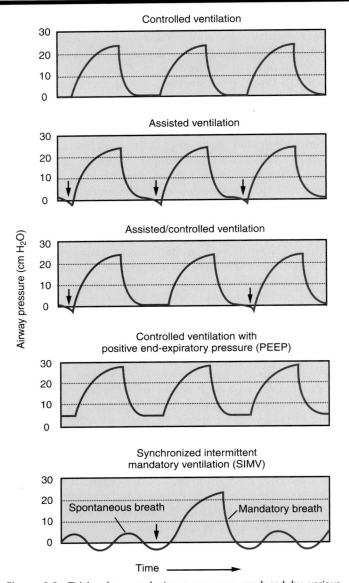

Figure 9-8 • Tidal volume and airway pressures produced by various modes of ventilation delivered through an endotracheal tube. *Arrows* indicate initiation of a spontaneous breath by the patient who triggers the ventilator to deliver a mechanically assisted breath.

Pressure-Cycled Ventilation Pressure-cycled ventilation provides gas flow into the lungs until a preset airway pressure is reached. Tidal volume is the dependent variable. Tidal volume varies with changes in lung compliance and airway resistance.

Management of Patients Receiving Mechanical Support of Ventilation

Critically ill patients who require mechanical ventilation may benefit from continuous infusion of sedative drugs to treat anxiety and agitation and to facilitate coordination with ventilator-delivered breaths. Inadequate sedation or agitation can lead to life-threatening problems such as self-extubation, acute deterioration in gas exchange, and barotrauma. The need for neuromuscular blockade is reduced by the optimum use of sedation. However, when acceptable sedation without hemodynamic compromise cannot be achieved, it may be necessary to produce skeletal muscle paralysis to ensure appropriate ventilation and oxygenation.

Sedation Benzodiazepines, propofol, and narcotics are the drugs most commonly administered to decrease anxiety, produce amnesia, increase patient comfort, and provide analgesia during mechanical ventilation. Newer approaches to mechanical ventilation involving the use of permissive hypercapnia ($Paco_2$ may reach 50 mm Hg) can cause substantial discomfort and necessitate deep sedation. Continuous infusion of drugs rather than intermittent injection provides a more constant and desirable level of drug effect. Daily interruption of sedative infusions and allowing the patient to "awaken" may facilitate evaluation of mental status and ultimately shorten the period of mechanical ventilation. For this practice, continuous infusion of propofol is uniquely attractive, as the brief context-sensitive half-life of this drug is not influenced by the duration of the infusion, and rapid awakening is predictable. Likewise, prompt recovery from the effects of remifentanil is not influenced by the duration of the intravenous drug infusion.

Paralysis When sedation is inadequate or hypotension accompanies the administration of drugs used for sedation, the administration of nondepolarizing neuromuscular-blocking drugs to produce skeletal muscle relaxation may be necessary to permit optimal mechanical ventilation. The dependence of certain of these drugs on renal clearance should be considered. It is better to use intermittent rather than continuous skeletal muscle paralysis to be able to periodically assess the adequacy of sedation and the need for ongoing paralysis. Monitoring of neuromuscular blockade and titration of muscle relaxant doses so that a twitch response remains present is prudent. A risk of prolonged drug-induced skeletal muscle paralysis is accentuation of the diffuse polyneuropathy that may accompany critical illness.

Complications

Infection In mechanically ventilated patients with acute respiratory failure, tracheal intubation is the single most important predisposing factor for developing nosocomial pneumonia (ventilator-associated pneumonia). The major pathogenic mechanism is microaspiration of contaminated secretions around the tracheal tube cuff. Diagnosis of pneumonia in the presence of acute respiratory failure may be difficult since fever and pulmonary infiltrates may already be present with the acute respiratory failure.

Nosocomial sinusitis is strongly related to the presence of a nasotracheal tube. Treatment of nosocomial sinusitis includes antibiotics, replacement of nasal tubes with oral tubes, and use of decongestants and head elevation to facilitate sinus drainage.

Alveolar Overdistention Alveolar overdistention due to large tidal volumes (10–12 mL/kg) and high airway pressures (>50 cm H_2O) may result in alveolar rupture and alveolar hemorrhage. In the presence of acute lung injury and ARDS, a ventilator-delivered breath preferentially follows the path of least resistance and travels to better aerated lungs or regions, putting these alveoli at risk of overdistention. These alveoli may collapse and reopen repeatedly, and this could be responsible for ventilator-induced lung injury. A gentler form of mechanical ventilation using tidal volumes of 5 to 8 mL/kg and airway pressures not exceeding 30 cm H_2O may be indicated for treating acute respiratory failure and ARDS. However, use of this form of ventilation may require acceptance of some degree of hypercarbia and respiratory acidosis and often a PaO_2 of less than 60 mm Hg.

Permissive hypercapnia or controlled hypoventilation may accompany the reduction in tidal volume and airway pressure designed to minimize or prevent alveolar overdistention. The increased respiratory drive associated with permissive hypercapnia causes discomfort, making deep sedation, skeletal muscle paralysis, or both necessary. Permissive hypercapnia is not recommended in patients with increased intracranial pressure, cardiac dysrhythmias, or pulmonary hypertension.

Barotrauma Barotrauma may present as subcutaneous emphysema, pneumomediastinum, pulmonary interstitial emphysema, pneumoperitoneum, pneumopericardium, arterial gas embolism, or tension pneumothorax. These examples of extraalveolar air almost always reflect dissection or passage of air from overdistended and ruptured alveoli. Infection also increases the risk of barotrauma presumably by weakening pulmonary tissue. Tension pneumothorax is the most common life-threatening manifestation of ventilator-induced barotrauma. Hypotension, worsening hypoxemia, and increased airway pressure suggest the presence of a tension pneumothorax.

Atelectasis Atelectasis is a common cause of hypoxemia that develops during mechanical ventilation. Migration of the tracheal tube into the left or right mainstem bronchus or development of mucus plugs should be considered when abrupt worsening of oxygenation occurs in the absence of hypotension. Arterial hypoxemia due to atelectasis is not responsive to an increase in FIO_2. Other causes of sudden hypoxemia in mechanically ventilated patients include tension pneumothorax and pulmonary embolism, but in contrast to atelectasis, these are usually accompanied by hypotension. Bronchoscopy may be necessary to remove mucus plugs responsible for persistent atelectasis.

Critical Illness Myopathy Patients who undergo mechanical ventilation for treatment of acute respiratory failure are at risk of neuromuscular weakness that persists long after the cause of the respiratory failure has resolved. A common cause of diffuse skeletal muscle weakness is polyneuropathy of critical illness, an axonal disorder that occurs in the presence of sepsis and multiple system organ failure. Prolonged administration of nondepolarizing neuromuscular-blocking drugs may contribute to the development of an acute myopathy, particularly in patients who undergo concomitant therapy with corticosteroids. The duration of drug-induced paralysis rather than the specific neuromuscular blocker used seems to be more important in development of persistent

weakness. Decreased clearance of active metabolites of nondepolarizing neuromuscular blocking drugs owing to renal and/or hepatic dysfunction is also a consideration when persistent weakness follows prolonged administration of these drugs.

Monitoring of Treatment

Monitoring the progress of the treatment of acute respiratory failure includes evaluation of pulmonary gas exchange (arterial and venous blood gases, pHa) and cardiac function (cardiac output, cardiac filling pressures, intrapulmonary shunt). A pulmonary artery catheter is useful for accomplishing many of these measurements.

Weaning from the Ventilator Mechanical ventilatory support can be withdrawn when a patient can maintain oxygenation and carbon dioxide elimination without assistance. When considering whether patients can be safely weaned from mechanical ventilation and will tolerate extubation, it is important that patients be alert and cooperative and able to tolerate a trial of spontaneous ventilation without excessive tachypnea, tachycardia, or obvious respiratory distress. Some of the guidelines that have been proposed for indicating the feasibility of discontinuing mechanical ventilation include (1) vital capacity more than 15 mL/kg; (2) $PAO_2 - PaO_2$ less than 350 cm H_2O while breathing 100% oxygen; (3) PaO_2 more than 60 mm Hg with FIO_2 less than 0.5; (4) negative inspiratory pressure greater than −20 cm H_2O; (5) normal pHa; (6) respiratory rate less than 20 breaths per minute; and (7) dead-space ventilation/tidal volume ratio (V_D/V_T) less than 0.6. Breathing at rapid rates and with low tidal volumes usually signifies an inability to tolerate extubation. Ultimately, the decision to attempt withdrawal of mechanical ventilation is individualized, considering not only pulmonary function but also the presence of co-existing abnormalities such as anemia, hypokalemia, and hypovolemia.

When a patient is ready for a trial of withdrawal from mechanical support of ventilation, three options may be considered: (1) synchronized intermittent mandatory ventilation, which allows spontaneous breathing amid progressively fewer mandatory breaths per minute until the patient is breathing unassisted; (2) intermittent trials of total removal of mechanical support and breathing through a T piece; and (3) use of decreasing levels of pressure-support ventilation. Overall, correcting the underlying condition responsible for the need for mechanical support of ventilation seems to be more important for successful extubation than the weaning method. Deterioration in oxygenation after withdrawal of mechanical ventilation may reflect progressive alveolar collapse, which can be responsive to treatment with continuous positive airway pressure rather than reinstitution of mechanical ventilation. Presumably continuous positive airway pressure helps maintain FRC.

Several things may interfere with successful withdrawal from mechanical ventilation and extubation. Respiratory alkalosis and persistent sedation may depress ventilatory drive. Excessive workload on the respiratory muscles imposed by hyperinflation, copious secretions, bronchospasm, increased

TABLE 9–14 Mechanisms of Arterial Hypoxemia

Mechanism	Pa_{O_2}	Pa_{CO_2}	$PA_{O_2} - Pa_{O_2}$	Response to Supplemental Oxygen
Low inspired oxygen concentration (altitude)	Decreased	Normal to decreased	Normal	Improved
Hypoventilation (drug overdose)	Decreased	Increased	Normal	Improved
Ventilation-to-perfusion mismatching (COPD, pneumonia)	Decreased	Normal to decreased	Increased	Improved
Right-to-left shunt (pulmonary edema)	Decreased	Normal to decreased	Increased	Poor to none
Diffusion impairment (pulmonary fibrosis)	Decreased	Normal to decreased	Increased	Improved

COPD, chronic pulmonary obstructive disease; $PA_{O_2} - Pa_{O_2}$, alveolar-arterial difference in partial pressure of oxygen.

lung water or increased carbon dioxide production from fever, or parenteral nutrition greatly decreases the likelihood of successful tracheal extubation.

Tracheal Extubation Tracheal extubation should be considered when patients tolerate 2 hours of spontaneous breathing during T-tube weaning or when a synchronized intermittent mandatory ventilation rate of 1 to 2 breaths per minute is tolerated without deterioration of arterial blood gases, mental status, or cardiac function. The Pa_{O_2} should remain above 60 mm Hg while breathing less than 50% oxygen. Likewise, Pa_{CO_2} should remain less than 50 mm Hg, and the pH_a should remain above 7.30. Additional criteria for tracheal extubation include the need for less than 5 cm H_2O PEEP, spontaneous breathing rates of less than 30 breaths per minute, and vital capacity of more than 15 mL/kg. Patients should be alert with active laryngeal reflexes and the ability to generate an effective cough and clear secretions. Protective glottic closure function may be impaired following tracheal extubation, resulting in an increased risk of aspiration.

Supplemental Oxygen Supplemental oxygen is often needed after tracheal extubation. This need reflects the persistence of ventilation-to-perfusion mismatching. Weaning from supplemental oxygen is accomplished by gradually decreasing in the inspired concentration of oxygen, as guided by measurements of Pa_{O_2} and monitoring of Sp_{O_2} by pulse oximetry.

Oxygen Exchange and Arterial Oxygenation Adequacy of oxygen exchange across alveolar-capillary membranes is reflected by the Pa_{O_2}. The efficacy of this exchange is paralleled by the differences between the calculated Pa_{O_2} and measured Pa_{O_2}. Calculation of $PA_{O_2} - Pa_{O_2}$ is useful for evaluating, the gas-exchange function of the lungs and for distinguishing among various mechanisms of arterial hypoxemia (**Table 9-14**).

Significant desaturation of arterial blood occurs only when the Pa_{O_2} is less than 60 mm Hg. Ventilation-to-perfusion mismatching, right-to-left intrapulmonary shunting and hypoventilation are the principal causes of arterial hypoxemia (see Table 9-14). Increasing the inspired oxygen concentration is likely to improve Pa_{O_2} in all these conditions, with the exception of a right-to-left intrapulmonary shunt exceeding 30% of cardiac output.

Compensatory responses to arterial hypoxemia vary. As a general rule, these responses are stimulated by an acute decrease in Pa_{O_2} below 60 mm Hg. They are also present in chronic hypoxemia when the Pa_{O_2} is less than 50 mm Hg. Compensatory responses to arterial hypoxemia include (1) carotid body–induced increase in alveolar ventilation, (2) regional pulmonary artery vasoconstriction (hypoxic pulmonary vasoconstriction) to divert pulmonary blood flow away from hypoxic alveoli, and (3) increased sympathetic nervous system activity to enhance tissue oxygen delivery by increasing cardiac output. With chronic hypoxemia, there is also an increase in erythrocyte mass to improve the oxygen-carrying capacity of blood.

Carbon Dioxide Elimination The adequacy of alveolar ventilation relative to the metabolic production of carbon dioxide is reflected by the Pa_{CO_2} (**Table 9-15**). The efficacy of carbon dioxide transfer across alveolar-capillary membranes is reflected by the V_D/V_T. This ratio depicts areas in the lungs that receive adequate ventilation but inadequate or no pulmonary blood flow. Ventilation to these alveoli is described as "wasted ventilation." Normally, the V_D/V_T is less than 0.3 but may increase to 0.6 or more when there is an increase in wasted ventilation. An increased V_D/V_T occurs in the presence of acute respiratory failure, decreased cardiac output (e.g., due

TABLE 9–15 Mechanisms of Hypercarbia

Mechanism	Pa_{CO_2}	V_D/V_T	$PA_{O_2} - Pa_{O_2}$
Drug overdose	Increased	Normal	Normal
Restrictive lung disease (kyphoscoliosis)	Increased	Normal to increased	Normal to increased
Chronic obstructive pulmonary disease	Increased	Increased	Increased
Neuromuscular disease	Increased	Normal to increased	Normal to increased

$PA_{O_2} - Pa_{O_2}$, alveolar-arterial difference in partial pressure of oxygen; V_D/V_T, deadspace ventilation/tidal volume ratio.

to anesthetic drugs or hypovolemia), and pulmonary embolism.

Hypercarbia is defined as Pa_{CO_2} greater than 45 mm Hg. Permissive hypercapnia is the strategy of allowing the Pa_{CO_2} to increase up to 55 mm Hg in spontaneously breathing patients to avoid or delay the need for tracheal intubation and mechanical ventilation. Symptoms and signs of hypercarbia depend on the rate of increase and the ultimate level of Pa_{CO_2}. Acute increases in Pa_{CO_2} are associated with increased cerebral blood flow and increased intracranial pressure. Extreme increases in the Pa_{CO_2} to more than 80 mm Hg may result in central nervous system depression and seizures.

Mixed Venous Partial Pressure of Oxygen The mixed venous partial pressure of oxygen (Pv_{O_2}) and the arterial-to-venous oxygen difference ($Ca_{O_2} - Cv_{O_2}$) reflect the overall adequacy of the oxygen transport system (cardiac output) relative to tissue oxygen extraction. For example, a decrease in cardiac output that occurs in the presence of unchanged tissue oxygen consumption causes the Pv_{O_2} to decrease and the $Ca_{O_2} - Cv_{O_2}$ to increase. These changes reflect the continued extraction of the same amount of oxygen by the tissues during a time of decreased tissue blood flow. A Pv_{O_2} less than 30 mm Hg or a $Ca_{O_2} - Cv_{O_2}$ higher than 6 mL/dL indicates the need to increase the cardiac output to facilitate tissue oxygenation. A pulmonary artery catheter permits sampling of mixed venous blood, measurement of Pv_{O_2}, and calculation of Cv_{O_2}.

Arterial pH Measurements of pH_a are necessary to detect acidemia or alkalemia. Metabolic acidosis predictably accompanies arterial hypoxemia and inadequate delivery of oxygen to tissues. Acidemia due to respiratory or metabolic derangements is associated with dysrhythmias and pulmonary hypertension.

Alkalemia is often associated with mechanical hyperventilation and diuretic use leading to loss of chloride and potassium ions. The incidence of dysrhythmias may be increased by metabolic or respiratory alkalosis. The presence of alkalemia in patients recovering from acute respiratory failure can delay or prevent successful weaning from mechanical ventilation because of the compensatory hypoventilation that will occur in an effort to correct the pH disturbance.

Intrapulmonary Shunt Right-to-left intrapulmonary shunting occurs when there is perfusion of alveoli that are not ventilated. The net effect is a decrease in Pa_{O_2}, reflecting dilution of oxygen in blood exposed to ventilated alveoli with blood containing less oxygen coming from unventilated alveoli. Calculation of the shunt fraction provides a reliable assessment of ventilation-to-perfusion matching and serves as a useful estimate of the response to various therapeutic interventions during treatment of acute respiratory failure.

Physiologic shunt normally comprises 2% to 5% of the cardiac output. This degree of right-to-left intrapulmonary shunting reflects the passage of pulmonary arterial blood directly to the left side of the circulation through the bronchial and thebesian veins. It should be appreciated that determination of the shunt fraction in patients breathing less than 100% oxygen reflects the contribution of ventilation-to-perfusion mismatching and the right-to-left intrapulmonary shunt. Calculation of the shunt fraction from measurements obtained with patients breathing 100% oxygen eliminates the contribution of ventilation-to-perfusion mismatching.

PULMONARY EMBOLISM

Surgery predisposes patients to pulmonary embolism even as late as 1 month postoperatively and despite significant advances in the prophylaxis and diagnosis of deep vein thrombosis, the mortality and recurrence rate of pulmonary embolism remain high.

Diagnosis

Accurate detection of pulmonary embolism remains difficult, and the differential diagnosis is extensive (**Table 9-16**). Pulmonary embolism can accompany as well as mimic other cardiopulmonary illnesses. Clinical manifestations of pulmonary embolism are nonspecific, and the diagnosis is often difficult to establish on clinical grounds alone (**Table 9-17**). The most consistent symptom of acute pulmonary embolism is acute dyspnea. Pleuritic or substernal chest pain, cough, or hemoptysis suggest pulmonary infarction due to a small embolism near the pleural surface. Tachypnea and tachycardia are the most common signs of pulmonary embolism but are also nonspecific. Other physical findings include wheezing, fever, rales, a pleural rub, a loud pulmonic component of the second heart sound, a right ventricular lift, and bulging neck veins. Arterial blood gases can be normal and arterial hypoxemia and hypocapnia (stimulation of airway irritant receptors causes hyperventilation) are not specific for pulmonary embolism. In the presence of a patent foramen ovale or atrial septal defect, paradoxical embolization may occur and interatrial right-to-left shunting of blood may cause severe hypoxemia. Electrocardiographic findings in the majority of patients with acute pulmonary embolism include ST-T wave changes and right-axis deviation. Peaked P waves, atrial fibrillation and right bundle branch block may be present if the pulmonary embolism is sufficiently large to cause acute cor pulmonale. The principal utility of the electrocardiogram is to help

TABLE 9-16 Differential Diagnosis of Pulmonary Embolism
Myocardial infarction
Pericarditis
Congestive heart failure
Chronic obstructive pulmonary disease
Pneumonia
Pneumothorax
Pleuritis
Thoracic herpes zoster
Anxiety/hyperventilation syndrome
Thoracic aorta dissection
Rib fractures

TABLE 9-17 Signs and Symptoms of Pulmonary Embolism	
Sign/Symptom	Incidence (%)
Acute dyspnea	75
Tachypnea (>20 breaths per minute)	70
Pleuritic chest pain	65
Rales	50
Nonproductive cough	40
Tachycardia (>100 bpm)	30
Accentuation of pulmonic component of second heart sound	25
Hemoptysis	15
Fever (38°–39°C)	10
Homans' sign	5

distinguish between pulmonary embolism and acute myocardial infarction or other alternative diagnoses.

Transthoracic echocardiography is particularly useful in critically ill patients suspected of having pulmonary embolism and can help identify right ventricular pressure overload as well as myocardial infarction, dissection of the aorta, and pericardial tamponade, which may mimic pulmonary embolism.

Manifestations of pulmonary embolism during anesthesia are nonspecific and often transient. Changes suggestive of pulmonary embolism during anesthesia include unexplained arterial hypoxemia, hypotension, tachycardia, and bronchospasm. The electrocardiogram and central venous pressure may indicate the onset of pulmonary hypertension and right ventricular dysfunction.

Capnography will demonstrate a decrease in end-tidal carbon dioxide and an increased alveolar-to-arterial difference for carbon dioxide. This represents an increase in dead-space ventilation. Transesophageal echocardiography may show acute dilation of the right atrium and right ventricle, pulmonary arterial hypertension, and occasionally even thrombus in the main pulmonary arteries.

Laboratory testing that aids in the diagnosis of acute pulmonary embolism includes the D-dimer test. A positive D-dimer test means that a pulmonary embolism is possible. A negative D-dimer test strongly suggests that thromboembolism is absent (negative predictive value > 99%). Troponin levels may also be elevated and may represent right ventricular myocyte damage due to acute right ventricular strain.

Spiral computed tomography scanning with contrast is useful for diagnosing both acute and chronic pulmonary embolism and has replaced ventilation-perfusion scanning in many centers. It is most useful in detecting clot in the main, lobar, and segmental arteries and is much less sensitive in detecting emboli in smaller blood vessels. However, it is these larger emboli that are most important clinically.

Pulmonary arteriography is the gold standard for the diagnosis of pulmonary embolism. It is used when pulmonary embolism must be diagnosed or excluded and other preliminary testing has been inconclusive.

Ventilation-perfusion lung scanning and ultrasonography of leg veins are other noninvasive tests that can aid in the diagnosis of deep vein thrombosis and/or pulmonary embolism.

Treatment

Treatment options for acute pulmonary embolism include anticoagulation, thrombolytic therapy, inferior vena caval filter placement, and surgical embolectomy.

Heparin remains the cornerstone of treatment for acute pulmonary embolism. An intravenous bolus of unfractionated heparin (5,000–10,000 units) followed by a continuous intravenous infusion should be administered immediately to any patient considered to have a high clinical likelihood of pulmonary embolism. An alternative is low molecular weight heparin given subcutaneously. The optimal duration of anticoagulation after pulmonary embolism remains uncertain, but it is known that a treatment period of 6 months prevents far more recurrences than a treatment period of 6 weeks. This extended anticoagulation is usually accomplished with warfarin in a dose that maintains an international normalized ratio of 2.0 to 3.0.

Patients who cannot be anticoagulated, have significant bleeding while being anticoagulated, or have recurrent pulmonary emboli despite being anticoagulated may require insertion of a vena caval filter to prevent lower extremity thrombi from becoming pulmonary emboli.

Thrombolytic therapy may be considered to hasten dissolution of pulmonary emboli especially if there is hemodynamic instability or severe hypoxemia. Hemorrhage is the principal adverse effect of thrombolytic therapy, and so this treatment is contraindicated in patients at high risk of bleeding.

The hypotension caused by a pulmonary embolism may require treatment with inotropes such as dopamine and dobutamine or a vasoconstrictor such as norepinephrine. A pulmonary vasodilator may be needed to help control pulmonary hypertension. Tracheal intubation and mechanical ventilation may be necessary. Analgesics to treat the pain associated with pulmonary embolism are important but must be administered very carefully because of the underlying cardiovascular instability. Pulmonary artery embolectomy is reserved for patients with a massive pulmonary embolism who are unresponsive to medical therapy and cannot receive thrombolytic therapy.

Management of Anesthesia

Management of anesthesia for the surgical treatment of life-threatening pulmonary embolism is designed to support vital organ function and to minimize anesthetic-induced myocardial depression. Patients typically arrive in the operating room intubated and mechanically ventilated, often with a high FIO_2. Monitoring of intra-arterial pressure and cardiac filling pressures is necessary. Right atrial filling pressure can be a guide to intravenous fluid administration in an effort to optimize right ventricular filling pressure and stroke volume in the presence of a marked increase in right ventricular afterload. It may be necessary to support cardiac output with inotropic drugs. Catecholamines such as dopamine and dobutamine may increase myocardial contractility but have little effect on pulmonary vascular resistance. The phosphodiesterase inhibitors amrinone and milrinone increase myocardial contractility and are excellent pulmonary artery vasodilators. This combination of effects may be specifically useful in this situation.

Induction and maintenance of anesthesia must avoid any accentuation of arterial hypoxemia, systemic hypotension, and pulmonary hypertension. Anesthesia can be maintained with any drug or combination of drugs that does not produce significant myocardial depression. Nitrous oxide is not a likely selection, considering the need to administer high concentrations of oxygen and the potential for this drug to increase pulmonary vascular resistance. A nondepolarizing neuromuscular-blocking drug that does not release histamine is best in this situation.

Removal of embolic fragments from the distal pulmonary artery may be facilitated by the application of positive pressure while the surgeon applies suction through the arteriotomy in the main pulmonary artery. Although the cardiopulmonary status of these patients is perilous prior to surgery, significant hemodynamic improvement usually occurs postoperatively.

FAT EMBOLISM

The syndrome of fat embolism typically appears 12 to 72 hours (lucid interval) after long-bone fractures, especially of the femur or tibia. Fat embolism syndrome has also been observed in association with acute pancreatitis, cardiopulmonary bypass, parenteral infusion of lipids, and liposuction. The triad of hypoxemia, mental confusion, and petechiae in patients with tibia or femur fractures should arouse suspicion of fat embolism. Associated pulmonary dysfunction may be limited to arterial hypoxemia (always present) or it may be fulminant, progressing from tachypnea to alveolar capillary leak and acute respiratory distress syndrome. Central nervous system dysfunction ranges from confusion to seizures and coma. Petechiae, especially over the neck, shoulders, and chest, occur in at least 50% of patients with clinical evidence of fat embolism and are thought to be caused by embolic fat rather than by thrombocytopenia or other disorders of coagulation. An increased serum lipase concentration or the presence of lipiduria is suggestive of fat embolism but may also occur after trauma in the absence of a fat embolism. Significant fever and tachycardia are often present. Magnetic resonance imaging can show the characteristic cerebral lesions during the acute stage of fat embolism syndrome.

The source of fat producing a fat embolism most likely represents disruption of the adipose architecture of bone marrow. The pathophysiology of fat embolism syndrome relates to obstruction of blood vessels by fat particles and the deleterious effects of free fatty acids released from the fat particles as a result of lipase activity. These free fatty acids can cause an acute, diffuse vasculitis especially of the cerebral and pulmonary vasculature. Treatment of fat embolism syndrome includes management of acute respiratory distress syndrome and immobilization of long-bone fractures. Prophylactic administration of corticosteroids for patients at risk may be useful, but the efficacy of corticosteroids for the established syndrome has not been documented. Conceptually, corticosteroids could decrease the incidence of fat embolism syndrome by limiting the endothelial damage caused by free fatty acids.

LUNG TRANSPLANTATION

The four principal approaches to lung transplantation are (1) single-lung transplantation, (2) bilateral sequential lung transplantation, (3) heart-lung transplantation, and (4) transplantation of lobes from living donors. **Table 9-18** lists the typical indications for lung transplantation.

The presence of cor pulmonale is not an indication for heart-lung transplantation because recovery of right ventricular function is typically rapid and complete after lung transplantation alone. In patients with pulmonary hypertension, high vascular resistance in the remaining native lung requires the allograft to handle nearly the entire cardiac output. This could result in reperfusion pulmonary edema and poor allograft function in the immediate postoperative period. Fibrotic

TABLE 9–18 Indications for Lung Transplantation
1. Chronic obstructive pulmonary disease
2. Cystic fibrosis
3. Idiopathic pulmonary fibrosis
4. Primary pulmonary hypertension
5. Bronchiectasis
6. Eisenmenger's syndrome
7. Retransplantation
Adapted from Singh H, Bossard RF: Perioperative anaesthetic considerations for patients undergoing lung transplantation. Can J Anaesth 1997;44:284–299.

lung disease responds well to single lung transplantation because both ventilation and perfusion are distributed preferentially to the transplanted lung. Bilateral sequential lung transplantation involves the sequential performance of two single-lung transplants at one time. In the absence of severe pulmonary hypertension, cardiopulmonary bypass can usually be avoided by ventilating the contralateral lung during each implantation. The primary indications for double lung transplantation are cystic fibrosis and other forms of bronchiectasis. Immunosuppression is initiated intraoperatively and continued for life.

Management of Anesthesia

Management of anesthesia for lung transplantation invokes the same principles followed when pneumonectomy is performed.

Preoperative

Physiologically, patients selected for lung transplantation most often have restrictive lung disease and a large $P_{AO_2} - Pa_{O_2}$. These patients generally have irreversible and progressive pulmonary disease. (Malignancy is regarded as a contraindication to transplantation because of the risk of cancer recurrence with immunosuppression.) Mild to moderate degrees of pulmonary hypertension and some degree of right heart failure are often present. Smokers should have quit smoking at least 6 to 12 months before transplantation. The ability of the right ventricle to maintain an adequate stroke volume in the presence of the acute increase in pulmonary vascular resistance produced by clamping the pulmonary artery before pneumonectomy needs to be evaluated. Evaluation of oxygen dependence, steroid use, hematologic and biochemical analyses, and tests of lung and other major organ system function are also required.

Intraoperative

Posterolateral thoracotomy is performed for single lung transplantation and bilateral anterothoracosternotomy for bilateral/sequential single lung transplantation. Cardiopulmonary bypass may be needed if cardiac or respiratory instability develops. The lung with poorer perfusion is removed for single lung transplantation. Monitoring includes intra-arterial and pulmonary artery catheters. Pulmonary artery pressure monitoring is especially important. During surgery, care must be taken to make sure that the pulmonary artery catheter is withdrawn from the pulmonary artery to be stapled and refloated to the nonoperative lung. Transesophageal echocardiographic monitoring can be used to evaluate right and left ventricular function and fluid balance. There are no specific recommendations regarding drugs for induction and maintenance of anesthesia and skeletal muscle paralysis for lung transplantation. Drug-induced histamine release is undesirable, whereas drug-induced bronchodilation is useful.

The trachea is intubated with a double-lumen endobronchial tube, and its proper placement is verified by fiberoptic bronchoscopy. Intraoperative problems may include arterial hypoxemia, especially during one-lung ventilation. Continuous positive airway pressure to the nondependent lung, PEEP to the dependent lung, or some form of differential lung ventilation may be needed to minimize intrapulmonary shunting. Severe pulmonary hypertension and right ventricular failure can occur when the pulmonary artery is clamped. Infusion of a pulmonary vasodilator such as prostacyclin or inhalation of nitric oxide may be helpful for controlling pulmonary hypertension. In extreme cases, support with partial cardiopulmonary bypass is required. Connection of the donor lung to the recipient is usually in the sequence of pulmonary veins to the left atrium anastomosis of the pulmonary artery and finally bronchial anastomosis, often with an omental wrap.

Postoperative

Postoperative mechanical ventilation is continued as needed. The principal causes of mortality with lung transplantation are bronchial dehiscence and respiratory failure due to sepsis or rejection. The denervated donor lung deprives patients of normal cough reflexes from the lower airways and predisposes to the development of pneumonia. In the absence of rejection, pulmonary function tests are usually normal.

Physiologic Effects of Lung Transplantation

Single or bilateral lung transplantation in patients with end-stage lung disease can dramatically improve lung function. Peak improvement is usually achieved within 3 to 6 months. Arterial oxygenation rapidly returns to normal, and supplemental oxygen is no longer needed. In patients with pulmonary vascular disease, both single and bilateral lung transplantation result in immediate and sustained normalization of pulmonary vascular resistance and pulmonary artery pressure. This is accompanied by a prompt increase in cardiac output and a gradual remodeling of the right ventricle with a decrease in ventricular wall thickness. Exercise capacity improves sufficiently to permit most lung transplant patients to resume an active lifestyle.

The innervation, lymphatics, and bronchial circulation are disrupted when the donor pneumonectomy is performed. The principal effect of lung denervation is loss of the cough reflex, which places patients at risk of aspiration and pulmonary infection. Mucociliary clearance is impaired during the early postoperative period. Lymphatic drainage disrupted by transection of the trachea and bronchi may be reestablished during the first 2 to 4 weeks postoperatively. Often a blunted ventilatory response to carbon dioxide persists even though pulmonary function improves. Denervation of the heart is another consideration in patients undergoing heart-lung transplantation.

Complications of Lung Transplantation

Mild transient pulmonary edema is common in a newly transplanted lung. However, in some patients, pulmonary edema is sufficiently severe to cause a form of acute respiratory failure termed *primary graft failure.* The diagnosis is confirmed by infiltrates seen on chest radiographs and severe hypoxemia during the first 72 hours postoperatively. Treatment is supportive and includes mechanical ventilation. Mortality is high.

Dehiscence of the bronchial anastomosis mandates immediate surgical correction or retransplantation. Stenosis of the bronchial anastomosis is the most common airway complication and typically occurs several weeks after transplantation. Evidence of clinically significant airway stenosis includes focal wheezing, recurrent lower respiratory tract infection, and suboptimal pulmonary function.

The rate of infection in lung-transplant recipients is several times higher than that in recipients of other transplanted organs and is most likely related to exposure of the allograft to the external environment. Bacterial infection of the lower respiratory tract is the most common manifestation of pulmonary infection. A ubiquitous organism acquired by inhalation is *Aspergillus*, which frequently colonizes the airways of lung-transplant recipients. Clinical infection with *Aspergillus* develops in only a small number of these patients, however.

Acute rejection of a lung allograft is a common event and is usually seen during the first 100 days following transplantation. Clinical manifestations are nonspecific and include malaise, low-grade fever, dyspnea, impaired oxygenation, and leukocytosis. Transbronchial lung biopsy is needed for a definitive diagnosis. Treatment of acute rejection consists of intravenous methylprednisolone. Most patients have a prompt clinical response, although histologic evidence of rejection may persist even in the absence of clinical symptoms and signs.

Chronic rejection is manifested as bronchiolitis obliterans, a fibroproliferative process that targets the small airways and leads to submucosal fibrosis and luminal obliteration. Bronchiolitis obliterans is uncommon during the first 6 months following transplantation, but its incidence exceeds 60% in patients who survive at least 5 years. The onset of this syndrome is insidious and is characterized by dyspnea, cough, and colonization of the airways with *Pseudomonas aeruginosa*, which produces recurrent bouts of purulent tracheobronchitis. The overall prognosis is poor. Retransplantation is the only definitive treatment for severe bronchiolitis obliterans.

Anesthetic Considerations in Lung Transplant Recipients

Anesthetic considerations in patients requiring surgery following lung transplantation should focus on (1) the function of the transplanted lung, (2) the possibility of rejection or infection in the transplanted lung, (3) the effect of immunosuppressive therapy on other organ systems and the effect of other organ system dysfunction on the transplanted lung, (4) the disease in the native lung, and (5) the planned surgical procedure and its likely effects on the lungs.

Preoperative

Evaluation before surgery includes eliciting a history suggestive of rejection or infection, auscultation of the lungs (normally clear), and evaluation of pulmonary function tests, arterial blood gases, and chest radiographs. If rejection or infection is suspected, elective surgery should be postponed.

The side effects of immunosuppressive drugs should be noted. Hypertension and renal dysfunction related to cyclosporine are present in many patients.

Because transplanted lungs may have ongoing rejection that can adversely affect pulmonary function, it is recommended that spirometry be performed preoperatively. It may be difficult to differentiate between chronic rejection and infection. With chronic rejection, the FEV_1, vital capacity, and total lung capacity decrease and arterial blood gases show an increased alveolar-to-arterial oxygen gradient, but carbon dioxide retention is rare. Bronchiolitis obliterans usually presents as a nonproductive cough developing after the third month following transplantation. Symptoms can mimic URI and include fever and fatigue. Dyspnea occurs within months and is followed by a clinical course similar to that of COPD. Chest radiography shows peribronchial and interstitial infiltrates.

Premedication is acceptable if pulmonary function is adequate. Hypercarbia is common during the early posttransplantation period. This is an increased sensitivity to opioids. Antisialagogues can be useful since secretions can be excessive. Supplemental corticosteroids may be needed for long, stressful surgical procedures. A major cause of morbidity and mortality in transplant recipients is infection. Prophylactic antibiotics are indicated, and strict aseptic technique is required for placement of intravascular catheters. Lung denervation has limited effects on the pattern of breathing, but bronchial hyperreactivity and bronchoconstriction are common. Denervation ablates afferent sensation below the level of the tracheal anastomosis. Patients lose the cough reflex and are prone to retention of secretions and silent aspiration. Response to carbon dioxide rebreathing is normal.

Intraoperative

Because lung transplant recipients lack a cough reflex below the tracheal anastomosis, they do not clear secretions unless they are awake. Because of the diminished cough reflex, the potential for bronchoconstriction, and the increased risk of pulmonary infection, it is recommended that regional anesthesia be selected whenever possible. Epidural and spinal anesthesia are acceptable. However, depression of intercostal muscle function may have special implications in these patients. The performance of any nerve block carries a risk of introducing infection. The importance of sterile technique in this high-risk population cannot be overemphasized. Fluid preloading before a spinal or epidural block may be risky in patients with a transplanted lung because disruption of the lymphatic drainage in the transplanted lung causes interstitial fluid accumulation. This is particularly problematic during the early posttransplantation period.

In heart-lung transplant recipients, fluid management may be a particular challenge because the heart requires adequate preload to maintain cardiac output, but the lungs have a lower threshold for developing pulmonary edema. In this situation, invasive monitoring may be very useful, but the benefits must be balanced against the risk of infection. Transesophageal echocardiography can be useful for monitoring volume status and cardiac function. If a central venous catheter is inserted via the internal jugular vein, it is prudent to select the internal jugular vein on the side of the native lung. Cardiac denervation is another consideration in patients who have undergone heart-lung transplantation. These patients may develop intraoperative bradycardia that does not respond to atropine. Epinephrine and/or isoproterenol may be required to increase the heart rate.

An important goal of anesthetic management is prompt recovery of adequate respiratory function and early tracheal extubation. Volatile anesthetics are well tolerated, and nitrous oxide is acceptable in the absence of bullous disease. Immunosuppressive drugs may interact with neuromuscular-blocking drugs, and the impaired renal function caused by immunosuppressive drugs may prolong the effects of certain muscle relaxants. The effects of nondepolarizing neuromuscular blockers are routinely antagonized pharmacologically because even minimal residual weakness can compromise ventilation in these patients.

When positioning an endotracheal tube, it is best to place the cuff just beyond the vocal cords to minimize the risk of traumatizing the tracheal anastomosis. Inadvertent endobronchial intubation of the native or transplanted lung must be avoided. If the surgical procedure requires a double-lumen endobronchial tube, it is preferable to place the endobronchial portion of the tube in the native bronchus, thus avoiding contact with the tracheal anastomosis. Positive-pressure ventilation in the presence of a single-lung transplant may be complicated by differences in lung compliance between the native and transplanted lung.

KEY POINTS

- Patients with preoperative respiratory disease are at increased risk of both intraoperative and postoperative respiratory complications.

- The anesthetic management of patients with a recent URI should be focused on reducing secretions and limiting manipulation of a potentially hyperresponsive airway.

- Asthma treatment has two components. The first is the use of controller treatments, which modify the airway environment such that acute airway narrowing occurs less frequently. Controller treatments include inhaled and systemic corticosteroids, theophylline, and antileukotrienes. The other component of asthma treatment is the use of reliever or rescue agents for acute bronchospasm. Reliever treatments include β-adrenergic agonists and anticholinergics drugs.

- In asthmatic patients, the goal during induction and maintenance of anesthesia is to depress airway reflexes sufficiently to avoid bronchoconstriction in response to mechanical stimulation of the airway.

- Cessation of smoking and long-term oxygen therapy are the only two therapeutic interventions that may favorably alter the natural progression of COPD associated with hypoxemia.

- Pulmonary function tests have limited value in predicting the likelihood of postoperative pulmonary complications, and the results of pulmonary function tests alone should not be used to deny patients surgery.

- Patients with COPD need to be ventilated with slow respiratory rates to allow sufficient time for exhalation to occur. This minimizes the risk of air-trapping and auto-PEEP.

- In patients with COPD, prophylaxis against the development of postoperative pulmonary complications is based on restoring diminished lung volumes, especially FRC, and facilitating production of an effective cough to remove airway secretions.

- The most effective treatment for aspiration pneumonitis is delivery of supplemental oxygen and institution of PEEP.

- The acute phase of ARDS manifests as the rapid onset of respiratory failure accompanied by arterial hypoxemia refractory to treatment and radiographic findings indistinguishable from those of cardiogenic pulmonary edema. This acute phase usually resolves completely, but in some patients, it may progress to fibrosing alveolitis with persistent arterial hypoxemia and decreased pulmonary compliance. The recovery or resolution phase of ARDS is characterized by gradual resolution of the hypoxemia and improved lung compliance.

- Treatment options for acute pulmonary embolism include anticoagulation, thrombolytic therapy, inferior vena caval filter placement, and surgical embolectomy.

- The principal effect of lung denervation as a result of lung transplantation is loss of the cough reflex, which places patients at risk of aspiration and pulmonary infection.

- In heart-lung transplant recipients, fluid management is a challenge as the heart requires adequate preload to maintain cardiac output, but the lungs have a low threshold for developing pulmonary edema.

REFERENCES

Arcasoy SM, Kotloff RM: Lung transplantation. N Engl J Med 1999;340:1081–1091.

Barrera R, Shi W, Amar D, et al: Smoking and timing of cessation: Impact on pulmonary complications after thoracotomy. Chest 2005;127:1977–1983.

Benumof J (ed): Anesthesia for Thoracic Surgery. Philadelphia, WB Saunders, 1995.

Bishop MJ, Cheney FW: Anesthesia for patients with asthma: Low risk but not no risk. Anesthesiology 1996;85:455–456.

Campbell NN: Respiratory tract infection and anesthesia. *Haemophilus influenzae* pneumonia that developed under anaesthesia. Anaesthesia 1990;45:561–562.

Goldhaber SZ, Elliott CG: Acute pulmonary embolism: Part I: Epidemiology, pathophysiology and diagnosis. Circulation 2003;108:2726–2729.

Goldhaber SZ, Elliott CG: Acute pulmonary embolism: Part II: Stratification, treatment and prevention. Circulation 2003;108:2834–2838.

Heikkinen T, Järvinen A: The common cold. Lancet 2003;361:51–59.

Kain ZN: Myths in pediatric anesthesia. ASA Refresher Courses Anesthesiol 2004;32:121–134.

Kostopanagiotou GMDP, Smyrniotis VMDP, Arkadopoulos NMD, et al: Anesthetic and perioperative management of adult transplant recipients in nontransplant surgery. Anesth Analg 1999;89:613–622.

Kroenke K, Lawrence VA, Theroux JF, et al: Postoperative complications after thoracic and major abdominal surgery in patients with and without obstructive lung disease. Chest 1993;104:1445–1451.

Mellor A, Soni N: Fat embolism. Anaesthesia 2001;56:145–154.

Pullerits J, Holzman R: Anaesthesia for patients with mediastinal masses. Can J Anesth 1989;36:681–688.

Qaseem A, Snow V, Fitterman N, et al: Risk assessment for and strategies to reduce perioperative pulmonary complications for patients undergoing noncardiothoracic surgery: A guideline from the American College of Physicians. Ann Intern Med 2006;144:575–580.

Ramsey BW: Management of pulmonary disease in patients with cystic fibrosis. N Engl J Med 1996;335:179–188.

Schreiner MS, O'Hara I, Markakis DA, Politis GD: Do children who experience laryngospasm have an increased risk of upper respiratory tract infection? Anesthesiology 1996;85:475–480.

Singh H, Bossard RF: Perioperative anaesthetic considerations for patients undergoing lung transplantation. Can J Anesth 1997;44:284–299.

Smetana GW: Preoperative pulmonary evaluation. N Engl J Med 1999;340:937–944.

Smetana GW, Lawrence VA, Cornell JE: Preoperative pulmonary risk stratification for noncardiothoracic surgery: A systematic review for the American College of Physicians. Ann Intern Med 2006;144:581–595.

Smith AD, Cowan JO, Brassett KP, et al: Use of exhaled nitric oxide measurements to guide treatment in chronic asthma. N Engl J Med 2005;352:2163–2173.

Steinbrook R: How best to ventilate? Trial design and patient safety in studies of the acute respiratory distress syndrome. N Engl J Med 2003;348:1393–1401.

Tait AR: Anesthetic management of the child with an upper respiratory tract infection. Curr Opin Anesthesiol 2005;18:603–607.

The National Heart Lung and Blood Institute Acute Respiratory Distress Syndrome Clinical Trials Network: Efficacy and safety of corticosteroids for persistent acute respiratory distress syndrome. N Engl J Med 2006;354:1671–1684.

Ware LB, Matthay MA: Acute pulmonary edema. N Engl J Med 2005;353:2788–2796.

Warner DO: Helping surgical patients quit smoking: Why, when, and how. Anesth Analg 2005;101:481–487

Diseases Affecting the Brain

Jeffrey J. Pasternak
William L. Lanier, Jr.

Neuro-ocular Disorders
- Leber's Optic Atrophy
- Retinitis Pigmentosa
- Kearns-Sayer Syndrome

- Ischemic Optic Neuropathy
- Cortical Blindness
- Retinal Artery Occlusion
- Ophthalmic Venous Obstruction

Patients with diseases affecting the brain and central nervous system may undergo surgery to treat the disease or its associated conditions, whereas in others, the need for surgery is unrelated to the nervous system disease. Regardless of the reason for surgery, co-existing nervous system diseases often have important implications when selecting anesthetic drugs, techniques, and monitors. Concepts of cerebral protection and resuscitation may assume unique importance in these patients. This chapter reviews these issues plus various diseases of the retina and optic nerve.

CEREBRAL BLOOD FLOW, BLOOD VOLUME, AND METABOLISM

Generally, cerebral blood flow (CBF) is governed by cerebral metabolic rate, cerebral perfusion pressure (CPP) (defined as the difference between the mean arterial pressure [MAP] and intracranial pressure [ICP]), arterial blood carbon dioxide ($Paco_2$) and oxygen (Pao_2) tensions, the influence of various drugs, and intracranial pathology. CBF is normally autoregulated or is constant over a given range of CPPs. In a healthy adult, CBF is approximately 50 mL/100 g brain tissue per minute over a CPP range of 50 to 150 mm Hg.

Normal cerebral metabolic rate, generally measured as rate of oxygen consumption ($CMRO_2$), is 3.0 to 3.8 mL O_2/100 g brain tissue per minute. It can be decreased by temperature reductions and various anesthetic agents and increased by temperature increases and seizures.

Anesthetic and intensive care management of neurologically impaired patients relies heavily on manipulating intracranial volume and pressure. These, in turn, are influenced by CBV, but not directly, as often assumed, by CBF. Indeed, CBF and CBV do not always change in parallel. For example, vasodilatory anesthetics and hypercapnia may produce parallel increases in CBF and CBV. Conversely, moderate systemic hypotension can produce reductions in CBF, but as a result of compensatory vessel dilation, increases in CBV. Similarly, partial occlusion of an intracranial artery (e.g., as occurs in embolic stroke) may reduce regional CBF. However, vessel dilation distal to the occlusion, which is an attempt to restore circulation, can produce increases in CBV.

Arterial Carbon Dioxide Partial Pressure

Variations in $Paco_2$ produce corresponding changes in CBF (**Fig. 10A-1**). As a guideline, CBF (normal ~50 mL/100 g brain tissue per minute) increases 1 mL/100 g per minute for every 1 mm Hg increase in the $Paco_2$. A similar decrease occurs during hypocarbia, such that CBF is decreased approximately 50% when the $Paco_2$ is acutely lower to 20 mm Hg. The impact of $Paco_2$ on CBF is mediated by variations in cerebrospinal fluid (CSF) pH around the walls of arterioles. Decreased CSF pH causes cerebral vasodilation, and increased CSF pH results in vasoconstriction. Corresponding changes in resistance to blood flow exerts predictable effects on CBF. $Paco_2$ also modulates CBV, with the extent of CBV reduction dependent on the background anesthetic. In general, vasoconstricting anesthetics tend to attenuate the effects of $Paco_2$ on CBV.

The ability of hypocapnia to acutely decrease CBF, CBV, and ICP is fundamental to the practice of clinical neuroanesthesia. Concern that cerebral hypoxia due to vasoconstriction can occur when the $Paco_2$ is lowered to less than 20 mm Hg has not been substantiated. The ability of hypocapnia to decrease CBV, and thus ICP, is attenuated by the return of CSF pH to normal after prolonged periods of hypocapnia. This reduces the effectiveness of induced hypocapnia as a means of long-term control of intracranial hypertension. This adaptive change, which reflects active transport of bicarbonate ions into or from the CSF, requires approximately 6 hours to return the CSF pH to normal.

Arterial Oxygen Partial Pressure

Decreased Pao_2 does not significantly affect CBF until a threshold value of approximately 50 mm Hg is reached (see Fig. 10A-1). Below this threshold, there is abrupt cerebral vasodilation, and the CBF increases. Furthermore, the combination of arterial hypoxemia and hypercarbia exerts a synergistic effect, with increases in CBF that exceed the increase that would be produced by either factor alone.

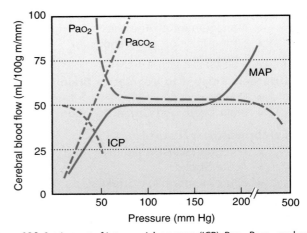

Figure 10A-1 • Impact of intracranial pressure (ICP), Pao_2, $Paco_2$, and mean arterial pressure (MAP) on cerebral blood flow.

Cerebral Perfusion Pressure and Cerebral Autoregulation

The ability of the brain to maintain CBF at constant levels, despite changes in CPP, is known as autoregulation (see Fig. 10A-1). Autoregulation is an active vascular response characterized by (1) arterial constriction when the blood pressure is increased and (2) arterial dilation in response to decreases in systemic blood pressure. For example, in normotensive patients, the lower limit of CPP associated with autoregulation is believed to be approximately 50 mm Hg, although the exact value is controversial. Below this threshold, cerebral blood vessels are maximally vasodilated and the CBF decreases, becoming directly related to CPP (i.e., pressure-dependent blood flow). Indeed, at a CPP of 30 to 45 mm Hg, symptoms of cerebral ischemia may appear in the form of nausea, dizziness, and slow cerebration. Autoregulation of CBF also has an upper limit, above which the flow becomes directly proportional to the CPP. This upper limit of autoregulation in normotensive patients is believed to be a CPP of approximately 150 mm Hg. Above this threshold, the cerebral blood vessels are maximally constricted, and thereafter CBF increases, becoming pressure dependent. This results in overdistention of the walls of the cerebral blood vessels. As a result, fluid may be forced across vessel walls into the brain tissue, producing cerebral edema.

Autoregulation of CBF is altered in the presence of chronic hypertension. Specifically, the autoregulation curve is displaced to the right, such that pressure dependence of CBF occurs at a higher CPP at both the upper and lower thresholds of autoregulation. The adaptation of cerebral vessels to increased blood pressure requires some time. Indeed, acute hypertension, as seen in children with acute-onset glomerulonephritis or in patients with short-duration pregnancy-induced hypertension, often produces signs of central nervous system dysfunction at MAP elevations tolerated by patients who are chronically hypertensive. Likewise, in previously normotensive patients, acute hypertensive episodes associated with stimulation produced by direct laryngoscopy or surgery may cause a break down of autoregulation. The lower limit of autoregulation is also shifted upward in chronically hypertensive patients, such that decreases in systemic blood pressure are not tolerated to the same low levels as in normotensive patients. As such, rapid lowering of blood pressure to population-normal values in patients who have been chronically hypertensive (e.g., with the use of vasodilating drugs) can, if excessive, precipitate a stroke. After gradual decreases in systemic blood pressure over time due to antihypertensive drug therapy, however, the tolerance of the brain to hypotension may improve as the autoregulation curve shifts back toward its original position.

Autoregulation of CBF may be lost or impaired in a variety of conditions, including the presence of intracranial tumors or head trauma and the administration of volatile anesthetics. The loss of autoregulation in the blood vessels surrounding intracranial tumors reflects acidosis leading to maximum vasodilation, such that blood flow becomes pressure dependent.

Venous Blood Pressure

Venous blood pressure probably has very little, if any, effect on CPP or CBF, but may profoundly affect CBV. In order for blood to continue to flow out of the cranial vault, ICP must be greater than central venous pressure. Since increases in central venous pressure (CVP) can lead to increases in CBV, increased venous pressure can contribute to increased brain bulk and bleeding during intracranial surgery. Other causes of increased intracranial venous pressure include venous sinus thrombosis or jugular compression due to improper neck positioning such as extreme flexion or rotation. In other situations where chronic elevations in venous pressure exist, such as superior vena cava syndrome, concomitant increases in CBV and ICP will also exist, as intracranial blood attempts to leave the cranial vault and flow down the pressure gradient. In the setting of coughing, where increases in intrathoracic pressure result in increases in CVP, transient cessation of cerebral venous drainage may exist, but this is a brief process. If such patients have tracheal intubation at the time that they attempt to cough or "buck," changes in mean intrathoracic pressure and CVP usually do not occur, given that the glottis is stented open by the presence of the endotracheal tube. In such a setting, ICP can still increase, but as a result of increases in CBF and CBV resulting from muscle afferent–mediated stimulation of the brain, CVP does not increase.

Anesthetic Drugs

During normal physiology, changes in $CMRO_2$ usually lead to concomitant changes in CBF, a concept known as CBF/$CMRO_2$ coupling. In contrast, volatile anesthetics, such as isoflurane, sevoflurane, and desflurane, particularly when administered in concentrations greater than 0.6 to 1.0 minimum alveolar concentration (MAC), are often potent direct cerebral vasodilators that produce dose-dependent increases in CBF despite concomitant decreases in cerebral metabolic oxygen requirements. Below 1 MAC, volatile anesthetics alter CBF minimally, in part because any direct effect of the anesthetic are counterbalanced by CBF/$CMRO_2$ coupling. When volatile anesthetic-induced $CMRO_2$ depression is maximized (i.e., concomitant with maximal depression of cerebral electrical activity), larger doses of volatile anesthetic will continue to dilate cerebral blood vessels. This can lead to increases in CBF, CBV, and possibly ICP. With halothane, which at clinically relevant doses does not induce the extent of $CMRO_2$ depression as seen with other volatile anesthetics (i.e., isoflurane, sevoflurane, desflurane), direct vasodilatory effects predominate, leading to greater increases in CBV at equipotent doses compared to other commonly used volatile agents. This, therefore, can lead to increased ICP, making halothane a less-than-ideal volatile anesthetic agent for neurosurgical procedures in which CBV and ICP management is critical. With all volatile anesthetics, the institution of arterial hypocapnia may help minimize increases in CBV that might accompany administration of these drugs at normocarbia. The same CBV- and ICP-attenuating effects can also be achieved with supplemental vasoconstricting anesthetics (e.g., thiopental or propofol).

In contrast to volatile anesthetics, nitrous oxide has less effect on CBF and does not appear to interfere with autoregulation of CBF. The effect of nitrous oxide on cerebral hemodynamics remains elusive probably because of a wide range of interspecies differences in the MAC of nitrous oxide as well as the presence of other drugs used to maintain general anesthesia in human studies. The initiation of nitrous oxide after closure of the dura may contribute to the development of a tension pneumocephalus given that there is likely air in the intracranial vault following dural closure and nitrous oxide has greater solubility in air than nitrogen, thereby leading to increases in gas volume. Clinically, tension pneumocephalus usually presents as a delayed emergence from general anesthesia following craniotomy.

Like the volatile anesthetics, ketamine has been considered to be a cerebral vasodilator. In contrast to volatile anesthetics and possibly ketamine, barbiturates, etomidate, propofol, and opioids are classified as cerebral vasoconstrictors, provided the patient is not permitted to develop respiratory depression and hypercapnia. Drugs that produce cerebral vasoconstriction predictably decrease CBV and ICP.

Propofol and barbiturates, such as thiopental, are potent cerebral vasoconstrictors capable of decreasing CBF, CBV, and ICP. Opioids are considered cerebral vasoconstrictors, assuming that opioid-induced ventilatory depression is not permitted to manifest as an increase in $Paco_2$.

Administration of nondepolarizing neuromuscular blocking drugs is unlikely to meaningfully alter ICP. However, in addition to adequate general anesthesia, muscle relaxation may help prevent acute increases in ICP due to movement or coughing during direct laryngoscopy. Nevertheless, drug-induced histamine release, as occurs with atracurium, d-tubocurarine, and metocurine, could theoretically produce cerebral vasodilation with associated increases in CBV and ICP, particularly if the drugs are given in large doses and infused rapidly. The use of succinylcholine in the setting of increased ICP may further, but temporarily, increase ICP. The mechanism for this effect is most likely due to increases in muscle afferent activity, a process somewhat independent of visible muscle fasciculations. This can lead to cerebral arousal, as manifested on the electroencephalogram, and corresponding increases in CBF and CBV.

INCREASED INTRACRANIAL PRESSURE

The intracranial and spinal vault contains neural tissue (i.e., brain and spinal cord), blood, and CSF, and is enclosed by the dura mater and bone. The pressure within this space is referred to as the ICP. Under normal conditions, brain tissue, intracranial CSF, and intracranial blood have a combined volume of approximately 1200 to 1500 mL, and normal ICP is usually 5 to 15 mm Hg. Any increase in one component of

intracranial volume must be offset by a decrease in another component to prevent an increase in ICP. Normally, these changes are well compensated; however, eventually a point is reached where even a small change in intracranial contents results in a large change in ICP (**Fig. 10A-2**). This condition is known as increased intracranial elastance. Since CPP depends on ICP, initially homeostatic mechanisms work to increase MAP in an effort to overcome the increase in ICP; however, eventually, this compensatory mechanism can fail, resulting in cerebral ischemia.

Factors leading to alterations in CSF flow or its absorption into the vasculature can often lead to increased ICP. CSF is produced by two mechanisms: (1) ultrafiltration and secretion by the cells of the choroid plexus and (2) via the passage of water, electrolytes, and other substances across the blood-brain barrier. CSF is, therefore, a direct extension of the extracellular fluid compartment of the central nervous system. CSF is produced at a constant rate of 500 to 600 mL/day in adults and is contained within the ventricular system of the brain, the central canal of the spinal cord, and the subarachnoid space, as well as the extracellular compartment of the central nervous system. CSF is absorbed from microscopic arachnoid villi and macroscopic arachnoid granulations within the dura mater, bordering venous sinusoids, and sinuses.

It is important to note that the intracranial vault is considered to be compartmentalized. Specifically, there are various meningeal barriers within the intracranial vault that functionally separate the contents: the falx cerebri (a reflection of dura mater that separates the two cerebral hemispheres) and the tentorium cerebelli (a reflection of dura mater that lies rostral to the cerebellum and marks the border between the supratentorial and infratentorial spaces). Increases in the contents of one region of brain may cause regional increases in ICP

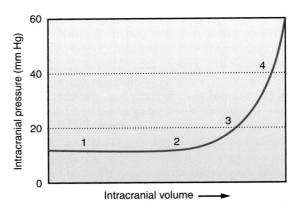

Figure 10A-2 • The intracranial elastance curve depicts the impact of increasing intracranial volume on intracranial pressure (ICP). As intracranial volume increases from point 1 to 2, ICP does not increase because cerebrospinal fluid is shifted from the cranium into the spinal subarachnoid space. Patients on the rising portion of the curve (point 3) can no longer compensate for increases in intracranial volume; the ICP begins to increase and is likely to be associated with clinical symptoms. Additional increases in intracranial volume at this point (point 3), as produced by anesthetic drug-induced increases in cerebral blood volume, can precipitate abrupt increases in ICP (point 4).

increases and cerebral perfusion is limited, decreased levels of consciousness and possibly coma can be observed. Finally, acute increases in ICP may not be tolerated as well as chronic intracranial hypertension.

Increased ICP is often diagnosed clinically based on the symptoms described above, by radiographic means, and by directly measuring ICP. Typically, computed tomography (CT) or magnetic resonance imaging (MRI) will demonstrate different findings depending on the cause. For example, a large mass or hematoma may be evident. If aqueductal stenosis is present, the third, but not fourth, ventricle is enlarged.

Multiple methods are currently available to measure and monitor ICP. The choice of technique depends on the clinical situation. Pressure transducers can be placed under aseptic conditions into the subdural space (known as a subdural bolt), brain parenchyma, or ventricle. This last technique, also known as a ventriculostomy, has the advantage that, in addition to pressure monitoring, it allows the withdrawal of CSF. This is a major benefit in that the drainage system can be organized such that CSF will only drain if the ICP is above a selected value. Such an approach allows some control over ICP. A second advantage of the ventriculostomy is that CSF can be easily obtained for laboratory analysis. A lumbar subarachnoid catheter is another available modality. It offers similar advantages to the ventriculostomy in that CSF can be withdrawn or allowed to passively drain if the ICP increases above a set value. The disadvantage of this technique over the ventriculostomy is related to the compartmentalization of the intracranial contents in that lumbar CSF pressure may not accurately reflect ICP in all circumstances. Of note, there is a risk of tonsillar herniation in certain clinical settings (i.e., tumor) with drainage of CSF via the lumbar subarachnoid approach.

A normal ICP wave is pulsatile and varies with the cardiac impulses and spontaneous breathing. The mean ICP should remain below 15 mm Hg. Abrupt increases in ICP to as high as 100 mm Hg observed during continuous monitoring are characterized as *plateau waves*. During this increase in ICP, patients may become symptomatic of inadequate cerebral perfusion, and spontaneous hyperventilation or changes in mental status may occur. Anxiety and painful stimulation can initiate abrupt increases in ICP.

Methods to Decrease Intracranial Pressure

Methods to decrease ICP include elevating the head; hyperventilating the patient's lungs; CSF drainage; administering hyperosmotic drugs, diuretics, corticosteroids, and cerebral vasoconstricting anesthetics (e.g., barbiturates, propofol); and surgical decompression. It is not possible to identify reliably the level of ICP than can interfere with regional CBF or alter cerebral function and well-being in individual patients. Therefore, a frequent recommendation is to treat any sustained increase in ICP that exceeds 20 mm Hg. Treatment may be indicated when the ICP is less than 20 mm Hg if the appearance of occasional plateau waves suggests the presence of increased intracranial elastance.

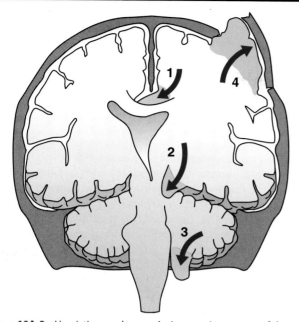

Figure 10A-3 • Herniation syndromes. An increase in contents of the supratentorial space by masses, edema, or hematoma can lead to herniation of (1) the cingulate gyrus under the falx leading to subfalcine herniation, (2) contents over the tentorium cerebelli causing transtentorial herniation, and (3) herniation of the cerebellar tonsils out through the foramen magnum, (4) herniation of brain contents out of a traumatic defect in the cranial cavity. *(Adapted from Fishman RA: Brain edema. N Engl J Med 1975;293:706.)*

and, in extreme instances, the contents of that compartment to move, or herniate, into a different compartment. Various types of herniation syndromes are categorized based on the region of brain affected (**Fig 10A-3**). Herniation of cerebral hemispheric contents under the falx cerebri is referred to a subfalcine herniation. Typically, this condition leads to compression of branches of the anterior cerebral artery and is evident on radiographic imaging as midline shift. Herniation of the supratentorial contents past the tentorium cerebelli is referred to as transtentorial herniation, where evidence of brainstem compression occurs in a rostral to caudal manner resulting in altered consciousness, defects in gaze, afferent ocular reflexes, and, finally, hemodynamic and respiratory compromise followed by death. The uncus (i.e., the medial portion of the temporal lobe) may herniate over the tentorium cerebelli, resulting in a subtype of transtentorial herniation referred to as uncal herniation. A specific sign is ipsilateral oculomotor nerve dysfunction because the oculomotor nerve is compressed against the brainstem, resulting in pupillary dilatation, ptosis, and lateral deviation of the affected eye, which occurs prior to evidence of brainstem compression and death. Herniation of the cerebellar tonsils can occur in the setting of elevated infratentorial pressure, resulting in extension of these cerebellar structures through the foramen magnum. Typical signs involve evidence of medullary dysfunction including cardiorespiratory instability and subsequently death.

Nonspecific signs and symptoms of increased ICP include headache, nausea, vomiting, and papilledema. As ICP

Posture is important for ensuring optimal venous drainage from the brain. For example, elevating the patient's head to approximately 30 degrees above heart level encourages venous outflow from the brain and lowers the ICP. Extreme flexion or rotation of the patient's head can further obstruct the jugular veins and restrict venous outflow from the brain. The head-down position is avoided, as this position can increase the ICP.

Hyperventilation, and hence lowering the $PaCO_2$, is an effective method for rapidly reducing the ICP. In adults a frequent recommendation is to maintain the $PaCO_2$ near 30 to 35 mm Hg. Lowering $PaCO_2$ more may not meaningfully decrease ICP further, yet may result in the accrual in adverse changes in systemic physiology. The optimal $PaCO_2$-related reduction in ICP will be influenced by whether the patient is receiving a background vasodilating versus vasoconstricting anesthetic. Regardless of the anesthetic, the effects of hyperventilation will diminish with time and wane after 6 to 12 hours. When prolonged hyperventilation is discontinued, rebound increases in ICP are a potential problem, especially if normocapnia is rapidly restored.

Draining of CSF from the lateral cerebral ventricles or the lumbar subarachnoid space decreases the intracranial volume and ICP. Lumbar CSF drainage via a catheter is usually reserved for operations in which surgical exposure is difficult, such as surgery on the pituitary gland or intracranial aneurysms. Lumbar CSF drainage is not routinely useful for the treatment of baseline intracranial hypertension, particularly that related to mass lesions, for fear that pressure gradients induced by drainage could result in cerebral herniation. If the cause of increased ICP is chronic, shunting of CSF from an intracranial ventricle is preferred. With chronic treatment, CSF is typically drained to the right atrium (ventriculoatrial shunt) or the peritoneal cavity (ventriculoperitoneal shunt).

Infusion of hyperosmotic drugs, such as mannitol, are effective in decreasing ICP. These drugs produce transient increases in the osmolarity of plasma, which act to draw water from tissues, including the brain. With osmotic diuretics, diuresis and a reduction in systemic blood volume, similar to that occurring with loop diuretics, are important secondary effects. With mannitol (and any other diuresing drug), care should be taken to avoid significant systemic hypovolemia and hypotension as excessive fluid loss can result in hypotension and jeopardize maintenance of adequate CPP. In addition, urinary losses of electrolytes, particularly potassium, may occur, requiring careful monitoring and replacement. Moreover, an intact blood-brain barrier is necessary, so mannitol can exert maximum beneficial effects on brain size. If the blood-brain barrier is disrupted, these drugs may cross into the brain, causing cerebral edema and increases in brain size. The brain eventually adapts to sustained increases in plasma osmolarity, such that long-term use of hyperosmotic drugs is likely to become less effective.

Mannitol is ideally administered in doses of 0.25 to 0.5 g/kg IV over 15 to 30 minutes. Larger initial doses may have little incremental effect on ICP, yet may predispose the patient to rebound increases in ICP. Hence, it is better to give an initial dose of 0.25 to 0.5 g/kg IV, and, if the desired effect is not achieved, either administer another dose or use another type of therapy. Under ideal settings, mannitol results in removal of approximately 100 mL of water from the patient's brain. After administration, decreases in ICP are seen within 30 minutes, and maximum effects occur within 1 to 2 hours. Urine output can reach 1 to 2 L within 1 hour after initiating the administration of mannitol. Appropriate infusion of crystalloid and colloid solutions is often necessary to prevent adverse changes in the plasma concentrations of electrolytes and intravascular fluid volume due to the brisk drug-induced diuresis. Conversely, mannitol can initially increase the intravascular fluid volume, emphasizing the need to carefully monitor those patients who have limited cardiac reserve, such as those with congestive heart failure. Mannitol also has direct vascular vasodilating properties. Interestingly, mannitol can transiently contribute to increased CBV and ICP in those with normal ICP, but in those with intracranial hypertension, mannitol will not further increase ICP. The duration of hyperosmotic effects produced by mannitol is approximately 6 hours.

Loop diuretics, particularly furosemide, have been used to promote decreases in ICP. Furosemide is particularly useful when there is evidence of increased vascular fluid volume and pulmonary edema or in patients who, due to various co-existing diseases such as congestive heart failure and nephrotic syndrome, will not tolerate the initial increase in intravascular volume associated with mannitol. In this instance, promotion of diuresis and systemic dehydration may improve arterial oxygenation along with concomitant decreases in ICP. Furosemide affects plasma osmolarity much less than mannitol, but it can also produce hypokalemia.

Corticosteroids, such as dexamethasone or methylprednisolone, are effective in lowering increased ICP reduction caused by the development of localized vasogenic cerebral edema around brain tumors. The precise mechanism of action is unknown but may involve stabilization of capillary membranes and decreased production of CSF. Patients with brain tumors often exhibit improved neurologic status and disappearance of headache within 12 to 36 hours after initiating therapy. Corticosteroids are also effective in treating increased ICP in patients with pseudotumor cerebri (i.e., benign intracranial hypertension). Conversely, corticosteroids are not effective in reducing ICP with some other forms of intracranial hypertension, such as closed head injury. Of concern, corticosteroids can increase blood glucose concentration, which may adversely affect outcome if ongoing cerebral ischemia is present. As such, corticosteroids are a poor choice for the nonspecific treatment of increased ICP.

Barbiturates in high doses are particularly effective for treating increased ICP that develops after an acute head injury. Propofol may also be useful in this situation. However, patients receiving prolonged propofol infusions, particularly pediatric patients, should be monitored for drug-associated metabolic acidosis, which can be fatal.

Specific Causes of Increased Intracranial Pressure

Increased ICP is typically a sign of underlying intracranial pathology and less commonly produces brain dysfunction independently. Therefore, one should seek the cause of increased ICP in addition to instituting treatment. Causes of increased ICP are many. Tumors can lead to increased ICP either (1) directly because of their size, (2) indirectly by causing edema in normal surrounding brain tissue, or (3) by causing obstruction of CSF flow as is commonly seen with tumors involving the third ventricle. Intracranial hematomas can cause increased ICP in a manner similar to mass lesions. Further, blood in the CSF, as is seen in subarachnoid hemorrhage, may lead to obstruction of CSF reabsorption at the arachnoid villi and granulations and may further exacerbate increased ICP. Infection, such as meningitis or encephalitis, can lead to edema or obstruction of CSF reabsorption. Some causes of intracranial hypertension not discussed elsewhere in this chapter follow.

Aqueductal Stenosis

Stenotic central nervous system lesions that impede CSF flow can lead to increased ICP. Aqueductal stenosis, one of the more common causes of obstructive hydrocephalus, is caused by congenital narrowing of the cerebral aqueduct that connects the third and fourth ventricles. Obstructive hydrocephalus can develop during infancy, when the narrowing is severe. Lesser obstruction results in slowly progressive hydrocephalus, which may not be evident until adulthood. Symptoms of aqueductal stenosis are the same as those seen with other forms of intracranial hypertension. Seizure disorders are present in approximately one third of these patients. CT is useful to confirm the presence of obstructive hydrocephalus. Symptomatic aqueductal stenosis is treated by ventricular shunting. Management of anesthesia for ventricular shunt placement must focus on existing intracranial hypertension.

Benign Intracranial Hypertension

Benign intracranial hypertension (pseudotumor cerebri) is a syndrome characterized by ICP greater than 20 mm Hg, normal CSF composition, normal sensorium, and absence of local intracranial lesions. This disorder typically occurs in obese women with menstrual irregularities. CT scan indicates a normal or even small cerebral ventricular system. Headaches and bilateral visual disturbances typically occur. Of note, symptoms may be exaggerated during pregnancy. Interestingly, no identifiable cause of increased ICP is found in most patients. However, the prognosis is usually excellent.

Acute treatment of benign intracranial hypertension includes removal of 20 to 40 mL of CSF via a needle or catheter placed in the lumbar subarachnoid space, as well as the administration of acetazolamide to decrease formation of CSF. Patients also respond to treatment with corticosteroids. The principal indication for treatment is loss of visual acuity. Initial treatment is often repeated lumbar puncture to remove CSF, which also facilitates measurement of the ICP.

Furthermore, continued leakage of CSF through the dural puncture site may be therapeutic. Chronic administration of acetazolamide can result in acidemia, presumably reflecting inhibition of hydrogen ion secretion by renal tubules. Surgical therapy, most often a lumboperitoneal shunt, is indicated only after medical therapy has failed and the patient's vision has begun to deteriorate. Optic nerve sheath fenestration is another surgical alternative to CSF shunting.

The anesthesia management for lumboperitoneal shunt placement involves avoiding exacerbation of intracranial hypertension and ensuring an adequate CPP. Hypoxia and hypercarbia should be rigorously avoided. Spinal anesthesia may be beneficial in parturients, as continued leakage of CSF is acceptable. In the presence of lumboperitoneal shunts, there is a theoretical possibility that injection of local anesthetic solutions into the subarachnoid space could escape into the peritoneal cavity, resulting in inadequate anesthesia. Therefore, general anesthesia may be a more logical choice in this patient population.

Normal Pressure Hydrocephalus

This disorder usually presents as the triad of dementia, gait changes, and urinary incontinence that develops over a period of weeks to months. The mechanism is thought to be related to compensated but impaired CSF absorption from a previous insult such as subarachnoid hemorrhage, meningitis, or head trauma; however, in most cases, the cause is never identified. Lumbar puncture usually reveals normal or low CSF pressure, yet CT or MRI will often demonstrate large ventricles. Treatment usually involves drainage of CSF, usually via ventriculoperitoneal or venticuloatrial shunting.

INTRACRANIAL TUMORS

Intracranial tumors may be classified as primary (those arising from the brain and its coverings) or metastatic. Tumors can originate from virtually any cell type within the central nervous system. Supratentorial tumors are more common in adults and often present with headache, seizures, or new neurologic deficits, whereas infratentorial tumors are more common in children and often present with obstructive hydrocephalus and ataxia. Treatment and prognosis depend both on the tumor type and location. Treatment may consist of surgical resection or debulking, chemotherapy, or radiation. Gamma knife irradiation differs from traditional radiation therapy in that multiple radiation sources are used, and by addressing the tumor from multiple angles, radiation to the tumor can be maximized while radiation dose to any single area of surrounding brain can be diminished. This same approach can be accomplished with the use of radiation produced by a linear accelerator.

Tumor Types

Astrocytoma

Astrocytes are the most prevalent neuroglial cell in the central nervous system and give rise to many types of infra- and supratentorial tumors. Well-differentiated (low-grade) gliomas are the least aggressive class of astrocytic-derived tumors. They often present in young adults with new-onset seizures. Upon imaging, they generally show minimal enhancement with contrast. Surgical or radiation treatment of low-grade gliomas usually results in symptom-free long-term survival.

Pilocytic astrocytomas usually affect children and young adults. They often arise in the cerebellum (cerebellar astrocytoma), cerebral hemispheres, hypothalamus, or optic pathways (optic glioma). The tumor usually appears as a contrast-enhancing, well-demarcated lesion with minimal to no surrounding edema. Because of its benign pathologic characteristics, prognosis following surgical resection is generally very good; however, the location of the lesion, such as within the brainstem, may preclude resection.

Anaplastic astrocytomas are poorly differentiated, usually appear as a contrast-enhancing lesion on imaging due to disruption of the blood-brain barrier, and usually evolve into glioblastoma multiforme. Treatment usually involves resection, radiation, or chemotherapy. Prognosis is intermediate between low-grade gliomas and glioblastoma multiforme.

Gliobastoma multiforme (grade IV glioma) accounts for 30% of all primary brain tumors in adults. Imaging usually reveals a ring-enhancing lesion due to central necrosis as well as surrounding edema. Treatment typically involves debulking combined with radiation and chemotherapy. Due to microscopic infiltration of normal brain by tumor cells, resection alone is usually inadequate. Instead, treatment usually consists of surgical debulking combined with chemotherapy and radiation and is aimed at palliation, not cure. Despite treatment, life expectancy is usually on the order of weeks.

Oligodendroglioma

Arising from myelin-producing cells within the central nervous system, oligodendrogliomas account for only 6% of primary intracranial tumors. Classically, seizures usually predate the appearance of tumor on imaging, often by many years. Calcifications within the tumor are common and are visualized on CT imaging. The tumor usually consists of a mixture of both oligodendrocytic and astrocytic cells. Treatment and prognosis depend on the pathologic features. Initial treatment involves resection since, early in the course, the tumor typically consists of primarily oligodendrocytic cells, which are radioresistant. Because of the presence of astrocytic cells, these tumors commonly behave more like anaplastic astrocytomas or glioblastoma multiforme later in their course.

Ependymoma

Arising from cells lining the ventricles and central canal of the spinal cord, ependymomas commonly present in childhood and young adulthood. Their most common location is the floor of the fourth ventricle. Symptoms include obstructive hydrocephalus, headache, nausea, vomiting, and ataxia. Treatment consists of resection and radiation. Tumor infiltration into surrounding tissues may preclude complete resection. Prognosis usually depends on the extent of resection.

Primitive Neuroectodermal Tumor

Primitive neuroectodermal tumor represents a diverse class of tumors including retinoblastoma, medulloblastoma, pineoblastoma, and neuroblastoma, all believed to arise from primitive neuroectodermal cells. Medulloblastoma is the most common pediatric primary malignant brain tumor and may disseminate via the CSF to encompass the spinal cord. Presentation of medulloblastoma is similar to ependymoma. Treatment usually involves a combination of resection and radiation given its high radiosensitivity. Prognosis is very good in children, if there is disappearance with treatment of both tumor on MRI and tumor cells within the CSF.

Meningioma

Meningiomas are usually extra-axial (arising outside of the brain proper), slow-growing, well-circumscribed, benign tumors arising from arachnoid cap cells, not the dura mater. Because of their slow-growing nature, they can be very large at the time of diagnosis. They can occur anywhere arachnoid cap cells exist, but are most common near the sagittal sinus, falx cerebri, and cerebral convexity. Tumors are usually apparent on plain radiographs and CT due to the presence of calcifications. On MRI and conventional angiography, these tumors often receive their blood supply from the *external* carotid artery. Surgical resection is the mainstay of treatment. Prognosis is usually excellent; however, some tumors may be recurrent and require additional resection. Malignant meningiomas are rare.

Pituitary Tumors

Pituitary adenomas usually arise from cells of the anterior pituitary gland. They may occur along with tumors of the parathyroids and pancreatic islet cells as part of multiple endocrine neoplasia type 1. Tumors are usually divided into functional (i.e., hormone secreting) and nonfunctional. The former usually present as a result of an endocrinologic disturbance related to the hormone secreted by the tumor. Functional tumors are usually smaller (<1 cm in diameter) at the time of diagnosis; hence, they are often called microadenomas. Macroadenomas are usually nonfunctional, present with symptoms related to their mass (i.e., headache or visual changes due to compression of the optic chiasm), and are larger at the time of diagnosis, usually greater than 1 cm in diameter. Panhypopituitarism may be caused by either tumor type due to compression of the normal functioning pituitary gland. Pituitary tumors may also present as apoplexy, which is the abrupt onset of headache, visual changes, ophthalmoplegia, and altered mental status secondary to hemorrhage, necrosis, or infarction within the tumor. Finally, tumors can invade the cavernous sinus or internal carotid artery or compress various cranial nerves, causing an array of symptoms. Treatment well may depend on tumor type. Prolactinomas are often initially treated medically with bromocriptine.

Surgical resection via the transsphenoidal or open craniotomy approach is often curative for most pituitary tumors.

Acoustic Neuroma

Usually the result of a benign schwannoma involving the vestibular component of cranial nerve VIII within the internal auditory canal, an acoustic neuroma typically occurs as a single mass. However, bilateral tumors may occur as part of neurofibromatosis type 2. Common presenting symptoms include hearing loss, tinnitus, and disequilibrium. Larger tumors, which grow out of the internal auditory canal and into the cerebellopontine angle, may cause symptoms related to compression of cranial nerves, most commonly the facial nerve (cranial nerve VII) as well as the brainstem. Treatment usually consists of surgical resection with or without radiation therapy. Surgery usually involves intraoperative cranial nerve monitoring with electromyography or brainstem auditory evoked potentials. Prognosis is usually very good; however, recurrence of tumor is not uncommon.

Central Nervous System Lymphoma

This is a rare tumor that can arise as a primary brain tumor, also known as a microglioma, or via metastatic spread from a systemic lymphoma. Primary central nervous system lymphoma can occur anywhere within the brain but is most common in supratentorial locations, especially in deep gray matter or the corpus callosum. Primary central nervous system lymphoma is thought to be associated with a variety of systemic disorders including systemic lupus erythematosus, Sjögren's syndrome, rheumatoid arthritis, immunosuppressed states, and infection with Epstein-Barr virus. Symptoms depend on the location of the tumor. Diagnosis is made by imaging as well as biopsy. During biopsy, it may be reasonable to wait to administer corticosteroids, such as dexamethasone, until after pathologic findings are obtained since these tumors may be sensitive to steroids. As such, steroid-associated tumor lysis prior to performing a biopsy may result in failure to obtain an adequate sample to make the diagnosis. The mainstay of treatment is chemotherapy (including intraventricularly delivered drugs) and whole-brain radiation. Prognosis is poor despite treatment.

Metastatic Tumor

Metastatic brain tumors originate most often from primary sites in the lungs or breasts. Malignant melanoma, hypernephroma, and carcinoma of the colon are also likely to spread to the brain. Metastatic brain tumor is the likely diagnosis when more than one intracranial lesion is present.

Management of Anesthesia

Anesthetic management of patients undergoing tumor resection can be challenging since it may involve patients of any age group as well as a variety of intraoperative patient positions. Further, some procedures may be conducted with electrophysiologic monitoring, which may have implications for anesthetic choice and the use of muscle relaxants.

Some procedures may even be conducted in awake patients to facilitate resection of a mass located near an eloquent region of brain, such as the motor cortex. Major goals during anesthesia include (1) maintenance of adequate perfusion and oxygenation of normal brain, (2) optimizing operative conditions to facilitate resection, (3) ensuring a rapid emergence from anesthesia at the conclusion of the procedure to facilitate neurologic assessment, and, when appropriate, (4) accommodating intraoperative electrophysiologic monitoring.

Preoperative Management

Preoperative evaluation of a patient with an intracranial tumor is directed toward identifying the presence or absence of increased ICP. Symptoms of increased ICP include nausea and vomiting, altered levels of consciousness, mydriasis and decreased reactivity of pupils to light, papilledema, bradycardia, systemic hypertension, and breathing disturbances. Evidence of midline shifts (>0.5 cm) on CT or MRI suggests the presence of increased ICP.

Patients with intracranial pathology may be extremely sensitive to the central nervous system depressant effects of opioids and sedatives. Drug-induced hypoventilation can lead to accumulation of arterial carbon dioxide and further increases in ICP. Likewise, drug-induced sedation can mask alterations in the levels of consciousness that accompany intracranial hypertension. Conversely, preoperative sedation can unmask subtle neurologic deficits that may not usually be apparent. This is thought to be a result of increased sensitivity of injured neurons to the depressant effects of various anesthetic and sedative agents. Considering all the potential adverse effects of preoperative medication, it is an inescapable conclusion that pharmacologic premedication should be used sparingly, if at all, in patients with intracranial tumors. Preoperative depressant drugs are particularly best avoided in patients with diminished levels of consciousness. In alert adult patients with intracranial tumors, benzodiazepines in small doses can provide anxiety relief without meaningfully affecting ventilation. Decisions to administer anticholinergic drugs or H_2-receptor antagonists are not influenced by the presence or absence of increased ICP.

Induction of Anesthesia

Anesthesia induction is achieved with drugs (e.g., thiopental, etomidate, propofol) that produce a rapid, reliable onset of unconsciousness without increasing ICP. This is often followed by a nondepolarizing muscle relaxant to facilitate tracheal intubation. Administration of succinylcholine may be associated with modest, transient increases in ICP. Mechanical hyperventilation of the patient's lungs is initiated with the goal of decreasing the Pa_{CO_2} to near 35 mm Hg. Adequate depth of anesthesia and profound skeletal muscle paralysis should be achieved prior to laryngoscopy, as noxious stimulation or patient movement can abruptly increase CBF, CBV, and ICP.

Direct laryngoscopy for tracheal intubation is accomplished during profound skeletal muscle paralysis as confirmed by the absence of electrically evoked neuromuscular transmission.

Additional doses of intravenous induction drugs, lidocaine 1.5 mg/kg IV, or potent short-acting opioids may blunt the responses laryngoscopy or other forms of intraoperative stimulation (e.g., placement of pinions, skin incision).

Abrupt, sustained increases in systemic blood pressure, particularly in areas of impaired cerebrovascular tone, may be accompanied by undesirable increases in CBF, CBV, and ICP, and followed by cerebral edema. Sustained hypotension must also be avoided, as brain ischemia can occur in the presence of decreased CPP. Skeletal muscle responses during tracheal intubation typically reflect inadequate anesthesia or incomplete skeletal muscle paralysis, both of which may confound management of ICP and brain volume. New-onset seizures or repeat episodes of seizures are another possible origin of unexpected movement. Following tracheal intubation, the patient's lungs are ventilated at a rate and tidal volume that maintain the $PaCO_2$ near 35 mm Hg. Positive end-expiratory pressure has a highly variable effect on ICP, resulting in increases, decreases, or no change in ICP. Hence, it should be used with caution, with attention paid to the ICP, MAP, and CPP effects of the intervention.

Maintenance of Anesthesia

The maintenance of anesthesia in patients undergoing surgical resection of supratentorial brain tumors is often achieved by combining drugs of various classes, including nitrous oxide, volatile anesthetics, opioids, barbiturates, and propofol. Although modest cerebrovascular differences can be demonstrated among different combinations of drugs, there is no evidence that any particular combination is significantly different from another in terms of effects on ICP and short-term patient outcome.

The use of nitrous oxide is controversial if there is any potential for venous air embolism (e.g., operations performed with patients in the sitting position). Despite theoretical concerns, the incidence of venous air embolism in sitting patients is not influenced by nitrous oxide use. Once a venous air embolism has been detected, nitrous oxide use must be discontinued out of concern that the embolus volume will expand, exacerbating the physiologic consequences. Both nitrous oxide and the potent volatile anesthetics have the potential to increase CBV and ICP as a result of direct cerebral vasodilation. However, low concentrations of volatile anesthetics (0.6–1.0 MAC) may be useful for preventing or treating increases in systemic blood pressure related to noxious surgical stimulation. Additionally, volatile anesthetic–associated increases in anesthetic depth and diminution of the physiologic responses to noxious stimuli will help preserve CBV and ICP. Administration of peripheral vasodilating drugs, such as nitroprusside or nitroglycerin, may increase CBV and ICP despite accompanying decreases in systemic blood pressure. This, in turn, can dramatically reduce CPP, which is dependent on both MAP and ICP. For this reason, vasodilating drugs are best used after craniotomy and opening of the dura.

Spontaneous movement by patients undergoing surgical resection of brain tumors must be prevented. Such movement

could result in dangerous increases in ICP, herniation of the brain, or bleeding at the operative site, making surgical exposure difficult. Therefore, in addition to adequate depths of anesthesia, skeletal muscle paralysis is typically maintained during intracranial surgery.

Fluid Therapy

Relatively iso-osmolar solutions (e.g., 0.9% saline, lactated Ringer's solution) do not adversely affect brain water or edema formation, provided there is an intact blood-brain barrier and they are used in modest doses. In contrast, free water in hypo-osmolar solutions (e.g, 0.45% sodium chloride) is rapidly distributed throughout body water, including brain water, and may adversely affect ICP management. Hyperosmolar solutions, such as 3% sodium chloride, initially tend to decrease brain water by increasing the osmolarity of plasma. Regardless of the crystalloid solutions selected, any solution administered in large amounts can increase CBV and ICP in patients with brain tumors. Therefore, the rate of fluid infusion should be titrated to maintain euvolemia with measures taken to avoid hypervolemia. Intravascular fluid volume depletion due to blood loss during surgery should be corrected with packed red blood cells or colloid solutions supplemented with balanced salt solutions. Glucose-containing solutions should be used with caution since hyperglycemia, in the setting of central nervous system ischemia, will exacerbate neuronal injury and worsen outcome.

Monitoring

The insertion of a peripheral arterial catheter is useful for continuous monitoring of systemic blood pressure and repetitive blood sampling. Capnography can facilitate ventilation and $PaCO_2$ management as well as detecting venous air embolism (see "Sitting Position and Venous Air Embolism"). Continuous ICP monitoring, although not routine, is of obvious value. Nasopharyngeal or esophageal temperature is monitored to prevent hyperthermia or uncontrolled hypothermia. A bladder catheter has utility for managing perioperative fluid volume. It is necessary if drug-induced diuresis is planned; in patients who have diabetes insipidus, syndrome of inappropriate antidiuretic hormone, or other aberrations of salt or water physiology; or if a lengthy surgical procedure is anticipated and bladder distention is a concern.

Intravenous access with large-bore catheters should be obtained, given the likelihood of bleeding and the need for transfusion or rapid administration of fluids. Central venous catheterization can be useful as reliable means of large-bore intravenous access, as well as a monitor of fluid status. Central venous cannulation also has utility during cases performed in the sitting position as a means to aspirate intracardiac air following venous air embolism. Transesophageal echocardiography can also be useful in sitting position cases to identify intravenous air and help assess cardiac function. Pulmonary artery catheterization should be considered in patients with cardiac disease.

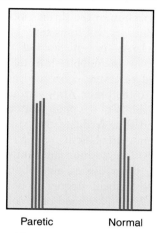

Figure 10A-4 • Train-of-four ratio recorded from the paretic extremity (0.6) is higher than that from the normal arm (0.3), reflecting resistance of the paretic arm to the effects of nondepolarizing muscle relaxants. *(Adapted from Moorthy SS, Hilgenberg JC: Resistance to nondepolarizing muscle relaxants in paretic upper extremities of patients with residual hemiplegia. Anesth Analg 1980;59:624–627.)*

Paretic   Normal

A peripheral nerve stimulator is helpful for monitoring the persistence of drug-induced skeletal muscle weakness or paralysis. If paresis or paralysis of an extremity is associated with the brain tumor, it is important to appreciate resistance (decreased sensitivity) to nondepolarizing muscle relaxants in the paretic extremity, compared with the normal extremity (**Fig. 10A-4**). Therefore, monitoring skeletal muscle paralysis on the paretic limb may be misleading. For example, the evoked response may be erroneously interpreted as inadequate skeletal muscle paralysis. Likewise, at the conclusion of surgery, the same response could be assumed to reflect recovery from the muscle relaxant when substantial neuromuscular block persists. In these instances, the altered muscle response to relaxants may reflect the proliferation of acetylcholine-responsive cholinergic receptors that can occur after denervation.

Monitoring the electrocardiographic activity is necessary to detect responses related to intracranial tumors or from surgery. Electrocardiographic changes can reflect increased ICP or, more importantly, surgical retraction or manipulation of the brainstem or cranial nerves. Indeed, the cardiovascular centers, respiratory control areas, and nuclei of the lower cranial nerves lie in close proximity in the brainstem. Manipulation of the brainstem may produce systemic hypertension and bradycardia or hypotension and tachycardia. Cardiac arrhythmias range from acute sinus arrhythmias to ventricular premature beats or ventricular tachycardia.

Postoperative Management

Ideally, the effects of anesthetics and muscle relaxants are dissipated or pharmacologically reversed at the conclusion of intracranial surgery. This facilitates monitoring the neurologic status and recognizing any adverse effects of the surgery. It is important to limit reaction to the tracheal tube as patients are awakening. Intraoperative use of narcotics and the optimal timing of extubation are of value. Lidocaine, 0.5 to 1.5 mg/kg IV, may also attenuate the physiologic response to the tracheal tube. However, it must be appreciated that this local anesthetic has general anesthetic properties and can produce central nervous system depression and reduce the activity of protective upper airway reflexes. If consciousness was depressed preoperatively or new-onset neurologic deficits are anticipated as a result of the surgical course, it may be best to delay tracheal extubation until return of airway reflexes are confirmed and spontaneous ventilation is sufficient to prevent CO_2 retention. Hypothermia must be considered a possible cause of slow postoperative awakening. Other causes of delayed emergence from anesthesia include residual neuromuscular block, residual effects of drugs with sedative effects (i.e., narcotics, benzodiazepines, volatile anesthetics), or a primary central nervous system event such as ischemia, hematoma, and tension pneumocephalus.

Following anesthesia, preexisting neurologic deficits may be exacerbated by the sedative effects of anesthetic agents making a subtle preoperative deficit appear more severe. This differential awakening is thought to be due to increased sensitivity of injured neurons to the depressant effects of anesthetic agents. Often, these deficits will disappear and neurologic function will return to its baseline state with time. Any persistent new deficit that does not quickly resolve should be further investigated.

Sitting Position and Venous Air Embolism

Craniotomy to remove a supratentorial tumor is usually performed in the supine position with the patient's head elevated 10 to 15 degrees to facilitate cerebral venous drainage. Infratentorial tumors have more unusual patient positioning requirements and may be performed in the lateral, prone, or sitting position.

The sitting position deserves special attention since, other than for surgery on the shoulder and thyroid, it is rarely used for non-neurosurgical cases and has a variety of anesthetic implications. The sitting position is often used for exploration of the posterior cranial fossa, which may be necessary to resect intracranial tumors, clip aneurysms, decompress cranial nerves, or implant electrodes for cerebellar stimulation, as well as for surgery on the cervical spine and posterior cervical musculature. Advantages of the sitting position include excellent surgical exposure and enhanced cerebral venous and CSF drainage, thereby minimizing blood loss and reducing ICP. These advantages are offset by the decreases in systemic blood pressure and cardiac output produced by this position, and the potential hazard of venous air embolism. For these reasons, the lateral or prone position may be selected as an alternative. However, as long as no contraindication to the sitting position exists (i.e., patent foramen ovale), the outcome of patients managed in the sitting versus horizontal position is similar or superior to that of other positions. If the sitting position is used, it is mandatory to maintain a high index of suspicion for venous air embolism.

The postoperative complications that may occur after posterior fossa craniotomy include apnea due to hematoma formation, tension pneumocephalus, or cranial nerve injuries. Macroglossia is also a possibility and is presumed due to impaired venous drainage from the tongue. This is sometimes associated with excessive neck flexion and may be influenced by the use of multiple oral instruments (e.g., endotracheal tube, oral airway, esophageal stethoscope, transesophageal echocardiography probe) simultaneously.

Venous air embolism is a potential hazard whenever the operative site is above the level of the patient's heart, such that pressures in the exposed veins are subatmospheric. Although this complication is most often associated with neurosurgical procedures, venous air embolism may also occur during operations involving the neck, thorax, abdomen, and pelvis and during open heart procedures, repair of liver and vena cava lacerations, obstetric and gynecologic procedures, and total hip replacement. Patients undergoing intracranial surgery are at increased risk not only because the operative site is usually above the level of the patient's heart but also because veins in the skull may not collapse when cut, owing to their attachment to bone or dura. Indeed, the cut edge of cranial bone, including that associated with burr holes, is a common site for the entry of air into veins.

Presumably, when air enters the right atrium and ventricle, there is interference with right-sided cardiac output and blood flow into the pulmonary artery. Air that eventually enters the pulmonary artery may trigger pulmonary edema and reflex bronchoconstriction. Death is usually secondary to a vapor lock causing right-sided cardiac output to plummet, acute cor pulmonale, or arterial hypoxemia from combined cardiac and pulmonary insults.

Small quantities of air can sometimes pass through pulmonary vessels to reach the coronary and cerebral circulations; large quantities of air can travel directly to the systemic circulation through right-to-left intracardiac shunts created by a patent foramen ovale or true septal defects. This passage of air from the right to left circulation is known as paradoxical air embolism. For that reason, known foramen ovale or other cardiac defects that could possibly result in a right-to-left shunt are relative contraindications to use of the sitting position.

Fatal cerebral embolism, subsequent to entrainment of systemic venous air, has occurred even in the absence of identifiable shunt mechanisms or intracardiac defects. This may occur because of failure of contrast echocardiography to detect an existing patent foramen ovale or septal defect. There are many theoretical reasons for this failure of detection. One is that Valsalva or other provocative maneuvers are not always successful in mimicking the physiologic changes that occur during general anesthesia and true venous air embolus and, as such, may underestimate the potential for venous air to pass from the right to left circulations. Paradoxical air embolism can occur even in the absence of any detectable elevations of mean right atrial pressure compared to that of the left atrium. This occurs as a result of small differences in

the timing of contraction of the various heart chambers. As a result, pressure gradients will transiently reverse, making the shunt bidirectional. An extremely brief right-to-left shunt could introduce a few air bubbles into the left-sided cardiac chambers and lead to severe consequences if those bubbles were to embolize to the brain. Also, various anesthetic drugs may diminish the ability of the pulmonary circulation to filter out air emboli and thus facilitate the passage of venous air emboli to the arterial circulation.

The use of the sitting position inherently predisposes neurosurgical patients to paradoxical air embolism, as the normal interatrial pressure gradient frequently becomes reversed in this position. When the likelihood of venous air embolism is increased, it is useful, but not mandatory, to place a right atrial catheter before beginning surgery. Death due to paradoxical air embolism results from obstruction of the coronary arteries by air, leading to myocardial ischemia and ventricular fibrillation. Neurologic damage may follow air embolism to the brain.

Early detection of venous air embolism is important for successful treatment. A Doppler sonography transducer placed over the right-sided cardiac structures is one of the most sensitive indicators of intracardiac air. Indeed, the small amount of air detected by the transducer is often clinically unimportant. In this regard, the transducer does not provide information as to the volume of air that has entered the venous circulation. Transesophageal echocardiography, by comparison, is also useful for both detecting and quantifying intracardiac air. A sudden decrease in the end-expired $Paco_2$ may reflect increased alveolar dead space and/or diminished cardiac output resulting from air embolus. An increase in right atrial and pulmonary artery pressures reflects acute cor pulmonale and correlates with abrupt decreases in the end-expired CO_2. Although these changes are less sensitive indicators of the presence of air than Doppler sonography or transesophageal echocardiography, they reflect the size of the venous air embolism. Increased end-expired nitrogen concentrations identify and partially quantify venous air embolism. Changes in end-expired nitrogen concentrations often precede decreased end-expired $Paco_2$ or increased pulmonary artery pressures. During controlled ventilation of the lungs, sudden attempts by patients to initiate spontaneous breaths ("gasp reflex") may be the first indication of venous air embolism. Hypotension, tachycardia, cardiac arrhythmias, and cyanosis are late signs of venous air embolism. Certainly detection of the characteristic "millwheel" murmur, as heard through an esophageal stethoscope, is a late sign of catastrophic venous air embolism.

Upon detection of venous air, the surgeon should flood the operative site with fluid, apply occlusive material to all bone edges, and attempt to identify any other sources of air entry (e.g., perforation of a venous sinus). Aspiration of air should be attempted through the right atrial catheter. The ideal location of the right atrial catheter tip is controversial, but evidence suggests that the junction of the superior vena cava with the right atrium is preferable, as this position appears to provide the most rapid aspiration of air. Right atrial multi-orifice catheters permit aspiration of larger amounts of air than do single-orifice catheters. Because of its small lumen size and slow speed of blood return, a pulmonary artery catheter is not as useful for aspirating air but may provide additional evidence that venous air embolism has occurred by virtue of increased pulmonary artery pressures. Nitrous oxide is promptly discontinued to avoid increasing the size of any venous air bubbles. Indeed, elimination of nitrous oxide from the inhaled gases after detecting a venous air embolism often results in decreased pulmonary artery pressures. At the same time oxygen is substituted for nitrous oxide, it may be helpful to apply positive end-expiratory pressure or direct jugular venous compression to increase venous pressure at the surgical site. Despite the logic of this maneuver, the prophylactic use of positive end-expiratory pressure is not of value in preventing venous air embolism.

Extreme hypotension may require the support of perfusion pressure using sympathomimetic drugs. Likewise, marked decreases in cardiac output may require the infusion of β-adrenergic agonists such as dopamine or dobutamine. Bronchospasm is treated with β2-adrenergic agonists by aerosol (metered-dose inhaler) or the intravenous route. The traditional admonition to treat venous air embolism by placing the patient in the lateral position with the right chest uppermost is rarely possible or safe during intracranial operations. It is likely that valuable time, better spent aspirating air and supporting circulation, could be lost attempting to attain this position.

After successful treatment of small or modest venous air embolism, the surgical procedure can be resumed. However, the decision to reinstitute administration of nitrous oxide must be individualized. If it is decided not to use nitrous oxide, maintenance of an adequate depth of anesthesia requires administration of larger doses of volatile or intravenous anesthetics. If nitrous oxide is added to the inhaled gases, it is possible that residual air in the circulation could again produce symptoms.

Hyperbaric therapy may be useful in the treatment of both severe venous as well as paradoxical air embolism. Transfer of patients to a hyperbaric chamber in an attempt to decrease the size of air bubbles and to improve blood flow is likely to be helpful only if the transfer can be accomplished within 8 hours.

DISORDERS RELATED TO VEGETATIVE BRAIN FUNCTION

Coma

Coma is a state of profound unconsciousness produced by drugs, disease, or injury affecting the central nervous system. It is usually caused by dysfunction of regions of the brain that are responsible for maintaining consciousness, such as the pontine reticular activating system, midbrain, or cerebral hemispheres. The causes of coma are many and can be

divided into two groups: structural lesions (i.e., tumor, stroke, abscess, intracranial bleeding) or diffuse disorders (i.e., hypothermia, hypoglycemia, hepatic or uremic encephalopathy, postictal state following seizures, encephalitis, drug effects). The most common means used to assess the overall severity of coma is by using the Glasgow Coma Scale (**Table 10A-1**).

The initial management of any comatose patient involves establishing a patent airway and ensuring the adequacy of oxygenation, ventilation, and circulation. One should then attempt to determine the cause of coma. This should begin by obtaining a medical history from family members or caretakers, if possible, and a physical examination followed by diagnostic studies. Vital signs are important as they might suggest a cause such as hypothermia. Respiratory patterns can also aid in diagnosis. Irregular breathing patterns may reflect an abnormality at a specific site in the central nervous system (**Table 10A-2**). Ataxic breathing is characterized by a completely random pattern of tidal volumes that results from the disruption of medullary neural pathways by trauma, hemorrhage, or compression by tumors. Lesions in the pons may result in apneustic breathing characterized by prolonged end-inspiratory pauses maintained for as long as 30 seconds. Occlusion of the basilar artery leading to pontine infarction is a common cause of apneustic breathing. Cheyne-Stokes breathing is characterized by breaths of progressively increasing and then decreasing volume (crescendo-decrescendo pattern), followed by periods of apnea lasting 15 to 20 seconds. Arterial blood gases typically also fluctuate in cyclic patterns. This pattern of breathing may reflect brain injury in the cerebral hemispheres, basal ganglia, or due to arterial hypoxemia and congestive heart failure. In the presence of congestive heart failure, the delay in circulation time from the pulmonary

TABLE 10A-1 Glasgow Coma Scale	
Response	Score
Eye Opening	
Spontaneous	4
To speech	3
To pain	2
Nil	1
Best Motor Response	
Obeys	6
Localizes	5
Withdraws (flexion)	4
Abnormal flexion	3
Extensor response	2
Nil	1
Verbal Responses	
Oriented	5
Confused conversation	4
Inappropriate words	3
Incomprehensible sounds	2
Nil	1

TABLE 10A-2 Abnormal Patterns of Breathing

Abnormality	Pattern	Site of Lesion
Ataxic (Biot's breathing)	Unpredictable sequence of breaths varying in rate and tidal volume	Medulla
Apneustic breathing	Repetetive gasps and prolonged pauses at full inspiration	Pons
Cheyne-Stokes breathing	Cyclic crescendo-decrescendo tidal volume pattern interrupted by apnea	Cerebral hemispheres Congestive heart failure
Central neurogenic hypoventilation	Hypocarbia	Cerebral thrombosis or embolism
Posthyperventilation apnea	Awake apnea following moderate decreases in Pa_{CO_2}	Frontal lobes

capillaries to the carotid bodies is presumed to be responsible for Cheyne-Stokes breathing. Central neurogenic hyperventilation is most often due to acute neurologic insults that are associated with cerebral thrombosis, embolism, or closed head injury. Hyperventilation is spontaneous and may be so severe the Pa_{CO_2} is decreased to less than 20 mm Hg. The basic neurologic examination can be the key to diagnosis and should, at least, include examination of the pupils and pupillary responses to light, function of the extraocular muscles via reflexes, and gross motor responses in the extremities (**Table 10A-3**).

Under normal conditions, pupils are usually 3 to 4 mm in diameter and equal bilaterally and react briskly to light, but approximately 20% of the general population normally have physiologic anisocoria (i.e., <1 mm difference in the diameter of their pupils). Compression of the diencephalon or thalamic structures leads to small (2 mm) but reactive pupils, probably due to interruption of descending sympathetic fibers.

Unresponsive midsize pupils (5 mm) usually indicate midbrain compression. A fixed and dilated pupil (>7 mm) usually indicates oculomotor nerve compression and can be seen in herniation as well as either anticholinergic or sympathomimetic drug intoxication. Pinpoint pupils (1 mm) usually indicate opioid or organophosphate intoxication as well as focal pontine lesions or neurosyphilis.

Evaluation of the function of the extraocular muscles will allow testing of the brainstem function via assessment of the function of the oculomotor, trochlear, and abducens nerves (cranial nerves III, IV, and VI). In the comatose patient, this can be performed by means of passive head rotation (oculocephalic reflex or doll's head maneuver) or by cold water irrigation of the tympanic membrane (oculovestibular reflex or cold caloric testing). In unresponsive patients with normal brainstem function, oculocephalic maneuvers will demonstrate full conjugate horizontal eye movements, and eliciting the oculovestibular reflex will result in tonic conjugate eye

TABLE 10A-3 Neurologic Findings on Compression of the Brainstem during Transtentorial Herniation

Region of Compression	Pupillary Examination	Response to Oculocephalic or Cold Caloric Testing	Gross Motor Findings
Diencephalon	Small pupils (2 mm) but reactive to light	Normal	Purposeful, semipurposeful, or decorticate (flexor) posturing
Midbrain	Midsize pupils (5 mm) and unreactive to light	May be impaired	Decerebrate (extensor) posturing
Pons or medulla oblongata	Midsize pupils (5 mm) and unreactive to light	Absent	No response

In the early stages, the diencephalon (i.e., hypothalamic region) is compressed. Small pupils are the result of interrupted sympathetic innervation from hypothalamic compression. Reflex eye movements are intact, and motor responses may be purposeful or semipurposeful (i.e., localizes to painful stimuli) early in the course but may progress to decerebrate posturing in response to stimuli. During midbrain compression, oculomotor nerve dysfunction leads to loss of the pupillary response to light. As the midbrain nuclei of cranial nerves, which innervate extraocular muscles (i.e, oculomotor and trochlear) become affected, there is impaired response to oculocephalic and cold caloric testing. Further, decerebrate posturing is seen at this stage. As compression progresses, such as to affect the pons or medulla oblongata, pupils are unresponsive, response to testing of reflexes involving eye movement is absent, and the patient is generally unresponsive to stimuli.
Adapted from Aminoff MJ, Greenberg DA, Simon RP: Clinical Neurology, 3rd ed. Stamford, CT, Appleton and Lange, 1996, p 291.

movement toward the side of cold water irrigation into the external auditory canal. Unilateral oculomotor nerve or midbrain lesions will result in failed adduction but intact contralateral abduction. Complete absence of responses can indicate pontine lesions or diffuse disorders.

Evaluation of motor responses to painful stimuli can also be helpful in localizing the cause of coma. Those with mild to moderate diffuse brain dysfunction above the level of the diencephalon will usually react with purposeful or semipurposeful movements toward the painful stimulus. Unilateral reactions may indicate unilateral lesions such as stroke or tumor. Decorticate responses to pain consist of flexion of the elbow, adduction of the shoulder, and extension of the knee and ankle and are usually indicative of diencephalic dysfunction. Decerebrate responses consist of extension of the elbow, internal rotation of the forearm, and leg extension and usually imply more severe brain dysfunction. Patients with pontine or medullary lesions often exhibit no response to painful stimuli.

In cases where the cause of coma is unknown, useful discriminatory laboratory tests include blood electrolytes and glucose to assess for disorders of sodium and glucose. Liver and renal function tests help evaluate hepatic or uremic encephalopathy. Drug and toxicology screens may help to identify exogenous intoxicants. A complete blood count and coagulation studies may suggest intracranial bleeding (i.e., thrombocytopenia or coagulopathy). CT or MRI may suggest a structural cause such as tumor or stroke. A lumbar puncture can be performed if meningitis or subarachnoid hemorrhage is suspected.

Patient outcome from comatose states will depend on multiple factors but is usually related to the cause and extent of injury to brain tissue.

Management of Anesthesia

Comatose patients may present to the operating suite either for treatment of the cause of their coma (e.g., burr hole drainage of an intracranial hematoma), or for treatment of injuries which resulted from their comatose state (e.g., bone fractures due to a motor vehicle accident in an intoxicated patient). It is important for the anesthesia provider to be aware of the likely cause of the coma since anesthetic management will vary depending on the cause as well as the type of planned surgery. Primary overall goals should be to safely establish an airway, provide adequate cerebral perfusion and oxygenation, and optimize operating conditions. One should pay careful attention to avoid increases in ICP during stimulating events. Means should be instituted to decrease elevations in baseline ICP, and intracranial monitoring may be helpful. Arterial catheterization will be useful for blood pressure optimization as well as management of hyperventilation, if needed. Anesthetic agents that increase ICP, such as halothane and ketamine, should be avoided, but other potent volatile agents such as isoflurane, sevoflurane, and desflurane, used at low doses (<1 MAC), as well as intravenous cerebral vasoconstrictive anesthetics, are acceptable. Nitrous oxide should be avoided if the patient has known or suspected pneumocephalus

(e.g., after recent intracranial surgery, basilar skull fracture). Nondepolarizing muscle relaxants help to facilitate tracheal intubation and patient positioning; however, succinylcholine is best avoided since it may transiently increase ICP.

Brain Death and Organ Donation

Brain death is defined as the permanent cessation of total brain function. The traditional criteria used to define brain death, which are an adaptation of the original Harvard Criteria established in 1968, are as follows:

1. Coma of an established and irreversible cause. All tests and reflexes listed should be performed after all possible reversible causes of coma have been ruled out.
   a. Lack of spontaneous movement bearing in mind that spinal reflexes may remain intact.
   b. Lack of all cranial nerve reflexes and function. This would include the failure of heart rate to increase by more than five beats per minute in response to intravenously, and preferably centrally, administered 0.04 mg/kg atropine, suggesting loss of vagal nuclear—and thus tonic vagal nerve function.
   c. Positive apnea test indicating lack of function of the respiratory control nuclei in the brainstem. The test is performed by initially ensuring a Pa_{CO_2} of 40 ± 5 mm Hg and an arterial pH of 7.35 to 7.45. The patient is then ventilated with 100% oxygen for more than 10 minutes, and while monitoring vital signs and insufflating the trachea with 100%, mechanical ventilation is discontinued for 10 minutes. Arterial blood gases are obtained at 5 and 10 minutes following the cessation of mechanical ventilation and the patient is observed for signs of spontaneous respiration. Given that hypercarbia (where the $Pa_{CO_2} > 60$ mm Hg) is a potent stimulus for ventilation, if no respiratory activity is noted, the apnea test is deemed positive.

Other confirmatory tests include isoelectricity demonstrated with electroencephalography and absence of CBF as demonstrated by various techniques including transcranial Doppler ultrasonography, cerebral angiography, and magnetic resonance angiography.

Following the establishment of the diagnosis of brain death and discussions with family, legal guardian, or next of kin, the decision is made to either withdraw artificial means of support or proceed to organ harvesting if that was the wish of the patient, family, or legal guardian.

Management of Anesthesia

The major goal in patients presenting for multiorgan harvesting is to attempt to optimize oxygenation and perfusion of the organs to be harvested. It is important to be aware of the various physiologic sequelae of brain death because it is useful to direct management of physiologic parameters with the needs of the organ recipient, not the donor, in mind. Due to loss of central hemodynamic regulatory mechanisms (i.e., neurogenic shock), brain dead patients are often hypotensive. Hypovolemia due to diabetes insipidus, third space losses, or drugs (e.g., mannitol, contrast dyes) can contribute to hypotension. Aggressive fluid resuscitation should be considered, with efforts made to avoid hypervolemia, which could lead to pulmonary edema, cardiac distension, or hepatic congestion. Peripheral vasoconstrictive agents should be avoided when considering pharmacologic treatment of hypotension. Inotropic agents such as dopamine and dobutamine should be first-line agents for the treatment of hypotension in euvolemic patients, with low-dose epinephrine as a second-line agent. For those in whom the heart is to be harvested, catecholamine doses should be minimized because of a theoretical risk of catecholamine-induced cardiomyopathy. Electrocardiographic abnormalities such as ST- and T-wave changes, as well as arrhythmias, can occur. Possible causes include electrolyte abnormalities, loss of vagal nerve function, increased ICP, and cardiac contusion (if death was trauma related). Arrhythmias should be treated pharmacologically or by electrical pacing.

Hypoxemia can occur due to diminished cardiac output or multiple pulmonary factors such as aspiration, edema, contusion, and atelectasis. Inspired oxygen concentration and ventilatory parameters should be adjusted in an attempt to maintain normoxia and normocapnia. Excessive positive end-expiratory pressure should be avoided due to its effect on cardiac output as well as the risk of barotrauma in the setting of possible trauma-related lung injury. Oxygen delivery to tissues should be optimized by treating coagulopathy and anemia with blood products.

Diabetes insipidus frequently occurs in brain dead patients and, if not treated, can lead to hypovolemia, hyperosmolality, and electrolyte abnormalities that could contribute to hypotension and cardiac arrhythmias. Treatment should initially include volume replacement with hypotonic solutions titrated to volume status and electrolyte concentrations. In severe cases, patients may need inotropic support, and either vasopressin (0.04–0.1U/hr IV) or desmopressin (0.3 μg/kg IV) should be used. Due to its vasoconstrictive properties, vasopressin use should be minimized to avoid end-organ ischemia. Various vasodilators, such as nitroprusside, may be coadministered to avoid vasopressin-induced hypertension and excessive vasoconstriction to end organs.

Finally, due to loss of temperature regulatory mechanisms, brain dead patients tend to become poikilothermic and may require aggressive measures to avoid hypothermia. Despite mild hypothermia possibly providing some degree of organ protection, it can also result in cardiac arrhythmias, coagulopathy, and reduced oxygen delivery to tissue, thus causing harm to the organs to be harvested. A good rule of thumb for the management of patients for organ donation is the rule of 100s: systolic blood pressure greater than 100 mm Hg, urine output greater than 100 mL/hr, PaO2 greater than 100 mm Hg, and hemoglobin greater than 100 g/L.

CEREBROVASCULAR DISEASE

Stroke is characterized by sudden neurologic deficits due to ischemia (88%) or hemorrhage (12%) (**Table 10A-4**). Ischemic stroke is described by the area of the brain affected and the etiologic mechanisms. Hemorrhagic strokes are classified as intracerebral (15%) or subarachnoid (85%).

Stroke is the third leading cause of death in the United States, and survivors of stroke represent the leading cause of major disability. The pathogenesis of stroke may differ among ethnic groups. Extracranial carotid artery disease and heart disease–associated embolism more commonly cause ischemic stroke in non-Hispanic whites, whereas intracranial thromboembolic disease is more common in African Americans. Women have lower stroke rates than men at all ages except 75 years and older, when stroke rates are at their highest. Overall, stroke-related mortality has decreased over the past several decades, probably due to better control of co-existing diseases (e.g., hypertension, diabetes), smoking cessation, and greater awareness of stroke and its risk factors.

Other disorders of the cerebrovascular system include atherosclerotic disease of the carotid artery, cerebral aneurysms, arteriovenous malformations (AVMs), and moyamoya disease.

Cerebrovascular Anatomy

Blood supply to the brain (20% of the cardiac output) is via two pairs of vessels: the internal carotid arteries and the vertebral arteries (**Fig. 10A-5**). These vessels join on the inferior surface of the brain to form the circle of Willis. Each internal carotid artery gives rise to an anterior cerebral artery and continues on to become a middle cerebral artery. These vessels arising from the carotid arteries comprise the anterior

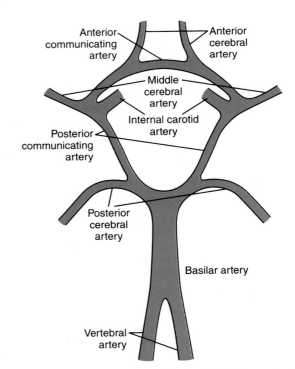

Figure 10A-5 • Cerebral circulation and circle of Willis. The cerebral blood supply is from the vertebral arteries (arising from the subclavian arteries) and the internal carotid arteries (arising from the common carotid arteries).

TABLE 10A-4 Characteristics of Stroke Subtypes

Parameter	Systemic Hypoperfusion	Embolism	Thrombosis	Subarachnoid Hemorrhage	Intracerebral Hemorrhage
Risk factors	Hypotension Hemorrhage Cardiac arrest	Smoking Ischemic heart disease Peripheral vascular disease Diabetes mellitus White men	Smoking Ischemic heart disease Peripheral vascular disease Diabetes mellitus White men	Often absent Hypertension Coagulopathy Drugs Trauma	Hypertension Coagulopathy Drugs Trauma
Onset	Parallels risk factors	Sudden	Often preceded by a TIA	Sudden, often during exertion	Gradually progressive
Signs and symptoms	Pallor Diaphoresis Hypotension	Headache	Headache	Headache Vomiting Transient loss of consciousness	Headache Vomiting Decreased level of consciousness Seizures
Imaging	CT (black) MRI	CT (black) MRI	CT (black) MRI	CT (white) MRI	CT (white) MRI

CT, computed tomography; MRI, magnetic resonance imaging; TIA, transient ischemic attack.
Adapted from Caplan LR: Diagnosis and treatment of ischemic stroke. JAMA 1991;266:2413–2418.

TABLE 10A-5 Clinical Features of Cerebrovascular Occlusive Syndromes

Occluded Artery	Clinical Features
Anterior cerebral artery	Contralateral leg weakness
Middle cerebral artery	Contralateral hemiparesis and hemisensory deficit (face and arm more than leg) Aphasia (dominant hemisphere) Contralateral visual field defect
Posterior cerebral artery	Contralateral visual field defect Contralateral hemiparesis
Penetrating arteries	Contralateral hemiparesis Contralateral hemisensory
Basilar artery	Oculomotor deficits and/or ataxia with "crossed" sensory and motor deficits
Vertebral artery	Lower cranial nerve deficits and/or ataxia with crossed sensory deficits

Adapted from Morgenstern LB, Kasner SE: Cerebrovascular disorders. Sci Am Med 2000:1–15.

circulation and ultimately supply the frontal, parietal, and lateral temporal lobes; the basal ganglia; and most of the internal capsule. The vertebral arteries each give rise to a posterior-inferior cerebellar artery before converging at the level of the pons to form the basilar artery. The basilar artery generally gives rise to two anterior-inferior and two superior cerebellar arteries before dividing to become the paired posterior cerebral arteries. Vessels which receive their predominant blood supply from this vertebral-basilar system comprise the posterior circulation and typically supply the brainstem, occipital lobes, cerebellum, medial portions of the temporal lobes, and most of the thalamus. The anterior and posterior circulations communicate via the posterior communicating artery, and the left and right anterior cerebral arteries communicate via the anterior communicating artery. Occlusion of specific arteries distal to the circle of Willis results in predictable clinical neurologic deficits (**Table 10A-5**).

Acute Stroke

Patients who present with the sudden onset of neurologic dysfunction or describe neurologic signs and symptoms evolving over minutes to hours are most likely experiencing a stroke. A transient ischemic attack is a sudden vascular-related focal neurologic deficit that resolves promptly (within 24 hours). A transient ischemic attack is not considered a separate entity but, rather, evidence of an impending ischemic stroke. It is important to recognize that stroke represents a medical emergency and that the patient's prognosis often depends on the time elapsed from the onset of symptoms to thrombolytic intervention if thrombosis is cause of their symptoms. Patients who receive early treatment to restore cerebral perfusion have better outcomes.

Systemic hypertension is the most significant risk factor for acute ischemic stroke, and long-term treatment of systolic or diastolic hypertension dramatically reduces the risk of a first stroke. Additionally, cigarette smoking, hyperlipidemia, diabetes mellitus, excessive alcohol consumption, and increased serum homocysteine concentrations all increase the risk of acute ischemic stroke.

In patients with suspected stroke, the brain should first be imaged using a noncontrast CT, which reliably distinguishes acute intracerebral hemorrhage from ischemia. This distinction is important as treatment of hemorrhagic stroke is substantially different from that of ischemic stroke. CT is relatively insensitive to ischemic changes (hyperdense vessels, loss of gray matter-white matter boundaries) during the first few hours after a stroke, but is very sensitive for detecting intracranial bleeding.

Conventional angiography is useful in demonstrating arterial occlusion. The vasculature can also be visualized noninvasively using CT or magnetic resonance angiography. Alternatively, transcranial Doppler sonography can provide indirect evidence of major vascular occlusion and offers the advantage of real-time bedside monitoring in patients undergoing thrombolytic therapy.

Acute ischemic strokes most likely reflect embolism occurring from a cardiac source, for example, atrial fibrillation, ventricular akinesis following myocardial infarction, dilated cardiomyopathy, valvular heart disease, large-vessel atherothromboembolism (atherosclerotic narrowing, especially at major arterial branches such as the carotid bifurcation in the neck), and small-vessel occlusive disease (lacunar infarction). Patients with long-standing diabetes mellitus or systemic hypertension are most likely to experience acute ischemic stroke due to small-vessel occlusive disease. Echocardiography is useful for evaluating the patient's cardiac status and looking for anatomic or vascular anomalies that could result in embolization.

Management of Acute Ischemic Stroke

Aspirin is often recommended as initial therapy for patients with an acute ischemic stroke and for the prevention of recurrent strokes. Intravenous recombinant tissue plasminogen activator is used in patients who meet specific eligibility requirements if treatment can be initiated within 3 hours of the onset of acute symptoms. Direct infusion of thrombolytic drugs (prourokinase or recombinant tissue plasminogen activator) into occluded blood vessels is a potential alternative or adjunctive therapy to intravenous recombinant tissue plasminogen activator. Despite advances in the treatment of acute ischemic stroke, most patients will have residual neurologic dysfunction. The initial stroke severity is a strong predictor of outcome, and early evidence of recovery is a good prognostic sign.

Management of the patient's airway, oxygenation, ventilation, systemic blood pressure, blood glucose concentrations, and body temperature are part of the initial global medical management. In the most critically ill stroke patients, cerebral edema and increased ICP may complicate the clinical course. The expanding infarction may cause focal and diffuse mass effects that typically peak 2 to 5 days following stroke onset. Large hemispheric strokes may be characterized by the malignant middle cerebral artery syndrome in which the edematous infarcted tissue causes compression of the anterior and posterior cerebral arteries, resulting in secondary infarctions. Similarly, infarction of the cerebellum may result in basilar artery compression and brainstem ischemia. Mortality rates for both middle cerebral artery syndrome and infarction of the cerebellum approach 80%.

Surgical decompression has a potential role in a small number of stroke patients. Craniotomy with cerebellar resection is a lifesaving intervention for acute cerebellar stoke by virtue of preventing secondary brainstem and vascular compression. The malignant middle cerebral artery syndrome may be similarly amenable to hemicraniectomy.

Respiratory function must be evaluated promptly in all stroke patients. Ventilatory drive is usually intact except after medullary or massive hemispheric infarction. The ability to protect the lungs against aspiration may be impaired in the acute setting, necessitating tracheal intubation. In most patients, supplemental oxygen administration without endotracheal intubation is sufficient to maintain arterial oxygen saturation at more than 95%.

Maintenance of adequate systemic blood pressure is critically important as blood flow to ischemic regions is dependent on CPP. Systemic hypertension is common at the time of initial stroke presentation, and rapid lowering of systemic blood pressure can impair CBF and worsen the ischemic injury. Increased systemic blood pressure often gradually decreases during the first few days following the acute stroke. Antihypertensive drug therapy (e.g., small intravenous doses of labetalol) may be used when necessary to maintain the systemic blood pressure at less than 185/110 mm Hg in an attempt to lessen myocardial work and irritability. Appropriate intravascular volume replacement in patients with acute stroke improves cardiac output and cerebral perfusion. Hypervolemic hemodilution may be considered in attempts to increase CBF while decreasing blood viscosity without causing significant decreases in oxygen delivery.

Hyperglycemia appears to parallel the poor outcome in patients experiencing acute ischemic stroke. During periods of cellular hypoxia or anoxia, as occur with stroke, glucose is metabolized to lactic acid, resulting in tissue acidosis and increased tissue injury. Normalization of blood glucose concentrations is recommended, using insulin when appropriate, and the administration of parenteral glucose should be avoided or kept to a minimum.

Based on animal data, hypothermia may improve outcome following acute ischemic stroke in patients as a result of its ability to decrease neuronal oxygen demands, cerebral edema, and neurotransmitter toxicity. There are few human studies evaluating the effectiveness of hypothermia for the reduction of morbidity and mortality from acute stroke. As such, hypothermia in this setting continues to be a debated treatment modality. However, fever should be avoided in patients with acute stroke. Even mild increases in body temperature are known to be deleterious, and normothermia should be maintained in previously febrile patients having acute ischemic stroke using antipyretics or cooling blankets.

Prophylaxis to prevent deep vein thrombosis is initiated early in the treatment of patients experiencing acute ischemic stroke. Heparin, 5000 units subcutaneously every 12 hours, is the most common intervention. Patients with acute hemorrhage who cannot be given heparin are treated with pneumatic compression stockings.

Acute Hemorrhagic Stroke

Acute hemorrhagic stroke results from either intracerebral hemorrhage or subarachnoid hemorrhage.

Intracerebral Hemorrhage

Intracerebral hemorrhage is four times more likely than ischemic stroke to cause death and most notably affects African Americans. Acute hemorrhagic stroke cannot be reliably distinguished from ischemic stroke based on clinical criteria alone. A noncontrast CT evaluation is needed to detect the presence of blood. The estimated volume of blood and the level of consciousness are the two most reliable predictors of outcome. Patients with intracerebral hemorrhage often deteriorate clinically as cerebral edema worsens during the first 24 to 48 hours following the acute bleed. Late hematoma evacuation is ineffective in decreasing mortality, whereas the efficacy of earlier surgical evacuation of the hematoma to decrease surrounding ischemic tissue injury and edema remains unclear. Intravenous administration of recombinant activated factor VIIA within 4 hours of onset of symptoms has been shown not only to decrease hematoma volume, but may also improve clinical outcome. Intraventricular hemorrhage is a particularly ominous complication as blood will occlude the CSF drainage, and prompt ventricular drainage should be performed to treat any signs of hydrocephalus. Sedation (with propofol infusion, barbiturates, or benzodiazepines), with or without drug-induced skeletal muscle paralysis, is often helpful for managing patients who require tracheal intubation. An ICP monitor is often recommended for patients who are obtunded. Systemic blood pressure management in patients who experience intracerebral hemorrhage is controversial, as there is concern about decreasing CPP in those with increased ICP. In patients with co-existing essential hypertension, a goal may be to keep the MAP at less than 130 mm Hg.

Subarachnoid Hemorrhage

Spontaneous subarachnoid hemorrhage most commonly results from rupture of intracranial aneurysms. Various pathologic conditions such as systemic hypertension, coarctation of the aorta, polycystic kidney disease, and fibromuscular dysplasia, as well as the occurrence of cerebral aneurysms in first-degree relatives, are associated with the presence of cerebral aneurysms. The risk of aneurysm rupture depends on the size of the aneurysm with a 6% risk of rupture occurring in aneurysms of at least 25 mm in diameter during the first year. Other risk factors for rupture include systemic hypertension, cigarette smoking, cocaine abuse, female sex, and use of oral contraceptives.

The diagnosis of subarachnoid hemorrhage is based on clinical symptoms (e.g., "worst headache of my life") and CT demonstration of subarachnoid blood. MRI is not as sensitive as CT for detecting acute hemorrhage, especially with thin layers of subarachnoid blood, although this technique may be useful for demonstrating subacute or chronic subarachnoid hemorrhage or infarction after CT findings have returned to normal. In addition to severe headache, the rapid onset of photophobia, stiff neck, decreased level of consciousness, and focal neurologic changes suggest subarachnoid hemorrhage. Establishing the diagnosis promptly followed by treatment of the aneurysm can decrease morbidity and mortality. Two of the most common methods used to grade the severity of subarachnoid hemorrhage are the Hunt and Hess classification and the World Federation of Neurologic Surgeons grading system (**Table 10A-6**). These grading systems are useful in that, not only do they help predict severity and outcome, but they also function as a metric to evaluate the efficacy of various therapies.

Changes on the electrocardiogram are common following subarachnoid hemorrhage (e.g., inversion of T waves and ST-segment depression). These changes are most often noted within 48 hours following hemorrhage and have been attributed to catecholamine release. The same catecholamine release that may result in cardiac arrhythmias may also be responsible for producing pulmonary edema. As demonstrated by echocardiography, temporary depression of myocardial contractility, independent of coronary artery disease, can also occur in subarachnoid hemorrhage. Of note, apical cardiac function may be preserved, a phenomenon attributed to the paucity of sympathetic innervation at the cardiac apex.

Treatment of subarachnoid hemorrhage involves localizing the aneurysm with conventional or magnetic resonance angiography and surgically excluding the aneurysmal sac from the intracranial circulation while preserving the parent artery. Outcome is optimal when treatment is performed within the first 72 hours after bleeding. Surgically, placing a clip across the neck of the intracranial aneurysm is the most definitive treatment. For larger or fusiform aneurysms that lack a definitive neck, surgical options include wrapping the exterior of

TABLE 10A-6	Common Grading Systems for Subarachnoid Hemorrhage	
HUNT & HESS CLASSIFICATION		
Score	**Neurologic Finding**	**Mortality**
0	Unruptured aneurysm	0%–2%
1	Ruptured aneurysm with minimal headache and no neurologic deficits	2%–5%
2	Moderate to severe headache, no deficit other than cranial nerve palsy	5%–10%
3	Drowsiness, confusion, or mild focal motor deficit	5%–10%
4	Stupor, significant hemiparesis, early decerebration	25%–30%
5	Deep coma, decerebrate rigidity	40%–50%
WORLD FEDERATION OF NEUROLOGIC SURGEONS GRADING SYSTEM		
Score	**GCS**	**Presence of Major Focal Deficit**
0		Intact, unruptured aneurysm
1	15	No
2	13–14	No
3	13–14	Yes
4	7–12	Yes or no
5	3–6	Yes or no

GCS, Glasgow Coma Scale.
Adapted from Lam AM: Cerebral aneurysms: Anesthetic considerations. In Cottrell JE, Smith DS (eds): Anesthesia and Neurosurgery, 4th ed. St. Louis, Mosby Inc., 2001.

the aneurysm or aneurysm trapping. In the latter procedure, a clip is placed on the artery both proximal and distal to the aneurysm, after the artery distal to the aneurysm is bypassed, usually by means of the superficial temporal artery. Endovascular techniques consisting of placing soft metallic coils in the lumen of the aneurysm may serve as an alternative to surgical therapy, but may not be an option for the treatment of all aneurysms, specifically those with a large neck or those that lack a neck. Due to the immense morbidity and mortality associated with surgical treatment of basilar tip aneurysms, endovascular treatment is preferred.

Surgery is often delayed in patients with severe symptoms such as coma. In these patients, other options, including interventional radiographic procedures, may be used. Anticonvulsants are administered should seizure activity occur. Systemic blood pressure is controlled, recognizing that hypertension increases the risk of rebleeding. Hydrocephalus is common after subarachnoid hemorrhage and is treated with ventricular drainage. Any change in mental status is promptly evaluated by CT to look for signs of rebleeding or hydrocephalus.

Following subarachnoid hemorrhage with or without surgical or radiographic treatment of the aneurysm, the goal is to prevent vasospasm (intracranial arterial narrowing) and its consequences. Development of vasospasm is likely triggered by many mechanisms, the most important being the contact of free hemoglobin with the abluminal surface of cerebral arteries. Not surprisingly, the incidence and severity of vasospasm correlate with the amount of subarachnoid blood seen on CT. Vasospasm typically occurs 3 to 15 days after subarachnoid hemorrhage. For this reason, daily transcranial Doppler sonographic examinations are performed to detect vasospasm, and once identified, triple H therapy (hypertension, hypervolemia, passive hemodilution) is initiated. Specifically, colloid and crystalloid therapy is used, and pressor support may be needed. Nimodipine, a calcium channel blocker, has been shown to improve outcome when initiated on the first day and continued for 21 days after subarachnoid hemorrhage, presumably reflecting a protective effect from the consequences of vasospasm. This benefit by nimodipine occurs without angiographic evidence of vessel luminal enlargement. Cerebral angiographic techniques can also be employed as a safe means to mechanically (via balloons) or chemically (via intra-arterial papaverine) dilate vasospastic arteries.

Management of Anesthesia

The goals of anesthesia during intracranial aneurysm surgery are to limit the risks of aneurysm rupture, prevent cerebral ischemia, and facilitate surgical exposure.

The goal during the induction of anesthesia is to prevent increases in the transmural pressure of the aneurysmal sac, which could increase the risk of aneurysmal rupture. Therefore, one should try to avoid significant increases in systemic blood pressure. Also, in those patients with cerebral aneurysms without associated increased ICP, as in those with unruptured aneurysms, it is reasonable to avoid excessive decreases in ICP prior to dural opening, as seen with hyperventilation, such as not to decrease the tamponading force on the external surface of the aneurysm. Patients presenting with an increased ICP prior to surgery represent a challenge, as they may not tolerate an MAP decrease used to protect against aneurysm rupture without the risk of developing cerebral ischemia. Patients with vasospasm pose a similar quandary in that systemic hypertension may improve flow through vasospastic vessels but may increase the risk of aneurysm rebleeding. Aneurysm clipping during the time period in which the patient is at high risk of vasospasm is associated with increased mortality. Given this, in patients with vasospasm who require anesthetic care, CPP should be kept elevated in order to maintain blood flow through vasospastic arteries.

Monitoring the systemic blood pressure via an intra-arterial catheter is desirable to observe the adequacy of systemic blood pressure control during direct laryngoscopy. Prophylaxis against systemic hypertension during direct laryngoscopy may be achieved by previous intravenous administration of the short-acting β-adrenergic antagonist esmolol, lidocaine, propofol, barbiturates, or short-acting opioids (fentanyl, sufentanil, remifentanil). Loss of consciousness is achieved with intravenous administration of thiopental, propofol, or etomidate. In these situations, nondepolarizing neuromuscular blocking drugs are most often selected to facilitate tracheal intubation.

Placing a CVP catheter is useful, considering the likely presence of hypovolemia, the large intraoperative fluid shifts associated with osmotic and loop diuretics, the potential for intraoperative aneurysm rupture, and the need for fluid resuscitation. A pulmonary artery catheter and a transesophageal echocardiography may be considered when patients have known cardiac disease. Electrophysiologic monitoring (electroencephalography, somatosensory or motor evoked potentials) may be helpful to identify intraoperative cerebral ischemia, but their complexity limits routine use.

The goals of anesthesia maintenance include providing a depth of anesthesia appropriate to the level of surgical stimulation, facilitating surgical exposure through optimal brain relaxation, maintaining CPP, reducing transmural pressure in the aneurysm during clipping of the aneurysm, and prompt awakening of the patient at the end of the procedure to permit neurologic assessment. Drugs, fluid, and blood must be immediately available to manage resuscitation should the aneurysm rupture intraoperatively. Generally, the risk of intraoperative rupture is approximately 7% and most commonly occurs during the late stages of surgical dissection. Anesthetic management or rupture consists of aggressive volume resuscitation to maintain normovolemia combined with controlled hypotension (e.g., with nitroprusside) to temporarily limit hemorrhage and permit the neurosurgeon to gain control of the aneurysm. If a temporary clip on the feeding vessel is used to gain control of a ruptured aneurysm, systemic blood pressure is then returned to a normal or to a slightly elevated level to improve collateral blood flow.

Anesthesia is most often maintained with volatile anesthetics (isoflurane, desflurane, sevoflurane) with or without the addition of nitrous oxide, which may be supplemented with intermittent (fentanyl) or continuous infusion of opioids (remifentanil). Alternatively, a total intravenous anesthetic maintenance technique (propofol and short-acting opioid) can be used. Cerebral vasoconstricting anesthetics (e.g., barbiturates, propofol) help reduce brain volume and, in the case of barbiturates and possibly propofol, may provide some degree of neuronal protection against ischemia. Muscle paralysis is critical to prevent movement during clipping.

In view of the trend for earlier surgical intervention in patients with subarachnoid hemorrhage due to rupture of intracranial aneurysms, it is predictable that many patients will manifest intraoperative brain edema. For this reason, optimization of brain relaxation is an important part of anesthetic maintenance and combinations of lumbar CSF drainage, mild hyperventilation of the patient's lungs, administration of loop and/or osmotic diuretics, and proper patient positioning to facilitate cerebral venous drainage can help to optimize surgical exposure. Intraoperative fluid administration is guided by blood loss, urine output, and measurement of cardiac filling pressures. Normovolemia is the goal, which is best achieved by intravenous administration of balanced salt solutions. Intravenous solutions containing glucose are not recommended for fear of exacerbating injury from focal and global cerebral ischemia. Despite convincing evidence of the cerebral protection by mild hypothermia in animal models and some clinical trials of resuscitation after cardiac arrest, current best evidence suggests no benefit if intraoperative hypothermia is used in patients undergoing aneurysm clipping. However, hyperthermia and fever should be avoided as they increase $CMRO_2$ and CBV.

Traditionally, drug-induced controlled hypotension has been used to decrease transmural pressure in the aneurysm, thereby decreasing the risk of aneurysm rupture during microscopic isolation and clipping. However, the use of controlled hypotension has decreased based on the impairment of autoregulation that follows subarachnoid hemorrhage, the unpredictable cerebrovascular responses to drug-induced hypotension, and the risk of global ischemia. Alternatively, regional controlled hypotension produced by placing a vascular clamp on the parent artery supplying the aneurysm provides protection against aneurysm rupture without the risk of global cerebral ischemia. Ideally, temporary occlusion of the parent artery does not exceed 10 minutes; but if longer periods of occlusion are needed, the administration of metabolic suppressant anesthetics (particularly barbiturates) may provide protection against regional cerebral ischemia and infarction. During temporary clamping of the feeding vessel, systemic blood pressure should be maintained toward the higher end of the patient's normal blood pressure range to encourage collateral circulation.

At the conclusion of the surgical procedure, prompt emergence from anesthesia is desirable to facilitate immediate neurologic evaluation of the patient. The use of short-acting inhaled and injected anesthetic drugs enhances success.

Incremental doses of antihypertensive drugs such as labetalol or esmolol may be needed as the patient emerges from anesthesia. In some patients, a systolic blood pressure up to 180 mm Hg may be tolerated, in part because, by this point, the aneurysm has been removed from the circulation. Lidocaine may be administered intravenously to suppress airway reflexes and the associated responses to the presence of a tracheal tube. Tracheal extubation immediately after surgery is acceptable and encouraged in patients who are awake with adequate spontaneous ventilation and protective upper airway reflexes. Patients who were obtunded preoperatively are likely to require continued tracheal intubation and support of ventilation during the postoperative period. Likewise, patients who experience intraoperative rupture of intracranial aneurysms may recover slowly and benefit from postoperative airway and ventilation support.

The neurologic status is assessed at frequent intervals in the postanesthesia care unit or intensive care unit. Occasionally, patients manifest delayed emergence or focal neurologic deficits following intracranial aneurysm resection, and it may be difficult to distinguish between drug-induced (e.g., differential awakening) and surgical (e.g., ischemic or mechanical brain injury) causes. However, the appearance of a new focal deficit should raise suspicion of a surgical cause as anesthetic drugs would be expected to cause primarily global effects. Unequal pupils that were not present preoperatively are also likely to reflect a surgical event. CT or angiography may be necessary when the patient does not awaken promptly during the postoperative period. Successful surgical therapy may be followed hours to days later by delayed deficits due to cerebral vasospasm. This, in turn, requires aggressive therapy (e.g., hypertension, hypervolemia, passive hemodilution, invasive radiographic interventions).

For patients undergoing angiographically guided cerebral aneurysm coil placement, the anesthetic goals are similar to those employed for aneurysm clip placement. Typically, these procedures are performed using mild sedation or under general anesthesia. Advantages of mild sedation include the ability to perform intraprocedural neurologic examination; however, patient movement during the procedure poses the risk of aneurysm rupture or inappropriate coil dislodgment resulting in coil embolization. For this reason, general anesthesia is preferred during actual coil placement. Anesthetic goals include ICP control, maintenance of adequate cerebral perfusion without excessive hypertension (which could increase the risk of aneurysm rupture), and facilitation of a rapid postprocedural assessment of neurologic function.

VASCULAR MALFORMATIONS

There are five types of vascular malformations affecting the central nervous system; all are non-neoplastic.

Arteriovenous Malformation

AVMs are abnormal collections of blood vessels where multiple direct arterial-to-venous connections exist without intervening capillaries. In addition, there is no neural tissue within the nidus. They typically represent high-flow, low-resistance shunts with vascular intramural pressure being less that systemic arterial pressure; thus, rupture does not appear to be clinically associated with acute or chronic hypertensive episodes. These are believed to be congenital in nature and commonly present in adulthood as either hemorrhage or new-onset seizures. The cause of AVM-associated seizures is unknown but is attributed to either steal (e.g., shunting of blood away from normal brain tissue toward the low-resistance AVM) or gliosis due to hemosiderin deposits from previous hemorrhage. The majority of AVMs occur supratentorially. There is a 4% to 10% incidence of cerebral aneurysms associated with AVMs. AVMs presenting in the neonatal or childhood period usually involve the vein of Galen, and presenting symptoms include hydrocephalus or macrocephaly, prominence of forehead veins, as well as evidence of a high-output cardiac state or heart failure. Diagnosis is made by either MRI or angiography.

Prior to the advent of focused, high-dose radiation and cerebral angiography, the historical treatment of AVMs was associated with a high morbidity and mortality. Currently, treatment may involve a combination of surgical resection, highly focused (gamma knife) radiation (see "Intracranial Tumors"), or angiographically guided embolization. With smaller AVMs, patients may respond completely to radiation or embolization therapy alone; however, with larger AVMs, these two techniques are often useful adjunctive therapy prior to surgery in order to decrease the size of the AVM nidus and reduce both the complexity and risks of surgery. Prognosis and perioperative outcome can be estimated using the Spetzler-Martin AVM grading system and involves grading the AVM based on three features (**Table 10A-7**).

Venous Angioma

Venous angiomas or malformations consist of tufts of veins. Often, they are occult lesions found during the evaluation of other disease states, appearing during cerebral angiography or MRI; however, some rarely present as either hemorrhage or new-onset seizures. These low-flow, low-pressure lesions usually contain intervening brain parenchyma within the nidus and are therefore only treated if bleeding or intractable seizures occur.

Cavernous Angioma

Also known as cavernous hemangiomas or cavernomas, these benign lesions consist of vascular channels without large feeding arteries or large veins. Brain parenchyma is not found within the nidus of the lesion. These low-flow, well-circumscribed lesions often present as new-onset seizures but occasionally as hemorrhage. They may appear on CT or MRI and typically appear as a flow void on cerebral angiography. Treatment usually involves surgical resection for symptomatic lesions. They do not respond to radiation nor are they amenable to embolization, since they are angiographically silent.

TABLE 10A-7 Spetzler-Martin Arteriovenous Malformation Grading System

Graded Feature	Points Assigned
Nidus Size	
Small (<3 cm)	1
Medium (3–6 cm)	2
Large (>6 cm)	3
Eloquence of Adjacent Brain*	
Noneloquent	0
Eloquent	1
Pattern of Venous Drainage	
Superficial only	0
Deep only or deep and superficial	1

SURGICAL OUTCOME BASED ON SPETZLER-MARTIN AVM GRADING SYSTEM

Grade	Percent of Patients With No Postoperative Neurologic Deficit
1	100
2	95
3	84
4	73
5	69

*Eloquent brain refers to sensory, motor, language, or visual areas as well as hypothalamus, thalamus, internal capsule, brainstem cerebellar peduncles, and deep nuclei.
AVM, arteriovenous malformations.
Adapted from Spetzler RF, Martin NA: A proposed grading system for arteriovenous malformations. J Neurosurg 65:476;1986.

Capillary Telangiectasia

Capillary telangiectasias represent low-flow, enlarged capillaries and are probably one of the least understood vascular lesions of the central nervous system. They are angiographically silent and difficult to diagnose premortem. The risk of hemorrhage is low, except for lesions occurring in the brainstem. They are often found incidentally on autopsy and are often associated with other disorders including Osler-Weber-Rendau syndrome and Sturge-Weber syndrome. These lesions are usually not treatable.

Arteriovenous Fistula

Arteriovenous (AV) fistulas are direct communications between an artery and a vein without an intervening nidus of vessels. They commonly occur between meningeal vessels within the dura mater or between the carotid artery and venous sinuses within the cavernous sinus. Some AV fistulas are thought to spontaneously occur. Many others are associated with a previous traumatic injury or, in the case of carotid-cavernous fistulas, are associated with previous (presumably silent) rupture of an intracavernous carotid artery aneurysm. Dural AV fistulas commonly present with pulsatile tinnitus or headache, and of note, an occipital bruit can be appreciated in 24% of cases given that the occipital artery is a common arterial feeder. Treatment options include angiographically guided embolization or surgical ligation, bearing in mind the risk of rapid blood loss associated with surgical treatment.

Patients with carotid-cavernous AV fistulas often present with orbital or retro-orbital pain, arterialization of the conjunctiva, or visual changes. Diagnosis is made by magnetic resonance or conventional angiography. Embolization is usually an effective option for treatment.

Management of Anesthesia

Surgical resection of low-flow vascular malformations (i.e., venous angiomas and cavernous angiomas) is generally not associated with the degree of both intraoperative and postoperative complications as associated with the resection of high-flow vascular lesions (i.e., AVMs and AV fistulas). Further, since AVMs are often associated with multiple feeding and draining vessels, unlike AV fistulas which involve a single feeding and a single draining vessel, surgical resection of AVMs often pose great clinical challenges during resection and postoperative care.

Preoperatively, the patient with an intracranial vascular malformation should be evaluated for evidence of cerebral ischemia or increased ICP. The nature of the malformations, such as size, location, mechanism of venous drainage, presence of associated aneurysms, and a history of treatment, should be elicited since these factors may help one to anticipate perioperative complications such as the risk of intraoperative bleeding as well as postoperative complications. Adjunct medications, including antiepileptics (if the patient has a concurrent seizure disorder), should be administered. Patients exposed to preoperative angiography may experience fluid and electrolyte abnormalities secondary to the administration of hypertonic contrast material.

In addition to standard monitors, an arterial catheter placed prior to the induction of anesthesia may be helpful in that it will allow rapid evaluation of systemic blood pressure. Blood pressure control is critical, given that hypotension may result in ischemia in hypoperfused areas and hypertension may increase the risk of rupture of an associated aneurysm, worsen intraoperative bleeding, or worsen intracranial hypertension. For embolization or surgical resection of a vascular malformation in an eloquent region of brain, monitored anesthesia care is an attractive option. For cases requiring general anesthesia, a smooth, hemodynamically stable induction of general anesthesia is paramount. Thiopental, propofol, or etomidate are all effective and safe induction agents. Muscle relaxation should be accomplished with a nondepolarizing neuromuscular blocking agent such as succinylcholine may induce further increases in ICP as well as cause hyperkalemia if motor deficits are present. Techniques to blunt the hemodynamic responses to stimulating events such as laryngoscopy, pinion placement, and incision, should be used. These may include the administration of lidocaine, short-acting β-adrenergic antagonists (i.e., esmolol), and nitroprusside or deepening the anesthetic state with either

higher concentrations of volatile anesthetics, small doses of induction agents, short-acting opioids, or intravenous lidocaine. Given the risk of severe and rapid intraoperative hemorrhage, especially with AVMs and AV fistulas, adequate intravenous access is essential. Further, central venous access may be useful in these cases to monitor volume status or for rapid administration of large volumes of fluids or blood products. A pulmonary artery catheter or transesophageal echocardiography can be useful in patients with cardiac disease.

With large or high-flow vascular malformations, frequent communication with the surgeon is of paramount importance because impressions of the lesions and the surgical and anesthetic requirements for safe resection may change during the operation. This is due, in part, to somewhat less than definitive imaging assessment preoperatively or changing surgical requirements during various stages of resection of a large, complex lesion. Hemodynamic stability, optimal surgical conditions, and rapid emergence at the end of surgery are appropriate goals when selecting maintenance techniques. Both intravenous and volatile-based techniques are appropriate and agents should be selected on a case-by-case basis.

Hypotonic and glucose-containing solutions should be avoided, given that the former can exacerbate cerebral edema and the latter can worsen the outcome from neurologic ischemia. Mild hyperventilation (Pa_{CO_2} of 30–35 mm Hg) will help facilitate surgical exposure. Lumbar CSF drainage may also help to decrease intracranial volume and improve exposure. Cerebral edema can be a significant problem during AVM treatment. Because AVMs represent a high-flow, low-resistance vascular lesion, as arterial feeders are ligated during resection or embolization, blood flow is thus directed toward normal brain tissue, resulting in possible cerebral edema. Mechanisms to be considered for the treatment of cerebral edema include moderate hyperventilation as a temporizing measure, diuretics such as mannitol and furosemide, and blood pressure reductions. In extreme cases, high-dose barbiturate or propofol anesthesia, or temporary craniectomy, with postoperative ventilatory support, may be useful.

Most patients, however, should respond quite well to surgical resection, and emergence from anesthesia should be smooth and rapid. Agents such as β-adrenergic antagonists as well as lidocaine or nitroprusside can be used to control short-term hypertensive events. Prompt neurologic assessment should follow emergence.

MOYAMOYA DISEASE

Progressive stenosis of intracranial vessels with the secondary development of an anastomotic capillary network is the hallmark of moyamoya disease. *Moyamoya* is the Japanese term for "puff of smoke" and refers to the angiographic finding of a cluster of small abnormal blood vessels. There seems to be a familial tendency toward the development of this disease; however, it may be seen following head trauma or in association with other disorders such as neurofibromatosis, tuberous sclerosis, and fibromuscular dysplasia.

Affected arteries have a thickened intima and a thin media. Since similar pathologic findings may be found in other organs, central nervous system abnormalities may be the manifestations of a systemic disease. Intracranial aneurysms occur with increased frequency in those with moyamoya disease. Symptoms of ischemia, such as transient ischemic attacks and infarcts, are common initial findings in children, whereas hemorrhagic complications are usually the presenting symptoms in adults. The diagnosis is typically made by conventional or magnetic resonance angiography, demonstrating a cluster of small abnormal blood vessels. However, conventional MRI and CT imaging will demonstrate a tissue void or hemorrhage, respectively.

Medical treatment is usually aimed at decreasing ischemic symptoms and usually consists of a combination of vasodilators and anticoagulants. Surgical options include direct anastomosis of the superficial temporal artery to the middle cerebral artery (also known as an extracranial-intracranial bypass) as well as various indirect revascularization procedures that may be combined with an extracranial-intracranial bypass. These techniques include an encephalomyosynangiosis (laying the temporalis muscle directly on the brain surface) and encephaloduroarteriosynangiosis (suturing the superficial temporal artery to the dura mater). Despite treatment, the overall prognosis is not good; only approximately 58% of patients ever attain normal neurologic function.

Management of Anesthesia

Preoperative assessment of the patient with moyamoya disease should involve the documentation of preexisting neurologic deficits and evaluation for history of hemorrhage or the concurrent presence of an intracranial aneurysm. Anticoagulants or antiplatelet drug should be discontinued, if possible, to avoid bleeding complications intraoperatively.

The goals of induction and maintenance of anesthesia include (1) ensuring hemodynamic stability because hypotension could lead to ischemia in the distribution of the abnormal vessels and hypertension may cause hemorrhagic complications, (2) avoiding factors that lead to cerebral or peripheral vasoconstriction (e.g., hypocapnia and phenylepherine), which can compromise blood flow in the feeding or recipient vessels, and (3) facilitating a rapid emergence from anesthesia so that neurologic function can be assessed. In addition to standard monitoring, intra-arterial catheterization is essential to rapidly assess changes in blood pressure. If possible, this should be instituted prior to induction of anesthesia to help ensure a hemodynamically stable induction sequence. Central venous catheterization is not essential, but can be useful to guide fluid management and can also provide access for administering vasoactive agents or blood products. With the exception of ketamine, any intravenous induction agent can be used safely. Inhalational induction with sevoflurane is an option for children. Succinylcholine should be used with caution in patients with preexisting neurologic deficits due to the risk of hyperkalemia. As with intraoperative management of aneurysms and AVMs, the hemodynamic response to stimulating events should be blunted. A volatile anesthetic-based technique may have the theoretical advantage in that it would enhance cerebral vasodilation. Excessive hyperventilation should be avoided due to its cerebral vasoconstrictive effect. Regarding the treatment of hypotension, hypovolemia should be treated with colloid or nonhypotonic crystalloid. Dopamine and ephedrine are reasonable options for the pharmacologic treatment of hypotension as they will avoid some of the adverse effects on the cerebral vasculature that might result from the use of a pure vasoconstrictor. Anemia should be avoided to prevent ischemia in already compromised brain regions.

Postoperative complications include stroke, seizure, and hemorrhage. Any of these may present as a delay in or failure to emerge from anesthesia, or, in those who do awaken, a new neurologic deficit.

TRAUMATIC BRAIN INJURY

Traumatic brain injury is the leading cause of disability and death in young adults in the United States. Brain injury may be caused by both closed head injury and penetrating injuries such as by bullets or foreign objects. Associated injuries, including cervical spine injury and thoracoabdominal trauma, frequently accompany acute head injury. Brain injury can be further exacerbated by systemic conditions related to trauma, including hypotension and hypoxia related to excessive bleeding, pulmonary contusion, aspiration, or adult respiratory distress syndrome.

Initial management of acute head injury patients includes immobilization of the cervical spine, establishment of a patent upper airway, and protection of the patient's lungs from aspiration of gastric contents, as well as maintaining perfusion of brain tissue by treating hypotension. The most useful diagnostic procedure, in terms of simplicity and rapidity, is CT, which should be performed as soon as possible. In this regard, CT has greatly facilitated identification of epidural or subdural hematomas. Routine CT may not be needed in patients with minor head trauma who meet the following criteria: no headache or vomiting, younger than 60 years of age, no intoxication, no deficits in short-term memory, no physical evidence of trauma above the clavicles, and no seizures.

It is not unusual for patients with traumatic brain injury who initially are stable and awake or in light coma to deteriorate suddenly. Delayed hematoma formation or cerebral edema is often responsible for these changes. Uncontrolled brain swelling that may not respond to conventional management may also cause sudden neurologic deterioration. Delayed secondary injury at the cellular level is an important contributor to brain swelling and subsequent irreversible brain damage.

The Glasgow Coma Scale score provides a reproducible method for assessing the seriousness of brain injury (scores of < 8 points indicate severe injury) and for following the patient's neurologic status (see Table 10A-1). Head injury patients with scores less than 8 are by definition in coma, and approximately 50% of these patients die or remain in vegetative states. Type of head injury and age are important determinants of outcome in the presence of low scores. For example, patients with acute subdural hematomas have a poorer prognosis than do patients with diffuse brain contusion injury. Mortality in children with severe head injury is less than in adults.

Perioperative Management

Perioperative management of patients with acute head trauma, such as those following motor vehicle accidents, must consider the risks of secondary injury due to cerebral ischemia as well as injuries affecting organ systems other than the brain. CBF is usually initially decreased and then gradually increases with time. Factors contributing to poor outcome in head injury patients are increased ICP and systolic blood pressures less than 70 mm Hg. Normal autoregulation of CBF is often impaired in patients with acute head injury, but carbon dioxide reactivity is usually preserved. Control of increased ICP with mannitol or furosemide is indicated, and in some patients craniectomy is necessary. Hyperventilation, although effective in controlling ICP, may contribute to cerebral ischemia in head injury patients, and for this reason, it is a common recommendation to *avoid hyperventilation* unless necessary. Barbiturate coma may be useful in some patients as a means to control intracranial hypertension when other more conservative means have failed. In adults, induced mild hypothermia in patients with acute head injury has not been shown to improve outcome. Administration of hypertonic saline and mannitol may decrease brain volume. Associated lung injuries may impair oxygenation and ventilation in these patients and necessitate mechanical ventilation. Neurogenic pulmonary edema may also contribute to acute pulmonary dysfunction. The exact mechanism for this disorder is unknown but is thought to be related to hyperactivity of the sympathetic nervous system, which results in alterations in Starling forces in the lung and pulmonary edema. Coagulopathy occurs in head injury patients and may be enhanced by hypothermia and the need for massive blood transfusions. Disseminated intravascular coagulation can occur following severe head injury. It is thought to be related to the release of brain thromboplastin into the systemic circulation. This protein is known to activate the coagulation cascade. Replacement of clotting factors may also be necessary.

Management of Anesthesia

Patients with traumatic brain injury may require anesthesia for neurosurgical interventions such as hematoma drainage, decompressive craniectomy for cerebral edema, or spinal stabilization. Anesthesia may also be required for the treatment of a variety of non-neurologic problems such as the repair of limb fractures and intra-abdominal injuries. Management of anesthesia includes efforts to optimize CPP, minimize the occurrence of cerebral ischemia, and avoid drugs and techniques that could increase ICP. CPP is maintained above 70 mm Hg if possible, and hyperventilation is not used unless it is needed as a temporizing measure to control ICP. During

surgical evacuation of acute epidural or subdural hematomas, systemic blood pressure may decrease precipitously at the time of surgical decompression and require aggressive resuscitation. Patients with severe head injury may experience impaired oxygenation and ventilation that complicates the intraoperative period. Adequate fluid resuscitation and replacement are important. Hypertonic crystalloid solutions, such as 3% saline, increase the plasma osmotic pressure and thus remove water from the brain's interstitial space. Hypotonic crystalloid solutions are avoided, as they decrease plasma osmotic pressure and increase cerebral edema even in normal brains. Glucose-containing solutions should be avoided unless specifically indicated (e.g., the treatment of laboratory-diagnosed hypoglycemia), out of concern for exacerbating neuronal injury in the setting of hyperglycemia.

Induction and Maintenance of Anesthesia

In hemodynamically stable patients, the induction of anesthesia with intravenous induction drugs and nondepolarizing muscle relaxants is acceptable. Fiberoptic intubation or tracheostomy should be considered in patients when there is added concern of either the inability to safely perform tracheal intubation via direct laryngoscopy, that a neurologic deficit may be further exacerbated (i.e., cervical spine fracture), or there is already evidence of airway compromise. In moribund patients, the establishment of a safe and effective airway takes priority over concerns for anesthetic selection, as drugs may not be needed. One should also be aware of the possible presence of hidden extracranial injuries (i.e., bone fractures, pneumothorax) as they may lead to problems such as excessive blood loss and perturbations in ventilation and circulation. Maintenance of anesthesia often includes continuous infusions of intravenous drugs or low-dose volatile anesthetics, keeping in mind the goal to optimize CPP and prevent increases in ICP. Nitrous oxide should be avoided because of the risk of pneumocephalus and concern for non-neurologic injuries such as pneumothorax. Among the volatile anesthetics, low-dose sevoflurane may be unique in minimally impairing cerebral autoregulation, although low-dose isoflurane is also a good choice. If acute brain swelling develops, correctable causes such as hypercapnia, arterial hypoxemia, systemic hypertension, and venous obstruction must be considered and corrected if present. Intra-arterial monitoring of systemic blood pressure is helpful, whereas time constraints may limit the use of CVP or pulmonary artery catheter monitoring.

Postoperative Period

During the postoperative period, it is common to maintain skeletal muscle paralysis to facilitate mechanical ventilation. Continuous monitoring of ICP is also useful in many patients.

Hematomas

Hematoma formation can result from head trauma. Typically, four major types of intracranial hematoma are described based on their location: epidural, subarachnoid, subdural, and intraparenchymal.

Epidural Hematoma

Epidural hematoma results from arterial bleeding into the space between the skull and dura. The cause is usually a tear in a meningeal artery and may be associated with a skull fracture. Classically, patients experience loss of consciousness in association with head injury, followed by return of consciousness and a variable lucid period. Hemiparesis, mydriasis, and bradycardia then suddenly develop a few hours after the head injury, reflecting uncal herniation and brainstem compression. If an epidural hematoma is suspected on CT, the treatment is prompt drainage.

Traumatic Subarachnoid Hematoma

Blood in the subarachnoid space most commonly follows rupture of an intracranial aneurysm; however, it can also be seen following trauma when it is usually caused by bleeding from cortical blood vessels. It has been found to occur in up to 40% of patients who suffered moderate or severe head injury. These lesions can evolve with time, due to further bleeding and, like subarachnoid hemorrhage associated with aneurysmal rupture, are also associated with the development of cerebral vasospasm.

Subdural Hematoma

Subdural hematoma results from lacerated or torn bridging veins that bleed into the space between the dura and arachnoid. Examination of the CSF reveals clear fluid as subdural blood does not typically have access to the subarachnoid CSF. Diagnosis of a subdural hematoma is confirmed by CT. Head trauma is the most common cause of a subdural hematoma. Patients may view the causative head trauma as trivial, and it may have been forgotten by the patient. This presentation is especially prevalent in elderly patients. Occasionally, subdural hematoma formation is spontaneous, as in patients on hemodialysis or those being treated with anticoagulants.

Signs and symptoms of a subdural hematoma characteristically evolve gradually over several days (in contrast to epidural hematomas) because the hematoma that results is due to slow venous bleeding. Headache is a universal complaint. Drowsiness and obtundation are characteristic findings, but the magnitude of these changes may fluctuate from hour to hour. Lateralizing neurologic signs eventually occur, manifesting as hemiparesis, hemianopsia, and language disturbances. Elderly patients may have unexplained progressive dementia.

Conservative medical management of subdural hematomas may be acceptable for patients whose condition stabilizes. Nevertheless, the most likely treatment is surgical evacuation of the clot, as the prognosis is poor if coma develops. Generally, most subdural hematomas can be drained via burr holes, which can be performed either under general anesthesia, local anesthesia, or monitored anesthesia care. If the subdural hematoma is either large or chronic and consists of clotted blood, drainage may require a craniotomy. Because venous bleeding in usually the cause of a subdural hematoma, following evacuation of the hematoma, normocapnia is usually the goal to allow for a larger brain volume in an attempt to tamponade any sites of venous bleeding.

Intraparenchymal Hematoma

An abnormal collection of blood located within the brain tissue proper is referred to as intraparenchymal hematoma. These lesions can be difficult to treat given their location and often acutely increase in size. As such, conservative management is often opted for unless the size or rate of growth of the hematoma is likely to cause impending herniation.

CONGENITAL ANOMALIES OF THE BRAIN

Congenital anomalies of the nervous system reflect defects in the development or architecture of the nervous system. Often a hereditary pattern is responsible for these disorders. Pathologic processes may be diffuse or may involve only those neurons that are anatomically and functionally related.

Chiari Malformation

Chiari malformations are a group of disorders consisting of congenital displacement of the cerebellum. A Chiari I malformation consists of downward displacement of the cerebellar tonsils over the cervical spinal cord, whereas Chiari II consist of downward displacement of the cerebellar vermis and are often associated with a meningomyelocele. Chiari III malformations are extremely rare and represent displacement of the cerebellum into an occipital encephalocele.

Signs and symptoms of Chiari I malformation appear at any age. The most common complaint is an occipital headache, often extending into the shoulders and arms, with corresponding cutaneous dysesthesias. Pain is aggravated by coughing or moving the head. Visual disturbances, intermittent vertigo, and ataxia are prominent symptoms. Signs of syringomyelia are present in approximately 50% of patients with this disorder. Chiari II malformations usually present in infancy with obstructive hydrocephalus plus lower brainstem and cranial nerve dysfunction.

Treatment of Chiari malformation consists of surgical decompression by freeing adhesions and enlarging the foramen magnum. Management of anesthesia must consider the possibility of associated increases in ICP as well as significant intraoperative blood loss, especially in the case of Chiari II malformations.

Tuberous Sclerosis

Tuberous sclerosis (Bourneville's disease) is an autosomal dominant disease characterized by mental retardation, seizures, and facial angiofibromas. Pathologically, tuberous sclerosis can be viewed as a condition in which a constellation of benign hamartomatous proliferative lesions and malformations occur in virtually every organ of the body. Brain lesions include cortical tubers and giant cell astrocytomas. Cardiac rhabdomyoma, although rare, is the most common benign cardiac tumor associated with tuberous sclerosis, and both echocardiography and MRI are useful for detecting cardiac tumors. An association of Wolff-Parkinson-White syndrome with tuberous sclerosis has also been described. Co-existing angiomyolipomas and cysts of the kidney may result in renal failure. Oral lesions such as nodular tumors, fibromas, or papillomas may be present on the tongue, palate, pharynx, and larynx. The prognosis of patients with tuberous sclerosis depends on the organ systems involved, ranging from no symptoms to life-threatening complications.

Anesthesia management considers the likely presence of mental retardation and treatment of seizures with antiepileptic drugs. Upper airway abnormalities are determined preoperatively. Cardiac involvement may be associated with intraoperative cardiac arrhythmias. Impaired renal function may have implications when selecting drugs that depend on renal clearance mechanisms. Although experience is limited, these patients seem to respond normally to inhaled and injected drugs, including opioids.

Von Hippel-Lindau Disease

Von Hippel-Lindau disease is familial, transmitted by an autosomal dominant gene with variable penetrance. It is characterized by retinal angiomas, hemangioblastomas, and central nervous system (typically cerebellar) and visceral tumors. Although benign, these tumors can cause symptoms secondary to pressure on surrounding structures or by virtue of hemorrhage. The incidence of pheochromocytoma, renal cysts, and renal cell carcinoma is increased with this syndrome. These patients may require intracranial surgery for resection of hemangioblastomas.

Management of anesthesia in patients with von Hippel-Lindau disease must consider the possible presence of pheochromocytomas. Preoperative treatment with antihypertensive drugs is indicated when a pheochromocytoma is identified. The possibility of spinal cord hemangioblastomas may limit the use of spinal anesthesia, although epidural anesthesia has been described for cesarean section. Exaggerated systemic hypertension, especially during direct laryngoscopy, or sudden changes in the intensity of surgical stimulation, may require intervention with esmolol, labetalol, or sodium nitroprusside (or a combination of these drugs).

Neurofibromatosis

Neurofibromatosis is due to an autosomal dominant mutation that is not limited to racial or ethnic origin. Both genders are affected with equal frequency and severity. Expressivity is variable, but penetrance of the trait is virtually 100%. Manifestations are classified as classic (von Recklinghausen's disease), acoustic, or segmental.

The diversity of clinical features of neurofibromatosis emphasizes the protean nature of this disease (**Table 10A-8**). One feature common to all patients is progression of the disease with time.

Café au lait spots (abnormal cutaneous pigmentation) are present in more than 99% of affected individuals; six or more spots larger than 1.5 cm in diameter are considered diagnostic of neurofibromatosis. Café au lait spots are usually present at birth and continue to increase in number and size during the first decade of life; they vary in size from 1 mm to more than 15 cm. Distribution of spots is random, except for disproportionately small numbers on the face. Other than an adverse cosmetic effect, café au lait spots per se pose no direct threat to health.

Neurofibromas virtually always involve the skin, but they can also occur in the deeper peripheral nerves and nerve roots and in or on viscera or blood vessels innervated by the autonomic nervous system. These neurofibromas may be nodular and discrete or diffuse with extensive interdigitations into surrounding tissues. Although neurofibromas are histologically benign, functional compromise and cosmetic disfigurement may result. The patient's airway may be compromised when neurofibromas develop in the laryngeal, cervical, or mediastinal regions. Neurofibromas may be highly vascular. Pregnancy or puberty can lead to increases in their number and size.

Intracranial tumors occur in 5% to 10% of patients with neurofibromatosis and account for a major portion of the associated morbidity and mortality. CT to rule out the presence of intracranial tumors is indicated when the diagnosis of neurofibromatosis is considered. The bilateral presence of acoustic neuromas in patients with café au lait spots establishes the diagnosis of neurofibromatosis.

Congenital pseudoarthrosis (i.e., a spontaneous fracture that progresses to nonunion) is commonly due to neurofibromatosis. The tibia is involved most often, with the radius the second most frequent site. Ordinarily, only a single site is involved in any one patient. The severity of pseudoarthrosis ranges from an asymptomatic radiographic presentation to the need for amputation. Kyphoscoliosis occurs in approximately 2% of patients afflicted with neurofibromatosis. Cervical and thoracic vertebrae are most often involved. Paravertebral neurofibromas are often present; but their role, if any, is not well understood in the development of kyphoscoliosis. Untreated, kyphoscoliosis often progresses, leading to cardiorespiratory

TABLE 10A-8 Manifestations of Neurofibromatosis
Café au lait spots
Neurofibromas (cutaneous, neural, vascular)
Intracranial tumor
Spinal cord tumor
Pseudarthrosis
Kyphoscoliosis
Short stature
Cancer
Endocrine abnormalities
Learning disability
Seizures
Congenital heart disease (pulmonic stenosis)

and neurologic compromise. Short stature is a recognized feature of neurofibromatosis.

There is an increased incidence of cancer in patients with neurofibromatosis. Associated cancers include neurofibrosarcoma, malignant schwannoma, Wilms' tumor, rhabdomyosarcoma, and leukemia. Other cancers, including neuroblastoma, medullary thyroid carcinoma, and pancreatic adenocarcinoma, are less often associated with neurofibromatosis.

It is a misconception that neurofibromatosis entails diffuse endocrine dysfunction. Associated endocrine disorders, however, include pheochromocytomas, disturbances in reaching puberty, medullary thyroid carcinoma, and hyperparathyroidism. Pheochromocytomas occur with a frequency of probably less than 1% in adults with neurofibromatosis and are virtually unknown in children with neurofibromatosis.

Intellectual impairment occurs in approximately 40% of patients with neurofibromatosis. Mental retardation is less frequent than learning disability. The intellectual handicap is usually apparent by school age and does not progress with time. Major and minor seizures are known complications of neurofibromatosis. Seizures may be idiopathic or may reflect the presence of intracranial tumors.

Treatment of neurofibromatosis consists of symptomatic drug therapy, such as antiepileptic drugs, and appropriately timed surgery. Surgical removal of cutaneous neurofibromas is reserved for those that are particularly disfiguring or functionally compromising. Progressive kyphoscoliosis is best treated with surgical stabilization. Surgery is indicated for symptoms due to nervous system involvement by neurofibromas or to associated endocrine dysfunction.

Management of Anesthesia

The anesthesia management for patients with neurofibromatosis includes consideration of the multiple clinical presentations of the disease. Although rare, the possible presence of pheochromocytomas should be considered during the preoperative evaluation. Signs of increased ICP may reflect expanding intracranial tumors. Airway patency may be jeopardized by expanding laryngeal neurofibromas. Patients with neurofibromatosis and scoliosis are also likely to have cervical spine defects that could influence positioning for direct laryngoscopy and the subsequent surgical procedure. Responses to muscle relaxants are variable, as these patients have been described as both sensitive and resistant to succinylcholine and sensitive to nondepolarizing muscle relaxants. Selection of regional anesthesia must recognize the possible future development of neurofibromas involving the spinal cord. Nevertheless, epidural analgesia is an effective method for producing analgesia during labor and delivery.

DEGENERATIVE DISEASES OF THE BRAIN

Degenerative diseases of the central nervous system usually involve neuronal malfunction or loss within specific anatomic regions and represent a diffuse group of disease states.

Alzheimer's Disease

Alzheimer's disease is a chronic neurodegenerative disorder. It is the most common cause of dementia in patients older than 65 years of age, and the fourth most common cause of death from disease in patients older than 65. Diffuse amyloid-rich senile plaques and neurofibrillary tangles are the hallmark pathologic findings. There are also changes in synapses and the activity of multiple major neurotransmitters, especially involving acetylcholine and central nervous system nicotinic receptors. Two types of Alzheimer's disease have been described: early onset and late onset. Early-onset Alzheimer's disease usually presents before age 60 and is thought to be due to missense mutations on up to three genes leading to an autosomal dominant mode of transmission. Late-onset Alzheimer's disease usually develops after age 60, and genetic transmission appears to play a relatively minor role in the risk of developing this disorder. With both forms of the disease, patients typically develop progressive cognitive impairment that can consist of problems with memory as well as apraxia, aphasia, and agnosia. Definitive diagnosis is usually made on postmortem examination, usually making premortem diagnosis of Alzheimer's disease one of exclusion. There is currently no cure for Alzheimer's disease, and treatment usually focuses on control of symptoms. Pharmacologic options include cholinesterase inhibitors, such as tacrine, donepezil, rivastigmine, and galantamine. Pharmacologic therapy should be combined with nonpharmacologic therapy including caregiver education and family support. Despite treatment, the prognosis for patients with Alzheimer's disease is poor.

Patients with Alzheimer's disease may present for a variety of surgical interventions that are common in the elderly population. Patients are often confused and sometimes uncooperative, making monitored anesthesia care or regional anesthesia challenging. However, there is probably no one single anesthesia technique or agent that is superior in this group of patients. Shorter acting sedative/hypnotic drugs, anesthetic agents, and narcotics are preferred since they may allow a more rapid return to baseline mental status. Finally, one should be aware of potential drug interactions, especially prolongation of the effect of succinylcholine and relative resistance to nondepolarizing muscle relaxants due to the use of cholinesterase inhibitors.

Parkinson's Disease

Parkinson's disease is a neurodegenerative disorder of unknown cause. Increasing age is the single most important risk factor in the development of this disease; however, an association between manganese exposure in welders as well as a variety of genetic associations have recently been identified. There is a characteristic loss of dopaminergic fibers normally present in the basal ganglia, and, as a result, regional dopamine concentrations are depleted. Dopamine is presumed to inhibit the rate of firing of the neurons that control the extrapyramidal motor system. Depletion of dopamine results in diminished inhibition of these neurons and unopposed stimulation by acetylcholine.

The classic triad of major signs of Parkinson's disease consists of skeletal muscle tremor, rigidity, and akinesia. Skeletal muscle rigidity first appears in the proximal muscles of the neck. The earliest manifestations may be loss of associated arm swings when walking and absence of head rotation when turning the body. Facial immobility is characterized by infrequent blinking and by a paucity of emotional responses. Tremors are characterized as rhythmic, alternating flexion and extension of the thumbs and other digits at a rate of four or five movements per second ("pill-rolling tremor"). Tremors are most prominent in resting limbs but tend to disappear during the course of voluntary movement. Seborrhea, oily skin, diaphragmatic spasms, and oculogyric crises are frequent. Dementia and depression are often present.

Treatment of Parkinson's disease is designed to increase the concentration of dopamine in the basal ganglia or to decrease the neuronal effects of acetylcholine. Replacement therapy with the dopamine precursor levodopa combined with a decarboxylase inhibitor, which prevents peripheral conversion of levodopa to dopamine and optimizes the amount of levodopa available to enter the central nervous system, is the standard medical treatment. Indeed, levodopa is the most effective treatment for Parkinson's disease, and early treatment with this drug prolongs life. Levodopa is also associated with a number of side effects including dyskinesias (i.e., the most serious side effect, developing in 80% of patients after 1 year of treatment) and psychiatric disturbances (including agitation, hallucinations, mania, and paranoia). Increased myocardial contractility and heart rate in treated patients may reflect increased levels of circulating dopamine converted from levodopa. Orthostatic hypotension may be prominent in treated patients. Gastrointestinal side effects of levodopa therapy include nausea and vomiting, most likely reflecting stimulation of the medullary chemoreceptor trigger zone.

Amantadine, an antiviral agent, is reported to help control the symptoms of Parkinson's disease; however, the mechanism for this effect is not fully understood. The type B monoamine oxidase inhibitor selegiline can also help control the symptoms of Parkinson's disease by inhibiting the catabolism of dopamine in the central nervous system. Selegiline has an advantage over nonspecific monoamine oxidase inhibitors since they are only weak inhibitors of type A monoamine oxidase, the isoenzyme found primarily in the gastrointestinal tract. Therefore, selegiline is not associated with tyramine-associated hypertensive crisis, which results when foods containing tyramine (i.e., cheese, wine) are consumed by those in whom type A monoamine oxidase is pharmacologically inhibited. Entry of tyramine into the systemic circulation in the setting of pharmacologically inhibited type A monoamine oxidase results in a hyperadrenergic state due to the inherent sympathomimetic activities of tyramine.

Surgical treatment of Parkinson's disease is reserved for disabling and medically refractory symptoms. Stimulation of the subthalamic nuclei via an implanted deep brain stimulator device may relieve or help to control tremor. Pallidotomy is associated with significant improvement in levodopa-induced dyskinesias, although the improvement may be short-lived. Fetal tissue transplantation for treatment of Parkinson's disease is based on the demonstration that implanted embryonic dopaminergic neurons can survive in recipients; however, the effectiveness of this treatment is currently not known.

Management of Anesthesia

Management of anesthesia in patients with Parkinson's disease is based on an understanding of the treatment of this disease and the associated potential adverse drug effects. The elimination half-time of levodopa and the dopamine it produces is brief, so interruption of therapy for more than 6 to 12 hours can result in an abrupt loss of therapeutic effects. Abrupt drug withdrawal can lead to skeletal muscle rigidity, which interferes with lung ventilation. In this regard, levodopa therapy, including the usual morning dose on the day of surgery, should be continued during the perioperative period. Oral levodopa can be administered approximately 20 minutes before inducing anesthesia and may be repeated intraoperatively and postoperatively via an oro- or nasogastric tube to minimize the likelihood of exacerbations.

The possibility of hypotension and cardiac arrhythmias must be considered during administration of anesthesia to patients treated with levodopa. Further, one must consider the ability of butyrophenones (e.g., droperidol, haloperidol) to antagonize the effects of dopamine in the basal ganglia. An acute dystonic reaction following administration of alfentanil has been speculated to reflect opioid-induced decreases in central dopaminergic transmission. Use of ketamine is questionable because of the possible provocation of exaggerated sympathetic nervous system responses. Nevertheless, ketamine has been administered safely to patients treated with levodopa. The choice of muscle relaxants does not seem to be influenced by the presence of Parkinson's disease.

Hallervorden-Spatz Disease

Hallervorden-Spatz disease is a rare autosomal recessive disorder of the basal ganglia. It follows a slowly progressive course from its onset during late childhood to death in approximately 10 years. No specific laboratory tests are diagnostic for this condition, and no effective treatment is known. Dementia and dystonia with torticollis, as well as scoliosis, are commonly present. Dystonic posturing is likely to disappear with the induction of anesthesia, although skeletal muscle contractures and bony changes may accompany the chronic forms of the disease, leading to immobility of the temporomandibular joint and cervical spine, even in the presence of deep general anesthesia or drug-induced skeletal muscle paralysis.

Management of anesthesia must consider the possibility of being unable to position these patients optimally for tracheal intubation following the induction of anesthesia. Noxious stimulation, as produced by attempted awake tracheal intubation, can intensify dystonia. For these reasons, induction of anesthesia may be achieved by inhalation and maintenance of spontaneous ventilation. Administration of succinylcholine is questionable, as skeletal muscle wasting and diffuse axonal changes in the brain, which may involve the upper motor neurons, could accentuate the release of potassium; however, succinylcholine has been reported to have been used safely. Offsetting this centrally mediated propensity for muscle wasting may be that chronic muscle hyperactivity produces muscular and cardiovascular effects similar to that of a trained athlete. Any required skeletal muscle relaxation is probably best provided by increased concentrations of volatile anesthetics or administration of nondepolarizing neuromuscular blocking drugs. Emergence from anesthesia is predictably accompanied by return of dystonic posturing.

Huntington's Disease

Huntington's disease is a premature degenerative disease of the central nervous system characterized by marked atrophy of the caudate nucleus and, to a lesser degree, the putamen and globus pallidus. Biochemical abnormalities include deficiencies in the basal ganglia of acetylcholine (and its synthesizing enzyme choline acetyltransferase) and γ-aminobutyric acid. Selective loss of γ-aminobutyric acid may decrease inhibition of the dopamine nigrostriatal system. This disease is transmitted as an autosomal dominant trait, but its delayed appearance until 35 to 40 years of age interferes with effective genetic counseling. Identification of the genetic defect may be useful for disease risk prediction in those who have inherited the defective gene, as applied to both prenatal and postnatal (including adult) testing.

Manifestations of Huntington's disease consist of progressive dementia combined with choreoathetosis. Chorea is usually considered the first sign of Huntington's disease; hence, the former designation of this disease as Huntington's chorea. Behavioral changes (e.g, depression, aggressive outbursts, mood swings) may precede the onset of involuntary movement by several years. Involvement of the pharyngeal muscles makes these patients susceptible to pulmonary aspiration. The disease progresses over several years, and accompanying mental depression makes suicide a frequent cause of death. The duration of Huntington's disease, from clinical onset to death, averages 17 years.

Treatment of Huntington's disease is symptomatic and is directed at decreasing the choreiform movements. Haloperidol and other butyrophenones may be administered to control the chorea and emotional lability associated with the disease. The most useful therapy for controlling involuntary movements is with drugs that interfere with the neurotransmitter effects of dopamine either via antagonism (i.e., haloperidol, fluphenazine) or via depletion of dopamine stores (i.e., reserpine, tetrabenazine).

Experience with the management of anesthesia in patients with Huntington's chorea is too limited to recommend specific anesthetic drugs or techniques. Preoperative sedation using butyrophenones such as droperidol or haloperidol may be helpful in controlling choreiform movements. The increased likelihood of pulmonary aspiration must be considered if pharyngeal muscles are involved. Nitrous oxide and volatile anesthetic use is acceptable. Thiopental, succinylcholine, and mivacurium have been administered without adverse effects, but decreased plasma cholinesterase activity, with prolonged responses to succinylcholine, has been observed. Likewise, it has been suggested that these patients may be sensitive to the effects of nondepolarizing muscle relaxants.

Torticollis

Torticollis is thought to result from disturbances of basal ganglia function. The most common mode of presentation is spasmodic contraction of nuchal muscles, which may progress to involvement of limb and girdle muscles. Hypertrophy of the sternocleidomastoid muscles may be present. Spasm may involve the muscles of the vertebral column, leading to lordosis, scoliosis, and impaired ventilation. Treatment is not particularly effective, but a bilateral anterior rhizotomy at C1 and C3, with a sectioning of the spinal accessory nerve, may be attempted. This operation may cause postoperative paralysis of the diaphragm, resulting in respiratory distress. Selective peripheral denervation of affected cervical musculature is also a surgical option. There are no known problems relative to the selection of anesthetic drugs, but spasm of nuchal muscles can interfere with maintenance of a patent upper airway before institution of skeletal muscle paralysis. Furthermore, awake tracheal intubation may be necessary if chronic skeletal muscle spasm has led to fixation of the cervical vertebrae. Surgery may be performed with the patient in the sitting position. If so, anesthetic considerations for the sitting position should come into play. (see "Sitting Position and Venous Air Embolism") Sudden appearance of torticollis after administration of anesthetic drugs has been reported, and administration of diphenhydramine, 25 to 50 mg IV, produces a dramatic reversal of this drug-induced torticollis.

Transmissible Spongiform Encephalopathies

The human transmissible spongiform encephalopathies are Creutzfeldt-Jakob disease (CJD), kuru, Gerstmann-Sträussler-Scheinker syndrome, and fatal familial insomnia. These noninflammatory diseases of the central nervous system are caused by transmissible slow infectious protein pathogens known as *prions*. Prions differ from viruses in that they lack RNA and DNA and fail to produce a detectable immune reaction. Transmissible spongiform encephalopathies are diagnosed on the basis of clinical and neuropathologic findings (diffuse or focally clustered small, round vacuoles that may become confluent). Familial progressive subcortical gliosis and some inherited thalamic dementias may also be spongiform encephalopathies. Bovine spongiform encephalopathy (mad cow disease) is a transmissible spongiform encephalopathy that occurs in animals. Infectivity has not been detected in skeletal muscles, milk, or blood.

CJD is the most common transmissible spongiform encephalopathy, with an estimated incidence of one case per million worldwide. Transmission of the prion and the development of clinical disease are still poorly understood. In fact, a significant proportion of the population are probably carriers of the CJD prion, but most do not develop clinical disease. Further, approximately 10% to 15% of persons with CJD have a family history of the disease; therefore, infectious and genetic factors probably both play a role in disease development. The time interval between infection and development of symptoms is measured in months to years. The disease develops by accumulation of an abnormal protein thought to act as a neurotransmitter in the central nervous system. This prion protein is encoded by a specific gene, and sporadic and random mutations may result in variants of CJD. Rapidly progressive dementia with ataxia and myoclonus suggests the diagnosis, although confirmation may require a brain biopsy because there are no reliable, noninvasive, diagnostic tests. Alzheimer's disease poses the most difficult differential diagnosis. In contrast to toxic and metabolic disorders, myoclonus is rarely present at the onset of CJD, and seizures, when they occur, are a late phenomenon. No vaccines or treatments are effective.

Universal infection precautions (e.g., as used for patients with hepatitis B or human immunodeficiency virus infection) are recommended when caring for patients with CJD, but other precautions are not necessary. Handling CSF calls for special precautions (double gloves, protective glasses, specimen labeled "infectious"), as this has been the only body fluid shown to result in transmission to primates. Biopsies and autopsies require similar precautions, although the risk of communicable infection is less than that created by similar procedures in those who are seropositive for hepatitis B virus or human immunodeficiency virus. Nevertheless, the main risk of transmitting CJD is during cerebral biopsy for diagnostic confirmation of the disease. Instruments should be disposable or should be decontaminated by soaking in sodium hypochlorite or autoclaving.

Human-to-human transmission has occurred inadvertently in association with surgical procedures (corneal transplantation, stereotactic procedures with previously used electrodes, contaminated neurosurgical instruments, and human cadaveric dura mater transplantation). Transmission has been attributed to treatment with growth hormone and gonadotropic hormones. Although the injection or transplantation of human tissues may result in transmission of infectious prions, the hazards of transmission through human blood are debatable as this disease is not observed more frequently in hemophiliacs as in the general population. Nevertheless, transfusion of blood from individuals known to be infected is not recommended.

Management of anesthesia includes the use of universal infection precautions, disposable equipment, and sterilization of any reusable equipment (laryngoscope blades) using sodium hypochlorite. Surgery in patients known or suspected to be infected may be better performed at the end of the day to allow thorough cleansing of equipment and the operating room before the next use. Personnel participating in anesthesia and surgery are kept to a minimum, and they should wear protective gowns, gloves, and face masks with transparent protective visors to protect the eyes. Given that a proportion of the general population are probably carriers of the prion thought to cause CJD and that both infectious and genetic

factors probably both play a role in the development of clinical symptoms, the likelihood of contracting and developing CJD after coming in contact with the CJD prion is probably very low. However, one should still exercise standard precautionary measures.

Multiple Sclerosis

Multiple sclerosis is an autoimmune disease affecting the central nervous system that seems to occur in genetically susceptible persons. Although there is a high rate of concordance among twins and an increased risk if one has a first-degree relative with the disease as well as a geographic association (e.g., highest incidence in northern Europe, southern Australia, and North America), no clear genetic, environmental, or infectious causes have been identified. There is also no clear understanding of the immunopathogenic processes that determine the sites of tissue damage in the central nervous system, the variations in natural history, or the severity of disability caused by the disease. It is twice as common in women as in men. In women with multiple sclerosis, the rate of relapse decreases during pregnancy, especially in the third trimester, and increases during the first 3 months postpartum. Exposure to viral illnesses may trigger relapses. Pathologically, multiple sclerosis is characterized by diverse combinations of inflammation, demyelination, and axonal damage in the central nervous system. The loss of myelin covering the axons is followed by formation of demyelinative plaques. Peripheral nerves are not affected by multiple sclerosis.

Clinical manifestations of multiple sclerosis reflect its multifocal involvement. Its course may be subacute, with relapses followed by remissions, or chronic and progressive. Manifestations of multiple sclerosis reflect sites of demyelination in the central nervous system and spinal cord. For example, inflammation of the optic nerves (optic neuritis) causes visual disturbances, involvement of the cerebellum leads to gait disturbances, and lesions of the spinal cord cause limb paresthesias and weakness as well as urinary incontinence and sexual impotence. Optic neuritis is characterized by diminished visual acuity and defective pupillary reaction to light. Ascending spastic paresis of the skeletal muscles is often prominent. Intramedullary disease of the cervical cord is suggested by an electrical sensation that runs down the back into the legs in response to flexion of the neck (Lhermitte's sign). Typically, symptoms develop over the course of a few days, remain stable for a few weeks, and then improve. Because remyelination in the central nervous system probably does not occur, remission of symptoms most likely results from correction of transient chemical and physiologic disturbances that have interfered with nerve conduction in the absence of complete demyelination. Further, increases in body temperature can cause exacerbation of symptoms due to further alterations in nerve conduction in regions of demyelination. There is an increased incidence of seizure disorders in patients with multiple sclerosis.

The course of multiple sclerosis is characterized by exacerbations and remissions of symptoms at unpredictable intervals over a period of several years. Residual symptoms eventually persist during remissions, leading to severe disability from visual failure, ataxia, spastic skeletal muscle weakness, and urinary incontinence. Nevertheless, the disease in some patients remains benign, with infrequent, mild episodes of demyelination, followed by prolonged, occasionally permanent remissions. The onset of multiple sclerosis after 35 years of age is typically associated with slow disease progression.

The diagnosis of multiple sclerosis can be established with different degrees of confidence (e.g., probable or definite) on the basis of clinical features alone or clinical features in combination with oligoclonal abnormalities of immunoglobulins in the CSF, prolonged latency of evoked potentials reflecting slowing of nerve conduction due to demyelination, and signal changes in white matter seen on cranial MRI.

No treatment is curative for multiple sclerosis. Instead, treatment is directed at both symptom control and methods to slow the progression of disease. Corticosteroids, the principal treatment for acute relapses of multiple sclerosis, have immunomodulatory and anti-inflammatory effects that restore the blood-brain barrier, decrease edema, and possibly improve axonal conduction. Treatment with corticosteroids shortens the duration of the relapse and accelerates recovery, but whether the overall degree of recovery or progression of the disease is altered is not known. Interferon-β is the treatment of choice for patients with relapsing-remitting multiple sclerosis. The most common side effect of interferon-β therapy is transient influenza-like symptoms for 24 to 48 hours after injection. Slight increases in serum aminotransferase concentrations, leukopenia, or anemia may be present, and co-existing depression may be exaggerated. Glatiramer acetate is a mixture of random synthetic polypeptides synthesized to mimic myelin basic protein. This drug is an alternative to interferon-β and may be most useful for patients who become resistant to interferon-β treatment owing to serum interferon-β-neutralizing activity. Mitoxantrone is an immunosuppressive agent that functions by inhibiting lymphocyte proliferation. Because of severe cardiac toxicity, its use is limited to patients with rapidly progressive disease. Azathioprine is a purine analogue that depresses both cell-mediated and humoral immunity. Treatment with this drug may decrease the rate of relapses in multiple sclerosis but has no effect on the progression of disability. Azathioprine is considered when patients do not respond to therapy with interferon-β or glatiramer acetate. Low-dose methotrexate is relatively nontoxic and inhibits both cell-mediated and humoral immunity as a result of its anti-inflammatory effects. Patients with secondary progressive multiple sclerosis may benefit most from treatment with this drug.

Management of Anesthesia

Management of anesthesia in patients with multiple sclerosis must consider the impact of surgical stress on the natural progression of the disease. For example, regardless of the anesthetic technique or drugs selected for use during the perioperative period, it is possible that symptoms of multiple sclerosis will be exacerbated postoperatively. This may be due to factors such as infection and fever. In this regard, any increase in body temperature (e.g., as little as 1°C) that follows surgery may be more likely than drugs to be responsible for exacerbations of multiple sclerosis. It is possible that increased body temperature results in complete block of conduction in demyelinated nerves. Of note, the unpredictable cycle of clinical exacerbations and remissions could lead to erroneous conclusions that there are cause-and-effect relationship between disease severity and drugs or events present during the perioperative period.

The changing and unpredictable neurologic presentation in patients with multiple sclerosis during the perioperative period must be appreciated when selecting regional anesthetic techniques. Indeed, spinal anesthesia has been implicated in postoperative exacerbations of multiple sclerosis, whereas exacerbations of the disease after epidural anesthesia or peripheral nerve blocks have not been described. The mechanism by which spinal anesthesia might differ from epidural anesthesia is unknown but might reflect local anesthetic neurotoxicity. Specifically, it is speculated that the demyelination associated with multiple sclerosis renders the spinal cord more susceptible to the neurotoxic effects of local anesthetics. Epidural anesthesia may be less of a risk than spinal anesthesia because the concentration of local anesthetics in the white matter of the spinal cord is lower than after spinal anesthesia. Nevertheless, both epidural anesthesia and spinal anesthesia have been used in parturients with multiple sclerosis.

General anesthesia is the most often used technique in patients with multiple sclerosis. There are no unique interactions between multiple sclerosis and the drugs used to provide general anesthesia, and there is no evidence to support use of one inhaled or injected anesthetic drug over another. When selecting muscle relaxants, one should consider the possibility of exaggerated release of muscle potassium, causing hyperkalemia, following administration of succinylcholine to these patients. Prolonged responses to the paralyzing effects of nondepolarizing muscle relaxants would be consistent with co-existing skeletal muscle weakness (myasthenia-like) and decreased skeletal muscle mass. Conversely, resistance to the effects of nondepolarizing muscle relaxants has been observed, perhaps reflecting proliferation of extrajunctional cholinergic receptors characteristic of upper motor neuron lesions.

Corticosteroid supplementation during the perioperative period may be indicated in patients being treated long-term with these drugs. Efforts must be made to recognize and prevent even modest increases in body temperature (more than 1°C), as this change might exacerbate symptoms. Periodic neurologic evaluation during the postoperative period may be useful for detecting exacerbations.

Postpolio Sequelae

Poliomyelitis is caused by an enterovirus that initially infects the reticuloendothelial system. In a minority of patients, the virus enters the central nervous system and preferentially targets motor neurons in the brainstem and anterior horn of the spinal cord. The worldwide incidence of poliomyelitis has significantly decreased since the institution of vaccination against this disease; however, various locations, such as India, Pakistan, and Nigeria still represent major reservoirs for the virus. In the United States, only six cases of poliomyelitis have been reported since 1979, and all were vaccine associated. Given that poliomyelitis is so rare, from the clinician's point of view, patients with postpolio sequelae are much more common than those with acute polio. Postpolio sequelae manifest as fatigue, skeletal muscle weakness, joint pain, cold intolerance, dysphagia, and sleep and breathing problems (i.e., obstructive sleep apnea) that presumably reflect neurologic damage from the original poliovirus infection. Poliovirus may damage the reticular activating system, accounting for the fact that these individuals may exhibit exquisite sensitivity to sedative effects of anesthetics as well as delayed awakening from anesthesia. Sensitivity to nondepolarizing muscle relaxants is common. Severe back pain following surgery may be due to co-existing skeletal muscle atrophy and scoliosis. Postoperative shivering may be profound, as these individuals are highly sensitive to cold. Postoperative pain sensitivity seems to be increased and is presumed to be related to poliovirus damage to endogenous opioid-secreting cells in the brain and spinal cord. Outpatient surgery may not be appropriate for many postpolio patients as they are at increased risk of complications, especially secondary to respiratory muscle weakness and dysphagia.

SEIZURE DISORDERS

Seizures are caused by transient, paroxysmal, and synchronous discharge of groups of neurons in the brain. Seizure is one of the most common neurologic disorders and may occur at any age, with more than 10% of the population experiencing seizures at some time during their life. Clinical manifestations depend on the location and number of neurons involved in the seizure discharge and its duration. Transient abnormalities of brain function, such as occurs with hypoglycemia, hyponatremia, hyperthermia, and drug toxicity, typically result in a single seizure; treatment of the underlying disorder usually is curative. Conversely, epilepsy is defined as recurrent seizures resulting from congenital or acquired (e.g., cerebral scarring) factors; it affects approximately 0.6% of the population.

Current classification of epileptic seizures is based on the 1981 revision of a method described by the Commission on Classification and Terminology of the International League Against Epilepsy. Seizures are currently classified based on two factors: loss of consciousness and focus of seizure activation. Simple seizures involve no loss of consciousness, whereas altered levels of consciousness are seen in complex seizures. Partial seizures appear to originate from a limited population of neurons in a single hemisphere, whereas generalized seizures appear to initially involve diffuse activation of neurons in both cerebral hemispheres. A partial seizure may be initially evident in one region of the body (i.e., the right arm) and may subsequently become generalized, involving both hemispheres, a process known as the jacksonian march.

MRI is the preferred method for studying brain structure in patients with epilepsy. Standard electroencephalography is used to identify the location or locations of seizure foci as well as characterize their electrical properties. The use of videography in addition to electroencephalography allows for the simultaneous documentation of electrical and clinical seizure activity. Electrocorticography, where electrodes are surgically placed directly on the cerebral cortex, not only permits more accurate focus identification but also allows for mapping electrical events in the context of identifiable brain surface anatomy (a feature that will be valuable during surgical resection). Further, stimulation of various electrocorticographic electrodes will help identify eloquent brain areas prior to seizure focus resection, such that those areas can be avoided during surgery.

Pharmacologic Treatment

Seizures are treated initially with antiepileptic drugs starting with a single drug and achieving seizure control by increasing the dose as necessary. Drug combinations may be considered when monotherapy fails. Changes in drug dose are guided by the patient's clinical response (e.g., effects versus side effects) rather than by serum drug concentrations. Monitoring serum drug levels is usually not necessary for patients who are experiencing adequate seizure control without evidence of toxicity. Effective antiepileptic drugs appear to decrease neuronal excitability or enhance neuronal inhibition. Drugs effective for the treatment of *partial* seizures include carbamazepine, phenytoin, and valproate. *Generalized* seizure disorders can be managed with carbamazepine, phenytoin, valproate, barbiturates, gabapentin, or lamotrigine. Except for gabapentin, all the useful antiepileptic drugs are metabolized in the liver before undergoing renal excretion. Gabapentin appears to have no in vivo metabolism and is excreted unchanged by the kidneys. Carbamazepine, phenytoin, and barbiturates cause enzyme induction, and long-term treatment with these drugs can alter the rate of their own metabolism and that of other drugs. Pharmacokinetic and pharmacodynamic drug interactions are considerations in patients being treated with antiepileptic drugs.

Dose-dependent neurotoxic effects are the most common adverse responses evoked by antiepileptic drugs. All antiepileptic drugs can cause depression of cerebral function with symptoms of sedation.

Phenytoin has many side effects including hypotension, cardiac arrhythmias, gingival hyperplasia, and aplastic anemia. It is associated with various cutaneous manifestations including erythema multiforme and Stevens-Johnson syndrome. Extravasation or intra-arterial injection of phenytoin can induce significant vasoconstriction, resulting in purple glove syndrome, which can lead to skin necrosis, compartment syndrome, and gangrene. These side effects make fosphenytoin, a phosphorylated prodrug that does not share the same toxicity profile as phenytoin, a more attractive option for intravenous antiepileptic administration.

Valproate produces hepatic failure in approximately one in every 10,000 patients. The mechanism of this hepatotoxicity is unknown but may reflect an idiosyncratic hypersensitivity reaction. Pancreatitis also has been observed during valproate therapy. Long-term use of valproate is associated with increased surgical bleeding, especially in children. The mechanism is currently unknown but is thought to be due to a combination of thrombocytopenia as well as valproate-induced decreases in von Willebrand factor and factor VIII.

Carbamazepine can cause diplopia, dose-related leukopenia, and hyponatremia (which is usually clinical unimportant) as well as alterations in the hepatic metabolism of various drugs.

Adverse hematologic reactions associated with antiepileptic drugs range from mild anemia to aplastic anemia and are most commonly associated with the use of carbamazepine, phenytoin, and valproate.

Surgical Treatment

Surgical treatment of seizure disorders is a consideration in patients who do not respond to antiepileptic drugs. Surgery is now being performed much earlier than in the past, particularly in young patients, to avoid social retardation resulting from medication side effects and persistent seizures. Partial seizures may respond to resection of a pathologic region within the brain (e.g., to remove a tumor, hamartoma, or scar tissue). Corpus callosotomy may help to prevent the generalization of partial seizures to the alternate hemisphere. Finally, hemispherectomy is sometimes needed for persistent catastrophic seizures.

In preparation for surgery, the seizure focus is first located by electrocorticography and information obtained from MRI studies. The most common operation is temporal lobectomy. Permanent hemiparesis is a potential adverse effect of this surgery. A more conservative surgical approach to medically intractable seizures involves the implantation of a left vagal nerve stimulator. The left side is chosen since the right vagal nerve usually has significant cardiac innervation, which could lead to severe bradyarrhythmias. The mechanism by which vagal nerve stimulation produces its effects is unclear. Patients tolerate this well except for hoarseness in some cases, reflecting the vagal innervation of the larynx.

Status Epilepticus

Status epilepticus is a life-threatening condition that manifests as continuous seizure activity or two or more seizures occurring in sequence without recovery of consciousness between them.

The goal of treatment of status epilepticus is prompt establishment of venous access and subsequent pharmacologic suppression of seizure activity combined with support of the patient's airway, ventilation, and circulation. Hypoglycemia can be ruled out as a cause within minutes using rapid bedside glucose assessment techniques. If present, it can be corrected by intravenous administration of 50 mL of 50% glucose. Routine use of glucose infusion prior to confirming preexisting hypoglycemia is not recommended as hyperglycemia can exacerbate brain injury. Tracheal intubation may be needed to protect the patient's lungs from aspiration and to optimize delivery of oxygen and removal of carbon dioxide. Long-acting muscle relaxants should be avoided if muscle movement, independent of electrophysiologic monitoring, is the principal endpoint for assessing therapy effectiveness. Usually, administration of an antiepileptic anesthetic, such as propofol or thiopental, will temporarily halt seizure activity during tracheal intubation. Monitoring arterial blood gases and pH may be useful for confirming the adequacy of oxygenation and ventilation. Metabolic acidosis is a common sequela of ongoing seizure activity. In such instances, intravenous sodium bicarbonate may be needed to treat extreme acid-base abnormalities. Hyperthermia associated with muscle hyperactivity and increased brain metabolism occurs frequently during status epilepticus and necessitates active cooling.

Management of Anesthesia

Management of anesthesia in patients with seizure disorders includes considering the impact of antiepileptic drugs on organ function and the effect of anesthetic drugs on seizures. Co-existing sedation produced by antiepileptic drugs may have additive effects with anesthetic drugs, whereas drug-induced enzyme induction could alter the pharmacokinetics and pharmacodynamics of other drugs.

When selecting anesthetic induction and maintenance drugs, one must consider their effects on central nervous system electrical activity. For example, methohexital can activate epileptic foci and has been recommended as a method for delineating these foci during electrocorticography in patients undergoing surgical treatment of epilepsy. Similarly, alfentanil, ketamine, enflurane, isoflurane, and sevoflurane can cause epileptiform spike-and-wave electroencephalographic activity in patients without a history of seizures, but are also known to suppress epileptiform and epileptic activity. Seizures and opisthotonos have rarely been observed following propofol anesthesia, suggesting caution when administering this drug to patients with known seizure disorders. When selecting muscle relaxants, the central nervous system–stimulating effects of laudanosine, a proconvulsant metabolite of atracurium and cisatracurium, may merit consideration. Various antiepileptic drugs, specifically phenytoin and carbamazepine, via both pharmacokinetic and pharmacodynamic means, shorten the duration of action of nondepolarizing muscle relaxants. Topiramate may cause unexplained metabolic acidosis, given its ability to inhibit carbonic anhydrase.

Most inhaled anesthetics, including nitrous oxide, have been reported to produce seizure activity. The presence of halogen atoms is an important determinant of the convulsant properties of volatile anesthetics, with fluorine being incriminated as epileptogenic.

It seems reasonable to avoid administering potentially epileptogenic drugs to patients with epilepsy. Instead, thiobarbiturates, opioids, and benzodiazepines are preferred. Isoflurane, desflurane, and sevoflurane seem to be acceptable choices in patients with seizure disorders. Regardless of the drugs used for anesthesia, it is important to maintain treatment with the existing antiepileptic drugs throughout the perioperative period.

NEURO-OCULAR DISORDERS

Disorders involving the visual system discussed in the following section are limited to those affecting the retina, optic nerve, and intracranial optic system. Degenerative diseases of this part of the visual system include Leber's optic atrophy, retinitis pigmentosa, and the Kearns-Sayer syndrome. The most common cause of blindness during the postoperative period is ischemic optic neuropathy. Other causes of postoperative visual defects are cortical blindness, retinal artery occlusion, and ophthalmic vein obstruction.

Leber's Optic Atrophy

Leber's optic atrophy, or Leber's hereditary optic neuropathy, is characterized by degeneration of the retina and atrophy of the optic nerves culminating in blindness. This disorder was the first human disorder for which a mitochondrial pattern of inheritance was definitively described. This rare disorder usually presents as loss of central vision in adolescence or early adulthood and is often associated with other neuropathology including multiple sclerosis and dystonia.

Retinitis Pigmentosa

Retinitis pigmentosa describes a genetically and clinically heterogeneous group of inherited retinopathies characterized by degeneration of the retina. These debilitating disorders collectively represent a common form of human visual handicap, with an estimated prevalence of approximately 1 in 3000. Examination of the retina shows areas of pigmentation, particularly in the peripheral regions. Vision is lost from the periphery of the retina toward the center until total blindness develops.

Kearns-Sayer Syndrome

Kearns-Sayer syndrome is characterized by retinitis pigmentosa associated with progressive external ophthalmoplegia, typically manifesting before 20 years of age. Cardiac conduction abnormalities, ranging from bundle branch block to complete atrioventricular heart block, are common. The latter can occur abruptly, leading to sudden death. Generalized degeneration of the central nervous system has been observed. This finding and the often increased concentrations of protein in the CSF suggest a viral etiology. Although Kearns-Sayer syndrome is rare, it is possible that these patients will require anesthesia for placement of implantable cardiac pacemakers.

Management of anesthesia requires a high index of suspicion for, and previous preparation to treat, new-onset third-degree atrioventricular heart block. Transthoracic pacing is the initial treatment of choice for high-degree heart block. Experience is too limited to recommend specific drugs for induction and maintenance of anesthesia. Presumably, the response to succinylcholine and nondepolarizing muscle relaxants is not altered, as this disease does not involve the neuromuscular junctions.

Ischemic Optic Neuropathy

Ischemic optic neuropathy should be suspected in patients who complain of visual loss during the first week following surgery of any form. Ischemic injury to the optic nerve can result in loss of both central and peripheral vision.

The optic nerve can be functionally divided into an anterior and a posterior segment based on difference in blood supply (**Fig. 10A-6**). Blood supply to the anterior portion is derived from both the central retinal artery as well as from small branches of the ciliary artery. In contrast, blood supply to the posterior segment of the optic nerve is derived from small branches of the ophthalmic and central retinal arteries. Baseline blood flow to the posterior segment of the optic nerve is significantly less than that of the anterior segment. Because of this difference, ischemic events in the anterior and posterior segments of the optic nerve have different risk factors and physical findings; however, the prognosis, in terms of improvement of vision, is poor in either case. If ischemic optic neuropathy is suspected, urgent ophthalmologic consultation should be obtained as other more treatable causes of perioperative blindness should be ruled out.

Anterior Ischemic Optic Neuropathy

The visual loss associated with anterior ischemic optic neuropathy is due to infarction within the watershed perfusion zones between the small branches of the short posterior ciliary arteries. The usual presentation involves sudden, painless, monocular visual deficits varying in severity from slight decreases in visual acuity to blindness. Asymptomatic optic disk swelling may be the earliest sign. A congenitally small optic disk is often present. The prognosis varies, but the most common outcome is minimal recovery of visual function.

The nonarteritic form of anterior ischemic optic neuropathy is more likely than the arteritic form to manifest during the postoperative period. It is usually attributed to decreased oxygen delivery to the optic disk in association with hypotension and/or anemia. This form of visual loss has been associated with hemorrhagic hypotension (gastrointestinal hemorrhage), anemia, cardiac surgery, head and neck surgery, cardiac arrest, and hemodialysis and may occur spontaneously. Arteritic anterior ischemic optic neuropathy, which is less common than the nonarteritic form, is associated with inflammation and thrombosis of the short posterior ciliary arteries. The diagnosis is confirmed by demonstration of giant cell arteritis on a biopsy sample of the temporal artery. High-dose corticosteroids are used to treat arteritic anterior ischemic optic

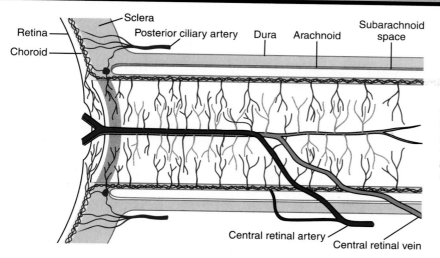

Figure 10A-6 • Blood supply to retina and optic nerve. Note the greater supply to the anterior portion of the optic nerve via the central retinal artery. Blood flow to the posterior portion of the optic nerve is supplied by pial perforators and is much less than blood flow to the anterior segment. *(Adapted from Hayreh SS: Anatomy and physiology of the optic nerve head. Trans Am Acad Ophthalmol Otolaryngol 1974;78:240–254.)*

neuropathy and as prophylaxis against disease manifestations in the contralateral eye.

Posterior Ischemic Optic Neuropathy

Posterior ischemic optic neuropathy presents as acute loss of vision and visual field defects similar to anterior ischemic optic neuropathy. It is presumed to be caused by decreased oxygen delivery to the posterior portion of the optic nerve between the optic foramen and the central retinal artery's point of entry. Spontaneous occurrence is less frequent than for anterior ischemic optic neuropathy; however, posterior ischemic optic neuropathy is more common than anterior ischemic optic neuropathy as a cause of visual loss in the perioperative period. There may be no abnormal ophthalmoscopic findings initially, reflecting retrobulbar involvement of the optic nerve. Mild disk edema is present after a few days, and CT of the patient's orbits may reveal enlargement of the intraorbital optic nerve.

The etiology of postoperative ischemic optic neuropathy appears to be multifactorial and may include hypotension, anemia, congenital absence of the central retinal artery, altered optic disk anatomy, air embolism, venous obstruction, and infection. It has been described following prolonged spine surgery performed in the prone position, cardiac surgery, radical neck dissection, and hip arthroplasty. Associated nonsurgical, but potentially contributory, factors include cardiac arrest, acute treatment of malignant hypertension, blunt trauma, and severe anemia (e.g., related to gastrointestinal hemorrhage). It is speculated that the risk of posterior ischemic optic neuropathy can be reduced by avoiding anemia, hypotension, and excessive fluid administration, although such speculation has not yet been proven.

Cortical Blindness

Cortical blindness may follow profound hypotension or circulatory arrest (e.g., as accompanies resuscitation from cardiac arrest) as a result of hypoperfusion and infarction of watershed areas in the parietal or occipital lobes. This form of blindness has been observed following diverse surgical procedures (e.g., cardiac surgery, craniotomy, laryngectomy, cesarean section) and may also result from air or particulate emboli during cardiopulmonary bypass. Cortical blindness is characterized by loss of vision, but retention of pupillary reactions to light and normal funduscopic examinations. Patients may not be aware of focal vision loss, which usually improves with time. CT or MRI abnormalities in the parietal or occipital lobes confirm the diagnosis.

Retinal Artery Occlusion

Central retinal artery occlusion presents as painless monocular blindness and occlusion of a branch of the retinal artery that results in limited visual field defects or blurred vision. Visual field defects are often severe initially but, unlike ischemic optic neuropathy, improve with time. Ophthalmoscopic examination reveals a pale edematous retina. Unlike ischemic optic neuropathy, central retinal artery occlusion is often caused by emboli from an ulcerated atherosclerotic plaque of the ipsilateral carotid artery. Most retinal artery occlusions due to emboli during open heart surgery resolve promptly. Vasospasm or thrombosis may also cause central retinal artery occlusion following radical neck surgery complicated by hemorrhage and hypotension. The condition can also occur following intranasal injection of α-adrenergic agonists. Stellate ganglion block improves vision in some of these patients.

Ophthalmic Venous Obstruction

Obstruction of venous drainage from the eyes may occur intraoperatively when patient positioning results in external pressure on the orbits. The prone position and use of headrests during neurosurgical procedures require careful attention to ensure that the patient's orbits are free from external compression. Ophthalmoscopic examination reveals engorgement of the veins and edema of the macula.

REFERENCES

Adams H, Adams R, Del Zoppo G, Goldstein LB: Guidelines for the early management of patients with ischemic stroke: 2005 guidelines update a scientific statement from the Stroke Council of the American Heart Association/American Stroke Association. Stroke 2005;36:916–923.

Black S, Cucchiara RF, Nishimura RA, Michenfelder JD: Parameters affecting occurrence of paradoxical air embolism. Anesthesiology 1989;71:235–241.

Browne TR, Holmes GL: Epilepsy. N Engl J Med 2001;344: 1145–1151.

Centers for Disease Control and Prevention (CDC): Paralytic poliomyelitis—United States, 1980–1994. MMWR Morb Mortal Wkly Rep 1997;46:79–83.

Clifton GL, Miller ER, Choi SC, et al: Lack of effect of induction of hypothermia after acute brain injury. N Engl J Med 2001;344:556–563.

Dodson BA: Interventional neuroradiology and the anesthetic management of patients with arteriovenous malformations. In Cottrell JE, Smith DS (eds): Anesthesia and Neurosurgery, 4th ed. St. Louis, Mosby, 2001:401.

Endovascular versus surgical treatment in patients with carotid stenosis in the Carotid and Vertebral Artery Transluminal Angioplasty Study (CAVATAS): A randomised trial. Lancet 2001;357:1729–1737.

Gupta R, Jovin TG, Krieger DW: Therapeutic hypothermia for stroke: Do new outfits change an old friend? Expert Rev Neurother 2005;5:235–246.

Ho VT, Newman NJ, Song S, et al: Ischemic optic neuropathy following spine surgery. J Neurosurg Anesthesiol 2005;17: 38–44.

Homocysteine and risk of ischemic heart disease and stroke: A meta-analysis. JAMA 2002;288:2015–2022.

Huang Y, Cheung L, Rowe D, Halliday G: Genetic contributions to Parkinson's disease. Brain Res Brain Res Rev 2004;46:44–70.

Jankovic J: Searching for a relationship between manganese and welding and Parkinson's disease. Neurology 2005;64:2021–2028.

Konstas AA, Choi JH, Pile-Spellman J: Neuroprotection for ischemic stroke using hypothermia. Neurocrit Care 2006;4:168–178.

Lambert DA, Giannouli E, Schmidt BJ: Postpolio syndrome and anesthesia. Anesthesiology 2005;103:638–644.

Lanier WL, Weglinski MW: Intracranial pressure. In Cucchiara RF, Michenfelder JD (eds): Clinical Neuroanesthesia. New York, Churchill Livingstone, 1990:77–115.

Lanier WL, Milde JH, Michenfelder JD: Cerebral stimulation following succinylcholine in dogs. Anesthesiology 1986;64:551–559.

Lee LA, Roth S, Posner KL, et al: The American Society of Anesthesiologists Postoperative Visual Loss Registry: Analysis of 93 spine surgery cases with postoperative visual loss. Anesthesiology 2006;105:652–659.

Leipzig TJ, Morgan J, Horner TG, et al: Analysis of intraoperative rupture in the surgical treatment of 1694 saccular aneurysms. Neurosurgery 2005;56:455–468.

Lusseveld E, Brilstra EH, Nijssen PC, et al: Endovascular coiling versus neurosurgical clipping in patients with a ruptured basilar tip aneurysm. J Neurol Neurosurg Psychiatry 2002;73:591–593.

Mayer SA, Brun NC, Begtrup K, et al: Recombinant activated factor VII for acute intracerebral hemorrhage. N Engl J Med 2005;352:777–785.

Mendelow AD, Gregson BA, Fernandes HM, et al: Early surgery versus initial conservative treatment in patients with spontaneous supratentorial intracerebral haematomas in the International Surgical Trial in Intracerebral Haemorrhage (STICH): A randomised trial. Lancet 2005;365:387–397.

Muth CM, Shank ES: Gas embolism. N Engl J Med 2000;342: 476–482.

Myers MA, Hamilton SR, Bogosian AJ, et al: Visual loss as a complication of spine surgery. A review of 37 cases. Spine 1997;22:1325–1329.

Nagele P, Hammerle AF: Sevoflurane and mivacurium in a patient with Huntington's chorea. Br J Anaesth 2000;85:320–321.

Nichols WC, Pankratz N, Hernandez D, et al: Genetic screening for a single common LRRK2 mutation in familial Parkinson's disease. Lancet 2005;365:410–412.

Noseworthy JH, Lucchinetti C, Rodriguez M, Weinshenker BG: Multiple sclerosis. N Engl J Med 2000;343:938–952.

Practice advisory for perioperative visual loss associated with spine surgery: A report by the American Society of Anesthesiologists Task Force on Perioperative Blindness. Anesthesiology 2006;104:1319–1328.

Qureshi AI, Tuhrim S, Broderick JP, et al: Spontaneous intracerebral hemorrhage. N Engl J Med 2001;344:1450–1460.

Sirven JI: Antiepileptic drug therapy for adults: When to initiate and how to choose. Mayo Clin Proc 2002;77:1367–1375.

Stocchetti N, Maas AI, Chieregato A, van der Plas AA: Hyperventilation in head injury: A review. Chest 2005;127: 1812–1827.

Thom T, Haase N, Rosamond W: Heart disease and stroke statistics—2006 update: A report from the American Heart Association Statistics Committee and Stroke Statistics Subcommittee. Circulation 2006;113:85–151.

Todd MM, Hindman BJ, Clarke WR, Torner JC: Mild intraoperative hypothermia during surgery for intracranial aneurysm. N Engl J Med 2005;352:135–145.

Ueki K, Meyer FB, Mellinger JF: Moyamoya disease: The disorder and surgical treatment. Mayo Clin Proc 1994;69:749–757.

Wass CT, Lanier WL: Glucose modulation of ischemic brain injury: review and clinical recommendations. Mayo Clin Proc 1996;71:801–812.

Zaroff JG, Rordorf GA, Ogilvy CS, Picard MH: Regional patterns of left ventricular systolic dysfunction after subarachnoid hemorrhage: Evidence for neurally mediated cardiac injury. J Am Soc Echocardiogr 2000;13:774–779.

Spinal Cord Disorders

Jeffrey J. Pasternak
William L. Lanier, Jr.

The most common cause of acute spinal cord injury is trauma. However, various disease processes, including tumors and congenital and degenerative diseases of the spinal cord and vertebral column, can also cause cord injury.

ACUTE TRAUMATIC SPINAL CORD INJURY

The mobility of the cervical spine makes it vulnerable to injury, especially hyperextension injury, during impact accidents. In this regard, it is estimated that cervical spine injury occurs in 1.5% to 3.0% of all major trauma victims. Further, there is a correlation between head injury and acute spinal cord injury such that injury to the cervical spine occurs in 2% of patients with head injury who survive to reach the hospital. Trauma can injure both the thoracic and lumbar spinal cord segments.

Acute spinal cord transection initially produces flaccid paralysis, with total absence of sensation below the level of the spinal cord injury. Although the cord is not usually anatomically transected, complete or nearly complete neuronal dysfunction may occur below a sentinel dermatomal level. Thus, from a functional standpoint, the spinal cord may appear transected. The extent of physiologic effects from spinal cord injury depends on the level of injury, with the most severe physiologic derangements occurring with injury to the cervical cord and lesser perturbations occurring with more caudal cord injuries. There is loss of temperature regulation and spinal cord reflexes below the level of the injury. Reductions in systemic blood pressure are common, especially with cervical cord injury, and are influenced by (1) loss of sympathetic nervous system activity and diminution of systemic vascular resistance and (2) bradycardia due to loss of the T1-T4 sympathetic innervation to the heart. Hypotension can also occur with thoracic and lumbar cord injuries, although typically less severe than with cervical injuries. These hemodynamic perturbations are collectively known as *spinal shock* and, in survivors, typically last 1 to 3 weeks. With cervical and upper thoracic cord injury, the major cause of morbidity and mortality is alveolar hypoventilation combined with an inability to clear bronchial secretions. Respiratory muscles are not affected with lumbar and low thoracic injuries; therefore, minimal respiratory impairment can be expected in these cases. Aspiration of gastric fluid or contents and pneumonia and pulmonary embolism are constant threats during spinal shock.

ACUTE CERVICAL SPINAL CORD INJURY

Cervical spine radiographs are obtained in a large fraction of patients who present with various forms of trauma for fear of missing occult cervical spine injuries. Nevertheless, the probability of cervical spine injury is minimal in patients who meet the following five criteria: (1) no midline cervical spine tenderness, (2) no focal neurologic deficits, (3) normal sensorium, (4) no intoxication, and (5) no painful distracting injury. Patients who meet these criteria *do not* require routine imaging studies to rule out occult cervical spine injury.

An estimated two thirds of trauma patients have multiple injuries that can interfere with cervical spine evaluation. Evaluation usually includes computed tomography or magnetic resonance imaging. Nevertheless, routine imaging may not be practical in some, considering the risk of transporting unstable patients. For this reason, standard radiographic views of the patient's cervical spine, often taken with a portable x-ray machine, are frequently relied on to evaluate the presence of cervical spine injury and associated instability. Regardless of the form of cervical spine imaging employed, the entire cervical spine including the body of the first thoracic vertebra must be seen and evaluated. Alignment of the vertebrae (lateral view), fractures (all views), and evaluation of disc and soft-tissue spaces are analyzed on the radiographic examination. The sensitivity of plain radiographs is less than 100%, and therefore the likelihood of cervical spine injury must be interpreted in conjunction with other clinical symptoms and risk factors. If there is any doubt, it is prudent to treat all acute cervical spinal injuries as potentially unstable.

Treatment of a cervical fracture dislocation entails immediate immobilization to limit neck flexion and extension. In addition, soft neck collars have almost no effect on limiting neck flexion, and neck extension is only modestly limited. Hard neck collars limit neck flexion and extension by only approximately 25%. Immobilization and traction as provided by halo-thoracic devices are most effective in preventing cervical spine movement. Manual in-line stabilization

(the assistant's hands are placed on each side of the patient's face with the fingertips resting on the mastoid process with downward pressure against a firm table surface to hold the head immobile in a neutral position) is recommended to help minimize cervical spine flexion and extension during direct laryngoscopy for tracheal intubation.

Cervical spine movement during direct laryngoscopy is likely to be concentrated at the occipitoatlantoaxial area, suggesting an increased risk of spinal cord injury at this level in vulnerable patients, even with the use of manual in-line stabilization.

In addition to mechanical deformation of the spinal cord produced by movement of the neck in the presence of cervical spine injury, there is perhaps an even greater risk of compromise of the blood supply to the spinal cord produced by neck motion that elongates the cord, with resultant narrowing of the longitudinal blood vessels. In fact, maintenance of perfusion pressure may be more important than positioning for preventing spinal cord injury in the presence of cervical spine injury.

Management of Anesthesia

Patients with acute spinal cord transections often require special precautions during airway management. The key principle when performing direct laryngoscopy is to minimize neck movements during the procedure. However, fear of possible spinal cord compression (from an unstable cervical spine injury) must not prevent necessary airway intervention. Extensive clinical experience seems to support the use of direct laryngoscopy for orotracheal intubation provided that (1) maneuvers are taken to stabilize the head during the procedure (avoiding hyperextension of the patient's neck) and (2) evaluation of the patient's airway did not suggest the likelihood of any associated technical difficulty.

Topical anesthesia and awake fiberoptic laryngoscopy are an alternative to direct laryngoscopy if patients are cooperative and airway trauma—with ensuing blood, secretions, and anatomic deformities—does not preclude visualization with the fiberscope. Of note, coughing during both topicalization of the airway and fiberoptic intubation may result in cervical spine movement. It is reasonable to have an assistant maintain manual in-line stabilization of the cervical spine during both interventions. Another alternative is rapid-sequence induction of anesthesia with intravenous anesthetics and a muscle relaxant. When the cervical spine is unstable or there is a high index of suspicion for the presence of cervical spine injury, it is important to proceed carefully, as neck hyperextension could further damage the spinal cord. Nevertheless, there is no evidence of increased neurologic morbidity after elective or emergency orotracheal intubation of anesthetized or awake patients who have an unstable cervical spine if appropriate and safe steps are taken to minimize neck movement. Awake tracheostomy is reserved for the most challenging airway conditions, in which neck injury, combined with facial fractures or other severe anomalies of airway anatomy, make safely securing the airway by nonsurgical means difficult or unsafe. All factors considered, airway management in the presence of cervical spine injury should be dictated by common sense, not dogmatic approaches. Certainly, clinical experience supports the safety of a variety of techniques just described.

The absence of compensatory sympathetic nervous system responses makes patients with cervical or high thoracic spinal cord injury particularly vulnerable to dramatic decreases in systemic blood pressure following acute changes in body posture, blood loss, or positive airway pressure. To minimize these effects, liberal intravenous infusion of crystalloid solutions may be necessary to replete intravascular volume, which has been abruptly compromised by vasodilation. Likewise, acute blood loss should be replaced promptly. Electrocardiogram abnormalities are common during the acute phase of spinal cord injury, especially with cervical cord injuries. Breathing is best managed by mechanical ventilation, as abdominal and intercostal muscle weakness or paralysis, exacerbated by general anesthesia, increases the chances of respiratory failure with ensuing hypoxia and hypercapnia. Body temperature should be monitored and manipulated as patients tend to become poikilothermic below the spinal cord transection. Anesthetic maintenance is targeted at ensuring physiologic stability and facilitating tolerance of the tracheal tube. Volatile or injected anesthetics are satisfactory for this purpose. Nitrous oxide should be used with caution, given concerns for co-existing trauma and air entrainment in closed spaces (e.g., as occurs with basilar skull fracture or rib fracture, which could potentially contribute to pneumocephalus or pneumothorax, respectively). Arterial hypoxemia is common following spinal cord injury, emphasizing the need for continuous pulse oximetry and delivery of supplemental oxygen.

Muscle relaxant use should be determined by the operative site and the level of spinal cord transection. If muscle relaxants are necessary, the sympathomimetic effects of pancuronium makes this drug an attractive choice; however, other nondepolarizing muscle relaxants can be used safely. Succinylcholine is unlikely to provoke excessive release of potassium during the first few hours after spinal cord transection. Even in these instances, the benefits of succinylcholine, which include rapid onset of action and short duration of relaxation, should be weighed against potential side effects. Use of a nondepolarizing relaxant, with mask ventilation while employing cricoid pressure, is another alternative to airway management during anesthesia induction and prior to laryngoscopy. Benefits of the latter approach are that once the endotracheal tube is placed, the longer duration of the nondepolarizing relaxant has utility during patient positioning.

CHRONIC SPINAL CORD INJURY

Sequelae of chronic spinal cord injury include impaired alveolar ventilation, cardiovascular instability manifesting as autonomic hyperreflexia, chronic pulmonary and genitourinary

tract infections, anemia, and altered thermoregulation (Table 10B-1). As in the acute phase, injuries that occur more rostral along the spinal cord tend to have more significant systemic effects. Chronic urinary tract infections reflect the patient's inability to empty the bladder completely and predispose to calculus formation. As a result, renal failure may occur and is a common cause of death in patients with chronic spinal cord transection. In addition, prolonged immobility leads to osteoporosis, skeletal muscle atrophy, and decubitus ulcers. Importantly, immobility can also predispose patients to deep venous thrombosis; therefore, prophylactic measures such as compression stockings, low-dose anticoagulation, and inferior vena cava filters may be indicated. Pathologic fractures can occur when moving these patients. Pressure points should be well protected and padded to minimize the likelihood of trauma to the skin and the development of decubitus ulcers.

Depression and chronic pain are common problems following spinal cord injury. Nerve root pain is localized at or near the level of the transection. Visceral pain is produced by distention of the bladder or bowel. Phantom body pain can occur in areas of complete sensory loss. As a result of mental depression or the presence of pain, these patients may be treated with drugs such as antidepressants and potent

TABLE 10B-1 Early and Late Complications in Patients with Spinal Cord Injury	
Complication	Incidence (%)
2 Years after injury	
Urinary tract infection	59
Skeletal muscle spasticity	38
Chills and fever	19
Decubitus ulcer	16
Autonomic hyperreflexia	8
Skeletal muscle contractures	6
Heterotopic ossification	3
Pneumonia	3
Renal dysfuntion	2
Postoperative wound infection	2
30 Years after Injury	
Decubitus ulcers	17
Skeletal muscle or joint pain	16
Gastrointestinal dysfunction	14
Cardiovascular dysfunction	14
Urinary tract infection	14
Infectious disease or cancer	11
Visual or hearing disorders	10
Urinary retention	8
Male genitourinary dysfunction	7
Renal calculi	6

opiates that require consideration when planning anesthesia management.

Several weeks after acute spinal cord transection, the spinal cord reflexes gradually return, and patients enter a more chronic stage characterized by overactivity of the sympathetic nervous system and involuntary skeletal muscle spasms. In these patients, baclofen, which potentiates the inhibitory effects of γ-aminobutyric acid, is a useful modality for treating spasticity. Abrupt cessation of baclofen therapy, as may occur with hospitalization for unrelated problems, may result in dramatic withdrawal reactions including seizures. Diazepam and other benzodiazepines also facilitate the inhibitory effects of γ-aminobutyric acid and may have utility in patient management of a patient receiving baclofen. Spasticity refractory to pharmacologic suppression may necessitate treatment with surgery via dorsal rhizotomy or myelotomy or implantation of a spinal cord stimulator or subarachnoid baclofen pump.

Spinal cord transection at or above the fifth cervical vertebra may result in apnea due to denervation of the diaphragm (C3-C5 innervation). When function of the diaphragm is intact, the tidal volume is likely to remain adequate. Nevertheless, in those with cervical or thoracic cord injury, the ability to cough and clear secretions from the airway is often impaired because of decreased expiratory reserve volume due to denervation of intercostal and abdominal muscles. Indeed, acute spinal cord transection at the cervical level is accompanied by marked decreases in vital capacity. Furthermore, arterial hypoxemia is a consistent early finding following cervical spinal cord injury. Tracheobronchial suctioning has been associated with bradycardia and cardiac arrest in these patients, emphasizing the importance of establishing optimal arterial oxygenation before undertaking this procedure.

Management of Anesthesia

Anesthetic management in patients with chronic transection of the spinal cord should focus on preventing autonomic hyperreflexia. When general anesthesia is selected, muscle relaxants have utility for facilitating tracheal intubation and preventing reflex skeletal muscle spasms in response to surgical stimulation. Nondepolarizing muscle relaxants are the primary choice in this circumstance, as succinylcholine is likely to provoke hyperkalemia, particularly during the initial 6 months (or perhaps longer) following spinal cord transection. All factors considered, it seems reasonable to avoid the use of succinylcholine in patients with a spinal cord injury of greater than 24-hour duration.

AUTONOMIC HYPERREFLEXIA

Autonomic hyperreflexia appears following spinal shock and in association with return of spinal cord reflexes. This reflex response can be initiated by cutaneous or visceral stimulation below the level of spinal cord transection. Distention of a hollow viscus, such as the bladder and rectum, and surgery are common stimuli.

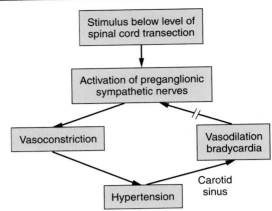

Figure 10B-1 • Sequence of events associated with clinical manifestations of autonomic hyperreflexia. Because the afferent impulses that produce vasodilation cannot reach the neurologically isolated portion of the spinal cord, vasoconstriction develops below the level of the spinal cord transection, resulting in systemic hypertension.

Stimulation below the level of spinal cord transection initiates afferent impulses that enter the spinal cord (**Fig. 10B-1**). Due to reflexes entirely within the spinal cord proper/parenchyma, these impulses elicit increases in sympathetic nervous system activity over the splanchnic outflow tract. In neurologically intact patients, this outflow is modulated by inhibitory impulses from higher centers in the central nervous system. In the presence of a spinal cord transection, however, this outflow below the lesion is isolated from inhibitory impulses from above, so generalized vasoconstriction persists below the level of the spinal cord injury.

Systemic hypertension and reflex bradycardia are the hallmarks of autonomic hyperreflexia, as stimulation of the carotid sinus manifests as bradycardia. Reflexive cutaneous vasodilation occurs above the level of the spinal cord transection. Nasal stuffiness reflects this pattern of vasodilation. Patients may complain of headache and blurred vision as evidence of severe hypertension. Precipitous increases in systemic blood pressure can result in cerebral, retinal, or subarachnoid hemorrhages as well as increased operative blood loss. In addition, loss of consciousness and seizures may occur and cardiac arrhythmias are often present. In this patient, pulmonary edema reflects acute left ventricular failure due to increased cardiac afterload.

The incidence of autonomic hyperreflexia depends on the level of spinal cord transection. For example, approximately 85% of patients with spinal cord transections above T6 exhibit this reflex, yet it is unlikely to be associated with spinal cord transections below T10 (**Fig. 10B-2**). Since the greater, lesser, and least splanchnic nerves typically receive innervation from T5-T9, T10-T11, and T12, respectively, loss of input from higher centers to these nerves and to the sympathetic chain will result in greater regions of the body at risk of increased autonomic reflexes. Specifically, spinal cord lesions above T5-T6 will completely isolate the splanchnic nerves from higher centers of control, whereas lesions to lumbar levels of the cord will result in a grossly intact peripheral sympathetic nervous system.

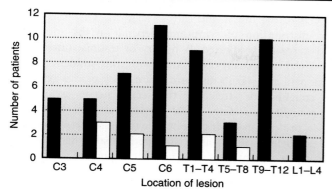

Figure 10B-2 • Autonomic hyperreflexia did not occur in any patient with a spinal cord transection below T9 and undergoing extracorporeal shock-wave lithotripsy. *Shaded bars* represent the number of patients with spinal cord transections (*n* = 52); *open bars* represent the patients developing autonomic hyperreflexia (*n* = 9). (*Adapted from Stowe DF, Bernstein JS, Madsen KE, et al: Autonomic hyperreflexia in spinal cord injured patients during extracorporeal shock wave lithotripsy. Anesth Analg 1989;68:788–791.*)

Management of at-risk patients should begin with efforts to *prevent* the development of autonomic hyperreflexia. Patients who have a negative history for this reflex are still at risk of its occurrence during surgery, simply because of the intense stimulus that surgery provides. Prior to surgical or other stimulation in locations that lack sensory innervation, general, neuraxial, or regional anesthesia should be instituted. Epidural anesthesia has been described for the treatment of autonomic hyperreflexia provoked by uterine contractions during labor. However, epidural anesthesia may be less effective than spinal anesthesia in preventing autonomic hyperreflexia because of the relative sparing of the sacral segments with the former technique. Blocking afferent pathways with topical local anesthetics applied to the urethra, as for a cystoscopic procedure, often does not prevent autonomic hyperreflexia, as this form of anesthesia does not block the bladder muscle proprioceptors, which are stimulated on bladder distention.

Regardless of the technique selected for anesthesia, vasodilator drugs with short half-life (e.g., sodium nitroprusside) should be readily available to treat sudden-onset systemic hypertension. Persistence of systemic hypertension requires continuous intravenous infusions of short-acting vasodilators, perhaps supplemented with longer acting agents (e.g., hydralazine). Of note, autonomic hyperreflexia may first manifest postoperatively when the effects of the anesthetic drugs begin to wane.

SPINAL CORD TUMORS

Spinal cord tumors can be divided into two broad categories. *Intramedullary* tumors are located within the spinal cord proper and account for approximately 10% of tumors affecting the spinal column, with gliomas and ependymomas accounting for the vast majority of intramedullary tumors.

Extramedullary tumors can be either intradural or extradural. Neurofibromas and meningiomas account for most of the intradural tumors. In contrast, metastatic lesions, usually from lung, breast, or prostate cancer, as well as myeloma, are the most common causes of extradural lesions. Other mass lesions of the spinal cord, including abscesses and hematomas, share many of the clinical signs and symptoms seen with tumors.

Spinal cord tumors typically present with symptoms of cord compression. Pain is a common finding and is usually aggravated by coughing or straining. Motor symptoms and sphincter disturbances may also occur. Sometimes spinal tenderness may be present. Diagnosis is usually based on symptoms and imaging of the spinal cord; magnetic resonance imaging is the technique of choice. Treatment and prognosis depend of the nature of the lesion and may include corticosteroids, radiation therapy, chemotherapy, or surgical decompression or excision.

Management of anesthesia involves ensuring adequate spinal cord oxygenation and perfusion. This is achieved by ensuring adequate Pao_2 and by avoiding hypotension and anemia. Specifics of management will depend on the level of the lesion and the extent of neurologic impairment.

Tumors involving the cervical spinal cord may influence the approach used to secure the airway. Significant motion of the cervical spine could lead to further cord compromise via compression and decreased cord perfusion. With any form of disease that places the cervical spine in jeopardy for new injury, airway management should be similar to that discussed in the management of acute spinal cord injury. This may include in-line stabilization during direct laryngoscopy or awake fiberoptic intubation. If the approach to patient management is uncertain, it is useful, prior to administering sedatives or narcotics, to have the patient placed in position for airway management (e.g., on the operating room table) and then carefully move through the anticipated variations of head and neck movement prior to actual airway manipulation or induction of anesthesia. Exacerbation or induction of symptoms upon movement should tip the clinician toward fiberoptic laryngoscopy (with the head held in neutral position) or other options that would less likely cause movement-associated harm to the cord. For example, a light-wand or Bullard laryngoscope may facilitate intubation of the trachea without significant neck extension.

Safe resection of a tumor may require the use of intraoperative electrophysiologic monitoring of neurologic function. Techniques such as electromyography, somatosensory evoked potentials, and motor evoked potential monitoring have a variety of anesthetic implications. The preferred approach may vary from institution to institution. We refer readers to a variety of review articles discussing the intraoperative use of these monitoring modalities.

Succinylcholine should be used with caution in patients with spinal cord tumors given the risk of associated hyperkalemia. Also, neuromuscular monitoring with train-of-four should be performed on a neurologically intact extremity.

Evidence of upper motor neuron impairment may lead to an up-regulation of acetylcholine receptors, thus making the extremity relatively resistant to nondepolarizing blockade. If there are any concerns regarding the possibility of altered responsiveness to neuromuscular block due to tumor-induced spinal cord dysfunction, monitoring train-of-four on the facial nerve is a reasonable option. However, one should be careful to monitor evoked muscle twitches, not direct muscle stimulation.

INTERVERTEBRAL DISC DISEASE

Low back pain ranks second only to upper respiratory tract disease as one of the most common reasons for office visits to physicians. An estimated 70% of adults experience low back pain at some time in their life. Among chronic conditions, low back pain is the most common cause for limitation of activity in patients younger than 45 years of age. Primary or metastatic cancer is the most common systemic disease affecting the vertebral bodies, although it accounts for fewer than 1% of all episodes of low back pain.

One of the most common causes of back pain is intervertebral disc disease. The intervertebral disc is composed of a compressible nucleus pulposus surrounded by a fibrocartilaginous annulus fibrosis. The disc acts as a shock absorber between vertebral bodies. Trauma or degenerative changes lead to changes in the intervertebral disc. Nerve root or spinal cord compression results when the nucleus pulposus protrudes through the annulus fibrosis. With compression of a single nerve root, patients usually complain of pain in a single dermatomal distribution or localized muscle weakness. Spinal cord compression can lead to complex sensory, motor, and autonomic symptoms at and below the level of the insult. There are signs of spinal cord compression if protrusion occurs in the cervical or thoracic regions, whereas signs of cauda equina compression appear if protrusion is into the lumbar region. Computed tomography or magnetic resonance imaging confirms the diagnosis and the location of intervertebral disc herniation.

Cervical Disc Disease

Lateral protrusion of a cervical disc usually occurs at the C5-C6 or C6-C7 intervertebral spaces. Protrusion can be secondary to trauma or can occur spontaneously. Symptoms are commonly aggravated by coughing. The same symptoms can be due to osteophytes that compress nerve roots in the intervertebral foramina.

Initial treatment of cervical disc protrusion is usually conservative involving rest, pain control, and possible epidural steroids. Surgical decompression is necessary if symptoms do not abate with conservative treatment.

Lumbar Disc Disease

The most common site for lumbar disc protrusion is the L4-L5 and L5-S1 intervertebral spaces. Both sites produce low back pain, which radiates down the posterior and lateral aspects of the thighs and calves (sciatica). The exact pattern and distribution of symptoms depend on the spinal level and nerve roots affected. A history of trauma, often viewed as trivial, is usually associated with the sudden onset of back pain and signals disc protrusion. Back pain is aggravated by coughing or stretching the sciatic nerve, as produced by straight-leg raising. These mechanical signs help distinguish protrusion from peripheral nerve disorders. For example, diabetes mellitus–associated peripheral neuropathy may share the symptoms, but not the signs, of a ruptured lumbar disc.

Treatment of acute lumbar disc protrusion has historically included bed rest, analgesics, and centrally acting muscle relaxants. Among patients with acute low back pain, continuing ordinary activities within the limits permitted by the pain leads to more rapid recovery than either bed rest or back-mobilizing exercises. When neurologic symptoms persist despite conservative medical management, surgical laminectomy or microdiscectomy can be considered to decompress the affected nerve roots. Epidural steroids (e.g., triamcinolone, methylprednisolone) are an alternative to surgery in select patients. They act by decreasing inflammation and edema around the nerve roots. Suppression of the hypothalamic-pituitary-adrenal axis is a consideration in treated patients and may have implications for anesthetic management. Exogenous corticosteroid coverage may be indicated should these patients undergo surgery. Although epidural steroid injections may result in short-term alleviation of symptoms due to sciatica, this treatment offers no significant functional benefit nor does it decrease the need for surgery.

CONGENITAL ANOMALIES AND DEGENERATIVE DISEASES OF THE VERTEBRAL COLUMN

Spina bifida occulta is a common form of congenital vertebral column disease, and spondylosis and spondylolisthesis are forms of degenerative diseases. It is not uncommon for multiple types of the degenerative changes to occur concomitantly, leading to more rapid progression of neurologic symptoms and the need for surgical intervention.

Spina bifida occulta (incomplete formation of a single lamina in the lumbosacral spine without other abnormalities) is a congenital defect that is present in an estimated 20% of individuals. Given that it usually produces no symptoms, it is often discovered as an incidental finding on radiographic examination during evaluation of some other unrelated disease process. Because there are usually no underlying abnormalities, an increased risk with spinal anesthesia is not expected, and large numbers of these patients have received spinal anesthesia safely. However, a variant of spina bifida occulta known as occult *spinal dysraphism* exists in which the bony defect may involve more than one lamina. A significant number of these defects are associated with a tethered spinal cord (cord ending below the L2-L3 interspace), which may be responsible for progressive neurologic symptoms. Up to 50% of individuals with a tethered spinal cord have cutaneous manifestations overlying the anomaly, including tufts of hair, hyperpigmented areas, cutaneous lipomas, and skin dimples. Performance of spinal anesthesia in patients with a tethered spinal cord may increase the risk of cord injury.

Spondylosis is a common noncongenital disorder that leads to osteophyte formation and degenerative disc disease. The term spondylosis is used synonymously with spinal stenosis. There is narrowing of the spinal canal and compression of the spinal cord by transverse osteophytes or nerve root compression by bony spurs in the intervertebral foramina. Spinal cord dysfunction may also reflect ischemic infarction secondary to bony compression of the spinal arteries. Symptoms typically develop insidiously after approximately the age of 50. With cervical spondylosis, neck pain and radicular pain in the arms and shoulders are accompanied by sensory loss and skeletal muscle wasting. Later, sensory and motor signs appear in the legs, producing an unsteady gait. Lumbar spondylosis usually leads to radicular pain and wasting in the lower extremities. Sphincter disturbances are uncommon regardless of the location of spondylosis. Radiographs of the spine often demonstrate osteoarthritic changes, but these changes correlate poorly with neurologic symptoms. Surgery may be necessary to arrest progression of the symptoms, especially motor loss.

Spondylolisthesis refers to anterior subluxation of one vertebral body on another. This most commonly occurs at the lumbosacral junction. Radicular symptoms usually involve the nerve root inferior to the pedicle of the anteriorly subluxed vertebra. Treatment usually involves analgesics, anti-inflammatory medications, and physical therapy if the low back pain is the only symptom. Surgery is usually reserved for patients who present with myelopathy, radiculopathy, or neurogenic claudication.

CONGENITAL ANOMALIES AND DEGENERATIVE DISEASES OF THE SPINAL CORD

Syringomyelia

Syringomyelia, also known as syrinx, is a disorder in which there is cystic cavitation of the spinal cord. The etiology is often congenital, but this condition can occur following spinal cord trauma or in association with various neoplastic conditions (e.g., gliomas). Rostral extension into the brainstem is called syringobulbia. Two main forms of syringomyelia occur depending on whether there is communication of the cystic regions with the subarachnoid space or central canal. In communicating syringomyelia, there is either only dilatation of the central canal of the cord, known as hydromyelia, or there is communication between the abnormal cystic lesions in the spinal cord proper and the cerebrospinal fluid spaces. Communicating syringomyelia is usually associated with either a history of basilar arachnoiditis or Chiari malformations. In contrast, the presence of cysts that have no connection to the cerebrospinal fluid spaces is called noncommunicating syringomyelia and is often associated with a history of trauma, neoplasms, or arachnoiditis.

Signs and symptoms of syringomyelia usually begin during the third or fourth decade of life. Early complaints are those of sensory impairment involving pain and temperature in the upper extremities. This reflects destruction of pain and temperature neuronal pathways that cross within the spinal cord near the central canal. As cavitation of the spinal cord progresses, destruction of lower motor neurons ensues, with the development of skeletal muscle weakness with wasting plus loss of reflexes. Thoracic scoliosis may result from weakness of paravertebral muscles. Syringobulbia is characterized by paralysis of the palate, tongue, and vocal cords, and loss of sensation over the face. Magnetic resonance imaging is the preferred diagnostic procedure.

No known treatment is effective in arresting the progressive degeneration of the spinal cord or medulla. Surgical procedures designed to restore normal cerebrospinal fluid flow have not been predictably effective.

Management of anesthesia in patients with syringomyelia or syringobulbia should be made considering the neurologic deficits associated with this disease. Thoracic scoliosis can contribute to ventilation-to-perfusion mismatching. The presence of lower motor neuron disease leading to skeletal muscle wasting suggests the possibility that hyperkalemia could develop after administration of succinylcholine. Likewise, exaggerated responses to nondepolarizing muscle relaxants can be observed. Thermal regulation may be impaired. Selection of drugs for induction and maintenance of anesthesia is not influenced by this disease. With syringobulbia, any decreased or absent protective airway reflexes may influence the timing of tracheal tube removal postoperatively.

Amyotrophic Lateral Sclerosis

Amyotrophic lateral sclerosis (ALS) is a degenerative disease involving (1) the lower motor neurons in the anterior horn gray matter of the spinal cord and (2) the corticospinal tracts (i.e., the primary descending upper motor neurons). Therefore, this disease process produces both upper and lower motor neuron degeneration. It most commonly afflicts men 40 to 60 years of age. When the degenerative process is limited to the motor cortex of the brain, the disease is called primary lateral sclerosis; limitation to the brainstem nuclei is known as pseudobulbar palsy. Werdnig-Hoffmann disease resembles ALS, except that manifestations of this disease occur during the first 3 years of life. Although the cause of ALS is unknown, occasionally a genetic pattern is present. A viral etiology is also a consideration.

Signs and symptoms of ALS reflect upper and lower motor neuron dysfunction and electromyographically sometimes resemble changes seen with myasthenia gravis. Frequent initial manifestations include skeletal muscle atrophy, weakness, and fasciculations, often beginning in the intrinsic muscles of the hands. With time, atrophy and weakness involve most of the patient's skeletal muscles, including the tongue, pharynx, larynx, and chest. Early symptoms of bulbar involvement include fasciculations of the tongue plus dysphagia leading to pulmonary aspiration. For reasons that are not clear, the ocular muscles are spared. Autonomic nervous system dysfunction manifests as orthostatic hypotension and resting tachycardia. Inability to control emotional responses is characteristic. Complaints of cramping and aching sensations, particularly in the legs, are common. Carcinoma of the lung has been associated with ALS. Plasma creatine kinase concentrations are normal, distinguishing this disease from chronic polymyositis. ALS has no known treatment, and death is likely within 6 years after the onset of clinical symptoms, usually due to respiratory failure.

General anesthesia in patients with ALS may be associated with exaggerated ventilatory depression. ALS patients are also vulnerable to hyperkalemia following administration of succinylcholine, as a result of lower motor neuron disease. Furthermore, these patients may show prolonged responses to nondepolarizing muscle relaxants. Bulbar involvement with dysfunction of pharyngeal muscles may predispose to pulmonary aspiration. There is no evidence that specific anesthetic drugs or combinations of drugs are best for patients with this disease. Regional anesthesia is often avoided for fear of exacerbating disease symptoms. Nevertheless, epidural anesthesia has been successfully administered to patients with ALS without neurologic exacerbation or impairment of pulmonary function.

Friedreich's Ataxia

Friedreich's ataxia is an autosomal recessive inherited condition characterized by degeneration of the spinocerebellar and pyramidal tracts. Cardiomyopathy is present in 10% to 50% of patients with this disease. Kyphoscoliosis, producing a steady deterioration of pulmonary function, is present in nearly 80% of affected patients. Ataxia is the typical presenting symptom. Dysarthria, nystagmus, skeletal muscle weakness and spasticity, and diabetes mellitus may be present. Friedreich's ataxia is usually fatal by early adulthood, often due to cardiac failure.

Management of anesthesia for Friedreich's ataxia is similar to that described for ALS. If cardiomyopathy is present, the negative inotropic effects of anesthetic drugs should be considered when selecting a technique. Although experience is limited, the response to muscle relaxants seems normal. Kyphoscoliosis may make epidural anesthesia technically difficult, whereas spinal anesthesia has been used successfully. The likelihood of postoperative ventilatory failure may be increased, especially in the presence of kyphoscoliosis.

KEY POINTS

- Major goals when caring for patients with spinal cord diseases or undergoing surgical procedures involving the spinal cord or vertebral column include maintenance of adequate oxygen delivery, optimization of operative conditions, and facilitation of a rapid, smooth anesthesia emergence to allow for immediate assessment of neurologic function.

- Succinylcholine should be used with caution in patients with spinal cord injury because of the potential risk of hyperkalemia in the setting of diseases that cause an up-regulation of acetylcholine receptors at the neuromuscular junction.

- In acute spinal cord injury, major goals include support of airway, breathing, and circulation. Care must be taken during airway manipulation to avoid excessive neck movement. Succinylcholine can be used without significant risk of hyperkalemia in the first 24 hours following injury.

- Patients with cervical and thoracic spinal cord injuries are at risk of developing autonomic hyperreflexia in response to various stimuli, including surgery, bowel distention, and bladder distention. Prevention is usually the goal, and both general and spinal anesthesia are effective in blocking the afferent limb of the pathway. Topical anesthesia for cystoscopic procedures as well as epidural anesthesia may not be reliably effective for preventing autonomic hyperreflexia.

REFERENCES

Agusti M, Adalia R, Fernandez C, Gomar C: Anaesthesia for caesarean section in a patient with syringomyelia and Arnold-Chiari type I malformation. Int J Obstet Anesth 2004;13:114–116.

Bird TM, Strunin L: Hypotensive anesthesia for a patient with Friedreich's ataxia and cardiomyopathy. Anesthesiology 1984;60:377–380.

Calder I: Spinal cord injury in patients with undiagnosed cervical spine fractures. Anesthesiology 1998;88:1411–1412.

Carette S, Leclaire R, Marcoux S, et al: Epidural corticosteroid injections for sciatica due to herniated nucleus pulposus. N Engl J Med 1997;336:1634–1640.

Deyo RA, Rainville J, Kent DL: What can the history and physical examination tell us about low back pain? JAMA 1992;268:760–765.

Ditunno JF Jr, Formal CS: Chronic spinal cord injury. N Engl J Med 1994;330:550–556.

Gugino V, Chabot RJ: Somatosensory evoked potentials. Int Anesthesiol Clin 1990;28:154–164.

Hara K, Sakura S, Saito Y, et al: Epidural anesthesia and pulmonary function in a patient with amyotrophic lateral sclerosis. Anesth Analg 1996;83:878–879.

Hastings RH, Marks JD: Airway management for trauma patients with potential cervical spine injuries. Anesth Analg 1991;73:471–482.

Hoffman JR, Mower WR, Wolfson AB, et al: Validity of a set of clinical criteria to rule out injury to the cervical spine in patients with blunt trauma. National Emergency X-Radiography Utilization Study Group. N Engl J Med 2000;343:94–99.

Holland NR: Intraoperative electromyography. J Clin Neurophysiol 2002;19:444–453.

Kubal K, Pasricha SK, Bhargava M: Spinal anesthesia in a patient with Friedreich's ataxia. Anesth Analg 1991;72:257–258.

Lambert DH, Deane RS, Mazuzan JE Jr: Anesthesia and the control of blood pressure in patients with spinal cord injury. Anesth Analg 1982;61:344–348.

Lennarson PJ, Smith D, Todd MM, et al: Segmental cervical spine motion during orotracheal intubation of the intact and injured spine with and without external stabilization. J Neurosurg 2000;92:201–206.

Lotto ML, Banoub M, Schubert A. Effects of anesthetic agents and physiologic changes on intraoperative motor evoked potentials. J Neurosurg Anesthesiol 2004;16:32–42.

Malmivaara A, Hakkinen U, Aro T, et al: The treatment of acute low back pain—bed rest, exercises, or ordinary activity? N Engl J Med 1995;332:351–355.

McLeod AD, Calder I: Spinal cord injury and direct laryngoscopy—the legend lives on. Br J Anaesth 2000;84:705–709.

Meschino A, Devitt JH, Koch JP, et al: The safety of awake tracheal intubation in cervical spine injury. Can J Anaesth 1992;39:114–117.

O'Malley KF, Ross SE: The incidence of injury to the cervical spine in patients with craniocerebral injury. J Trauma 1988;28:1476–1478.

Ravindran RS, Cummins DF, Smith IE: Experience with the use of nitroprusside and subsequent epidural analgesia in a pregnant quadriplegic patient. Anesth Analg 1981;60:61–63.

Rosenbaum KJ, Neigh JL, Strobel GE: Sensitivity to nondepolarizing muscle relaxants in amyotrophic lateral sclerosis: Report of two cases. Anesthesiology 1971;35:638–641.

Suderman VS, Crosby ET, Lui A: Elective oral tracheal intubation in cervical spine-injured adults. Can J Anaesth 1991;38:785–789.

Diseases of the Autonomic and Peripheral Nervous Systems

Jeffrey J. Pasternak
William L. Lanier, Jr.

Autonomic Disorders
- Shy-Drager Syndrome
- Orthostatic Intolerance Syndrome
- Glomus Tumors of the Head and Neck
- Carotid Sinus Syndrome

Diseases of the Peripheral Nervous System
- Idiopathic Facial Paralysis (Bell's Palsy)
- Trigeminal Neuralgia (Tic Douloureux)

- Glossopharyngeal Neuralgia
- Charcot-Marie-Tooth Disease
- Brachial Plexus Neuropathy
- Guillain-Barré Syndrome (Acute Idiopathic Polyneuritis)
- Entrapment Neuropathies
- Diseases Associated with Peripheral Neuropathies

The peripheral nervous system consists of nerve elements outside the brain and spinal cord. It encompasses both the autonomic nervous system and peripheral nerves. Disorders of the autonomic nervous system can result in significant hemodynamic changes as well as abnormal responses to drugs that work via adrenergic receptors. Diseases affecting peripheral nerves often have implications for perioperative patient management, including the choice of muscle relaxants and control of neuropathic pain.

AUTONOMIC DISORDERS

Shy-Drager Syndrome

Shy-Drager syndrome belongs to a group of heterogeneous disorders known as multiple-system atrophy. Multiple-system atrophy includes three conditions that, in years past, were thought to be unrelated: striatonigral degeneration, olivopontocerebellar atrophy, and Shy-Drager syndrome. The hallmark of multiple-system atrophy is degeneration and dysfunction of various central nervous system structures such as the basal ganglia, cerebellar cortex, locus ceruleus, pyramidal tracts, inferior olives, vagal motor nucleus, and the spinocerebellar tracts. The extent of differential degeneration among these structures dictates signs and symptoms. Shy-Drager syndrome is characterized by autonomic nervous system dysfunction due predominantly to degeneration of nervous system structures important for autonomic function, such as the locus ceruleus, intermediolateral column of the spinal cord, and peripheral autonomic neurons. It is important to note that other regions of the central nervous system described above may also be affected, but to a lesser degree; hence, characteristics of striatonigral degeneration (e.g., parkinsonism) and olivopontocerebellar atrophy (e.g., ataxia) may also be present in patients with Shy-Drager syndrome. Idiopathic orthostatic hypotension, rather than Shy-Drager syndrome, is thought to be present when autonomic nervous system dysfunction occurs in the absence of central nervous system degeneration.

Signs and symptoms of Shy-Drager syndrome are related to autonomic nervous system dysfunction, manifested by orthostatic hypotension, urinary retention, bowel dysfunction, and sexual impotence. Postural hypotension is often severe enough to produce syncope. Plasma norepinephrine concentrations fail to show a normal increase after standing or exercise. Pupillary reflexes may be sluggish and control of breathing abnormal. Further evidence of autonomic nervous system dysfunction is failure of baroreceptor reflexes to produce increases in heart rate or vasoconstriction in response to hypotension.

Treatment of orthostatic hypotension is symptomatic and includes elastic stockings, a high-sodium diet to expand the intravascular fluid volume, and administration of vasoconstricting α_1-adrenergic agonists, such as midodrine or α_2-adrenergic antagonists, such as yohimbine. These drugs are intended to facilitate continued release of norepinephrine from postganglionic adrenergic neurons. Death usually occurs within 8 years of the diagnosis, most often due to cerebral ischemia from prolonged hypotension. Levodopa is administered to decrease parkinsonian symptoms, but it is usually poorly effective.

Management of Anesthesia

Perioperative evaluation may disclose autonomic nervous system dysfunction manifested as orthostatic hypotension and the absence of beat-to-beat variability in heart rate associated with deep breathing. Management of anesthesia is based on understanding the impact of decreased autonomic nervous system activity on the cardiovascular responses to such events such as changes in body position, positive airway pressure, and acute blood loss. The negative inotropic effects of anesthetic drugs should also be considered.

Despite the obvious physiologic vulnerability of these patients to perioperative events, clinical experience has shown that most tolerate general and regional anesthesia without undue risk. The keys to management include continuous monitoring of the systemic blood pressure and prompt correction of hypotension by infusion of crystalloid or colloid solutions. If vasopressors are needed, these patients may exhibit exaggerated responses to indirect-acting drugs that provoke the release of norepinephrine. Instead, a direct-acting vasopressor such as phenylephrine is preferred. Small doses should be used initially until the response of the individual patient can be confirmed. This is because the up-regulated expression of α-adrenergic receptors in Shy-Drager syndrome (i.e., due to chronic relative autonomic denervation) can produce an exaggerated physiologic response to a small dose of drug. A continuous infusion of phenylephrine may be used to maintain systemic blood pressure during general anesthesia in affected patients. Spinal or epidural anesthesia can be considered, although concerns for blood pressure reduction demand diligence and caution by the anesthesiologist. Volatile anesthetics can diminish cardiac contractility and output, resulting in exaggerated hypotension. This is because compensatory responses such as vasoconstriction or tachycardia are unlikely in view of absent carotid sinus activity. Bradycardia, which contributes to hypotension, is best treated with atropine or glycopyrrolate. Signs of deep anesthesia may be less apparent in these patients because of decreased responses of the sympathetic nervous system to noxious stimulation. Administration of a muscle relaxant having less effect on the systemic circulation, such as vecuronium, is preferred. Thiopental or propofol dose and rate of administration should be adjusted to accommodate the patient's diminished compensatory responses. Conversely, the possibility of accentuated systemic blood pressure increases following ketamine administration is a theoretical possibility.

Orthostatic Intolerance Syndrome

Orthostatic intolerance syndrome is a chronic idiopathic disorder of primary autonomic system failure characterized by episodic or postural tachycardia occurring independent of alterations in systemic blood pressure. Orthostatic intolerance syndrome probably represents a variety of other entities including postural tachycardia syndrome, effort syndrome, hyperdynamic β-adrenergic state, hyperdynamic orthostatic tachycardia, idiopathic hypovolemia, irritable heart, mitral valve prolapse syndrome, neurocirculatory asthenia, and others. It is most often observed in young women. Symptoms often include palpitations, tremulousness, light-headedness, fatigue, and syncope. The pathophysiology of the orthostatic intolerance syndrome is unclear, although possible explanations include enhanced sensitivity of β_1-adrenergic receptors, hypovolemia, excessive venous pooling during standing, primary dysautonomia, and lower extremity sympathetic nervous system denervation.

Medical treatment of patients with orthostatic intolerance syndrome includes attempts to increase the intravascular fluid volume (increased sodium and water intake, administration of mineralocorticoids) in order to increase venous return. Long-term administration of α_1-adrenergic agonists, such as midodrine, may compensate for decreased sympathetic nervous system activity in the patient's lower extremities and blunt heart rate responses to standing by activating baroreceptor reflexes.

Management of anesthesia in patients with orthostatic intolerance syndrome includes preoperative administration of crystalloid solutions to expand the patient's intravascular fluid volume. Low-dose phenylephrine infusions may be cautiously administered, recognizing that lower extremity sympathetic nervous system denervation may cause up-regulation of α_1-adrenergic receptors and contribute to receptor hypersensitivity. The combination of volume expansion and low-dose phenylephrine infusions should augment peripheral vascular tone, maintain systemic blood pressure, and decrease autonomic nervous system lability in the presence of vasodilating anesthetic drugs (volatile anesthetics) or techniques (epidural or spinal anesthesia). Neuraxial opioids have utility for postoperative pain management. β-Adrenergic antagonists may be useful for blunt tachycardia; however, care should be taken to avoid excessive hypotension, which might result from the use of these drugs.

Glomus Tumors of the Head and Neck

Glomus tumors are paragangliomas that arise embryologically from neural crest cells. These tumors appear clinically in the head and neck within neuroendocrine tissue that lies along the carotid artery, aorta, glossopharyngeal nerve, and middle ear. When a glomus tumor is present, it is likely a second craniocervical paraganglioma; usually a carotid body tumor also exists. These tumors are rarely malignant.

Tumor location determines signs and symptoms, which most often reflect middle ear and cranial nerve invasion. Unilateral pulsatile tinnitus, conductive hearing loss, aural fullness, and a bluish red mass behind the tympanic membrane are characteristic of middle ear involvement, whereas facial paralysis, dysphonia, hearing loss, and pain typify cranial nerve invasion. Recurrent aspiration, dysphagia, and upper airway obstruction may also accompany cranial nerve involvement. Invasion of the posterior fossa may obstruct the aqueduct of Sylvius, causing hydrocephalus. It is common for glomus jugulare tumors to invade the internal jugular vein.

Glomus jugulare tumors can secrete a variety of hormonal substances. The most common secretory product is norepinephrine, producing symptoms that mimic pheochromocytoma. Cholecystokinin secretion is thought to play a role in the high incidence of postoperative ileus following tumor resection. Release of serotonin or kallikrein can mimic a carcinoid-like constellation of symptoms such as bronchoconstriction, diarrhea, headache, flushing, and hypertension. Finally, release of histamine or bradykinin can cause bronchoconstriction and hypotension.

Small glomus tumors are most often treated with radiation, as either an independent treatment or a component of radiation or embolization adjunct treatment prior to surgery. Surgery is recommended if bony destruction is present.

Preoperative determination of serum norepinephrine and catecholamine metabolite (i.e., metanephrine, vanillylmandelic acid) concentrations may be used to recognize patients likely to respond as if a pheochromocytoma were present. However, unlike pheochromocytomas, glomus tumors do not secrete epinephrine because they lack the transferase necessary to convert norepinephrine to epinephrine. Administration of phenoxybenzamine or prazosin may be used preoperatively to lower blood pressure and facilitate volume expansion in patients with increased serum norepinephrine concentrations. Patients with increased serum 5-hydroxyindoleacetic acid concentration, especially those with symptoms similar to those of carcinoid syndrome, should receive preoperative octreotide, often administered subcutaneously.

Management of Anesthesia

Anesthesia management is a formidable challenge in these patients. Anesthetic risks include catecholamine secretion, producing symptoms resembling pheochromocytomas; serotonin secretion, producing symptoms of carcinoid syndrome; aspiration after tumor resection due to cranial nerve dysfunction; impaired gastric emptying due to vagal nerve dysfunction; threat of venous air embolism; and massive blood loss. Intraoperatively, histamine and bradykinin released during surgical manipulation can cause profound hypotension. Cranial nerve deficits may be present preoperatively (vagus, glossopharyngeal, hypoglossal nerves) or may occur as a result of tumor resection. Airway obstruction is a risk after cranial nerve injury. Unilateral vocal cord paralysis, which in adults usually does not result in complete airway obstruction, can produce airway obstruction in combination with airway edema or laryngeal distortion.

During anesthesia, invasive arterial and venous pressure monitoring is indicated, and urinary output is monitored with a urinary bladder catheter. Given the risk of pheochromocytoma-like and carcinoid-like signs occurring intraoperatively, drugs used to treat both hypertension (i.e., sodium nitroprusside, phentolamine) and carcinoid-like signs (i.e., octreotide) should be immediately available. An internal jugular vein involved by tumor should not be cannulated in an attempt to place a right atrial or pulmonary artery catheter.

Venous air embolism is a risk, especially if the internal jugular vein is opened to remove the tumor. It is also a risk if excision of a tumor that has invaded temporal bone results in exposure of veins that cannot collapse because of bony attachments. Appropriate monitors for detecting venous air are indicated when venous air embolism is considered a risk (see "Venous Air Embolism and Sitting Position" in Chapter 10A). Sudden, unexplained cardiovascular collapse and death during resection of these tumors may reflect the presence of a venous air or tumor embolism. If the surgeon finds it necessary to identify the facial nerve, profound skeletal muscle paralysis should be avoided so that a visible twitch response can be maintained. The choice of anesthetic drugs is not uniquely influenced by the presence of glomus jugulare tumors, although the potential adverse effects of nitrous oxide have implications if venous air embolism occurs.

Carotid Sinus Syndrome

Carotid sinus syndrome is an uncommon entity caused by exaggeration of normal activity of the baroreceptors in response to mechanical stimulation. For example, stimulation of the carotid sinus by external massage, which in normal individuals produces modest decreases in heart rate and systemic blood pressure, can produce syncope in those exhibiting carotid sinus syndrome. Affected individuals have an increased incidence of peripheral vascular disease. Carotid sinus syndrome is a recognized complication following carotid endarterectomy.

Two distinct cardiovascular responses may be noted in the presence of carotid sinus hypersensitivity. In approximately 80% of affected individuals, a cardioinhibitory reflex, mediated by the vagus nerve, produces profound bradycardia. In approximately 10% of affected individuals, a vasodepressor reflex, mediated by inhibition of sympathetic nervous system vasomotor tone, produces decreases in systemic vascular resistance and profound hypotension. The remaining 10% exhibit components of both reflexes.

Carotid sinus syndrome may be treated with drugs, a demand-type artificial cardiac pacemaker, or ablation of the carotid sinus. Anticholinergic and vasopressor drug use is limited by their side effects and rarely effective in patients with vasodepressor or mixed forms of carotid sinus hypersensitivity. Because most patients have the cardioinhibitory type of carotid sinus syndrome, implantation of an artificial cardiac pacemaker is the usual initial treatment. Denervation of the carotid sinus may be attempted in patients in whom the vasodepressor reflex response is refractory to cardiac pacing. Since the glossopharyngeal nerve provides the afferent limb of the reflex that produces symptoms in carotid sinus syndrome, block of this nerve may be an alternative therapy in patients refractory to artificial cardiac pacing or drug therapy. The nerve is approached with a stimulating needle as it passes anterior to the styloid process. Successful identification of its location is noted when the patient complains of a vague sensation in the region supplied by this nerve (e.g., external ear and pharynx) upon electrical nerve stimulation. Initially, a test block is performed with local anesthetic, and if the desired effect of reduced symptoms upon carotid massage is obtained, the nerve is ablated with ethanol.

Management of Anesthesia

Anesthetic management in patients with carotid sinus syndrome is often complicated by hypotension, bradycardia, and cardiac arrhythmias. Infiltration of a local anesthetic-containing solution around the carotid sinus before dissection usually improves hemodynamic stability, but may also interfere with determining the completeness of the ablation. Drugs such as atropine, isoproterenol, and epinephrine electrical cardiac pacing may be a more effective option in many circumstances.

DISEASES OF THE PERIPHERAL NERVOUS SYSTEM

Idiopathic Facial Paralysis (Bell's Palsy)

Idiopathic facial paralysis is characterized by the rapid onset of motor weakness or paralysis of all the muscles innervated by the facial nerve. Often the onset is first noted on arising in the morning and looking into a mirror. Additional symptoms can include the loss of taste sensation over the anterior two thirds of the tongue as well as hyperacusis and diminished salivation and lacrimation. The absence of cutaneous sensory loss emphasizes that the trigeminal nerve supplies cutaneous sensory innervation to the face. The cause of idiopathic facial paralysis is presumed to be inflammation and edema of the facial nerve, most often in the facial canal of the temporal bone. A viral inflammatory mechanism (perhaps herpes simplex virus) may be the cause. Indeed, the onset of this cranial mononeuropathy is often preceded by a viral prodrome. During pregnancy, there is an increased incidence of idiopathic facial paralysis. The presence of idiopathic facial paralysis does not influence the choice of anesthetic technique.

Spontaneous recovery usually occurs over approximately 12 weeks. If no recovery is seen in 16 to 20 weeks, the clinical signs and symptoms are probably not due to idiopathic facial paralysis. Prednisone (1 mg/kg orally each day for 5 to 10 days, depending on the extent of facial nerve paralysis) dramatically relieves pain and decreases the number of patients experiencing complete denervation of the facial nerve. If blinking is not possible, the patient's affected eye should be covered to protect the cornea from dehydration.

Surgical decompression of the facial nerve may be needed for persistent or severe cases of idiopathic facial paralysis or for facial paralysis secondary to trauma. Trauma to the facial nerve can reflect a stretch injury produced by excessive traction on the angle of the mandible during maintenance of the upper airway in unconscious patients. Uveoparotid fever (Heerfordt syndrome) is a variant of sarcoidosis characterized by bilateral anterior uveitis, parotitis, and mild pyrexia as well as the presence of facial nerve paralysis in 50% to 70% of patients. Facial nerve paralysis associated with postoperative uveoparotid fever may be erroneously attributed to mechanical pressure over the nerve during general anesthesia.

Facial nerve palsy has been described following placement of an extradural blood patch to treat postdural puncture headaches. Sudden increases in intracranial pressure were speculated to have transiently compromised the blood flow to the facial nerve.

Trigeminal Neuralgia (Tic Douloureux)

Trigeminal neuralgia is characterized by the sudden onset of brief but intense unilateral facial pain triggered by local sensory stimuli to the affected side of the face. Trigeminal neuralgia can be diagnosed based on purely clinical signs and symptoms. Patients report brief, stabbing pain or clusters of stabbing pains in the face or mouth that are restricted to one or more divisions of the trigeminal nerve, most often the mandibular division. Trigeminal neuralgia most often develops in otherwise healthy individuals during late middle age. The appearance of this neuralgia at an earlier age should arouse suspicion of multiple sclerosis. Although the pathophysiology of the pain associated with trigeminal neuralgia is uncertain, compression of the root, i.e., the location where central myelin (produced by oligodendrocytes) changes to peripheral myelin (produced by Schwann cells) by an abnormal blood vessel, is a possibility with the most common offending blood vessel being a branch of the superior cerebellar artery. Antiepileptic drugs are useful for treating trigeminal neuralgia; however, there are few clinical trials supporting their use for this indication. The anticonvulsant carbamazepine is the drug treatment of choice, but baclofen and lamotrigine are also effective. Surgical therapy (selective radiofrequency destruction of trigeminal nerve fibers, transection of the sensory root of the trigeminal nerve, microsurgical decompression of the trigeminal nerve root) is recommended for individuals who develop pain refractory to drug therapy.

There are no special considerations for management of anesthesia in patients with trigeminal neuralgia. Patients undergoing surgical therapy, however, may experience significant increases in systemic blood pressure during destruction of nerve fibers, necessitating treatment with antihypertensive agents. The potential enzyme-inducing effects of anticonvulsant drugs must be considered when predicting drug effects. Carbamazepine can cause altered hepatic function and produce leukopenia and thrombocytopenia.

Glossopharyngeal Neuralgia

Glossopharyngeal neuralgia is characterized by episodes of intense pain in the throat, neck, tongue, and ear. Swallowing, chewing, coughing, or talking can trigger the pain. This neuralgia may also be associated with severe bradycardia and syncope, presumably reflecting activation of the motor nucleus of the vagus nerve. Hypotension, seizures due to cerebral ischemia, and even cardiac arrest may manifest in some patients.

Glossopharyngeal neuralgia is usually idiopathic but has been described in patients with cerebellopontine angle vascular anomalies and tumors, vertebral and carotid artery occlusive disease, arachnoiditis, and extracranial tumors arising in the area of the pharynx, larynx, and tonsils. The presence of glossopharyngeal neuralgia is supported by pain in the distribution of the glossopharyngeal nerve and relief of pain by topical anesthesia of the oropharynx, usually at the tonsillar pillar and fossa. Trigger zones are rare.

In the absence of pain, cardiac symptoms associated with glossopharyngeal neuralgia may be confused with sick sinus syndrome or carotid sinus syndrome. Sick sinus syndrome can be discounted by the absence of characteristic changes on the electrocardiogram. Failure of carotid sinus massage to produce cardiac symptoms rules out carotid sinus hypersensitivity. Glossopharyngeal nerve block is useful for differentiating glossopharyngeal neuralgia from atypical trigeminal neuralgia. This nerve block does not differentiate glossopharyngeal neuralgia from the carotid sinus syndrome, as afferent pathways of both syndromes are mediated by the glossopharyngeal nerve.

Glossopharyngeal neuralgia-associated cardiac symptoms should be aggressively treated as there is a risk of sudden death. Cardiovascular symptoms are treated acutely with atropine, isoproterenol, an artificial external cardiac pacemaker, or a combination of these modalities. Pain associated with this syndrome is managed by chronic administration of anticonvulsant drugs such as carbamazepine and phenytoin. Prevention of cardiovascular symptoms and provision of predictable pain relief are achieved by intracranial surgical transection of the glossopharyngeal nerve and the upper two roots of the vagus nerve. Although permanent pain relief is possible after repeated glossopharyngeal nerve blocks, this neuralgia is sufficiently life-threatening to justify intracranial transection of the nerve in patients not responsive to medical therapy.

Management of Anesthesia

Preoperative evaluation of patients with glossopharyngeal neuralgia is directed at assessing the patient's intravascular fluid volume and cardiac status. Hypovolemia may be present, as these patients avoid oral intake and its associated pharyngeal stimulation in attempts to avoid triggering the pain attacks. Furthermore, drooling and loss of saliva can contribute to decreased intravascular fluid volume. A preoperative history of syncope or documented bradycardia, concurrent with the episodes of pain, introduces the possible need for prompt transcutaneous cardiac pacing or placement of a prophylactic transvenous cardiac pacemaker before the induction of anesthesia. Continuous monitoring of electrocardiographic activity and of systemic blood pressure (via an intra-arterial catheter) is useful. Topical anesthesia of the oropharynx with lidocaine is helpful for preventing bradycardia and hypotension, which may occur in response to stimulation from direct laryngoscopy. Intravenous administration of atropine or glycopyrrolate just before initiating laryngoscopy may be recommended.

Cardiovascular changes should be expected in response to surgical manipulation and intracranial transection of glossopharyngeal and vagus nerve roots. For example, bradycardia and hypotension are likely during manipulation of the vagus nerve. Anticholinergic drugs should be promptly available to treat vagus nerve–mediated responses. Systemic hypertension, tachycardia, and ventricular premature beats may occur after surgical transection of the glossopharyngeal nerve and the upper two roots of the vagus nerve. These events may reflect the sudden loss of sensory input from the carotid sinus. Systemic hypertension is usually transient but, due to an overall increase in sympathetic nervous system activity, can persist into the postoperative period. In this setting, hydralazine may be useful. Experience is too limited to permit recommendations for specific anesthetic drugs or muscle relaxants. The possible development of vocal cord paralysis following vagal nerve transection should be considered if airway obstruction follows tracheal extubation.

Charcot-Marie-Tooth Disease

The most common inherited cause of chronic motor and sensory peripheral neuropathy, Charcot-Marie-Tooth disease type 1A (CMT1A or peroneal muscle disease) has an estimated incidence of 1 in 2500 individuals. An autosomal dominant mode of inheritance is most common; however, an X-linked variant is known to exist. This disorder manifests as distal skeletal muscle weakness, wasting, and loss of tendon reflexes, which usually become evident by the middle teenage years. Classically, this neuropathy is described as being restricted to the lower one third of the legs, producing foot deformities (high pedal arches and talipes) and peroneal muscle atrophy ("stork-leg" appearance). The disease may slowly progress to include wasting of the quadriceps muscles and the muscles of the hands and forearms. Mild to moderate stocking-glove sensory loss occurs in many patients. Pregnancy may be associated with exacerbations of CMT1A.

Treatment of CMT1A is limited to supportive measures, including splints, tendon transfers, and various arthrodeses. Although life span is not decreased, many individuals with CMT1A experience long-term disability.

Management of anesthesia in patients with CMT1A is influenced by concerns about the responses to neuromuscular blocking drugs and the possibility of postoperative respiratory failure due to weakness of the muscles responsible for respiration. Cardiac manifestations attributed to this neuropathy, including conduction disturbances (atrial flutter) and cardiomyopathy, have not been observed consistently. Drugs known to trigger malignant hyperthermia have been used safely in patients with CMTD, although there has been a single reported case of malignant hyperthermia in the perioperative period in a patient with CMT1A. However, this concurrence probably represents a chance phenomenon of malignant hyperthermia susceptibility independent of CMT1A. The responses to neuromuscular blocking drugs seem to be predictable in patients with CMT1A. It appears reasonable to avoid succinylcholine based on theoretical concerns about exaggerated potassium release following administration of this drug to individuals with neuromuscular diseases. Nevertheless, succinylcholine has been used safely in some patients without producing hyperkalemia or triggering malignant hyperthermia. Use of epidural anesthesia for labor has been described.

Brachial Plexus Neuropathy

Brachial plexus neuropathy (idiopathic brachial neuritis, Parsonage-Turner syndrome, shoulder-girdle syndrome) is characterized by the acute onset of severe pain in the upper arm with its maximum intensity at the onset of the neuropathy. As the pain diminishes, there is the appearance of a patchy paresis or paralysis of the skeletal muscles innervated by branches of the brachial plexus. Skeletal muscle wasting, particularly involving the shoulder girdle and arm, is common. Brachial plexus neuropathy is more common on the right, although the involvement and pain are bilateral in 10% to 30% of afflicted individuals, with both sides becoming involved simultaneously or sequentially. Although this neuropathy seems to have a predilection for the upper trunks of the brachial plexus (axillary, suprascapular, long thoracic nerves), it may involve a variety of nerves in the upper extremity. An estimated 70% of afflicted individuals have involvement of the axillary nerve.

Diagnosis of brachial plexus neuropathy and demonstration of the multifocal pattern of denervation is best evaluated by electrodiagnostic studies. Muscle fibrillations and slowing of nerve conduction velocity are observed. Skeletal muscles most often affected, in decreasing order, are the deltoid, supraspinatus, infraspinatus, serratus anterior, biceps, and triceps. The diaphragm may also be affected. Sensory disturbances occur in most patients, but tend to be minimal and generally resolve with time. The incidence of this neuropathy is two to three times higher in males than females. Overall, recovery may take 24 to 36 months but is nearly always complete. The annual incidence of brachial plexus neuropathy is an estimated 1.64 cases per 100,000 population.

Nerve biopsy of individuals having hereditary brachial plexus neuropathy and Parsonage-Turner syndrome suggests that these brachial plexopathies have an inflammatory-immune pathogenesis. Autoimmune neuropathies may also occur during the postoperative period independent of the site of surgery. It is possible that the stress of surgery activates an unidentified dormant virus in the nerve roots, a circumstance similar to the onset of herpes zoster after surgery. Additionally, strenuous exercise or pregnancy may be inciting events for brachial plexus neuropathy. A hereditary form of this peripheral neuropathy has also been described.

Guillain-Barré Syndrome (Acute Idiopathic Polyneuritis)

Guillain-Barré syndrome is characterized by sudden onset of skeletal muscle weakness or paralysis that typically manifests initially in the legs and spreads cephalad over the ensuing days to involve skeletal muscles of the arms, trunk, and face. With the virtual elimination of poliomyelitis, this syndrome has become the most common cause of acute generalized paralysis, with an annual incidence of 0.75 to 2.0 cases per 100,000 population. Bulbar involvement most frequently manifests as bilateral facial paralysis. Difficulty swallowing due to pharyngeal muscle weakness and impaired ventilation due to intercostal muscle paralysis are the most serious symptoms of this process. Because of lower motor neuron involvement, paralysis is flaccid, and corresponding tendon reflexes are diminished. Sensory disturbances (e.g., paresthesias) generally precede the onset of paralysis and are most prominently in the distal extremities. Pain often exists in the form of headache, backache, or tenderness of skeletal muscles to deep pressure.

Autonomic nervous system dysfunction is a prominent finding in patients with Guillain-Barré syndrome and is usually manifested as wide fluctuations in systemic blood pressure, sudden profuse diaphoresis, peripheral vasoconstriction,

TABLE 10C-1	Diagnostic Criteria for Guillain-Barré Syndrome

Features Required for Diagnosis
Progressive bilateral weakness in legs and arms
Areflexia

Features Strongly Supporting the Diagnosis
Progression of symptoms over 2–4 weeks
Symmetry of symptoms
Mild sensory symptoms or signs (definitive sensory level makes diagnosis doubtful)
Cranial nerve involvement (especially bilateral facial weakness)
Spontaneous recovery beginning 2–4 weeks after progression ceases
Autonomic nervous system dysfunction
Absence of fever at onset
Increased concentrations of protein in the cerebrospinal fluid

resting tachycardia, and cardiac conduction abnormalities. Orthostatic hypotension may be so severe that elevating the patient's head on a pillow leads to syncope. Thromboembolism occurs with increased frequency. Sudden death associated with this disease is most likely due to autonomic nervous system dysfunction.

Complete spontaneous recovery from acute idiopathic polyneuritis can occur within a few weeks, when segmental demyelination is the predominant pathologic change. Axonal degeneration (as detected by electromyography screening) may result in slower recovery over several months, with some degree of permanent weakness remaining. The mortality rate associated with Guillain-Barré syndrome is 3% to 8%, and death is most often due to sepsis, acute respiratory failure, pulmonary embolism, and cardiac arrest (the last likely related to autonomic nervous system dysfunction).

The diagnosis of Guillain-Barré syndrome is based on clinical signs and symptoms (**Table 10C-1**), supported by findings of increased protein concentrations in the cerebrospinal fluid. Cerebrospinal fluid cell counts typically remain within a normal range. Support of a viral etiology or mycoplasma infection is based on the observation that this syndrome develops after respiratory or gastrointestinal infections in approximately one half of patients.

Treatment of Guillain-Barré syndrome is mainly symptomatic. The vital capacity is monitored, and when it drops to less than 15 mL/kg, mechanical support of the patient's ventilation is considered. Arterial blood gas measurements help assess the adequacy of ventilation and oxygenation. Pharyngeal muscle weakness, even in the absence of ventilatory failure, may require a cuffed endotracheal tracheal tube or tracheostomy to protect the lungs from aspiration of secretions and gastric fluid. Autonomic nervous system dysfunction may require treatment of systemic hypertension or hypotension. Corticosteroids are not considered useful therapy for this syndrome. Plasma exchange or infusion of γ-globulin may benefit some patients.

Management of Anesthesia

Altered function of the autonomic nervous system and the presence of lower motor neuron lesions are the two major factors in the developing a management plan for anesthesia in patients with Guillain-Barré syndrome. Compensatory cardiovascular responses may be absent, resulting in profound hypotension in response to changes in posture, blood loss, or positive airway pressure. Conversely, noxious stimulation, such as during direct laryngoscopy, could manifest as exaggerated increases in systemic blood pressure, reflecting the autonomic nervous system lability. In view of these unpredictable changes in systemic blood pressure, it seems prudent to monitor the systemic blood pressure continuously with an intra-arterial catheter. Patients may exhibit exaggerated responses to indirect-acting vasopressors likely due to up-regulation of postsynaptic receptors.

Succinylcholine should not be administered to these patients, as there is a risk of excessive potassium release from denervated skeletal muscles. A nondepolarizing muscle relaxant with minimal circulatory effects, such as cisatracurium or vecuronium, seems to be a logical choice. Even if spontaneous ventilation is present preoperatively, it is likely that depression from anesthetic drugs will necessitate mechanical ventilation during surgery. Similarly, continued support of ventilation is often necessary during the postoperative period.

Entrapment Neuropathies

Entrapment neuropathies occur at anatomic sites where peripheral nerves pass through narrow passages (median nerve and carpal tunnel at the wrist, ulnar nerve and cubital tunnel at the elbow), making compression a possibility. Peripheral nerves are probably more sensitive to compressive (ischemic) injury in patients who also have generalized polyneuropathies (e.g., as occurs with diabetes mellitus or hereditary peripheral neuropathies). A peripheral nerve may also be more susceptible to compression if the same fibers have been partially damaged proximally (double crush hypothesis). In this regard, spinal nerve root compression (cervical radiculopathy) may increase the vulnerability of nerve fibers at distal entrapment sites, such as the carpal tunnel at the wrist. Alternatively, osteoarthritis may explain symptoms attributed to the double crush phenomenon. Peripheral nerve damage resulting from compression depends on the severity of the compression and the anatomy of the nerve. In most instances, the outermost nerve fibers (i.e., those that innervate more proximal tissues) are more vulnerable to ischemia from compression than the fibers lying more deeply in the bundle of the nerve. Differing damage to fascicles in the peripheral nerve makes it difficult to localize the site of nerve injury precisely, although nerve conduction studies are useful. Focal demyelination of nerve fibers causes slowing or blocking of nerve impulse conduction through the damaged area. Electromyography studies are adjuncts to nerve conduction studies, showing the presence of denervation impulses and ultimately reinnervation of muscle fibers by surviving axons.

Carpal Tunnel Syndrome

Carpal tunnel syndrome is the most common entrapment neuropathy. It results from compression of the median nerve between the transverse carpal ligament forming the roof of the carpal tunnel and the carpal bones at the wrist. This compression neuropathy most often occurs in otherwise healthy women (three times more frequent in women than men) and is often bilateral, although the dominant hand is typically involved initially. Patients describe repeated episodes of pain and paresthesias in the wrist and hand following the distribution of the median nerve (thumb and index and middle fingers), often occurring during sleep or on waking. Population-based studies reveal that approximately 3% of adults have symptomatic electrodiagnostically confirmed carpal tunnel syndrome.

The cause of carpal tunnel syndrome is often unknown, although afflicted individuals may engage in occupations that require repetitive movements of the hands and fingers. Nerve conduction studies are the definitive method for confirming the diagnosis. In previously asymptomatic patients who acquire symptoms of carpal tunnel syndrome shortly after an unrelated surgery, it is likely that the accumulation of third space fluid, resulting in increased tissue pressure, may have caused compression of the nerve. In such patients, subsequent neurologic examination and neurophysiologic testing often discover preexisting carpal tunnel syndrome that was asymptomatic during the preoperative evaluation. Pregnancy and associated peripheral edema may also precipitate the initial manifestations of carpal tunnel syndrome. Cervical radiculopathy may produce similar symptoms unilaterally but rarely bilaterally.

Immobilizing the wrist with a splint is a common treatment for carpal tunnel syndrome that is likely to be transient (pregnancy) or due to a medically treatable disease (hypothyroidism, acromegaly). Injection of corticosteroids into the carpal tunnel may relieve symptoms, but is seldom curative. Definitive treatment of carpal tunnel syndrome is decompression of the median nerve by surgical division of the transverse carpal ligament.

Cubital Tunnel Entrapment Syndrome

Compression of the ulnar nerve after it passes through the condylar groove and enters the cubital tunnel may result in clinical symptoms considered typical of ulnar nerve neuropathy. It may be difficult to differentiate clinical symptoms of ulnar nerve neuropathy due to compression in the condylar groove from symptoms related to entrapment in the cubital tunnel. Surgical treatment of cubital tunnel entrapment syndrome (by tunnel decompression and transposition of the nerve) may be helpful for relieving symptoms, but may also make symptoms worse, perhaps by interfering with the nerve's blood supply.

Diseases Associated with Peripheral Neuropathies

Diabetes Mellitus

Diabetes mellitus is commonly associated with peripheral polyneuropathies, with the incidence increasing with the duration of the disease and perhaps the extent of hypoinsulinemia. Up to 7.5% of patients with non–insulin-dependent diabetes mellitus have clinical neuropathy at the time of diagnosis. Electromyograms may show evidence of denervation, and nerve conduction velocity is likely to be slowed. The most common neuropathy is distal, symmetrical, and predominantly sensory. The principal manifestations are unpleasant tingling, numbness, burning, and aching in the lower extremities; skeletal muscle weakness; and distal sensory loss. Occasionally, an isolated sciatic neuropathy suggests the presence of a herniated intervertebral disc. Sciatic neuropathy in patients with diabetes mellitus is not associated with pain in response to straight-leg raising, serving to distinguish this peripheral neuropathy from lumbar disc disease. Discomfort is prominent at night and is often relieved by walking. Symptoms often progress and may extend to the upper extremities. Impotence, urinary retention, gastroparesis, resting tachycardia, and postural hypotension are common and reflect autonomic nervous system dysfunction. For reasons that are not understood, the peripheral nerves of patients with diabetes mellitus are more vulnerable to ischemia due to compression or stretch injury (such as may occur during intraoperative and postoperative positioning), despite accepted padding and positioning during these periods.

Alcohol Abuse

Polyneuropathy of chronic alcoholism is nearly always associated with nutritional and vitamin deficiencies. Symptoms characteristically begin in the lower extremities, with pain and numbness in the feet. Weakness and tenderness of the intrinsic muscles of the feet, absent Achilles tendon reflexes, and hypalgesia in a stocking-glove distribution are early manifestations. Restoration of a proper diet, abstinence from alcohol, and multivitamin therapy promote slow but predictable resolution of the neuropathy.

Vitamin B$_{12}$ Deficiency

The earliest neurologic symptoms of vitamin B$_{12}$ deficiency resemble the neuropathy typically seen in patients who abuse alcohol. Paresthesias in the legs with sensory loss in a stocking distribution plus absent Achilles tendon reflexes are characteristic findings. Similar neurologic findings have been reported in dentists who are chronically exposed to nitrous oxide and in individuals who chronically inhale nitrous oxide for nonmedical purposes. Nitrous oxide is known to inactivate certain vitamin B$_{12}$–dependent enzymes, which could lead to symptoms of altered nerve function.

Uremia

Distal polyneuropathy with sensory and motor components often occurs in the extremities of patients with chronic renal failure. Symptoms tend to be more prominent in the legs than in the arms. Presumably, metabolic abnormalities are responsible for axonal degeneration and segmental demyelination, which accompany the neuropathy. Slowing of nerve conduction has been correlated with increased plasma concentrations of parathyroid hormone and myoinositol, a component of myelin. Improved nerve conduction velocity often occurs within a few days after renal transplantation. Hemodialysis does not appear to be equally effective for reversing the polyneuropathy.

Cancer

Peripheral sensory and motor neuropathies occur in patients with a variety of malignancies, especially those involving the lung, ovary, and breast. Polyneuropathy that develops in elderly patients should always arouse suspicion of undiagnosed cancer. Myasthenic (Eaton-Lambert) syndrome may be observed in patients with carcinoma of the lung. This paraneoplastic syndrome results from the abnormal production of an antibody against presynaptic calcium channels located on cholinergic neurons. As a result of calcium channel blockade, decreased quantities of acetylcholine are released from nerve terminals at the neuromuscular junction, resulting in weakness. It can lead to increased sensitivity to both depolarizing and nondepolarizing neuromuscular blocking agents. Invasion of the lower trunks of the brachial plexus by tumors in the apex of the lungs (Pancoast syndrome) produces arm pain, paresthesias, and weakness of the hands and arms.

Collagen Vascular Diseases

Collagen vascular diseases are commonly associated with peripheral neuropathies. The most common conditions are systemic lupus erythematosus, polyarteritis nodosa, rheumatoid arthritis, and scleroderma. Detection of multiple mononeuropathies suggests vasculitis of nerve trunks and should stimulate a search for the presence of collagen vascular diseases.

Sarcoidosis

Sarcoidosis is a disorder of unknown etiology whereby noncaseating granulomas occur in multiple organ systems, most commonly the lung, lymphatics, bone, liver, and nervous system. Polyneuropathy, due to the presence of granulomatous lesions in peripheral nerves, is a frequent finding in patients with sarcoidosis. Unilateral or bilateral facial nerve paralysis may result from sarcoid involvement of this nerve in the parotid gland and is often one of the first manifestations of sarcoidosis.

Refsum's Disease

Refsum's disease is a multisystem disorder that manifests as polyneuropathies, ichthyosis, deafness, retinitis pigmentosa, cardiomyopathy, and cerebellar ataxia. Metabolic defects responsible for this disease reflect a failure to oxidize phytic acid, a fatty acid that subsequently accumulates in excessive concentrations.

KEY POINTS

- When caring for patients with diseases affecting the autonomic nervous system, one should carefully monitor for and be prepared to treat rapid-onset, and sometimes extreme, changes in heart rate and blood pressure.

- In the setting of autonomic disorders, changes in catecholamine release and adrenergic receptor density may occur. Therefore, one should take care to titrate direct-acting adrenergic drugs and avoid indirect-acting adrenergic drugs if possible.

- Succinylcholine should be used with caution in patients with neurologic disease affecting the peripheral nervous system because of the risk of hyperkalemia in the setting of diseases that cause an up-regulation of acetylcholine receptors at the neuromuscular junction.

- Some diseases affecting the peripheral nervous system may be associated with significant neuropathic pain. Both narcotics and non-narcotic pain management options should be considered.

REFERENCES

Antognini JF: Anaesthesia for Charcot-Marie-Tooth disease: a review of 86 cases. Can J Anaesth 1992;39:398–400.

Atroshi I, Gummesson C, Johnsson R, et al: Prevalence of carpal tunnel syndrome in a general population. JAMA 1999;282: 153–158.

Bergoffen J, Scherer SS, Wang S, et al: Connexin mutations in X-linked Charcot-Marie-Tooth disease. Science 1993;262: 2039–2042.

D'Arcy CA, McGee S: The rational clinical examination. Does this patient have carpal tunnel syndrome? JAMA 2000;283:3110–3117.

Dorsey DL, Camann WR: Obstetric anesthesia in patients with idiopathic facial paralysis (Bell's palsy): A 10-year survey. Anesth Analg 1993;77:81–83.

Fibuch EE, Mertz J, Geller B: Postoperative onset of idiopathic brachial neuritis. Anesthesiology 1996;84:455–458.

Fields HL: Treatment of trigeminal neuralgia. N Engl J Med 1996;334:1125–1126.

Greenberg RS, Parker SD: Anesthetic management for the child with Charcot-Marie-Tooth disease. Anesth Analg 1992;74: 305–307.

Horlocker TT, O'Driscoll SW, Dinapoli RP: Recurring brachial plexus neuropathy in a diabetic patient after shoulder surgery and continuous interscalene block. Anesth Analg 2000;91: 688–690.

Jackson CG, Gulya AJ, Knox GW, et al: A paraneoplastic syndrome associated with glomus tumors of the skull base? Early observations. Otolaryngol Head Neck Surg 1989;100:583–587.

Jacob G, Costa F, Shannon JR, et al: The neuropathic postural tachycardia syndrome. N Engl J Med 2000;343:1008–1014.

Jensen NF: Glomus tumors of the head and neck: Anesthetic considerations. Anesth Analg 1994;78:112–119.

Klein CJ, Dyck PJ, Friedenberg SM, et al: Inflammation and neuropathic attacks in hereditary brachial plexus neuropathy. J Neurol Neurosurg Psychiatry 2002;73:45–50.

Lupski JR, Chance PF, Garcia CA: Inherited primary peripheral neuropathies. Molecular genetics and clinical implications of CMT1A and HNPP. JAMA 1993;270:2326–2330.

McHaourab A, Mazzeo AJ, May JA, Pagel PS: Perioperative considerations in a patient with orthostatic intolerance syndrome. Anesthesiology 2000;93:571–573.

Niquille M, Van Gessel E, Gamulin Z: Continuous spinal anesthesia for hip surgery in a patient with Shy-Drager syndrome. Anesth Analg 1998;87:396–399.

Osborne PJ, Lee LW: Idiopathic orthostatic hypotension, midodrine, and anaesthesia. Can J Anaesth 1991;38:499–501.

Partanen J, Niskanen L, Lehtinen J, et al: Natural history of peripheral neuropathy in patients with non–insulin-dependent diabetes mellitus. N Engl J Med 1995;333:89–94.

Pogson D, Telfer J, Wimbush S: Prolonged vecuronium neuromuscular blockade associated with Charcot Marie Tooth neuropathy. Br J Anaesth 2000;85:914–917.

Robertson D, Robertson RM: Cardiovascular Manifestations of Autonomic Disorders. Braunwald's Heart Disease: A Textbook of Cardiovascular Medicine. 7th ed, Philadelphia, WB Saunders, 2005:2180–2182.

Ropper AH: The Guillain-Barre syndrome. N Engl J Med 1992;326:1130–1136.

Scrivani SJ, Mathews ES, Maciewicz RJ: Trigeminal neuralgia. Oral Surg Oral Med Oral Pathol Oral Radiol Endod 2005;100: 527–538.

Scull T, Weeks S: Epidural analgesia for labour in a patient with Charcot-Marie-Tooth disease. Can J Anaesth 1996;43: 1150–1152.

Vaghadia H: Facial paresis after general anesthesia. Report of an unusual case: Heerfordt's syndrome. Anesthesiology 1986; 64:513–514.

Warner MA, Warner DO, Matsumoto JY, et al: Ulnar neuropathy in surgical patients. Anesthesiology 1999;90:54–59.

CHAPTER 11

Diseases of the Liver and Biliary Tract

Katherine E. Marschall

Diseases of the liver and biliary tract can be categorized as parenchymal liver disease (hepatitis and cirrhosis) and cholestasis with or without obstruction of the extrahepatic biliary pathway.

ACUTE HEPATITIS

Acute hepatitis is most often due to a virus but can also be caused by drugs and toxins. Acute viral hepatitis is typically caused by one of five viruses: hepatitis A virus (HAV), hepatitis B virus (HBV), hepatitis C virus (HCV), hepatitis D virus (HDV), or hepatitis E virus (HEV). In the United States, approximately 50% of cases of acute viral hepatitis in adults are due to HAV infection, 35% to HBV infection, and 15% to HCV infection. HDV infection is rare (< 1% of cases), and only imported cases of HEV have been seen. Chronic infection may result from HBV, HCV, and HDV infection. Viruses that cause systemic illness and also affect the liver include cytomegalovirus and Epstein-Barr virus.

Viral Hepatitis

All types of viral hepatitis are similar and cannot be distinguished reliably by clinical features or routine laboratory tests (**Table 11-1**). Infection may be asymptomatic or associated with flulike symptoms; some patients develop jaundice. The diagnostic laboratory abnormality of acute hepatitis is a markedly increased aminotransferase level. The specific etiology of viral hepatitis is determined by serologic testing.

Classification

Hepatitis A HAV is a picornavirus similar to poliovirus and rhinovirus. Shed virus is present in the serum and stool of patients with HAV. The antigenic composition of HAV is such that immunoglobulin and HAV vaccine provide protection. Immunoglobulin M (IgM) antibodies to HAV (IgM anti-HAV) are detectable at the onset of clinical illness and may persist for several months. Immunoglobulin G (IgG) antibodies achieve high titers during convalescence and persist indefinitely, thereby conferring immunity. Nearly one half of the U.S. population has serum antibodies to HAV.

Hepatitis A is highly contagious, being transmitted via the fecal-oral route especially if there are poor sanitary conditions. It may result from person-to-person exposure or to fecal contamination of food or water. High-risk groups for acquiring hepatitis A include travelers to underdeveloped areas, children in day care centers, persons in institutions, homosexual men, and intravenous drug users. Viremia is present for several days prior to the onset of clinical symptoms. The virus is shed in the stool for 14 to 21 days before the onset of jaundice. The virus continues to be shed for the first 7 to 14 days of clinical illness but patients are no longer infectious by three weeks. Hepatitis A is invariably a self-limiting infection and does not lead to chronic infection or to cirrhosis.

Hepatitis B Hepatitis B is transmitted primarily by the parenteral route or by intimate personal contact. It is endemic in many areas of the world. In the United States, it is the second most common cause of acute hepatitis. HBV is present in the serum and body secretions of most patients early in the course of acute hepatitis B. Hepatitis B is common among intravenous drug users, homosexual men, and heterosexuals with multiple partners. Maternal-infant transmission is another important mode of transmission. Blood transfusion and plasma products are now rarely infectious because of screening procedures for HBV antigens and antibodies.

The surface coat of the hepatitis B virion is composed of a polypeptide that acts as the major hepatitis B surface antigen (HBsAg). A large proportion of the population has serum antibodies to HBsAg, which confer immunity to hepatitis B.

Hepatitis C HCV is transmitted predominantly by the parenteral route. At present, hepatitis C is usually due to intravenous drug use (60%), sexual exposure (15%–20%), and,

TABLE 11–1	Characteristic Features of Viral Hepatitis			
Parameter	**Type A**	**Type B**	**Type C**	**Type D**
Mode of transmission	Fecal-oral Sewage-contaminated shellfish	Percutaneous Sexual	Percutaneous	Percutaneous
Incubation period	20–37 days	60–110 days	35–70 days	60–110 days
Results of serum antigen and antibody tests	IgM early and IgG appears during convalescence	HBsAg and anti-HBc early and persists in carriers	Anti-HCV in 6 weeks to 9 months	Anti-HDV late and may be short-lived
Immunity	Antibodies in 45%	Antibodies in 5%–15%	Unknown	Protected if immune to type B
Course	Does not progress to chronic liver disease	Chronic liver disease develops in 1%–5% of adults and 80%–90% of children	Chronic liver disease develops up to 75%	Co-infection with type B
Prevention after exposure	Pooled γ-globulin Hepatitis A vaccine	Hepatitis B immuno-globulin Hepatitis B vaccine	? Interferon	Unknown
Mortality	< 0.2%	0.3%–1.5%	Unknown	Acute icteric hepatitis: 2%–20%

HBc, hepatitis B core antigen; HBsAg, hepatitis B surface antigen.
Adapted from Keefe EB: Acute hepatitis. Sci Am Med 1999;1–9.

much less commonly, maternal-infant spread, blood transfusion, or occupational exposure to blood or blood products or needlestick injury. The ability to screen for HCV has essentially eliminated HCV as a cause of posttransfusion hepatitis. Recipients of organs from donors with antibodies to HCV have a high likelihood of becoming infected with HCV.

The major complication of acute hepatitis due to HCV is development of chronic hepatitis and cirrhosis. Hepatitis C has emerged as the predominant liver disease in the United States. Progression of chronic hepatitis C to cirrhosis may be slow, but end-stage liver disease due to HCV-associated cirrhosis is the most common indication for liver transplantation and HCV-associated cirrhosis is responsible for an increasing incidence of hepatocellular cancer.

Hepatitis D HDV is a unique virus that requires HBV for replication. Therefore, hepatitis D occurs only in patients with hepatitis B and is transmitted via the parenteral route or sexually. Co-infection with HBV and HDV may produce more severe acute hepatitis and more severe chronic hepatitis and cirrhosis than infection with HBV alone.

Hepatitis E HEV is spread by the fecal-oral route, usually due to contaminated water and poor hygienic conditions. It is less contagious than HAV and is rarely found in the United States.

Diagnosis

The diagnosis of viral hepatitis is dependent on clinical signs and symptoms, laboratory findings, serologic assays, and occasionally liver biopsy.

Signs and Symptoms The onset of viral hepatitis may be gradual or sudden and most often manifests as dark urine, fatigue, anorexia, and nausea (**Table 11-2**). Low-grade fever is common. Right upper quadrant pain or generalized abdominal discomfort may be present. Approximately one half of patients complain of myalgias or arthralgias, especially with hepatitis B. Many of the initial symptoms abate when jaundice develops. Hepatomegaly and splenomegaly may be present. If viral hepatitis is severe, there may be evidence of

acute liver failure including confusion, asterixis, peripheral edema, and ascites.

Laboratory Tests Serum aminotransferase concentrations (aspartate aminotransferase [AST], alanine aminotransferase [ALT]) are sensitive indicators of liver cell injury. AST and ALT concentrations increase 7 to 14 days before the appearance of jaundice and begin to decrease shortly after jaundice develops. The degree of aminotransferase increase does not necessarily parallel the severity of the hepatitis, but concentrations less than 500 IU/L usually reflect mild hepatitis.

Anemia and lymphocytosis are typically present. Serum bilirubin concentration rarely exceeds 20 mg/dL. Alkaline phosphatase is not increased unless cholestasis develops at a later phase of the acute hepatitis. Severe acute hepatitis may impair the synthetic capacity of the liver and result in hypoalbuminemia and/or a prolonged prothrombin time.

Serologic Markers Serologic markers are used to identify each type of viral hepatitis. IgM anti-HAV appears early in the course of the disease and is specific for acute hepatitis A. The antibody persists for approximately 120 days and is then replaced by IgG anti-HAV, which confers lasting immunity to HAV infection.

Hepatitis B surface antigen (HBsAg) is present in the serum as early as 7 to 14 days after infection and may persist for several months. Detection of HBsAg indicates that HBV is actively replicating and that the blood of these individuals is infectious. The antibody to HBsAg usually appears in the blood 60 to 240 days after infection by which time the surface antigen is undetectable. The antibody to HBsAg is a long-lasting antibody and is associated with immunity. The antibody to the core antigen of HBV appears promptly after infection and persists for 6 to 12 months. High titers of IgM antibody to the core antigen of HBV may be the only marker of acute hepatitis B if HBsAg is no longer detectable.

Detection of antibodies to HCV (anti-HCV) is the most reliable way to diagnose acute and chronic hepatitis C. The detection of HCV RNA confirms the presence of viremia.

HDV infection is diagnosed by detecting anti-HDV, HBsAg, and IgM antibody to the core antigen of HBV in serum. The diagnosis of hepatitis E can be made by the finding of anti-HEV antibody.

Liver Biopsy Liver biopsy is not often necessary to confirm the diagnosis of acute hepatitis. Serologic and biochemical measurements are usually sufficient. Spotty necrosis of hepatocytes and widespread parenchymal inflammation are the typical histologic findings of acute viral hepatitis. Fibrosis is absent. There are no reliable histologic findings that separate the five kinds of viral hepatitis from each other.

Clinical Course

Hepatitis typically produces symptoms for 7 to 14 days before the appearance of dark urine and jaundice. As jaundice increases, the appetite begins to return and malaise decreases. Serum bilirubin concentration increases for 10 to 14 days and then decreases during the next 14 to 28 days. Aminotransferase concentrations usually begin to decrease just before peak

TABLE 11-2 Incidence of Signs and Symptoms in Acute Viral Hepatitis	
Symptom/Sign	Incidence (%)
Dark urine	94
Fatigue	91
Anorexia	90
Nausea	87
Fever	76
Emesis	71
Headache	70
Abdominal discomfort	65
Light-colored stools	52
Pruritus	42
Adapted from Keefe EB: Acute hepatitis. Sci Am Med 1999;1–9.	

jaundice occurs and then they decrease rapidly. The clinical course is typically uneventful, and the return to normal liver function is complete.

In a small percentage of patients, especially elderly patients or those with HBV or HCV infection, acute viral hepatitis may run a protracted course with full recovery taking as long as a year. Rarely, acute viral hepatitis results in fulminant liver failure and death. Some patients never recover from the initial acute viral infection and chronic hepatitis develops. Chronic hepatitis does not occur after hepatitis A or E but develops in 2% to 7% of patients infected with HBV and in 60% to 75% of patients infected with HCV. The development of cirrhosis and primary hepatocellular carcinoma are risks of chronic hepatitis B or C, although decades may pass before these adverse effects occur.

Treatment

Treatment of acute viral hepatitis is symptomatic, with restriction of physical activity and sensible nutrition. Significant nausea and vomiting may require intravenous fluids and electrolyte replacement. Abstinence from alcohol during acute viral hepatitis is recommended. Liver transplantation is a consideration if fulminant hepatic failure develops.

Prevention

Prevention of viral hepatitis includes avoidance of exposure to the virus, passive immunization with γ-globulin, and active immunization with a specific vaccine. Pooled γ-globulin administered intramuscularly as soon as possible after known exposure dramatically decreases the incidence of hepatitis A. Administration of γ-globulin more than 14 days after exposure to HAV is not protective. Individuals exposed to HBV by percutaneous or mucous membrane routes should receive hepatitis B immunoglobulin and hepatitis B vaccine within 24 hours.

Hepatitis A Vaccine An inactivated hepatitis A vaccine is highly effective in eliciting an antibody response. Compared with short-term protection afforded by immunoglobulin, inactivated HAV vaccine provides protection for 10 years or longer. Travelers to endemic regions, neonatal intensive care unit staff, food handlers, children in day care centers, and military personnel represent high-risk groups for hepatitis A and should receive this vaccine.

Hepatitis B Vaccine Hepatitis B vaccine is highly effective in producing antibodies to HBV and preventing HBV infection in infants, children, and adults. The vaccine is recommended for individuals at increased risk of HBV infection, including health care workers with frequent exposure to blood products, homosexual men, intravenous drug users, recipients of certain blood products, and infants born to HBsAg-positive mothers. After successful vaccination, titers of antibody to HBsAg decline. In 5 years, 20% to 30% of people lack protective antibody levels. These persons respond promptly to a booster dose of vaccine.

Additional Viruses That Cause Hepatitis

In addition to the classic hepatitis viruses, acute hepatitis may be due to viruses that cause systemic illness and also affect the liver.

Cytomegalovirus

Cytomegalovirus is a herpesvirus that is ubiquitous. Approximately 80% of adults have serum complement-fixation reactivity for cytomegalovirus. This virus can produce a disease similar to infectious mononucleosis but without adenopathy or tonsillopharyngeal involvement. Liver dysfunction caused by cytomegalovirus may mimic common forms of viral hepatitis but is usually mild and does not progress to chronic liver disease. Diagnosis requires demonstration of the virus following inoculation of an appropriate tissue culture.

Epstein-Barr Virus

Epstein-Barr virus usually produces mild hepatitis associated with nausea and vomiting. Jaundice occurs in 10% to 20% of patients. Serum aminotransferase concentrations are moderately increased. In most instances, the hepatitis is part of the typical clinical syndrome of infectious mononucleosis. In rare instances, hepatic dysfunction is severe and may be fatal, especially in immunosuppressed patients. Epstein-Barr virus appears to be transmitted during oral-oral contact through infected saliva but may also be transmitted parenterally. The incubation period is approximately 28 days. An increase in the titer of specific antibodies to Epstein-Barr virus confirms the diagnosis.

Drug-Induced Hepatitis

Many drugs (analgesics, volatile anesthetics, antibiotics, antihypertensives, anticonvulsants, tranquilizers) can cause hepatitis indistinguishable histologically from acute viral hepatitis. Most of these drug reactions are idiosyncratic, that is, they are rare, unpredictable, and not dose dependent. Clinical signs of liver dysfunction usually occur 2 to 6 weeks after initiation of the drug therapy but can occur immediately or up to 6 months later. Failure to discontinue the offending drug may result in progressive hepatitis and death. In some patients, the disease progresses despite withdrawal of the drug.

Acetaminophen Overdose

Acetaminophen overdose produces profound hepatocellular necrosis in most persons (see discussion of acetaminophen poisoning in Chapter 22). Cell injury occurs because the liver produces toxic metabolites that are usually rendered harmless by conjugation with glutathione. When the acetaminophen dose is high, hepatic glutathione stores are depleted and toxic metabolites accumulate and destroy liver cells. Oral *N*-acetylcysteine given within 8 hours of an acetaminophen overdose can dramatically decrease the risk of hepatotoxicity. Acetaminophen can also cause hepatotoxicity in normal clinical doses if hepatic glutathione levels are decreased as a result of long-term alcohol use or fasting.

Volatile Anesthetics

Volatile anesthetics may produce mild, self-limiting postoperative liver dysfunction that likely reflects anesthetic-induced alterations in hepatic oxygen supply relative to demand. Any anesthetic that decreases hepatic blood flow could interfere with adequate hepatocyte oxygenation. Indeed, α glutathione-S-transferase concentration (a sensitive marker of hepatocellular damage) increases transiently after administration of isoflurane, desflurane, and sevoflurane.

Immune-Mediated Hepatotoxicity

A rare but life-threatening form of hepatic dysfunction following administration of volatile anesthetics (most often halothane) likely reflects an immune-mediated hepatotoxicity in genetically susceptible individuals. The most compelling evidence of an immune-mediated mechanism is the presence of circulating IgG antibodies in the majority of patients with the diagnosis of halothane hepatitis. These antibodies are directed against microsomal proteins on the surface of hepatocytes that have been covalently modified by the reactive oxidative trifluoroacetyl halide metabolite of halothane to form neoantigens. This acetylation of liver proteins, in effect, changes these proteins from self to nonself (neoantigens), resulting in the formation of antibodies against this new protein and a form of autoimmune hepatitis. To detect the IgG anti–trifluoroacetyl antibodies, synthetic trifluoroacetylated rabbit serum albumin is used as the antigen in the enzyme-linked immunosorbent assay. The anti-trifluoroacetyl antibody testing procedure is highly specific since these antibodies do not appear in any other form of liver disease or in the presence of drugs other than certain volatile anesthetics. It is presumed that the subsequent antigen-antibody interactions are responsible for the rare (estimated incidence 1:10,000–1:30,000 in adult patients receiving halothane) liver injury characterized as halothane hepatitis.

Like halothane, the fluorinated volatile anesthetics enflurane, isoflurane, and desflurane may form trifluoroacetyl metabolites resulting in cross-sensitivity with halothane. The incidence of hepatitis after these anesthetics, however, is very much lower than after halothane because the degree of anesthetic metabolism is substantially less. It is possible that genetically susceptible patients could become sensitized to one volatile anesthetic (most likely halothane) and experience drug-induced hepatitis later in life when exposed to isoflurane or desflurane. Indeed, suspected isoflurane hepatitis with associated anti-trifluoroacetyl IgG antibodies has been described in a patient with a history of halothane hepatitis.

The chemical structure of sevoflurane is such that it does not undergo metabolism to trifluoroacetylated metabolites. Therefore, unlike the other fluorinated volatile anesthetics, sevoflurane would not be expected to produce immune-mediated hepatotoxicity or to cause cross-sensitivity in patients previously exposed to halothane.

Differential Diagnosis of Postoperative Hepatic Dysfunction

When postoperative hepatic dysfunction (jaundice) occurs, an analysis of historical data, clinical signs and symptoms, serial liver function tests, and a search for extrahepatic causes of hepatic dysfunction facilitate development of a differential diagnosis. The causes of hepatic dysfunction can be categorized as prehepatic, intrahepatic (hepatocellular), or posthepatic (cholestatic) based on measurement of serum bilirubin, aminotransferases, and alkaline phosphatase (**Table 11-3**). Postoperative hepatic dysfunction is often multifactorial. The following steps may be helpful in determining the etiology of postoperative hepatic dysfunction. It is important to do a systematic review of the situation rather than to assume that the history of an anesthetic establishes a cause-and-effect relationship between hepatic dysfunction and the volatile anesthetic.

TABLE 11-3 Causes of Hepatic Dysfunction Based on Liver Function Tests

Hepatic Dysfunction	Bilirubin	Aminotransferase Enzymes	Alkaline Phosphatase	Causes
Prehepatic	Increased unconjugated fraction	Normal	Normal	Hemolysis Hematoma resorption Bilirubin overload from blood transfusion
Intrahepatic (hepatocellular)	Increased conjugated fraction	Markedly increased	Normal to slightly increased	Viral Drugs Sepsis Hypoxemia Cirrhosis
Posthepatic (cholestatic)	Increased conjugated fraction	Normal to slightly increased	Markedly increased	Biliary tract stones Sepsis

1. Review all drugs administered (analgesics, antibiotics, over-the-counter preparations) because many drugs have the potential for liver injury. Administration of catecholamines or vasoconstrictors can cause sufficient splanchnic vasoconstriction to interfere with adequate hepatic blood flow and hepatocyte oxygenation.

2. Check for sources of sepsis. The development of jaundice is common in patients with severe infection.

3. Evaluate the possibility of an increased exogenous bilirubin load. Transfusion of one unit of blood contains approximately 250 mg of bilirubin. The bilirubin load of a unit of blood increases as the age of the transfused blood increases. Patients with normal hepatic function can be given large amounts of blood without an appreciable increase in bilirubin concentration but this response may be different in patients with co-existing liver disease.

4. Rule out occult hematomas. Resorption of large hematomas may produce hyperbilirubinemia for several days. Furthermore, patients with Gilbert syndrome have limited ability to conjugate bilirubin and even a small increase in the bilirubin load may lead to jaundice (see "Gilbert Syndrome").

5. Rule out hemolysis. A decrease in hematocrit or increase in reticulocyte count may indicate hemolysis.

6. Review perioperative records. Evidence of hypotension, arterial hypoxemia, hypoventilation, and hypovolemia can be etiologic factors for postoperative hepatic dysfunction.

7. Consider extrahepatic abnormalities (congestive heart failure, respiratory failure, pulmonary embolism, renal insufficiency) as possible causes of postoperative hepatic dysfunction.

8. Consider the possibility of benign postoperative intrahepatic cholestasis, an entity associated with extensive surgery, hypotension, hypoxemia, and massive blood transfusion (see "Benign Postoperative Intrahepatic Cholestasis").

9. Consider the possibility of immune-mediated hepatotoxicity. This is a diagnosis of exclusion based on the clinical history of a recent anesthetic that included a volatile anesthetic. It may be possible to confirm the diagnosis by documenting the presence of circulating anti-trifluoroacetyl antibodies.

CHRONIC HEPATITIS

Chronic hepatitis encompasses a diverse group of diseases characterized by long-term elevation of liver chemistries and evidence of inflammation on liver biopsy. Chronic hepatitis is generally defined as disease that has lasted 6 months or longer. The most common diseases that cause chronic hepatitis are autoimmune hepatitis and chronic viral hepatitis (HBV with or without HDV co-infection, infection with HCV). Chronic hepatitis may also be caused by drugs, Wilson's disease, α_1-antitrypsin (α_1AT) deficiency,

or the early stages of primary biliary cirrhosis and primary sclerosing cholangitis.

Signs and Symptoms

The signs and symptoms of chronic hepatitis vary and range from asymptomatic disease characterized by a mildly increased serum aminotransferase concentration to rapidly progressive illness with fulminant hepatic failure. The most common symptoms of chronic hepatitis are fatigue, malaise, and abdominal pain. Extrahepatic manifestations of chronic hepatitis are common and include arthralgias, arthritis, glomerulonephritis, skin rashes, amenorrhea, and thyroiditis.

Laboratory Tests

The ALT and AST concentrations are characteristically increased in patients with chronic hepatitis, and serum bilirubin concentrations are typically normal in patients with chronic viral hepatitis but increased in patients with autoimmune hepatitis. A characteristic feature of autoimmune hepatitis, but not of chronic viral hepatitis, is an increased serum γ-globulin concentration. With the most severe forms of chronic hepatitis, hepatic synthetic function is impaired, as reflected by a decreased serum albumin concentration and a prolonged prothrombin time. Imaging studies of the abdomen reveal variable degrees of hepatomegaly with or without splenomegaly. The specific etiology of chronic hepatitis can usually be determined by clinical evaluation combined with immunologic and serologic testing, but liver biopsy can help confirm the presence of certain diseases such as Wilson's disease or α_1AT deficiency.

Autoimmune Hepatitis

Autoimmune hepatitis is characterized by a wide spectrum of clinical symptoms and immunoserologic manifestations. Hypergammaglobulinemia, increased serum aminotransferase concentrations, and antinuclear antibodies are characteristic. Other autoimmune diseases may be present concurrently. Treatment with corticosteroids prolongs survival. However, treatment with corticosteroids for longer than 18 months is associated with diabetes mellitus, hypertension, psychosis, infection, and osteoporosis in many patients. To prevent these side effects of corticosteroid therapy, autoimmune hepatitis is often treated with corticosteroids plus azathioprine. This therapy is usually continued indefinitely. The distinction between autoimmune hepatitis and chronic hepatitis C may be difficult but is important because autoimmune hepatitis responds to immunosuppressive drugs but can be exacerbated by treatment with interferon.

Chronic Hepatitis B

Chronic HBV infection is present in 5% of the world's population and an estimated 0.5% of the U.S. population are carriers of HBsAg. In patients with chronic HBV infection, HBsAg remains detectable for more than 6 months. Persons who continue to test positive for HBsAg but who are asymptomatic and have normal serum aminotransferase concentrations are termed HBsAg carriers. Other chronically infected HBsAg-positive individuals who have clinical or laboratory evidence of chronic hepatic disease are diagnosed with chronic hepatitis B.

Age at the time of the initial HBV infection is a major determinant of chronicity; 90% of infected neonates become carriers. Another important risk factor for the development of chronic hepatitis B is the presence of intrinsic or iatrogenic immunosuppression. Women are more likely than men to clear HBsAg, and, as a result, men are more likely to be HBsAg carriers. Persistent HBV infection is an important risk factor for development of hepatocellular carcinoma.

The goal of treatment of chronic hepatitis B is to eradicate HBV infection and prevent the development of cirrhosis or hepatocellular cancer. Currently available therapies can suppress HBV replication and lead to improvement in the clinical, biochemical, and histologic features of chronic hepatitis B. Therapy with lamivudine and/or adefovir, nucleotide analogues, may dramatically suppress HBV replication. Liver transplantation can be performed for liver failure associated with chronic hepatitis B, but HBV will infect the allograft in nearly all recipients. Posttransplantation prophylaxis with lamivudine and hepatitis B immunoglobulin reduces the reinfection rate to approximately 10%.

Chronic Hepatitis C

Chronic HCV infection follows acute HCV infection in up to 75% of patients, and an estimated 1.8% of the U.S. population are carriers of HCV. Therefore, chronic HCV infection is more prevalent than chronic HBV infection.

The diagnosis of chronic hepatitis C is based on persistently or intermittently increased serum aminotransferase concentrations in association with the presence of anti-HCV antibody. The natural history of chronic hepatitis C may span several decades, progressing insidiously with the ultimate development of cirrhosis or hepatocellular cancer after 10 to 20 years. Factors associated with a more rapid rate of progression to cirrhosis include age older than 40 years at the time of initial infection, significant daily alcohol consumption, male gender, and co-infection with other hepatic viruses or human immunodeficiency virus.

Interferon reduces or normalizes serum ALT concentration and decreases inflammation as indicated by liver biopsy in approximately 40% of patients with chronic hepatitis C, but a sustained response to interferon therapy is uncommon. However, the combination of interferon with the antiviral drug ribavirin significantly increases the percentage of patients who have a sustained virologic response. Chronic hepatitis C with liver failure is one of the most common indications for liver transplantation. Although HCV reinfects the allograft, the subsequent illness is usually mild and rarely progresses to liver failure.

Less Common Causes of Chronic Hepatitis

Several liver diseases must be distinguished from autoimmune and chronic viral hepatitis as causes of chronic hepatitis.

In most instances, these diseases can be identified on the basis of clinical, biochemical, and histologic evidence.

Drug-induced chronic hepatitis is seen in a small group of patients. Methyldopa, trazodone, and isoniazid are recognized causes of drug-induced chronic hepatitis. In addition, some patients treated with sulfonamides, acetaminophen, aspirin, and phenytoin may develop drug-induced chronic hepatitis. Treatment consists of discontinuation of the suspected drug as soon as the chronic hepatitis is diagnosed or suspected. If the chronic hepatitis is due to the drug, liver function abnormalities and the clinical course usually improve after drug discontinuation.

In the absence of associated neurologic symptoms, Wilson's disease mimics chronic hepatitis. The diagnosis is confirmed by liver biopsy and determination of hepatic copper content. Treatment is with penicillamine.

α_1-AT deficiency is associated with a liver disease that can progress to cirrhosis. Liver disease due to α_1-AT deficiency can be differentiated from chronic hepatitis by decreased α_1-globulin on protein electrophoresis or by specific serum assays for α_1-AT.

Primary biliary cirrhosis may be indistinguishable from chronic viral hepatitis on liver biopsy. Characteristic hyperpigmentation, pruritus, and extreme increases in serum alkaline phosphatase concentration are helpful in the differential diagnosis.

Primary sclerosing cholangitis can mimic chronic viral hepatitis. A marked increase in serum alkaline phosphatase concentration and accompanying inflammatory bowel disease distinguish this illness from chronic viral hepatitis.

CIRRHOSIS

Cirrhosis can result from a large variety of chronic, progressive liver diseases. Most often cirrhosis is the result of excessive chronic alcohol ingestion or chronic viral hepatitis due to HBV or HCV infection. Scarring of the liver results in disruption of normal liver architecture, and regenerating parenchymal nodules are typically seen. The pattern of scarring seldom permits determination of a specific etiology, but other histologic features may provide clues as to the cause of the cirrhosis.

Diagnosis

Percutaneous liver biopsy establishes the diagnosis of cirrhosis. Computed tomography, magnetic resonance imaging, and hepatic ultrasonography with Doppler flow studies may reveal findings consistent with cirrhosis (splenomegaly, ascites, irregular liver surface). Upper gastrointestinal endoscopy can establish the presence of esophagogastric varices.

Signs and Symptoms

Fatigue and malaise are common with all forms of cirrhosis as well as with almost all forms of acute and chronic liver disease. Characteristic but nondiagnostic physical findings of cirrhosis include palmar erythema, spider angiomata, gynecomastia, testicular atrophy, and evidence of portal hypertension (splenomegaly, ascites). Decreased hepatic blood flow resulting from increased intrahepatic resistance to flow through the portal vein (portal hypertension) reflects the fibrotic process associated with cirrhosis. Portal hypertension results in a decrease in the proportion of hepatic blood flow delivered from the portal vein and an increase in the proportion of hepatic blood flow from the hepatic artery. The cirrhotic liver is often enlarged and is typically palpable below the costal margin. A decreased serum albumin concentration and a prolonged prothrombin time are characteristic of cirrhosis. An increase in serum aminotransferase and alkaline phosphatase concentration is common.

Specific Forms of Cirrhosis

Specific forms of cirrhosis include alcoholic cirrhosis, postnecrotic cirrhosis, primary biliary cirrhosis, hemochromatosis, Wilson's disease, α_1-AT deficiency, and nonalcoholic steatohepatitis.

Alcoholic Cirrhosis

Alcoholic cirrhosis is directly attributable to chronic ingestion of large quantities of alcohol. Women may develop cirrhosis after consumption of lesser amounts of alcohol than men. Daily alcohol consumption of approximately three to four drinks per day for 10 to 15 years is associated with alcoholic liver disease in women, whereas consumption of five to six drinks per day for this time period is required for alcoholic cirrhosis to develop in men. The development of alcoholic cirrhosis does not require concomitant malnutrition, although this condition is frequently present (substitution of alcohol for normal dietary calories).

The diagnosis of alcohol abuse can be difficult because many patients conceal information about alcohol use. However, the diagnosis of alcoholic hepatitis is supported by an AST/ALT ratio of at least 2:1, reflecting increased synthesis as well as secretion of mitochondrial AST into plasma and selective loss of ALT activity because of the pyridoxine deficiency that is common in alcoholism. Alkaline phosphatase concentration is often mildly increased. A decreased serum albumin concentration (<3.5 g/dL) and a prolonged prothrombin time are common.

The only effective therapy for patients with alcoholic liver disease is cessation of alcohol ingestion. Vigorous nutritional support may improve survival.

Postnecrotic Cirrhosis

Postnecrotic cirrhosis is characterized by a shrunken liver containing regenerating nodules. The most common causes of this condition are chronic viral hepatitis, autoimmune hepatitis, and cryptogenic (cause unknown) hepatitis. The distinguishing clinical features of postnecrotic cirrhosis include its predominance in women and an increase in serum γ-globulin concentration. Postnecrotic cirrhosis may progress insidiously. The usual cause of death is gastrointestinal hemorrhage or hepatic failure. Primary liver cell cancer develops in 10% to

15% of patients who have postnecrotic cirrhosis. Treatment is supportive and related to symptom control. Corticosteroids may be useful if the cirrhosis is associated with autoimmune hepatitis.

Primary Biliary Cirrhosis

Primary biliary cirrhosis occurs most often in women 30 to 50 years of age and the presence of antimitochondrial antibodies suggests an immune mechanism in the pathogenesis of this disorder. In addition, primary biliary cirrhosis is commonly associated with autoimmune diseases such as rheumatoid arthritis, CREST syndrome, thyroiditis, pernicious anemia, Sjögren's syndrome, and renal tubular acidosis. There is progressive destruction of intrahepatic bile ducts.

Presenting complaints are fatigue and generalized pruritus. Jaundice may not develop for years after the onset of pruritus. Symptoms and signs resulting from malabsorption of fat-soluble vitamins may be present. Osteoporosis is common and may be associated with bone pain and spontaneous fractures. Alkaline phosphatase concentrations are increased, as are serum cholesterol and IgM concentrations.

Treatment includes administration of a hydrophilic bile acid, ursodeoxycholic acid, which is presumed to decrease the concentration of toxic bile acids in the hepatic pool. Corticosteroids do not alter the course of primary biliary cirrhosis. Cholestyramine may alleviate the pruritus. Fat-soluble vitamin supplements and bisphosphonates are often required.

Hemochromatosis

Hereditary hemochromatosis is an autosomal recessive disorder associated with iron deposition in various body tissues. The iron accumulation is progressive from birth but rarely causes symptoms before age 40. The disease is delayed further in women because of the loss of iron in menses and a lower dietary intake of iron. The disease occurs 10 times more often in men. Iron deposits in the pancreas and heart muscle are associated with development of diabetes mellitus and congestive heart failure. There is bronze discoloration of the skin. Hepatomegaly is found in 75% of patients even if they are asymptomatic. Signs of portal hypertension eventually develop in most patients. Primary hepatocellular cancer occurs in 15% to 20% of patients with hemochromatosis.

Laboratory evaluation reveals an increase in serum iron and ferritin concentration and an increase in transferrin saturation. Computed tomography and magnetic resonance imaging may demonstrate signs of iron overload. The diagnosis of hemochromatosis is confirmed by a liver biopsy specimen, which shows hemosiderin granules in hepatocytes and bile duct cells. Mild increases in serum alkaline phosphatase and aminotransferase concentration are common but jaundice is unusual.

Treatment of hemochromatosis consists of removal of excess iron by phlebotomy. If patients are identified before cirrhosis develops and total body iron depletion is accomplished, life expectancy approaches normal. Treated patients with cirrhosis are at increased risk of development of primary hepatocellular carcinoma even after total body iron stores are normalized. Hepatocellular cancer is the leading cause of death in patients with hemochromatosis. Normalization of total body iron stores is associated with a decrease in the signs of liver and cardiac disease, but endocrine abnormalities and arthropathy persist.

Wilson's Disease

Wilson's disease (hepatolenticular degeneration) is an autosomal recessive disorder due to a defect in the gene that codes for copper binding. The subsequent excretion of copper into bile is defective, leading to total body copper accumulation. Neurologic dysfunction (tremors, gait disturbances, slurring of speech) and hepatic dysfunction (fatigue, jaundice, ascites, splenomegaly, gastroesophageal varices) develop. Associated hemolytic anemia is another clue to the diagnosis as is the Kayser-Fleischer ring, a thin brown crescent of pigmentation at the periphery of the cornea. Laboratory findings include a decreased serum ceruloplasmin concentration and increased urinary copper excretion.

Treatment of Wilson's disease entails copper chelation with trientine or penicillamine. These drugs bind copper and promote urinary copper excretion. Penicillamine may be associated with nausea, vomiting, leukopenia, and thrombocytopenia that can progress to aplastic anemia. Pyridoxine is administered weekly to offset the pyridoxine antagonist effects of penicillamine. Copper chelation improves survival but does not reverse the cirrhosis.

α_1-Antitrypsin Deficiency

Homozygous α_1AT deficiency is associated with a rare syndrome of progressive cirrhosis. Adult patients usually have accompanying pulmonary emphysema. The liver disease is not due to α_1AT deficiency but rather to accumulation of abnormal α_1AT in the liver. The presence of hepatomegaly, mild derangements on liver function tests, and the absence of α_1AT on protein electrophoresis makes the diagnosis likely. The only treatment for cirrhosis due to α_1AT deficiency is liver transplantation. After transplantation, the α_1AT in the serum assumes the phenotype of the liver donor.

Nonalcoholic Steatohepatitis

Nonalcoholic steatohepatitis (fatty liver) is fat accumulation in the liver leading to cirrhosis. It is more common in women and is associated with obesity, hyperlipidemia, and diabetes mellitus. Hepatomegaly may be marked, but evidence of hepatic dysfunction is mild. The mechanism of hepatic damage is not known, although the onset of the disorder often follows poor control of diabetes mellitus or rapid weight loss. Disease progression is gradual, and therapies include *gradual* weight loss, exercise, better control of diabetes mellitus, and treatment of hyperlipidemia.

Complications of Cirrhosis

Hepatic and extrahepatic complications of hepatic cirrhosis develop predictably in patients afflicted with progressive

TABLE 11-4 Complications of Cirrhosis
Portal hypertension
Esophagogastric varices
Ascites
Hyperdynamic circulation
Cardiomyopathy
Anemia
Coagulopathy
Arterial hypoxemia
Hepatorenal syndrome
Hypoglycemia
Duodenal ulcer
Gallstones
Spontaneous bacterial peritonitis
Hepatic encephalopathy
Primary hepatocellular carcinoma

liver scarring (**Table 11-4**). Alcoholic cirrhosis is the prototype of these complications. Acute hepatic failure is characterized by an increased expression of these complications.

Portal Hypertension

Portal hypertension usually develops several years after the first attack of alcoholic hepatitis. The resulting increase in resistance to blood flow through the portal venous system, combined with hypoalbuminemia and increased secretion of antidiuretic hormone, contributes to the development of ascites. Physical examination will demonstrate hepatomegaly with or without ascites.

Gastroesophageal Varices

Gastroesophageal varices are dilated submucosal veins that permit passage of splanchnic venous blood from the high-pressure portal venous system to the low-pressure azygos and hemiazygous veins. Not all patients with cirrhosis develop esophageal varices and not all patients with varices bleed from them. When bleeding does occur, variceal hemorrhage is usually from the distal esophagus or proximal stomach and is often hemodynamically significant. Bleeding esophageal varices are most reliably identified by upper gastrointestinal endoscopy.

Endoscopic therapy with variceal banding, ligation, or sclerotherapy (injection of a sclerosing substance into the varices) is the treatment for immediate control of esophageal variceal bleeding. Banding or sclerotherapy is also effective for long-term control of recurrent esophageal variceal hemorrhage. Tracheal intubation may be performed to prevent pulmonary aspiration of blood and to facilitate endoscopic evaluation of the bleeding site. Complications of sclerotherapy include esophageal ulceration, pleural effusion, and esophageal stricture or perforation. Respiratory distress may occur 24 to 48 hours after sclerotherapy. Bleeding from gastric varices is less common than bleeding from esophageal varices but

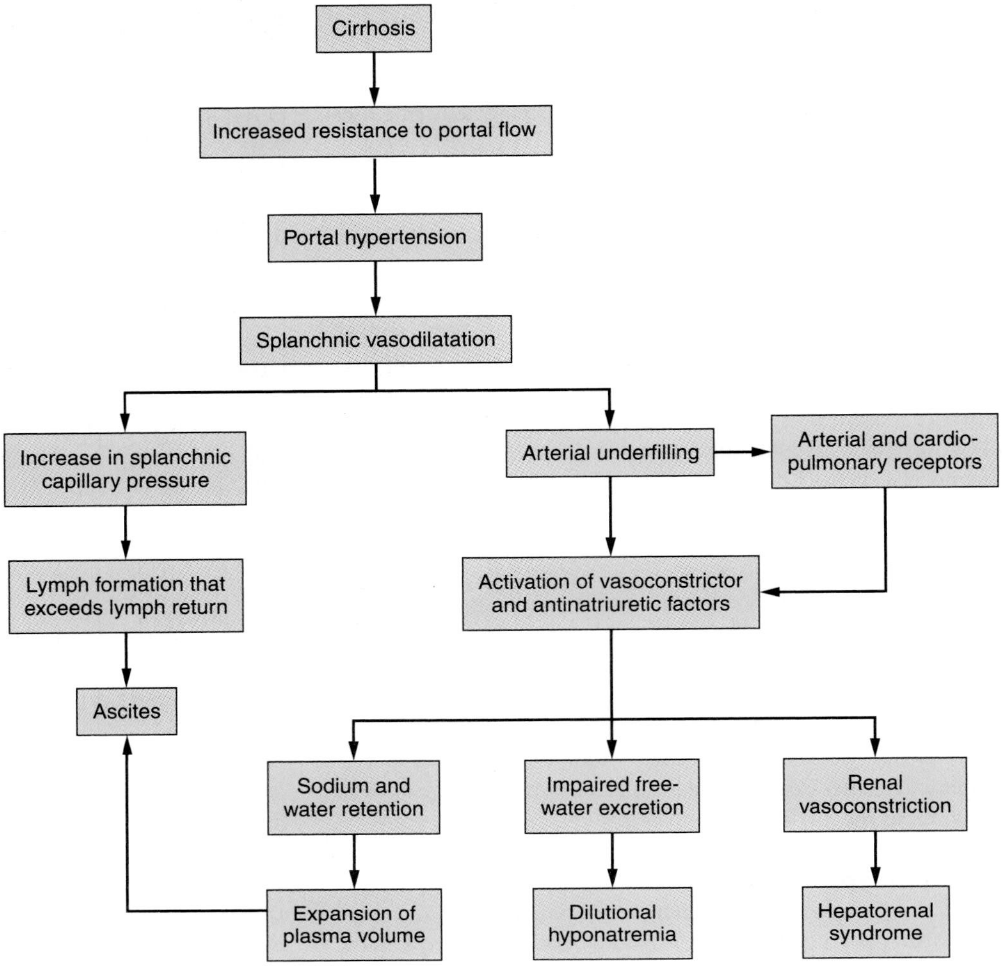

Figure 11-1 • Pathogenesis of ascites. Vasoconstrictor and antinatriuretic factors include norepinephrine, angiotensin II, aldosterone, and antidiuretic hormone. *(Reproduced with permission from Gines P, Cardenas A, Arroyo V, Rades J: Management of cirrhosis and ascites. N Engl J Med 2004;350:1646–1654. Copyright 2004 Massachusetts Medical Society. All rights reserved.)*

is more difficult to treat. Bleeding from varices accounts for one third of all deaths due to cirrhosis.

If variceal bleeding persists or recurs and is life-threatening, transjugular intrahepatic portosystemic shunting has supplanted balloon tamponade (via Blakemore-Sengstaken tube) and emergent surgical portal decompression. Transjugular intrahepatic portosystemic shunting consists of an angiographically inserted shunt between a hepatic vein and a portal vein to decompress the portal circulation. It can control variceal bleeding by dramatically decreasing the pressure gradient between the portal vein and the inferior vena cava. Hepatic encephalopathy develops in some patients following this procedure.

Recurrent or continued bleeding from esophageal varices may indicate the need for a portosystemic shunt. This operation has a very high mortality rate when performed emergently, and mortality and morbidity are still substantial when this operation is performed electively. Portosystemic shunts may not prolong survival, but they do prevent variceal bleeding.

Propranolol produces a sustained decrease in portal venous pressure in patients with cirrhosis. Propranolol can reduce the risk of a first variceal hemorrhage as well as the risk of rebleeding.

Ascites

Ascites is a common sequela of many forms of cirrhosis. Factors that contribute to the formation of ascites include portal hypertension, hypoalbuminemia, and sodium and water retention (**Fig. 11-1**). Any patient presenting with new ascites should undergo evaluation of hepatic, cardiac, and renal function as well as analysis of the ascitic fluid (**Table 11-5**).

Drug-induced diuresis with an aldosterone antagonist such as spironolactone is an effective treatment for removing ascitic fluid. Maximum diuresis of ascitic fluid should not exceed 1 L daily. More rapid diuresis can lead to hypovolemia and azotemia. Spironolactone decreases renal excretion of potassium, and this can be problematic in patients with renal insufficiency. Long-term treatment with spironolactone often produces gynecomastia.

Ascites that does not respond to diuretic therapy may be treated by insertion of a LeVeen shunt that routes ascitic fluid subcutaneously from the peritoneal cavity to the internal jugular vein through a one-way valve. Complications of shunt placement include low-grade disseminated intravascular coagulation and infection. These complications limit the use of this shunt. Large-volume paracentesis (4–6 L/day) is an alternative

TABLE 11-5 Evaluation of Patients with Cirrhosis and Ascites

Evaluation of Liver Disease
Liver function and coagulation tests
Standard hematologic tests
Abdominal ultrasonography and computed tomography
Endoscopy of the upper gastrointestinal tract (assessment of varices)
Liver biopsy in selected patients

Evaluation of Renal and Circulatory Function
Measurement of serum creatinine and electrolytes
Measurement of urinary sodium
Measurement of urinary protein
Arterial blood pressure

Evaluation of Ascitic Fluid
Cell count
Bacterial culture
Measurement of total protein
Other tests (measurement of albumin, glucose, lactate dehydrogenase, amylase, triglycerides; acid-fast smear; cytologic examination)

From Gines P, Cardenas A, Arroyo V, Rades J: Management of cirrhosis and ascites. N Engl J Med 2004; 350:1646–1654.

to diuretic therapy in some patients. Placing a transjugular intrahepatic portosystemic shunt is more effective than medical therapy or paracentesis in controlling ascites.

Spontaneous Bacterial Peritonitis

Spontaneous bacterial peritonitis, which consists of fever, leukocytosis, abdominal pain, and decreased bowel sounds, may develop in patients with advanced cirrhosis. Ascitic fluid should be analyzed whenever the clinical condition of a patient with ascites deteriorates suddenly. The ascitic fluid with spontaneous bacterial peritonitis is often turbid because of leukocytosis and bacterial growth. The pathogenesis of spontaneous bacterial peritonitis may relate to an increase in gut wall permeability, a large volume of peritoneal fluid conducive to bacterial growth, or impaired capacity of hepatic or splenic macrophages to clear portal bacteremia. Despite antibiotic therapy, the mortality associated with spontaneous bacterial peritonitis is substantial. Two-year survival after spontaneous bacterial peritonitis is less than 50%.

Hepatorenal Syndrome

Hepatorenal syndrome is functional renal failure associated with severe liver disease without an intrinsic abnormality of the kidneys. The prognosis is very poor. More than 95% of patients die within a few weeks of the development of azotemia. Typically, these patients have ascites. The pathogenesis of hepatorenal syndrome is uncertain, but decreased renal blood flow and glomerular filtration rate due to dehydration or variceal hemorrhage often precede the onset of this syndrome. Recovery of renal function is rare.

Malnutrition

Almost all patients with cirrhosis have protein-calorie malnutrition, which leads to salt and water retention, defective immune responses, and delayed recovery of liver function. In

some critically ill patients, nutrition must be provided parenterally. Megaloblastic anemia is common and due to folate antagonism by alcohol or dietary folate deficiency.

Hyperdynamic Circulation

Cirrhosis is often associated with a hyperdynamic circulation with an increased cardiac output due to peripheral and splanchnic vasodilation, increased intravascular fluid volume, decreased blood viscosity as a result of anemia, and arteriovenous communications, especially in the lungs. Occasionally, cardiomyopathy and congestive heart failure occur in a patient with alcoholic cirrhosis.

Arterial Hypoxemia

Pa_{O_2} values of 60 to 70 mm Hg are common in patients with cirrhosis. Possible explanations for this low Pa_{O_2} include impaired movement of the diaphragm due to accumulation of ascitic fluid, right-to-left intrapulmonary shunting as a result of portal hypertension, cigarette smoking, and chronic obstructive pulmonary disease. Arterial hypoxemia may also be due to pneumonia, a frequent occurrence in alcoholic patients. Vulnerability to pneumonia may reflect the ability of alcohol to inhibit phagocytic activity in the lungs. As a result, bacteria inhaled into the respiratory tract can more easily produce pneumonia. Also, regurgitation of gastric contents is more likely because of an alcohol-induced decrease in lower esophageal sphincter tone. Indeed, most lung abscesses are found in chronic alcoholic patients.

Hypoglycemia

Hypoglycemia is a constant threat in patients with hepatic cirrhosis, especially in those abusing alcohol. Hypoglycemia reflects glycogen depletion due to malnutrition plus alcohol-induced interference with gluconeogenesis. The liver is responsible for clearing lactic acid from the systemic circulation and then converting lactate to glucose. Severe cirrhosis may impair this function, contributing not only to hypoglycemia but to the development of metabolic acidosis as well.

Impaired Immune Defenses

Alcohol ingestion suppresses immune defense mechanisms rendering alcoholic patients vulnerable to bacterial and viral infection, tuberculosis, and cancer. The patient using alcohol to excess, either episodically or on a regular basis, should be viewed as immunocompromised.

Hepatic Encephalopathy

Hepatic encephalopathy is a neuropsychiatric disorder caused by hepatic insufficiency. There may be changes in cognition, personality, motor function, or consciousness. Mental obtundation and asterixis (a flapping tremor of the hands at the wrists) may be present. Slowing or flattening of brain waves on the electroencephalogram verifies encephalopathy. The cause of hepatic encephalopathy may be multifactorial, but, in most instances, a precipitating event such as gastrointestinal hemorrhage, an electrolyte abnormality, an acid-base disorder, arterial hypoxemia, sepsis, administration of diuretics, sedatives or opiates, excessive dietary protein intake, or creation of a portosystemic shunt can be identified.

Treatment of hepatic encephalopathy requires identification and removal of any precipitating factors. Standard therapy includes dietary protein restriction to decrease production of endogenous neuroactive toxins such as ammonia. Nonabsorbable disaccharides such as lactulose and nonabsorbable antibiotics such as neomycin are effective in decreasing ammonia production and/or absorption from the gastrointestinal tract.

Liver transplantation has improved the prognosis for many forms of end-stage liver disease. Contraindications to liver transplantation include acquired immunodeficiency syndrome, extrahepatic malignancy, sepsis, advanced cardiopulmonary disease, and active alcohol or substance abuse.

Management of Anesthesia

It is estimated that 5% to 10% of patients with cirrhosis require surgery in the last 2 years of life. Many trauma beds are occupied by patients who were injured while under the influence of alcohol. In those patients who abuse alcohol, the presence of ascites, sepsis, and chronic obstructive pulmonary disease preoperatively is associated with increased postoperative morbidity and mortality. Postoperative morbidity includes pneumonia, bleeding, sepsis, poor wound healing, and deterioration in liver function. The pathogenic mechanisms of these complications often includes subclinical cardiorespiratory insufficiency and immune incompetence. The complications of alcohol withdrawal can also affect perioperative morbidity.

Preoperative Preparation

Certain preoperative criteria correlate with surgical risk and postoperative outcome in patients with cirrhosis undergoing major surgery (**Table 11-6**). Identifying co-existing problems that can be optimized preoperatively (cardiorespiratory function, coagulation status, renal function, intravascular fluid volume, electrolyte balance, nutrition) may decrease morbidity and mortality associated with elective surgery in patients with severe liver disease. Coagulation status should be evaluated and parenteral vitamin K administered if the prothrombin time is prolonged. Failure of parenteral vitamin K to improve synthesis of prothrombin suggests the presence of severe hepatocellular disease. Impaired prothrombin production due to biliary obstruction and the absence of bile salts that facilitate gastrointestinal absorption of vitamin K is promptly reversed by parenteral vitamin K therapy. Thrombocytopenia, which often accompanies severe liver disease, may require treatment. Hypoglycemia may be present, and administration of a glucose solution is a consideration perioperatively. There should be proper hydration and urine output prior to surgery. Hepatic blood flow is predictably decreased in patients with cirrhosis, and any further decrease due to anesthetic-induced depression of cardiac output or blood pressure could jeopardize hepatocyte oxygenation.

Chronic alcohol ingestion has been demonstrated to increase anesthetic requirements (MAC) for isoflurane most likely due to cross-tolerance. Accelerated metabolism of drugs in the presence of alcohol-induced microsomal enzyme induction can also alter the amount of anesthetic drug needed to achieve a certain anesthesia depth. Decreased protein binding of drugs in the presence of hypoalbuminemia could increase

TABLE 11-6	Prediction of Perioperative Risk in the Patient with Liver Disease		
Parameter	Low Risk	Moderate Risk	High Risk
Bilirubin (mg/dL)	<2	2–3	>3
Albumin (g/dL)	>3.5	3.0–3.5	<3
Prothrombin time (seconds prolonged)	1–4	4–6	>6
Encephalopathy	None	Moderate	Severe
Nutrition	Excellent	Good	Poor
Ascites	None	Moderate	Marked
Adapted from Strunin I: Preoperative assessment of the patient with liver dysfunction. Br J Anaesth 1978;50:25–34.			

the pharmacologically active fraction of intravenous anesthetic drugs. Alcohol-induced cardiomyopathy could make patients unusually sensitive to the cardiac depressant effects of volatile anesthetics. There may be decreased responsiveness to catecholamines.

Intoxicated Alcoholic Patients

In contrast to a chronic but sober alcoholic patient, the acutely intoxicated patient requires *less* anesthetic because there are additive depressant effects from the alcohol and the anesthetic drugs. Acutely intoxicated patients are also ill equipped to withstand stress and acute surgical blood loss. Furthermore, alcohol may decrease the tolerance of the brain to hypoxia. Intoxicated patients may be more vulnerable to regurgitation of gastric contents since alcohol delays gastric emptying and decreases lower esophageal sphincter tone. Surgical bleeding may reflect alcohol-induced interference with platelet aggregation. Alcohol, even in moderate doses, causes increased plasma catecholamine concentrations, most likely reflecting inhibition of neurotransmitter uptake back into presynaptic nerve endings.

Intraoperative Management

Optimal anesthetic drug choices or techniques in the presence of liver disease are unknown. It is important to remember, however, that a constant feature of chronic liver disease is decreased hepatic blood flow due to portal hypertension. As a result, hepatic blood flow and hepatocyte oxygenation are more dependent on hepatic artery blood flow than normally. The hepatic artery may provide more than 50% of the oxygen supply by vasodilating during periods of decreased portal vein blood flow. Hepatic blood flow and hepatocyte oxygenation seem to be well maintained during administration of isoflurane, desflurane, and sevoflurane but not halothane. However, the ability of the hepatic artery to vasodilate in response to a decrease in portal vein blood flow can be blunted by volatile anesthetics, especially halothane and especially in high concentrations. It is prudent to limit the dose of volatile anesthetic to minimize the likelihood of a persistent decrease in mean arterial pressure because intraoperative hypotension may be associated with increased postoperative morbidity and mortality. Intravenous anesthetic drugs are valuable adjuncts to volatile anesthetics with or without nitrous oxide, but cumulative drug effects are likely if liver disease is severe enough to slow metabolism of the intravenous anesthetics. Regardless of the drugs selected for anesthesia, postoperative liver dysfunction is likely to be exaggerated in patients with chronic liver disease, presumably due to the effects of anesthetic drugs and/or stress-induced activation of the sympathetic nervous system on hepatocyte oxygenation. Regional anesthesia can be useful in patients with advanced liver disease if the coagulation status is acceptable.

Muscle Relaxants Hepatic clearance of muscle relaxants must be considered when selecting a particular neuromuscular blocker for administration to patients with cirrhosis.

Succinylcholine or mivacurium are acceptable, although severe liver disease may decrease plasma cholinesterase activity and prolong the duration of action of these drugs. The increased volume of distribution that accompanies cirrhosis, especially with ascites, will result in the need for a larger initial dose of nondepolarizing muscle relaxant to produce the required plasma concentration. However, subsequent doses may be smaller due to decreased hepatic clearance and metabolism. Hepatic dysfunction does not alter the elimination half-time of atracurium or cisatracurium. The elimination half-time of vecuronium is not increased until the dose exceeds 0.1 mg/kg, consistent with the dependence of this drug on hepatic clearance. Altered protein binding of muscle relaxants is insignificant as a mechanism of an altered response in patients with cirrhosis.

Monitoring Monitoring of arterial blood gases and urine output is often necessary. The need for invasive intraoperative monitoring is determined by the extent and urgency of the surgery. Management of anesthesia for surgical creation of a portocaval shunt includes monitoring arterial pressure and cardiac filling pressures. Fluid administration must be carefully titrated to an endpoint such as central venous pressure, pulmonary artery occlusion pressure, and urine output. Intraoperative maintenance of an acceptable urine output may help decrease the risk of postoperative acute renal failure. When blood replacement is necessary, the stored blood should be administered as slowly as possible to compensate for the decreased clearance of citrate by the cirrhotic liver. Infusion of glucose may be necessary during the perioperative period to prevent hypoglycemia. A practical point is avoidance of unnecessary esophageal instrumentation (esophageal stethoscope, orogastric or nasogastric tube) in patients with known esophageal varices.

Postoperative Management

Regardless of the drugs selected for anesthesia, postoperative liver dysfunction/jaundice is likely in patients with chronic liver disease. Cholestasis and sepsis can also be causes of postoperative jaundice. Manifestations of alcohol withdrawal usually appear 24 to 72 hours after cessation of drinking and can constitute a medical emergency in the postoperative period.

HYPERBILIRUBINEMIA

Bilirubin is the degradation product of hemoglobin and myoglobin. Unconjugated bilirubin formed in the periphery is transported to the liver where it is conjugated to mono- and diglucoronides by the action of the enzyme glucoronosyl transferase. This greatly increases the water solubility of bilirubin, which enhances its elimination from the body while simultaneously decreasing its ability to cross biological membranes including the blood-brain barrier. *Unconjugated hyperbilirubinemia* will occur with an increase in bilirubin production, decreased hepatic uptake of bilirubin, or decreased conjugation of bilirubin. *Conjugated hyperbilirubinemia* occurs with decreased canalicular transport of bilirubin, acute or chronic hepatocellular dysfunction, or obstruction of the bile ducts.

Gilbert Syndrome

The most common example of a hereditary hyperbilirubinemia (present in varying degrees in 7% to 12% of the general population) is Gilbert syndrome, inherited as an autosomal dominant trait with variable penetrance. The primary defect is a mutation in the glucoronosyl transferase enzyme, but usually there is approximately one third of normal enzyme activity. Plasma bilirubin concentrations seldom exceed 5 mg/dL but will increase two- to threefold with fasting or illness.

Crigler-Najjar Syndrome

Crigler-Najjar syndrome is a rare hereditary form of severe unconjugated hyperbilirubinemia that results from a mutation in the glucuronosyl transferase enzyme. Typically glucoronosyl transferase activity is reduced to less than 10% of normal. Children who lack effective enzyme function are jaundiced in the perinatal period. Kernicterus can develop. Optimal treatment for a neurologically intact child includes exchange transfusion in the neonatal period, daily phototherapy throughout childhood, and early liver transplantation before brain damage develops. Chronic phenobarbital therapy may decrease jaundice by stimulating activity of glucoronosyl transferase.

Bilirubin phototherapy lights should be available for anesthetic management of children with this syndrome. Fasting should be minimized because this stress is known to increase plasma bilirubin concentration. Morphine is metabolized by a glucuronosyl transferase enzyme system different from that deficient in Crigler-Najjar syndrome. Therefore, morphine can be safely administered to these patients. Barbiturates, inhaled anesthetics, and muscle relaxants are acceptable choices in these patients.

Dubin-Johnson Syndrome

Dubin-Johnson syndrome is due to decreased ability to transport organic ions from hepatocytes into the biliary system resulting in conjugated hyperbilirubinemia. Despite the conjugated hyperbilirubinemia, these patients are not cholestatic. Inheritance of this syndrome is autosomal recessive. The prognosis is benign.

Benign Postoperative Intrahepatic Cholestasis

Benign postoperative intrahepatic cholestasis may occur when surgery is prolonged, especially if it is complicated by hypotension, hypoxemia, and the need for blood transfusion. The hyperbilirubinemia may be caused by an increase in bilirubin production (breakdown of transfused red cells or resorption of a hematoma) and/or decreased hepatic clearance of bilirubin. Jaundice with conjugated hyperbilirubinemia is usually apparent within 24 to 48 hours. Liver function tests other than bilirubin and alkaline phosphatase are usually normal or only mildly abnormal. This condition typically resolves in tandem with improvement in the underlying surgical or medical condition.

Progressive Familial Intrahepatic Cholestasis

Progressive familial intrahepatic cholestasis is a rare hereditary metabolic disease presenting as cholestasis in infancy and end-stage cirrhosis before adulthood. Pruritus may be severe. The precise metabolic defect responsible for this disease has not been identified. Liver transplantation is the only curative treatment. Management of anesthesia in patients with progressive familial intrahepatic cholestasis/cirrhosis is influenced by malnutrition, portal hypertension, coagulation abnormalities, hypoalbuminemia, and chronic hypoxemia.

ACUTE LIVER FAILURE

Acute hepatic failure is characterized by jaundice, hypoalbuminemia, coagulopathy, malnutrition, susceptibility to infection, and renal dysfunction in the clinical setting of acute hepatic disease. Fulminant hepatic failure refers to acute liver failure with superimposed hepatic encephalopathy that develops within 2 to 8 weeks of the onset of illness in a patient without preexisting liver disease. Viral hepatitis and drug-induced liver injury account for most cases of acute liver failure (Table 11-7).

Signs and Symptoms

Regardless of cause, acute liver failure presents with clinical features that distinguish it from chronic hepatic insufficiency. Typically, nonspecific symptoms such as malaise or nausea develop in a previously healthy individual. This is followed by jaundice, altered mental status, and even coma. The progression of symptoms is rapid. Altered mentation and a prolonged prothrombin time are hallmarks of acute liver failure. Supportive laboratory findings include increased serum aminotransferase concentrations, hypoglycemia, and evidence of respiratory alkalosis. Cerebral edema is often present, manifesting as hypertension and bradycardia. Hypotension and decreased systemic vascular resistance are common, and oliguric renal failure (hepatorenal syndrome) occurs in many patients. These patients are also at increased risk of development of bacterial and fungal infection.

Acute fatty liver of pregnancy is characterized by accumulation of fat in hepatocytes. Approximately one half of patients have evidence of pregnancy-induced hypertension, and many have laboratory evidence of HELLP syndrome (hemolysis,

TABLE 11-7	Some Causes of Acute Liver Failure

Viral hepatitis
Drug-induced hepatitis, e.g., acetaminophen
Toxin-induced hepatitis, e.g., carbon tetrachloride
Hepatic ischemia
Acute fatty liver of pregnancy
Reye's syndrome

elevated liver enzymes, and low platelet count occurring in association with preeclampsia). Symptoms of acute fatty liver of pregnancy typically begin during the third trimester. The initial manifestations are nonspecific (nausea and vomiting, right upper quadrant pain, virus-like syndrome with malaise and anorexia) followed in 7 to 14 days by the appearance of jaundice. Treatment entails prompt termination of pregnancy. Untreated, acute fatty liver of pregnancy typically progresses to acute liver failure and death.

Treatment

There are no specific treatments for managing acute liver failure. Efforts to elucidate the cause are important, as antidotes must be administered early for acetaminophen or mushroom poisoning. Glucose is indicated in the presence of hypoglycemia. Invasive hemodynamic monitoring may be helpful for management of intravascular volume replacement. Vasopressors and inotropes are relatively ineffective in treating the hypotension associated with liver failure. Cerebral edema requires aggressive intervention in the hope of preventing brain herniation. When survival seems unlikely, the only curative treatment is liver transplantation.

Management of Anesthesia

Only surgery necessary to correct life-threatening problems should be considered in patients with acute liver failure. Preoperative correction of coagulation abnormalities with fresh frozen plasma may be indicated. Low doses of volatile anesthetics or even nitrous oxide alone may be sufficient to provide analgesia and amnesia in these critically ill patients. Intravenous anesthetics may have prolonged effects due to the marked reduction in metabolism of these drugs. Muscle relaxants may be needed to facilitate operative exposure or manage ventilation. When choosing a muscle relaxant, one must consider the impact of decreased hepatic function and associated renal dysfunction on the clearance of the drug. Because the plasma half-life of pseudocholinesterase is 14 days, it is unlikely that acute liver failure would be associated with a prolonged response to succinylcholine or mivacurium.

Administration of glucose is important, and plasma glucose measurement to confirm the absence of hypoglycemia is prudent. Blood should be administered as slowly as possible to minimize the likelihood of citrate intoxication. Monitoring arterial blood gases and electrolyte concentrations is helpful since these patients are vulnerable to development of arterial hypoxemia, metabolic acidosis, hypokalemia, hypocalcemia, and hypomagnesemia. Hypotension and its adverse effect on hepatic blood flow and hepatocyte oxygenation must be considered. Urine output is maintained with intravenous infusion of crystalloid or colloid and, if necessary, diuretic administration. Invasive monitoring is helpful for guiding overall hemodynamic management. These patients are vulnerable to infection, emphasizing the importance of aseptic technique during insertion of intravascular catheters. Lactulose therapy during the preoperative period may decrease the ammonia load and help prevent development of hepatic encephalopathy.

LIVER TRANSPLANTATION

Liver transplantation is the only curative therapy for patients with severe acute liver failure or end-stage liver disease with cirrhosis. In 2006, 6650 liver transplantations were performed in the United States, 40% of these for liver disease related to hepatitis C. At present, the typical 1-year survival rate for liver transplant recipients is approximately 85% and the 5-year survival rate is approximately 70%.

More than 90% of livers for transplantation are cadaveric organs. Live donor liver transplantation, which usually involves removal of an entire lobe of the liver (especially the right lobe) produces excellent results in children. However, adult-to-adult live donor liver transplantation is often more problematic due to size mismatching. The small-for-size syndrome is not uncommon and manifests as liver dysfunction within the first week after surgery. It appears that cirrhotic patients do better with a donor liver at least as large if not larger than their native liver.

Management of Anesthesia

Candidates for liver transplantation may present with severe multiorgan dysfunction. Many of the physiologic derangements, such as the coagulopathy, are not correctable until after successful liver transplantation. The likely presence of HBV or HBC in the transplant recipient must be considered by the health care providers.

The pharmacokinetics and pharmacodynamics of many drugs used in anesthesia are altered by severe liver disease. Changes in drug metabolism, protein binding, and volume of distribution are common. Induction of anesthesia can be affected by the presence of ascites compromising lung volumes and delaying gastric emptying. Hypoxemia and pulmonary aspiration are significant risks. Anesthesia can be maintained with opioids and/or inhaled anesthetics combined with muscle relaxants that are not dependent on hepatic clearance mechanisms (atracurium, cisatracurium). Nitrous oxide is usually avoided because of concerns regarding bowel distention that can compromise surgical exposure. Fluid warming devices and rapid infusion systems designed to deliver warmed fluids or blood products at rates exceeding 1 L per minute are routinely employed. Invasive monitoring of systemic blood pressure and cardiac filling pressures and placement of several large-bore intravenous catheters to optimize fluid replacement are important parts of anesthetic management. Surgery for removal of the native liver and implantation of the donor liver is characterized by three phases: the dissection phase, the anhepatic phase, and the reperfusion or neohepatic phase.

The *dissection phase* involves mobilizing the vascular structures around the liver (hepatic artery, portal vein, supra- and infrahepatic vena cava), isolating the common bile duct, and removing the native liver. Cardiovascular instability due to hemorrhage, venous pooling as a result of decreases in intra-abdominal pressure, and impaired venous return due to surgical retraction are not uncommon during this phase.

The *anhepatic stage* begins when the blood supply to the native liver is interrupted by clamping of the hepatic artery and portal vein. To avoid a marked decrease in venous return and cardiac output as well as splanchnic venous congestion during occlusion of the inferior vena cava, a venovenous bypass system is often used. Placement of the donor liver may require vigorous retraction near the diaphragm, leading to possible compromise of ventilation and oxygenation. Because of the lack of liver metabolic function during the anhepatic phase, metabolic acidosis, decreased drug metabolism, and citrate intoxication are likely. A calcium infusion may be needed to treat hypocalcemia.

The *reperfusion or neohepatic phase* begins after reanastomosis of the major vascular structures to the donor liver. Before removal of the vascular clamps, the allograft is flushed to remove air, debris, and preservative solutions. Despite this step, subsequent unclamping can cause significant hemodynamic instability, dysrhythmias, severe bradycardia, hypotension, and hyperkalemic cardiac arrest. Once the allograft begins to function, hemodynamic and metabolic stability are gradually restored and urine output increases. Recovery of the capacity to metabolize drugs occurs soon after reperfusion of the graft. Clotting parameters usually normalize with administration of clotting factors. Postoperative support of ventilation and oxygenation may be required.

Anesthetic Considerations in the Patient after Liver Transplantation

Potential adverse effects (systemic hypertension, anemia, thrombocytopenia) and drug interactions related to chronic immunosuppressive therapy are considered when planning the management of anesthesia in liver transplant recipients. Certainly these patients are at increased risk of infectious complications of any kind. If regional anesthesia or invasive hemodynamic monitoring are undertaken, strict aseptic technique is essential.

Liver function tests return to normal following successful liver transplantation. Liver transplantation also results in reversal of the hyperdynamic circulation that characterizes liver failure. Oxygenation improves, although intrapulmonary shunts may persist and contribute to ventilation-to-perfusion abnormalities. Normal physiologic mechanisms that protect hepatic blood flow are blunted after liver transplantation. The liver is normally an important source of autotransfusion of blood volume in shock states via a vasoconstrictive response, and this mechanism may be impaired after liver transplantation.

There is no evidence of an increased risk of developing hepatitis after administration of volatile anesthetics to liver transplant recipients.

DISEASES OF THE BILIARY TRACT

Cholelithiasis and inflammatory biliary tract disease constitute major health problems in the United States. Approximately 30 million Americans have gallstones. The prevalence of gallstones is significantly higher in women than men. Furthermore, the prevalence increases with age, obesity, rapid weight loss, and pregnancy. Gallstone formation is most likely related to abnormalities in the physicochemical characteristics of the various components of bile. Approximately 90% of gallstones in countries with a Western diet high in protein and fat are radiolucent, composed primarily of cholesterol. The remaining gallstones are usually radiopaque and are typically composed of calcium bilirubinate. These gallstones develop most often in patients with cirrhosis or hemolytic anemia.

Cholelithiasis and Cholecystitis

Patients who have gallbladder or biliary tract stones can exhibit no symptoms (silent disease), acute symptomatic disease, or chronic intermittently symptomatic disease. Obstruction of the cystic duct or common bile duct by a gallstone causes acute inflammation.

Acute Cholecystitis

Obstruction of the cystic duct, which is nearly always due to a gallstone, produces acute inflammation of the gallbladder. Cholelithiasis is present in 95% of patients with acute cholecystitis.

Signs and Symptoms Signs and symptoms of acute cholecystitis include nausea, vomiting, fever, abdominal pain, and right upper quadrant tenderness. Severe pain that begins in the mid-epigastrium, moves to the right upper quadrant, and may radiate to the back and is caused by a stone lodged in a duct is designated *biliary colic*. This pain is extraordinarily intense and usually begins abruptly and subsides gradually. Patients may notice dark urine and scleral icterus. Most jaundiced patients have stones in the common bile duct at the time of surgery. Laboratory testing commonly demonstrates leukocytosis.

Diagnosis Ultrasonography is the principal diagnostic procedure used in patients with suspected gallstones and acute cholecystitis. In addition to detecting gallstones, ultrasonography can identify other causes of right upper quadrant pain, such as abscess and malignancy, and it may reveal biliary tract obstruction. Radionuclide scanning (hepatoiminodiacetic acid [HIDA] scan) is the most specific test for diagnosing acute cholecystitis. The radiolabeled material is normally taken up by the liver, excreted into bile, and concentrated in the gallbladder. When a gallstone obstructs the cystic duct, the gallbladder fails to fill with hepatoiminodiacetic acid. Gallstones may also be detected by computed tomography and magnetic resonance imaging, but these techniques are much more expensive and less sensitive than ultrasonography.

Differential Diagnosis Acute pancreatitis may be nearly impossible to distinguish from acute cholecystitis (**Table 11-8**). Patients with a penetrating duodenal ulcer may experience severe epigastric pain, and free air may be evident on a plain film of the abdomen if the ulcer has perforated. Acute appendicitis may produce symptoms similar to those

TABLE 11–8 Differential Diagnosis of Acute Cholecystitis

Pancreatitis
Penetrating duodenal ulcer
Appendicitis
Acute viral hepatitis
Alcoholic hepatitis
Pyelonephritis
Right lower lobe pneumonia
Acute myocardial infarction

of acute cholecystitis, particularly if the appendix is retrocecal. Acute pyelonephritis of the right kidney, right lower lobe pneumonia, and acute myocardial infarction may also produce pain similar to the pain that occurs with acute cholecystitis.

Treatment Patients with a clinical diagnosis of acute cholecystitis are treated with intravenous fluids and opioids to manage the pain. Febrile patients with leukocytosis are given antibiotics. Surgery is typically considered when the patient's condition has stabilized. Laparoscopic cholecystectomy has almost completely replaced open cholecystectomy. Laparoscopic cholecystectomy is associated with less postoperative pain, fewer pulmonary complications, and more rapid convalescence. In approximately 5% of patients, laparoscopic cholecystectomy must be converted to an open cholecystectomy because inflammation obscures the anatomy. Cholangiography can be performed during surgery, and common duct stones can be removed concurrently or subsequently by endoscopic retrograde cholangiopancreatography (ERCP). Operative common bile duct exploration and stone removal may occasionally be needed. Patients with septic shock, peritonitis, pancreatitis, or coagulopathy may undergo open cholecystectomy or ultrasonography-guided percutaneous cholecystostomy.

Complications The principal complications of acute cholecystitis are related to severe inflammation and necrosis of the gallbladder. Localized perforation and abscess formation are likely if symptoms persist for several days. Free perforation occurs in 1% to 2% of patients and is associated with a significant mortality. Severe abdominal pain lasting longer than 7 days could be the result of empyema of the gallbladder. Mortality in this situation approaches 25% and is most often due to sepsis. Gallstone ileus results from obstruction of the small bowel, often at the ileocecal valve, by a large gallstone.

Management of Anesthesia Anesthetic considerations for laparoscopic cholecystectomy are similar to those for other laparoscopic procedures. Insufflation of the abdominal cavity (pneumoperitoneum) with carbon dioxide results in increased intra-abdominal pressure that may interfere with the adequacy of ventilation and venous return. Changes in cardiovascular function due to insufflation of the abdomen are characterized by an immediate decrease in venous return and cardiac output and an increase in mean arterial pressure and systemic vascular resistance. During the next several minutes, there is partial restoration of cardiac output, but blood pressure and heart rate usually remain unchanged. This pattern of cardiovascular responses is most likely the result of interactions caused by increased abdominal pressure, neurohumoral responses, and absorbed carbon dioxide.

The reverse Trendelenburg position favors movement of abdominal contents away from the operative site and may improve ventilation. Mechanical ventilation is recommended to prevent atelectasis, to ensure adequate ventilation in the presence of increased intra-abdominal pressure, and to offset the effects of systemic absorption of carbon dioxide. High intra-abdominal pressure may increase the risk of reflux of gastric contents. Endotracheal intubation with a cuffed tube minimizes the risk of pulmonary aspiration should reflux occur. Intraoperative decompression of the stomach with a nasogastric or orogastric tube may decrease the risk of visceral puncture during needle insertion to produce the pneumoperitoneum. Carbon dioxide embolism may be responsible for cardiovascular collapse. Capnography is important for recognizing carbon dioxide embolism. Cardiac dysrhythmias may occur due to hypercarbia. Hemorrhage or liver injury require intervention via open laparotomy. There is no evidence that nitrous oxide significantly expands bowel gas or interferes with surgical working conditions during laparoscopic cholecystectomy. Subcutaneous emphysema associated with pneumomediastinum and pneumothorax has been observed in patients undergoing laparoscopic cholecystectomy.

The use of opioids during anesthesia for this operation is controversial because these drugs can cause spasm of the sphincter of Oddi. Despite these concerns, opioids have been used in many instances without adverse effects, emphasizing that not all patients respond to opioids with sphincter of Oddi spasm. It has been suggested that the incidence of opioid-induced sphincter spasm is so low (<3%) that this response should not influence the selection of these drugs. In addition, it is possible to antagonize this spasm with intravenous administration of glucagon or naloxone. Nitroglycerin may also be effective in treating spasm of the sphincter of Oddi.

Emergency surgery for acute cholecystitis or common bile duct obstruction in patients who have been vomiting necessitates fluid and electrolyte replacement. Many of these patients have an ileus and should be considered at increased risk of pulmonary aspiration of gastric contents.

Chronic Cholecystitis

Chronic cholelithiasis is usually accompanied by evidence of chronic cholecystitis. The wall of the gallbladder may be thickened, fibrotic, and inflexible, thereby preventing normal contraction and expansion. Chronic cholecystitis typically follows a series of attacks of acute cholecystitis.

Signs and Symptoms Signs and symptoms are often nonspecific and include complaints of flatulence, heartburn, and postprandial distress. Physical examination is often normal. Routine laboratory tests are usually normal.

Diagnosis Ultrasonography is used to diagnose chronic cholecystitis. When the sonogram is nondiagnostic, oral cholecystography may be used. Failure of the contrast dye to cause opacification of the gallbladder is highly suggestive of chronic cholecystitis and cholelithiasis. Computed tomography and magnetic resonance imaging may also detect gallstones, but these techniques are unlikely to demonstrate stones not detected by ultrasonography.

Treatment Elective cholecystectomy is indicated for patients who have symptomatic gallstones and/or chronic cholecystitis. Alternative forms of therapy for cholelithiasis include oral dissolution therapy and extracorporeal biliary lithotripsy.

Oral Dissolution Therapy. Ursodeoxycholic acid administered orally for 6 to 12 months results in dissolution of up to 90% of small cholesterol stones that are floating in a normally functioning gallbladder. This situation is present in approximately 15% of symptomatic patients. Recurrence of cholesterol stones after discontinuation of ursodeoxycholic acid is common. Overall, dissolution therapy has limited value except in patients who are very poor candidates for surgery.

Extracorporeal Shock-Wave Lithotripsy. Fragmentation of larger stones in the gallbladder or common bile duct can be produced by carefully focused shock waves. The administration of ursodeoxycholic acid after fragmentation of stones increases the percentage of patients who are free of gallbladder stones several months after lithotripsy. The success of laparoscopic cholecystectomy has limited the use of lithotripsy for treatment of biliary stones.

Choledocholithiasis

Choledocholithiasis indicates that gallstones are present in the common bile duct. Stones typically lodge at the point of insertion of the duct into the ampulla of Vater.

Signs and Symptoms

Patients with choledocholithiasis may present with signs of cholangitis (fever, shaking chills, jaundice, right upper quadrant pain) or jaundice alone and a history of pain suggestive of cholecystitis. Not all stones obstruct the common duct. Some

pass into the duodenum or into a pancreatic duct resulting in acute pancreatitis. Serum bilirubin and alkaline phosphatase concentrations typically increase markedly and abruptly when a stone obstructs the common bile duct. Aminotransferase concentrations are only modestly increased.

Diagnosis

Ultrasonography may reveal a dilated common bile duct, although this finding is not present in a significant number of patients with proven choledocholithiasis. Computed tomography is no more sensitive than ultrasonography. Cholescintigraphy may reveal common bile duct obstruction. The biliary tract can also be visualized radiographically using endoscopic retrograde cholangiopancreatography or percutaneous transhepatic cholangiography.

Differential Diagnosis

Acute obstruction of the common bile duct by a stone may mimic ureterolithiasis because of the similarities in location and severity of the pain, but liver function tests distinguish between these two conditions. Acute inflammation of the head of the pancreas may produce obstruction of the common bile duct. Computed tomography or ERCP helps distinguish pancreatitis from choledocholithiasis. Symptoms of an acute myocardial infarction or viral hepatitis may produce abdominal pain that is similar to that of biliary tract disease. The epigastric pain may be similar to that in patients with pancreatic carcinoma. Acute intermittent porphyria can also cause severe abdominal pain, but alkaline phosphatase and bilirubin concentrations are normal in this condition.

Treatment

Endoscopic sphincterotomy is the initial treatment for the patient with choledocholithiasis. ERCP can be used to identify the cause of common bile duct obstruction and can also be used to remove a stone or place a stent. Sphincterotomy is also the recommended treatment for patients with retained bile duct stones after gallbladder or biliary tract surgery. Operative exploration of the common bile duct is reserved for the few patients in whom endoscopic sphincterotomy is unsuccessful.

KEY POINTS

- Acute hepatitis is most often a result of viral infection but can also be caused by drugs and toxins. Acute viral hepatitis is typically caused by one of five viruses: HAV, HBV, HCV, HDV, or HEV. In the United States, approximately 50% of acute viral hepatitis in adults is due to HAV infection, 35% to HBV infection, and 15% to HCV infection. Hepatitis D infection is rare and HEV is not endemic in this country.

- The major complication of acute hepatitis C is development of chronic hepatitis and cirrhosis. Hepatitis C is currently the predominant liver disease in the United States. End-stage liver disease due to HCV-associated cirrhosis is the most common indication for liver transplantation and HCV-associated cirrhosis is responsible for an increasing incidence of hepatocellular cancer.

- Many drugs (analgesics, volatile anesthetics, antibiotics, antihypertensives, anticonvulsants, tranquilizers) can cause hepatitis indistinguishable histologically from acute viral hepatitis. Many of these drug reactions are idiosyncratic, that is, they are rare, unpredictable,

KEY POINTS—cont'd

and not dose dependent. Failure to discontinue the offending drug may result in progressive hepatitis and even death.

- A rare form of hepatic dysfunction can follow administration of volatile anesthetics, especially halothane, in genetically susceptible individuals. IgG anti–trifluoroacetyl antibodies are directed against microsomal proteins on the surface of hepatocytes that have been modified by the trifluoroacetyl halide metabolite of halothane to form neoantigens. Formation of antibodies against these proteins produces a form of autoimmune hepatitis.

- Enflurane, isoflurane, and desflurane can form trifluoroacetyl metabolites resulting in cross-sensitivity with halothane. However, the incidence of hepatitis after these anesthetics is much lower than after halothane because the degree of anesthetic metabolism is substantially less. Sevoflurane does not undergo metabolism to trifluoroacetylated metabolites. Therefore, unlike the other fluorinated volatile anesthetics, sevoflurane does not produce immune-mediated hepatotoxicity.

- Chronic hepatitis is characterized by long-term elevation of liver chemistries and evidence of inflammation on liver biopsy. Chronic hepatitis is generally defined as disease that lasts 6 months or longer. The most common diseases that cause chronic hepatitis are autoimmune hepatitis and chronic viral hepatitis (HBV with or without hepatitis D virus co-infection, infection with HCV).

- Portal hypertension is the result of an increase in resistance to blood flow through the portal venous system as a result of the fibrotic cirrhotic process. Portal hypertension combined with hypoalbuminemia and increased secretion of vasoconstrictor and antinatriuretic factors and antidiuretic hormone causes development of ascites.

- Chronic alcohol ingestion increases anesthetic requirements (MAC) most likely due to cross-tolerance. In contrast to a chronic but sober alcoholic patient, the acutely intoxicated patient requires less anesthetic because there are additive depressant effects between the alcohol and the anesthetic drugs. Accelerated metabolism of drugs in the presence of alcohol-induced microsomal enzyme induction can also alter the amount of anesthetic drug needed to achieve a certain anesthetic depth. Decreased protein binding of drugs in the presence of hypoalbuminemia could increase the pharmacologically active fraction of intravenous anesthetic drugs.

- Bilirubin is the degradation product of hemoglobin and myoglobin. Unconjugated bilirubin formed in the periphery is transported to the liver where it is conjugated to mono- and diglucoronides by glucoronosyl transferase. Unconjugated hyperbilirubinemia will occur with an increase in bilirubin production, decreased hepatic uptake of bilirubin, or decreased conjugation of bilirubin. Conjugated hyperbilirubinemia occurs with decreased canalicular transport of bilirubin, acute or chronic hepatocellular dysfunction, or obstruction of the bile ducts.

- More than 90% of livers for transplantation are cadaveric organs. Live donor liver transplantation involves transplantation of one entire lobe of the liver. This technique produces excellent results in children but adult-to-adult live donor liver transplantation is often problematic due to size mismatching. The small-for-size syndrome is not uncommon and manifests as liver dysfunction within the first week after surgery.

- Surgery for liver transplantation is characterized by three phases: the dissection phase, the anhepatic phase, and the reperfusion or neohepatic phase. The dissection phase involves mobilizing the vascular structures around the liver (hepatic artery, portal vein, supra- and infrahepatic vena cava), isolating the common bile duct and removing the native liver. The anhepatic stage begins when the blood supply to the native liver is interrupted by clamping of the hepatic artery and portal vein. The reperfusion or neohepatic phase begins after reanastomosis of the major vascular structures to the donor liver.

- Cardiovascular instability due to hemorrhage, venous pooling, and impaired venous return due to surgical retraction are not uncommon during the dissection phase. A marked decrease in venous return and cardiac output and splanchnic venous congestion can occur during occlusion of the inferior vena cava during the anhepatic phase. In addition, because of the lack of liver metabolic function during the anhepatic phase, metabolic acidosis, decreased drug metabolism, and citrate intoxication are likely. After removal of the vascular clamps, the reperfusion phase can be complicated by significant hemodynamic instability, dysrhythmias, severe bradycardia, hypotension, and hyperkalemic cardiac arrest. Once the allograft begins to function, hemodynamic and metabolic stability are gradually restored.

- Anesthetic considerations for laparoscopic cholecystectomy are similar to those for other laparoscopic procedures. Insufflation of the abdominal cavity with carbon dioxide results in increased intra-abdominal pressure that may interfere with ventilation. Changes in cardiovascular function due to insufflation are characterized by an immediate decrease in venous return and cardiac output and an increase in mean arterial pressure and systemic vascular resistance.

KEY POINTS—cont'd

- The use of opioids during anesthesia for gallbladder or common bile duct surgery is controversial because these drugs can cause spasm of the sphincter of Oddi. However, it is possible to antagonize this spasm with intravenous administration of glucagon, nitroglycerin, or naloxone.

REFERENCES

Adachi T: Anesthetic principles in living donor liver transplantation at Kyoto University Hospital: Experiences of 760 cases. J Anesth 2003;17:116–124.

Brundage SC, Fitzpatrick AN: Hepatitis A. Am Fam Physician 2006;73:2162–2168.

Faust TW, Reddy KR: Postoperative jaundice. Clin Liver Dis 2004;8:151–166.

Ganem D, Prince AM: Hepatitis B virus infection—natural history and clinical consequences. N Engl J Med 2004;350:1118–1129.

Garcia-Tsao G: Portal hypertension. Curr Opin Gastroenterol 2006;22:254–262.

Gines P, Cardenas A, Arroyo V, Rades J: Management of cirrhosis and ascites. N Engl J Med 2004;350:1646–1654.

Kostopanagiotou G, Smyrniotis V, Arkadopoulos N, et al: Anesthetic and perioperative management of adult transplant recipients in nontransplant surgery. Anesth Analg 1999;89:613–622.

Laver GM, Walker BD: Hepatitis C virus infection. N Engl J Med 2001;345:41–52.

Merritt WT: Perioperative concerns in acute liver failure. Int Anesthesiol Clin 2006;44:37–57.

Njoku D, Laster MJ, Gong DH, et al: Biotransformation of halothane, enflurane, isoflurane, and desflurane to trifluoroacetylated liver proteins: Association between protein acylation and hepatic injury. Anesth Analg 1997;84:173–178.

Schafer DF, Sorrell MF: Conquering hepatitis C, step by step. N Engl J Med 2000;343:1723–1724.

Spies CD, Rommelspacher H: Alcohol withdrawal in the surgical patient: Prevention and treatment. Anesth Analg 1999;88:946–954.

Steadman RH: Anesthesia for liver transplant surgery. Anesthesiol Clin North Am 2004;4:687–711.

Suttner SW, Schmidt CC, Boldt J, et al: Low-flow desflurane and sevoflurane anesthesia minimally affect hepatic integrity and function in elderly patients. Anesth Analg 2000;91:206–212.

Ziser A, Plevak DJ, Wiesner RH, et al: Morbidity and mortality in cirrhotic patients undergoing anesthesia and surgery. Anesthesiology 1999;90:42–53.

CHAPTER 12

Diseases of the Gastrointestinal System

Hossam Tantawy

The principal function of the gastrointestinal (GI) tract is to provide the body with a continual supply of water, nutrients, and electrolytes. Each division of the GI tract—esophagus, stomach, small and large intestines—is adapted for specific functions, such as passage, storage, and digestion of food. Impairment of any part of GI tract may significantly affect the patient. Therefore, preoperative assessment of patient's serum electrolytes, acid base, and volume status is crucial.

ESOPHAGEAL DISEASES

Dysphagia is the classic symptom of all disorders of the esophagus. To evaluate dysphagia, a barium contrast study is recommended, followed by esophagoscopy, which permits direct viewing as well as recovery of biopsy and cytology specimens.

Diffuse Esophageal Spasm

Diffuse esophageal spasm occurs most often in elderly patients and is most likely due to dysfunction of the autonomic nervous system. Pain produced by esophageal spasm may mimic angina pectoris and frequently even responds favorably to treatment with nitroglycerin, making it even a more confusing clinical scenario. Nifedipine and isosorbide, which decrease lower esophageal sphincter (LES) pressure, may also relieve pain produced by esophageal spasm.

Gastroesophageal Reflux Disease
Physiology and Pathophysiology

Currently, gastroesophageal reflux disease is described as "reflux of gastric contents (into the esophagus) associated with symptoms" (esophageal or extraesophageal). Generally, the LES opens on swallowing and closes afterward to prevent gastric acid in the stomach from refluxing into the esophagus. At rest, the LES typically exerts a pressure high enough to prevent reflux. With inappropriate relaxation or weakness of the LES, gastric acid re-enters the esophagus, causing irritation (**Table 12-1**).

Antireflux mechanisms consist of the LES, the crural diaphragm, and the anatomic location of the gastroesophageal junction below the diaphragmatic hiatus. The primary underlying defect leading to esophagitis seems to be a decrease in the resting tone of the LES (average 13 mm Hg versus 29 mm Hg in normal patients) Reflux occurs only when the gradient of pressure between the LES and the stomach is lost.

Factors that contribute to the likelihood of aspiration include the urgency of surgery, airway problems, inadequate depth of anesthesia, use of the lithotomy position, autonomic neuropathy, insulin-dependent diabetes mellitus, pregnancy, depressed consciousness, increased severity of illness, and obesity as well as increased intra-abdominal pressure. Chronic peptic esophagitis is caused by reflux of acidic gastric fluid into the esophagus, producing retrosternal discomfort ("heartburn"). Reflux into the pharynx, larynx, and tracheobronchial tree can result in chronic cough, bronchoconstriction, pharyngitis, laryngitis, bronchitis, or pneumonia. Morning hoarseness may also be noted. Recurrent

TABLE 12–1	Effect of Agents on Lower Esophageal Sphincter Tone	
Increase	**Decrease**	**No Change**
Metoclopramide	Atropine	Propranlol
Domeperidone	Glycopyrrolate	Oxprenolol
Prochlorperazine	Dopamine	Cimetidine
Cyclizine	Sodium nitropusside	Ranitidine
Edrophonium	Ganglion blockers	Atracurium
Neostigmine	Thiopental	?Nitrous
Succinylcholine	Tricyclic antidepressants	oxide
Pancuronium	β–adrenergic stimulants	
Metoprolol	Halothane	
α–adrenergic	Enflurane	
stimulants	Opioids	
Antacids	?Nitrous oxide	
	Propofol	

pulmonary aspiration can also result in aspiration pneumonia, pulmonary fibrosis, or chronic asthma. Persistent dysphagia suggests development of a peptic stricture.

Incidence

Reflux esophagitis is a common clinical problem, with more than one third of healthy adults experiencing symptoms of heartburn at least once every 30 days. In 1986, a study of Scandinavian Teaching Hospitals suggested that the incidence of aspiration varied between 0.7 and 4.7 per 10,000 general anesthetics. A report published one decade later suggested that the incidence was 2.9 per 10,000 at a Norwegian hospital. Studies from the Mayo Clinic in 1993 indicated that the incidence of aspiration is similar in adults (3.1 per 10,000).

By extrapolation from early studies in the rhesus monkey on direct administration of aspirate into the lungs, it is commonly held that patients are at risk of aspiration pneumonitis if there is a minimum gastric volume of 0.4 mL/kg and the pH of the gastric contents is less than 2.5.

Complications

Other than the natural concern among anesthesiologists with patients having gastroesophageal reflux disease in whom aspiration is a natural concern, other complications from the natural disease process could also affect the anesthetic management such as *mucosal* complications, such as esophagitis and stricture, where stricture could cause esophageal dilatation and another risk for aspiration, and *extraesophageal* or respiratory complications, such as laryngitis, recurrent pneumonia, and progressive pulmonary fibrosis. It is increasingly recognized that a significant proportion of patients with gastroesophageal reflux will have either primary respiratory symptoms or respiratory symptoms in association with more prominent heartburn and regurgitation. Up to 50% of patients with asthma have either endoscopic evidence of esophagitis or increased esophageal acid exposure on 24-hour ambulatory pH monitoring.

Prophylaxis and Treatment

The decision to include anticholinergic drugs in the preoperative medication must be balanced against the known ability of these drugs to decrease LES tone. Theoretically, anticholinergic drugs, by decreasing LES pressure, can increase the likelihood of silent regurgitation and the possibility of pulmonary aspiration. However, this potential adverse effect has not been documented. Succinylcholine increases LES pressure, but the barrier pressure (LES pressure minus gastric pressure) is unchanged, as fasciculations are associated with increased gastric pressure.

Depending on the nature of planned surgery and the type of anesthetic anticipated, prophylactic medications may be given preoperatively. Cimetidine and ranitidine decrease gastric acid secretion and increase gastric pH. Cimetidine's effect begins in 1 to 1.5 hours, lasts for 3 hours, and is cost-effective. Ranitidine is four to six times more potent than cimetidine

and has fewer side effects. Famotidine and nizatidine, also given intravenously, are similar to ranitidine but have a longer duration. If protein pump inhibitors are used, they should generally be given orally the night before surgery and again on the morning of surgery. However, if protein pump inhibitors are used as a single dose, then rabeprazole and lansoprazole should be given on the morning of surgery. Omeprazole, as a single dose, should be given the night before surgery. Sodium citrate is an oral nonparticulate antacid that increases gastric pH. It should be given with a gastrokinetic agent such as intravenous metoclopramide and should be restricted to those who are diabetic, morbidly obese, or pregnant.

Cricoid pressure compresses the lumen of the pharynx between the cricoid and cervical vertebrae. It is usually applied by an assistant under direction of the anesthesia provider and maintained until successful endotracheal intubation is verified. The force applied should be sufficient to prevent aspiration but not so great as to cause airway obstruction or allow the possibility of esophageal rupture in the event of vomiting.

Tracheal intubation is clearly the gold standard for protecting the airway from aspiration in anesthetized patients. Despite the observed leak of methylene blue in studies of intubated patients around the cuff, a new cuff under evaluation, termed the pressure-limited tracheal tube cuff, showed no detectable leak in any of the patients tested.

Hiatal Hernia

A *hiatal hernia* is a herniation of part of the stomach into the thoracic cavity through the esophageal hiatus in the diaphragm. A *sliding hiatal hernia* is one in which the gastroesophageal junction and fundus of the stomach slide upward. This type of hernia can be seen in approximately 30% of patients undergoing upper GI radiographic examination. Although the current belief is that many of these patients may be asymptomatic (i.e., no clinical symptoms of reflux). It may result from weakening of the anchors of the gastroesophageal junction to the diaphragm, from longitudinal contraction of the esophagus, or from increased intra-abdominal pressure. A *paraesophageal hernia* is one in which the esophagogastric junction remains fixed in its normal location and a pouch of stomach is herniated beside the gastroesophageal junction through the esophageal hiatus. Based on the assumption that the hiatal hernia predisposes to the development of peptic esophagitis, surgical repair of the hernia may be recommended. Nevertheless, most patients with hiatal hernia do not have symptoms of reflux esophagitis, emphasizing the importance of the integrity of the LES.

Esophageal Diverticula

Diverticuli are outpouchings of the wall of the esophagus. *Zenker's diverticulum* appears in the natural zone of weakness in the posterior hypopharyngeal wall (Killian's triangle) and causes halitosis and regurgitation of saliva and food particles consumed up to several days previously. When it becomes large and filled with food, such a diverticulum can compress the esophagus and cause dysphagia or complete obstruction. Nasogastric tube and echocardiography probe insertion should be performed with utmost care in these patients since it may cause perforation of the diverticulum. A mid-esophageal diverticulum may be caused by traction from old adhesions or by propulsion associated with esophageal motor abnormalities. An epiphrenic diverticulum may be associated with achalasia. Small- or medium-sized diverticula and mid-esophageal and epiphrenic diverticula are usually asymptomatic.

Treatment

Symptomatic Zenker's diverticuli are treated by cricopharyngeal myotomy with or without diverticulectomy. Large symptomatic esophageal diverticuli are removed surgically.

Mucosal Tear (Mallory-Weiss Syndrome)

This tear is usually caused by vomiting, retching, or vigorous coughing. The tear usually involves the gastric mucosa near the squamocolumnar mucosal junction. Patients present with upper GI bleeding. In most patients, bleeding ceases spontaneously. Continued bleeding may respond to vasopressin therapy or angiographic embolization. Surgery is rarely needed.

PEPTIC ULCER DISEASE

Classically speaking, burning epigastric pain exacerbated by fasting and improved with meals is a symptom complex associated with peptic ulcer disease (PUD). Lifetime prevalence of PUD in the United States is approximately 12% in men and 10% in women. Moreover, an estimated 15,000 deaths per year occur as a consequence of complicated PUD. Bleeding, peritonitis, and dehydration together with sepsis in cases of perforation, especially in elderly debilitated malnourished patients, impose the greatest anesthetic challenge

The Protective Function of the Gastric Lining

The *mucus-bicarbonate layer* serves as a physicochemical barrier to multiple agents including hydrogen ions. Gastroduodenal surface epithelial cells secrete mucus. The mucous gel impedes diffusion of ions and molecules such as pepsin. Bicarbonate, secreted by surface epithelial cells of the gastroduodenal mucosa into the mucous gel, forms a pH gradient ranging from 1 to 2 at the gastric luminal surface and reaching 6 to 7 along the epithelial cell surface. Bicarbonate secretion is stimulated by calcium, prostaglandins, cholinergic input, and luminal acidification.

Surface epithelial cells provide the next line of defense through several factors, including mucus production, epithelial cell ionic transporters that maintain intracellular pH and bicarbonate production, and intracellular tight junctions. If the preepithelial barrier was breached, gastric epithelial cells bordering a site of injury can migrate to restore a damaged region.

Prostaglandins play a central role in gastric epithelial defense and repair. These metabolites of arachidonic acid are formed by the cyclooxygenase. The cyclooxygenase-1 present in the stomach, platelets, kidneys, and endothelial cells regulating the release of mucosal bicarbonate and mucus and inhibiting parietal cell secretion and are important in maintaining mucosal blood flow and epithelial cell restitution. In contrast, the expression of cyclooxygenase-2 is inducible by inflammatory stimuli and is expressed in macrophages, leukocytes, fibroblasts, and synovial cells. The beneficial effects of nonsteroidal anti-inflammatory drugs (NSAIDs) on tissue inflammation are due to inhibition of cyclooxygenase-2.

Causes of Injury

Hydrochloric acid and pepsinogen are the two principal gastric secretory products capable of inducing mucosal injury. Acid secretion occurs under basal and stimulated conditions. Basal acid production occurs in a circadian pattern, with the highest levels occurring during the night and the lowest levels during the morning hours. Cholinergic input via the vagus nerve and histaminergic input from local gastric sources are the principal contributors to basal acid secretion. Stimulated gastric acid secretion occurs primarily in three phases based on the site where the signal originates (cephalic, gastric, and intestinal). Sight, smell, and taste of food are the components of the cephalic phase, which stimulates gastric secretion via the vagus nerve. The gastric phase is activated once food enters the stomach. Distention of the stomach wall also leads to gastrin release and acid production. The last phase of gastric acid secretion is initiated as food enters the intestine, mediated by luminal distention. This observation explains why blocking one receptor type (H_2) decreases acid secretion stimulated by agents that activate a different pathway (gastrin, acetylcholine).

Helicobacter pylori

Many lines of circumstantial evidence establish *H. pylori* as a factor in the pathogenesis of duodenal ulceration: Infection is virtually always associated with a chronic active gastritis, but only 10% to 15% of infected individuals develop frank peptic ulceration. Studies indicate that most of these secretory abnormalities are a direct consequence of *H. pylori* infection. Ironically, the earliest stages of *H. pylori* infection are accompanied by a marked decrease in gastric acid secretion. *H. pylori* infection might induce increased acid secretion through both direct and indirect actions of *H. pylori* and proinflammatory cytokines (interleukin [IL]-8, tumor necrosis factor, and IL-1) on G, D, and parietal cells. *H. pylori* also decreases duodenal mucosal bicarbonate production.

Complications
Bleeding

Hemorrhage is the leading cause of death associated with PUD, and the incidence of this complication has not changed since the introduction of H_2-receptor antagonists. The lifetime risk of hemorrhage for patients with duodenal ulcer who have not had surgery and did not receive continuing maintenance drug therapy is approximately 35%. The contemporary risk of mortality from bleeding is 10% to 20%.

Perforation

The lifetime risk of perforation in patients with duodenal ulceration who do not receive therapy is approximately 10%. Perforation is usually accompanied by sudden and severe epigastric pain caused by the spillage of highly caustic gastric secretions into the peritoneum. The mortality of emergent ulcer operations is correlated with preoperative shock, co-existing medical illness, and perforation for more than 48 hours.

Obstruction

Gastric outlet obstruction can occur acutely or chronically in patients with duodenal ulcer disease; hence, they probably should be considered as full stomach when they present for surgery. Acute obstruction is caused by edema and inflammation in the pyloric channel and the first portion of the duodenum. Pyloric obstruction is suggested by recurrent vomiting, dehydration, and hypochloremic alkalosis due to loss of gastric secretions. Treatment consists of nasogastric suction, rehydration, and intravenous administration of antisecretory agents. In most instances, acute obstruction resolves with these supportive measures within 72 hours. However, repeated episodes of ulceration and healing often lead to pyloric scarring and a subsequent fixed stenosis with chronic gastric outlet obstruction. Operative management of gastric outlet obstruction should include treatment of the underlying ulcer disease and relief of any anatomic abnormality. Truncal vagotomy with antrectomy and truncal vagotomy with drainage have both been used with success in this circumstance.

Gastric Ulcer

Benign gastric ulcers are a form of PUD, occurring with one third the frequency of benign duodenal ulceration (**Table 12-2**).

Stress Gastritis

Major trauma accompanied by shock, sepsis, respiratory failure, hemorrhage, transfusion requirement of more than 6 units, or multiorgan injury is often accompanied by the development of acute stress gastritis. Acute stress gastritis is particularly prevalent after thermal injury, which involves

greater than 35% total surface area, central nervous system injury, or intracranial hypertension. The major complication of stress gastritis is hemorrhage. The following clinical conditions have been associated with the greatest risk of hemorrhage: coagulopathy (platelet count < 50,000/ mm^3), international normalized ratio greater than 1.5, and partial thromboplastin time greater than two times normal.

Treatment
Antacids

They are rarely, if ever, used as the primary therapeutic agents but instead are often used by patients for symptomatic relief of dyspepsia. The most commonly used agents are mixtures of aluminum hydroxide and magnesium hydroxide. Aluminum hydroxide can produce constipation and phosphate depletion; magnesium hydroxide may cause loose stools. Many of the commonly used antacids (e.g., Maalox, Mylanta) have a combination of both aluminum and magnesium hydroxide in order to avoid these side effects. Neither magnesium- nor aluminum-containing preparations should be used in patients with chronic renal failure. The former can cause hypermagnesemia and the latter chronic neurotoxicity in patients with renal failure. The other potent antacids are calcium carbonate and sodium bicarbonate. The long-term use of calcium carbonate can lead to milk-alkali syndrome (hypercalcemia and hyperphosphatemia) with possible development of renal calcinosis and progression to renal insufficiency. Sodium bicarbonate may induce systemic alkalosis.

H$_2$-Receptor Antagonists

Four are currently available (cimetidine, ranitidine, famotidine, and nizatidine), and their structures share homology with histamine. All will significantly inhibit basal and stimulated acid secretion. This class of drugs has been shown to be effective for the treatment of active ulcer (4–6 weeks) and as an adjuvant (with antibiotics) for the management of *H. pylori*. Cimetidine was the first H$_2$-receptor antagonist used for the treatment of acid peptic disorders with healing rates approaching 80% at 4 weeks. Ranitidine, famotidine, and nizatidine are more potent H$_2$-receptor antagonists than cimetidine. Cimetidine and ranitidine, but not famotidine and nizatidine, bind to hepatic cytochrome P-450. Therefore, careful monitoring of drugs such as warfarin, phenytoin, and theophylline is indicated with long-term use. Additional rare,

TABLE 12–2	Various Classifications of Gastric Ulcers	
Type of Gastric Ulcer	**Location**
Type I	Along the lesser curvature close to incisura; no acid hypersecretion
Type II	2 ulcers, first on the body, second is duodenal; usually acid hypersecretion
Type III	Prepyloric with acid hypersecretion
Type IV	At lesser curvature near gastroesophageal junction; not acid hypersecretion
Type V	Anywhere in the stomach, usually with nonsterodial anti-inflammatory drugs ingestion

reversible systemic toxicities reported with H_2-receptor antagonists include pancytopenia, neutropenia, anemia, and thrombocytopenia.

Proton Pump (H^+-K^+-ATPase) Inhibitors

Omeprazole, esomeprazole, lansoprazole, rabeprazole, and pantoprazole are substituted benzimidazole derivatives that covalently bind and irreversibly inhibit H^+-K^+-ATPase. These are the most potent acid inhibitory agents available. Proton pump inhibitors potently inhibit all phases of gastric acid secretion. Onset of action is rapid, with a maximum effect between 2 and 6 hours following administration with a duration of inhibition lasting up to 72 to 96 hours. As with any agent that leads to significant hypochlorhydria, proton pump inhibitors may interfere with absorption of drugs such as ketoconazole, ampicillin, iron, and digoxin. Hepatic cytochrome P-450 may also be inhibited by the earlier proton pump inhibitors (omeprazole, lansoprazole).

Prostaglandin Analogues

In view of their central role in maintaining mucosal integrity and repair, stable prostaglandin analogues were developed for the treatment of PUD. At present, the prostaglandin E_1 derivative misoprostol is the only agent of this class approved by the U.S. Food and Drug Administration for clinical use in the prevention of NSAID-induced gastroduodenal mucosal injury. Prostaglandin analogues enhance mucosal bicarbonate secretion, stimulate mucosal blood flow, and decrease mucosal cell turnover. The most common toxicity noted with this drug is diarrhea. Other major toxicities include uterine bleeding and contractions. Therefore, misoprostol is contraindicated in women who may be pregnant, and women of child-bearing age must be made clearly aware of this potential drug toxicity. Prevention of NSAID-induced ulceration can be accomplished by misoprostol 200 μg four times daily.

Cytoprotective Agents

Sucralfate is a complex sucrose salt in which the hydroxyl groups have been substituted by aluminum hydroxide and sulfate. It may act by several mechanisms. In the gastric environment, aluminum hydroxide dissociates, leaving the polar sulfate anion, which can then bind to positively charged tissue proteins found within the ulcer bed. This process provides a physicochemical barrier impeding further tissue injury by acid and pepsin. It may also induce a trophic effect by binding growth factors such as endothelial growth factor, enhance prostaglandin synthesis, stimulate mucous and bicarbonate secretion, and enhance mucosal defense and repair. Toxicity from this drug is rare, with constipation being the most common one. It should be avoided in patients with chronic renal insufficiency to prevent aluminum-induced neurotoxicity. Standard dosing of sucralfate is 1 g four times daily.

Bismuth-containing preparations as colloidal bismuth subcitrate and bismuth subsalicylate (Pepto-Bismol) are of the most widely used preparations. The mechanism by which these agents induce ulcer healing is unclear. Potential mechanisms include ulcer coating, prevention of further pepsin/HCl-induced damage, binding of pepsin, and stimulation of prostaglandins, bicarbonate, and mucus secretion. Long-term use with high doses, especially as observed with the avidly absorbed colloidal bismuth subcitrate, may lead to neurotoxicity.

Miscellaneous Drugs

Anticholinergics, designed to inhibit activation of the muscarinic receptor in parietal cells, had limited success due to their relatively weak acid-inhibiting effect and significant side effects (dry eyes, dry mouth, urinary retention). Tricyclic antidepressants have been suggested by some, but again the toxicity of these agents in comparison to the safe, effective drugs already described precludes their utility.

Treatment of *Helicobacter pylori*

The National Institutes of Health Consensus Development, American Digestive Health Foundation International Update Conference, European Maastricht Consensus, and Asia Pacific Consensus Conference recommendation is that *H. pylori* should be eradicated in patients with PUD. Documented eradication is associated with a dramatic decrease in ulcer recurrence. No single agent is effective in eradicating the organism. Combination therapy for 14 days provides the greatest efficacy. The agents used with the greatest frequency include amoxicillin, metronidazole, tetracycline, clarithromycin, and bismuth compounds.

Triple Therapy Treatment protocols combine a proton pump inhibitor, usually omeprazole, with two antibiotics, clarithromycin and metronidazole or amoxicillin. The most feared complication with amoxicillin is pseudomembranous colitis, but this occurs in less than 1% to 2% of patients.

Surgical Treatment

Operative intervention is reserved for the treatment of the most complicated ulcer disease. Most common complications requiring surgery are hemorrhage, perforation, and obstruction as well as failure of a recurrent ulcer to respond to medical therapy and/or the inability to exclude malignant disease. The first goal of any surgical treatment should be removal of the ulcer diathesis so that ulcer healing is achieved and recurrence is minimized. The second goal is treatment of co-existing anatomic complications, such as pyloric stenosis or perforation. The third major goal should be patient safety and freedom from undesirable chronic side effects.

Three procedures, truncal vagotomy and drainage, truncal vagotomy and antrectomy, and proximal gastric vagotomy, have been most widely used for the operative treatment of peptic ulcer disease. With increasing frequency, surgical treatment is directed exclusively at correcting the immediate problem (e.g., closure of duodenal perforation) without gastric denervation. Division of both vagal trunks at the esophageal hiatus-truncal vagotomy denervates the acid-producing fundic mucosa as well as the remainder of the vagally supplied viscera. Because denervation can result in impairment of gastric emptying, truncal vagotomy must be combined with a procedure to eliminate pyloric sphincteric function, usually a pyloroplasty. Truncal vagotomy can also be combined with resection of the gastric antrum, resulting in even further reduction in acid secretion, presumably by removing antral source of gastrin. Restoration of GI continuity is achieved by gastroduodenostomy (Billroth I). Proximal gastric vagotomy (or parietal cell vagotomy) differs from truncal vagotomy in that only the nerve fibers to the acid-secreting fundic mucosa are divided. Vagotomy also diminishes parietal cell responsiveness to gastrin and histamine. Basal acid secretion is reduced by approximately 80% in the immediate postoperative period.

ZOLLINGER-ELLISON SYNDROME

In 1955, Robert M. Zollinger, Sr., and Edwin H. Ellison described two patients with gastroduodenal and intestinal ulceration together with gastric hypersecretion and non–beta islet cell tumor of the pancreas. The incidence of Zollinger-Ellison syndrome varies from 0.1% to 1% of individuals presenting with PUD. Men are affected more than women, with the majority of patients presenting between ages 30 and 50.

Pathophysiology

Gastrin stimulates acid secretion through gastrin receptors on parietal cells and by inducing histamine release. It also exerts a trophic action on gastric epithelial cells. Long-standing hypergastrinemia leads to markedly increased gastric acid secretion through both parietal cell stimulation and increased parietal cell mass. This increased gastric acid output leads to the peptic ulcer disease, erosive esophagitis, and diarrhea.

Clinical Manifestations

Abdominal pain and peptic ulceration are seen in up to 90% of patients, diarrhea in 50% of patients, with 10% having diarrhea as their only symptom. Gastroesophageal reflux is seen in up to half of the patients. Initial presentation and ulcer location (duodenal bulb) may be indistinguishable from common PUD, but unusual locations (second part of the duodenum and beyond), ulcers refractory to standard medical therapy, and ulcer recurrence after acid-reducing surgery, ulcers presenting with frank complications (bleeding, obstruction, and perforation) create the suspicion of a gastrinoma. Gastrinomas can develop in the presence of multiple endocrine neoplasia type I (MEN I) syndrome, a disorder involving primarily three organ sites: the parathyroid glands (80%–90%), pancreas (40%–80%), and pituitary gland (30%–60%). In view of the stimulatory effect of calcium on gastric secretion, the hyperparathyroidism and hypercalcemia seen in MEN I patients may have a direct effect on ulcer disease. Resolution of hypercalcemia by parathyroidectomy reduces gastrin and gastric acid output in gastrinoma patients. An additional distinguishing

TABLE 12-3 Causes of Increased Fasting Serum Gastrin

Hypo- and achlorhydria (± pernicious anemia)	*Helicobacter pylori*
	Retained gastric antrum
	Gastric outlet obstruction
G-cell hyperplasia	Massive small bowel obstruction
Renal insufficiency	Vetiligo, diabetes mellitus
Rheumotoid arthritis	Patients on antisecretory drugs
Pheochromocytomas	Diabetes mellitus

feature in Zollinger-Ellison syndrome patients with MEN I is the higher incidence of gastric carcinoid tumor development compared to patients with sporadic gastrinomas.

Diagnosis

The first step in the evaluation of a patient with suspected ZES is to obtain a fasting gastrin level (**Table 12-3**). Multiple processes can lead to an elevated fasting gastrin level. Gastric acid induces feedback inhibition of gastrin release. A decrease in acid production will subsequently lead to failure of the feedback inhibitory pathway, resulting in net hypergastrinemia. Up to 50% of patients will have metastatic disease at the time of initial diagnosis.

Treatment

Patients with duodenal ulcers as part of the Zollinger-Ellison syndrome are initially treated with proton pump inhibitors followed by a maintenance dose guided by gastric acid measurements. Curative surgical resection of the gastrinoma is indicated in the absence of evidence of MEN I syndrome and metastatic disease.

Management of anesthesia for surgical excision of a gastrinoma takes into account the presence of gastric hypersecretion and the likely presence of large gastric fluid volumes at the time of anesthesia induction. Esophageal reflux is common in these patients despite the ability of gastrin to increase LES tone. Depletion of intravascular fluid volume and electrolyte imbalance (hypokalemia, metabolic alkalosis) may accompany profuse watery diarrhea. Associated endocrine abnormalities (MEN I syndrome) could also influence the management of anesthesia in these patients. Antacid prophylaxis with proton pump inhibitors and H_2-receptor antagonists is maintained until surgery. A preoperative coagulation screen and liver function test may be recommended, as alterations in fat absorption could influence clotting factors and hepatic function may be impaired by liver metastases. Intravenous administration of ranitidine is useful for preventing gastric acid hypersecretion during surgery.

POSTGASTRECTOMY SYNDROMES

A number of syndromes have been described following gastric operations performed for peptic ulcer or gastric neoplasm. The overall occurrence of severe postoperative symptoms is fortunately low, perhaps 1% to 3% of cases, but the disturbances can be disabling. The two most common postgastrectomy syndromes are dumping and alkaline reflux gastritis.

Dumping

The precise cause of dumping is not known but is believed to relate to the unmetered entry of ingested food into the proximal small bowel after vagotomy accompanied by either resection or division of the pyloric sphincter. Early dumping symptoms occur immediately after a meal and include nausea, epigastric discomfort, palpitations, and, in extreme cases, dizziness or syncope. Late dumping symptoms follow a meal by 1 to 3 hours and can include reactive hypoglycemia in addition to the aforementioned symptoms. Octreotide has been reported to improve dumping symptoms when 50 to 100 mg is administered subcutaneously before a meal. The beneficial effects of somatostatin on the vasomotor symptoms of dumping are postulated to occur as a result of pressor effects of the compound on splanchnic vessels. In addition, somatostatin analogues inhibit the release of vasoactive peptides from the gut, decrease peak plasma insulin levels, and slow intestinal transit.

Alkaline Reflux Gastritis

This syndrome is identified by the occurrence of the clinical triad of postprandial epigastric pain often associated with nausea and vomiting, evidence of reflux of bile into the stomach, and an associated histologic evidence of gastritis. There is no perfect solution for the treatment of alkaline reflux gastritis. Antacids, H_2-receptor antagonists, bile acid chelators, and dietary manipulations have not been demonstrated definitely to be beneficial. The only proved treatment for alkaline reflux gastritis is the operative diversion of intestinal contents from contact with the gastric mucosa. The most common surgical procedure used for this purpose is a Roux-en-Y gastrojejunostomy.

IRRITABLE BOWEL SYNDROME

Patients with irritable bowel syndrome (spastic or mucous colitis) often complain of generalized bowel discomfort, usually confined to the left lower quadrant. Commonly, the frequency of stools is increased and the stool is covered with mucus. Many patients have associated symptoms of vasomotor instability, including tachycardia, hyperventilation, fatigue, diaphoresis, and headaches. Air trapped in the splenic flexure may produce pain in the left shoulder, radiating down the left arm (splenic flexure syndrome). Despite the frequent occurrence of irritable bowel syndrome, there is no known specific etiologic agent or structural or biochemical defect.

INFLAMMATORY BOWEL DISEASE

Inflammatory bowel diseases are the second most common chronic inflammatory disorders after rheumatoid arthritis. The diagnosis of ulcerative colitis (UC) and Crohn's disease (CD), and the differentiation between them is based on nonspecific clinical and histologic patterns often obscured by intercurrent infections or iatrogenic events or that are altered by medications or surgery. The incidence rates of UC and CD in the United States are approximately 11 per 100,000 and 7 per 100,000. The peak age at onset of UC and CD is between 15 and 30 years and between the ages of 60 and 80, respectively. The male-to-female ratio for UC is 1:1 and is 1.1:1.8 for CD.

Ulcerative Colitis

UC is a mucosal disease for which treatment involves the rectum and extends proximally to involve all or part of the colon. Approximately 40% to 50% of patients will have disease limited to the rectum and rectosigmoid, 30% to 40% have disease extending beyond the sigmoid but not involving the whole colon, and 20% have a total colitis. Proximal spread occurs in continuity without areas of spared mucosa. In more severe disease, the mucosa is hemorrhagic, edematous, and ulcerated. In long-standing disease, inflammatory polyps (pseudopolyps) may be present. In patients with many years of disease, the mucosa appears atrophic and featureless and the entire colon narrows and shortens. The major symptoms of UC are diarrhea, rectal bleeding, tenesmus, passage of mucus, and crampy abdominal pain. Other symptoms in moderate to severe disease include anorexia, nausea, vomiting, fever, and weight loss. Active disease can be associated with an increase in acute-phase reactants (C-reactive protein, orosomucoid levels), platelet count, erythrocyte sedimentation rate, and a decrease in hemoglobin. In severely ill patients, the serum albumin level will fall rather quickly, and leukocytosis may be present.

Complications

Catastrophic illness is an initial presentation of only 15% of patients with UC. In 1% of patients, a severe attack may be accompanied by massive hemorrhage, which usually stops with treatment of the underlying disease. However, if the patient requires six to eight units of blood within 24 to 48 hours, colectomy is frequently the treatment of choice. Toxic megacolon is defined as a dilated transverse colon with loss of haustration. It occurs in approximately 5% of attacks and can be triggered by electrolyte abnormalities and narcotics. Approximately 50% of all acute dilatations will resolve with medical therapy alone, but urgent colectomy is required for those that do not improve with conservative treatment. Perforation is the most dangerous of the local complications (mortality rate is approximately 15%), and the physical signs of peritonitis may not be obvious, especially if the patient is receiving glucocorticoids. Some patients can develop toxic colitis and such severe ulcerations that the bowel may perforate without first dilating. Obstructions caused by benign stricture formation occur in 10% of patients.

Crohn's Disease

Although CD usually presents as acute or chronic bowel inflammation, the inflammatory process evolves toward one of two patterns of disease: a penetrating-fistulous pattern or an obstructing pattern, each with different treatments and prognoses.

ILEOCOLITIS

The most common site of inflammation is the terminal ileum; therefore, the usual presentation of ileocolitis is a chronic history of recurrent episodes of right lower quadrant pain and diarrhea. Sometimes the initial presentation mimics acute appendicitis with pronounced right lower quadrant pain, a palpable mass, fever, and leukocytosis. A high-spiking fever suggests intra-abdominal abscess formation. Weight loss is common, typically 10% to 20% of body weight, and develops as a consequence of diarrhea, anorexia, and fear of eating. An inflammatory mass may be palpated in the right lower quadrant of the abdomen. Extension of the mass can cause obstruction of the right ureter or bladder inflammation, manifested by dysuria and fever. Bowel obstruction may take several forms. In the early stages of disease, bowel wall edema and spasm produce intermittent obstructive manifestations and increasing symptoms of postprandial pain. Over several years, persistent inflammation gradually progresses to fibrostenotic narrowing and stricture. Diarrhea will decrease and be replaced by chronic bowel obstruction. Severe inflammation of the ileocecal region may lead to localized wall thinning, with microperforation and fistula formation to the adjacent bowel, the skin, the urinary bladder, or to an abscess cavity in the mesentery.

JEJUNOILEITIS

Extensive inflammatory disease is associated with a loss of digestive and absorptive surfaces, resulting in malabsorption and steatorrhea. Nutritional deficiencies can also result from poor intake and enteric losses of protein and other nutrients causing hypoalbuminemia, hypocalcemia, hypomagnesemia, coagulopathy, and hyperoxaluria with nephrolithiasis. Vertebral fractures are caused by a combination of vitamin D deficiency, hypocalcemia, and prolonged glucocorticoid use. Pellagra from niacin deficiency can occur in extensive small-bowel disease, and malabsorption of vitamin B_{12} can lead to a megaloblastic anemia and neurologic symptoms.

Diarrhea is a sign of active disease due to bacterial overgrowth in obstructive stasis or fistulization, bile-acid malabsorption due to a diseased or resected terminal ileum, and intestinal inflammation with decreased water absorption and increased secretion of electrolytes.

COLITIS AND PERIANAL DISEASE

Patients with colitis present with low-grade fevers, malaise, diarrhea, crampy abdominal pain, and sometimes hematochezia. Gross bleeding is not as common as in UC and appears in approximately half of patients with exclusively colonic disease. Only 1% to 2% bleed massively. Pain is caused by passage of fecal material through narrowed and inflamed segments of large bowel. Toxic megacolon is rare but may be seen with severe inflammation and short-duration disease. Stricturing can produce symptoms of bowel obstruction. Colonic disease may fistulize into the stomach or duodenum, causing feculent vomiting, or to the proximal or mid small bowel, causing malabsorption by "short circuiting" bacterial overgrowth.

GASTRODUODENAL DISEASE

Symptoms and signs of upper GI tract disease include nausea, vomiting, and epigastric pain. Patients usually have a *H. pylori*–negative gastritis. The second portion of the duodenum is more commonly involved than the bulb. Patients with advanced gastroduodenal CD may develop a chronic gastric outlet obstruction.

Extraintestinal Manifestations

Up to one third of patients have at least one. Patients with perianal CD are at higher risk of developing extraintestinal manifestations (**Table 12-4**).

Treatment

CD is a recurring disorder that cannot be cured with surgical resection. As such, surgery is intended to provide palliation. Current surgical alternatives for treatment of obstructing CD include resection of the diseased segment and strictureplasty. A diverting colostomy may help heal severe perianal disease or rectovaginal fistulas, but disease almost always recurs with reanastomosis. Often, these patients require a total proctocolectomy and ileostomy. Resection of one half to two thirds of the small bowel represents the upper limit of safety. Fortunately, only in rare instances does a true short-gut syndrome occur. In many such cases, the short-gut syndrome can be managed with dietary manipulations. Less than 1% of patients with CD require long-term total parenteral nutrition.

Surgical Treatment

Nearly half of patients with extensive chronic UC undergo surgery within the first 10 years of their illness. The indications for surgery are listed. Morbidity is approximately 20% in elective, 30% in urgent, and 40% in emergency proctocolectomy. The risks are primarily hemorrhage, sepsis, and neural injury. Although single-stage total proctocolectomy with ileostomy has traditionally been the operation of choice, newer operations maintain continence while surgically removing the involved rectal mucosa (**Table 12-5**).

Medical Treatment

Sulfasalazine is the mainstay of therapy for mild to moderate disease. It was originally developed to deliver both antibacterial (sulfapyridine) and anti-inflammatory (5-acetylsalicylic acid) therapy into the connective tissues of joints and the colonic mucosa. 5-Acetylsalicylic acid agents are effective in

TABLE 12–4 Extraintestinal Manifestation of Inflammatory Bowel Disease

Dermatologic	Erythema nodosum in 10%–15% of IBD; pyoderma gangrenosum in 1%–12%
Rheumatologic	Peripheral arthritis develops in 15% to 20% of IBD
Ocular	1%–10% of IBD; conjunctivitis, anterior uveitis/iritis, and episcleritis
Hepatobiliary	Approximately 50% of IBD; hepatomegaly; fatty liver due to chronic debilitating illness, malnutrition, and glucocorticoid therapy; cholelithiasis caused by malabsorption of bile acids; primary sclerosing cholangitis leading to biliary cirrhosis and hepatic failure
Urologic	Calculi in 10%–20%; ureteral obstruction
Others	Thromboembolic disease (pulmonary embolism, cerebrovascular accidents, and arterial emboli) due to thrombocytosis; increased levels of fibrinopeptide A, factor V, factor VIII, and fibrinogen; accelerated thromboplastin generation; antithrombin III deficiency due to increased gut losses or increased catabolism; free protein S deficiency, endocarditis, myocarditis, pleuropericarditis, and interstitial lung disease, secondary/reactive amyloidosis

IBD, inflammatory bowel disease.

TABLE 12–5 Surgical Indications: Inflammatory Bowel Disease

Ulcerative Colitis
Massive hemorrhage, perforation, toxic megacolon obstruction, intractable and fulminant disease, cancer

Crohn's Disease
Stricture, obstruction, hemorrhage, abscess, fistulas, intractable and fulminant disease, cancer and unresponsive perianal disease

inducing remission in both UC and CD and in maintaining remission in UC. Up to 30% of patients experience allergic reactions or intolerable side effects such as headache, anorexia, nausea, and vomiting that are attributable to the sulfapyridine moiety. Hypersensitivity reactions, independent of sulfapyridine levels, include rash, fever, hepatitis, agranulocytosis, hypersensitivity pneumonitis, pancreatitis, worsening of colitis, and impairment of folate absorption. Newer sulfa-free aminosalicylate preparations deliver increased amounts of the pharmacologically active ingredients, of sulfasalazine (5-acetylsalicylic acid, mesalamine), to the site of active bowel disease while limiting systemic toxicity. The most commonly used drugs besides sulfasalazine in the United States are Asacol and Pentasa (mesalamine). Asacol is an enteric-coated form of mesalamine, but it has a slightly different release pattern, with 5-acetylsalicylic acid liberated at a pH greater than 7.0.

The majority of patients with moderate to severe UC benefit from oral or parenteral glucocorticoids. Prednisone is usually started at doses of 40 to 60 mg/day for active UC that is unresponsive to sulfa therapy. Parenteral glucocorticoids or corticotropin is occasionally preferred for glucocorticoid-naive patients despite a risk of adrenal hemorrhage. Topically applied glucocorticoids are also beneficial for distal colitis and may serve as an adjunct in those who have rectal involvement plus more proximal disease. These glucocorticoids are significantly absorbed from the rectum and can lead to adrenal suppression with prolonged administration. Glucocorticoids are also effective for treatment of moderate to severe CD. Controlled ileal-release budesonide has been nearly equal to prednisone for ileocolonic CD with fewer glucocorticoid side effects. Steroids play no role in maintenance therapy in either UC or CD. Once clinical remission has been induced, they should be tapered and discontinued.

Antibiotics have no role in the treatment of active or quiescent UC. However, pouchitis, which occurs in approximately one third of UC patients after colectomy, usually responds to treatment with metronidazole or ciprofloxacin. These two antibiotics should be used as second-line therapy in active CD after 5-acetylsalicylic acid agents and as first-line drugs in perianal and fistulous CD.

Azathioprine and 6-mercaptopurine are purine analogues commonly used in the management of glucocorticoid-dependent irritable bowel syndrome. Azathioprine is rapidly absorbed and converted to 6-mercaptopurine, which is then metabolized to thioinosinic acid, an inhibitor of purine ribonucleotide synthesis and cell proliferation. Efficacy is typically seen within 3 to 4 weeks. Pancreatitis occurs in 3% to 4% of patients, typically within the first few weeks of therapy, and is completely reversible when the drug is stopped. Other side effects include nausea, fever, rash, and hepatitis. Bone marrow suppression (particularly leukopenia) is dose related and often delayed.

Methotrexate inhibits dihydrofolate reductase, resulting in impaired DNA synthesis. Additional anti-inflammatory properties may be related to decreased IL-1 production. Potential toxicities include leukopenia, hepatic fibrosis, hypersensitivity, and pneumonitis.

Cyclosporine alters the immune response by acting as a potent inhibitor of T cell–mediated responses. Although cyclosporine acts primarily via inhibition of IL-2 production from T helper cells, it also decreases recruitment of cytotoxic T cells and blocks other cytokines, including IL-3, IL-4, interferon-γ, and tumor necrosis factor. It has a more rapid onset of action than 6-mercaptopurine and azathioprine. Renal function should be monitored frequently. Hypertension, gingival hyperplasia, hypertrichosis, paresthesias, tremors, headaches, and electrolyte abnormalities are common side effects. Creatinine elevation calls for dose reduction or discontinuation.

PSEUDOMEMBRANOUS ENTEROCOLITIS

Pseudomembranous enterocolitis is attributable to unknown causes, although it is often associated with antibiotic therapy (especially clindamycin and lincomycin), bowel obstruction, uremia, congestive heart failure, and intestinal ischemia. Clinical manifestations include fever, watery diarrhea, dehydration, hypotension, cardiac dysrhythmias, skeletal muscle weakness, intestinal ileus, and metabolic acidosis.

CARCINOID TUMORS

The incidence of clinically significant carcinoids is seven to 13 cases per million per year. Carcinoid tumors can occur in almost any GI tissue. However, at present, most (70%) originate from one of three sites: bronchus, jejuno-ileum, or colon/rectum. For common produced substances, see **Table 12-6**.

Carcinoid Tumors without Carcinoid Syndrome

Carcinoid tumors (**Table 12-7**) are usually found incidentally during surgery for suspected appendicitis. Because of the vagueness of the symptoms, the diagnosis is usually delayed approximately 2 years from the onset of the symptoms.

Carcinoid Tumors with Systemic Symptoms Due to Secreted Products

Carcinoid tumors can contain numerous GI peptides including gastrin, insulin, somatostatin, motilin, neurotensin, tachykinins (substance K, substance P, neuropeptide K), glucagon, gastrin-releasing peptide, vasoactive intestinal peptide, pancreatic peptide, other biologically active peptides (corticotropin, calcitonin, growth hormone), prostaglandins, and bioactive amines (serotonin). These substances may or may not be released in sufficient amounts to cause symptoms. Foregut carcinoids are more likely to produce various GI peptides than midgut carcinoids.

Carcinoid Syndrome

The syndrome occurs in approximately 20% of patients with carcinoids as a result of the massive amounts of circulating hormones reaching the systemic circulation. The two most common symptoms are flushing and diarrhea. The characteristic flush is of sudden onset. Physically it appears as a deep red blush, especially in the neck and face, often associated with a feeling of warmth, and occasionally associated with pruritus, lacrimation, diarrhea, or facial edema. Flushes may be precipitated by stress, alcohol, exercise, certain foods such as cheese, or agents such as catecholamines, pentagastrin, and serotonin reuptake inhibitors. Cardiac manifestations may occur and are due to fibrosis involving the endocardium, primarily on the right side. Left side lesions can occur with pulmonary involvement or through a right-to-left intracardiac shunt. Pulmonic stenosis is usually predominant, whereas the tricuspid valve is often fixed open, resulting in regurgitation. Carcinoid triad is cardiac involvement with flushing and diarrhea. Other clinical manifestations include wheezing or asthma-like symptoms and pellagra-like skin lesions. In addition, increased fibrous tissue may be seen including retroperitoneal fibrosis causing urethral obstruction.

In 90% to 100% of patients with carcinoid syndrome, serotonin is overproduced and is thought to be predominantly responsible for the diarrhea through its effects on gut motility and intestinal secretion. Serotonin receptor antagonists (especially 5-HT$_3$ antagonists) relieve the diarrhea in most patients. Serotonin does not appear to be involved in the flushing. In patients with gastric carcinoids, the red, patchy pruritic flush is likely due to histamine release and can be prevented by H$_1$- and H$_2$-receptor antagonists. Both histamine and serotonin may be responsible for the bronchial constriction. Atrial natriuretic peptide overproduction is also reported in patients with cardiac disease, but its precise role in the pathogenesis is unknown.

One of the most life-threatening complications of the carcinoid syndrome is the development of a carcinoid crisis. Clinically, this is represented as an intense flushing, diarrhea, abdominal pain, and cardiovascular manifestations including tachycardia, hypertension, or hypotension. If not adequately treated, it can be fatal. The crises may occur spontaneously or be provoked by stress, chemotherapy, or a biopsy. For drugs involved with crisis, see **Table 12-8**.

TABLE 12–6 Substances Produced by Carcinoid Tumors at Various Locations			
	Foregut	**Midgut**	**Hindgut**
Serotonin (5-HT)	Low	High	Rarely
Other substances	ACTH, 5-HTP, GRF	Tachykinins (substance P, neuropeptide K, substance K); rarely 5HTP, ACTH	Rarely 5HTP, ACTH; contains numerous peptides
Carcinoid syndrome	Atypical	Typical	Rare
ACTH, corticotropin; GRF, growth hormone releasing factor; 5-HTP, 5–hydroxy–L–tryptophan.			

TABLE 12–7 Location and Presentation of Carcinoid Tuncas	
Carcinoid Location	**Presentation**
Small intestine	Abdominal pain (51%), intestinal obstruction (31%), tumor (17%), gastrointestinal bleed (11%)
Rectal	Bleeding (39%), constipation (17%), diarrhea (17%)
Bronchial	Asymptomatic (31%)
Thymic	Anterior mediastinal masses
Ovarian and testicular	Masses discovered on physical examination or ultrasonography
Metastatic	In the liver; frequently presents as hepatomegaly

TABLE 12–8 Pharmacologic Agents Associated with Carcinoid Crisis
Drugs That May Provoke Mediator Release
Succinylcholine, mivacurium, atracurium, d-tubocurarine Epinephrine, norepinephrine, dopamine, isoproterenol, and thiopental
Drugs Not Known to Release Mediators
Propofol, etomidate, vecuronium, cisatracurium, rocuronium, sufentanil, alfentanil, fentanyl, remifentanil. All inhalation agents; desflurance may be the better choice in patients with liver metastasis because of its low rate of metabolism

The diagnosis of carcinoid syndrome relies on measurement of urinary or plasma serotonin or its metabolites in the urine. The measurement of 5-hydroxyindoleacetic acid is most frequently used. False-positive elevations may occur if the patient is eating serotonin-rich foods, such as bananas, pineapple, walnuts, pecans, avocados, and hickory nuts or taking certain medications, such as cough syrup containing guaifenesin, acetaminophen, salicylates, or L-dopa.

Management of Anesthesia

Increased levels of serotonin have been associated with delayed awakening. Administration of octreotide prior to manipulation of the tumor will attenuate most adverse hemodynamic responses. Use of epidural analgesia in patients who have been adequately treated with octreotide is a safe technique provided the local anesthetic is administered in a graded manner accompanied by careful hemodynamic monitoring. The sympathetic blockade produced by epidural or spinal anesthesia may worsen hypotension, which can be minimized by dosing the epidural catheter with opioids or dilute local anesthetic solutions. Ondansetron, a serotonin antagonist, is a useful and logical antiemetic choice. Invasive arterial blood pressure monitoring may be necessary during the intraoperative management of patients with carcinoid syndrome because of rapid changes in hemodynamic variables.

Treatment

Treatment includes avoiding conditions that precipitate flushing, dietary supplementation with nicotinamide, treatment of heart failure, treatment of wheezing, and controlling the diarrhea with antidiarrheal agents such as loperamide or diphenoxylate. If patients still have symptoms, serotonin receptor antagonists or somatostatin analogues are the drugs of choice. They have a very short half-life of approximately 3 minutes and therefore must be given as infusions. There are 14 subclasses of serotonin receptors and antagonists for most

are not available. The 5-HT$_1$ and 5-HT$_2$ receptor antagonists methysergide, cyproheptadine, and ketanserin have all been used to control diarrhea but usually do not decrease flushing. The use of methysergide is limited because it can cause or enhance retroperitoneal fibrosis. 5-HT$_3$ receptor antagonists (ondansetron, tropisetron, alosetron) can control diarrhea and nausea in majority of patients and occasionally ameliorate the flushing. A combination of histamine H$_1$- and H$_2$-receptor antagonists (i.e., diphenhydramine and cimetidine or ranitidine) may be useful in controlling the flushing in patients with foregut carcinoids.

Synthetic analogues of somatostatin octreotide controls symptoms in more than 80% of patients. Lanreotide is now the most widely used agent to control the symptoms of patients with carcinoid syndrome. These drugs are effective in relieving symptoms and decreasing urinary 5-hydroxyacetic acid levels. In patients with carcinoid crises, somatostatin analogues are effective in both treating the condition as well as preventing its development during known precipitating events such as surgery, anesthesia, chemotherapy, and stress. Octreotide (150–250 μg SC every 6 to 8 hours) should be administered 24 to 48 hours before anesthesia and then continued throughout the procedure. Short-term side effects occur in 40% to 60% of patients receiving subcutaneous somatostatin analogues. Pain at the injection site and side effects related to the GI tract (59% discomfort, 15% nausea) are the most common. Important long-term side effects include gallstone formation, steatorrhea, and deterioration in glucose tolerance. Aprotinin has been used for hypotension if octreotide treatment is not effective. Interferon-alfa controls symptoms of the carcinoid syndrome either alone or combined with hepatic artery embolization. Hepatic artery embolization alone or with chemotherapy (chemoembolization) has been used to control the symptoms of carcinoid syndrome. Parachlorophenylanine can inhibit tryptophan hydroxylase and therefore the conversion of tryptophan to 5-hydroxy-L-tryptophan. However, its severe side effects, including psychiatric disturbances, make it intolerable for long-term use. α-Methyldopa inhibits the conversion of 5-hydroxy-L-tryptophan to serotonin. Its effects are only partial.

Surgery is the only potentially curative therapy for nonmetastatic carcinoid tumors.

ACUTE PANCREATITIS

Acute pancreatitis is characterized as an inflammatory disorder of the pancreas in which normal pancreatic function is restored once the primary cause of the acute event is resolved. Pancreatic autodigestion is the most likely explanation for the pathogenesis of acute pancreatitis. The incidence of acute pancreatitis has increased 10-fold since the 1960s, perhaps reflecting increased alcohol abuse and/or improved diagnostic techniques.

Etiology

Gallstones and alcohol abuse are etiologic factors in 60% to 80% of patients with acute pancreatitis. Gallstones are believed to cause pancreatitis by transiently obstructing the ampulla of Vater, leading to pancreatic ductal hypertension. Acute pancreatitis is common in patients with acquired immunodeficiency syndrome and those with hyperparathyroidism and associated hypercalcemia. Trauma-induced acute pancreatitis is usually associated with blunt trauma rather than penetrating injury to the upper abdomen, reflecting compression of the pancreas against the spine. Postoperative pancreatitis has been described after abdominal and thoracic surgery, especially with the use of cardiopulmonary bypass. Clinical pancreatitis develops in 1% to 2% of patients following endoscopic retrograde cholangiopancreatography.

Signs and Symptoms

Excruciating, unrelenting mid-epigastric abdominal pain that radiates to the back occurs in almost every patient who develops acute pancreatitis. Patients find that sitting and leaning forward decreases the pain. Nausea and vomiting occur at the peak of the pain. Abdominal distention with ileus often develops. Dyspnea may reflect the presence of pleural effusions or ascites. Fever may appear despite the absence of an identifiable infection, and shock occurs in nearly half of these patients. Obtundation and psychosis often reflect delirium tremens associated with alcohol withdrawal. Development of tetany may reflect hypocalcemia. Most patients with acute pancreatitis have a benign course.

Diagnosis

The hallmark of acute pancreatitis is an increased serum amylase concentration. Contrast-enhanced computed tomography is the best noninvasive test for documenting the morphologic changes associated with acute pancreatitis. Endoscopic retrograde cholangiopancreatography is useful for evaluating traumatic pancreatitis (localization of injury) and severe gallstone pancreatitis (endoscopic drainage). The differential diagnosis of acute pancreatitis includes a perforated duodenal ulcer, acute cholecystitis, mesenteric ischemia, and bowel obstruction. Acute myocardial infarction may cause severe abdominal pain, but the serum amylase concentrations are

usually not increased. Patients with pneumonia may present with severe epigastric pain and fever.

Ranson Criteria
- Age older than 55
- White blood cell count more than $16 \times 10{-9}/L$
- Blood urea more than 16 mmol/L
- Aspartate transaminase more than 250 U/L
- Arterial Po_2 less than 8 kPa (60 mm Hg)
- Fluid deficit more than 6L
- Blood glucose more than 200 mg/dL, no history of DM
- Lactate dehydrogenase more than 350 IU/L
- Corrected calcium less than 8 mg/dL
- Decreasing hematocrit more than 10
- Metabolic acidosis with base deficit more than 4 mmol/L
(Note that the serum amylase value is not one of the criteria.)
   The mortality per positive criterion:
- Number of positive criteria:
- 0 to 2: less than 5% mortality
- 3 to 4: 20% mortality
- 5 to 6: 40% mortality
- 7 to 8: 100% mortality

Complications

Nearly 25% of the patients who develop acute pancreatitis experience significant complications. Shock develops early in the course of severe acute pancreatitis and is a major risk factor for death. Sequestration of large volumes of fluid in the peripancreatic space, hemorrhage, and decreased systemic vascular resistance contribute to hypotension. Arterial hypoxemia is often present early in the course of the disease; acute respiratory distress syndrome is seen in 20% of patients. Renal failure occurs in 25% of patients and is associated with a poor prognosis. GI hemorrhage and coagulation defects from disseminated intravascular coagulation may occur. Pancreatic infection is a serious complication associated with more than 50% mortality.

Treatment

Aggressive intravenous fluid administration (up to 10 L of crystalloid) is necessary as significant hypovolemia occurs even in patients with mild pancreatitis. Colloid replacement may be necessary if there is significant bleeding or albumin loss into interstitial spaces. Oral intake is stopped on the presumption that it "rests" the pancreas and accompanying ileus. Further attempts to suppress pancreatic secretions with nasogastric suction or administration of H_2-receptor antagonists provide no additional benefit. Nasogastric suction is needed only to treat persistent vomiting or ileus. Opioids administered intravenously are likely to be necessary to manage the severe pain. Prophylactic antibiotic therapy may be instituted in patients with necrotizing pancreatitis. Endoscopic removal of obstructing gallstones is indicated within the first 24 to 72 hours of the onset of symptoms to decrease the risk of cholangitis. Parenteral feeding is indicated if it is anticipated that patients will experience a protracted course.

CHRONIC PANCREATITIS

The true incidence of chronic pancreatitis is difficult to determine as the disease may be clinically asymptomatic or abdominal pain is attributed to other causes. The chronic inflammation characteristic of chronic pancreatitis leads to irreversible damage to the pancreas.

Etiology

Chronic pancreatitis is most often due to chronic alcohol abuse, accounting for 80% to 90% of affected patients. Diets high in protein seem to predispose alcoholic patients to the development of chronic pancreatitis. Idiopathic chronic pancreatitis is the second most common form of this disease. Chronic pancreatitis occasionally occurs in association with cystic fibrosis or hyperparathyroidism (hypercalcemia) or as a hereditary disease transmitted by an autosomal dominant gene.

Signs and Symptoms

Chronic pancreatitis, often characterized by epigastric abdominal pain that radiates to the back and often postprandial, is nevertheless painless in 10% to 30% of patients. Steatorrhea is present when at least 90% of the pancreas is destroyed. Diabetes mellitus eventually manifests, although the development of ketoacidosis is uncommon. Pancreatic calcifications develop in most alcohol-induced chronic pancreatitis.

Diagnosis

The diagnosis of chronic pancreatitis may be based on the history of chronic alcohol abuse and demonstration of pancreatic calcifications. Patients who develop chronic pancreatitis are often thin and appear emaciated; serum amylase concentrations are usually normal. Once exocrine secretions are decreased to the point that enzymes entering the duodenum are 10% to 20% of normal; maldigestion of proteins and fats is evident. An abdominal radiograph may reveal pancreatic calcifications. Ultrasonography is useful for documenting the presence of an enlarged pancreas or identifying a fluid-filled pseudocyst. Computed tomography in patients with chronic pancreatitis demonstrates dilated pancreatic ducts and changes in the size of the pancreas. Endoscopic retrograde cholangiopancreatography is the most sensitive imaging test for detecting early changes in the pancreatic ducts caused by chronic pancreatitis.

Treatment

Treatment of chronic pancreatitis includes management of pain, malabsorption, and diabetes mellitus. Opioids may be required for adequate pain control, and in some patients, celiac plexus block may be considered. An internal surgical drainage procedure (pancreaticojejunostomy) or endoscopic placement of stents and extraction of stones may be helpful in patients who are otherwise resistant to medical management of pain. Enzyme supplement (lipase) is administered to permit fat digestion.

MALABSORPTION AND MALDIGESTION

Malabsorption of nutrients is reflected by impaired absorption of fat (steatorrhea), although other substances (iron, calcium, bile salts, specific amino acids, saccharides) may be selectively poorly absorbed in the absence of steatorrhea. Steatorrhea is most likely due to small bowel disease, liver or biliary tract disease, or pancreatic exocrine insufficiency. Patients with small bowel disease may develop hypoalbuminemia due to a protein leak through diseased intestinal mucosa. Fat-soluble vitamin deficiencies (vitamins A, D, E, K), hypocalcemia, and hypomagnesemia may be present in patients with liver and biliary tract disease.

Gluten-Sensitive Enteropathy

Gluten-sensitive enteropathy (previously termed celiac disease in children or nontropical sprue in adults) is a disease of the small intestine resulting in malabsorption (steatorrhea), weight loss, abdominal pain, and fatigue. Treatment is removal of gluten (wheat, rye, barley) from the diet.

Small Bowel Resection

Massive small bowel resection (mesenteric ischemia, volvulus, CD) may result in malabsorption if the small intestinal surface area that remains for absorption is decreased below critical levels. Clinical manifestations of the resulting short bowel syndrome include diarrhea, steatorrhea, trace element deficiencies, and electrolyte imbalance (hyponatremia, hypokalemia). Total parenteral nutrition is needed only if multiple small feedings are not effective.

GASTROINTESTINAL BLEEDING

GI bleeding (**Table 12-9**) most often originates from the upper GI tract (peptic ulcer) and is a common reason for hospital admission. Bleeding from the lower GI tract (diverticulosis) accounts for 10% to 20% of all cases of GI bleeding and primarily affects elderly patients.

Upper Gastrointestinal Bleeding

Patients with acute upper GI bleeding may experience hypotension and tachycardia if blood loss exceeds approximately 25% of the total blood volume (1500 mL in adults). Most patients with evidence of acute hypovolemia (orthostatic hypotension characterized by decreases in systolic blood pressure of 10 to 20 mm Hg and corresponding increases in heart rate) have hematocrits less than 30%. The hematocrit may be normal early in the course of acute hemorrhage because of the insufficient time for equilibration of the plasma volume. Melena usually indicates that bleeding has occurred at a site above the cecum.

TABLE 12–9	Causes of Upper and Lower Gastrointestinal Bleeding	
Causes		**Incidence (%)**
Upper gastrointestinal bleeding		
Peptic ulcer		
Duodenal ulcer		36
Gastric ulcer		24
Mucosal erosive disease		
Gastritis		6
Esophagitis		6
Esophageal varices		6
Mallory-Weiss tear		3
Malignancy		2
Lower gastrointestinal bleeding		
Colonic diverticulosis		42
Colorectal malignancy		9
Ischemic colitis		9
Acute colitis of unknown causes		5
Hemorrhoids		5

Adapted from Young HS: Gastrointestinal bleeding. Sci Am Med 1998;1–10.

The blood urea nitrogen concentration is usually higher than 40 mg/dL because of the absorbed nitrogen load in the small intestine. Elderly individuals with esophageal variceal bleeding, those with malignancy, and those who develop bleeding after hospitalization for other comorbid diseases have an acute mortality rate higher than 30%. Multiple organ system failure, rather than hemorrhage, is the usual cause of death in these patients. Endoscopy following hemodynamic stabilization is the diagnostic procedure of choice in patients with acute upper GI bleeding.

For patients with bleeding peptic ulcers, endoscopic coagulation (thermotherapy, injection with epinephrine or a sclerosant) is indicated when active bleeding is visible. Patients receiving anticoagulants can be safely treated with endoscopic coagulation. Perforation occurs in approximately 0.5% of patients undergoing endoscopic coagulation. Endoscopic ligation of bleeding esophageal varices is as effective as sclerotherapy. A transjugular intrahepatic portosystemic shunt may be used in patients with esophageal variceal bleeding resistant to control by endoscopic coagulation or sclerotherapy and can lead to worsening of encephalopathy and liver ischemia due to increased shunting. Surgical treatment of nonvariceal upper GI bleeding (oversewing an ulcer, gastrectomy for diffuse hemorrhagic gastritis) is used in patients who continue to bleed despite optimal supportive therapy and in whom endoscopic coagulation is unsuccessful.

Lower Gastrointestinal Bleeding

Lower GI (colonic) bleeding usually occurs in elderly patients and typically presents as abrupt passage of bright red blood and clots. In contrast to those with upper GI bleeding, the BUN concentration is not likely to be significantly increased in these patients.

Sigmoidoscopy to exclude anorectal lesions is indicated as soon as patients are hemodynamically stable. Colonoscopy can be performed only after the bowel has been purged with polyethylene glycol solution. If bleeding is persistent and brisk, angiography and possibly embolic therapy may be attempted. Up to 15% of patients with lower GI bleeding require surgical intervention to control it.

Occult Gastrointestinal Bleeding

Occult GI bleeding may present as unexplained iron deficiency anemia or as intermittent positive tests for blood in the patient's feces. Peptic ulcer disease and colonic neoplasm are the most common causes of occult GI bleeding. The site of occult bleeding is determined by upper GI endoscopic examination or colonoscopy. Others can be diagnosed by tagged red blood cell bleeding scan and angiography.

DIVERTICULOSIS AND DIVERTICULITIS

Colonic diverticula, herniations of the mucosa and submucosa through the muscularis propria, occur most often in individuals who consume low-fiber diets. Diverticulitis occurs with inflammation of one or more diverticula, mostly in sigmoid or descending colon. Mild diverticulitis typically manifests with fever, lower abdominal pain, and lower abdominal tenderness. Nausea, vomiting, constipation, diarrhea, dysuria, tachycardia, and an elevated white blood cell count with a left shift may be noted. Right-sided colonic diverticulitis is usually indistinguishable from appendicitis. Severe diverticulitis is characterized by development of a diverticular abscess that may rupture and produce purulent peritonitis. Fistula formation, when it occurs, is most commonly from the sigmoid colon to the bladder. Abdominal computed tomography is the most useful study for early evaluation of suspected diverticulitis.

Treatment for mild distress in a patient tolerating oral hydration should include 7 to 10 days of oral broad-spectrum antimicrobial therapy, which includes anaerobic coverage. Most patients with diverticulitis severe enough to require hospitalization can be treated with intravenous fluids, bowel rest, broad-spectrum antibiotics, and analgesics. If, despite maximal therapy, the patient does not improve within 48 hours, complications of diverticulitis probably exist and further therapy is necessary. Surgical treatment of acute diverticulitis is resection of the diseased segment of colon. Although reversal of nondepolarizing muscle relaxants with anticholinesterase drugs increases GI intraluminal pressure, there is no evidence that it results in a risk of colon suture line dehiscence (**Fig. 12-1**).

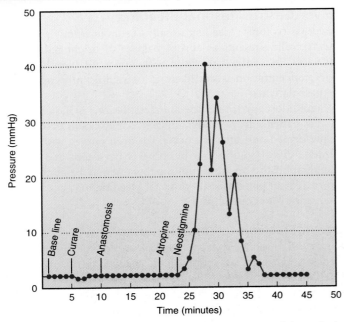

Figure 12-1 • Intraluminal colonic pressure was measured in a single anesthetized dog after division of the colon and a standard two-layer anastomosis. There was no evidence that the neostigmine-induced increase in intracolonic pressure caused disruption of the freshly completed bowel anastomosis. *(Adapted from Yellin YE, Newman J, Donovan AJ: Neostigmine-induced hyperperistalsis: Effects of security of colonic anastomoses. Arch Surg 1973;106:779–781.)*

APPENDICITIS

Incidence and Epidemiology

The peak incidence of acute appendicitis is in the second and third decades of life. It is relatively rare at the extremes of age. Perforation is more common in infancy and in the aged, during which periods mortality rates are highest. The mortality rate has decreased steadily in Europe and the United States from 8.1 per 100,000 of the population in 1941 to less than 1 per 100,000 in 1970 and subsequently. The overall incidence of appendicitis is much lower in underdeveloped countries, especially parts of Africa, and in lower socioeconomic groups.

Pathogenesis

Luminal obstruction can be identified in only 30% to 40% of cases, and ulceration of the mucosa is the initial event in the majority. Obstruction, when present, is most commonly caused by a fecalith. Enlarged lymphoid follicles associated with viral infections (e.g., measles), inspissated barium,

worms (e.g., pinworms, ascaris, tinea) and tumors (e.g., carcinoid, carcinoma) may also obstruct the lumen. Luminal bacteria multiply and invade the appendiceal wall as venous engorgement, and subsequent arterial compromise results from the high intraluminal pressures. Finally, gangrene and perforation can occur. Although infrequently, if the process evolves slowly, adjacent organs such as the terminal ileum, cecum, and omentum may wall off the appendiceal area so that a localized abscess will develop, whereas rapid progression of vascular impairment may cause perforation with free access to the peritoneal cavity.

Clinical Manifestations

The history and sequence of symptoms are important diagnostic features of appendicitis. The initial symptom is almost invariably mild abdominal pain of the visceral type, often cramping, resulting from appendiceal contractions or distention of the lumen. It is usually poorly localized in the periumbilical or epigastric region with an accompanying urge to defecate or pass flatus, neither of which relieves the distress. As inflammation spreads to the parietal peritoneal surfaces, the pain becomes somatic, steady, and more severe, aggravated by motion or cough and usually located in the right lower quadrant. Anorexia is very common; a hungry patient probably does not have acute appendicitis. Nausea and vomiting occur in 50% to 60% of cases. Urinary frequency and dysuria occur if the appendix lies adjacent to the bladder. The temperature is usually normal or slightly elevated (37.2°–38°C [99°–100.5°F]), but a temperature higher than 38.3°C (101°F) should suggest perforation. Perforation is rare before 24 hours after onset of symptoms, but the rate may be as high as 80% after 48 hours. Moderate leukocytosis of 10,000 to 18,000 cells/μL is frequent (with a concomitant left shift), and the absence of leukocytosis does not rule out acute appendicitis. Leukocytosis of more than 20,000 cells/μL suggests probable perforation. Infants younger than 2 years of age have a 70% to 80% incidence of perforation and generalized peritonitis. In the elderly, pain and tenderness are often blunted, and thus the diagnosis is frequently delayed and leads to a 30% incidence of perforation in patients older than 70. Appendicitis occurs approximately once in every 1000 pregnancies and is the most common extrauterine condition requiring abdominal surgery.

For differential diagnosis, see **Table 12-10**.

Treatment

Early surgery and appendectomy is performed as soon as the patient can be prepared. The only circumstance in

TABLE 12-10 Differential Diagnosis: Appendicitis		
Mesenteric lymphadenitis	Ureteral calculus	Pelvic inflammatory disease
Ruptured grafian follicle	Acute cholecystitis	Corpus luteum cyst
Acute pancreatitis	Acute gastroenteritis	Strangulating intestinal obstruction
Perforated ulcer	Acute diverticulitis	No organic disease

which operation is not indicated is the presence of a palpable mass 3 to 5 days after the onset of symptoms; such patients treated with broad-spectrum antibiotics, parenteral fluids, and rest usually show resolution of the mass and symptoms within 1 week. Interval appendectomy should be done safely 3 months later.

PERITONITIS

Peritonitis is an inflammation of the peritoneum (**Table 12-11**). It may be localized or diffuse in location, acute or chronic in natural history, and infectious or aseptic in pathogenesis. Acute peritonitis is most often infectious and is usually related to a perforated viscus (and called secondary peritonitis). When no bacterial source is identified, infectious peritonitis is called primary or spontaneous.

Etiology

Infectious agents gain access to the peritoneal cavity through a perforated viscus, a penetrating wound of the abdominal wall, or external introduction of a foreign object that is or becomes infected (e.g., a chronic peritoneal dialysis catheter). In the absence of immune compromise, host defenses are capable of eradicating small contaminations. For the conditions that most commonly result in the introduction of bacteria into the peritoneum, see Table 12-11. Bacterial peritonitis can also occur in the apparent absence of an intraperitoneal source of bacteria (primary or spontaneous bacterial peritonitis). This condition occurs in the setting of ascites and liver cirrhosis, usually in patients with ascites with low protein concentration (<1 g/L). Spontaneous bacterial peritonitis is characterized by the spontaneous infection of ascitic fluid in the absence of an intra-abdominal source of infection. Spontaneous bacterial peritonitis is diagnosed when there are 250 or more polymorphonuclear cells/mm^3 in ascitic fluid. Bacterascites is diagnosed when there are positive ascitic fluid cultures and the neutrophil count is less than 250 cells/mm^3. Spontaneous bacterial peritonitis develops secondary to translocation of bacteria from the intestinal lumen to regional lymph nodes with subsequent bacteremia and infection of the ascitic fluid.

Aseptic peritonitis may be due to peritoneal irritation by the abnormal presence of physiologic fluids (e.g., gastric juice, bile, pancreatic enzymes, blood, urine) or sterile foreign bodies (e.g., surgical sponges or instruments, starch from surgical gloves) in the peritoneal cavity or as a complication of rare systemic diseases such as lupus erythematosus, porphyria, or familial Mediterranean fever.

Clinical Features

The cardinal manifestations of peritonitis are acute abdominal pain and tenderness, usually with fever. Generalized peritonitis is associated with widespread inflammation and diffuse abdominal tenderness and rebound. Rigidity of the abdominal wall is common in both localized and generalized peritonitis. Bowel sounds are usually absent. Tachycardia, hypotension, and signs of dehydration are common. Leukocytosis and acidosis are common laboratory findings. When ascites is present, diagnostic paracentesis with cell count (>250 neutrophils/μL is usual in peritonitis), protein, and lactate dehydrogenase levels, and culture is essential. In elderly and immunosuppressed patients, signs of peritoneal irritation may be more difficult to detect.

Therapy and Prognosis

Treatment relies on rehydration, correction of electrolyte abnormalities, antibiotics, and surgical correction of the underlying defect. Mortality rates are less than 10% for uncomplicated peritonitis in an otherwise healthy person. Mortality rates of 40% or higher have been reported for elderly people, those with underlying illnesses, and when peritonitis has been present for more than 48 hours.

ACUTE COLONIC PSEUDO-OBSTRUCTION

Acute colonic pseudo-obstruction is a clinical syndrome characterized by massive dilation of the colon in the absence of mechanical obstruction. The disorder is characterized by the loss of effective colonic peristalsis and subsequent distention of the proximal colon. This syndrome generally develops in ill patients, hospitalized initially for other significant medical problems, and is also observed in surgical patients after a variety of non-GI operations. If left untreated, massive colonic dilation can result in ischemia of the right colon and cecum with associated perforation. A current hypothesis invokes an imbalance in neural input to the colon distal to the splenic flexure with an excess of sympathetic stimulation and a paucity of parasympathetic input, resulting in a spastic contraction of the distal colon and functional obstruction. Plain films of the abdomen, associated with the finding of proximal dilation of the colon associated with a decompressed distal colon with some gas in the rectosigmoid region, are highly suggestive of acute colonic pseudo-obstruction. For patients with a cecal diameter less than 14 cm, an initial trial of conservative

---

TABLE 12-11 Peritonitis Causes

Bowel Perforation
Trauma, iatrogenic, endoscopic perforation, ischemia, anastomotic leak, catheter perforation, ingested foreign body, inflammatory bowel disease, vascular, embolus, strangulated hernias, volvulus, intussusception

Other Organ Leak
Pancreatitis, cholecystitis, salpingitis, bile leak after biopsy, urinary bladder rupture

Peritoneal Disruption
Peritoneal dialysis, intraperitoneal chemotherapy, postoperative foreign body, penetrating-fistulous pattern, trauma

therapy is indicated and includes correction of electrolyte disorders, avoidance of narcotic and anticholinergic agents, hydration, mobilization, tap water enemas, and placement of a nasogastric tube. Seventy percent of the cases that resolve with conservative therapy do so within 2 days, suggesting that a 48-hour trial in stable patients is warranted. However, patients who fail conservative therapy for more than 48 hours should be considered for active intervention with the first-line treatment consisting of intravenous administration of the cholinesterase inhibitor neostigmine. Intravenous

neostigmine at a dose of 2.0 to 2.5 mg given over 3 to 5 minutes results in immediate colonic decompression in 80% to 90% of patients. Because symptomatic bradycardia is a serious side effect of neostigmine, all patients being treated with the drug require cardiac monitoring. Decompressive colonoscopy is the next line of therapy. Approximately 40% of cases require multiple colonoscopies. For findings suggestive of colonic ischemia or those who fail colonoscopic decompression, surgical therapy with either resection or a stoma is necessary, although it is associated with a 30% to 50% mortality rate.

KEY POINTS

- Antireflux mechanisms consist of the LES, the crural diaphragm, and the anatomic location of the gastroesophageal junction below the diaphragmatic hiatus.

- Factors that contribute to the likelihood of aspiration include the urgency of surgery, airway problems, inadequate depth of anesthesia, use of the lithotomy position, insulin-dependent diabetes mellitus, autonomic neuropathy, pregnancy, depressed consciousness, increased severity of illness, and obesity as well as increased intra-abdominal pressure.

- Patients with silent aspirations may present with bronchial asthma.

- Most patients with paraesophageal hernia do not have symptoms of reflux esophagitis, emphasizing the importance of the integrity of the LES.

- Patients with esophageal diverticulum may have halitosis and may experience regurgitation of saliva and food particles consumed several days previously.

- Major trauma accompanied by shock, sepsis, respiratory failure, hemorrhage, transfusion requirement above 6 units, or multiorgan injury is often also accompanied by the development of acute stress gastritis.

- Cimetidine and rantidine, not famotidine and nizatidine, bind to hepatic cytochrome P450. Careful monitoring of drugs such as warfarin, phenytoin, and theophylline is indicated with long-term usage.

- Cardiac manifestations of carcinoid may occur and are due to fibrosis involving the endocardium, primarily on the right side. Left-side lesions can occur with pulmonary involvement or through a right-to-left shunt. Pulmonic stenosis is usually predominant, whereas the tricuspid valve is often fixed open, resulting in regurgitation.

REFERENCES

Aitkenhead AR: Anaesthesia and bowel surgery. Br J Anaesth 1984;56:95–101.

Cortinez FLI: Refractory hypotension during carcinoid resection surgery. Anaesthesia 2000;55:505.

Dierdorf SF: Carcinoid tumor and carcinoid syndrome. Curr Opin Anaesthesiol 2003;16:343.

Hunter AR: Colorectal surgery for cancer: The anaesthetist's contribution? Br J Anaesth 1986;58:825–826.

Kasper DL, Fauci AS, Longo DL (eds): Harrison's Principles of Internal Medicine, 16th ed. New York, McGraw-Hill, 2005.

Mulholland MW, Lillemoe KD, Doherty GM. Greenfield's Surgery: Scientific Principles and Practice. Philadelphia, Lippincott Williams & Wilkins, 2006.

Ng A, Smith G: Gastroesophageal reflux and aspiration of gastric contents in anesthetic practice. Anesth Analg 2001;93:494–513.

Redmond MC: Perianesthesia care of the patient with gastroesophageal reflux disease. J Perianesthesia Nurs 2003;18:535–544; quiz 345-347.

Sontag SJ, O'Connell S, Khandewal S, et al: Most asthmatics have gastroesophageal reflux with or without bronchodilator therapy. Gastroenterology 1990;99:613.

Steinberg W, Tenner S: Acute pancreatitis. N Engl J Med 1994;330:1198–1210.

Young HS: Diseases of the pancreas. Sci Am Med 1997;1–16.

Young HS: Gastrointestinal bleeding. Sci Am Med 1998;1–10.

CHAPTER 13

Nutritional Diseases and Inborn Errors of Metabolism

Hossam Tantawy

Obesity
- Pathogenesis
- Physiologic Disturbances Associated with Obesity
- Management of Anesthesia
- Treatment
- Surgical Treatment

Eating Disorders
- Anorexia Nervosa
- Bulimia Nervosa
- Binge-Eating Disorder

Malnutrition and Vitamin Deficiencies
- Malnutrition
- Vitamin Deficiencies

Inborn Errors of Metabolism
- Porphyrias
- Gout
- Lesch-Nyhan Syndrome
- Disorders of Carbohydrate Metabolism
- Disorders of Amino Acid Metabolism

The presence of nutritional disorders or inborn errors of metabolism will significantly influence the management of anesthesia (**Table 13-1**). The pathophysiology and the associated anesthetic implications of the most frequently encountered nutritional diseases are highlighted in this chapter. In addition, the clinical anesthetic application of inborn errors of metabolism is reviewed and discussed.

OBESITY

In 1999, National Health and Nutrition Examination Survey (NHANES 1999) found that 34% of adults in the United States older than the age of 20 are overweight and 27% of these individuals are obese. This is an approximately 100% increase in the prevalence of obesity from 15% previously reported in 1976 to 1980. Overweight is defined as body mass index (BMI) of 25 to 29.9 kg/m^2 and obese defined as a BMI of 30 kg/m^2 or more. Obesity (body weight $\geq$ 20% above ideal weight) is a disorder of energy balance and is associated with increased morbidity and mortality and a wide spectrum of medical and surgical diseases (**Tables 13-2** and **13-3**). A BMI greater than 28 is associated with an increase in morbidity due to stroke, ischemic heart disease, and diabetes that is three to four times the risk in the general population. A central distribution of body fat is associated with a higher risk of morbidity and mortality than a peripheral distribution of body fat and may be a better indicator of the risk of morbidity than absolute body fat mass (see "Fat Storage").

TABLE 13-1 Nutritional Disorders and Inborn Errors of Metabolism

Nutritional Disorders

Obesity
Malnutrition
Anorexia nervosa
Bulimia nervosa
Binge-eating disorder
Vitamin imbalance disorders

Inborn Errors of Metabolism

Porphyria
Gout
Pseudogout
Hyperlipidemia
Carbohydrate metabolism disorders
Amino acid disorders
Mucopolysaccharidoses
Gangliosidoses

TABLE 13-2 Medical and Surgical Conditions Associated with Obesity

Organ System	Side Effects
Respiratory system	Obstructive sleep apnea
	Obesity hypoventilation syndrome
	Restrictive lung disease
Cardiovascular system	Systemic hypertension
	Cardiomegaly
	Congestive heart failure
	Ischemic heart disease
	Cerebrovascular disease
	Peripheral vascular disease
	Pulmonary hypertension
	Deep vein thrombosis
	Pulmonary embolism
	Hypercholesterolemia
	Hypertriglyceridemia
	Sudden death
Endocrine system	Diabetes mellitus
	Cushing syndrome
	Hypothyroidism
Gastrointestinal system	Hiatal hernia
	Inguinal hernia
	Gallstones
	Fatty liver infiltration
Musculoskeletal system	Osteoarthritis of weight-bearing joints
	Back pain
Malignancy	Breast
	Prostate
	Cervical
	Uterine
	Colorectal

Adapted from Adams JP, Murphy PG: Obesity in anaesthesia and intensive care. Br J Anaesth 2000;85:91–108.

TABLE 13-3 Calculation of Body Mass Index

$$\text{Body mass index (BMI)} = \frac{\text{weight (kg)}}{\text{height}^2 \text{ (m)}}$$

Example: A 150 kg, 1.8 m tall man has a BMI of 47 (more than 100% above ideal body weight). A similar patient weighing 80 kg has a BMI of 25.

Pathogenesis

Obesity is a complex, multifactorial disease (mechanisms of fat storage, genetic, psychological). However, most simply, it occurs when net energy intake exceeds net energy expenditure over a prolonged period of time. Energy expenditure is determined by the energy costs of maintaining the integrated bodily functions (resting metabolic rate), thermic effect of activity, and heat produced by food digestion, absorption, and storage. The resting metabolic rate accounts for about 60% of total energy expenditure. The thermic effect of activity accounts for about 20% of total energy expenditure in the average sedentary individual. This component can be increased by exercise. Exercise can increase the resting metabolic rate for as long as 18 hours after increased activity. It is likely that caloric restriction (dieting) initiates a defense mechanism that decreases energy expenditure, which leads to slower weight loss during periods of caloric restriction and more rapid weight gain during periods of increased caloric intake.

The primary form in which potential chemical energy is stored in the body is fat (triglyceride). The high caloric density and hydrophobic nature of triglycerides permits efficient energy storage without adverse osmotic effects. The amount of triglycerides in adipose tissues is the cumulative sum of the differences between energy (food) intake and energy expenditure (resting metabolism and physical activity) over time. If daily energy intake exceeds energy expenditure by 2%, the cumulative effect after 1 year is approximately a 2.3-kg increase in body weight. Although there is great interest in dietary composition, it is unlikely that these factors alone (i.e., fats, carbohydrates, protein) play a major role in the pathogenesis of obesity. Protein and carbohydrate can be metabolically converted to fat, and there is no evidence that changing the relative proportion of protein, carbohydrate, and fat in the diet without reducing caloric intake promotes weight loss.

Fat Storage

Surplus calories are converted to triglycerides and stored in adipocytes. This storage is regulated by the enzyme lipoprotein lipase. The activity of this enzyme varies in different parts of the body, being more active in abdominal fat and less active in hip fat. The increased morbidity and mortality associated with obesity depends on both the amount of fat and its anatomic distribution. Central or android distribution of fat, which is more common in men, manifests as abdominal obesity. Abdominal fat deposits are metabolically more active than peripheral or gynecoid fat distribution (hips, buttocks, thighs) and are thus associated with a higher incidence of metabolic complications (dyslipidemias, glucose intolerance and diabetes mellitus, ischemic heart disease, congestive heart failure, stroke). For example, a waist-to-hip ratio higher than 1.0 in women and 0.8 in men increases the risk of ischemic heart disease, stroke, diabetes mellitus, and death independent of total body fat. Because men tend to accumulate abdominal fat, which is broken down by the more active form of lipoprotein lipase, they generally lose weight more readily than women, who accumulate hip fat. Environmental facts such as stress and cigarette smoking stimulate cortisol production, which may facilitate deposition of excess calories as abdominal fat.

When triglycerides are deposited in fat cells, the cells initially increase in size until a maximum size is reached, at which point the cells divide. Moderate degrees of obesity (BMI < 40) are likely to result in increased fat cell size, whereas extreme obesity (BMI > 40) is likely to result in adipocyte proliferation.

Metabolic Effects of Weight Change

The responses of both lean and obese individuals to experimental weight change support the notion that body fat content is regulated, meaning it is unlikely that behavior alone is the sole determinant of obesity. The 24-hour energy expenditure per unit of lean body mass is similar in lean and obese individuals. Small decreases in body weight result in decreased energy expenditures that persist despite a caloric intake that is sufficiently decreased to maintain the lower weight. Thus, a formerly obese person requires approximately 15% fewer calories to maintain normal body weight than persons of the same body composition who have never been obese. Should formerly obese patients return to the previous level of caloric intake, the resulting weight gain exceeds that previously lost because energy expenditures have been decreased, perhaps due to changes in the efficiency with which skeletal muscles convert chemical energy to mechanical work. Indeed, in both obese and lean subjects who lose weight, there is an almost inevitable recidivism, with the lost weight rapidly regained. It is likely that obese patients who report failure to lose weight despite dieting in fact greatly underestimate their caloric intake and overestimate their physical activity.

Genetic Factors

The importance of energy stores for survival and the ability to conserve energy in the form of adipose tissue at one time may have conferred a survival advantage. For this reason, humans are presumably enriched with genes that favor energy storage and diminish energy expenditure. However, the combination of easy access to calorically dense foods and a sedentary lifestyle have made the metabolic consequences of these genes maladaptive. Furthermore, the increasing prevalence of obesity and the inverse relationship between obesity and social class confirm the co-existing importance of environmental factors in the development of obesity.

Physiologic Disturbances Associated with Obesity

Obesity has potential detrimental effects on multiple organ systems, particularly the patient's respiratory and cardiovascular systems (see Table 13-2). Respiratory derangements associated with obesity include obesity hypoventilation syndrome and effects on lung volumes and gas exchange. Cardiovascular disease is a dominant cause of morbidity and mortality in obese individuals and may manifest itself as ischemic heart disease, systemic hypertension, and congestive heart failure.

Morbidly obese individuals have limited mobility and may therefore appear to be asymptomatic even in the presence of significant respiratory and cardiovascular impairment. Exertional dyspnea and/or angina pectoris, although infrequent, may accompany periods of physical activity. Many obese individuals choose to sleep sitting up in a chair to avoid symptoms of orthopnea and paroxysmal nocturnal dyspnea. A history of this sleep pattern should raise concerns regarding the patient's cardiovascular status.

Obstructive Sleep Apnea

Obstructive sleep apnea is definitively diagnosed using polysomnography in a sleep laboratory (defined as observed episodes of apnea during sleep). Obstructive sleep apnea is defined as airflow cessation of more than 10 seconds and characterized by frequent episodes of apnea or hypopnea during sleep. Hypopnea is defined as airflow decreased below a given percentage of the surrounding baseline and may also require the presence of some degree of oxyhemoglobin desaturation. The severity of obstructive sleep apnea is measured by the average number of incidents per hour; more than five incidents per hour is considered sleep apnea syndrome. Airway obstruction is often manifested as snoring, daytime somnolence due to repeated episodes of fragmented sleep during the night, and physiologic changes that include arterial hypoxemia, arterial hypercarbia, polycythemia, systemic hypertension, pulmonary hypertension, and right ventricular failure. This syndrome is present in 2% to 4% of middle-aged adults, especially men. An estimated 5% of obese subjects develop obstructive sleep apnea. In obese individuals, increased adipose tissue in the neck and pharyngeal tissues is thought to predispose to airway narrowing and lead to sleep apnea. Nonobese patients who develop obstructive sleep apnea often have tonsillar hypertrophy or craniofacial skeletal abnormalities (retrognathia) that predispose to airway narrowing or closure during sleep.

Pathogenesis Apnea occurs when the pharyngeal airways collapse. Pharyngeal patency depends on the action of dilator muscles that prevent upper airway collapse. This pharyngeal muscle tone is decreased during sleep and in many individuals leads to a significant narrowing of the airway resulting in turbulent airflow and snoring. Administration of even light general anesthesia, combined with sedatives, can lead to airway obstruction in narrowed upper airways of many obese patients. In patients with obstructive sleep apnea, the depressant effect of anesthetics on the muscle tone of the pharynx is potentiated. Although most current employed anesthetic drugs are relatively short acting in patients without obstructive sleep apnea, there can be some residual respiratory depressant effects during the first 12 to 24 hours after surgery. Increased inspiratory effort and the response to arterial hypoxemia and hypercarbia result in arousal, which in turn restore upper airway tone. The individual then falls asleep again, and the cycle repeats.

Risk Factors The main predisposing factors for the development of obstructive sleep apnea are male gender, middle age, and obesity (BMI > 30), with other factors such as evening alcohol consumption or drug-induced sleep compounding the problem. For example, in addition to physiologic sleep, drugs, especially alcohol, may decrease pharyngeal muscle tone. Sleep fragmentation is the most likely explanation for daytime somnolence, which is associated with impaired concentration, memory problems, and motor vehicle accidents. In addition, patients may complain of morning headaches due to nocturnal carbon dioxide retention and cerebral vasodilation.

Treatment Positive airway pressure, delivered through a nasal mask, is the initial treatment of choice for clinically significant obstructive sleep apnea. The level of positive pressure required to sustain the patency of the patient's upper airway during sleep must be determined in a sleep laboratory. Patients treated with positive airway pressure demonstrate improved neuropsychiatric function and a lessening of daytime somnolence. Patients with mild sleep apnea who do not tolerate positive airway pressure may benefit from nighttime application of oral appliances designed to enlarge the airway by keeping the tongue in an anterior position or by displacing the mandible forward. The use of drugs to treat obstructive sleep apnea (protriptyline, fluoxetine) has not shown to be reliably effective in most severe cases of obstructive sleep apnea. Nocturnal oxygen therapy is a consideration for individuals who experience severe arterial oxygen desaturation.

Surgical treatment of obstructive sleep apnea includes tracheostomy (patients with severe apnea who do not tolerate positive airway pressure), palatal surgery (laser-assisted uvulopalatopharyngoplasty), although the efficacy of this procedure is now questioned, and maxillofacial surgical procedures to enhance upper airway patency during sleep (genioglossal advancement). Patients with obstructive sleep apnea who have significant craniofacial abnormalities or who have had unsuccessful genioglossal advancement, with or without uvulopalatopharyngoplasty, may benefit from maxillomandibular advancement.

Management of Anesthesia Management of anesthesia in patients with a history of obstructive sleep apnea poses significant risks. These patients may be exquisitely sensitive to all central nervous system depressant drugs, with a potential for upper airway obstruction or apnea occurring with even minimal doses of these agents. For these reasons, preoperative medication with sedatives including benzodiazepines and opioids must be used sparingly if at all.

Induction and Maintenance Upper airway abnormalities (decreased anatomic space to accommodate anterior displacement of the tongue) that predispose to difficult exposure of the glottic opening during direct laryngoscopy may also predispose to obstructive sleep apnea. When awake, these patients appear to compensate for compromised airway anatomy by increasing their craniocervical angulation, which increases the space between the mandible and cervical spine and elongates the tongue and soft tissues of the neck. This postural compensation is lost when these patients are rendered unconscious and paralyzed. Indeed, difficult tracheal intubation is a predictable problem in patients with a history of obstructive sleep apnea.

When selecting an intraoperative anesthetic plan, short-acting inhaled agents (sevoflurane, desflurane, nitrous oxide) are the primary agents of choice. It is important to note, however, that obesity increases uptake of these agents in two ways. The greater fat burden increases the blood flow directed to bulk fat, and uptake by the fat group, therefore, increases. Obesity also may increase fat surfaces accessible by intertissue diffusion (e.g., intra-abdominal fat and fat intercalated in muscle), and this, too, results in increased uptake. Nitrous oxide should be avoided in the presence in patients with a history of co-existing pulmonary hypertension. Neuromuscular blocking drugs characterized by rapid spontaneous recovery are most often selected. When feasible, regional anesthesia using a catheter to provide continuous anesthesia is often a useful option. Perioperative monitoring for apnea, arterial oxygen desaturation, and the development of cardiac dysrhythmias is recommended. Tracheal extubation must not be considered until patients are fully conscious with intact upper airway reflexes and undertaken only under controlled conditions in a monitored environment.

Postoperative Management Patients with a history of obstructive sleep apnea are at increased risk of developing arterial hypoxemia during the postoperative period. Episodic arterial hypoxemia may occur both early (first 24 hours) and late (2–5 days postoperatively). Early episodic arterial hypoxemia may be a reflection of opioid use either intraoperatively or as a therapy employed to manage postoperative pain. The sitting position may be a useful postoperative posture to improve arterial oxygenation, especially in morbidly obese patients. Routine administration of oxygen during the postoperative period is controversial, as oxygen could increase the duration of apnea by delaying the arousal effect produced by arterial hypoxemia. Therefore, it may be preferable to provide supplemental oxygen only when arterial oxygen desaturation is indicated by pulse oximetry.

Management of postoperative pain in patients with obstructive sleep apnea must consider the exquisite sensitivity of these patients to the ventilatory depressant effects of opioids. Even neuraxial opioids have been associated with unexpected degrees of ventilatory depression. Regional analgesia is associated with a low incidence of both apnea and arterial hypoxemia, making this approach an attractive technique for providing postoperative analgesia.

Nonsteroidal anti-inflammatory drugs have considerable analgesic effects and are useful agents in this patient population.

Specialized Surgical Procedures Upper airway surgical procedures used to treat patients with obstructive sleep apnea, especially in situations where multiple procedures are needed concomitantly to address multiple levels of airway obstruction, may involve several operative visits. In these situations, a general anesthetic with muscle relaxants is often selected. The specifics of the anesthetic delivery system is influenced by the need for the surgeon to have complete access to the patient's head. A tracheostomy is mandatory before any surgery that involves the base of the tongue. Tracheostomy may be exceedingly difficult in markedly obese patients with short necks. A cuffed armored nasotracheal tube is often used for mandibular and maxillomandibular surgery to permit occlusion of the mouth (intermaxillary fixation). Postoperatively, patients undergoing extensive corrective surgery should be managed in a monitored care setting with the inclusion of supplemental oxygen, appropriate analgesics, and pulse oximetry monitoring.

Uvulopalatopharyngoplasty is performed with the patient supine position with the head slightly elevated to enhance venous drainage. Worsening of upper airway obstruction is possible during the early postoperative period due to the residual effects of anesthetic drugs or surgically induced upper airway edema. Acute upper airway obstruction may occur immediately following tracheal extubation. A nasopharyngeal airway may be left in place to facilitate maintenance of airway patency following tracheal extubation. Continuous positive airway pressure and supplemental oxygen may be added following tracheal extubation. Postoperative analgesia with nonsteroidal antiinflammatory drugs is most often recommended. The adequacy of ventilation should be assessed and monitored for 24 to 48 hours postoperatively.

Obesity Hypoventilation Syndrome

Obesity hypoventilation syndrome is the long-term consequence of obstructive sleep apnea. Obstructive sleep apnea is initially limited to nocturnal sleep with correction of respiratory acidosis occurring during waking hours. As the obesity hypoventilation syndrome develops, there is evidence of nocturnal alterations in the control of breathing manifesting as central apneic events (apnea without respiratory efforts). These nocturnal episodes of central apnea reflect progressive desensitization of the respiratory centers to nocturnal hypercarbia. At its extreme, obesity hypoventilation syndrome culminates in the pickwickian syndrome, which is characterized by obesity, daytime hypersomnolence, arterial hypoxemia, polycythemia, hypercarbia, respiratory acidosis, pulmonary hypertension, and right ventricular failure.

Derangement in the Pulmonary System

Lung Volumes Obesity imposes a restrictive ventilatory defect as a result of the weight added to the thoracic cage and the abdomen. This added weight impedes the motion of the diaphragm, especially with assumption of the supine position.

This added weight and associated splinting of the diaphragm result in decreases in functional residual capacity (FRC), expiratory reserve volume, and total lung capacity, with the FRC declining exponentially with increasing BMI. The FRC may be decreased to the point that small airway closure occurs with resulting ventilation-to-perfusion mismatching, right-to-left shunting, and arterial hypoxemia. General anesthesia will accentuate these changes such that a 50% decrease in FRC occurs in obese anesthetized patients compared with a 20% decrease in nonobese individuals (**Fig. 13-1**). In these situations, the application of positive end-expiratory pressure improves the FRC and arterial oxygenation but at the expense of cardiac output and oxygen delivery.

The decrease in FRC impairs the ability of obese patients to tolerate periods of apnea, such as during direct laryngoscopy for tracheal intubation. Obese individuals are likely to experience arterial oxygen desaturation following induction of anesthesia despite preoxygenation. It reflects a decreased oxygen reservoir in their decreased FRC and an increase in oxygen consumption.

Gas Exchange Morbidly obese individuals usually have only modest decreases in arterial oxygenation and increases in the alveolar-to-arterial oxygen difference, presumably reflecting ventilation-to-perfusion mismatching. Nevertheless, arterial oxygenation may deteriorate markedly on induction of anesthesia, and increased concentrations of delivered oxygen are needed to maintain an acceptable Pa_{O_2}. In contrast to the likely decrease in Pa_{O_2}, the Pa_{CO_2} and ventilatory response to carbon dioxide remain within a normal range in obese patients, reflecting the high diffusing capacity and favorable characteristics of the dissociation curve for carbon dioxide.

Lung Compliance and Resistance Increasing BMI is associated with exponential decreases in respiratory compliance and resistance. This decrease in lung compliance reflects the accumulation of fat tissue in and around the chest wall and the effects of increased pulmonary blood volume. Decreased lung compliance is associated with decreases in FRC and impaired gas exchange. These changes in lung compliance and resistance result in rapid, shallow breathing patterns and increased work

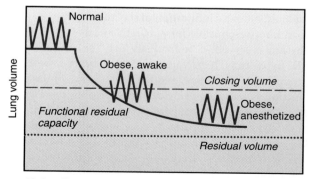

Figure 13-1 • Effects of severe obesity on functional residual capacity (FRC). Anesthesia and obesity are associated with decreases in FRC resulting in small airway closure, ventilation-to-perfusion mismatching, and impaired arterial oxygenation. *(Adapted from Adams JP, Murphy PG: Obesity in anaesthesia and intensive care. Br J Anaesth 2000;85:91–108.)*

of breathing that is most marked when obese individuals assume the supine position.

Work of Breathing Oxygen consumption and carbon dioxide production are increased in obese individuals as a result of the increased metabolic activity of the excess fat and the increased workload on supportive tissues. Normocapnia is maintained usually by increased minute ventilation, which results in increased oxygen cost (work) of breathing. Obese patients typically breathe rapidly and shallowly, as this pattern results in the least oxygen cost of breathing.

Cardiovascular Issues

Systemic Hypertension Mild to moderate systemic hypertension is present in 50% to 60% of obese patients. Increased extracellular fluid volume resulting in hypervolemia and increased cardiac output is characteristic of obesity-induced hypertension. These changes are predictable, considering that each kilogram of fat contains 3000 m of blood vessels. Cardiac output is estimated to increase 0.1 L/min for each kilogram of weight gain related to adipose tissue. Cardiomegaly and systemic hypertension most likely reflect increased cardiac output. Hyperinsulinemia, which is characteristic of obesity, contributes to systemic hypertension by activating the sympathetic nervous system and causing sodium retention. Insulin resistance may be responsible for the enhancement of pressor activity of norepinephrine and angiotensin II.

Pulmonary hypertension is common in obese patients and most likely reflects the impact of chronic arterial hypoxemia or increased pulmonary blood volume (or both).

Ischemic Heart Disease Obesity seems to be an independent risk factor for the development of ischemic heart disease and is more common in obese individuals with central distributions of fat. Other factors, such as systemic hypertension, diabetes mellitus, and hypercholesterolemia, which are common in obese individuals, compound the likely development of ischemic heart disease.

Congestive Heart Failure Systemic hypertension leads to concentric left ventricular hypertrophy and a progressively noncompliant left ventricle, which, when combined with hypervolemia, increases the risk of congestive heart failure (**Fig. 13-2**). Increases in epicardial fat are common in obese individuals, but fatty infiltration of the myocardium is uncommon and not responsible for congestive heart failure. Cardiac dysrhythmias in obese individuals may be precipitated by arterial hypoxemia, hypercarbia, ischemic heart disease, obese hypoventilation syndrome, and fatty infiltration of the cardiac conduction system. Left ventricular hypertrophy demonstrated by echocardiography is frequently seen in obese patients. Obesity-induced cardiomyopathy is associated with hypervolemia and increased cardiac output (see Fig. 13-2). Of note, ventricular hypertrophy and dysfunction worsen with increasing duration of obesity. In addition, the increased demands placed on the cardiovascular system by obesity decrease the reserve of the cardiovascular system and limit exercise tolerance.

Morbidly obese patients tolerate exercise poorly, with any increase in cardiac output being achieved by increasing the heart rate without an increase in stroke volume or ejection fraction. Likewise, changing position from the sitting to the supine position is associated with increases in cardiac output, pulmonary capillary wedge pressure, and mean pulmonary artery pressure, together with decreases in heart rate and systemic vascular resistance.

Gastrointestinal and Metabolic Derangement

Gastric Emptying The notion that obese patients are at increased risk of aspiration and development of aspiration pneumonitis based on increased intra-abdominal pressure, delayed gastric emptying, and the increased incidence of hiatal hernia and gastroesophageal reflux is questionable. In fact, obese patients without symptoms of gastroesophageal reflux have resistance gradients between the stomach and gastroesophageal junction similar to those in nonobese individuals in both the sitting and supine positions. Furthermore, although gastric volume is greater in obese individuals, gastric emptying may be more rapid in these subjects than in nonobese subjects. Nevertheless, because of the larger gastric capacity, the residual volume is larger in obese individuals.

Diabetes Mellitus Glucose tolerance curves are often abnormal, and the incidence of diabetes mellitus is increased several-fold in obese patients. This finding is consistent with the resistance of peripheral tissues to the effects of insulin in the presence of increased adipose tissue. Indeed, obesity is an important risk factor for the development of non–insulin-dependent diabetes mellitus (NIDDM). In obese patients with NIDDM, the catabolic response to surgery may necessitate the use of exogenous insulin during the perioperative period.

Hepatobiliary Disease Abnormal liver function tests and fatty liver infiltration are frequent findings in obese patients. Despite evidence that volatile anesthetics are defluorinated to a greater extent in obese patients, there is no evidence of exaggerated anesthetic-induced hepatic dysfunction. The risk of developing gallbladder and biliary tract disease is increased threefold in obese patients, perhaps reflecting abnormal cholesterol metabolism.

Thromboembolic Disease

The risk of deep vein thrombosis in obese patients undergoing surgery is approximately double that of nonobese individuals. The increased risk of thromboembolic disease in obese patients presumably reflects the effects of polycythemia, increased abdominal pressure, and immobilization leading to venous stasis and increased abdominal pressure in deep veins. The use of low molecular weight heparin has been advocated to decrease thromboembolic complications in the postoperative period. When using these agents, a current suggestion is to use total body weight as it better correlated with drug clearance and therefore preferable to lean body weight for dose calculations.

Pharmacokinetics of Drugs

The physiologic changes associated with obesity may lead to alterations in the distribution, binding, and elimination of many drugs. The volume of distribution of drugs in obese

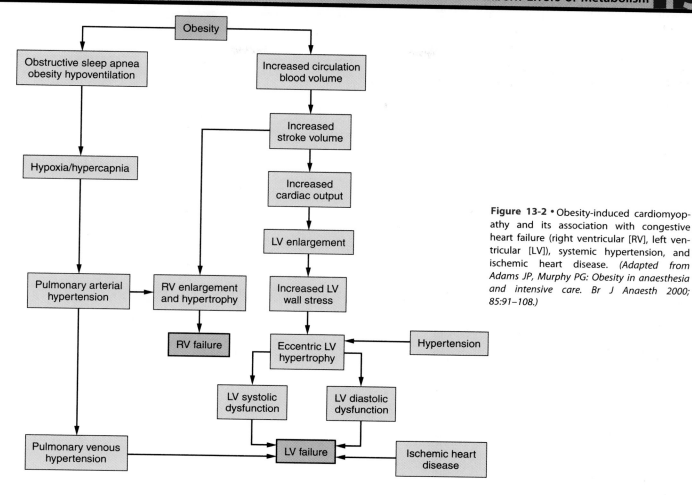

Figure 13-2 • Obesity-induced cardiomyopathy and its association with congestive heart failure (right ventricular [RV], left ventricular [LV]), systemic hypertension, and ischemic heart disease. (*Adapted from Adams JP, Murphy PG: Obesity in anaesthesia and intensive care. Br J Anaesth 2000; 85:91–108.*)

individuals may be influenced by a variety of factors including increase in blood volume and cardiac output, decrease in total body water (fat contains less water than other tissues), altered protein binding of drugs, and the lipid solubility of the drug being administered. The effect of obesity on protein binding of drugs, if any, is variable and not always predictable. Despite the occasional presence of liver dysfunction, hepatic clearance of drugs is not usually altered in obese individuals. Congestive heart failure and decreased hepatic blood flow could slow elimination of drugs that are highly dependent on liver clearance. Renal clearance of drugs may increase in obese individuals because of increased renal blood flow and glomerular filtration rate.

The impact of obesity on the selection of appropriate dose of injected drugs is difficult to predict. Total blood volume is likely to be increased, which would tend to decrease the plasma concentrations achieved following rapid intravenous injection of drugs. Conversely, fat has a low blood flow such that the increased doses calculated based on body weight could result in excessive plasma concentrations. The most clinically applicable approach is to calculate the initial dose of injected drug for administration to obese patients based on "ideal" body weight (reflects lean body mass) rather than actual body weight, which in obese patients overestimates

the lean body mass. Subsequent doses are determined based on the pharmacologic response to the initial dose. Repeated injections of drugs, however, can result in cumulative drug effects and prolonged responses, reflecting storage of drugs in fat and subsequent release from this inactive depot into the systemic circulation as the plasma concentration of drug declines. It is important to note that oral absorption of drugs is not influenced by obesity.

The notion that slow emergence of morbidly obese patients from the effects of general anesthesia reflects delayed release of the volatile anesthetic from fat stores is not accurate (see "Maintenance of Anesthesia"). Poor total fat blood flow limits the delivery of volatile anesthetics for storage such that slow emergence, if real, most likely reflects a central nervous system effect. Overall, recovery times are often comparable in obese and lean individuals undergoing surgery that requires anesthesia less than 4 hours. The impact of absorption on the dosing of a specific agent is displayed in **Table 13-4**.

Management of Anesthesia
Induction of Anesthesia
A detailed assessment of the obese patient's upper airway must be performed before induction of anesthesia. Difficulties with mask ventilation and tracheal intubation may be

TABLE 13-4 Medication Dosing in Obesity

Drug	Dosing	Comments
Propofol	IBW Maintenance: TBW	Systemic clearance and V_D at steady-state correlates well with TBW. High affinity for excess fat and other well-perfused organs. High hepatic extraction and conjugation relates to TBW.
Thiopental	TBW	Increased V_D, increased blood volume, cardiac output, and muscle mass. Increased absolute dose. Prolonged duration of action.
Midazolam	TBW	Central V_D increases in line with body weight. Increased absolute dose. Prolonged sedation because larger initial doses are needed to achieve adequate serum concentrations.
Succinylcholine	TBW	Plasma cholinesterase activity increases in proportion to body weight. Increased absolute dose.
Vecuronium	IBW	Recovery may be delayed if given according to TBW because of increased V_D and impaired hepatic clearance.
Rocuronium	IBW	Faster onset and longer duration of action. Pharmacokinetics and pharmacodynamics are not altered in obese subjects.
Atracurium, cisatracurium	TBW	Absolute clearance, V_D, and elimination half-life do not change. Unchanged dose per unit body weight without prolongation of recovery because of organ-independent elimination.
Fentanyl Sufentanil	TBW TBW Maintenance: IBW	Increased V_D and elimination half-time, which correlates positively with the degree of obesity. Distributes as extensively in excess body mass as in lean tissues. Dose should account for total body mass.
Remifentanil	IBW	Systemic clearance and V_D corrected per kilogram of TBW—significantly smaller in the obese. Pharmacokinetics are similar in obese and nonobese patients. Age and lean body mass should be considered for dosing.

IBW, ideal body weight; TBW, total body weight; V_D, volume of distribution.

considerable based on the presence of the following anatomic features: fat face and cheeks, short neck, large tongue, excessive palatal and pharyngeal soft tissue, restricted mouth opening, limited cervical and mandibular mobility, large breasts. Obese patients are traditionally presumed to be at increased risk of pulmonary aspiration during the induction of anesthesia. Perhaps the greater risk of pulmonary aspiration is related to the potential for technically difficult tracheal intubation. Pharmacologic intervention with H_2-receptor antagonists (e.g., cimetidine, ranitidine, famotidine), nonparticulate antacids (e.g., sodium bicitrate), and proton pump inhibitors (e.g., omeprazole, lansoprazole, rabeprazole) will reduce gastric volume, acidity, or both, thereby reducing the risk and complications of aspiration. In selected patients, awake tracheal intubation using fiberoptic laryngoscopy may be the most appropriate method for securing the airway. Neither absolute obesity nor increasing BMI has been shown to be consistently associated with problematic intubation in morbidly obese patients. However, problematic intubation was associated with increasing neck circumference and a Mallampati score of 3 or higher.

The low FRC associated with obesity means that rapid decreases in arterial oxygenation may be seen with direct laryngoscopy and tracheal intubation (**Fig. 13-3**). The risk of potential arterial oxygen desaturation emphasizes the importance of maximizing the oxygen content in the lungs before initiating direct laryngoscopy and monitoring arterial oxygen saturation continuously with pulse oximetry. Decreased FRC also leads to decreased mixing time for inhaled drugs, accelerating the rate of increase of the drug's alveolar concentration.

Maintenance of Anesthesia

Positioning Specially designed tables or two regular tables joined together may be required for safe anesthesia for bariatric surgery. Regular operating room tables have a maximum weight limit of approximately 205 kg, but operating tables capable of holding up to 455 kg, with a little extra width to accommodate the extra girth, are now available. Particular care should be paid to protecting pressure areas because pressure sores and neural injuries are more common in this group, especially in the superobese and any obese patients with diabetes. Brachial plexus and sciatic and ulnar nerve palsies have been reported in patients with increased BMI. A retrospective study by Warner and colleagues documented such an association because 29% of patients with ulnar neuropathy in their series had a BMI of more than 38 kg/m² compared with only 1% of the control subjects.

Laparoscopy Pneumoperitoneum causes systemic changes during laparoscopy. The gas most often used for this purpose is carbon dioxide. Positioning, such as Trendelenburg, can worsen the systemic changes of pneumoperitoneum. The degree of intra-abdominal pressure determines its effects on

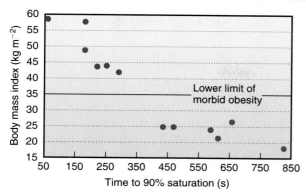

Figure 13-3 • Arterial oxygen saturation decreases to 90% more rapidly in morbidly obese patients, as quantitated by the body mass index. *(Adapted from Berthoud MC, Peacock JE, Reilly CS: Effectiveness of preoxygenation in morbidly obese patients. Br J Anaesth 1991;67:464–466.)*

venous return and myocardial performance. There is a biphasic cardiovascular response to increases in intra-abdominal pressure. At an intra-abdominal pressure of approximately 10 mm Hg, there is an increase in venous return, probably from a reduction in splanchnic sequestration of blood, with a subsequent increase in cardiac output and arterial pressure. Hypovolemia, however, blunts this response. Compression of the inferior vena cava occurs at an intra-abdominal pressure of approximately 20 mm Hg, with decreased venous return from the lower body and consequent decreased cardiac output. Increased renal vascular resistance at an intra-abdominal pressure of 20 mm Hg decreases renal blood flow and glomerular filtration rate. Femoral venous blood flow can be reduced by both pneumoperitoneum and Trendelenburg positioning, with an increased risk of lower extremity thrombosis. Absorption of carbon dioxide can worsen hypercarbia and acidosis, which can be offset by hyperventilation as well as increasing the pulmonary artery pressure. Anesthetized obese patients undergoing laparoscopy have higher left ventricular end systolic wall stress before pneumoperitoneum (due to increased end-systolic left ventricular dimensions) and during pneumoperitoneum (due to more pronounced increases in blood pressure). Since higher left ventricular end systolic wall stress is a determinant of myocardial oxygen demand, more aggressive control of blood pressure (ventricular afterload) in morbidly obese patients may be warranted to optimize the myocardial oxygen requirements.

Monitoring As is the case with all patients, the extent of surgery and concomitant comorbid disease process should be the primary factors that determine the need for and the extent of monitoring. With respect to obese patients, the obesity itself is not an indication for the incorporation of any additional measure monitors (i.e., arterial line, central venous pressure, pulmonary artery catheter, echocardiography). However, there will be patients whose cardiovascular status may warrant these modalities. In such cases, the technical difficulty of placing these monitors may be increased by the presence of obesity. Invasive arterial monitoring should be used for the morbidly obese with severe cardiopulmonary

disease and for those patients in whom a poor fit of the non-invasive blood pressure cuff is seen because of the severe conical shape of the upper arms or unavailability of appropriately sized cuffs. In these situations, blood pressure measurements can be falsely increased if the cuff is too small for the arm used. Cuffs with bladders that encircle a minimum of 75% of the upper arm circumference or, preferably, the entire arm, should be used. Intravenous access also becomes problematic and central line may be the only available option.

Pharmacokinetics There is one regimen for selection of drugs or techniques that is best for the maintenance of anesthesia in obese patients. An increased incidence of fatty liver infiltration suggests caution when selecting drugs that have been associated with postoperative liver dysfunction. Increased defluorination of volatile anesthetics in obese patients, however, has not been shown to result in hepatic or renal dysfunction. This increased defluorination observed after the administration of certain volatile anesthetics to obese patients does not seem to accompany the administration of sevoflurane to these patients. Awakening of obese patients is more prompt after exposure to desflurane or sevoflurane than after administration of either isoflurane or propofol. The rapid elimination of nitrous oxide is useful, but the frequent need for increased supplemental concentrations of oxygen may limit the usefulness of this inhaled drug in obese patients. Dexmedetomidine may be a useful anesthetic adjunct for patients who are susceptible to narcotic-induced respiratory depression. In a case report using dexmedetomidine to reduce postoperative narcotic, a patient self-administered 48 mg of morphine via patient-controlled analgesia, while receiving a dexmedetomidine infusion during the first 24 hours following surgery. After 24 hours, the dexmedetomidine infusion was stopped, and during the next 24-hour period, the patient required a total of 148 mg of morphine via patient-controlled analgesia to obtain adequate pain relief. Clearly, dexmedetomidine may be a valuable option for managing pain in the obese patient.

Spinal and Epidural Anesthesia Spinal and epidural anesthesia may be technically difficult in obese patients, as bony landmarks are obscured. Local anesthetic requirements for spinal and epidural anesthesia in obese patients may be as much as 20% lower than in nonobese patients, presumably reflecting fatty infiltration and vascular engorgement caused by increased intra-abdominal pressure, which decreases the volume of the epidural space. As a result, it is difficult to predict reliably the sensory anesthesia level that will be achieved. In obese patients, it seems prudent to decrease the initial dose of local anesthetic administered for regional anesthesia when the body weight is greatly increased owing to excess adipose tissue.

Management of Ventilation As a result of peritoneal insufflation, there is decrease in respiratory system compliance that is partially improved by reverse Trendelenburg position, a significant increase in peak and plateau airway pressures at constant tidal volume. There are no data on which ventilation mode is better in the operating room; data from the intensive care unit could not be extrapolated to the operating room because of different ventilators in the intensive care unit as well as the lack of the pneumoperitoneum and patient position in the operating room.

Controlled ventilation of the obese patient's lungs using large tidal volumes is often applied in an attempt to offset the decreased FRC. Positive end-expiratory pressure may improve ventilation-to-perfusion matching and arterial oxygenation in obese patients, but adverse effects on cardiac output and oxygen delivery may offset these benefits. Using pressure control ventilation and changing the inspiration-to-exhalation ratio could help limit the airway pressure. The prone and head-down positions can further decrease chest wall compliance and Pa_{O_2} in obese patients. Acute assumption of the supine position by spontaneously breathing obese patients can decrease the Pa_{O_2} and lead to cardiac arrest. As a result, monitoring arterial oxygenation and ventilation is of increased importance in obese patients during the perioperative period.

Tracheal Extubation Tracheal extubation is considered when obese patients are fully recovered from the depressant effects of anesthetics. Ideally, obese patients are allowed to recover in a head-up to sitting position. A history of obstructive sleep apnea or obesity hypoventilation syndrome mandates intense postoperative monitoring to ensure maintenance of a patient's upper airway and acceptable oxygenation and ventilation. There are no specific studies to guide the practice of tracheal extubation in obese patients. However, reintubation is usually more difficult and more urgent than initial intubation; the use of tube exchanger could help in those patients and they usually tolerate it very well.

Postoperative Analgesia

Opioid depression of ventilation in obese patients is a concern, and the intramuscular route of administration may be unreliable owing to the unpredictable absorption of drugs. Patient-controlled analgesia is a commonly selected option for providing postoperative analgesia in obese patients. If this approach is used, doses of opioids used for patient-controlled analgesia are based on ideal body weight. Neuraxial opioids (continuous infusion of epidural solutions containing opioids and local anesthetics) comprise an effective method for producing postoperative analgesia in obese patients. Supplementation with oral analgesics such as nonsteroidal anti-inflammatory drugs has become an increasing option.

Postoperative Complications

Postoperative morbidity and mortality rates are higher in obese patients than in nonobese patients mostly due to the preexisting comorbidities and the risk of aspiration during intubation. Wound infection is twice as common in obese patients compared with their nonobese counterparts. Postoperative ventilation is more likely to be required in obese patients who have co-existing carbon dioxide retention and have undergone prolonged surgery, especially abdominal operations. The semisitting position is often used during the postoperative period in attempts to decrease the likelihood of arterial hypoxemia. The hazards and risk of obstructive sleep apnea and obesity hypoventilation syndrome may extend

several days into the postoperative period. Arterial oxygenation should be closely monitored and supplemental oxygen provided as indicated by pulse oximetry and/or blood gas analysis of the Pa_{O_2}. The maximum decrease in Pa_{O_2} typically occurs 2 to 3 days postoperatively. Weaning from mechanical ventilation may be difficult because of the increased work of breathing, decreased lung volumes, and ventilation-to-perfusion mismatching. The likelihood of deep vein thrombosis and pulmonary embolism is also increased, emphasizing the importance of early postoperative ambulation and the potential need for prophylactic anticoagulation. Obese patients tend not to be able to mobilize their fat stores during critical illnesses and tend to rely on carbohydrates. This increased carbohydrate use increases the respiratory quotient (further worsening ventilatory issues) and accelerates protein breakdown. If these patients are take nothing by mouth for prolonged periods, a protein malnutrition syndrome may be seen.

Treatment

The purpose of weight reduction should be to decrease morbidity rather than to meet a cosmetic standard of thinness. A weight loss of only 5 to 20 kg has been associated with a decrease in systemic blood pressure and plasma lipid concentrations and enhanced control of diabetes mellitus. Lifestyle alterations in the form of increased physical activity and/or decreased caloric intake must be continued indefinitely to sustain positive results. Agents designed to advance calorie intake consist of serotonin reuptake inhibitors (fenfluramine, phentermine) function as appetite suppressants but also produce unacceptable side effects (primary pulmonary hypertension) in some individuals. Sibutramine is an appetite suppressant that inhibits the reuptake of serotonin and norepinephrine, and orlistat is a lipase inhibitor that acts in the gastrointestinal tract and is not absorbed.

Surgical Treatment

Current strategies for surgically induced weight loss fall into two categories: gastric restriction and intestinal malabsorption.

Laparoscopic adjustable gastric banding and vertical banded gastroplasty are examples of restrictive procedures, in which a small gastric pouch with a small outlet (10–12 mm in diameter) is created. This results in early and prolonged satiety, thereby reducing caloric intake. Since the normal absorptive physiology of the entire small intestine is left intact, specific nutrient deficiencies are rare unless there is a significant change in eating habits or if complications, such as stomal stenosis, occur.

The biliopancreatic diversion (BPD) procedure, with or without duodenal switch, and the distal gastric bypass are considered malabsorptive procedures. These procedures typically combine gastric volume reduction with a bypass of various lengths of small intestine. After creation of a gastric pouch (200–250 mL in volume), the small bowel is divided 250 cm proximal to the ileocecal valve and connected directly to the gastric pouch, producing a gastroileostomy. The remaining proximal limb (biliopancreatic conduit) is anastomosed to the side of the distal ileum 50 cm proximal to the ileocecal valve. Hence, a common channel that allows for mixture of nutrients with digestive enzymes is created in the ileum, the length of which (typically 50–100 cm) determines the degree of malabsorption. Biliopancreatic diversion is considered a less preferred procedure because the extensive bypassing of small intestine (including the entire jejunum) is associated with a substantially increased risk of nutritional and metabolic complications.

The Roux-en-Y gastric bypass (RYGB) procedure involves both restrictive and malabsorptive components. The gastric volume is more reduced compared with BPD and distal gastric bypass. In the RYGB procedure, the surgeon typically creates a 15- to 50-mL proximal gastric pouch with a 75- to 150-cm Roux limb connected as an enteroenterostomy to the jejunum 30 to 50 cm from the ligament of Trietz. This bypassing of the distal stomach, duodenum, and proximal jejunum leads to diminished absorption of nutrients, similar to that which occurs in a patient with short-bowel syndrome. This loss of absorptive surface area causes a marked reduction in absorptive capacity of nutrients, electrolytes, and bile salts.

The adjustable gastric band is the most commonly performed bariatric procedure in Europe, Latin America, and Australia, and the U.S. Food and Drug Administration approved its use in the United States in 2001. This procedure is gaining popularity in the United States. The surgery entails the placement of an adjustable band around the upper end of the stomach, creating a small pouch and restrictive stoma that slow the passage of food into the distal gastrointestinal tract. This procedure requires no cutting of, or entry into, the stomach or small intestine and theoretically carries a lower complication rate. The gastric band is adjusted after surgery by injection into a subcutaneous port placed at the time of surgery to provide flexibility with respect to stoma size.

Adult bariatric surgery results in significant, sustained weight loss as well as a diminution of obesity-related comorbidities, especially hypertension and diabetes. In a recent meta-analysis of adult studies, the mean percentage of excess weight loss after a RYGB was 68% and 62% for gastric banding, as well as 77% reporting complete resolution of diabetes and 62% reporting resolution of hypertension.

Complications

Complications are most common in males and in patients with the highest BMIs. The most severe focus of these complications include anastomotic leaks or strictures, pulmonary embolism, sepsis, gastric prolapse, and bleeding. Less demonstrated complications such as wound dehiscence, hernia and seroma, lymphocele, lymphorrhea, and suture extrusion have also been reported. In addition, the RYGB procedure induces an undesirable "dumping syndrome."

After RYGB, there is a marked reduction in vitamin and mineral intake, which is often below the recommended daily allowance level for these compounds. The majority of patients after RYGB can maintain a relatively normal nutritional status, but deficiencies of iron, vitamin B_{12}, and folate are common. Some patients develop subclinical micronutrient deficiency.

Multivitamins with mineral supplements reduce but do not totally prevent development of iron, folate, or vitamin deficiencies. Some patients develop dumping syndrome, and others have major nutritional complications. Three of the most clinically significant are protein-calorie malnutrition, Wernicke's encephalopathy, and peripheral neuropathy. In the long term, patients are also at risk of metabolic bone disease. Pregnant women and adolescents are at higher risk of nutritional complications after RYGB because of the higher physiologic nutrition needs. Therefore, long-term nutritional follow-up care is essential to promote a healthy optimal life following weight loss surgery.

The death rate after RYGB is 0.5% to 1.5%. Weight loss after RYGB is typically greater than that after the gastric band as is the risk of nutritional deficiencies and the dumping syndrome.

Protein-Calorie Malnutrition Severe malnutrition is the most serious metabolic complication of bariatric surgery. Red meat is poorly tolerated after bariatric surgery as it is much harder to break down so that it will fit through the small stomach outlet. If the outlet gets plugged, vomiting will result, and if the patient does not consume enough alternative protein sources, such as milk, yogurt, eggs, fish, and poultry, protein malnutrition can develop. Protein-calorie malnutrition is more common with BPD and very rare with vertical banded gastroplasty, unless there are mechanical problems such as stomal stenosis. Protein-calorie malnutrition has a reported incidence of 7% to 12% in patients who have undergone BPD. This incidence is improved with the duodenal switch variation of the surgery. Hypoalbuminemia has been reported as early as 1 year after BPD. Revision of the common channel from 50 to 200 cm in the ileum has been shown to correct this hypoalbuminemia associated with excessive weight loss. In cases of severe malnutrition, enteral or parenteral nutrition therapy may be necessary. Mild to moderate cases usually respond to dietary counseling and increased compliance with clinical follow-up visits. More frequent monitoring may be necessary for patients prone to developing protein-calorie malnutrition.

Fat Malabsorption Fat-soluble vitamin malabsorption and fat malabsorption (evidenced by steatorrhea) are common with RYGB and very commonly associated with BPD. This phenomenon is the principal means by which BPD promotes weight loss. The length of the common channel in BPD regulates the degree of fat absorption (and malabsorption). A 100-cm common channel has been shown to be better tolerated than a 50-cm channel, is associated with less diarrhea and steatorrhea, and improves protein metabolism. Of note, problems with fat-soluble imbalance and fat malabsorption are rarely seen with vertical banded gastroplasty.

Extension of Bariatric Surgery into the Pediatric/ Adolescent Population

The appropriateness and extension of bariatric surgery options to adolescents with severe obesity is controversial.

Serious questions concerning the safety and effectiveness of this aggressive intervention need to be answered, including

1. Will adolescent bariatric treatment result in sustained weight loss or diminution of comorbidities as seen in adult surgery?
2. Will adolescents be capable of complying with the challenging dietary, nutritional, and medical requirements of surgery?
3. What are the long-term nutritional consequences to the adolescent, particularly in terms of growth, bone mineralization, and reproductive potential?

Obesity and Obstetrics

The prevalence of obesity is increasing at an alarming rate in both developed and developing countries. In pregnant women in the United States at the end of the last century, the prevalence ranged from 18.5% to 38.3% according to the cohort studied and the cutoff point used to define overweight. A Brazilian study at a similar time reported the prevalence of obesity in pregnancy to be 5.5%. The percentage of women with BMI greater than 30 increased from 12% in 1993 to 18.3% in 2002. Hormonal changes, through the relaxing effect of progesterone on smooth muscle, decreases airway resistance, thus reducing some of the negative effects of obesity on the respiratory system. Obstructive sleep apnea is not common in obese women who become pregnant. However, pregnancy has some protective effects on sleep apnea, despite the hyperemia of nasal passages. Early in pregnancy, the increased sensitivity of the respiratory center decreases apneic episodes and, in the later part of pregnancy, women tend to sleep on their side, thereby decreasing the likelihood of airway obstruction. Unlike the respiratory system, where pregnancy offers some favorable effects in obese patients, the cardiovascular system is often significantly stressed in obese parturients.

The extent of cardiovascular pathologic changes secondary to obesity is dependent on the duration of obesity and its severity. The heart rate increases in line with elevated cardiac output, thereby decreasing the diastolic interval and thus the time for myocardial perfusion. Impaired myocardial diastolic relaxation leads to diastolic dysfunction. If fat deposition occurs in myocardial tissue, then conduction and contractility can be seriously affected. Insulin resistance and dyslipidemias affect the vascular tree, and increased inflammatory mediators such as C-reactive protein, interleukin-6, and tumor necrosis factor α affect endothelial function has been observed. This endothelial dysfunction in pregnant women may predispose to the development of pregnancy-induced hypertension. The well-known effect of an enlarged uterus compressing abdominal major vessels and causing supine hypotension syndrome can also be seen in obese patients. This can be greatly exacerbated in obese parturients in whom a large panniculus adds to the uterine compression. Tseuda and colleagues reported two cases of sudden death on assuming the supine position in morbidly obese patients, which they attributed to circulatory changes brought about by changes in their position. Drenick and Fisler also reported cases of postoperative cardiac arrest in obese surgical patients. There was no pathology found at autopsy to explain the cardiac arrest (**Table 13-5**).

Gastrointestinal Changes Both anatomic and hormonal changes increase the incidence and severity of gastric reflux in obese and nonobese pregnant women in labor. It is important to note that the gastric volume in obese parturients is five times greater than in controls.

Maternal Morbidity The major maternal complications reported to be associated with obesity during pregnancy include hypertensive disease (chronic hypertension and preeclampsia), diabetes mellitus (pregestational and gestational), respiratory disorders (asthma and sleep apnea), thromboembolic disease, increased incidence of cesarean section, and infections, primarily urinary tract infections, wound infections, and endometritis. The association between obesity and hypertensive disorders of pregnancy, diabetes, delivery by cesarean section (both primary and repeat) is well documented. Although obese parturients are at significant risk of developing preeclampsia, they do not seem to be at increased risk of HELLP (hemolysis, elevated liver enzymes, and low platelet count occurring in association with preeclampsia) syndrome. Complications during labor such as intrapartum fetal distress, meconium aspiration, failure to progress, abnormal presentation, shoulder dystocia, and an increased rate of instrumental delivery are also more common in the obese parturient. Overall, the literature suggests that obese pregnant women have a 14% to 25% incidence of preeclampsia, a 6% to 14% incidence of gestational diabetes, and a 30% to 47% likelihood of cesarean delivery.

Airway The incidence of failed tracheal intubation is approximately 1 in 280 in the obstetric population compared with 1 in 2230 in the general surgical population. In the morbidly obese parturient (> 300 lb), difficult intubation was described in as high as one third of the patients, with a failure rate of as high as 6%. The difficulty in the obese population is mainly due to the short neck with large neck circumference and limited mobility as well as a high Mallampati score (≥ 3), large tongue, and large breasts rather than the weight or the BMI.

Anesthetic Management

Analgesia for Labor As obesity appears to increase the need for cesarean section, placing a functional epidural catheter for labor analgesia is advantageous should any operative intervention be required. Jordan and colleagues noted 74.4% of massively obese parturients needed more than a single attempt and 14% needed more than three attempts for successful epidural placement. The advantage of using subarachnoid block includes a dense reliable block of rapid onset. However, relevant issues include technical difficulties, potential for high spinal blockade, profound dense thoracic motor blockade leading to cardiorespiratory compromise, and inability to prolong the blockade. Proposed mechanisms for the enhanced neural blockade in pregnancy include hormone-related changes in the action of spinal cord

TABLE 13-5 Cardiopulmonary Changes with Pregnancy and Obesity

Parameter	Pregnancy	Obesity	Combined
Heart rate	↑	↑↑	↑↑
Stroke volume	↑↑	↑	↑
Cardiac output	↑↑	↑↑	↑↑↑
Cardiac index	↑ or ↔	↔	↔ or ↓
Hematocrit	↓↓	↑	↓
Blood volume	↑↑	↑	↑
Systemic vascular resistance	↓↓	↑	↔ or ↓
Mean arterial pressure	↑	↑↑	↑↑
Supine hypotension	Present	Present	↑↑
Left ventricular morphology	Hypertrophy	Hypertrophy and dilation	Hypertrophy and dilation
Sympathetic activity	↑	↑↑	↑↑↑
Systolic function	↔	↔ or ↓	↔ or ↓
Diastolic function	↔	↓	↓
Central venous pressure	↔	↑	↑↑
Pulmonary wedge pressure	↔	↑↑	↑↑
Pulmonary hypertension	Absent	May be present	May be present
Preeclampsia	↔	n/a	↑↑
Progesterone level	↑	↔	↑
Sensitivity to CO_2	↑	↓	↑
Tidal volume	↑	↓	↑
Respiratory rate	↑	↔ or ↑	↑
Minute volume	↑	↓ or ↔	↑
Inspiratory capacity	↑	↓	↑
Inspiratory reserve volume	↑	↓	↑
Expiratory reserve volume	↓	↓↓	↓
Residual volume	↓	↓ or ↔	↑
Functional residual capacity	↓↓	↓↓↓	↓↓
Vital capacity	↔	↓	↓
FEV_1	↔	↓ or ↔	↔
FEV_1/vital capacity	↔	↔	↔
Total lung capacity	↓	↓↓	↓
Compliance	↔	↓↓	↓
Work of breathing	↑	↑↑	↑
Resistance	↓	↑	↓
V/Q mismatch	↑	↑	↑↑
DL_{CO}	↑ or ↔	↔	↔
Pao_2	↓	↓↓	↓
$Paco_2$	↓	↑	↓

↑, increase; ↓, decrease; ↔, no change (multiple arrows represent the degree of intensity); DL_{CO}, diffusion capacity of lung for carbon monoxide; FEV_1, forced expiratory volume in 1 second; V/Q, ratio of ventilation to perfusion; $Paco_2$, partial pressure of carbon dioxide; Pao_2, partial pressure of oxygen.

neurotransmitters, potentiation of the analgesic effect of endogenous analgesic systems, increased permeability of the neural sheath, or other pharmacokinetic/dynamic differences. Both pregnancy and obesity increase intra-abdominal pressure and cause compression of the inferior vena cava, which leads to engorgement of the epidural venous plexus and increased epidural space pressure. Magnetic resonance imaging has confirmed decreased cerebrospinal fluid volume in obese parturients. Potential for an unanticipated difficult airway, difficult mask ventilation, and rapid desaturation emphasizes the need for an additional pair of experienced hands when administering general anesthesia. The nasal route is not recommended because of the characteristic engorgement of nasal mucosa during pregnancy.

Postoperative Care Obese parturients are at increased risk of postoperative complications such as hypoxemia, atelectasis and pneumonia, deep vein thrombosis and pulmonary embolism, pulmonary edema, postpartum cardiomyopathy, postoperative endometritis, and wound complications such as infection and dehiscence.

TABLE 13-6	Diagnostic Criteria for Eating Disorders
Anorexia Nervosa	
Body mass index < 17.5	
Fear of weight gain	
Inaccurate perception of body shape and weight	
Amenorrhea	
Bulimia Nervosa	
Recurrent binge eating (twice weekly for 3 months)	
Recurrent purging, excessive exercise, or fasting	
Excessive concern about body weight or shape	
Binge-Eating Disorder	
Recurrent binge eating (2 days per week for 6 months)	
Eating rapidly	
Eating until uncomfortably full	
Eating when not hungry	
Eating alone	
Feeling guilty after a binge	
No purging or excessive exercise	

Adapted from Becker AE, Grinspoon SK, Klibanski A, et al: Eating disorders. N Engl J Med 1999;340:1092–1098.

EATING DISORDERS

Eating disorders are traditionally classified as anorexia nervosa, bulimia nervosa, and binge-eating disorders (**Table 13-6**). Bulimia nervosa and binge-eating disorder are encountered clinically more often than anorexia nervosa. All these disorders are characterized by serious disturbances in eating (restriction or bingeing) and excessive concerns about body weight. Eating disorders typically occur in adolescent girls or young women, although 5% to 15% of cases of anorexia nervosa and bulimia nervosa and 40% of binge-eating disorders occur in boys and young men.

Anorexia Nervosa

Anorexia nervosa is a relatively rare disorder, having an incidence of five to 10 cases per 100,000 persons and a mortality rate of 5% to 10%. Approximately one half the deaths result from medical complications associated with malnutrition, and the remainder are due to suicide associated with depression. The disease is characterized by striking decreases in food intake and excessive physical activity in the obsessive pursuit of thinness. Bulimic symptoms may be part of the syndrome. Females are most often affected, and weight loss exceeds 25% of normal body weight with the patient's perception that they are still obese despite of this dramatic weight loss.

Signs and Symptoms

Marked, unexplained weight loss in adolescent girls is suggestive of anorexia nervosa. Among the more serious medical complications seen in patients with anorexia nervosa are those that affect the cardiovascular system. Cardiac changes include decreased cardiac muscle mass and myocardial contractility. Cardiomyopathy secondary to starvation and to the abuse of ipecac (used to induce vomiting) may be present.

Sudden death has been attributed to ventricular dysrhythmias in these patients, presumably reflecting the effects of starvation and associated hypokalemia. Other electrocardiographic findings include low QRS amplitude, nonspecific ST-T wave changes, sinus bradycardia and U wave, and prolonged QT interval that could be associated with sudden death. Hyponatremia, hypochloremia, and hypokalemia as well as the metabolic alkalosis result from vomiting and laxative and diuretic abuse.

Amenorrhea is often seen soon after the onset of the disorder. Physical examination reveals marked emaciation, dry skin that may be covered with fine body hair, and cold, cyanotic extremities. Decreased body temperature, orthostatic hypotension, bradycardia, and cardiac dysrhythmias may reflect alterations in autonomic nervous system activity. Bone density is decreased as a result of poor nutrition and low estrogen concentrations, and long bones or vertebrae may fracture as a result of osteoporosis. Gastric emptying may be slowed, leading to complaints of gastric distress after eating. In addition, starvation may impair cognitive function. Hypokalemia may occur in patients who induce self-vomiting or abuse diuretics and laxatives. Occasionally patients exhibit fatty liver infiltration and altered liver function tests. Renal complications may reflect long-term dehydration accompanied by hypokalemia resulting in irreversible damage to the renal tubules. Parturients are at increased risk of delivering low birth weight infants. These patients are anemic (30%), neutropenic (50%), and thrombocytopenic.

Treatment

Treatment of patients with anorexia nervosa is complicated by the patient's denial of the condition. Psychopharmacologic treatment, including tricyclic antidepressants, fluoxetine, lithium, and antipsychotic drugs, has not been predictably successful. Selective serotonin reuptake inhibitors (fluoxetine) that are effective in obsessive-compulsive disorders may have some value for treating patients with anorexia nervosa.

Management of Anesthesia

There is a paucity of information relating to the management of anesthesia of patients with this eating disorder. Preoperative evaluation is based on the known pathophysiologic effects evoked by starvation. The electrocardiogram is useful for detecting evidence of cardiac dysfunction. Electrolyte abnormalities (hypokalemia), hypovolemia owing to dehydration, and delayed gastric emptying are important preoperative considerations and need to be explored in this population. Development of cardiac dysrhythmias in patients with anorexia nervosa have been attributed to the presence of hypokalemia, prolonged QT intervals, and possible imbalance of the autonomic nervous system. Reversal of neuromuscular blockade and changes in Pa_{CO_2} could contribute to the potential for the development of cardiac dysrhythmias in these patients. Experience is too limited to permit recommendations regarding specific anesthetic drugs, muscle relaxants, or anesthetic techniques in the presence of anorexia nervosa.

Bulimia Nervosa

Bulimia nervosa is characterized by episodes of binge eating (a sense of loss of control over eating), purging, and dietary restriction. Binges are most often triggered by a negative emotional experience. Purging usually consists of self-induced vomiting that may be facilitated by laxatives and/or diuretics. In most patients, this disorder is chronic, with relapses and remissions. Depression, anxiety disorders, and substance abuse commonly accompany bulimia nervosa.

Signs and Symptoms

Findings on physical examination that suggest the presence of bulimia nervosa are dry skin, evidence of dehydration, and fluctuant hypertrophy of the salivary glands. Resting bradycardia is often present. The most common laboratory findings are increased serum amylase concentrations presumably of parotid gland origin. Metabolic alkalosis secondary to purging is frequently present with increased serum bicarbonate concentrations, hypochloremia, and occasionally hypokalemia. Dental complications including periodontal disease are likely.

Treatment

The most effective treatment of bulimia nervosa is cognitive-behavioral therapy. Pharmacotherapy with tricyclic antidepressants and selective serotonin reuptake inhibitors (fluoxetine) may be helpful. Potassium supplementation may be necessary in the presence of hypokalemia due to recurrent self-induced vomiting.

Binge-Eating Disorder

Binge-eating disorders resemble bulimia nervosa, but in contrast to patients with bulimia nervosa, these individuals do not purge and periods of dietary restriction are less striking. The diagnosis of binge-eating disorders should be suspected in morbidly obese patients, particularly obese patients with continued weight gain or marked weight cycling. The disease is chronic and accompanied by weight gain. Like anorexia nervosa and bulimia nervosa, this disorder is frequently accompanied by depression, anxiety disorders, and personality disorders. The principal medical complication of binge-eating disorders is morbid obesity and associated systemic hypertension, non–insulin-dependent diabetes mellitus, hypercholesterolemia, and joint disorders. As in patients with bulimia nervosa, antidepressant medications are useful for treating those with binge-eating disorders.

MALNUTRITION AND VITAMIN DEFICIENCIES

Malnutrition is a medically distinct syndrome that is responsive to caloric support provided by enteral or total parenteral nutrition (TPN) (hyperalimentation). Vitamin deficiencies are principally of historic interest but may still occur in severely malnourished patients.

Malnutrition

Signs and Symptoms

Malnourished patients are identified by the presence of serum albumin concentrations less than 3 g/dL and transferrin levels below 200 mg/dL and prealbumin levels (normally 16.0–35.0 mg/dL. Skin test anergy (immunosuppression) also accompanies malnutrition. Critically ill patients often experience negative caloric intake complicated by hypermetabolic states due to increased caloric needs produced by trauma, fever, sepsis, and wound healing. An estimated daily caloric intake of 1500 to 2000 calories is necessary to maintain basic energy requirements. An increase in body temperature of 1°C increases daily energy (caloric) requirements by approximately 15%. Multiple fractures increase energy needs by approximately 25% and major burns by approximately 100%. A large tumor, by virtue of its growth and metabolism, requires fuels that can exceed 100% of basic caloric requirements. Malnutrition is also associated with increased morbidity and mortality with impaired respiratory, cardiac, renal function as well as poor wound healing and immunosuppression. Postoperatively, patients experience increased protein breakdown and decreased protein synthesis.

Treatment

It is often recommended that patients who have lost more than 20% of their body weight be treated nutritionally before undergoing elective surgery. In this regard, provision of nutritional support for 7 days before surgery decreases postoperative complications, especially in patients with gastrointestinal cancer and elderly patients undergoing surgery for hip fractures. Patients who are unable to eat or absorb food after 7 days postoperatively also may require parenteral nutrition.

Enteral Nutrition When the gastrointestinal tract is functioning, enteral nutrition can be provided by means of nasogastric or gastrostomy tube feedings. Continuous drip infusion is the method most frequently used for administering enteral feedings. The exact rate and composition of the feeding solution will be individualized based on patient laboratory data. More recently, post-pyloric and nasojejunal tubes have been used more frequently with good results. The question when to stop post-pyloric feeding in patients requiring surgery is still not well studied, but if there is a naso- or orogastric tube, it should be suctioned prior to going to the operating room. Complications of enteral feedings are infrequent but may include hyperglycemia leading to osmotic diuresis and hypovolemia. Exogenous insulin administration is a consideration when blood glucose concentrations are elevated or exceed 110 mg/dL in the intensive care unit. The high osmolarity of elemental diets (550–850 mOsm/L) is often the cause of diarrhea.

Total Parenteral Nutrition TPN is indicated when the gastrointestinal tract is not functioning. Peripheral parenteral nutrition using an isotonic solution delivered through a peripheral vein is acceptable when patients require less than 900 mOsm/L and the anticipated need for nutritional support is less than 14 days. In TPN, when daily caloric requirements exceed 2000 calories or prolonged nutritional support is required, a catheter is traditionally placed in the subclavian vein to permit infusion of hypertonic parenteral solutions (approximately 1900 mOsm/L) in a daily volume of approximately 40 mL/kg.

Potential complications of TPN are numerous (**Table 13-7**). In patients receiving TPN, blood glucose concentrations are monitored, as hyperglycemia will require treatment with exogenous insulin, and hypoglycemia may occur if the TPN infusion is abruptly discontinued (mechanical obstruction in the delivery tubing) as increased circulating endogenous concentrations of insulin will persist. Hyperchloremic metabolic acidosis may occur because of the liberation of hydrochloric acid during the metabolism of amino acids present in most parenteral nutrition solutions. Parenteral feeding of patients with compromised cardiac function is associated with the risk of congestive heart failure as a result of fluid overload. Increased production of carbon dioxide resulting from metabolism of large amounts of glucose may result in the need to initiate mechanical ventilation of the lungs or failure to wean patients from long-term ventilator support.

Vitamin Deficiencies

Table 13-8 lists a number of vitamin deficiencies categorized by type.

INBORN ERRORS OF METABOLISM

Inborn errors of metabolism manifest as a variety of metabolic defects that may complicate the management of anesthesia (**Table 13-9**). In some instances, these defects are clinically asymptomatic and manifest only in response to specific triggering events, such as certain drugs or foods.

Porphyrias

Porphyrias are a group of inborn errors of metabolism characterized by the overproduction of porphyrins and their precursors. Porphyrins are essential for many vital physiologic functions including oxygen transport and storage. The synthetic pathway involved in the production of porphyrins is determined by a sequence of enzymes. A defect in any of these enzymes results in accumulation of the preceding intermediaries and produces a form of porphyria (**Fig. 13-4**). In human physiology, heme is the most important porphyrin being bound to proteins to form hemoproteins that include hemoglobin and cytochromes (P-450 isozymes, which are important for drug metabolism). Production of heme is controlled by the activity of aminolevulinic acid (ALA) synthetase, which is present in mitochondria. The formation of ALA synthetase is controlled by the endogenous concentration of heme, ensuring that the level of heme production parallels requirements (see Fig. 13-4). ALA synthetase is readily inducible and can respond rapidly to increased heme requirements such as those resulting from the administration of drugs that require P-450 for their metabolism. In the presence of porphyria, any increase in heme requirements results in accumulation of pathway intermediates immediately preceding the site of enzyme block (see Fig. 13-4).

Classification

Porphyrias are classified by the site of the enzyme defect hepatic or erythropoietic, reflecting the major sites of heme production in the liver and bone marrow, the enzyme defect itself, or whether it causes acute symptoms (**Table 13-10; see** also Fig. 13-4). Only acute forms of porphyria are relevant to the management of anesthesia, as they are the only forms of

TABLE 13-7 Other Complications of Total Parenteral Nutrition/Peripheral Parenteral Nutrition		
Hypokalemia	Hypomagnesemia	Hypocalcemia
Hypophosphatemia	Venous thrombosis	Infection/sepsis
Bacterial translocation from the gastrointestinal tract	Osteopenia	Elevated liver enzymes
Renal dysfunction	Hyperchloremic metabolic acidosis	Fluid overload
Nonketotic hyperosmolar hyperglycemic coma		Refeeding syndrome*

*Hemolytic anemia, respiratory distress, tetany, paresthesia, and cardiac arrhythmias. More common in anorexia, alcoholics, rapid refeeding, and associated with low phosphorus, potassium, magnesium.

TABLE 13-8 Vitamin Deficiencies

Vitamin	Laboratory Test	Causes of Deficiency	Signs of Deficiency
Thiamine (B_1) (beriberi)	Urinary thiamine	Chronic alcoholics due to decreased intake of thiamine	Low SVR, high CO, polyneuropathy (demyelination, sensory deficit, paresthesia), exaggerated decreased response to hemorrhage, change in body position, positive pressure ventilation
Riboflavin (B_2)	Urinary riboflavin	Almost always due to dietary deficiency, photodegradation of milk, other dairy products	Magenta tongue, angular stomatitis, seborrhea, cheilosis
Pantothenic acid (B_3)	Urinary pantothenic acid	Liver, yeast, egg yolks, and vegetables	Nonspecific and include gastrointestinal disturbance, depression, muscle cramps, paresthesia, ataxia, and hypoglycemia
Niacin (B_5) (pellegra)	Urinary niacin metabolite	Nicotinic acid is synthetized from tryptophan; carcinoid tumor uses tryptophan to form serotonin instead of nicotinic acid, making these patients more susceptible.	Mental confusion, irritability, peripheral neuropathy, achlorhydria, diarrhea, vesicular dermatitis, stomatitis, glossitis, urethritis, and excessive salivation
Pyridoxine (B_6)	Plasma B_6	Alcoholism, isoniazid	Seborrhea, glossitis, convulsions, neuropathy, depression, confusion, microcytic anemia
Folate (B_9)	Serum folate	Alcoholism, sulfasalazine, pyrimethamine, triamterene	Megaloblastic anemia, atrophic glossitis, depression, ↑homocysteine
Cyanocobalamine (B_{12})	Serum B_{12}	Gastric atrophy (pernicious anemia), terminal ileal disease, strict vegetarianism	Megaloblastic anemia, loss of vibratory and position sense, abnormal gait, dementia, impotence, loss of bladder and bowel control, ↑homocysteine, ↑methylmalonic acid
Biotin	Serum biotin	Liver, soy, beans, yeast, and egg yolks, egg white contains the protein avidin, which strongly binds the vitamin and reduces its bioavailability	Mental changes (depression, hallucinations), paresthesia, anorexia, and nausea; a scaling, seborrheic, and erythematous rash may occur around the eyes, nose, and mouth as well as on the extremities
Ascorbic acid (C) (scurvy)	Serum ascorbic acid	Smoking, alcoholism	Capillary fragility, petechial hemorrhage, joint and skeletal muscle hemorrhage, poor wound healing, catabolic state, loosened teeth and gangrenous alveolar margins, low potassium, iron
A	Plasma vitamin A	Dietary lack of leafy vegetables and animal liver or malabsorption	Loss of night vision, conjunctival drying, corneal destruction, anemia
D (rickets)	Plasma 25-dihydroxy vitamin D	Decreased vitamin D leads to less calcium absorption balanced by parathormone activity that increases due to low calcium, leading to increased osteoclastic activity and bone resorption	Thoracic kyphosis could lead to hypoventilation, normal to low serum calcium, low serum phosphate, high plasma alkaline phosphatase
E	Plasma α-tocopherol	Occurs only with fat malabsorption, or genetic abnormalities of vitamin E metabolism/transport	Peripheral neuropathy, spinocerebellar ataxia, skeletal muscle atrophy, retinopathy
K	Prothrombin time	Formed by intestinal bacteria that are eliminated by prolonged antibiotic therapy or failure of fat absorption	Bleeding

CO, cardiac output; SVR, systemic vascular resistance.

TABLE 13-9 Inborn Errors of Metabolism

Porphyria
Gout
Pseudogout
Hyperlipidemia
Carbohydrate metabolism disorders
Amino acid disorders
Mucopolysaccharidoses
Gangliosidoses

porphyria that may result in life-threatening reactions in response to certain drugs (see Table 13-10).

Acute Porphyrias Acute porphyrias, with the exception of the rare plumboporphyria, are inherited as non–sex-linked autosomal dominant conditions with variable expression. The enzyme defects in porphyria are deficiencies rather than absolute deficits. Although there is no direct influence of gender on the pattern of inheritance, attacks occur more frequently in women and are most frequent during the third and fourth decades of life. Attacks are rare before puberty or following the onset of menopause. Acute attacks of porphyria are most commonly precipitated by events that decrease heme concentrations, thus increasing the activity of ALA synthetase and stimulating the production of porphyrinogens (see Fig. 13-4). Enzyme-inducing drugs are the most important triggering factors for the development of acute porphyrias. These acute attacks may also be precipitated by physiologic hormonal fluctuations such as those that accompany menstruation, fasting (such as before elective surgery), dehydration, stress (such as that associated with anesthesia and surgery), and infection. Pregnancy in these patients is often associated with spontaneous abortion. Furthermore, pregnancy may be complicated by systemic hypertension and an increased incidence of low birth weight infants.

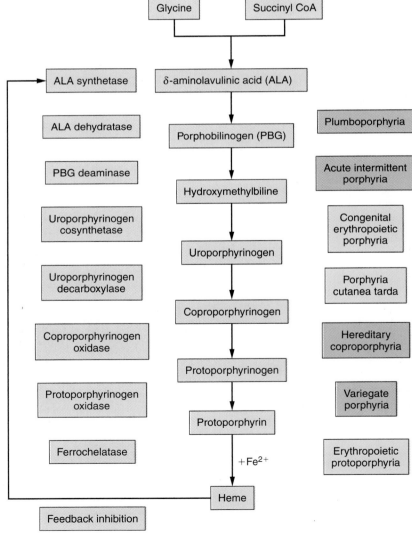
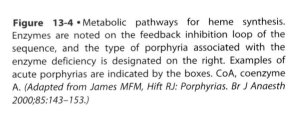

Figure 13-4 • Metabolic pathways for heme synthesis. Enzymes are noted on the feedback inhibition loop of the sequence, and the type of porphyria associated with the enzyme deficiency is designated on the right. Examples of acute porphyrias are indicated by the boxes. CoA, coenzyme A. *(Adapted from James MFM, Hift RJ: Porphyrias. Br J Anaesth 2000;85:143–153.)*

TABLE 13-10 Classification of Porphyrias

Acute
Acute intermittent porphyria
Variegate porphyria
Hereditary coproporphyria
Plumboporphyria

Nonacute
Porphyria cutanea tarda
Erythropoietic porphyrias
   Erythropoietic uroporphyria
   Erythropoietic protoporphyria

Adapted from James MFM, Hift RJ: Porphyrias. Br J Anaesth 2000;85:143–153.

Signs and Symptoms Acute attacks of porphyria are characterized by severe abdominal pain, autonomic nervous system instability, electrolyte disturbances, and neuropsychiatric manifestations ranging from mild disturbances to fulminating life-threatening events. Skeletal muscle weakness that may progress to quadriparesis and respiratory failure is the most potentially lethal neurologic manifestation of acute attacks of porphyria. Central nervous system involvement with upper motor neuron lesions, cranial nerve palsies, and involvement of the cerebellum and basal ganglia is seen less frequently as well as autonomic neuropathy that together with hypovolemia can exacerbate cardiovascular instability. Seizures may occur during an attack of acute porphyria. Psychiatric disturbances may develop, but it seems their incidence may have been overemphasized.

Gastrointestinal symptoms accompanying abdominal pain include vomiting and diarrhea. Despite severe abdominal pain (which may mimic acute appendicitis, acute cholecystitis, renal colic), clinical examination of the abdomen is typically normal. Abdominal pain is thought to relate directly to autonomic nervous system neuropathy. Dehydration and electrolyte disturbances involving sodium, potassium, and magnesium may be prominent in these patients. Tachycardia and systemic hypertension or less commonly hypotension are manifestations of cardiovascular instability.

Complete and prolonged remissions are likely between attacks, and many individuals with the genetic defect never develop symptoms. In this regard, patients at known risk of porphyria but previously asymptomatic (silent or latent porphyria) may experience their first symptoms in response to inadvertent administration of triggering drugs during the perioperative period. ALA synthetase concentrations are increased during all acute attacks of porphyria.

Triggering Drugs Drugs may trigger an acute attack of porphyria by inducing the activity of ALA synthetase or interfering with the negative feedback control as the final common pathway (see Fig. 13-4). It is not possible to predict which drugs will be porphyrinogenic, although chemical groupings such as the allyl groups present on barbiturates and certain steroid structures have been incriminated in the production of porphyria. Only the acute forms of porphyria are affected by drug-induced enzyme induction. It is not clear why the manifestations of nonacute porphyria are apparently not affected by enzyme-inducing drugs. For example, potent enzyme inducers of ALA synthetase, including the anticonvulsants, do not exacerbate or precipitate porphyria cutanea tarda or the erythropoietic porphyrias. The labeling of drugs as safe or unsafe for patients with porphyria is often based on anecdotal experience with the use of the drugs in porphyric patients and reports of the induction of acute attacks. Drugs may be tested in cell culture models for their ability to induce ALA synthetase activity or for their effects on porphyrin synthesis. Alternatively, the action of drugs on the porphyrin synthetic pathway can be investigated in animal models. Both cell culture and animal models tend to overestimate the porphyrinogenicity of drugs.

It is difficult to assess the porphyrinogenic potential of anesthetic drugs, as other factors such as sepsis or stress may precipitate a porphyric crisis coincidentally with administration of anesthesia. Any classification of anesthetic drugs with regard to their porphyrinogenicity is likely to be imperfect and arbitrary (**Table 13-11**). Particular care is needed when selecting drugs for patients with acute intermittent porphyria or clinically active forms of porphyria and when prescribing drugs in combination, as exacerbation of porphyria is more likely under these circumstances.

Acute Intermittent Porphyria Of all the acute porphyrias, acute intermittent porphyria affecting the central and peripheral nervous systems produces the most serious symptoms (systemic hypertension, renal dysfunction) and is the one most likely to be life-threatening. The defective enzyme is porphobilinogen deaminase, and the gene encoding this enzyme is located on chromosome 11 (see Fig. 13-4).

Variegate Porphyria Variegate porphyria is characterized by neurotoxicity and cutaneous photosensitivity in which bullous skin eruptions occur on exposure to sunlight as a result of the conversion of porphyrinogens to porphyrins. The enzyme defect is at the level of protoporphyrinogen oxidase, and the gene encoding this enzyme is on chromosome 1 (see Fig. 13-4). The incidence of variegate porphyria is highest in South Africa.

Hereditary Coproporphyria Acute attacks of hereditary coproporphyria are less common and severe than acute intermittent porphyria or variegate porphyria. As in patients with variegate porphyria, neurotoxicity and cutaneous hypersensitivity are characteristic, although they tend to be less severe. The defective enzyme is coproporphyrinogen oxidase, encoded by a gene on chromosome 9 (see Fig. 13-4).

Porphyria Cutanea Tarda Porphyria cutanea tarda is due to an enzymatic defect (decreased hepatic activity of uroporphyrinogen decarboxylase) transmitted as an autosomal dominant trait. ALA synthetase activity is not important, and drugs capable of precipitating attacks of other forms of porphyria do not provoke an attack of porphyria cutanea tarda. Likewise, neurotoxicity does not accompany this form of porphyria. Signs and symptoms of porphyria cutanea tarda most often appear as photosensitivity in men older than 35 years of age. Porphyrin accumulation in the liver is associated with

TABLE 13-11 Recommendations Regarding the Use of Anesthetic Drugs in the Presence of Acute Porphyrias

Drug	Recommendation	Drug	Recommendation
Inhaled Anesthetics		**Opioid Antagonists**	
Nitrous oxide	Safe	Naloxone	Safe
Isoflurane	Probably safe*		
Sevoflurane	Probably safe*	**Anticholinergics**	
Desflurane	Probably safe*	Atropine	Safe
		Glycopyrrolate	Safe
Intravenous Anesthetics		**Anticholinesterases**	
Propofol	Safe	Neostigmine	Safe
Ketamine	Probably safe*		
Thiopental	Avoid	**Local Anesthetics**	
Thiamylal	Avoid	Lidocaine	Safe
Methohexital	Avoid	Tetracaine	Safe
Etomidate	Avoid	Bupivacaine	Safe
		Mepivacaine	Safe
Analgesics		Ropivacaine	No data
Acetaminophen	Safe		
Aspirin	Safe	**Sedatives and Antiemetics**	
Codeine	Safe	Droperidol	Safe
Morphine	Safe	Midazolam	Probably safe*
Fentanyl	Safe	Lorazepam	Probably safe*
Sufentanil	Safe	Cimetidine	Probably safe*
Ketorolac	Probably avoid†	Ranitidine	Probably safe*
Phenacetin	Probably avoid†	Metoclopramide	Probably safe*
Pentazocine	Avoid	Ondansetron	Probably safe*
Neuromuscular Blocking Drugs		**Cardiovascular Drugs**	
Succinylcholine	Safe	Epinephrine	Safe
Pancuronium	Safe	α-Agonists	Safe
Atracurium	Probably safe*	β-Agonists	Safe
Cisatracurium	Probably safe*	β-Antagonists	Safe
Vecuronium	Probably safe*	Diltiazem	Probably safe*
Rocuronium	Probably safe*	Nitroprusside	Probably safe*
Mivacurium	Probably safe*	Nifedipine	Probably avoid†

*Although safety is not conclusively established, the drug is unlikely to provoke acute porphyria.
†Use only if expected benefits outweigh the risks.
Adapted from James MFM, Hift RJ: Porphyrias. Br J Anaesth 2000;85:143–153.

hepatocellular necrosis. Anesthesia is not a hazard in affected patients, although the choice of drugs should take into consideration the likely presence of co-existing liver disease.

Erythropoietic Uroporphyria Erythropoietic uroporphyria is a rare form of porphyria, transmitted as an autosomal recessive trait. In contrast to porphyrin synthesis in the liver, porphyrin synthesis in the erythropoietic system is responsive to changes in hematocrit and tissue oxygenation. Hemolytic anemia, bone marrow hyperplasia, and splenomegaly are often present. Repeated infections are common, and photosensitivity is severe. The urine of affected patients turns red when exposed to light. Neurotoxicity and abdominal pain do not occur, and administration of barbiturates does not adversely alter the course of the disease. Death usually occurs during early childhood.

Erythropoietic Protoporphyria Erythropoietic protoporphyria (**Table 13-12**) is a more common, but less debilitating, form of erythropoietic porphyria. Signs and symptoms include photosensitivity, vesicular cutaneous eruptions, urticaria, and edema. In occasional patients cholelithiasis develops secondary to increased excretion of protoporphyrin. Administration of barbiturates does not adversely affect the course of the disease, and survival to adulthood is common.

Management of Anesthesia

Anesthesia has been implicated in the triggering of acute attacks of porphyria, although recent reports are rare. Indeed, most patients with porphyria can be safely anesthetized assuming that appropriate precautions are taken. In this regard, patients with evidence of active porphyria or a history

TABLE 13-12   Summary of Major Biochemical Findings in the Acute Porphyrias

Disorder	Urinary ALA and PBG	Urinary Porphyrins	Fecal Porphyrins
Quiescent AIP	Increased	Mild increase	Normal
Acute AIP	Very high	Very high	As above
Quiescent HCP	Normal	Coproporphyrin III often increased	Increased coproporphyrin III
Acute HCP	High	Increased	As above
Quiescent VP	Normal	Normal	Increased pentacarboxylic porphyrin III, coproporphyrin III, and protoporphyrin IX
Acute VP	High	High	As above

Silent carriers will demonstrate no abnormality on urine and fecal testing, yet carry the gene and are at risk of an acute attack.
AIP, acute intermittent porphyria; ALA, aminolevulinic acid; HCP, hereditary coproporphyria; PBG, porphobilinogen.

of acute porphyric crises must be considered to be at increased risk. Short-acting drugs are presumed to be safe because their rapid elimination limits exposure time for enzyme induction to occur. Repeated or prolonged use (continuous intravenous infusions of propofol) could result in different responses. There are multiple case reports of successful use of intermittent propofol administration in patients with porphyria, although there are not enough data on continuous infusion to validate this technique. There is reason to believe that exposure to multiple potential enzyme-inducing drugs may be more dangerous than exposure to any one drug.

Preoperative Evaluation

Guidelines for drug selection:

1. There is evidence that single exposure to potent inducers is tolerated but not in acute attacks.
2. There are reasons to believe exposure to multiple potential agents is more dangerous than any new single agent.
3. Some drugs are listed based on animal or cell culture experiments and may not be true.
4. Case reports with adverse outcome are frequently unreliable

The principles of safe anesthetic management of patients with porphyria depend on the identification of susceptible individuals and the determination of potential porphyrinogenic triggering drugs. Laboratory identification of porphyric individuals is not easy, as many show only subtle or no biochemical abnormalities during asymptomatic phases. In the presence of a suggestive family history, determination of erythrocyte porphobilinogen activity is the most appropriate screening test for patients with suspected acute intermittent porphyria. In addition to a careful family history and thorough physical examination (often no clinical evidence or only subtle skin lesions), the presence or absence of peripheral neuropathy and autonomic nervous system instability is noted.

If an acute exacerbation of porphyria is suspected during the preoperative period, particular attention must be given to skeletal muscle strength and cranial nerve function, as symptoms related to these systems may predict impending respiratory failure and an increased risk of pulmonary aspiration. Cardiovascular examination may reveal systemic hypertension and tachycardia, which necessitate treatment before induction

of anesthesia. Postoperative ventilation of the patient's lungs may be required during an acute porphyric crisis. During an acute exacerbation, severe abdominal pain may mimic a surgical abdomen. Preoperative preparation in patients experiencing an acute porphyric crisis should include careful assessment of fluid balance and electrolyte status.

Preoperative starvation should be minimized, but if a prolonged fast is unavoidable, administration of a glucose-saline infusion during the preoperative period may be considered, as caloric restriction has been linked to the precipitation of acute porphyria attacks. In view of the frequency with which hyponatremia is encountered during acute attacks of porphyria, intravenous fluids containing only glucose are not recommended.

Preoperative Premedication Benzodiazepines are commonly selected for preoperative anxiolysis. Aspiration prophylaxis that includes antacids and/or H_2-receptor antagonists is acceptable. Cimetidine has been recommended for treatment of acute porphyric crises, as this drug may decrease heme consumption and inhibit ALA synthetase activity. Cimetidine does not appear to be effective prophylactically.

Prophylactic Therapy No specific prophylactic therapy has been shown to be of proven benefit. However, because carbohydrate administration can suppress porphyrin synthesis, administering oral carbohydrate supplements (20 g/hr) preoperatively may be recommended. If oral feedings are not acceptable, 10% glucose in saline is an option. Hematin has not been evaluated as prophylactic therapy.

Regional Anesthesia There is no absolute contraindication to the use of regional anesthesia in patients with porphyria. If a regional anesthetic is considered, it is essential to perform a neurologic examination before initiating the block to minimize the likelihood that worsening of any preexisting neuropathy would be erroneously attributed to the regional anesthetic. Autonomic nervous system blockade induced by the regional anesthetic could unmask cardiovascular instability, especially in the presence of autonomic nervous system neuropathy, hypovolemia, or both. There is no evidence that any local anesthetic has ever induced an acute attack of porphyria or neurologic damage in porphyric individuals. Regional anesthesia has been safely administered to parturients with acute intermittent porphyria.

Regional anesthesia for patients experiencing acute intermittent porphyria, however, is not likely to be used because of concerns related to hemodynamic instability, mental confusion, and associated neuropathy.

General Anesthesia The total dose of drugs administered and the length of exposure may influence the risk of triggering a porphyric crisis in vulnerable patients (see Table 13-11). In this regard, the availability of short-acting anesthetic drugs has likely contributed to the safety of anesthesia in the presence of porphyria. Perioperative monitoring should consider the frequent presence of autonomic nervous system dysfunction and the possibility of labile systemic blood pressure.

Induction of Anesthesia Propofol has been used safely for induction of anesthesia in patients with porphyria, although the use of prolonged continuous infusions of this drug is of unproven safety. Ketamine has been used safely in the presence of quiescent acute intermittent porphyria. Use of etomidate is questionable, as it has been shown to be potentially porphyrinogenic in animal studies despite its safe use in this patient population. All barbiturates must be considered unsafe for anesthetic use despite numerous reports of their safe administration to porphyric patients during the quiescent phase. Conversely, worsening of symptoms has been observed when thiopental is administered in the presence of a porphyric crisis.

Maintenance of Anesthesia Nitrous oxide is well established as a safe inhaled anesthetic to administer to patients with porphyria. Safe use of isoflurane has been described. The short durations of action of sevoflurane and desflurane are desirable characteristics for drugs to be administered to patients with porphyria, but experience is too limited to make recommendations. Opioids have been administered safely to these patients. Neuromuscular blocking drugs do not seem to introduce a predictable risk when administered to these patients.

Cardiopulmonary Bypass Theoretically, cardiopulmonary bypass is a potential risk for patients with porphyria, as the additional stress introduced by hypothermia, pump-induced hemolysis, blood loss and its consequent increase in heme demand by the bone marrow, and the large number of drugs administered could increase the risk of developing a porphyric crisis. Nevertheless, clinical experience does not support an increased incidence of porphyric crises in these patients when undergoing cardiopulmonary bypass.

Treatment of a Porphyric Crisis

The first step in treating an acute porphyric crisis is removal of any known triggering factors. Adequate hydration and carbohydrates are necessary either via an enteral or parenteral route. Sedation using phenothiazine can be used; pain often necessitates treatment with opioids. Nausea and vomiting are treated with conventional antiemetics. β-Adrenergic blockers are administered to control tachycardia and systemic hypertension. Should seizures occur, traditional anticonvulsants are regarded as unsafe, necessitating the use of a benzodiazepine or case report describes propofol to terminate

the seizure. Electrolyte disturbances, including hypomagnesemia, are treated aggressively.

Hematin (3–4 mg/kg IV over 20 minutes) is the only specific form of therapy for an acute porphyric crisis. It is presumed that hematin supplements the intracellular pool of heme and thus suppresses ALA synthetase activity. Heme arginate is more stable than hematin and lacks the potential adverse effects associated with hematin (renal failure, coagulopathy, thrombophlebitis). Somatostatin decreases the rate of formation of ALA synthetase and combined with plasmapheresis may effectively decrease pain and induce remission.

Gout

Gout is a disorder of purine metabolism and may be classified as primary or secondary. Primary gout is due to an inherited metabolic defect that leads to overproduction of uric acid. Secondary gout is hyperuricemia due to an identifiable cause, such as chemotherapeutic drugs used to treat leukemia, leading to the rapid lysis of purine-containing cells. Gout is characterized by hyperuricemia with recurrent episodes of acute arthritis owing to deposition of urate crystals in joints. Deposition of urate crystals typically initiates an inflammatory response that causes pain and limited motion of the joints. At least one half of the initial attacks of gout are confined to the first metatarsophalangeal joint. Persistent hyperuricemia also results in deposition of urate crystals in extra-articular locations, manifested most often as nephrolithiasis. Urate crystal deposition can also occur in the myocardium, aortic valves, and extradural spinal regions. The incidence of systemic hypertension, ischemic heart disease, and diabetes mellitus are increased in patients with gout.

Treatment

Treatment of gout is designed to decrease the plasma concentrations of uric acid by administration of uricosuric drugs (probenecid) or inhibition of the conversion of purines to uric acid by xanthine oxidase (allopurinol). Colchicine, which lacks any effect on purine metabolism, is considered the drug of choice for management of acute gouty arthritis. It relieves joint pain presumably by modifying leukocyte migration and phagocytosis. The side effects of colchicine include vomiting and diarrhea. Large doses of colchicine also can produce hepatorenal dysfunction and agranulocytosis.

Management of Anesthesia

Management of anesthesia in the presence of gout focuses on prehydration to facilitate continued renal elimination of uric acid. Sodium bicarbonate to alkalinize the urine also facilitates excretion of uric acid. As lactate can decrease the renal tubular secretion of uric acid, the use of lactated Ringer's solution may be questioned, although this is an unproven concern. Despite appropriate precautions, acute attacks of gout may follow surgical procedures for no apparent reason in patients with a history of gout.

Extra-articular manifestations of gout and side effects of drugs used to control the disease deserve consideration when formulating the plan for anesthesia management. Renal function is evaluated, as clinical manifestations of gout usually increase with deteriorating renal function. Abnormalities detected on the electrocardiogram could reflect urate deposits in the myocardium. The increased incidence of systemic hypertension, ischemic heart disease, and diabetes mellitus in patients with gout is considered. Although rare, adverse renal and hepatic effects may be associated with probenecid and colchicine. Limited temporomandibular joint motion from gouty arthritis, if present, can make direct laryngoscopy for tracheal intubation difficult.

Lesch-Nyhan Syndrome

Lesch-Nyhan syndrome is a genetically determined disorder of purine metabolism that occurs exclusively in males. Biochemically, the defect is characterized by decreased or absent activity of hypoxanthine-guanine phosphoribosyl transferase, leading to excess purine production and increased uric acid concentrations throughout the body. Clinically, patients are often mentally retarded and exhibit characteristic spasticity and self-mutilation patterns. Self-mutilation usually involves trauma to perioral tissues, and subsequent scarification may present difficulties with direct laryngoscopy for tracheal intubation. Seizure disorders associated with this syndrome are often treated with benzodiazepines. Athetoid dysphagia may increase the likelihood of aspiration if vomiting occurs. Malnutrition is often present. Hyperuricemia is associated with nephropathy, urinary tract calculi, and arthritis. Death is often due to renal failure.

Management of anesthesia is influenced by co-existing renal dysfunction and possible impaired metabolism of drugs administered during anesthesia. The presence of a spastic skeletal muscle disorder suggests caution in using succinylcholine. The sympathetic nervous system response to stress is enhanced, suggesting caution in the administration of exogenous catecholamines to these patients.

Disorders of Carbohydrate Metabolism

Disorders of carbohydrate metabolism usually reflect genetically determined enzyme defects (**Table 13-13**). The defect can result in a deficiency or an excess of precursors or end-products of metabolism that are normally involved in the formation of glycogen from glucose. In some instances, an alternate metabolic pathway is used. Ultimately, signs and symptoms of specific disorders of carbohydrate metabolism reflect the effects produced by alterations in the amount of precursors or end-products of metabolism that result from the enzyme defects.

Glycogen Storage Disease Type 1a

Glycogen storage disease type 1a (von Gierke's disease) is due to the deficiency or lack of the enzyme glucose 6-phosphatase. As a result, glycogen cannot be hydrolyzed in hepatocytes, neutrophils, and possibly other cells, leading to its intracellular accumulation. Hypoglycemia can be severe, and oral feedings are required every 2 to 3 hours to maintain acceptable blood glucose concentrations. Chronic metabolic

TABLE 13-13 Disorders of Carbohydrate Metabolism
Glycogen storage disease type 1a (von Gierke's disease)
Glycogen storage disease type 1b
Pompe's disease
McArdle's disease
Galactosemia
Fructose 1,6-diphosphate deficiency
Pyruvate dehydrogenase deficiency
Mucopolysaccharidoses
Gangliosidoses

acidosis is present and may lead to osteoporosis. Mental retardation, growth retardation, and seizures due to hypoglycemia are likely. Hepatomegaly is due to accumulation of glycogen in the liver. Renal enlargement caused by accumulation of glycogen may manifest as chronic pyelonephritis. A hemorrhagic diathesis may be due to platelet dysfunction and manifest as recurrent epistaxis and bleeding after minor trauma and surgery. Facial and truncal obesity occurs. Survival beyond 2 years of age is unusual, although surgical creation of a portocaval shunt may benefit some patients.

Management of anesthesia includes provision of exogenous glucose to prevent potentially unrecognized intraoperative hypoglycemia. Monitoring of the arterial pH and blood glucose concentrations is helpful, as these patients often become acidotic owing to an inability to convert lactic acid to glycogen. In this regard, lactate-containing solutions for intravenous infusions are avoided to minimize the theoretic possibility of metabolic acidosis due to lactate administration during the perioperative period.

Glycogen Storage Disease Type 1b

Glycogen storage disease type 1b is a rare autosomal recessive disease in which glucose 6-phosphate, a product of metabolic cleavage of glycogen, cannot be transported to the inner surface of microsomes because of a deficiency in its transport system. As such, this disease is a variant of glycogen storage disease type 1a. In glycogen storage disease type 1b, glycogen accumulates in the liver, kidneys, and intestinal mucosa, and glucose availability to tissues is impaired. Hypoglycemia and lactic acidosis ensue. Clinical signs and symptoms resemble those described for glycogen storage disease type 1a. In addition, type 1b patients may experience recurrent infections owing to impaired neutrophil activity.

Preoperative fasting is minimized, and glucose-containing infusions are administered intravenously throughout the perioperative period. Strict asepsis is important, and preoperative normalization of blood glucose concentrations may improve platelet function, thereby decreasing the likelihood of intraoperative bleeding. Intraoperative monitoring of blood glucose concentrations is recommended, as hypoglycemia may be profound and difficult to recognize during general anesthesia. Lactic acidosis develops as a result of the incomplete conversion of glycogen. For this reason, monitoring the arterial pH is helpful; administration of lactate-containing solutions is not recommended. Iatrogenic hyperventilation of the patient's lungs and associated respiratory alkalosis may stimulate release of lactate from skeletal muscles and aggravate metabolic acidosis. Treatment of metabolic acidosis includes administration of intravenous sodium bicarbonate.

Disorders of Amino Acid Metabolism

Although there are more than 70 known disorders of amino acid metabolism, most are extremely rare. Classic manifestations include mental retardation, seizures, and aminoaciduria (Table 13-14). In addition, metabolic acidosis, hyperammonemia, hepatic failure, and thromboembolism can also occur.

Management of anesthesia in patients with disorders of amino acid metabolism is directed toward maintenance of intravascular fluid volume and acid-base homeostasis. Use of anesthetics that could evoke seizures may be questionable in view of the likely presence of seizure disorders in these patients.

Phenylketonuria

Phenylketonuria is the prototype of disorders attributable to abnormal amino acid metabolism. Phenylalanine accumulates owing to an enzymatic deficiency of phenylalanine hydroxylase. Clinical features include mental retardation and seizures. The skin may be friable and vulnerable to damage from pressure or friction created by adhesive materials. Also, these patients are more liable to vitamin B_{12} deficiency, especially with strict dietary control. If this is the case and the patient has B_{12} deficiency due to lack of supplementary treatment, nitric oxide should probably be avoided. They may also be more sensitive to narcotics.

Homocystinuria

Homocystinuria is due to failure of transsulfuration of precursors of cystine, an important constituent of cross linkages in collagen. Manifestations of the disease reflect weakened collagen and include dislocation of the lens, osteoporosis, kyphoscoliosis, brittle light-colored hair, and malar flush. Mental retardation may be a prominent finding in this disease. The diagnosis of homocystinuria is confirmed by demonstrating homocystine in the urine as evidenced by the development of a characteristic magenta color upon exposure to nitroprusside. Thromboembolism can be life-threatening and is presumed to reflect activation of the Hageman factor by homocystine, resulting in increased platelet adhesiveness. Attempts to minimize the likelihood of thromboembolism during the perioperative period should include administration of pyridoxine, which decreases platelet adhesiveness, preoperative hydration, infusion of dextran, and early ambulation.

Maple Syrup Urine Disease

Maple syrup urine disease is a rare inborn error of metabolism that results from defective carboxylation of branched-chain amino acids. In the absence of adequate enzyme activity, consumption of foods containing branched-chain amino acids results in the accumulation of these amino acids and ketoacids in tissues and blood. Increased concentrations of leucine are usually greater than those of isoleucine or valine, as leucine is the predominant amino acid in most proteins. These amino acids result in a maple syrup odor in the urine.

TABLE 13-14 Disorders of Amino Acid Metabolism							
Disorder	Mental Retardation	Seizures	Metabolic Acidosis	Hyper-ammonemia	Hepatic Failure	Thrombo-embolism	Other
Phenylketonuria	Yes	Yes	No	No	No	No	Friable skin
Homocystinuria	Yes/no	Yes	No	No	No	Yes	
Hypervalinemia	Yes	Yes	Yes	No	No	No	Hypoglycemia
Citrullinemia	Yes	Yes	No	Yes	Yes	No	
Branched-chain aciduria (maple syrup urine disease)	Yes	Yes	Yes	No		Yes	Hypoglycemia Neurologic deterioration during perioperative period
Methylmalonyl coenzyme A mutase deficiency			Yes	Yes			Acidosis intraoperatively Avoid nitrous oxide?
Isoleucinemia	Yes	Yes	Yes	Yes	Yes	No	Hypovolemia
Methioninemia	Yes	No	No	No	No	No	Thermal instability
Histidinuria	Yes	Yes/no	No	No	No	No	Erythrocyte fragility
Neutral aminoaciduria (Hartnup's disease)	Yes/no		Yes	No	No	No	Dermatitis
Arginemia	Yes		No	Yes	Yes	No	

Growth retardation and delayed psychomotor development are often a consequence of this chronic metabolic imbalance. Infection or fasting commonly results in acute metabolic decompensation, with increased plasma levels of branched-chain amino acids and ketoacids due to the breakdown of endogenous proteins. Increased plasma levels of ketoacids contributes to the production of metabolic acidosis. Hypoglycemia is a possibility, presumably reflecting the ability of increased plasma leucine concentrations to stimulate the release of insulin. A potentially fatal encephalopathy may accompany this disease.

Treatment is directed at decreasing the plasma levels of branched-chain amino acids and ketoacids with peritoneal dialysis or hemodialysis. Parenteral nutrition using preparations devoid of branched-chain amino acids may also be effective.

Surgery and anesthesia introduce a number of hazards for the perioperative management of patients with maple syrup urine disease. For example, catabolism of body proteins produced by surgery or infection could result in increased blood concentrations of branched-chain amino acids. Even blood in the gastrointestinal tract, as can occur following a tonsillectomy, produces an added metabolic load in patients with maple syrup urine disease. Accumulation of branched-chain amino acids in the circulation can produce neurologic deterioration during the perioperative period. The danger of hypoglycemia in affected patients is exacerbated by the period of fasting that precedes elective operations. Therefore, it is useful to initiate intravenous infusions of glucose-containing solutions intraoperatively. Measurement of arterial pH is helpful for detecting metabolic acidosis due to accumulation of ketoacids in these patients. Significant metabolic acidosis during the perioperative period may necessitate treatment with intravenous administration of sodium bicarbonate.

Methylmalonyl-Coenzyme A Mutase Deficiency

Methylmalonyl-coenzyme A mutase deficiency is an inborn error of metabolism that can result in the formation of methylmalonic acidemia. Acute treatment includes intravenous administration of crystalloid solutions containing sodium bicarbonate. Events during the perioperative period that increase protein catabolism (fasting, bleeding into the gastrointestinal tract, stress responses, tissue destruction) may predispose to acidosis.

Experience with anesthesia is limited, and recommendations are based more on theory than on clinical experience. For example, nitrous oxide may be avoided based on the theoretic concern that this inhaled anesthetic could predispose to methylmalonic acidemia in susceptible patients, reflecting nitrous oxide–induced inhibition of cobalamin coenzymes. The impact of preoperative fasting on amino acid metabolism and intravascular fluid volume is lessened by permitting clear fluid ingestion up to 2 hours before scheduled induction of anesthesia. Generous administration of intravenous fluids and glucose is also helpful for minimizing hypovolemia and protein catabolism.

KEY POINTS

- A BMI greater than 28 is associated as an increase in morbidity due to stroke, ischemic heart disease, and diabetes.

- The resting metabolic rate accounts for about 60% of total energy expenditure. Exercise can increase the resting metabolic rate for as long as 18 hours after increased activity.

- Morbidly obese individuals have limited mobility and may therefore appear to be asymptomatic even with significant respiratory and cardiovascular impairment.

- Obstructive sleep apnea is defined as airflow cessation of more than 10 seconds and is characterized by frequent episodes of apnea or hypopnea during sleep. The severity of OSA is measured by the average number of incidents per hour; more than 5 per hour is considered sleep apnea syndrome.

- In patients with OSA, the depressant effect of anesthetics on the muscle tone of the pharynx is potentiated.

- The level of positive pressure required to sustain the patency of the patient's upper airway during sleep must be determined in a sleep laboratory.

- Surgical treatment of obstructive sleep apnea includes palatal surgery (laser-assisted uvulopalatopharyngoplasty) or even tracheostomy (for patients with severe apnea who do not tolerate positive airway pressure).

- In the intraoperative anesthetic plan of OSA patients, short-acting inhaled agents (sevoflurane, desflurane, nitrous oxide) are the primary agent of choice. They are at increased risk for developing arterial hypoxemia in the postoperative period.

- Regional analgesia is associated with a low incidence of both apnea and arterial hypoxemia, making it an attractive technique for postoperative analgesia.

- Obesity imposes a restrictive ventilatory defect. The added weight and associated splinting of the diaphragm results in a decrease in functional residual capacity (FRC), expiratory reserve volume (ERV), and total lung capacity, with the FRC declining exponentially with increasing BMI.

- Morbidly obese patients tolerate exercise poorly; any increase in cardiac output is achieved by increasing the heart rate without an increase in stroke volume or ejection fraction.

Continued

KEY POINTS—cont'd

- Early in pregnancy, the increased sensitivity of the respiratory center decreases apnoeic episodes and, in the later part of pregnancy, women tend to sleep on their side, thereby decreasing the likelihood of airway obstruction.

- Development of cardiac dysrhythmias in patients with anorexia nervosa has been attributed to the presence of hypokalemia, prolonged QT intervals, and possible imbalance of the autonomic nervous system

- If TPN infusion is abruptly discontinued (e.g., a mechanical obstruction in the delivery tubing) as increased circulating endogenous concentrations of insulin persist, hypoglycemia will result. Dextrose-containing fluid should be started, with frequent glucose checks.

- Acute attacks of porphyria are characterized by severe abdominal pain, autonomic nervous system instability, electrolyte disturbances, and neuropsychiatric manifestations ranging from mild disturbances to fulminating life-threatening events.

- Skeletal muscle weakness that may progress to quadriparesis and respiratory failure is the most potentially lethal neurologic manifestation of acute attacks of porphyria. Seizures may occur during an attack of acute porphyria.

- Because carbohydrate administration can suppress porphyrin synthesis, carbohydrate supplements preoperatively may be recommended.

- In a phenylketonuria patient with B12 deficiency due to lack of supplementary treatment, nitrous oxide should probably be avoided.

REFERENCES

Adams JP, Murphy PG: Obesity in anaesthesia and intensive care. Br J Anaesth 2000;85:91–108.

Agras WS: The eating disorders. Sci Am Med 1998;1–7.

Becker AE, Grinspoon SK, Klibanski A, et al: Eating disorders. N Engl J Med 1999;340:1092–1098.

Berthoud MC, Peacock JE, Reilly CS: Effectiveness of preoxygenation in morbidly obese patients. Br J Anaesth 1991;67:464–466.

Brodsky JB, Lemmens HJ, Brock-Utne JG, et al: Morbid obesity and tracheal intubation. Anesth Analg 2002;94:3732–3736.

Brodsky JB, Lemmens HJ, Brock-Utne JG, et al: Anesthetic considerations for bariatric surgery: Proper positioning is important for laryngoscopy. Anesth Analg 2003;96:1841–1842; author reply, 1842.

Cannon BW, Meshier WT: Extremity amputation following radial artery cannulation in a patient with hyperlipoproteinemia type V. Anesthesiology 1982;56:222–223.

Deutzer J: Potential complications of obstructive sleep apnea in patients undergoing gastric bypass surgery. Crit Care Nurs Q 2005;28:3293–3299.

Diaz JH, Belani KG: Perioperative management of children with mucopolysaccharidoses. Anesth Analg 1993;77:1261–1270.

Dierdorf SF, McNiece WL: Anaesthesia and pyruvate dehydrogenase deficiency. Can Anaesth Soc J 1983;30:413–416.

Gross JB, Bachenberg KL, Benumof JL, et al: American Society of Anesthesiologists Task Force on Perioperative Management. Practice guidelines for the perioperative management of patients with obstructive sleep apnea: a report by the American Society of Anesthesiologists Task Force on Perioperative Management of patients with obstructive sleep apnea. Anesthesiology 2006;104:1081–1093; quiz 1117–1118.

Herrick IA, Rhine EJ: The mucopolysaccharidoses and anaesthesia: A report of clinical experience. Can J Anaesth 1988;35:67–73.

Hofer RE, Sprung J, Sarr MG, Wedel DJ: Anesthesia for a patient with morbid obesity using dexmedetomidine without narcotics. Can J Anaesth 2005;52:2176–2180.

Jensen NF, Fiddler DS, Striepe V: Anesthetic considerations in porphyrias. Anesth Analg 1995;80:591–599.

James MFM, Hift RJ: Porphyrias. Br J Anaesth 2000;85:143–153.

Juvin P, Vadam C, Malek L, et al: Postoperative recovery after desflurane, propofol, or isoflurane anesthesia among morbidly obese patients: A prospective, randomized study. Anesth Analg 2000;91:714–719.

Kadar AG, Ing CH, White PF, et al: Anesthesia for electroconvulsive therapy in obese patients. Anesth Analg 2002;94:2360–2361.

Lemmens HJ, Brodsky JB: The dose of succinylcholine in morbid obesity. Anesth Analg 2006;102:2438–2442.

Linstedt U, Maier C, Joehnk H, et al: Threatening spinal cord compression during anesthesia in a child with mucopolysaccharidosis VI. Anesthesiology 1994;80:227–229.

Malinowski SS: Nutritional and metabolic complications of bariatric surgery. Am J Med Sci 2006;331:4219–4225.

Roberts RB, Shirley MA: Reducing the risk of acid aspiration during cesarean section. Anesth Analg 1974;53:859–868.

Rowe RW, Helander E: Anesthetic management of a patient with systemic carnitine deficiency. Anesth Analg 1990;71:295–297.

Saravanakumar K, Rao SG, Cooper GM: Obesity and obstetric anaesthesia. Anaesthesia 2006;61:136–148.

Sharar SR, Haberkern CM, Jack R, et al: Anesthetic management of a child with methylmalonyl-coenzyme A mutase deficiency. Anesth Analg 1991;73:499–501.

Shibutani K, Inchiosa MAJr, Sawada K, et al: Accuracy of pharmacokinetic models for predicting plasma fentanyl concentrations in lean and obese surgical patients: Derivation of dosing weight (pharmacokinetic mass). Anesthesiology 2004;101:603–613.

Wilder RT, Belani KG: Fiberoptic intubation complicated by pulmonary edema in a 12 year old child with Hurler syndrome. Anesthesiology 1990;72:205–207.

Renal Disease

Susan Garwood

The kidneys are responsible for, or contribute to, a number of essential functions including water conservation, electrolyte homeostasis, acid base balance, and several neurohumoral or hormonal functions. When the kidneys are involved in a disease process, some or all of these functions may be affected.

Knowledge of how the kidneys perform these important functions aids in the understanding of the clinical presentation, signs and symptoms, and treatment of renal diseases.

Each kidney consists of approximately a million nephrons, each of which has distinct anatomic parts: Bowman's capsule, proximal tubule, loop of Henle, distal tubule, and collecting duct. A glomerulus, which is a tuft of capillaries, is surrounded by Bowman's capsule and is supplied by an afferent arteriole and drained by a slightly smaller efferent arteriole. The glomeruli filter the plasma at a rate of 180 L/day, allowing all but protein and polysaccharides to pass into the nephron. The glomerular filtration rate (GFR) is calculated from the clearance of either endogenous or exogenous substances (creatinine and inulin, respectively). Normal values for GFR are 125 mL/min but vary with gender, body weight, and age, and GFR decreases by approximately 1% per year after the age of 20. The GFR may be calculated from timed urine volumes plus urinary and serum creatinine concentrations (creatinine clearance), or, alternatively, a number of formulas exist that estimate the GFR from serum creatinine, As the plasma flows along the nephron, virtually all the fluid and solutes are reabsorbed by a number of active and passive transport systems.

The main function of the kidneys is water and sodium homeostasis, which is intimately linked and regulated by a number of feedback and hormonal systems.

CLINICAL ASSESSMENT OF RENAL FUNCTION

Table 14-1 discusses a number of tests used to evaluate renal function.

TABLE 14-1 Tests Used to Evaluate Renal Function	
Test	**Normal Value**
Glomerular Filtration Rate	
Blood urea nitrogen	10–20 mg/dL
Serum creatinine	0.7–1.5 mg/dL
Creatinine clearance	110–150 mL/min
Proteinuria (albumin)	<150 mg/day
Renal Tubular Function and/or Integrity	
Urine specific gravity	1.003–1.030
Urine osmolality	38–1400 mOsm/L
Urine sodium excretion	<40 mEq/L
Glucosuria	
Enzymuria	
N-Acetyl-β-glucosaminidase	
α-Glutathione-S-transferase	
Factors That Influence Interpretation	
Dehydration	
Variable protein intake	
Gastrointestinal bleeding	
Catabolism	
Advanced age	
Skeletal muscle mass	
Accurate timed urine volume measurement	

Glomerular Filtration Rate

The GFR is considered the best measure of renal function, as it parallels the various functions of the nephrons. Alterations in the GFR are associated with predictable changes in erythropoietic activity. Clinical manifestations of uremia generally appear when the GFR falls below 15 mL/min/1.73 m^2 (normal $\geq$ 90 mL/min/1.73 m^2). Because many drugs are excreted by kidney filtration, dose adjustments may be necessary to prevent cumulative effects when the GFR is decreased.

Blood Urea Nitrogen

Blood urea nitrogen (BUN) concentrations vary with the GFR. Nevertheless, the influence of dietary intake, co-existing disease, and intravascular fluid volume on BUN concentrations makes it a potentially misleading test of renal function. For example, production of urea is increased by high-protein diets or gastrointestinal bleeding, resulting in increased BUN concentrations despite a normal GFR. Other causes of increased BUN concentrations despite a normal GFR include dehydration and increased catabolism, as occurring during a febrile illness. Increased BUN concentrations in the presence of dehydration most likely reflect increased urea absorption owing to slow movement of fluid through the renal tubules. When the latter is responsible for increased BUN concentrations, the serum creatinine levels remain normal. BUN concentrations can remain normal in the presence of low-protein diets (hemodialysis patients) despite decreases in the GFR. Even with these extraneous influences, BUN concentrations higher than 50 mg/dL usually reflect a decreased GFR.

Serum Creatinine

Serum creatinine levels can be used as an estimate of the GFR. Normal serum creatinine concentrations range from 0.6 to 1.0 mg/dL in women and 0.8 to 1.3 mg/dL in men, reflecting differences in skeletal muscle mass. A number of factors (accelerated creatinine production, decreased tubular secretion of creatinine, presence of chromogens in the blood) can increase serum creatinine concentrations without there being a concomitant decrease in GFR. Conversely, small reductions in serum creatinine can reflect large decreases in GFR. The maintenance of normal serum creatinine concentrations in elderly patients with known decreases in the GFR reflects decreased creatinine production owing to the decreased skeletal muscle mass that accompanies aging. In this regard, mild increases in serum creatinine concentrations suggest significant renal disease. Serum creatinine values are slow to reflect acute changes in renal function. For example, if acute renal failure (ARF) occurs and the GFR decreases from 100 mL/min to 10 mL/min, serum creatinine values do not increase correspondingly for approximately 7 days.

Creatinine Clearance

Creatinine, an endogenous marker of renal filtration, is produced at a relatively constant rate by hepatic conversion of skeletal muscle creatine. Creatinine is freely filtered and is not reabsorbed. As a result, the creatinine clearance correlates with the GFR and is the most reliable measure of GFR. Creatinine clearance does not depend on corrections for age or the presence of a steady state. Preoperatively, patients with creatinine clearances between 10 and 25 mL/min must be considered at risk of developing prolonged or adverse responses to drugs (such as nondepolarizing muscle relaxants) that depend on renal excretion for their clearance from the plasma. The reliability of creatinine clearance is diminished by the variability in tubular secretion of creatinine and the inability of most patients to collect timed urine samples accurately.

Renal Tubular Function and Integrity

Renal tubular function is most often assessed by measuring the urine concentrating ability. The presence of proteinuria may reflect renal tubular damage. Enzymes present in the renal tubular cells (N-acetyl-β-glucosaminidase, α-glutathione-S-transferase) may be detectable in the urine following sevoflurane anesthesia, presumably reflecting transient drug-induced tubular dysfunction that is not accompanied by changes in the BUN or serum creatinine concentrations.

Urine Concentrating Ability

The diagnosis of renal tubular dysfunction is established by demonstrating that the kidneys do not produce appropriately concentrated urine in the presence of a physiologic stimulus for the release of antidiuretic hormone. In the absence of diuretic therapy or glycosuria, urine specific gravity higher than 1.018 suggests that the ability of renal tubules to concentrate urine is adequate. Treatment with diuretics or the presence of hypokalemia or hypercalcemia may interfere with the ability of renal tubules to concentrate urine. Although unlikely following the administration of sevoflurane, the inorganic fluoride resulting from metabolism of this anesthetic is capable of interfering with the urine-concentrating ability of the renal tubules.

Proteinuria

Proteinuria (transient, orthostatic, persistent) is relatively common, being present in 5% to 10% of tested adults during screening examinations. Transient proteinuria may be associated with fever, congestive heart failure, seizure activity, pancreatitis, and exercise. This form of proteinuria resolves with treatment of the underlying illness. Orthostatic proteinuria occurs in up to 5% of adolescents while in the upright position and resolves when the recumbent position is assumed. Generally, orthostatic proteinuria resolves spontaneously and is not associated with any deterioration in renal function. Persistent proteinuria generally connotes significant renal disease. Microalbuminuria is the earliest sign of diabetic nephropathy. Severe proteinuria may result in hypoalbuminemia, with associated decreases in plasma oncotic pressures and decreased protein binding of drugs.

Urinary Sodium Excretion

Urinary sodium excretion exceeding 40 mEq/L reflects decreased ability of the renal tubules to conserve sodium. Damage to the renal tubules by hypoxia results in increased loss of sodium in the urine, and the urine osmolarity is likely to be less than 350 mOsm/L. Minimal urinary sodium excretion (<15 mEq/L) occurs when normally functioning renal tubules conserve sodium in the presence of hypovolemia, and the urine osmolarity is likely to exceed 500 mOsm/L. Drug-induced diuresis is also associated with increased urinary excretion of sodium.

Urinalysis

Examination of the urine is useful for diagnosing urinary tract disease. Urinalysis is intended to detect the presence of protein, glucose, acetoacetate, blood, and leukocytes. The urine pH and solute concentrations (specific gravity) are determined, and sediment microscopy is used to determine the presence of cells, casts, microorganisms, and crystals. Hematuria may be caused by bleeding anywhere between the glomerulus and urethra. Microhematuria may be benign (focal nephritis) or may reflect glomerulonephritis, renal calculi, or cancer of the genitourinary tract. Joggers may experience hematuria, presumably as a result of trauma to the urinary tract. Sickle cell disease is a consideration in African Americans who exhibit hematuria. In the absence of proteinuria or red blood cell casts, glomerular disease as a cause of hematuria is unlikely. Red blood cell casts are pathognomonic of acute glomerulonephritis. White blood cell casts are most commonly seen with pyelonephritis.

ACUTE RENAL FAILURE/INSUFFICIENCY

ARF is characterized by deterioration of renal function over a period of hours to days, resulting in failure of the kidneys to excrete nitrogenous waste products and to maintain fluid and electrolyte homeostasis. Commonly used definitions of ARF include increases in serum creatinine concentrations of more than 0.5 mg/dL compared with the baseline value, a 50% decrease in the calculated creatinine clearance, or decreased renal function that results in the need for dialysis. ARF may be oliguric (urinary output < 400 mL/day) or nonoliguric (urinary output > 400 mL/day). Despite major advances in dialysis therapy and critical care, the mortality rate among patients with severe ARF (primarily ischemic in origin) requiring dialysis remains high and has not decreased greatly over the past 50 years. This observation can be explained by the fact that, compared with patients 50 years ago, patients today are often elderly and have multiple co-existing diseases. When ARF occurs in the setting of multiorgan failure, especially in patients with severe hypotension or respiratory failure, the mortality rate often exceeds 50%. The most common causes of death are sepsis, cardiovascular dysfunction, and pulmonary complications.

Incidence

The incidence of ARF depends on the definition used and the patient population studied. As a clinical entity, some degree of ARF is thought to affect 5% to 7% of all hospitalized patients. ARF is associated with a number of other systemic diseases,

TABLE 14-2 Etiology of Acute Renal Failure

Prerenal Azotemia (Decreased Renal Blood Flow)
Absolute decrease
Acute hemorrhage
Gastrointestinal fluid loss
Trauma
Surgery
Burns
Low output syndrome
Renal artery stenosis
Relative decrease
Sepsis
Hepatic failure
Allergic reaction

Renal Azotemia (Intrinsic)
Acute glomerulonephritis (5% of cases)
Interstitial nephritis (drugs, sepsis) (10% of cases)
Acute tubular necrosis (85% of cases)
   Ischemia (50% of cases)
   Nephrotoxic drugs (antibiotics, anesthetic drugs?)
     (35% of cases)
   Solvents (carbon tetrachloride, ethylene glycol)
   Radiographic contrast dyes
   Myoglobinuria

Postrenal (Obstructive)
Upper urinary tract obstruction (ureteral)
Lower urinary tract obstruction (bladder outlet)

Adapted from Klahr S, Miller SB: Acute oliguria. N Engl J Med 1998;338:671–675; and Thadhani R, Pascual M, Bonventre JV: Acute renal failure. N Engl J Med 1996;334:1148–1169.

TABLE 14-3 Characteristic Urinary Indices in Patients with Acute Oliguria Due to Prerenal or Renal Causes

Index	Prerenal Causes	Renal Causes
Urinary sodium concentration (mEq/L)	<20	>40
Fractional excretion of sodium (%)	<1	>1
Urine osmolarity (mOsm/L)	>400	250–300
Urine creatinine/ plasma creatinine	>40	<20
Urine/plasma osmolarity	>1.5	<1.1

Adapted from Klahr S, Miller SB: Acute oliguria. N Engl J Med 1998;338:671–675.

acute clinical conditions, drug treatments, and interventional therapies (**Table 14-2**). It almost invariably accompanies multiple organ failure syndromes in the critically ill patient population. Those at the highest risk of ARF in either the community or hospital population are elderly patients with diabetes and a degree of baseline renal insufficiency.

The etiology of ARF is classically divided into prerenal, intrarenal (or intrinsic), and postrenal causes (see Table 14-2). It is important to note that prolonged prerenal failure will lead to intrarenal injury.

Azotemia

Prerenal Azotemia

Prerenal azotemia accounts for nearly half of hospital-acquired cases of ARF. Sustained prerenal azotemia is the most common factor that predisposes patients to ischemia-induced acute tubular necrosis. Prerenal azotemia is rapidly reversible if the underlying cause (hypovolemia, congestive heart failure) is corrected. Elderly patients are uniquely susceptible to prerenal azotemia because of their predisposition to hypovolemia (poor fluid intake) and high incidence of renovascular disease. Among hospitalized patients, prerenal azotemia is often due to congestive heart failure, liver dysfunction, or septic shock. Reduced renal blood flow may be a result of anesthetic drug–induced decreases in perfusion pressure,

particularly in the presence of hypovolemia associated with the intraoperative period.

Assessment of blood volume status, hemodynamics, and drug therapy may result in identification of potential prerenal causes of acute oliguria. Invasive monitoring (central venous pressure, pulmonary artery catheter) may be necessary to assess the intravascular fluid volume. Renal ultrasonography is the best diagnostic test for determining the presence of obstructive nephropathy. Urinary indices may help distinguish prerenal from intrinsic ARF (**Table 14-3**). The use of urinary indices is based on the assumption that the ability of renal tubules to reabsorb sodium and water is maintained in the presence of prerenal causes of ARF, whereas these functions are impaired in the presence of tubulointerstitial disease or acute tubular necrosis. Blood and urine specimens for determination of urinary indices must be obtained before the administration of fluids, dopamine, mannitol, or other diuretic drugs.

Renal Azotemia

Intrinsic renal diseases that result in ARF are categorized according to the primary site of injury (renal tubules, interstitium, glomerulus, renal vasculature). Injury to the renal tubules is most often due to ischemia or nephrotoxins (aminoglycoside antibiotics, radiographic contrast agents). Prerenal azotemia and ischemic tubular necrosis present as a continuum with the initial decreases in renal blood flow leading to ischemia of the renal tubular cells. The principal functional derangements in patients with acute oliguria are sudden and profound decreases in the GFR that are sufficient to cause ARF manifesting as increased serum urea and creatinine concentrations, retention of sodium and water, and development of acidosis and hyperkalemia. Although some cases of ischemic ARF are reversible if the underlying cause is corrected, irreversible cortical necrosis can occur if the ischemia is severe or prolonged. Ischemia and toxins often combine to cause ARF in severely ill patients with conditions such as sepsis or AIDS. ARF due to acute interstitial nephritis is most often caused by allergic reactions to drugs.

Postrenal Azotemia

ARF occurs when urinary outflow tracts are obstructed, as with prostatic hypertrophy or cancer of the prostate or cervix. It is important to diagnose postrenal causes of ARF promptly because the potential for recovery is inversely related to the duration of the obstruction. Percutaneous nephrostomy can relieve the obstruction and may improve the outcome. Renal ultrasonography is the best diagnostic test for determining the presence of obstructive nephropathy.

Risk Factors for Development of Acute Renal Failure

Risk factors for the development of ARF include co-existing renal disease, advanced age, congestive heart failure, symptomatic cardiovascular disease that is likely to be associated with renovascular disease, and major operative procedures (cardiopulmonary bypass, abdominal aneurysm resection). Sepsis and multiple organ system dysfunction due to trauma introduce the risk of ARF. Iatrogenic components that predispose to ARF include inadequate fluid replacement, delayed treatment of sepsis, and administration of nephrotoxic drugs or dyes. The incidence of radiographic contrast dye-induced ARF may approach 50% in patients with diabetes mellitus or co-existing renal disease.

Appropriate hydration and optimal preservation of the intravascular fluid volume are essential to maintain adequate renal perfusion. It is also important to maintain adequate systemic blood pressure and cardiac output and to prevent peripheral vasoconstriction. Hypotension may result in inadequate renal perfusion and loss of renal autoregulation. Potentially nephrotoxic substances (nonsteroidal anti-inflammatory drugs, aminoglycosides, radiographic contrast dyes, angiotensin-converting [ACE] inhibitors, general anesthetics) are logically avoided in patients with prerenal oliguria, and diuretic therapy may be detrimental in these patients. Prophylactic administration of furosemide or mannitol prior to injection of radiographic contrast dyes may decrease renal function further rather than protect it. Conversely, prior administration of acetylcysteine, a thio-containing antioxidant that acts as a free radical scavenger, may provide protection against radiographic dye–induced nephropathy.

Complications Associated with Acute Renal Failure

Complications of ARF may manifest in the central nervous system, cardiovascular system, and gastrointestinal system. In addition, infections occur frequently in patients who develop ARF and are leading causes of morbidity and mortality. Drugs known to be excreted by the kidneys (cephalosporins, digoxin, diazepam, propranolol) should be avoided or the doses adjusted in proportion to the decrease in renal function.

Neurologic complications of ARF include confusion, asterixis, somnolence, and seizures. These changes may be ameliorated by dialysis.

Cardiovascular complications include systemic hypertension, congestive heart failure, and pulmonary edema principally as reflections of sodium and water retention. Hypotension is also commonly encountered. Cardiac dysrhythmias may occur. Pericarditis appears to be less common than in the past. The presence of systemic hypertension, congestive heart failure, or pulmonary edema suggests the need to decrease the intravascular fluid volume. ARF may be is accompanied by dilutional anemia with hematocrit values between 20% and 30%.

Gastrointestinal complications include anorexia, nausea, vomiting, and ileus. Gastrointestinal bleeding occurs in as many as one third of patients who develop ARF and may contribute to anemia in patients with ARF. Administration of H_2-receptor antagonists may decrease the risk of gastrointestinal bleeding.

Primary sites of *infection* include the respiratory and urinary tracts and sites where breaks in normal anatomic barriers have occurred owing to indwelling catheters. Impaired immune responses due to uremia may contribute to the increased likelihood of infections in patients who develop ARF.

Signs and Symptoms

Signs and symptoms of ARF are often absent in the early stages, and a high degree of suspicion is required to identify subtle changes that accompany the development of ARF. Patients may present with a generalized malaise or begin to show evidence of volume overload such as dyspnea, edema, and hypertension. As toxins accumulate, without treatment, patients become lethargic, nauseated, and confused. Salt and water excess leads to pulmonary edema and hypoxia, while hyperkalemia and acidosis affect cardiac rhythm and contractility. Encephalopathy, coma, seizures, and death may ensue.

Other signs and symptoms of ARF may be associated with the etiology, such as hypotension, jaundice, hematuria, and urinary retention.

Diagnosis

The diagnosis of ARF is usually made based on laboratory data demonstrating an acute increase in serum creatinine. Urinary output may or may not fall, and, depending on this, the terms oliguric and nonoliguric are used to qualify ARF. Again, there are a number of definitions of oliguria, the most commonly used being less than 0.5 mL/kg per minute or less than 400 mL/day. Anuria is defined as less than 100 mL/day, with complete anuria being very unusual.

Urinalysis may be helpful in diagnosing whether ARF is likely to be prerenal, intrarenal, or postrenal. The sensitivity and specificity of urinary sodium less than 20 mEq/L in differentiating prerenal azotemia from acute tubular necrosis are 90% and 82%, respectively (see Table 14-3).

Management/Treatment of Acute Renal Failure

There are no specific treatment modalities for ARF; management is essentially supportive and aimed at limiting further renal injury and correcting the water, electrolyte, and acid-base derangements. Underlying causes should be sought and terminated or reversed, if possible; specifically, hypovolemia, hypotension, and low cardiac output should be corrected and sepsis eliminated. A minimal arterial pressure of 80 mm Hg (or mean arterial pressure of 65 mm Hg) should be attained, but there is no evidence to support a better outcome with supraphysiologic values of either systemic pressures or cardiac output. Failure to maintain these pressures is associated with an independent risk of developing ARF (odds ratio = 15). In the interest of maintaining tissue oxygenation, some authors advocate increasing cardiac output rather than arterial pressure; however, it must be noted that urinary flow is pressure dependent.

Fluid resuscitation and the use of vasopressor therapy are universally emphasized in the prevention and treatment of ARF. Although the controversy regarding crystalloid versus colloid still rages on in the literature, it is agreed that the prompt and adequate correction of hypovolemia and hypotension is much more important than the type of fluid used. There is little to support the use of either in ARF. However, one randomized study showed that the use of high molecular weight hydroxyethyl starch was associated with a higher incidence of ARF in severe sepsis than gelatin, and another study demonstrated that renal dysfunction occurred more frequently in the recipients of renal grafts taken from brain-dead organ donors resuscitated with hydroxyethyl starch.

With regard to the use of vasopressors in ARF, concern has been expressed that renal vasoconstriction may be increased and the situation exacerbated. While it is true that norepinephrine reduces renal blood flow in healthy volunteers, the effect of norepinephrine in ARF depends on the balance of a variety of factors. The normal response of the renal vasculature during hypotension is vasoconstriction of the efferent arteriole to maintain filtration. An increase in systemic pressure is accompanied by reduced renal sympathetic tone and vasodilation, while improved renal perfusion pressure triggers an autoregulatory vasoconstrictive response if that autoregulatory response is intact. Direct α_1-mediated renal vasoconstriction is of minor importance when compared with the preceding two effects. It appears that the overall effect of using norepinephrine in septic patients is to increase the GFR and urinary output. Lower mortality rates were observed in a prospective observational trial of almost 100 septic patients who were treated with norepinephrine rather than other vasopressors (e.g., high-dose dopamine).

The use of dopamine to either treat or prevent ARF is not supported by the literature; in fact, dopamine use has been associated with a number of undesirable side effects. Similarly, the practice of trying to convert oliguric to nonoliguric ARF with the use of diuretics is also advised against; mortality rates and dialysis requirements are not changed by this practice. There are several reports of increased mortality and nonrecovery of renal function in critically ill patients with ARF treated with loop diuretics.

In contrast, in two specific scenarios, mannitol has been shown to be associated with improved renal outcome. The incidence of posttransplantation acute tubular necrosis is significantly lower in patients treated with mannitol plus hydration compared with hydration alone. Forced alkaline diuresis together with mannitol is generally accepted as preventing acute tubular necrosis in severe crush injury.

N-acetylcysteine, a reactive oxygen metabolite scavenger, has been advocated as a renal protection agent specifically in contrast-mediated nephropathy. A number of meta-analyses and systematic reviews exist in the literature, and it is probable that N-acetylcysteine reduces ARF in high-risk patients exposed to radiocontrast dye.

Various drugs purported to minimize the activation of the inflammatory response and fibrinolytic cascades that takes place in ARF have not met with clinical success other than activated protein C and steroid replacement (in those patients who demonstrate a steroid deficiency). These two latter strategies have been shown to reduce mortality in patients with severe sepsis and are now accepted as part of the adjunctive therapy armamentarium.

With regard to supportive therapy, dialysis (or hemofiltration) is still the mainstay of severe ARF. However, there remains significant controversy over dosing regimens, frequency of dialysis, and whether dialysis should be a continuous or intermittent therapy. A recent meta-analysis confirmed the lack of difference between continuous and intermittent therapy, but it has been recognized that either way, the dose is more important. Further points of agreement are that intermittent dialysis should at least be performed on a daily basis and that biocompatible membranes can improve survival numbers without changing renal outcome. A number of international committees and consensus panels have met and made their recommendations, but, in general, dialysis practices are governed by regional and individual preferences with no widely accepted trigger point for the initiation of therapy.

Prognosis

The overall prognosis for hospital-acquired ARF is poor, with current mortality rates no different than those of 40 years ago. Many ARF series report mortality rates of more than 20%, and once dialysis is required, mortality rates are invariably in excess of 50%. Those who succumb usually die of failure of other organ systems after prolonged and complex hospital courses. Approximately 15% of patients developing ARF will fully recover their renal function. Five percent of ARF patients will retain a degree of renal insufficiency that remains stable, while another 5% will experience continual deterioration of renal function throughout the remainder of their life. Fifteen percent will be left with stable renal insufficiency for a period but remain at high risk of developing chronic renal failure later in life.

Drug Dosing in Patients with Renal Impairment

Renal impairment affects most of the organ systems of the body, and consequently the pharmacology of many drugs may be dramatically changed in renal insufficiency.

TABLE 14-4 Renal Effects of Commonly Used Analgesics

Drug	Adjustment Method	GFR > 50 mL/min	GFR 10–50 mL/min	GFR < 10 mL/min
Acetaminophen	↑ interval	Q4hr	Q6hr	Q8hr
Acetylsalicylic acid	↑ interval	Q4hr	Q6–8hr	Avoid
Al/remi/sufentanil	↔ dose	100%	100%	100%
Codeine	↓ dose	100%	75%	50%
Fentanyl	↓ dose	100%	75%	50%
Ketorolac*	↓ dose	100%	50%	50%
Meperidine	↓ dose	100%	75%	50%
Methadone	↓ dose	100%	100%	50%–75%
Morphine	↓ dose	100%	75%	50%

*Usually avoided since this class of drug may be associated with worsening of renal function
↓, decreases; ↑, increases; ↔, no change; GFR, glomerular filtration rate; Q, every.
Adapted from Schrier RW: Manual of Nephrology, 6th ed. Philadelphia, Lippincott Williams & Wilkins, 2005, p 268.

The first step in tailoring drug dosing for patients with renal impairment is to establish the creatinine clearance since the rate of elimination of drugs excreted by the kidneys is proportional to the GFR. If the patient is oliguric, use 5 mL/min for creatinine clearance.

If the normal drug regimen starts with a loading dose to rapidly achieve therapeutic levels, use the following guidelines. If after clinical examination, the extracellular fluid volume looks normal, use the loading dose suggested for patients with normal renal function. If the extracellular fluid is contracted, reduce the loading dose; if the extracellular fluid is expanded, use a higher loading dose. There are formulas to calculate a loading dose that can be provided by the hospital pharmacy. Formulas also exist to calculate the maintenance doses and depend on either the fraction of drug excreted in the urine or the ratio of the half-life in normal patients to the half-life in patients with renal failure.

Drugs with wide therapeutic ranges or long plasma half-lives can be dose adjusted in renal failure by increasing the interval between doses. The other method of dose adjustment would be to reduce the amount prescribed per dose. This is more useful in medications with narrow therapeutic ranges and short plasma half-lives in patients with renal impairment. In reality, a combination of the two methods of dose adjustment is frequently used (e.g., analgesics, **Table 14-4**).

Drug removal by hemodialysis or peritoneal dialysis may be very efficient, particularly for drugs that weigh less than 500 Da, those that are less than 90% protein bound, and those that have a small volume of distribution. Usually these drugs are given at the end of the dialysis schedule to avoid the necessity of redosing.

The removal of drugs by other renal replacement therapies, such as continuous venovenous hemofiltration, is more dependent on the membrane characteristics, flow rate, and whether a dialysate is added to the circuit.

Anesthetic Management in Patients with Acute Renal Failure

The morbidity and mortality of ARF are so high that only life-saving surgery should be undertaken in such a patient. The principles guiding the management of anesthesia are the same as those that guide supportive treatment of ARF, namely, maintenance of an adequate mean systemic blood pressure and cardiac output and the avoidance of further renal insults including hypotension, hypovolemia, hypoxia, and nephrotoxic exposure. Invasive hemodynamic monitoring is mandatory, as are frequent blood gas analysis and electrolyte determination.

The administration of diuretics to maintain urine output in those patients who are not oliguric has not been shown to improve either renal outcome or patient survival except in crush injuries and other forms of pigmenturia where the administration of mannitol improves outcome. When a dilutional anemia has been caused by overzealous hydration, diuretics may allow administration of blood or blood products. For patients undergoing renal replacement therapy, institute postoperative dialysis/hemodialysis as soon as the patient has stable hemodynamics.

CHRONIC RENAL FAILURE

Chronic renal failure is the progressive, irreversible deterioration of renal function that results from a wide variety of diseases (**Table 14-5**) Diabetes mellitus is the leading cause of end-stage renal disease (ESRD) followed closely by systemic hypertension. The clinical manifestations of chronic renal failure are typically independent of the initial insult that damaged the kidneys and instead reflect the overall inability of the kidneys to excrete nitrogenous waste products, regulate fluid and electrolyte balance, and secrete hormones. In most patients with chronic renal disease, regardless of the etiology, a decrease in the GFR to less than 25 mL/min is characterized

TABLE 14-5 Causes of Chronic Renal Failure

Glomerulopathies
  Primary glomerular disease
  Focal glomerulosclerosis
  Membranous nephropathy
  Immunoglobulin A nephropathy
  Membranoproliferative glomerulonephritis
  Glomerulopathies associated with systemic disease
  Diabetes mellitus
  Amyloidosis
  Postinfectious glomerulonephritis
  Systemic lupus erythematosus
  Wegener's granulomatosis
Tubulointerstitial disease
  Analgesic nephropathy
  Reflux nephropathy with pyelonephritis
  Myeloma kidney
  Sarcoidosis
Heredity disease
  Polycystic kidney disease
  Alport syndrome
  Medullary cystic disease
Systemic hypertension
Renal vascular disease
Obstructive uropathy
Human immunodeficiency virus

Adapted from Tolkoff-Rubin NE, Pascual M: Chronic renal failure. Sci Am Med 1998;1–12.

one half million individuals. Prevalent counts continue to increase, partly because the general population itself is aging and patients with ESRD are surviving longer. However, the incidence of ESRD (which is the number of new cases) has started to slow and is quoted as 347 per million in 2005 or more than 106,000 individuals with a new diagnosis of ESRD that year.

Patients in the age group 45 to 64 years account for the largest proportion of new cases (36%), while those older than 65 years have the greatest prevalence (4000–5000 per million people in that age group). In 2005, more than 28,000 new patients older than age 75 began therapy for ESRD, while a total of almost 75,000 patients in this age group appeared on the census in the ESRD database.

Diabetes and/or hypertension account for the most of the etiology of ESRD. For 2005, diabetes was the cause of 53% of all new patients with ESRD (45% of the total number of ESRD patients). However, incident rates of diabetes and hypertension vary dramatically with age and race; one in two elderly people starting therapy for ESRD has a primary diagnosis of hypertension, while the rate of hypertension in African American patients is 15 times greater than that in their white counterparts.

There is a preponderance of white ESRD patients (currently two thirds of all ESRD patients), but this belies the incident rates within races. The incident rates for whites for 2005 was 268 per million, while for African Americans, it was 991. Asians living in the United State have an incident rate close to 1.5 times that of white patients, and Native Americans have an incident rate approximately 100% higher.

by progressive deterioration in renal function that eventually leads to end-stage renal failure requiring dialysis or transplantation (**Table 14-6**).

The best source of data on the incidence and etiology of chronic renal insufficiency (CRI) comes from the 2007 United States Renal Data System of the National Institutes of Health. This database has followed the course of patients with ESRD living in the United States since 1980, with the most recent data reported for 2005. Total patient counts for 2005 (point prevalence) reached 1569 patients per million, approximately

Pathogenesis of Chronic Renal Failure
Glomerular Hypertension, Hyperfiltration, Systemic Hypertension

Intrarenal hemodynamic changes (glomerular hypertension, glomerular hyperfiltration and permeability changes, glomerulosclerosis) are likely responsible for progression of renal disease. Systemic hypertension may be a primary cause of renal failure and is also a major risk factor for progression of renal disease. Genetic factors may be important in

TABLE 14-6 Stages of Chronic Renal Failure

Stage of Failure	Functioning Nephrons (% of Total)	Glomerular Filtration Rate (mL/min)	Signs	Laboratory Abnormalities
Normal	100	125	None	None
Decreased renal reserve	40	50–80	None	None
Renal insufficiency	10–40	12–50	Nocturia	Increased blood urea nitrogen Increased serum creatinine
Renal failure	10	<12	Uremia	Increased blood urea nitrogen Increased serum creatinine Anemia Hyperkalemia Increased bleeding time

determining whether renal disease develops in hypertensive patients. Decreases in glomerular hypertension and in systemic hypertension can be achieved by the administration of ACE inhibitors and/or angiotensin receptor blocker (ARB). In addition to beneficial effects on intraglomerular hemodynamics and systemic pressures, the renoprotective effects of ACE/ARB inhibitors manifest as reductions in proteinuria and slowing of the progression of glomerulosclerosis in patients with diabetic and nondiabetic nephropathy. Other antihypertensive drugs that lower the systemic pressure to similar degrees do not provide the renoprotective effects seen with ACE/ARB inhibitors.

Dietary Factors

In animal models, protein intake can influence the progression of renal disease, and new guidelines call for moderate protein restriction in all patients with renal insufficiency. There is no evidence in humans that restricting dietary phosphate or lipid intake slows the progression of renal disease.

Strict control of blood glucose concentrations (attempts to maintain hemoglobin A_{1c} [glycosylated hemoglobin] near normal) can delay the onset of proteinuria and slow the progression of nephropathy, neuropathy, and retinopathy.

Signs and Symptoms of Chronic Renal Failure

Signs and symptoms of CRI may be undetectable until the later stages of the disease (**Table 14-7**; see also Table 14-6) and even then often continue to be nonspecific and vague, appearing insidiously as fatigue, general malaise, and anorexia. Volume overload (peripheral edema and dyspnea) and electrolyte or acid base disturbances are late signs of CRI (see previously). CRI and cardiac disease are intimately linked, and as CRI progresses, coronary artery disease and congestive

TABLE 14-8 Manifestations of Chronic Renal Failure
Electrolyte imbalance
Hyperkalemia
Hypermagnesemia
Hypocalcemia
Metabolic acidosis
Unpredictable intravascular fluid volume status
Anemia
Increased cardiac output
Oxyhemoglobin dissociation curve shifted to the right
Uremic coagulopathies
Platelet dysfunction
Neurologic changes
Encephalopathy
Cardiovascular changes
Systemic hypertension
Congestive heart failure
Attenuated sympathetic nervous system activity due to treatment with antihypertensive drugs
Renal osteodystrophy
Pruritus

heart failure contribute to symptomatology. More than 70% of diabetic ESRD patients have congestive heart failure, while almost 70% have ischemic heart disease. In nondiabetic ESRD patients, congestive heart failure and ischemic heart disease occur less frequently, just more than 40% for both diagnoses. Seventy-five percent of older patients beginning ESRD therapy carry a diagnosis of five or more comorbidities, contributing to complex clinical presentation. It is well established that anemia develops in the course of chronic kidney disease and is nearly universal in patients with kidney failure. Other symptoms associated with CRI include cognitive impairment, peripheral neuropathy, infertility, and increased susceptibility to infection (**Table 14-8**).

Diagnosis

Again, diagnosis is usually made by laboratory testing. Oliguria does not set in until late in the disease and is an unreliable marker of disease progression. Most patients will have the diagnosis made during routine testing and follow-up of the primary disease or annual physical examinations. However, patients do present with CRI in the later stages of the disease, and, again, diagnosis is made from signs and symptoms of fluid overload and concomitant cardiac disease and confirmed by laboratory testing. Patients may be further categorized based on the presence and extent of proteinuria. Urinary sediment analysis is also helpful in the diagnosis of CRI.

TABLE 14-7 Classification of Chronic Renal Disease		
Stage	Description	GFR (mL/min/1.73 m^2)
1	Kidney damage with normal or ↑ GFR	≥90
2	Kidney damage with mild ↓ GFR	60–89
3	Moderate ↓ GFR	30–59
4	Severe ↓ GFR	15–29
5	Kidney failure	<15 or dialysis

CKD is defined as either kidney damage or a GFR less than 60 mL/min/1.73 m^2 for 3 months or more. Kidney damage is defined as a pathologic abnormality or markers of damage including abnormalities of the blood or on urine or imaging studies.
CKD, chronic kidney disease; GFR, glomerular filtration rate.
Adapted from National Kidney Foundation Clinical Practice Guidelines for Chronic Kidney Disease (CKD): Evaluation, Classification, and Stratification. Available at: www.kidney.org/professionals/kdoqi/guidelines_ckd/toc.htm, accessed January 10, 2008.

Adaptation to Chronic Renal Failure/ Insufficiency

The normally functioning kidneys precisely regulate the concentrations of solutes and water in the ECF despite large variations in daily dietary intake. Patients with chronic renal disease can still excrete solute and water loads without altering their diet, even when the GFR has been significantly decreased. Hence, patients with chronic renal failure may remain relatively asymptomatic until renal function is less than 10% of normal.

The kidneys demonstrate three stages of adaptation to progressive impairment of renal function. The first pattern includes substances such as creatinine and urea, which are dependent largely on the GFR for their urinary excretion. As the GFR decreases, the plasma concentrations of these substances begin to increase, but the increase is not directly proportional to the degree of GFR impairment. For example, early in the course of renal insufficiency, there are minimal changes in serum creatinine concentrations despite more than 50% decreases in GFR. Beyond this point, however, when the renal reserve has been exhausted, even minimal further decreases in the GFR can result in significant increases in the serum creatinine and urea concentrations.

The second stage of adaptation to progressive renal impairment is seen with solutes such as potassium. Serum potassium concentrations are maintained within normal limits until the decrease in GFR approaches 10% of normal, at which point hyperkalemia manifests. Normally, potassium is secreted by the distal renal tubules, and as nephrons are lost, the remaining nephrons increase their secretion of potassium through increased blood flow and increased sodium delivery to the collecting tubules. In addition, because aldosterone secretion increases in patients with renal failure, there is a greater loss of potassium through the gastrointestinal tract. This system of enhanced gastrointestinal secretion is an effective compensatory mechanism in the presence of normal dietary intake of potassium but can be easily overwhelmed by an acute exogenous potassium load (administration of potassium, such as during the perioperative period) or acute endogenous potassium load (hemolysis, tissue trauma such as that associated with surgery).

The third stage of adaptation is seen in sodium homeostasis and regulation of the ECF volume. In contrast to the levels of other solutes, sodium balance remains intact despite progressive deterioration in renal function and variations in dietary intake. Nevertheless, the system can be overwhelmed by abruptly increased sodium intake (resulting in volume overload) or decreased sodium intake (sodium restriction during the perioperative period leading to extracellular volume depletion).

Associated Clinical Conditions

Uremic Syndrome Uremic syndrome is a constellation of signs and symptoms (anorexia, nausea, vomiting, pruritus, anemia, fatigue, coagulopathy) that reflect the kidney's progressive inability to perform its excretory, secretory, and regulatory functions. Although it is questionable whether urea itself produces the signs and symptoms (except at high concentrations), the BUN concentration is a useful clinical indicator of the severity of the uremic syndrome and the patient's

response to therapy. In contrast, the serum creatinine concentration, correlates poorly with uremic symptoms. Traditional treatment of the uremic syndrome is dietary protein restriction based on the presumption that a low-protein diet results in decreased protein catabolism and urea production.

Renal Osteodystrophy Renal osteodystrophy is a complication of chronic renal failure, reflecting the complex interaction of secondary hyperparathyroidism and decreased vitamin D production by the kidneys. As the GFR decreases, there is a parallel decrease in phosphate clearance and an increase in the serum phosphate concentrations that result in reciprocal decreases in serum calcium concentrations. Hypocalcemia stimulates parathyroid hormone (PTH) secretion, which leads to bone resorption and calcium release. As a result of decreased renal production of vitamin D by the kidneys, intestinal absorption of calcium is impaired, which also leads to hypocalcemia, stimulation of PTH release, and bone resorption.

Hyperparathyroid bone disease is the most common form of uremic osteodystrophy. Radiographs demonstrate evidence of bone demineralization (clavicles, skull, middle phalanges of the middle and index fingers). Further evidence of bone resorption is the presence of increased serum alkaline phosphatase concentrations. The diagnosis of hyperparathyroidism is confirmed by documentation of increased serum PTH concentrations. Accumulation of aluminum in patients undergoing chronic renal dialysis, although decreasing in frequency, may result in bone pain, fractures, and weakness. Hyperparathyroidism seems to protect against aluminum-induced bone disease. Adynamic (aplastic) bone disease occurs in patients (often diabetics) with ESRD who are undergoing long-term renal dialysis and who do not have secondary hyperparathyroidism (after parathyroidectomy).

Treatment of renal osteodystrophy is intended to prevent skeletal complications by restricting dietary phosphate intake (antacids may be administered to bind phosphorus in the gastrointestinal tract), administration of oral calcium supplements, and vitamin D therapy. Magnesium-containing antacids introduce the risk of hypermagnesemia, and aluminum-containing antacids are equally undesirable. If aluminum toxicity is present, deferoxamine chelation therapy is helpful. Overzealous suppression of PTH by calcium and vitamin D may be undesirable, as PTH may be necessary to maintain bone mass in chronic renal failure patients. If medical therapies fail to control hypercalcemia and hyperparathyroidism, subtotal parathyroidectomy is often recommended.

Anemia Anemia frequently accompanies chronic renal failure and is presumed to be responsible for many of the symptoms (fatigue, weakness, decreased exercise tolerance) characteristic of the uremic syndrome. This anemia is primarily due to decreased erythropoietin production by the kidneys. Excess PTH appears to contribute to anemia by replacing bone marrow with fibrous tissue.

Treatment of the anemia of chronic renal disease is with recombinant human erythropoietin (epoetin), eliminating the need for blood transfusions and avoiding the symptoms of anemia in most patients. Blood transfusions are avoided if possible, as the resultant sensitization to HLA antigens makes kidney transplantation less successful. The goal of erythropoietin therapy is to maintain the hematocrit between 36% and 40%. Intermittent injections of parenteral iron are recommended to maximize the responses to erythropoietin. The development of systemic hypertension or exacerbation of co-existing systemic hypertension, necessitating further antihypertensive therapy, is a risk of erythropoietin administration.

Uremic Bleeding Patients with chronic renal failure have an increased tendency to bleed despite the presence of normal laboratory coagulation studies (platelet count, prothrombin time, plasma thromboplastin time). The bleeding time is the screening test that best correlates with the tendency to bleed. Hemorrhagic episodes (gastrointestinal bleeding, epistaxis, hemorrhagic pericarditis, subdural hematoma) remain major factors contributing to the morbidity and mortality associated with anemia.

Treatment of uremic bleeding may include the administration of cryoprecipitate to provide factor VIII–von Willebrand factor (vWF) complex (risk of transmission of viral diseases) or administration of 1-desamino-8-D-arginine vasopressin (DDAVP, desmopressin). DDAVP, an analogue of antidiuretic hormone, increases the circulating levels of factor VIII–von Willebrand factor complex and decreases the bleeding time. In patients with uremia, the intravenous infusion or subcutaneous injection of DDAVP decreases prolonged bleeding and is particularly useful for preventing clinical hemorrhage when invasive procedures such as surgery are planned. The maximal effect of DDAVP is present within 2 to 4 hours and lasts 6 to 8 hours. The effects of DDAVP appear to be attenuated by repeated doses. DDAVP may act by increasing or changing platelet membrane receptor binding of the factor VIII–von Willebrand factor complex or by inducing the appearance of a more active complex (**Table 14-9**).

Although cryoprecipitate and DDAVP can correct bleeding times so surgical procedures can be performed without excessive bleeding in patients with chronic renal failure, the effects of both drugs last for only a few hours. Conversely, conjugated estrogen administration may improve bleeding times for up to 14 days. It has also been observed that erythropoietin shortens bleeding times. It is of interest that prior to the availability of erythropoietin, it had been recognized that blood transfusions to increase the hematocrit to above 30% also corrected the bleeding times.

Neurologic Changes Neurologic changes may be early manifestations of progressive renal insufficiency. Initially, symptoms may be mild (impaired abstract thinking, insomnia, irritability), but as renal disease progresses, more significant changes (increased deep tendon reflexes, seizures, obtundation, uremic encephalopathy, coma) may develop. A disabling complication of advanced chronic renal failure is the development of a distal, symmetrical mixed motor and sensory polyneuropathy, paresthesias or hyperesthesias of the feet secondary to sensory neuropathy, or distal weakness of the lower extremities. The arms may also be affected, but the incidence is less than in the legs. Diabetic neuropathy may be superimposed on uremic peripheral neuropathy. Some aspects of uremic encephalopathy and the severity of peripheral neurologic symptoms may be improved by hemodialysis.

Cardiovascular Changes Systemic hypertension is the most significant risk factor accompanying chronic renal failure and contributes to the congestive heart failure, coronary artery disease, and cerebrovascular disease that occurs in these patients. Uncontrolled systemic hypertension speeds the progressive decrease in GFR. The pathogenesis of systemic hypertension in these patients reflects intravascular fluid volume expansion due to retention of sodium and water and activation of the renin-angiotensin-aldosterone system. Uremic pericarditis may occur in patients with severe chronic renal failure. Cardiac ultrasonography determines the size of an associated pericardial effusion and its effect on myocardial contractility. Atrial cardiac dysrhythmias are common in the presence of uremic pericarditis.

Dialysis is the indicated treatment of patients who are hypertensive because of hypervolemia (remove volume to attain "dry weight") and those who develop uremic pericarditis. Dialysis is less likely to control systemic hypertension due to activation of the renin-angiotensin-aldosterone system. Increasing doses of antihypertensive drugs are recommended in these patients. ACE inhibitors are used cautiously in patients in whom the GFR is dependent on increased efferent arteriolar vasoconstriction (bilateral renal artery stenosis, transplanted kidney with unilateral stenosis), which is mediated by angiotensin II. Administration of ACE inhibitors to these patients

TABLE 14-9 Treatment of Uremic Bleeding				
Drug	Dose	Onset of Effect	Peak Effect	Duration of Effect
Cryoprecipitate	10 units IV over 30 min	<1 hr	4–12 hr	12–18 hr
DDAVP (desmopressin)	0.3 µg/kg IV or SC	<1 hr	2–4 hr	6–8 hr
Conjugated estrogen	0.6 mg/kg/day IV for 5 days	6 hr	5–7 days	14 days
Adapted from Tolkoff-Rubin NE, Pascual M: Chronic renal failure. Sci Am Med 1998;1–12.				

can result in efferent arteriolar dilatation and decreased GFR, which results in sudden deterioration in renal function.

Cardiac tamponade and hemodynamic instability associated with uremic pericarditis and effusion is an indication for prompt drainage of the effusion, often via placement of a percutaneous pericardial catheter. In occasional patients, surgical drainage with creation of a pericardial window or pericardiectomy is necessary. The development of hypotension unresponsive to intravascular fluid volume replacement may be an important clue that cardiac tamponade is present.

Treatment of Chronic Renal Failure/Insufficiency

Treatment currently includes aggressive treatment of the underlying cause (diabetes or hypertension if present), pharmacologic therapy to delay the progress, and renal replacement therapy as ESRD ensues.

Since hypertension is both a cause and a consequence of CRI and is directly correlated with deterioration of renal function, blood pressure control is the mainstay of treatment aimed at slowing the decline of renal function. Hypertension in CRI is difficult to treat, and most patients will be on three or more antihypertensive agents given the current national and international recommendations for blood pressure control in patients with CRI.

Considering that a major driving force in the pathophysiology of CRI is the renin-angiotensin-aldosterone system, most guidelines recommend either ACE inhibitors or angiotensin receptor blockers, whether or not hypertension is present. For most patients, the first drug of choice is an ACE inhibitor, which is then titrated upward into the moderate- to high-dose range as tolerated. However, angiotensin receptor blockers are the preferred choice in those with type 2 diabetes with CRI and proteinuria. Treatment of CRI with ACE inhibitors and/or angiotensin receptor blockers has been shown in many clinical trials to slow the progression of renal dysfunction, reduce mortality and cardiac events, and decrease proteinuria. Great debate exists in the literature whether these two classes of drug have actions beyond their blood pressure–lowering effects, but the general opinion is that they do and it is unusual for a patient with a GFR less than 70 mL/min not to be on one or both of these drugs. Other classes of drug, particularly β-blockers (specifically carvedilol) are given as second- or third-line antihypertensive drugs and have been demonstrated to reduce cardiac events in this patient population. Calcium channel blockers are also useful adjuncts in blood pressure control but have not been shown to offer added benefit in terms of reducing cardiac events or slowing the decline in renal function in the absence of an ACE inhibitor or angiotensin receptor blocker.

The current guidelines for treatment of diabetes in CRI recommend a goal of less than 7% glycosylated hemoglobin. Long-term follow-up in diabetics with CRI have shown that euglycemia is associated with reversal of the typical lesions seen in diabetic nephropathy and a reduction in albuminuria. However, this is a long-term change and may take 5 to 10 years to achieve.

A number of studies in both diabetic and nondiabetic renal disease have addressed the question of dietary protein restriction. The multicenter Modification of Diet in Renal Disease study compared a normal protein intake (1 g/kg per day) with low (0.6 g/kg per day) and very low (0.28 g/kg per day) protein intake in nondiabetic patients and suggested that a prescribed dietary protein intake of 0.6 g/kg per day reduced the rate of progression of renal disease. Meta-analyses of other studies of protein restriction in CRI concur that a modest reduction in rate of progression occurs with dietary protein restriction. However, although it is desirable to restrict protein intake (to reduce the accumulation of toxic metabolites), many CRI patients experience chronic anorexia and have a poor nutritional status verging on protein-energy malnutrition and require intensive counseling and education or even specialized nutrition therapy.

With respect to anemia, the National Kidney Foundation Kidney Disease Outcomes Quality Initiative clinical practice guidelines state that hemoglobin, rather than hematocrit, is the preferred method for assessing anemia and while decreased hemoglobin often accompanies chronic kidney disease, there is no quantitative definition of anemia in chronic kidney disease. Instead, anemia is defined according to physiologic population norms. All patients with chronic kidney disease who have hemoglobin levels lower than physiologic norms are considered anemic. Thus, for males, anemia is defined as a hemoglobin level less than 13.0 g/dL, while in women, anemia is defined as a hemoglobin level less than 12.0 g/dL regardless of age or menopausal status. The low hemoglobin level that is often seen in chronic kidney disease should not lead to the acceptance of lower than normal hemoglobin levels as appropriate in patients with chronic kidney disease. Therefore, hemoglobin levels below 13.0 g/dL for men and 12.0 g/dL for women require treatment. Anemia is responsive to treatment with erythropoietin in all stages of chronic kidney disease.

Treatment of the failing kidney inevitably requires either preemptive transplantation or some form of dialysis to control volume overload and derangements of electrolytes, acid base balance, and uremia. Patients are counseled about options for renal replacement therapy when the GFR begins to approach 30 mL/min/1.73 m^2. The initiation of dialysis therapy remains a decision informed by a number of clinical factors, personal choices, regional preferences, as well as by outcome studies and the constraints of regulation and reimbursement. Although effective dialysis therapy offers increased survival, it has a major impact on quality of life and is not without its own specific risks. For some patients, conservative therapy, without dialysis or transplantation, is the appropriate option. In this case, dietary and pharmacologic therapy is used to minimize uremic symptoms and to maintain volume homeostasis.

By the time GFR is 15 mL/min/1.73 m^2, most patients who elect dialysis will have commenced therapy. The current Medicare guidelines of creatinine clearances of 15 mL/min and 10 mL/min or of serum creatinine concentrations of 6 mg/dL and 8 mg/dL for diabetics and nondiabetics, respectively, are often-used criteria for initiating hemodialysis. While the literature suggests some disagreement as to specific prescription, frequency, and length of time of hemodialysis, there is clear evidence that the dialysis dose is significantly correlated with survival. National guidelines recommend a minimal dialysis dose, which, if not achieved, has been shown to be associated with increased mortality. Since clinical signs and symptoms are not reliable indicators of hemodialysis adequacy, the delivered dose should be measured and monitored routinely. Dialysis dose can be calculated from a number of different formulae or models, but essentially measures the clearance of urea by estimating the difference in predialysis and postdialysis serum urea. Urea is used to calculate dialysis dose because it is a small, readily dialyzed solute that accounts for 90% of waste nitrogen that accumulates between hemodialysis treatments. Furthermore, the fractional clearance of urea has been shown to correlate with patient morbidity and mortality in dialysis patients.

Hemodialysis and Associated Clinical Challenges

Hemodialysis is used for treating patients in whom chronic renal failure would otherwise result in the uremic syndrome. Objectives when caring for patients who are undergoing hemodialysis include adequate dialysis, ensuring adequate nutrition, maintaining vascular access, correcting hormonal deficiencies, minimizing hospitalizations, and prolonging life while enhancing its quality. During hemodialysis, diffusion of solutes between the blood and dialysis solution results in removal of metabolic waste products and replenishment of body buffers.. The dose of dialysis, which depends on the length of treatment, the type of dialysis membrane, and solute clearance are the most important modifiable determinants of survival in patients with ESRD undergoing hemodialysis. Inadequate dialysis shortens survival and leads to malnutrition, anemia, and functional impairment, resulting in frequent hospitalizations and increased cost of care (**Table 14-10**). The annual mortality for patients on hemodialysis is nearly 25% and is most often attributed to cardiovascular causes or infection.

Vascular Access A surgically created vascular access site is necessary for effective hemodialysis. To preserve the blood vessels for vascular access, venipuncture should be avoided in the nondominant arm and the upper part of the dominant arm of patients with chronic renal failure. Despite the presence of coagulopathy in patients with uremia and the routine use of heparin during dialysis, thrombosis of the vascular access site is common. Native arteriovenous fistulas (cephalic vein anastomosed to the radial artery) are superior to polytetrafluoroethylene grafts as sites of vascular access because of their longer life span and lower incidence of thrombosis and infection. Native arteriovenous fistulas are the preferred vascular access sites in all patients undergoing hemodialysis. The most common access-related complication is intimal hyperplasia, which results in stenosis proximal to the venous anastomosis. Other complications related to access include infection, the

TABLE 14-10	Findings Suggestive of Inadequate Hemodialysis

Clinical
Anorexia, nausea, vomiting
Peripheral neuropathy
Poor nutritional status
Depressed sensorium
Pericarditis
Ascites
Minimal weight gain or weight loss between treatments
Fluid retention and systemic hypertension

Chemical
Decrease in blood urea nitrogen concentration during hemodialysis < 65%
Albumin concentration < 4 g/dL
Predialysis blood urea concentration < 50 mg/dL (a sign of malnutrition)
Predialysis serum creatinine concentration < 5 mg/dL (a sign of malnutrition)
Persistent anemia (hematocrit < 30%) despite erythropoietin therapy

Adapted from Ifudu O: Care of patients undergoing hemodialysis. N Engl J Med 1998;339:1054–1062.

formation of aneurysms, and ischemia of the arm. When dialysis is urgently required, vascular access is obtained with a double-lumen dialysis catheter, most often using the jugular or femoral vein.

Complications Associated with Hemodialysis Hypotension is the most common adverse event during hemodialysis and most likely reflects osmolar shifts and ultrafiltration-induced volume depletion. Hypotensive episodes may reflect myocardial ischemia, cardiac dysrhythmias, or pericardial effusion with cardiac tamponade. Most hypotensive episodes are successfully treated by slowing the rate of ultrafiltration and/or administering intravenous saline.

Hypersensitivity reactions to the ethylene oxide used to sterilize the dialysis machine may occur as an adverse reaction to the specific membrane material, polyacrylonitrile. Reactions to polyacrylonitrile occur most commonly in patients receiving ACE inhibitors. When blood comes in contact with the polyacrylonitrile membrane, the membrane's high negative surface charge stabilizes enzymes, which generate bradykinins. Normally, bradykinin is degraded by kinases, but ACE inhibitors block this response, and profound peripheral vasodilation and hypotension may occur.

Nutrition and Fluid Balance During progressive renal failure, catabolism and anorexia lead to loss of lean body mass, but concomitant fluid retention masks weight loss and may even lead to weight gain. There is no justification for stringent restriction of dietary potassium in patients undergoing hemodialysis. Patients with ESRD have decreased total body potassium and an inexplicable tolerance of hyperkalemia. The expected cardiac and neuromuscular responses to hyperkalemia are less pronounced in patients on hemodialysis than in those with normal renal function. Clearance of potassium by hemodialysis is efficient, and because most potassium is intracellular, it is likely that hypokalemia will be suggested by a blood sample obtained soon after completion of hemodialysis and before transcellular equilibration has occurred. Water-soluble vitamins are removed by hemodialysis and should be replaced. Between treatments, a weight gain of 3% to 4% of body mass in 2 days is appropriate.

Cardiovascular Disease Cardiovascular disease accounts for nearly 50% of all deaths in patients on hemodialysis.

Ischemic Heart Disease The increased incidence of ischemic heart disease and myocardial infarction among patients with ESRD is attributed to systemic hypertension, anemia, hyperlipidemia, hyperhomocysteinemia, accelerated atherosclerosis, and possibly impaired oxygen delivery to the myocardium due to uremic toxins. Chemical stress testing (dipyridamole or dobutamine) may be preferred to exercise stress testing, as patients in renal failure are often unable to exercise adequately. The baseline electrocardiogram may be altered by metabolic derangements. For unknown reasons, baseline serum creatinine kinase concentrations are increased in nearly one third of patients on hemodialysis. Because this increase is accounted for principally by the MM isoenzyme, the value of the MB fraction for diagnosis of an acute myocardial infarction remains intact. Medical management of ischemic heart disease in patients on hemodialysis is the same as for those with normal renal function.

Congestive Heart Failure Congestive heart failure in patients on hemodialysis is treated as in patients with normal renal function with the exception that diuretics are not administered. Protein-bound digoxin-like immunoreactive substances in the serum of patients on hemodialysis may interfere with the accuracy and interpretation of measurements of digoxin concentrations and the diagnosis of toxicity. Hemodialysis has beneficial effects on cardiac hemodynamics, as removal of fluid during hemodialysis provides symptomatic relief for patients in congestive heart failure.

Systemic Hypertension Fluid retention during progressive renal failure is the most likely explanation for the presence of systemic hypertension in most patients who present for hemodialysis. Failure to distinguish essential hypertension from that due to fluid retention in the presence of ESRD may lead to the inappropriate and ineffective use of antihypertensive drugs. The appropriate management of systemic hypertension is gradual removal of fluid by hemodialysis to achieve an ideal postdialysis body weight. Patients with associated essential hypertension also require treatment with antihypertensive drugs.

Pericarditis Pericarditis with pericardial effusion occurs infrequently in patients on hemodialysis and is often due to inadequate hemodialysis. Intensive heparin-free dialysis is the treatment for suspected uremic pericarditis. Persistent effusion despite intensive dialysis or early suspicion of infection is an indication for pericardiocentesis or pericardiotomy.

Bleeding Tendency Bleeding due to altered platelet function is partially correctable by hemodialysis. Heparin-free dialysis or administration of DDAVP is often sufficient to correct a bleeding tendency.

Infection Patients requiring hemodialysis have increased susceptibility to infection because of impaired phagocytosis and chemotaxis. Some of the factors resulting in impaired phagocytosis and chemotaxis may be partially reversed by hemodialysis. Some patients on hemodialysis have severe infection without a fever. Tuberculosis in patients on hemodialysis is usually extrapulmonary and often presents with atypical symptoms that mimic those of inadequate dialysis. Because anergy in response to skin testing is common, unexplained weight loss and anorexia, with or without persistent fever, should prompt further testing to rule out tuberculosis. All patients on hemodialysis are vaccinated against pneumococcus, and those who are not already immune receive hepatitis B vaccine. Malnutrition or inadequate dialysis may impair antibody response to vaccines.

Hepatitis B or C virus infection in patients on hemodialysis is often asymptomatic, and liver aminotransferase concentrations may not be increased. Patients with hepatitis B virus should undergo hemodialysis in isolation with a dedicated machine. A substantial proportion of patients on hemodialysis have antibodies to hepatitis C. Of note, dose adjustments of drugs used to treat acquired immunodeficiency syndrome is not required during hemodialysis. However, isolation of patients with acquired immunodeficiency syndrome or use of a dedicated hemodialysis machine is not necessary.

Miscellaneous Considerations Good glucose control, as evidenced by a glycosylated hemoglobin value less than 7%, is important in patients with diabetes mellitus requiring hemodialysis, as hyperglycemia may result in hyperkalemia or excessive weight gain. Decreased catabolism of insulin in many patients on hemodialysis may result in decreased insulin requirements compared with needs prior to the initiation of hemodialysis. The presentation of diabetic ketoacidosis may be atypical with respiratory acidosis and alkalosis but without metabolic acidosis and hypovolemia. Hypertriglyceridemia reflects diminished clearance in patients on hemodialysis. Depression is a potential risk in patients on hemodialysis and may be misdiagnosed as functional impairment due to renal failure. There is conflicting evidence on whether the risk of cancer is increased in patients on hemodialysis.

Peritoneal Dialysis

Peritoneal dialysis is simple to perform; it requires placing an anchored plastic catheter in the peritoneal cavity for infusion of a dialysis solution that remains in place for several hours. During that time, diffusive solute transport occurs across the peritoneal membrane until fresh fluid is exchanged for the old fluid. Automated peritoneal dialysis, in which a mechanized cycler infuses and drains peritoneal dialysate at night is used in many patients. Peritoneal dialysis may be selected over hemodialysis for patients with congestive heart failure or unstable angina who may not tolerate the rapid fluid shifts or systemic blood pressure changes that may accompany hemodialysis. Peritoneal dialysis is also indicated for patients with extensive vascular disease that prevents placing a catheter for vascular access. In patients with diabetes, insulin can be infused with the dialysate with resultant precise regulation of blood glucose concentrations. The presence of abdominal hernias or adhesions may interfere with the ability to use peritoneal dialysis effectively. Peritonitis presenting as abdomi-nal pain and fever is the most common serious complication of peritoneal dialysis. Treatment is with antibiotics, which may include cephalosporins, aminoglycosides, and vancomycin. Survival rates and annual costs are similar with peritoneal dialysis or hemodialysis, but hospitalization rates are higher among patients treated with peritoneal dialysis.

Drug Clearance in Patients Undergoing Dialysis

Patients who are undergoing dialysis may require special consideration with respect to drug dosing intervals and may require supplemental dosing with drugs that have been cleared by dialysis. When possible, scheduled doses of drugs are administered after completion of dialysis. Drug properties that influence clearance by dialysis include protein binding, water solubility, and molecular weight. In this regard, low molecular weight (<500 Da), water-soluble, nonprotein-bound drugs are readily cleared by dialysis. Continuous renal replacement therapies, such as continuous venovenous hemofiltration, and continuous arteriovenous hemofiltration, efficiently remove drugs unless they are bound to protein.

Role for Perioperative Hemodialysis

Patients should undergo adequate hemodialysis before elective surgery to minimize the likelihood of uremic bleeding, pulmonary edema, and impaired arterial oxygenation. Depending on the planned surgery, the use of heparin may be avoided or minimized during preoperative hemodialysis. Urgent hemodialysis is not required after radiocontrast dye studies in those who are undergoing regular hemodialysis. Although these dyes can be removed by hemodialysis, the volume administered in most studies does not result in pulmonary edema in patients with adequate dialysis, and nephrotoxicity is not a concern in patients with ESRD. Meperidine is avoided for postoperative analgesia because its metabolites may accumulate in patients with renal failure and result in seizures.

ANESTHETIC MANAGEMENT OF PATIENTS WITH CHRONIC RENAL DISEASE/INSUFFICIENCY

Management of anesthesia in patients with chronic renal disease requires an understanding of the pathologic changes that accompany renal disease, whether the renal disease is sufficient to require hemodialysis, and which drugs are affected by reduced renal function (**Table 14-11**). An important assessment is whether the renal disease is stable, progressing, or diminishing. This information is obtained by monitoring the serum creatinine concentrations.

Preoperative Evaluation

Preoperative evaluation of patients with chronic renal disease includes consideration of concomitant drug therapy and evaluation of the changes deemed characteristic of chronic renal failure (see Table 14-8). Blood volume status may be estimated by comparing body weight before and after hemodialysis, monitoring vital signs (orthostatic hypotension, tachycardia), and measuring atrial filling pressures. As diabetes is often seen in these patients, glucose management is of concern. Inappropriate signs of digitalis toxicity should be sought in treated patients, emphasizing the role of renal clearance for digitalis and other drugs.

Antihypertensive drug therapy is traditionally continued. Preoperative medication must be individualized, remembering that these patients may exhibit unexpected sensitivity to central nervous system depressant drugs. In addition to patients with preoperative renal dysfunction, it is important to recognize others who are at high risk of developing perioperative renal failure, even in the absence of co-existing renal disease. Preservation of renal function intraoperatively depends on maintaining an adequate intravascular fluid volume and minimizing drug-induced cardiovascular depression.

Patients on hemodialysis should undergo dialysis during the 24 hours preceding elective surgery. A common recommendation is that the serum potassium concentration should not exceed 5.5 mEq/L on the day of surgery. Anemia is evaluated preoperatively, but the introduction of recombinant human erythropoietin therapy has decreased the number of patients in renal failure who present for elective surgery with a hematocrit less than 30%. The preoperative presence of a coagulopathy may be treated with DDAVP.

TABLE 14-11 Drugs Used in Anesthesia Practice That Significantly Depand on Renal Elimination		
Class of Drug	**Action Terminated by Renal Excretion**	**Action Partially Terminated by Renal Excretion**
Induction agents	—	Barbiturates
Muscle relaxants	Gallamine, metocurine	Pancuronium, vecuronium
Cholinesterase inhibitors	—	Neostigmine, edrophonium
Cardiovascular drugs	Digoxin, inotropes	Atropine, glycopyrrolate, milrione, hydralazine
Antimicrobials	Aminoglycosides, vancomycin, cephalosporin, penicillin	Sulfonamides
Adapted from Malhotra V, Sudheendra V, Diwan S: Anesthesia and the renal and genitourinary systems. In Miller RD, Fleischer LA, Johns RA, et al (eds): Miller's Anesthesia, 6th ed. Philadelphia, Elsevier Churchill Livingstone, 2005.		

Induction of Anesthesia

Induction of anesthesia and tracheal intubation can be safely accomplished with intravenous drugs (propofol, etomidate, thiopental) plus a muscle relaxant such as succinylcholine, remembering that these patients may exhibit uremia-induced slowing of gastric emptying. Alternatively, if the possibility of increased gastric fluid volume does not mandate the rapid onset of skeletal muscle paralysis, administration of intermediate- or short-acting, nondepolarizing, neuromuscular-blocking drugs that are independent of renal clearance mechanisms is a consideration. Logic suggests slow injection of induction drugs to minimize the likelihood of drug-induced decreases in systemic blood pressure. Regardless of blood volume status, these patients often respond to induction of anesthesia as if they were hypovolemic. The likelihood of hypotension during induction of anesthesia may be increased if sympathetic nervous system function is attenuated by antihypertensive drugs or uremia. Attenuated sympathetic nervous system activity impairs compensatory peripheral vasoconstriction; thus, small decreases in blood volume, institution of positive-pressure ventilation of the patient's lungs, abrupt changes in body position, or drug-induced myocardial depression can result in an exaggerated decrease in systemic blood pressure. Patients being treated with ACE inhibitors may be at increased risk of experiencing intraoperative hypotension, especially with acute surgical blood loss.

Exaggerated central nervous system effects of anesthetic induction drugs may reflect uremia-induced disruption of the blood-brain barrier. Furthermore, decreased protein binding of drugs may result in the availability of more unbound drugs to act at receptor sites. Indeed, the amount of pharmacologically active unbound thiopental in plasma is increased in patients with chronic renal failure (see Table 14-11).

Potassium release following administration of succinylcholine is not exaggerated in patients with chronic renal failure, although there is a theoretical concern that those with extensive uremic neuropathies might be at increased risk. Likewise, caution is indicated when the preoperative serum potassium concentration is in the high-normal range, as this finding combined with maximum drug-induced potassium release (0.5–1.0 mEq/L) could result in dangerous hyperkalemia. It is important to recognize that small doses of nondepolarizing muscle relaxants administered before the injection of succinylcholine do not reliably attenuate the succinylcholine-induced release of potassium.

Maintenance of Anesthesia

In patients with chronic renal disease who are not dependent on hemodialysis or in those vulnerable to renal dysfunction because of advanced age or the need for major thoracic or abdominal vascular surgery, anesthesia is often maintained with nitrous oxide combined with isoflurane, desflurane, or short-acting opioids. Sevoflurane may be avoided because of concerns related to fluoride nephrotoxicity or production of compound A, although there is no evidence that patients with co-existing renal disease are at increased risk of renal dysfunction following administration of sevoflurane. Isoflurane or desflurane combined with nitrous oxide provides sufficient potency to suppress excessive increases in systemic blood pressure due to surgical stimulation, to avoid the controversy related to fluoride nephrotoxicity, and to decrease the dose of nondepolarizing muscle relaxants needed to produce skeletal muscle relaxation. Total intravenous anesthesia with remifentanil, propofol, and cisatracurium has been recommended for patients with end-stage renal failure.

Potent volatile anesthetics are useful for controlling intraoperative systemic hypertension and decreasing the doses of muscle relaxants needed for adequate surgical relaxation. The high incidence of associated liver disease in patients with chronic renal disease should be considered, however, when selecting these drugs. Furthermore, excessive depression of cardiac output is a potential hazard of volatile anesthetics. Decreases in tissue blood flow must be minimized in the presence of anemia to avoid jeopardizing oxygen delivery to the tissues. Opioids decrease the likelihood of cardiovascular depression and avoid the concern of hepatotoxicity or nephrotoxicity. Nevertheless, opioids do not reliably control intraoperative systemic blood pressure elevations. Furthermore, prolonged sedation and depression of ventilation from small doses of opioids have been described in anephric patients. Conceivably, pharmacologically active metabolites of opioids accumulate in the circulation and cerebrospinal fluid when renal function is absent.

Muscle Relaxants

Selection of nondepolarizing muscle relaxants for maintenance of skeletal muscle paralysis during surgery is influenced by the known clearance mechanisms of these drugs. Renal disease may slow excretion of vecuronium and rocuronium, whereas clearance of mivacurium, atracurium, and cisatracurium from plasma is independent of renal function. Renal failure may delay clearance of laudanosine, the principal metabolite of atracurium and cisatracurium. Laudanosine lacks effects at the neuromuscular junction, but at high plasma concentrations, it may stimulate the central nervous system. Regardless of the nondepolarizing, neuromuscular-blocking drug selected, it seems prudent to decrease the initial dose of the drug and administer subsequent doses based on the responses observed using a peripheral nerve stimulator.

The diagnosis of residual neuromuscular blockade after apparent reversal of nondepolarizing neuromuscular blockade with anticholinesterase drugs should be considered in anephric patients who manifest signs of skeletal muscle weakness during the early postoperative period. Renal excretion accounts for approximately 50% of the clearance of neostigmine and approximately 75% of the elimination of edrophonium and pyridostigmine. As a result, the elimination half-time of these drugs is greatly prolonged by renal failure. Even in anephric patients, there is some protection because renal elimination of anticholinesterase drugs is delayed as long as, if not longer than, that of the nondepolarizing neuromuscular blocking drugs. In addition, other explanations (antibiotics, acidosis, electrolyte imbalance, diuretics) should be considered when neuromuscular blockade persists or reappears in patients with renal dysfunction.

Fluid Management and Urine Output

Patients with severe renal dysfunction but not requiring hemodialysis and those without renal disease undergoing operations associated with a high incidence of postoperative renal failure may benefit from preoperative hydration with administration of balanced salt solutions. Indeed, most patients come to the operating room with a contracted ECF volume unless corrective measures are taken. Lactated Ringer's solution (potassium 4 mEq/L) or other potassium-containing fluids should not be administered to anuric patients. Administration of balanced salt solutions (3–5 mL/kg per hour IV), is often recommended to maintain acceptable urine output. Rapid infusion of a bolus of balanced salt solutions to restore circulating volume (500 mL IV) should increase urine output in the presence of hypovolemia. Stimulation of urine output with osmotic (mannitol) or tubular (furosemide) diuretics in the absence of adequate intravascular fluid volume replacement is discouraged. Indeed, the most likely etiology of oliguria is an inadequate circulating fluid volume, which can only be further compromised by drug-induced diuresis. Furthermore, although administration of mannitol or furosemide predictably increases urine output, there is no evidence of corresponding improvements in the GFR. Likewise, intraoperative urine output has not been shown to be predictive of postoperative renal insufficiency after abdominal vascular surgery.

Patients dependent on hemodialysis require special attention with respect to perioperative fluid management. An absence of renal function narrows the margin of safety between insufficient and excessive fluid administration to these patients. Noninvasive operations require replacement of only insensible water losses with 5% glucose in water (5–10 mL/kg IV). The small amount of urine output can be replaced with 0.45% sodium chloride. Thoracic or abdominal surgery can be associated with loss of significant intravascular fluid volume to the interstitial spaces. This loss is often replaced with balanced salt solutions or 5% albumin solutions. Blood transfusions may be considered if the oxygen-carrying capacity must be increased or if blood loss is excessive. Measuring the central venous pressure may be useful for guiding fluid replacement.

Monitoring

If invasive monitoring is required, there are a few issues to be considered. Any patient with CRI may require a(nother) fistula at some point in the future. While it is recommended that the radial and ulnar arteries should be avoided in case they are needed for an arteriovenous fistula in the future, the same may be said of the brachial and even the axillary arteries. Use of the femoral arteries carries the risk of line infection, particularly since these patients may be immunocompromised as part of their disease process or therapy. That leaves the dorsalis pedis or posterior tibial arteries, which may be inconvenient because of positioning or difficult to access because of edema and tissue induration. Whichever site is chosen, it is important to note that neither the arterial pressure nor the arterial blood gases will be accurate if the cannula is placed in the same extremity as a functioning or partially patent fistula.

Venous pressure monitoring is often extremely helpful, if not necessary, since a volume load is not well tolerated by patients with even modest decreases in renal function. The choice of right atrial (central venous pressure) or pulmonary artery (pulmonary artery occlusion pressure) pressure monitoring will be guided by the presence or otherwise of underlying cardiac disease or pulmonary edema. Strict asepsis must be adhered to when placing a central venous pressure or pulmonary artery occlusion pressure catheter; CRI patients are extremely prone to infection. Central venous access may be difficult in patients who have a tunneled Portacath or temporary dialysis catheter in situ or who have had many such catheters previously placed with subsequent stenosis of the veins. It is not unreasonable to use a temporary dialysis catheter for areas if other intravenous access proves difficult. However, it must be remembered that (1) the catheter must be accessed aseptically, just as it is at the time of dialysis, (2) the catheter is left heparinized and must be aspirated before connecting to an intravenous line or pressure transducer, (3) if it is to be disconnected at the end of the procedure, it must be reheparinized and sealed aseptically again.

Associated Concerns

Since many of these patients come to the operating room frequently, premedication may or may not be necessary. Some patients become accustomed to their many surgeries, while others find it extremely wearing and stressful. A small dose of oral or intravenous benzodiazepine is appropriate, while intramuscular injection of any predication should be avoided in consideration of low muscle mass and uremic platelet dysfunction.

Attention to patient positioning on the operating room table is important. Poor nutritional status renders the skin particularly prone to bruising and sloughing, and extra padding is required to protect vulnerable nerves around the elbow, knees, and ankles. Fistulas must be protected at all cost and be well padded to prevent pressure injury. If it is at all possible, the arm with the fistula should not be tucked but positioned so that the fistula thrill can be checked at intervals throughout the surgery.

Guidelines recommend that arm veins of the nondominant hand not be used for intravenous cannulas and to even advise patients to wear Medic Alert bracelets to this effect.

Regional Anesthesia

Brachial plexus block is useful for placing the vascular shunts necessary for chronic hemodialysis. In addition to providing analgesia, this form of regional anesthesia abolishes vasospasm and provides optimal surgical conditions by producing maximal vascular vasodilation. The suggestion that the duration of brachial plexus anesthesia is shortened in patients with chronic renal failure has not been confirmed in controlled studies. Adequacy of coagulation should be considered and the presence of uremic neuropathies excluded before regional anesthesia is performed in these patients. Co-existing metabolic acidosis may decrease the seizure threshold for local anesthetics.

Postoperative Management

A diagnosis of inadequate reversal of muscle relaxant should be considered in anephric patients who show signs of skeletal muscle weakness during the postoperative period.

Caution should be exercised in the use of parenteral opioids for postoperative analgesia in view of a potential for exaggerated central nervous system depression and hypoventilation after administration of even small doses of opioids. Administration of naloxone may be necessary if the depression of ventilation is severe. Continuous monitoring of the electrocardiogram is helpful for detecting cardiac dysrhythmias, such as those related to hyperkalemia. Continuation of supplemental oxygen into the postoperative period is a consideration, especially if anemia is present.

RENAL TRANSPLANTATION

Candidates for renal transplantation are selected from patients with ESRD who are on established programs of long-term hemodialysis. In adults, the most common causes of end-stage renal failure are diabetes mellitus, glomerulonephritis, polycystic kidney disease, and systemic hypertension. Despite concerns about the recurrence of disease in the donor kidney, it has generally been only slowly progressive. A kidney from a cadaver donor can be preserved by perfusion at low temperatures for up to 48 hours, making its transplantation a semielective surgical procedure. Attempts are made to match HLA and ABO blood groups between donor and recipient. Paradoxically, the presence of certain common shared HLA in blood administered to a potential transplant recipient has been observed to induce tolerance to donor antigens and thus improve graft survival. The donor kidney is placed in the lower abdomen and receives its vascular supply from the iliac vessels. The ureter is anastomosed directly to the bladder. Immunosuppressive therapy is instituted during the perioperative period.

Management of Anesthesia
General Anesthesia

Although both regional and general anesthesia have been successfully used for renal transplantation, general anesthesia is most often selected. General anesthesia provides the advantage of mechanically maintaining the patient's ventilation, which may become compromised by surgical retraction in the area of the diaphragm. Drug selection is influenced by known side effects of anesthetic drugs (bowel distention from nitrous oxide, metabolism of sevoflurane to inorganic fluoride). Renal function after kidney transplantation is not predictably influenced by the volatile anesthetic administered. A common approach is to combine volatile anesthetics (isoflurane or desflurane) with nitrous oxide or short-acting opioids. Decreased cardiac output due to negative inotropic effects of volatile anesthetics is minimized to avoid jeopardizing the adequacy of tissue oxygen delivery (especially if anemia is present) and to promote renal perfusion. A high normal systemic blood pressure is required in the presence of euvolemia to maintain adequate urine flow. The selection of muscle relaxants is influenced by the dependence of many of these drugs on renal clearance. In this regard, atracurium, cisatracurium, and mivacurium are attractive selections, as their clearance from the plasma is independent of renal function. A newly transplanted but functioning kidney is able to clear neuromuscular-blocking drugs and the anticholinesterase drugs used for their reversal at the same rate as normal patients.

Central venous pressure monitoring is useful for guiding the rate and volume of crystalloid infusions. Optimal hydration during the intraoperative period is intended to optimize renal blood flow and improve early function of the transplanted kidney. Diuretics are often administered to facilitate urine formation by the newly transplanted kidney. In this regard, osmotic diuretics such as mannitol facilitate urine output and decrease excess tissue and intravascular fluid. Unlike the loop diuretic furosemide, mannitol does not depend on renal tubular concentrating mechanisms to produce diuresis.

When the vascular clamps are released, renal preservative solution from the transplanted kidney and venous drainage from the legs are also released into the circulation. These effluents contain potassium and acid metabolites but, in adults, seem to have minimal systemic effects. Nevertheless, cardiac arrest has been described after completion of the arterial anastomosis to the transplanted kidney and release of the vascular clamp. This event is most likely due to sudden hyperkalemia caused by washout of the potassium-containing preservative solutions from the newly perfused kidney. Unclamping may also be followed by hypotension due to the abrupt addition of up to 300 mL to the capacity of the intravascular fluid space and the release of vasodilating chemicals from previously ischemic tissues. When hypotension results from this change, the treatment is most often intravenous infusion of fluids.

Regional Anesthesia

The advantages of regional anesthesia compared with general anesthesia are the absence of a need for tracheal intubation or administration of neuromuscular blocking drugs. These advantages are negated, however, if regional anesthesia must be extensively supplemented with injected or inhaled drugs. Furthermore, blockade of the peripheral sympathetic nervous system, as produced by regional anesthesia, can complicate control of systemic blood pressure, especially considering the unpredictable intravascular fluid volume status of many of these patients. The use of regional anesthesia, particularly epidural anesthesia, is controversial in the presence of abnormal coagulation.

Postoperative Complications

The newly transplanted kidney may suffer acute immunologic rejection, which manifests in the vasculature of the transplanted kidney. It can be so rapid that inadequate circulation is evident almost immediately after the blood supply to the kidney is established. The only treatment for this acute rejection reaction is removal of the transplanted kidney, especially if the rejection process is accompanied by disseminated intravascular coagulation. A hematoma also may arise in the graft postoperatively, causing vascular or ureteral obstruction.

Delayed signs of graft rejection include fever, local tenderness, and deterioration of urine output. Treatment with high doses of corticosteroids and antilymphocyte globulin may be helpful. The acute tubular necrosis that occurs in the transplanted kidney secondary to prolonged ischemia usually responds to hemodialysis. Cyclosporine toxicity may also cause ARF. Ultrasonography and needle biopsy are performed to differentiate between the possible causes of kidney malfunction.

Opportunistic infections owing to long-term immunosuppression are common after renal transplantation. Long-term survival is unsatisfactory in renal transplant recipients who are immunosuppressed and who also carry hepatitis B surface antigen. The frequency of cancer is 30 to 100 times higher in transplant recipients than in the general population, presumably reflecting the loss of protective effects due to immunosuppression. Large-cell lymphoma is a well-recognized complication of transplantation, occurring almost exclusively in patients with evidence of Epstein-Barr virus infections.

Anesthetic Considerations in Renal Transplant Recipients Presenting for Surgery

Renal transplant recipients are often elderly with co-existing cardiovascular disease and diabetes mellitus. The side effects of immunosuppressant drugs (systemic hypertension, lowered seizure thresholds, anemia, thrombocytopenia) must be considered when planning the management of anesthesia. Serum creatinine concentrations are likely to be normal in the presence of normally functioning renal transplants. Nevertheless, the GFR and renal blood flow are likely to be lower than those of healthy individuals, and the activity of drugs excreted by the kidneys may be prolonged. The presence of azotemia, proteinuria, and systemic hypertension may indicate chronic rejection of the kidney transplant.

Drugs that are potentially nephrotoxic or dependent on renal clearance are avoided. Diuretics are administered only with careful evaluation of the patient's intravascular fluid volume status. Decreases in renal blood flow from

hypovolemia are minimized. It is likely these patients will be receiving oral antihypertensive drugs.

PRIMARY DISEASES OF THE KIDNEYS

A number of pathologic processes can primarily involve the kidneys or occur in association with dysfunction of other organ systems. Knowledge of the associated pathology and characteristics of the renal disease may be important when planning management of these patients during the perioperative period.

Glomerulonephritis

Acute glomerulonephritis is usually due to deposition of antigen-antibody complexes in the glomeruli. The source of antigens may be exogenous (poststreptococcal infection) or endogenous (collagen diseases). Clinical manifestations of glomerular diseases include hematuria, proteinuria, hypertension, edema, and increased plasma creatinine concentrations. Red blood cell casts are suggestive of glomerular disease rather than of nonglomerular disease, such as nephrolithiasis or prostatic disease. Proteinuria reflects an increase in glomerular permeability. It is important to diagnose glomerulonephritis quickly because prompt use of immunosuppressive drugs may be efficacious.

Nephrotic Syndrome

Nephrotic syndrome is defined by daily urinary protein excretion exceeding 3.5 g associated with sodium retention, hyperlipoproteinemia, and thromboembolic and infectious complications. Diabetic nephropathy is the most common cause of nephrotic proteinuria. In the absence of diabetes, the most common cause of nephrotic syndrome in adults is membranous glomerulonephritis, which is frequently associated with neoplasia (carcinoma, sarcoma, lymphoma, leukemia). Human immunodeficiency virus nephropathy typically causes nephrotic proteinuria and renal insufficiency, which may be the first clinical manifestation of acquired immunodeficiency syndrome. Pregnancy-induced hypertension is often associated with nephrotic syndrome.

Signs and Symptoms

Sodium retention and edema formation in patients with nephrotic syndrome have been presumed to reflect decreased plasma oncotic pressure with resultant hypovolemia (**Table 14-12**). Increased tubular reabsorption of sodium was assumed to be a homeostatic response to hypovolemia. Nevertheless, there is evidence that the primary event is initial sodium retention by the kidneys that precedes proteinuria. Increased sodium reabsorption by the distal renal tubules may be due to an inappropriately low natriuretic response to atrial natriuretic peptide. Patients with nephrotic syndrome may experience hypovolemia with associated orthostatic hypotension, tachycardia, peripheral vasoconstriction, and occasionally even ARF in response to the administration of diuretics. The risk of ARF is increased in elderly patients

TABLE 14-12	Features of Nephrotic Syndrome
Hypertension+	
Proteinuria, hematuria+	
Sodium retention+	
Edema+	
Hypovolemia	
Thromboembolism	
Hyperlipidemia	
Infectious complications	
+, Also shared with the nephritic syndrome	

TABLE 14-13	Treatment of Nephrotic Syndrome
Antihypertensive therapy*	
ACE inhibitor or ARB (antiproteinuric)†	
Dietary counseling‡	
Dietary restriction of sodium	
Diuretic therapy	
Albumin infusions as required	
Anticoagulant therapy	
Statin therapy	
Pneumococcal vaccine	

ACE, angiotensin-converting enzyme; ARB, angiotensin receptor blocker.
*A mean systemic blood pressure below 90 mm Hg reduces proteinuria independent of class of antihypertensive
†ACE inhibitors and ARB drugs have antiproteinuric effects separate from their blood pressure lowering effects.
‡Some authorities advise dietary protein restriction to reduce proteinuria, but the safety of this therapy has not been established, particularly in patients with heavy proteinuria.

and those who receive nonsteroidal anti-inflammatory drugs. Infusion of albumin corrects the clinical signs of hypovolemia. Hyperlipidemia accompanies nephrotic syndrome and may be associated with an increased risk of vascular disease.

Thromboembolic Complications Thromboembolic complications manifesting as renal vein thrombosis are major risks of nephrotic syndrome, particularly in patients with membranous glomerulonephritis. Pulmonary embolism and deep vein thrombosis in other vascular beds are also hazards. Arterial thrombosis is less common than venous thrombosis, although the risk of acute myocardial infarction in these patients may be increased. Prophylactic administration of heparin and support stockings are used to protect against thromboembolic complications.

Infection Pneumococcal peritonitis has been responsible for fatalities in children with nephrotic syndrome. Viral infections may be more likely in immunosuppressed patients, whereas susceptibility to bacterial infections seems to be related to decreased levels of immunoglobulin G.

Protein Binding Plasma levels of vitamins and hormones may be decreased in patients with nephrotic syndrome as a result of proteinuria. Hypoalbuminemia decreases the available binding sites for drugs and increases the proportion of circulating free drug. In this regard, when plasma drug levels are monitored, low levels of highly protein-bound drugs do not necessarily indicate low therapeutic concentrations.

Nephrotic Edema

Generalized edema implies that total body sodium content is increased, and stimulation of a negative sodium balance by administering diuretics is enhanced by dietary decreases in sodium intake (**Table 14-3**). Potent loop diuretics such as furosemide are needed to offset the kidney's avidity to retain sodium. In addition, thiazide diuretics or potassium-sparing diuretics may be added to decrease sodium reabsorption in the distal nephrons. The goal is to decrease edema slowly, as abrupt natriuresis may cause hypovolemia and even ARF; it may also produce hemoconcentration, increasing the risk of thromboembolic complications. Administration of albumin solutions to expand the plasma volume is considered only if symptomatic hypovolemia is present. In particularly severe cases, plasma ultrafiltration may be considered.

Goodpasture Syndrome

Goodpasture syndrome is a combination of pulmonary hemorrhage and glomerulonephritis, occurring most often in young males. Antibodies account for renal lesions and apparently react also with similar antigens in the lungs, producing alveolitis, which results in hemoptysis. Typically, hemoptysis precedes clinical evidence of renal disease. The prognosis is poor, with no known effective therapy to prevent progression to renal failure usually within 1 year of the diagnosis.

Interstitial Nephritis

Interstitial nephritis has been observed as an allergic reaction to drugs, including sulfonamides, allopurinol, phenytoin, and diuretics. Other less common causes include autoimmune diseases (lupus erythematosus) and infiltrative diseases (sarcoidosis). Patients exhibit decreased urine-concentrating ability, proteinuria, and systemic hypertension. Renal failure due to acute interstitial nephritis is often reversible after withdrawal of the offending drug or treatment of the underlying disease. Corticosteroid therapy may be beneficial.

Hereditary Nephritis

Hereditary nephritis (Alport's syndrome) is often accompanied by hearing loss and ocular abnormalities. Males are afflicted more often, with the disease culminating in systemic hypertension and renal failure. Drug therapy has not proven successful, although lowering the intraglomerular pressure with ACE inhibitors may offer some protection.

Polycystic Renal Disease

Polycystic renal disease is inherited as an autosomal dominant trait. The disease typically progresses slowly until renal failure occurs during middle age. Mild systemic hypertension and proteinuria are common. Decreased urine concentrating ability develops early in the course of the disease. Cysts may also be present in the liver and in the central nervous system as intracranial aneurysms. Hemodialysis or renal transplantation is eventually necessary in most of these patients.

Fanconi Syndrome

Fanconi syndrome results from inherited or acquired disturbances of proximal renal tubular function, causing hyperaminoaciduria, glycosuria, and hyperphosphaturia. There is renal loss of substances normally conserved by proximal renal tubules, including potassium, bicarbonate, and water. The symptoms of Fanconi syndrome, which reflect the abnormality of the renal tubules, include polyuria, polydipsia, metabolic acidosis due to loss of bicarbonate ions, and skeletal muscle weakness related to hypokalemia. Dwarfism and osteomalacia, reflecting loss of phosphate, is prominent in these patients. Presentation as vitamin D–resistant rickets is common. Management of anesthesia includes evaluation of fluid and electrolyte disorders characteristic of this syndrome, and the recognition that left ventricular cardiac failure secondary to uremia is often present in the final stages.

Nephrolithiasis

Although the pathogenesis of renal stones (**Table 14-14**) is poorly understood, several predisposing factors are recognized for the five major types of stones. Most stones are composed of calcium oxalate, and the causes of hypercalcemia (hyperparathyroidism, sarcoidosis, cancer) must be considered in these patients. Urinary tract infections with urea-splitting organisms that produce ammonia favors the formation of magnesium ammonium phosphate stones. Formation of uric acid stones is favored by a persistently acidic urine (pH < 6.0) that decreases the solubility of uric acid. Approximately 50% of patients with uric acid stones have gout.

Stones in the renal pelvis are typically painless unless they are complicated by infection or obstruction. By contrast, renal stones passing down the ureter can produce intense flank pain, often radiating to the groin, associated with nausea and vomiting and mimicking an acute surgical abdomen. Hematuria is common during ureteral passage of stones, whereas ureteral obstruction may lead to signs and symptoms of renal failure.

Treatment

Treatment of renal stones depends on identifying the composition of the stone and correcting the predisposing factors, such as hyperparathyroidism, urinary tract infection, or gout. High fluid intake sufficient to maintain a daily urine output at 2 to 3 L is often part of the therapy. Extracorporeal shock wave lithotripsy is a noninvasive treatment for renal stones that destroys the stones by shock waves. As an alternative to percutaneous nephrolithotomy, this approach has the advantages of being associated with low morbidity and being performed on an outpatient basis.

Renal Hypertension

Renal disease is the most common cause of secondary systemic hypertension. Accelerated or malignant hypertension is likely to be associated with renal disease. Furthermore, the appearance of systemic hypertension in young patients suggests the diagnosis of renal rather than essential hypertension. Hypertension due to renal dysfunction reflects parenchymal disease of the kidneys or renovascular disease.

Chronic pyelonephritis and glomerulonephritis are parenchymal diseases often associated with systemic hypertension, particularly in younger patients. Less common forms of renal parenchymal disease that can cause systemic hypertension include diabetic nephropathy, cystic disease of the kidneys, and renal amyloidosis. Renovascular disease is characterized by atherosclerosis and accounts for only a small percentage of patients with systemic hypertension. However, the sudden onset of a marked increase in systemic blood pressure or the

TABLE 14-14 Composition and Characteristics of Renal Stones			
Type of Stone	**Incidence (%)**	**Radiographic Appearance**	**Etiology**
Calcium oxalate	65	Opaque	Primary hyperparathyroidism Idiopathic hypercalciuria Hyperoxaluria Hyperuricosuria
Magnesium ammonium phosphate (struvite)	20	Opaque	Alkaline urine (usually due to chronic bacterial infection)
Calcium phosphate	7.5	Opaque	Renal tubular acidosis
Uric acid	5	Lucent	Acid urine Gout Hyperuricosuria
Cystine	1.5	Opaque	Cystinuria

presence of hypertension before the age of 30 years should arouse suspicion of renovascular disease. A bruit may be audible on auscultation of the abdomen over the kidneys. Systemic hypertension due to renovascular disease does not respond well to treatment with antihypertensive drugs.

The mechanism that produces systemic hypertension in the presence of renal parenchymal or renovascular disease is not established. Stimulation of the renin-angiotensin-aldosterone system is a possible, but unproven, mechanism. Alternatively, the kidneys may function to some extent as antihypertensive organs, possibly producing substances with vasodepressor activity. Regardless of the mechanism, treatment of systemic hypertension due to renal parenchymal disease is usually with antihypertensive drugs, including β-adrenergic antagonist drugs, which inhibit the release of renin from the kidneys. Treatment of renovascular hypertension is with renal artery endarterectomy or nephrectomy.

Uric Acid Nephropathy

Acute uric acid nephropathy is distinct from gout. It occurs when uric acid crystals are precipitated in the renal collecting tubules or ureters, producing acute oliguric renal failure. This precipitation occurs when uric acid concentrations reach a saturation point in acidic urine. The condition is particularly likely to occur when uric acid production is greatly increased, as in patients with myeloproliferative disorders being treated for cancer with chemotherapeutic drugs. These patients are particularly vulnerable to uric acid nephropathy if they have good renal function and urine-concentrating ability and then become dehydrated or acidotic because of decreased caloric intake.

Hepatorenal Syndrome

Acute oliguria manifesting in patients with decompensated cirrhosis of the liver is designated hepatorenal syndrome. Indeed, cirrhosis of the liver is associated with decreased GFR and renal blood flow preceding overt renal dysfunction by several weeks. The typical patient is deeply jaundiced and moribund; ascites, hypoalbuminemia, and hypoprothrombinemia are present. Renal failure in these patients may reflect hypovolemia caused by vigorous attempts to treat ascites. Treatment is directed at intravascular fluid volume replacement, remembering that saline and albumin may aggravate ascites. Therefore, whole blood or packed red blood cells may be a more appropriate form of volume replacement. A peritoneal-to-venous shunt for the treatment of ascites may also be associated with improved renal function. In some patients, a circulating toxin may be responsible for extreme renal vasoconstriction and ARF. Nevertheless, hemodialysis has not been reliable for eliminating suspected hepatic toxins.

There is an increased incidence of postoperative ARF in patients with obstructive jaundice who undergo surgery. The cause of renal failure in these patients is unclear, but preoperative administration of mannitol may be recommended in the hope of providing some renoprotective effect.

Benign Prostatic Hyperplasia

Benign prostatic hyperplasia (BPH) is a nonmalignant enlargement of the prostate due to excessive cellular growth of both the glandular and stromal elements of the gland. BPH is common worldwide in men older than 40 years of age. The two components of BPH are a static component related to enlargement of the prostate and a dynamic component that reflects the tone of the smooth muscle in the prostate. α-Adrenergic receptors are present in the prostatic capsule and hyperplastic prostatic tissue. Transurethral resection of the prostate (TURP) and open prostatectomy have been the traditional treatments for men with symptomatic BPH. Surgery, however, may be associated with intraoperative complications (bleeding, hypervolemia from systemic absorption of the irrigating fluid) and postoperative problems (retrograde ejaculation, impotence, urinary incontinence). As a result, alternative treatments may be employed including medical management with androgen-deprivation drugs and minimally invasive surgical approaches.

Medical Therapy

The prostate gland is androgen sensitive such that androgen deprivation decreases the size of the prostate and the resistance to outflow through the prostatic urethra. Finasteride, an orally effective inhibitor of 5α-reductase, is moderately effective for symptomatic treatment of BPH by reducing the static component of this disease. Side effects of 5α-reductase inhibitors are minimal. α-Adrenergic antagonists (terazosin, doxazosin, tamsulosin) are administered to block adrenergic receptors in hyperplastic prostatic tissue, the prostatic capsule, and the bladder neck so the smooth muscle tone (dynamic component of BPH) of these structures is decreased. As a result, resistance to urinary flow through the bladder neck and the prostatic urethra decreases, and urinary flow increases. These drugs may also have antihypertensive effects, whereas undesirable side effects include orthostatic hypotension.

Minimally Invasive Treatments

The most commonly used minimally invasive treatment of BPH is transurethral incision of the prostate. This technique is effective in patients with bladder outlet obstruction and enlarged prostates weighing 30 g or less and in whom the primary obstruction is located at the bladder neck. As the incisions are deepened, the bladder neck and prostatic urethra "spring open," and the bladder outlet obstruction is relieved. The surgical procedure is accompanied by absorption of nonelectrolyte irrigating fluids (glycine, sorbitol, mannitol) used to distend the bladder and wash away blood and prostatic tissue. The irrigation fluid gains direct intravascular access through the prostatic venous plexus or is more slowly absorbed from the retroperitoneal and perivesical spaces. When irrigation fluid enters the intravascular space, the results are acute changes in intravascular fluid volume and plasma solute concentrations manifesting as cardiovascular and central nervous system complications known as *TURP syndrome.*

Regional or general anesthesia is used for this surgical procedure. Other minimally invasive treatments for BPH include placement of prostatic stents (primarily in patients who are poor surgical risks), and laser prostatectomy. Advantages of visual laser ablation of the prostate is a brief operating time (≤20 minutes) and the absence of perioperative hemorrhage.

TURP Syndrome

TURP syndrome (**Table 14-15**) is characterized by intravascular fluid volume shifts and plasma solute effects. Solute changes may alter neurologic function independent of volume-related effects. The risk of intravascular hemolysis is greatly reduced by use of osmotically active irrigating solutions rather than distilled water. Although monitoring serum sodium concentrations during TURP is common practice and is effective for assessing intravascular fluid absorption, there may be benefits from monitoring serum osmolality as well. Hypo-osmolality appears to be the principal factor that contributes to the neurologic and hypovolemic changes considered to reflect TURP syndrome. Supportive care remains the most important therapeutic approach for managing cardiovascular, central nervous system, and renal complications of TURP syndrome. The introduction of medical management and minimally invasive surgical procedures to treat BPH may decrease the risk of TURP syndrome in the future.

A disorder similar to TURP syndrome may occur in women undergoing endometrial ablation that uses irrigation fluids (saline, glycine, sorbitol) to improve surgical visualization. When 32% dextran 70 irrigation is used, the major risk is a reaction to dextran, whereas hypo-osmolality is not a problem as this solution is hyperosmolar.

Intravascular Fluid Volume Expansion and Other Clinical Conditions Associated with TURP

Rapid intravascular fluid volume expansion due to systemic absorption of irrigating fluids (absorption rates may reach 200 mL/min) can cause systemic hypertension and reflex bradycardia. Patients with poor left ventricular function may develop pulmonary edema owing to this acute circulatory volume overload. Factors that influence the amount of irrigating solution absorbed include the intravesicular pressure, which is determined by the height of the irrigation bag above the prostatic sinuses (limit height to 40 cm above the prostate) and the number of prostatic sinuses opened (limit resection time to 1 hour and leave a rim of tissue on the capsule). If intravesical pressures are maintained below 15 cm H_2O, absorption of irrigating fluids is minimal.

The most widely used indicator of intravascular fluid volume gain is hyponatremia. Before treating TURP syndrome with hypertonic saline, it is important to exclude the presence of hypervolemia with near-normal plasma sodium concentrations. Cardiovascular compromise and impaired arterial oxygenation due to pulmonary edema require aggressive intervention, which may include administration of inotropic drugs, diuretics, and even augmentation of intravascular fluid volume.

Intravascular Fluid Volume Loss

Perioperative hypotension during TURP is sometimes preceded by systemic hypertension. It is conceivable that

TABLE 14-15	Signs and Symptoms of Transurethral Resection of the Prostate Syndrome	
System	**Signs and Symptoms**	**Cause**
Cardiovascular	Hypertension, reflex bradycardia, pulmonary edema, cardiovascular collapse Hypotension ECG changes (wide QRS, elevated St segments, ventricular arrhythmias)	Rapid fluid absorption (reflex bradycardia may be secondary to hypertension or increased ICP) Third spacing secondary to hyponatremia and hypo-osmolality; cardiovascular collapse Hyponatremia
Respiratory	Tachypnea, oxygen desaturation, Cheyne-Stokes breathing	Pulmonary edema
Neurologic	Nausea, restlessness, visual disturbances, confusion, somnolence, seizures, coma, death	Hyponatremia and hypo-osmolality causing cerebral edema and increased ICP, hyperglycinemia (inhibitory neurotransmitter, potentiates NMDA receptor activity), hyperammonemia
Hematologic	Disseminated intravascular hemolysis	Hyponatremia and hypo-osmolality
Renal	Renal failure	Hypotension, hyperoxaluria (metabolite of glycine)
Metabolic	Acidosis	Deamination of glycine to glyoxylic acid and ammonia

ECG, electrocardiogram; ICP, intracranial pressure; NMDA, N-methyl-D-aminotransferase.

hyponatremia in association with systemic hypertension can result in water flux along osmotic and hydrostatic pressure gradients out of the intravascular space and into the lungs with resultant pulmonary edema and hypovolemic shock. Sympathetic nervous system blockade produced by regional anesthesia could compound the hypotension, as could intraoperative endotoxemia, which is common during TURP.

Hyponatremia

Acute hyponatremia due to intravascular absorption of sodium-free irrigating fluids may cause confusion, agitation, visual disturbances, pulmonary edema, cardiovascular collapse, and seizures. Changes on the electrocardiogram may accompany progressive decreases in serum sodium concentrations (see Table 14-14). Spinal anesthesia associated with hypotension may cause nausea and vomiting indistinguishable from that caused by acute hyponatremia. Nevertheless, some hyponatremic patients show no signs of water intoxication, and it is possible that hyponatremia may not be the sole or even the primary cause of the neurologic manifestations of the TURP syndrome.

Hypo-osmolality

Hypo-osmolality rather than hyponatremia is the crucial physiologic derangement leading to central nervous system dysfunction during TURP. This is predictable because the blood-brain barrier is essentially impermeable to sodium but freely permeable to water. Cerebral edema caused by acute hypo-osmolality can result in increased intracranial pressure with resultant bradycardia and hypertension.

Diuretics administered to treat hypervolemia during TURP may accentuate hyponatremia and hypo-osmolality. A patient's serum sodium concentration and osmolality may continue to decrease following TURP because of continued absorption of irrigating solutions from the perivesicular and retroperitoneal spaces. If the serum osmolality is near normal, no interventions to correct serum sodium concentrations are recommended for asymptomatic patients even in the presence of hyponatremia. The most feared complication of correcting hyponatremia is central pontine myelinolysis (osmotic demyelination syndrome), which has been observed after both rapid and slow correction of serum sodium concentrations in patients undergoing TURP. The safest treatment of hyponatremia and hypo-osmolality may be symptomatic, recognizing that the presence of symptoms is the single most important factor determining morbidity and mortality from hyponatremia. Instituting treatment in the absence of symptoms risks too rapid correction because the correction rate is difficult to control. Serum osmolality should be monitored and corrected aggressively with hypertonic saline only until symptoms resolve substantially; then correction should be continued slowly (serum sodium concentrations increase 1.5 mEq/L per hour).

Metabolic Acidosis

Mild metabolic acidosis has been observed in patients undergoing TURP. Moderate irrigating solution absorption during TURP leads to metabolic acidosis (TURP acidosis), and this derangement could be more severe should irrigating solution absorption be more profound.

Hyperammonemia

Hyperammonemia is the result of the use of glycine-containing irrigation solutions with subsequent systemic absorption of glycine and its oxidative deamination to glyoxylic acid and ammonia. Alterations in central nervous system function may accompany hyperammonemia, but its role in TURP syndrome remains unclear. Endogenous arginine in the liver prevents hepatic release of ammonia and facilitates conversion of ammonia to urea. The time necessary to deplete endogenous arginine stores may be as brief as 12 hours, which approximates the preoperative fasting time. Prophylactic administration of intravenous arginine blunts the increase in serum ammonia concentrations associated with the presence of glycine in the systemic circulation.

Hyperglycinemia

Glycine is an inhibitory neurotransmitter similar to γ-aminobutyric acid in the spinal cord and brain. Glycine is the most likely cause of visual disturbances including transient blindness during TURP syndrome, reflecting the role of glycine as an inhibitory neurotransmitter in the retina. Therefore, glycine likely affects retina physiology independent of cerebral edema caused by hyponatremia and hypo-osmolality. Vision returns to normal within 24 hours as serum glycine concentrations approach normal. Reassurance that unimpaired vision will return is probably the best treatment. In addition to glycine, benzodiazepines, by their actions on γ-aminobutyric acid receptors, may mediate some compromise of vision through activation of the retinal γ-aminobutyric acid receptor.

Glycine may lead to encephalopathy and seizures via its ability to potentiate the effects of N-methyl-D-aspartate, an excitatory neurotransmitter. Magnesium exerts a negative control on the N-methyl-D-aspartate receptor, and hypomagnesemia caused by dilution (due to systemic absorption of irrigating solutions during TURP or administration of loop diuretics) may increase the susceptibility to seizures. For this reason, a trial of magnesium therapy may be indicated in patients who develop seizures and in whom glycine-containing irrigating solutions were used.

Glycine may also exert toxic effects on the kidneys. Hyperoxaluria due to metabolism of glycine to oxalate and glycolate could compromise renal function in patients with co-existing renal disease as is often present in elderly patients undergoing TURP.

KEY POINTS

- The kidneys are involved in water conservation, electrolyte homeostasis, acid base balance, and several neurohumoral and hormonal functions. Some or all of these functions will be affected in renal disease.

- There is currently no specific preemptive treatment for ARF. Prevention hinges on providing an adequate blood pressure and cardiac output plus avoiding nephrotoxic exposure or injury.

- Treatment of ARF is supportive, aiming to limit further injury by continuing to provide an adequate blood pressure and cardiac output. Only in ARF complicating sepsis has specific therapy been proven to improve outcome (activated protein C and steroid replacement therapy).

- National guidelines advise that patients with renal impairment should be prescribed ACE inhibitors and/or angiotensin receptor blockers and should have their blood pressure maintained below 125/80, their diabetes controlled so that glycosylated hemoglobin in less than 7%, and anemia corrected to the normal level of hemoglobin as is appropriate for age and gender.

- Provision of anesthesia for patients with chronic renal impairment focuses on meticulous fluid and electrolyte management, acid base maintenance, and attention to drug disposition in renal failure. Preserve vessels of the forearm in patients with deteriorating renal function for future arteriovenous shunts.

REFERENCES

Abbott K, Basta E, Bakris GL: Blood pressure control and nephroprotection in diabetes. J Clin Pharmacol 2004;44:431–438.

Bellomo R, Bonventre J, Macias W, Pinsky M: Management of early acute renal failure: Focus on post-injury prevention. Curr Opin Crit Care 2005;11:542–547.

De Vries AS, Bourgeois M: Pharmacologic treatment of acute renal failure in sepsis. Curr Opin Crit Care 2003;9:474–480.

Eger EI, Gong D, Koblin DD, et al: Dose-related biochemical markers of renal injury after sevoflurane versus desflurane anesthesia in volunteers. Anesth Analg 1997;85:1154–1163.

Gravenstein D: Transuretheral resection of the prostate (TURP) syndrome: A review of the pathophysiology and management. Anesth Analg 1997;84:438–446.

Kellum JA, Leblanc M, Gibney RTN, et al: Primary prevention of acute renal failure in the critically ill. Curr Opin Crit Care 2005;11:537–541.

Koomans HA, Blankestijn PJ, Joles JA: Sympathetic hyperactivity in chronic renal failure: A wake up call. J Am Soc Nephrol 2004;15:524–537.

Kostopanagiotou G, Smyrniotis V, Arkadopoulos N, et al: Anesthetic and perioperative management of adult transplant recipients in nontransplant surgery. Anesth Analg 1999;89:613–622.

Lamiere NH, De Vries AS, Vanholder R: Prevention of nondialytic treatment of acute renal failure. Curr Opin Crit Care 2003;9:481–490.

Lamiere N, Hoste E: Reflections on the definition, classification and diagnostic evaluation of acute renal failure. Curr Opin Crit Care 2004;10:468–475.

Mazze RI: No evidence of sevoflurane-induced renal injury in volunteers. Anesth Analg 1998;86:228–235.

Mehta RL, Clark WC, Schetz M: Techniques for assessing and achieving fluid balance in acute renal failure. Curr Opin Crit Care 2002;8:535–543.

National Kidney Foundation: NKF-KDOQI Guidelines. Available at: http://www.kidney.org/professionals/KDOQI/guidelines.cfm, accessed January 10, 2008.

National Kidney Foundation: 25 Facts about Organ Donation and Transplantation. Available at: http://www.kidney.org/news/newsroom/fsitem.cfm?id=30, accessed January 10, 2008.

Oesterling JE: Benign prostatic hyperplasia: Medical and minimally invasive treatment options. N Engl J Med 1995;332:99–110.

Port FK, Pisoni RL, Bragg-Gersham JL, et al: DOPPS estimates of patient life years attributable to modifiable hemodialysis practices in the United States. Blood Purif 2004;22:175–180.

Safirstein R, Andrade L, Vieira JM: Acetylcysteine and nephrotoxic effects of radiographic contrast agents: A new use for an old drug. N Engl J Med 2000;343:310–312.

United States Renal Data System: USRDS 2007. Annual data report. Atlas of End-stage Renal Disease in the United States. Bethesda, MD, National Institutes of Health, National Institute of Diabetes and Digestive and Kidney Disease, 2007. Also at http://www.usrds.org/atlas.htm, accessed December 13, 2007.

Zeitlin GL, Roth RA: Effect of three anesthetic techniques on the success of extracorporeal shock wave lithotripsy. Anesthesiology 1988;68:272–276.

CHAPTER 15

Fluid, Electrolyte, and Acid-Base Disorders

Susan Garwood

Abnormalities of Water and Electrolyte Homeostasis

Disorders of Sodium
- Hyponatremia
- TURP Syndrome
- Hypernatremia

Disorders of Potassium
- Hypokalemia
- Hyperkalemia

Disorders of Calcium
- Hypocalcemia
- Hypercalcemia

Disorders of Magnesium
- Hypomagnesemia
- Hypermagnesemia

Acid-Base Disorders
- Respiratory Acidosis
- Respiratory Alkalosis
- Metabolic Acidosis
- Metabolic Alkalosis

Alterations of water and electrolyte content and distribution as well as acid-base disturbances can produce multiple organ system dysfunction during the perioperative period. Impairment of central nervous system, cardiac, and neuromuscular function is especially likely in the presence of water, electrolyte (sodium, potassium, calcium, magnesium), and acid-base disturbances. In addition, numerous perioperative events can initiate or aggravate fluid, electrolyte, and acid-base disturbances (**Table 15-1**). Management of patients manifesting water and electrolyte disturbances is based on an understanding of the distribution of total body water and electrolytes.

ABNORMALITIES OF WATER AND ELECTROLYTE HOMEOSTASIS

Total body water content is categorized as intracellular fluid and extracellular fluid (ECF), according to the location of the water relative to cell membranes (**Fig. 15-1**). The distribution and concentration of electrolytes differ greatly among fluid compartments. The electrophysiology of excitable cells is dependent on the intracellular and extracellular concentrations of sodium, potassium, and calcium. An inherent characteristic of excitable cells is their ability to maintain concentration gradients across their cell membranes. The resulting

TABLE 15-1 Etiology of Water, Electrolyte, and Acid Base Disturbances during the Perioperative Period

Disease states
　Endocrinopathies
　Nephropathies
　Gastroenteropathies
Drug therapy
　Diuretics
　Corticosteroids
Nasogastric suction
Surgery
　Transurethral resection of the prostate
　Translocation of body water due to tissue trauma
　Resection of portions of the gastrointestinal tract
Management of anesthesia
　Intravenous fluid administration
　Alveolar ventilation
　Hypothermia

unequal distribution of ions (more potassium inside and more sodium outside) produces electrochemical differences across the cell membrane. The electrophysiology of cells and the resulting action potentials are altered by changes in electrolyte concentrations.

Regulation of water balance by the kidney is dependent on its ability to excrete urine with an osmolality that

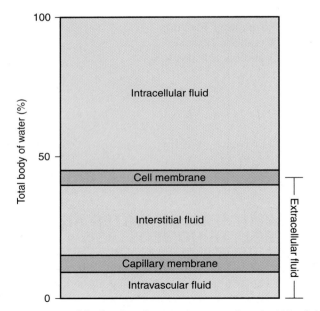

Figure 15-1 • Total body water (constituting approximately 60% of the total body weight in kilograms) is designated intracellular or extracellular fluid, depending on the location of water relative to cell membranes. Water in extracellular compartments is further subdivided into interstitial and intravascular fluid, depending on its location relative to cell membranes. Approximately 55% of total body water is intracellular, 37% is interstitial, and the remaining 8% is intravascular.

varies from maximal dilution to maximal concentration. The predominant regulators of water balance are osmolality sensors (which are neurons located in the anterior hypothalamus that stimulate thirst) and vasopressin (antidiuretic hormone). Vasopressin is stored as granules in the posterior pituitary and is released in response to an increase in serum osmolality. Vasopressin acts on the collecting ducts of the kidney causing water retention, which in turn corrects serum osmolality. Under normal circumstances, serum osmolality and therefore sodium concentration (since it is the predominant ion in ECF) are tightly regulated by water homeostasis. The normal range for serum osmolality is 280 to 290 mOsm/kg.

Vasopressin release plays an important role in the correction of disorders of fluid balance. Water losses sufficient to cause a contraction of ECF volume stimulate vasopressin release as do hypotension and a reduction in cardiac output. A number of conditions encountered in the perioperative period, including pain, nausea, and surgery itself also stimulate vasopressin release causing water retention and, consequently, a dilutional hyponatremia (**Table 15-2**).

DISORDERS OF SODIUM

Under normal circumstances, serum sodium concentration is regulated within narrow limits by the action of vasopressin on water homeostasis. Normal serum sodium concentration is 136 to 145 mmol/L. However, because serum sodium is measured as a *concentration*, serum sodium derangements can exist in the presence of increased, normal, or decreased total body sodium and/or increased, normal, or decreased total body water. It is important to recognize this fact because the diagnosis and treatment of serum sodium disorders will vary accordingly.

Hyponatremia

Hyponatremia exists when water retention or water intake exceeds the ability of the kidneys to excrete a dilute urine. Hyponatremia exists in approximately 15% of hospitalized patients and in this patient group is usually secondary to a dilutional effect. Hyponatremia in the outpatient setting is more likely to be caused by chronic disease.

Signs and Symptoms

The signs and symptoms of hyponatremia depend on the rate at which the hyponatremia has developed, being less pronounced in chronic cases. In addition, younger patients appear to tolerate a decrease in serum sodium better than elderly patients.

Anorexia, nausea, and general malaise may occur early, but central nervous system signs and symptoms predominate later in the course or in acutely deteriorating cases of hyponatremia (**Table 15-3**). As hyponatremia develops, extracellular hypotonicity allows water to move into brain cells, resulting in cerebral edema and increased intracranial pressure. Initial

TABLE 15-2 Factors and Drugs Affecting Vasopressin Secretion

Stimulation of Vasopressin Release	Inhibition of Vasopressin Release	Drugs That Stimulate Vasopressin Release and/or Potentiate the Renal Action of Vasopressin
Contracted ECF volume	Expanded ECF volume	Amitriptyline
Hypernatremia	Hyponatremia	Barbiturates
Hypotension	Hypertension	Carbamazepine
Nausea and vomiting		Chlorpropamide
Congestive heart failure		Clofibrate
Cirrhosis		Morphine
Hypothyroidism		Nicotine
Angiotensin II		Phenothiazines
Catecholamines		SSRIs
Histamine		
Bradykinin		

ECF, extracellular fluid; SSRIs, selective serotonin reuptake inhibitors.

compensation is afforded by the movement of ECF into the cerebrospinal fluid. Later compensation includes lowering intracellular osmolality by moving potassium and organic solutes out of brain cells. This reduces water movement into the intracellular space. However, when these adaptive mechanisms fail or hyponatremia progresses, central nervous system manifestations of hyponatremia present as a change in sensorium, seizures, brain herniation, and even death.

Diagnosis

Hyponatremia usually co-exists with hypo-osmolality except in two circumstances. The addition of osmotically active solutes that are unable to cross cell membranes easily, such as glucose, mannitol, and glycine, causes water to move from the intracellular space into the ECF with a resultant decrease in the serum sodium concentration. This decrease in serum sodium occurs without a change in total body sodium or total body water.

When the sodium concentration in measured in *plasma* and the solid phase of plasma is greatly increased as, for example, in severe hyperlipidemia or a paraproteinemic disorder, the measured sodium concentration will be falsely low. This is termed pseudohyponatremia. Measuring sodium concentration in *serum* avoids this problem.

Once these two causes of hyponatremia have been excluded, the approach to the diagnosis of hyponatremia is to first evaluate ECF volume from the clinical presentation. Then, urinary sodium concentration from a spot urine sample will further distinguish between etiologies (**Fig. 15-2**). Massive absorption of irrigating solutions that do not contain sodium, such as during transurethral resection of the prostate, is a relatively common cause of intraoperative hyponatremia.

Treatment

Treatment of hyponatremia involves withholding free water and encouraging free water excretion with a loop diuretic. Administration of saline is only necessary if significant symptoms are present. The rate of correction of hyponatremia depends primarily on whether the development of hyponatremia was acute, that is, occurred in less than 48 hours or was chronic.

Acute *symptomatic* hyponatremia must be treated promptly. Solute-free fluids are withheld and hypertonic saline (3% NaCl) plus furosemide is administered to enhance renal excretion of free water. Serum electrolytes should be checked frequently and this treatment continued until symptoms disappear, which may occur before the serum sodium concentration returns to normal.

Chronic *symptomatic* hyponatremia should be corrected slowly to avoid the risk of osmotic demyelination. During the development of chronic hyponatremia, brain cells retain their normal intracellular volume as the serum sodium decreases by exporting "effective osmoles." Approximately half of these effective osmoles are potassium ions and anions, and the remainder are small organic compounds. While hyponatremia is being corrected, brain cells must

TABLE 15-3 Symptoms and Signs of Hyponatremia

Symptoms	Signs
Anorexia	Abnormal sensorium
Nausea	Disorientation/agitation
Lethargy	Cheyne-Stokes breathing
Apathy	Hypothermia
Muscle cramps	Pathologic reflexes
	Pseudobulbar palsy
	Seizures
	Coma
	Death

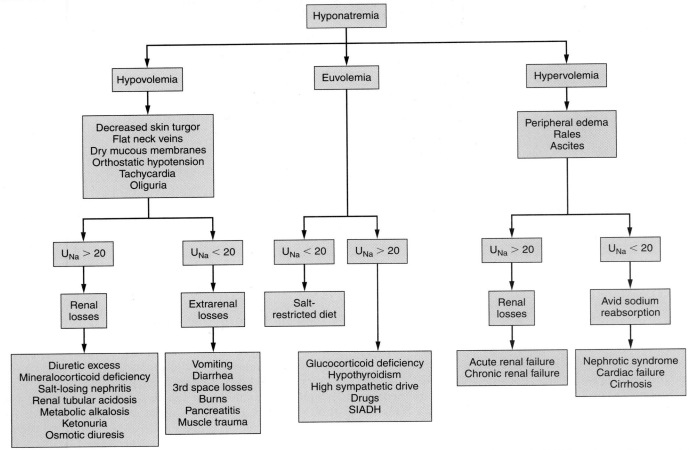

Figure 15-2 • Diagnostic algorithm for hyponatremia. Urinary sodium concentration (U_{Na}) (mEq/L) in a spot urine sample. SIADH, syndrome of inappropriate secretion of antidiuretic hormone. (*Adapted from Schrier RW: Manual of Nephrology, 6th ed. Philadelphia, Lippincott Williams & Wilkins, 2006.*)

reaccumulate these effective osmoles or water will move out of the cells into the now relatively hypertonic ECF, causing cell shrinkage. Such shrinkage triggers demyelination of pontine and extrapontine neurons and may result in quadriplegia, seizures, coma, and death. The risk of osmotic demyelination is higher in patients who are malnourished or potassium depleted. Guidelines for correction of chronic symptomatic hyponatremia call for an initial correction in the serum sodium of approximately 10 mEq/L. Thereafter, correction should not exceed 1 to 1.5 mEq/L per hour or a daily maximum increase of 12 mEq/L.

Treatment of chronic *asymptomatic* hyponatremia requires treating the underlying cause of the electrolyte disturbance and fluid restriction. Patients with hypervolemic hyponatremia secondary to congestive heart failure respond very well to a combination of angiotensin-converting enzyme inhibitor and loop diuretic.

Management of Anesthesia

If at all possible, hyponatremia, especially if symptomatic, should be corrected prior to surgery. If the surgery is urgent, then appropriate corrective treatment should continue throughout the surgery and into the postoperative period. Frequent measurement of serum sodium is necessary to

avoid overly rapid correction of hyponatremia with resultant osmotic demyelination or overcorrection resulting in hypernatremia. If the treatment of hyponatremia includes hypertonic sodium infusion during surgery, it may be appropriate to infuse this via a pump while replacing losses due to the surgery with lactated Ringer's solution, normal saline, colloid, or blood as required. Treatment of the underlying cause of the hyponatremia should also continue throughout the perioperative period.

Induction and maintenance of anesthesia in patients with hypovolemic hyponatremia are fraught with the risk of hypotension. In addition to fluid therapy, vasopressors and/or inotropes may be required to treat the hypotension and should be made available prior to the start of induction. Hypervolemic hyponatremic patients particularly those with heart failure may benefit from invasive hemodynamic monitoring to guide fluid therapy.

TURP Syndrome

Benign prostatic hyperplasia is often treated surgically by transurethral resection of the prostate (TURP). This involves resection via a cystoscope with continuous irrigation of the bladder to aid visualization while removing blood and resected material. The irrigating fluid is a nonelectrolyte fluid containing glycine, sorbitol, or mannitol, and this fluid may be absorbed rapidly via open venous sinuses in the prostate gland, causing volume overload, hyponatremia, and hypo-osmolality. This is known as TURP syndrome. This syndrome is more likely to occur if resection is prolonged (>1 hour), if the irrigating fluid is suspended more than 40 cm above the operative field, or if the pressure in the bladder is allowed to increase above 15 cm H_2O. TURP syndrome manifests principally with cardiovascular and neurologic signs and symptoms. Hypertension is common. Monitoring for development of this syndrome includes direct neurologic assessment in the patient under regional anesthesia or measurement of serum sodium concentration and osmolality in the patient under general anesthesia.

Treatment consists of terminating the surgical procedure so that no more fluid is absorbed, diuretics if needed for relief of cardiovascular symptoms, and hypertonic saline administration if severe neurologic symptoms are present or the serum sodium concentration is less than 120 mEq/L.

Hypernatremia

Hypernatremia, defined as a serum sodium greater than 145 mEq/L, is much less common than hyponatremia in the community because the thirst mechanism is very effective. Even in renal disorders of sodium retention or water loss, patients regulate their serum sodium within the normal range if they are able to drink water. Therefore, hypernatremia is much more likely to be seen in the very young, the elderly, and people who are debilitated, have altered mental status, or are unconscious. In the hospital setting, hypernatremia is most likely to be iatrogenic as a result of overcorrection of hyponatremia or treatment of acid-base disturbances with sodium bicarbonate. Sodium is a functionally impermeable solute; it contributes to osmolality and induces the movement of water across cell membranes. Hence, hypernatremia is invariably accompanied by hyperosmolality and always causes cellular dehydration and shrinkage.

Signs and Symptoms

Signs and symptoms of hypernatremia can vary from mild to life-threatening (**Table 15-4**). The earliest signs and symptoms include restlessness, irritability, and lethargy.

TABLE 15-4 Symptoms and Signs of Hypernatremia	
Symptoms	**Signs**
Polyuria	Muscle twitching
Polydipsia	Hyperreflexia
Orthostasis	Tremor
Restlessness	Ataxia
Irritability	Muscle spasticity
Lethargy	Focal and generalized seizures
	Death

As hypernatremia progresses, muscular twitching, hyperreflexia, tremors, and ataxia may develop. The signs and symptoms progress as the osmolality increases above 325 mOsm/kg. Muscle spasticity, seizures, and death may ensue. The very young and the very old and those with preexisting central nervous system disease exhibit more severe symptoms for any given serum sodium concentration or degree of hyperosmolality.

The most prominent abnormalities in hypernatremia are neurologic. Dehydration of brain cells occurs as water shifts out of the cells into the hypertonic interstitium. Capillary and venous congestion and venous sinus thrombosis have all been reported. As the brain cells shrink, cerebral blood vessels may stretch and tear, resulting in intracranial hemorrhage.

Usually the signs and symptoms are more severe in acute rather than chronic hypernatremia and when excessive elevations in serum sodium are present. Mortality rates up to 75% have been reported in adults with severe acute hypernatremia (serum sodium > 160 mEq/L), and survivors of severe acute hypernatremia often have permanent neurologic sequelae. During the development of chronic hypernatremia, brain cells generate "idiogenic osmoles" that restore intracellular water in spite of the ongoing hypernatremia and protect against brain cell dehydration. However, if chronic hypernatremia is corrected too rapidly, these idiogenic osmoles predispose to the development of cerebral edema.

Diagnosis

Hypernatremia may exist in the presence of normal, increased, or decreased total body water and normal, increased, or decreased total body sodium (**Fig. 15-3**).

In hypovolemic hypernatremia, the patient loses more water than sodium via renal or extrarenal routes. This may occur as a result of excessive diuresis or fluid losses from diarrhea, sweating, extensive burns, or gastrointestinal fistulas.

Patients with hypervolemic hypernatremia will show signs of ECF volume expansion, such as jugular venous distention, peripheral edema, and pulmonary congestion. Patients with hypernatremia secondary to water loss without concomitant salt loss appear euvolemic with a near-normal total body sodium. Water loss in the absence of concomitant sodium loss does not produce clinically overt volume contraction.

As with hyponatremia, a spot urine sample tested for sodium concentration and osmolality can help distinguish between the causes of hypernatremia (see Fig. 15-3).

Treatment

Treatment will be determined by the severity and rapidity of development of hypernatremia and whether the ECF volume is increased or decreased.

In hypovolemic hypernatremia, the water deficit is replaced with normal saline until the patient is euvolemic and then the plasma osmolality is corrected with hypotonic saline or 5% dextrose solution.

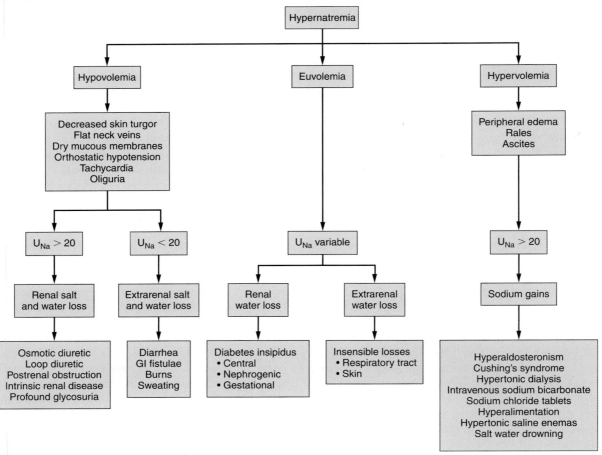

Figure 15-3 • Diagnostic algorithm for hypernatremia. GI, gastrointestinal; U_{Na}, urinary sodium concentration (mEq/L) in a spot urine sample. *(Adapted from Schrier RW: Manual of Nephrology, 6th ed. Philadelphia, Lippincott Williams & Wilkins, 2006.)*

In patients with hypervolemic hypernatremia, the primary treatment is diuresis with a loop diuretic, but if the cause of the hypervolemic hypernatremia is renal failure, then hemofiltration or hemodialysis may be needed.

The patient with euvolemic hypernatremia requires water replacement either orally or with 5% dextrose intravenously.

Acute hypernatremia should be corrected over several hours. However, to avoid cerebral edema, chronic hypernatremia should be corrected more slowly, over 2 to 3 days. Ongoing sodium and water losses should also be calculated and replaced.

Management of Anesthesia

If at all possible, surgery should be delayed until the hypernatremia has been corrected or at least until symptoms have abated. Frequent serum sodium measurements will be required perioperatively, and invasive hemodynamic monitoring may be useful. Hypovolemia will be exacerbated by induction and maintenance of anesthesia and prompt correction of hypotension with fluids, vasopressors, and/or inotropes may be required. The volume of distribution of drugs will be altered in hypovolemia and hypervolemia and drug administration must be adjusted accordingly.

DISORDERS OF POTASSIUM

Potassium is the major intracellular cation. The normal total body potassium content depends on muscle mass and is maximal in young adults and decreases progressively with age. Less than 1.5% of total body potassium is found in the extracellular space. Extracellular potassium concentration is controlled by factors that regulate transcellular potassium distribution, while total body potassium is regulated principally by the kidneys. More than 90% of the potassium taken in by diet is excreted in the urine, and the remainder is eliminated in the feces. As the glomerular filtration rate decreases in renal failure, the amount of potassium excreted by the gastrointestinal route increases.

Hypokalemia
Signs and Symptoms

Signs and symptoms of hypokalemia are generally restricted to the cardiac and neuromuscular systems and include dysrhythmias, muscle weakness, cramps, paralysis, and ileus.

Diagnosis

Hypokalemia is diagnosed by testing the serum potassium concentration, and the differential diagnosis requires determining whether the hypokalemia is acute and secondary to intracellular potassium shifts, such as might be seen with hyperventilation or alkalosis, or whether the hypokalemia is chronic and associated with depletion of total body potassium stores (Table 15-5). If the hypokalemia is suspected to be related to depletion of total body potassium stores, a spot urinary potassium will guide the diagnosis toward either renal or extrarenal causes. Renal potassium losses will be associated with a urinary potassium greater than 20 mEq/L, and inadequate potassium intake or gastrointestinal losses of potassium will be associated with a urinary potassium of less than 20 mEq/L. Hypokalemia without a change in total body potassium stores can be caused by familial hypokalemic periodic paralysis, treatment of megaloblastic anemia, and refeeding syndromes when malnourished patients are started on enteral feeding.

Treatment

Treatment of hypokalemia is dependent on the degree of potassium depletion and the underlying cause. If the hypokalemia is profound or associated with life-threatening signs, potassium must be administered intravenously. The amount of potassium to be given depends on whether there are associated decreases in total body potassium. Typically, 20 mEq of potassium can be administered over 30 to 45 minutes and repeated as needed. Such rapid repletion requires electrocardiographic monitoring.

Management of Anesthesia

The decision to treat hypokalemia prior to surgery depends on the chronicity and severity of the defect. If total body potassium stores are suspected to be low due to chronic potassium loss, then it is unlikely that the administration of small aliquots of potassium immediately prior to surgery will make any significant difference in potassium balance. However, it has been suggested that even small improvements in potassium balance may help normalize transmembrane potentials and reduce the incidence of perioperative dysrhythmias. Unfortunately, there are no prospective, randomized clinical trials of potassium repletion prior to surgery, so the risk of perioperative dysrhythmias in these patients remains unclear. It may be prudent to correct significant hypokalemia in patients with other risk factors for dysrhythmias such as those with congestive heart failure or on digoxin therapy. It is also important to avoid further decreases in serum potassium concentration, such as by the administration of insulin, glucose, β-adrenergic agonists, bicarbonate, and diuretics, or by hyperventilation and respiratory alkalosis.

Because of the effect of hypokalemia on skeletal muscle, there is the theoretical possibility of prolonged action of muscle relaxants. Doses of neuromuscular blockers should be guided by nerve stimulator testing.

Potassium levels should be measured frequently if repletion is ongoing or changes due to drug administration or ventilation are expected.

Hyperkalemia

Hyperkalemia is defined as a serum potassium concentration greater than 5.5 mEq/L. Hyperkalemia can be the result of changes in the transcellular movement of potassium or in total body potassium stores. In hospitalized patients, hyperkalemia is frequently the result of overzealous correction of hypokalemia (Table 15-6).

Signs and Symptoms

Signs and symptoms of hyperkalemia are dependent on the acuity of the increase. Chronic hyperkalemia is often asymptomatic, and dialysis-dependent patients can withstand considerable variations in serum potassium concentration between dialysis sessions (usually 2–3 days) with remarkably little symptomatology. Chronic hyperkalemia may be associated with nonspecific symptoms such as general malaise and mild gastrointestinal disturbances. More acute or significant increases in potassium manifest as cardiac and neuromuscular changes and include weakness, paralysis, nausea, vomiting, and bradycardia/asystole.

Diagnosis

The first step in the diagnosis of hyperkalemia is to rule out a spuriously high potassium level secondary to hemolysis of the specimen. A spuriously high potassium level may also

TABLE 15-5 Causes of Hypokalemia
Hypokalemia Due to Increased Renal Potassium Loss
Thiazide diuretics
Loop diuretics
Mineralocorticoids
High-dose glucocorticoids
High-dose antibiotics (penicillin, nafcillin, ampicillin)
Drugs associated with magnesium depletion (aminoglycosides)
Surgical trauma
Hyperglycemia
Hyperaldosteronism
Hypokalemia Due to Excessive Gastrointestinal Loss of Potassium
Vomiting and diarrhea
Zollinger-Ellison syndrome
Jejunoileal bypass
Malabsorption
Chemotherapy
Nasogastric suction
Hypokalemia Due to Transcellular Potassium Shift
β-Adrenergic agonists
Tocolytic drugs (ritodrine)
Insulin
Respiratory or metabolic alkalosis
Familial periodic paralysis
Hypercalcemia
Hypomagnesemia
Adapted from Gennari JF: Hypokalemia. N Engl J Med 1998;339: 451–458.

TABLE 15-6 Causes of Hyperkalemia

Increased Total Body Potassium Content
Acute oliguric renal failure
Chronic renal disease
Hypoaldosteronism
Drugs that impair potassium excretion
  Triamterene
  Spironolactone
  Nonsteroidal anti-inflammatory drugs
Drugs that inhibit the renin-angiotensin-aldosterone system

Altered Transcellular Potassium Shift
Succinylcholine
Respiratory or metabolic acidosis
Lysis of cells due to chemotherapy
Iatrogenic bolus

Pseudohyperkalemia
Hemolysis of blood specimen
Thrombocytosis/leukocytosis

occur with thrombocytosis and leukocytosis due to leakage of potassium from the cells in vitro.

Hyperkalemia due to extracellular potassium shifts may be a result of acidosis, rhabdomyolysis, or administration of drugs such as succinylcholine. If the increase in serum potassium is thought to be associated with increased total body potassium stores, then decreased renal excretion or increased extrarenal production of potassium is likely. The urinary potassium excretion rate can aid in the differential diagnosis of hyperkalemia.

Treatment

Immediate treatment of hyperkalemia is required if life-threatening dysrhythmias or electrocardiographic signs of severe hyperkalemia are present. This treatment is aimed at antagonizing the effects of a high potassium on the transmembrane potential and redistributing the potassium intracellularly. Calcium chloride or calcium gluconate is administered intravenously to stabilize cellular membranes. The onset of action is immediate. Potassium can be driven intracellularly by the action of insulin with or without glucose. This will be effective within 10 to 20 minutes. Other adjuvant therapies include sodium bicarbonate and hyperventilation to promote alkalosis and movement of potassium intracellularly. Potassium driven intracellularly will eventually move extracellularly again, usually after several hours, so therapy may need to be continued.

If the hyperkalemia is secondary to increased total body stores of potassium, then potassium must be eliminated from the body. This can be achieved by a loop diuretic such as furosemide, an infusion of saline to encourage diuresis, or an ion exchange resin. The primary potassium exchange resin in use is sodium polystyrene sulfonate (Kayexalate) given either orally or by enema. Dialysis may be required to remove potassium in patients with poor renal function.

Management of Anesthesia

It is recommended that the serum potassium concentration be below 5.5 mEq/L for elective surgery. It is preferable to correct hyperkalemia prior to surgery, but if this is not feasible, steps should be taken to lower the potassium immediately prior to induction of anesthesia by the methods indicated previously. Potassium levels do not influence the selection of drugs for induction and maintenance of anesthesia. Since succinylcholine increases serum potassium by approximately 0.5 mEq/L, it is best avoided. The effects of muscle relaxants may be exaggerated if there is muscle weakness from the hyperkalemia. Respiratory and metabolic acidosis must be avoided since either will exacerbate the hyperkalemia and its effects. Intravenous fluids should be potassium free. Avoid Ringer's lactated solution (contains 4 mEq/L of potassium) and Normosol (contains 5 mEq/L of potassium).

DISORDERS OF CALCIUM

Only 1% of total body calcium is present in the ECF. The remainder is stored in bone. Calcium in the ECF exists with 60% free or coupled with anions and thus filterable and the remaining 40% bound to proteins, mainly albumin. Only the ionized calcium in the extracellular space is physiologically active. Net calcium balance (zero in a healthy adult) equals absorption from the diet minus losses of calcium in feces and urine. Several hormones regulate calcium metabolism: parathyroid hormone, which increases bone resorption and renal tubular reabsorption of calcium; calcitonin, which inhibits bone resorption; and vitamin D, which augments intestinal absorption of calcium. The activity of these hormones is altered in response to changes in plasma ionized calcium concentration. Other hormones including thyroid hormone, growth hormone, and adrenal and gonadal steroids also affect calcium homeostasis, but their secretion is determined by factors other than plasma calcium concentration.

Hypocalcemia

Hypocalcemia is defined as a reduction in serum ionized calcium concentration. It is important to note that many blood chemistry analysis systems measure total calcium rather than ionized calcium. Several formulas exist to convert total calcium to ionized calcium, but none of these is totally reliable.

Binding of calcium to albumin is pH dependent, and acid-base disturbances can change the fraction and therefore the concentration of ionized calcium without changing total body calcium. Alkalosis reduces the ionized calcium concentration, so ionized calcium may be significantly reduced after bicarbonate administration or with hyperventilation.

Signs and Symptoms

The signs and symptoms of hypocalcemia depend on the rapidity and the degree of reduction in ionized calcium. Most of these signs and symptoms are evident in the cardiovascular and neuromuscular systems and include paresthesias, irritability, seizures, hypotension, and myocardial depression. Laryngospasm can be life threatening.

Diagnosis

The most common causes of hypocalcemia are due to a decrease in parathyroid hormone secretion, end-organ resistance to parathyroid hormone, or disorders of vitamin D metabolism. These are usually seen clinically as complications of thyroid or parathyroid surgery, magnesium deficiency, and renal failure.

Treatment

Acute symptomatic hypocalcemia with seizures, tetany, and/or cardiovascular depression must be treated immediately with intravenous calcium. The duration of treatment will be dependent on serial calcium measurements. Treatment of hypocalcemia in the presence of hypomagnesemia is ineffective unless magnesium is also replenished. Metabolic or respiratory *alkalosis* should be corrected. If metabolic or respiratory *acidosis* is present with hypocalcemia, then the calcium level should be corrected before the acidosis is treated because correcting an acidosis with bicarbonate or hyperventilation will only exacerbate the hypocalcemia.

Less acute and asymptomatic hypocalcemia may be treated with oral calcium supplementation and vitamin D.

Management of Anesthesia

Symptomatic hypocalcemia must be treated prior to surgery, and every effort must be made to minimize any further decrease in serum calcium intraoperatively. This might occur with hyperventilation or administration of bicarbonate. Ionized calcium levels may be decreased by massive transfusion of blood containing citrate or when the metabolism of citrate is impaired by hypothermia, liver disease, or renal failure.

Sudden decreases in ionized calcium levels may be seen in the early postoperative period after thyroidectomy or parathyroidectomy and may cause laryngospasm.

Hypercalcemia

Hypercalcemia results from increased calcium absorption from the gastrointestinal tract (milk alkali syndrome, vitamin D intoxication, granulomatous diseases such as sarcoidosis), decreased renal calcium excretion in renal insufficiency, and increased bone resorption of calcium (primary or secondary hyperparathyroidism, malignancy, hyperthyroidism, and immobilization).

Signs and Symptoms

Hypercalcemia is associated with neurologic and gastrointestinal signs and symptoms such as confusion, hypotonia, depressed deep tendon reflexes, lethargy, abdominal pain, and nausea and vomiting, especially if the increase in serum calcium is relatively acute. Chronic hypercalcemia is often associated with polyuria, hypercalciuria, and nephrolithiasis.

Diagnosis

Almost all patients with hypercalcemia have either hyperparathyroidism or cancer. Primary hyperparathyroidism is usually associated with a serum calcium concentration less than 11 mEq/L and no symptoms, whereas malignancy often presents with acute symptoms and a serum calcium level greater than 14 mEq/L.

Treatment

Treatment of hypercalcemia is directed toward increasing urinary calcium excretion and inhibiting bone resorption and further gastrointestinal absorption of calcium.

Since hypercalcemia is frequently associated with hypovolemia secondary to polyuria, volume expansion with saline not only corrects the fluid deficit but also increases urinary excretion of calcium. Loop diuretics will enhance urinary excretion of sodium and calcium.

Calcitonin, bisphosphonates, or mithramycin may be required in disorders associated with osteoclastic bone resorption. Hydrocortisone may reduce gastrointestinal absorption of calcium in granulomatous disease, vitamin D intoxication, lymphoma, and myeloma. Oral phosphate may also be given to reduce gastrointestinal uptake of calcium if renal function is normal. Dialysis may be required for life-threatening hypercalcemia. Surgical removal of the parathyroid glands may be necessary to treat primary or secondary hyperparathyroidism.

Management of Anesthesia

Management of anesthesia for emergency surgery in a patient with hypercalcemia is aimed at restoring intravascular volume prior to induction and increasing urinary excretion of calcium with loop diuretics (thiazide diuretics should be avoided as they increase renal tubular reabsorption of calcium). Ideally, surgery should be postponed until calcium levels have normalized.

Central venous pressure or pulmonary artery pressure monitoring may be advisable in some patients requiring fluid resuscitation and diuresis as part of their perioperative treatment of hypercalcemia. Dosing of muscle relaxants must be guided by neuromuscular monitoring if muscle weakness, hypotonia, or loss of deep tendon reflexes is present.

DISORDERS OF MAGNESIUM

Magnesium is predominantly found intracellularly and in mineralized bone. Sixty percent to 70% of serum magnesium is ionized, with 10% complexed to citrate, bicarbonate, or phosphate and approximately 30% bound to protein, mostly albumin. There is little difference between extracellular and intracellular ionized magnesium concentrations so there is only a small transmembrane gradient for ionized magnesium. It is the ionized fraction of magnesium that is associated with clinical outcome.

Magnesium is absorbed from and secreted into the gastrointestinal tract and filtered, reabsorbed, and excreted by the kidneys. Renal reabsorption and excretion are passive, following sodium and water.

Hypomagnesemia

Some degree of hypomagnesemia occurs in up to 10% of hospitalized patients. An even higher percentage of patients in intensive care units, especially those receiving parenteral nutritional or dialysis, have hypomagnesemia. Coronary care unit patients with hypomagnesemia have a higher mortality rate that those with normal levels of serum magnesium.

Signs and Symptoms

Signs and symptoms of hypomagnesemia are similar to those of hypocalcemia and involve mostly the cardiac and neuromuscular systems. Dysrhythmias, weakness, muscle twitching, tetany, apathy, and seizures can be seen. Hypokalemia and/or hypocalcemia that had been refractory to supplementation do respond after correction of hypomagnesemia.

Diagnosis

Hypomagnesemia is most commonly due to reduced gastrointestinal uptake (reduced dietary intake or reduced absorption from the gastrointestinal tract) or to renal wasting of magnesium. These entities can be differentiated by measuring the urinary magnesium excretion rate. Much less frequently, hypomagnesemia is due to intracellular shifts of magnesium with no overall change in total body magnesium, to the "hungry bone syndrome" after parathyroidectomy, or to cutaneous losses.

Treatment

Treatment of hypomagnesemia depends on the severity of the deficiency and the signs and symptoms that are present. If cardiac dysrhythmias or seizures are present, magnesium is administered intravenously as a bolus (2 g of magnesium sulfate equals 8 mEq of magnesium), and the dose is repeated until symptoms abate. After life-threatening signs have resolved, a slower infusion of magnesium sulfate can be continued for several days to allow for equilibration of intracellular and total body magnesium stores. If renal wasting is present, supplementation must be increased to account for the magnesium lost in the urine.

Hypermagnesemia is a potential side effect of the treatment of hypomagnesemia so the patient should be monitored for signs of hypotension, facial flushing, and loss of deep tendon reflexes.

Management of Anesthesia

Management of anesthesia in a patient with hypomagnesemia includes attention to the signs of magnesium deficiency, magnesium supplementation, and treatment of refractory hypokalemia or hypocalcemia if needed. If the hypomagnesemia is secondary to malnutrition or alcoholism, the anesthetic implications of these diseases must be considered.

Ventricular dysrhythmias should be anticipated and treated as necessary. Muscle relaxation should be guided by the use of a peripheral nerve stimulator since hypomagnesemia can be associated with both muscle weakness and muscle excitation. Fluid loading (particularly with sodium-containing solutions) and the use of diuretics should be avoided since the renal excretion of magnesium passively follows sodium excretion.

Hypermagnesemia

Hypermagnesemia (i.e., a serum magnesium concentration > 2.5 mEq/L) is much less common than hypomagnesemia because a magnesium load can be briskly excreted if renal function is normal. Even patients with renal failure rarely have symptomatic hypermagnesemia unless there is a significantly increased dietary intake. However, milder elevations of serum magnesium are frequently found in intensive care unit and dialysis patient populations. Hypermagnesemia may be a complication of magnesium sulfate therapy for preeclampsia/eclampsia.

Signs and Symptoms

Signs and symptoms of hypermagnesemia begin to occur at serum levels of 4 to 5 mEq/L and include lethargy, nausea and vomiting and facial flushing. At levels above 6 mEq/L, there are a loss of deep tendon reflexes and hypotension. Paralysis, apnea, and/or cardiac arrest are likely if the magnesium level exceeds 10 mEq/L.

Diagnosis

Evaluation of hypermagnesemia involves determining renal function (creatinine clearance) and detecting any source of excess magnesium intake, such as parenteral infusion, oral ingestion of antacids, and magnesium-based enemas or cathartics. Once these have been excluded, less common causes of hypermagnesemia including hypothyroidism, hyperparathyroidism, Addison's disease, and lithium therapy can be considered.

Treatment

Life-threatening signs of hypermagnesemia may be temporarily ameliorated with intravenous calcium administration but may require hemodialysis. Lesser degrees of hypermagnesemia can be treated with forced diuresis with saline and loop diuretics to increase renal excretion of magnesium.

Management of Anesthesia

Invasive cardiovascular monitoring may be necessary perioperatively to measure and treat the hypotension and vasodilation of hypermagnesemia and to guide fluid resuscitation and ongoing replacement of fluids during a forced diuresis. Acidosis exacerbates hypermagnesemia so careful attention must be paid to ventilation and arterial pH. Initial and subsequent doses of muscle relaxant should be reduced in the presence of muscle weakness and guided by a peripheral nerve stimulator. Hypermagnesemia and skeletal muscle weakness are not uncommon causes of failure to wean from mechanical ventilation in the intensive care setting, especially in patients with renal failure.

ACID-BASE DISORDERS

Acid-base balance is normally regulated within the range of 7.35 to 7.45, as measured by arterial pH, to ensure an optimal pH for cellular enzyme function. Values of arterial blood pH less than 7.35 are termed acidosis or acidemia, and values greater than 7.45 are termed alkalosis or alkalemia. Intracellular pH is maintained at a lower, but closely regulated level of 7.0 to 7.3. This acid-base regulation occurs under normal continuous production of acidic metabolites approximating 1 mEq/kg body weight per day and is accomplished by a system of intracellular and extracellular buffers. A number of buffer systems participate in the regulation of pH, most of which are closed systems, such as serum proteins, bone apatite, and phosphate ions. In closed buffer systems, neither form of the buffer pair can enter or leave the system, so the concentration of total buffer is fixed. Closed buffer systems may minimize changes in pH but cannot change overall acid or alkali content. The major buffer system of the body is the bicarbonate/carbon dioxide buffer pair, which is an open system. Carbon dioxide can enter or leave the system via the lungs, and bicarbonate may enter or leave the system via the kidneys. Changes in respiration regulate carbon dioxide tension, while renal regulation modifies bicarbonate concentration. While the respiratory system can provide some defense against acid-base disorders, the kidneys have a greater ability to normalize pH. Filtered bicarbonate may be reabsorbed from the proximal tubule or excreted into the urine, and hydrogen ions can be reabsorbed in the distal tubule and collecting duct or excreted into the urine. Excretion of hydrogen ions in the urine regenerates the bicarbonate originally consumed by buffering a hydrogen ion in the ECF. The excreted hydrogen ions are themselves buffered by titratable renal buffers (mainly ammonia) and lost in the urine.

The relationship between the pulmonary and renal regulation of pH by this buffer system is expressed by the Henderson-Hasselbalch equation: $pH = 6.1 + \log$ (serum bicarbonate concentration/$0.03 \times Pa_{CO_2}$).

Substitution of average values for pH 7.4 and Pa_{CO_2} (40 mm Hg) results in a calculated bicarbonate concentration of 24 mEq/L. Maintenance of a normal bicarbonate concentration relative to carbon dioxide tension results in an optimal ratio of approximately 20:1. Maintenance of this ratio of 20:1 allows for a relatively normal pH despite deviations from normal of either bicarbonate concentration or carbon dioxide tension.

Identification of an acid-base disturbance follows a series of steps:

1. Identify whether the pH is increased or decreased. An increase identifies an alkalosis and a decrease identifies an acidosis.
2. Identify the change in Pa_{CO_2} and bicarbonate from their normal levels of 40 mm Hg and 24 mEq/L, respectively.
3. If both Pa_{CO_2} and bicarbonate change in the same direction (i.e., both are increased or both are decreased), then there is a primary acid-base disorder with a compensatory secondary disorder that brings the ratio of bicarbonate/carbon dioxide tension back to 20:1.
4. If bicarbonate and Pa_{CO_2} change in opposite directions, there is a mixed acid-base disorder.
5. Determine the primary acid-base disorder by comparing the fractional change of the measured bicarbonate or carbon dioxide tension to the normal value.
6. There are equations and nomograms that calculate the expected change in one of the three parameters involved in acid-base determination (pH, bicarbonate, or carbon dioxide tension) for a given change in one of the other two parameters. If the actual change is markedly different from the expected change, then there is a mixed acid-base disorder.
7. Finally, calculate the anion gap to determine whether there is a hidden metabolic acidosis.

Figures 15-4, 15-5, and **15-6** provide an overview of the diagnostic approaches to acid-base disorders with a normal, high, or low pH.

Signs and Symptoms

Major adverse consequences of severe systemic acidosis (pH < 7.2) can occur independently of whether the acidosis is of respiratory, metabolic, or mixed origin (**Table 15-7**). The effects of acidosis are particularly detrimental to the cardiovascular system. Acidosis decreases myocardial contractility, although clinical effects are minimal until the pH decreases to less than 7.2, perhaps reflecting the effects of catecholamine release in response to the acidosis. When the pH is less than 7.1, cardiac responsiveness to catecholamines decreases and compensatory inotropic effects are diminished. The detrimental effects of acidosis may be accentuated in those with underlying left ventricular dysfunction or myocardial ischemia or in those in whom sympathetic nervous system activity is impaired, such as by β-adrenergic blockade or general anesthesia.

Major adverse consequences of severe systemic alkalosis (pH > 7.60) reflect impairment of cerebral and coronary

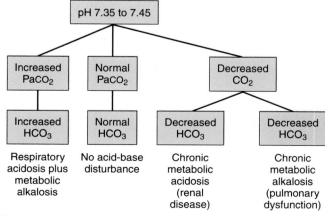

Figure 15-4 • Diagnostic approach to the interpretation of normal arterial pH based on Pa_{CO_2} and bicarbonate concentration.

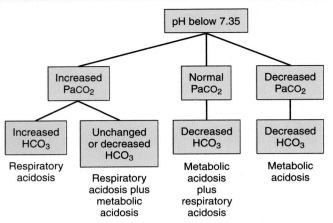

Figure 15-5 • Diagnostic approach to interpretation of an arterial pH less than 7.35 based on Pa_{CO_2} and bicarbonate concentration.

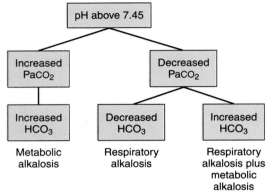

Figure 15-6 • Diagnostic approach to interpretation of an arterial pH greater than 7.45 based on Pa_{CO_2} and bicarbonate concentration.

TABLE 15-7	Adverse Consequences of Severe Acidosis

Nervous System
Obtundation
Coma

Cardiovascular System
Impaired myocardial contractility
Decreased cardiac output
Decreased arterial blood pressure
Sensitization to re-entrant cardiac dysrhythmias
Decreased threshold for ventricular fibrillation
Decreased responsiveness to catecholamines

Ventilation
Hyperventilation
Dyspnea
Fatigue of respiratory muscles

Metabolism
Hyperkalemia
Insulin resistance
Inhibition of anaerobic glycolysis

Adapted from Adrogué HJ, Madias NE: Management of life-threatening acid-base disorders. N Engl J Med 1998;338:26–34.

TABLE 15-8	Adverse Consequences of Alkalosis

Nervous System
Decreased cerebral blood flow
Seizures
Lethargy
Delirium
Tetany

Cardiovascular System
Arteriolar vasoconstriction
Decreased coronary blood flow
Decreased threshold for angina pectoris
Predisposition to refractory dysrhythmias

Ventilation
Hypoventilation
Hypercarbia
Arterial hypoxemia

Metabolism
Hypokalemia
Hypocalcemia
Hypomagnesemia
Hypophosphatemia
Stimulation of anaerobic glycolysis

Adapted from Adrogué JH, Madias NE: Management of life-threatening acid-base disorders. N Engl J Med 1998; 338:107–11.

blood flow due to arteriolar vasoconstriction (**Table 15-8**). Associated decreases in serum ionized calcium concentration probably contribute to the neurologic abnormalities associated with systemic alkalosis. Alkalosis predisposes patients, especially those with co-existing heart disease, to refractory ventricular dysrhythmias. Alkalosis depresses ventilation and can frustrate efforts to wean patients from mechanical ventilation. Hypokalemia accompanies both metabolic and respiratory alkalosis but is more prominent in the presence of metabolic alkalosis. Alkalosis stimulates anaerobic glycolysis and increases the production of lactic acid and ketoacids. Although alkalosis can decrease the release of oxygen to the tissues by tightening the binding of oxygen to hemoglobin, chronic alkalosis negates this effect by increasing the concentration of 2,3-diphosphoglycerate in erythrocytes.

Respiratory Acidosis

Respiratory acidosis is present when a decrease in alveolar ventilation results in an increase in the Pa_{CO_2} sufficient to decrease arterial pH to less than 7.35 (**Table 15-9**). Carbonic acid resulting from dissolved carbon dioxide is considered a respiratory acid. The most likely cause of respiratory acidosis during the perioperative period is drug-induced depression of ventilation from opioids and general anesthetics. Respiratory acidosis may be complicated by metabolic acidosis when renal perfusion is decreased to the extent that reabsorption mechanisms in the renal tubules are impaired. For example, cardiac output and renal blood flow may be so decreased in patients with chronic obstructive pulmonary disease and cor pulmonale as to lead to metabolic acidosis.

TABLE 15-9 Causes of Respiratory Acidosis

Drug-induced ventilatory depression
Permissive hypercapnia
Upper airway obstruction
Status asthmaticus
Restriction of ventilation (rib fractures/flail chest)
Disorders of neuromuscular function
Malignant hyperthermia
Hyperalimentation solutions

Respiratory acidosis is treated by correcting the disorder responsible for hypoventilation. Mechanical ventilation is necessary when the increase in $Paco_2$ is marked. It must be remembered that rapid lowering of chronically increased $Paco_2$ levels by mechanical ventilation decreases body stores of carbon dioxide much more rapidly than the kidneys can produce a corresponding decrease in serum bicarbonate concentration. The resulting metabolic alkalosis can cause neuromuscular irritability and excitation of the central nervous system manifesting as seizures. It is best to decrease the $Paco_2$ slowly to permit sufficient time for renal tubular elimination of bicarbonate.

Metabolic alkalosis may accompany respiratory acidosis when the body stores of chloride and potassium are decreased. For example, decreased serum chloride concentrations facilitate renal tubular reabsorption of bicarbonate, leading to metabolic alkalosis. Hypokalemia stimulates renal tubules to excrete hydrogen, which may produce metabolic alkalosis or aggravate a co-existing alkalosis due to chloride deficiency. Treatment of metabolic alkalosis associated with these electrolyte disturbances requires administration of potassium chloride.

Respiratory Alkalosis

Respiratory alkalosis is present when an increase in alveolar ventilation results in a decrease in $Paco_2$ sufficient to increase the pH to greater than 7.45 (**Table 15-10**). The most likely cause of acute respiratory alkalosis during the perioperative period is iatrogenic hyperventilation as may occur during general anesthesia. Respiratory alkalosis occurs normally during pregnancy and on ascent to high altitude.

TABLE 15-10 Causes of Respiratory Alkalosis

Iatrogenic (mechanical hyperventilation)
Decreased barometric pressure
Arterial hypoxemia
Central nervous system injury
Hepatic disease
Pregnancy
Salicylate overdose

Treatment of respiratory alkalosis is directed at correcting the underlying disorder responsible for alveolar hyperventilation. During anesthesia, this is most often accomplished by adjusting the ventilator to decrease alveolar ventilation. The hypokalemia and hypochloremia that may co-exist with respiratory alkalosis may also require treatment.

Metabolic Acidosis

A metabolic acid lowers blood pH, which stimulates the respiratory center to hyperventilate and lower carbon dioxide tension. Respiratory compensation does not in general fully compensate for increased acid production, but the pH will return *toward* normal.

Acidoses of metabolic origin are typically divided into those with a normal anion gap and those with a high anion gap. Normal anion gap acidosis is the result of a net increase in chloride concentration. Bicarbonate loss is counterbalanced by a net gain of chloride ions to maintain electrical neutrality. Therefore, a normal anion gap acidosis is often called a *hyperchloremic* metabolic acidosis. The most common causes of a normal anion gap acidosis are intravenous infusion of sodium chloride and gastrointestinal and renal losses of bicarbonate (diarrhea, renal tubular acidosis, early renal failure). A high anion gap occurs when a fixed acid is added to the extracellular space. The acid dissociates, the hydrogen ion combines with bicarbonate forming carbonic acid, and the decreased bicarbonate concentration produces an increased anion gap. Lactic acidosis, ketoacidosis, renal failure, and the acidoses associated with many poisonings are examples of acidoses with a high anion gap.

Signs and Symptoms

Since acidosis is secondary to an underlying disorder, the presentation of acidosis is complicated by the signs and symptoms of the causative disorder. Derangements of pH have wide-ranging effects on tissue, organ, and enzyme function, and the signs and symptoms attributable to an acidosis relate to these effects. The clinical features of metabolic acidosis depend also on the rate of development of the acidosis and are likely to be more dramatic in rapidly developing acidosis where compensatory respiratory or renal changes are not able to limit the fall in pH.

Diagnosis

Diagnosis depends on a high index of suspicion and laboratory testing. Most commonly, arterial blood is analyzed for pH, carbon dioxide tension, bicarbonate concentration, and anion gap. Common causes of metabolic acidosis are listed in **Table 15-11**.

Metabolic acidosis can be of renal or nonrenal origin. Metabolic acidosis of renal origin involves a primary disorder of renal acidification. This will happen if the kidneys are unable to regenerate sufficient bicarbonate to replace that lost by buffering normal endogenous acid production

TABLE 15-11 Causes of Metabolic Acidosis
Lactic acidosis
Diabetic ketoacidosis
Renal failure
Hepatic failure
Methanol and ethylene glycol intoxication
Aspirin intoxication
Increased skeletal muscle activity
Cyanide poisoning
Carbon monoxide poisoning

(distal renal tubular acidosis) or because an abnormally high fraction of filtered bicarbonate is not reabsorbed in the proximal tubule and is subsequently lost in the urine (proximal renal tubular acidosis or acetazolamide use). Combined defects occur in renal failure. The most common causes of extrarenal sources of a metabolic acidosis are gastrointestinal bicarbonate losses, ketoacidosis, and lactic acidosis.

Treatment

Treatment of metabolic acidosis includes treatment of the cause of the acidosis, for example, insulin and fluids for diabetic ketoacidosis and improvement in tissue perfusion in lactic acidosis. Administration of sodium bicarbonate for acute treatment of metabolic acidosis is very controversial. Many recommend that bicarbonate be given only if the pH is less than 7.1 or the bicarbonate concentration is less than 10 mEq/L. It is thought that the bicarbonate reacts with hydrogen ions, generating CO_2, which diffuses into cells lowering intracellular pH even more than before the bicarbonate treatment. It is also postulated that administration of bicarbonate to patients with chronic metabolic acidosis may result in transient tissue hypoxia. Acute changes in pH toward normal (or alkalosis) may negate the rightward shift of the oxyhemoglobin dissociation curve caused by academia (Bohr effect) and result in increased hemoglobin affinity for oxygen, thus reducing oxygen delivery at the tissue level.

The 2005 American Heart Association Guidelines for Cardiopulmonary Resuscitation and Emergency Cardiovascular Care do not recommend administering sodium bicarbonate routinely during cardiac arrest and cardiopulmonary resuscitation. However, sodium bicarbonate may be considered for life-threatening hyperkalemia or cardiac arrest associated with hyperkalemia or cardiac arrest associated with a preexisting metabolic acidosis.

Management of Anesthesia

Elective surgery should be postponed until an acidosis has been treated. For urgent surgery in a patient with a metabolic acidosis, invasive hemodynamic monitoring should be considered as a guide to fluid resuscitation and as a monitor of cardiac function in marked acidosis. Frequent laboratory measurement of acid-base parameters should be made throughout the perioperative period because pH can change rapidly and significantly depending on changes in ventilation, volume status, circulation, and drug administration.

Acidosis will affect the proportion of drug in the ionized and unionized states. Volume of distribution may also be affected in patients who have uncorrected hypovolemia.

Metabolic Alkalosis

Metabolic alkalosis is defined as an increase in pH, an increase in plasma bicarbonate concentration, and a compensatory increase in carbon dioxide tension. Common causes of metabolic alkalosis are noted in **Table 15-12**.

Metabolic alkalosis can be of renal or extrarenal origin and caused by either a net loss of hydrogen ions (such as loss of hydrochloric acid with vomiting) or a net gain of bicarbonate (such as due to tubular defects of bicarbonate reabsorption). Abnormal losses of chloride with or without hydrogen ion (e.g., in cystic fibrosis, villous adenoma) also induce increased renal bicarbonate reabsorption in an attempt to maintain electrical neutrality. Therefore, metabolic alkaloses can be characterized as chloride responsive or chloride resistant. Another classification of metabolic alkalosis is volume-depletion alkalosis (due to vomiting, diarrhea, or chloride losses) and volume-overload alkalosis (due to primary or secondary mineralocorticoid excess).

Metabolic alkalosis can also occur secondary to renal compensation for chronic respiratory disease with hypercarbia. In these patients, bicarbonate levels may be quite high and associated with urinary losses of chloride along with obligatory losses of sodium and potassium. If the respiratory disorder is treated with mechanical ventilation and the carbon dioxide tension reduced rapidly, a profound metabolic alkalosis may result.

Signs and Symptoms

There is progressively more binding of calcium to albumin as an alkalosis develops so the signs and symptoms of an alkalosis, especially those related to the neuromuscular and central nervous systems, may be very similar to those of hypocalcemia. Metabolic alkalosis may be accompanied by volume contraction, hypochloremia and hypokalemia, or volume overload and sodium retention depending on the etiology.

TABLE 15-12 Causes of Metabolic Alkalosis
Hypovolemia
Vomiting
Nasogastric suction
Diuretic therapy
Bicarbonate administration
Hyperaldosteronism
Chloride-wasting diarrhea

Diagnosis

As with metabolic acidosis, the diagnosis of a metabolic alkalosis is dependent on a high index of suspicion and laboratory testing. Metabolic alkaloses secondary to chloride losses are associated with low urinary chloride (typically < 10 mEq/L) and volume contraction. In contrast, metabolic alkaloses associated with mineralocorticoid excess are typically associated with volume overload and spot urine chloride greater than 20 mEq/L.

Treatment

Treatment rarely requires administration of an acid. Volume-depletion metabolic alkalosis is treated by replacement of chloride along with fluid resuscitation using saline. If the alkalosis has been caused by gastric losses of hydrochloric acid, then proton pump inhibitors can be given to stop the perpetuation of the alkalosis. Diuretic-associated metabolic alkalosis can be improved by addition or substitution of loop diuretics with potassium-sparing diuretics. In the case of volume-overload metabolic alkalosis, where excess mineralocorticoid is present, spironolactone plus potassium chloride may be useful if the source of mineralocorticoid secretion cannot be removed.

Management of Anesthesia

Anesthesia management is directed at judicious volume replacement and adequate supplementation with chloride, potassium, and magnesium as needed. Invasive monitoring may be helpful in some patients. Care must be taken not to exacerbate a compensatory metabolic alkalosis in patients with chronic lung disease and significant carbon dioxide retention.

KEY POINTS

- Total body water content is categorized as intracellular fluid and extra cellular fluid, according to the location of the water relative to cell membranes. The distribution and concentration of electrolytes differ greatly among fluid compartments. The electrophysiology of excitable cells is dependent on the intracellular and extracellular concentrations of sodium, potassium, and calcium.

- The predominant regulators of water balance are osmolality sensors (which are neurons located in the anterior hypothalamus that stimulate thirst) and vasopressin (antidiuretic hormone). Vasopressin is stored as granules in the posterior pituitary and is released in response to an increase in serum osmolality. Vasopressin acts on the collecting ducts of the kidney causing water retention, which in turn corrects serum osmolality.

- As hyponatremia develops, extracellular hypotonicity allows water to move into brain cells, resulting in cerebral edema and increased intracranial pressure. Initial compensation is afforded by the movement of ECF into the cerebrospinal fluid. Later compensation includes lowering intracellular osmolality by moving potassium and organic solutes out of brain cells. This reduces water movement into the intracellular space. However, when these adaptive mechanisms fail or hyponatremia progresses, central nervous system manifestations of hyponatremia occur.

- The volume overload, hyponatremia, and hypoosmolality that may accompany transurethral resection of the prostate is known as the TURP syndrome. This syndrome is more likely to occur if resection is prolonged (>1 hour), if the irrigating fluid is suspended more than 40 cm above the operative field, or if the pressure in the bladder is allowed to increase above 15 cm H_2O. TURP syndrome manifests principally with cardiovascular and neurologic signs and symptoms.

- Hypokalemia is diagnosed by testing the serum potassium concentration and the differential diagnosis requires determining whether the hypokalemia is acute and secondary to intracellular potassium shifts such as might be seen with hyperventilation or alkalosis, or whether the hypokalemia is chronic and associated with depletion of total body potassium stores.

- Immediate treatment of hyperkalemia is required if life-threatening dysrhythmias or electrocardiographic signs of severe hyperkalemia are present. This treatment is aimed at antagonizing the effects of a high potassium on the transmembrane potential and redistributing the potassium intracellularly. Calcium chloride or calcium gluconate is administered to stabilize cellular membranes. Hyperventilation, sodium bicarbonate administration, and insulin administration promote movement of potassium intracellularly.

- Binding of calcium to albumin is pH dependent, and acid base disturbances can change the fraction and therefore the concentration of ionized calcium without changing total body calcium. Alkalosis reduces the ionized calcium concentration, so ionized calcium may be significantly reduced after bicarbonate administration or with hyperventilation.

- Signs and symptoms of hypermagnesemia begin to occur at serum levels of 4 to 5 mEq/L and include lethargy, nausea and vomiting, and facial flushing. At levels above 6 mEq/L, there are a loss of deep tendon reflexes and hypotension. Paralysis, apnea, and/or cardiac arrest are likely if the magnesium level exceeds 10 mEq/L.

Continued

KEY POINTS—cont'd

- Major adverse consequences of severe systemic acidosis (pH < 7.2) can occur independently of whether the acidosis is of respiratory, metabolic, or mixed origin. Acidosis decreases myocardial contractility, although clinical effects are minimal until the pH decreases below 7.2, perhaps reflecting the effects of catecholamine release in response to the acidosis. When the pH is less than 7.1, cardiac responsiveness to catecholamines decreases and compensatory inotropic effects are diminished. The detrimental effects of acidosis may be accentuated in those with underlying left ventricular dysfunction or myocardial ischemia or in those in whom sympathetic nervous system activity is impaired, such as by β-adrenergic blockade or general anesthesia.

- Major adverse consequences of severe systemic alkalosis (pH > 7.60) reflect impairment of cerebral and coronary blood flow due to arteriolar vasoconstriction. Associated decreases in serum ionized calcium concentration contribute to the neurologic abnormalities associated with systemic alkalosis. Alkalosis predisposes patients, especially those with co-existing heart disease, to refractory ventricular dysrhythmias. Alkalosis also depresses ventilation.

REFERENCES

2005 American Heart Association guidelines for cardiopulmonary resuscitation and emergency cardiovascular care. Circulation 2005;112(24 suppl IV):1–203.

Adrogue HJ, Madias NE: Management of life-threatening acid-base disorders. N Engl J Med 1998;338:26–34, 107–111.

Adrogue HJ, Madias NE: Hyponatremia. N Engl J Med 2000;342:1581–1589.

Bilezikian JP: Management of acute hypercalcemia. N Engl J Med 1992;326:1196–1203.

Escuela MP, Guerra M, Anon JM, et al: Total and ionized serum magnesium in critically ill patients. Intensive Care Med 2005;31:151–156.

Gennari FJ: Hypokalemia. N Engl J Med 1998;339:451–458.

Kellum JA: Determinants of blood pH in health and disease. Crit Care 2000;4:6–14.

Lin SH, Hsu YJ, Chiu JS, et al: Master classes in medicine. Osmotic demyelination syndrome: A potentially avoidable disaster. QJM 2003;96:935–947.

Maccari C, Kamel KS, Davids MR, Halperin ML: Master classes in medicine. The patient with a severe degree of metabolic acidosis: A deductive analysis. QJM 2006;99:475–485.

Parham WA, Mehdirad AA, Biermann KM, Fredman CS: Hyperkalemia revisited. Tex Heart Inst J 2006;33:40–47.

Wahr JA, Parks R, Boisvert D, et al: Preoperative serum potassium levels and perioperative outcomes in cardiac surgical patients. JAMA 1999;281:2203–2210.

CHAPTER 16

Endocrine Disease

Russell T. Wall, III

DIABETES MELLITUS

Normal glucose physiology demonstrates a balance between glucose utilization and endogenous production or dietary delivery (**Fig. 16-1**). The liver is the primary source of endogenous glucose production via glycogenolysis and gluconeogenesis. Following a meal, plasma glucose increases, which stimulates an increase in plasma insulin (maximum insulin level is reached within 30 minutes) promoting glucose utilization. Late in the postprandial period (i.e., 2–4 hours after eating), when glucose utilization exceeds glucose production, the plasma glucose concentration decreases to below the fasting level before returning to preprandial values. A transition from exogenous glucose delivery to endogenous production then becomes necessary to maintain a normal plasma glucose

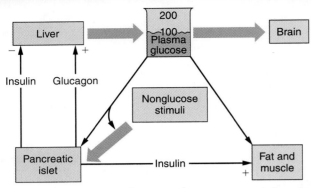

Figure 16-1 • The pancreatic islets act as glucose sensors to balance hepatic glucose release to insulin-insensitive tissues (brain) and insulin-sensitive tissues (fat, muscle). Insulin inhibits glucose release by the liver and stimulates glucose utilization by insulin-sensitive tissues. With hyperglycemia, insulin secretion increases. With hypoglycemia, the reverse occurs. (Adapted from Porte D Jr: Beta-cells in type II diabetes mellitus. Diabetes 1991;40:166–180.)

level. During the postabsorptive phase (i.e., 4–8 hours after eating) plasma glucose remains relatively stable with production and utilization rates being equal. At this time, 75% of glucose production results from hepatic glycogenolysis and 25% from hepatic gluconeogenesis. Approximately 70% to 80% of glucose released by the liver is metabolized by insulin-insensitive tissues such as the brain, gastrointestinal tract, and red blood cells. During this time, diminished insulin secretion is fundamental to the maintenance of a normal plasma glucose concentration. Hyperglycemia-producing hormones (glucagon, epinephrine, growth hormone, cortisol) constitute the glucose counterregulatory system and support glucose production. Glucagon plays a primary role by stimulating glycogenolysis, gluconeogenesis, and inhibiting glycolysis. Epinephrine predominates when glucagon secretion is deficient. Neural glucoregulatory factors (i.e., norepinephrine) and glucose autoregulation also support glucose production.

Humans require insulin for survival. Diabetes mellitus results from an inadequate supply of insulin and an inadequate tissue response to insulin, yielding increased circulating glucose levels with eventual microvascular and macrovascular complications. Type 1a diabetes is caused by an autoimmune destruction of beta cells within pancreatic islets resulting in complete absence or barely negligible circulating insulin levels. Type 1b diabetes is a rare disease with absolute insulin deficiency, although not immune mediated. Type 2 diabetes is not immune mediated and results from a relative deficiency of insulin coupled with an insulin receptor defect or defect(s) in its postreceptor intracellular signaling pathways.

Signs and Symptoms
Type 1 Diabetes
Five percent to 10% of all cases of diabetes are type 1. There are 1.4 million type 1 diabetics in the United States and 10 to 20 million globally. Currently, incidence is increasing by 3% to 5% per year. It is usually diagnosed before the age of 40 years and is one of the most common chronic childhood illnesses.

Type 1 diabetes is caused by a T cell–mediated autoimmune destruction of beta cells of the pancreas. The exact etiology is unknown, although environmental triggers such as viruses (especially enteroviruses), dietary proteins, and drugs/chemicals may initiate the autoimmune process in genetically susceptible hosts. A long preclinical period (9–13 years) characterized by antibodies to beta-cell antigens with loss of beta-cell function precedes the onset of clinical diabetes in the majority of patients. At least 80% to 90% of beta-cell function must be lost before hyperglycemia occurs. The autoimmune attack initially presents as islet inflammation (insulitis) with immune cells infiltrating pancreatic islets and releasing cytokines resulting in cytotoxicity and an impairment of insulin secretion and/or a functional inhibition of insulin release. Circulating antibodies signify islet cell injury. The presentation of clinical disease is often sudden and severe secondary to loss of a critical mass of beta cells. Patients demonstrate hyperglycemia over several days to weeks associated with fatigue, weight loss, polyuria, polydipsia, blurring of vision, and signs of intravascular volume depletion. The diagnosis is based on the following symptoms: a random blood glucose greater than 200 mg/dL and a hemoglobin (Hb) A_{1c} level greater than 7.0%. The presence of ketoacidosis indicates severe insulin deficiency and unrestrained lipolysis. Beta-cell destruction is complete within 3 years of diagnosis in most young children, with the process being slower in adults.

Type 2 Diabetes
Type 2 diabetes is responsible for 90% of all cases of diabetes mellitus in the world. In 2000, there were approximately 150 million type 2 diabetics globally with the number expected to double by 2025. Type 2 diabetics are typically in the middle to older age group and overweight, although there has been a significant increase in younger patients and even children over the past decade. Type 2 diabetes continues to be underrecognized and underdiagnosed because of its subtle presentation. It is estimated that most type 2 diabetics have had the disease for approximately 4 to 7 years before it is diagnosed.

Type 2 diabetes is characterized by relative beta-cell insufficiency and insulin resistance. In the initial stages of the disease, an insensitivity to insulin by peripheral tissues yields an increase in pancreatic insulin secretion to maintain normal plasma glucose levels. As the disease progresses and pancreatic cell function decreases, insulin levels are unable to compensate in peripheral tissues and hyperglycemia occurs. There are three important defects in type 2 diabetes: an increased rate of hepatic glucose release, impaired basal and stimulated insulin secretion, and inefficient use of glucose by peripheral tissues (i.e., insulin resistance) (**Fig. 16-2**). The increase in hepatic glucose release is caused by the reduction of insulin's normal inhibitory effects on the liver and abnormalities in regulation of glucagon secretion. Glucagon appears responsible for more than 50% of hepatic glucose production in type 2 diabetes. Although relative beta-cell insufficiency is significant, type 2 diabetes is characterized by insulin resistance in skeletal muscle, adipose tissue, and the liver. Insulin resistance is

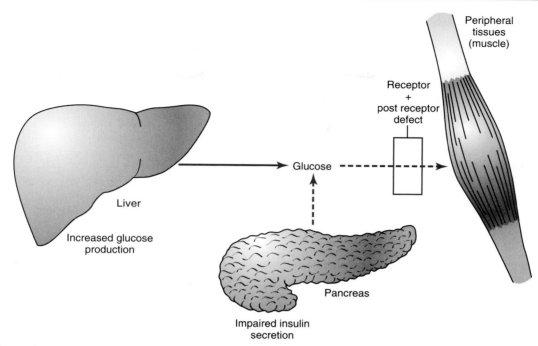

Figure 16-2 • Abnormalities in type 2 diabetes. *(Adapted from Inzucchi S [ed]: The Diabetes Mellitus Manual: A Primary Companion to Ellenberg and Rifkin's Sixth Edition. New York, McGraw-Hill, 2005, p 79.)*

defined as a less-than-normal biologic response to a given concentration of insulin. Causes of insulin resistance include an abnormal insulin molecule, circulating insulin antagonists including counterregulatory hormones, free fatty acids, anti-insulin and insulin receptor antibodies and cytokines, and target tissue defects at insulin receptors and/or postreceptor sites. Skeletal muscle is the prototypical peripheral insulin-sensitive target tissue. Postprandial hyperglycemia in type 2 diabetics is primarily due to glucose underuse by peripheral tissues, primarily muscle. It appears that insulin resistance is an inherited component of type 2 diabetes with obesity and sedentary lifestyle being acquired and contributing factors. The increasing prevalence of type 2 diabetes among children and adolescents appears related to obesity, with 85% of affected children being overweight or obese at the time of diagnosis. Obese patients exhibit a compensatory hyperinsulinemia to maintain normoglycemia. These increased insulin levels may desensitize target tissues causing a reduced response to insulin. The mechanism for hyperinsulinemia and insulin resistance from weight gain remains elusive. Insulin resistance appears rare in type 1 diabetics, although patients may have high titers of anti-insulin antibodies.

The transition from normal glucose tolerance to impaired glucose tolerance and then eventual diabetes has been studied extensively. Impaired glucose tolerance is associated with an increase in body weight, a decrease in insulin secretion, and a reduction in peripheral insulin action. The transition to clinical diabetes demonstrates these same factors plus an increase in hepatic glucose production.

The metabolic syndrome or insulin-resistance syndrome is a constellation of clinical and biochemical characteristics

TABLE 16-1 Metabolic Syndrome
At least three of the following
Fasting plasma glucose ≥ 110 mg/dL
Abdominal obesity (waist girth > 40 [in men], 35 [in women])
Serum triglycerides ≥ 150 mg/dL
Serum high-density lipoprotein cholesterol < 40 mg/dL (men), < 50 mg/dL (women)
Blood pressure ≥ 130/85 mm Hg
Adapted from Expert Panel on Detection, Evaluation, and Treatment of High Blood Cholesterol in Adults: Executive Summary of The Third Report of The National Cholesterol Education Program (NCEP) Expert Panel on Detection, Evaluation, and Treatment of High Blood Cholesterol in Adults (Adult Treatment Panel III). JAMA 2001;285:2486–2497.

frequently seen in patients with or at risk of type 2 diabetes (**Table 16-1**). It combines insulin resistance with hypertension, dyslipidemia, a procoagulant state, and obesity with premature atherosclerosis and subsequent cardiovascular disease. This syndrome affects at least 25% of people in the United States.

Diagnosis

In 1997 the American Diabetes Association established diagnostic criteria for diabetes mellitus (**Table 16-2**). A fasting plasma glucose is the recommended screening and diagnostic test for diabetes mellitus. In 2004, the American Diabetes Association reduced the normal fasting glucose threshold from 110 mg/dL to 100 mg/dL. A normal fasting plasma glucose is 70 to 100 mg/dL. Hyperglycemia not sufficient to meet the diagnostic criteria for diabetes is classified as either impaired fasting glucose or impaired glucose tolerance,

TABLE 16-2 Diagnostic Criteria for Diabetes Mellitus

Symptoms of diabetes (polyuria, polydipsia, unexplained weight loss) plus a random plasma glucose concentration $\geq$ 200 mg/dL
or
Fasting (no caloric intake for $\geq$ 8 hours) plasma glucose $\geq$ 126 mg/dL
or
2-hour plasma glucose > 200 mg/dL during an oral glucose tolerance test

depending on whether it is identified through a fasting plasma glucose or an oral glucose tolerance test. Any fasting glucose between 101 and 125 mg/dL is impaired fasting glucose. Glucose levels, especially in type 2 diabetics, usually increase over years to decades progressing from the normal range to the impaired glucose tolerance range and finally to clinical diabetes. Patients with impaired glucose tolerance are at risk of progressing to diabetes and also experiencing cardiovascular morbidity. Although rarely used in routine practice, the oral glucose tolerance test is recommended for diagnosis when glucose values are equivocal.

Random glucose measurements are not measures of overall glycemic control. Fasting glucose values also do not provide a total picture. The Hb A_{1c} test provides a valuable assessment of long-term glycemic control. Erythrocyte hemoglobin is nonenzymatically glycosylated by glucose that freely crosses red blood cell membranes. The percentage of hemoglobin molecules participating in this reaction is proportional to the average plasma glucose concentration during the preceding 60 to 90 days. The normal range for Hb A_{1c} is 4% to 6%. Increased risk of microvascular and macrovascular disease begins at a Hb A_{1c} of 6.5%.

Venous plasma or serum is the standard body fluid for glucose determinations, and values are essentially identical. Arterial and capillary blood yield glucose values approximately 7% higher than venous blood. Whole blood determinations are usually 15% lower than plasma or serum values. Urine glucose is a poor diagnostic test since the renal glucose threshold is not reached until the extracellular glucose concentration exceeds 180 mg/dL. Other emerging technologies include interstitial sensors that provide continuous monitoring of extracellular glucose concentrations.

Treatment

The cornerstones of therapy for type 2 diabetes are diet with weight loss, exercise therapy, and the oral antidiabetic agents. Reduction of body weight through diet and exercise is the first therapeutic measure to control type 2 diabetes. The initial decrease in fasting plasma glucose results from a decrease in hepatic glycogen stores and a decline in glycogenolysis. The decrease in adiposity improves hepatic and peripheral tissue insulin sensitivity, enhances postreceptor insulin action, and may possibly increase insulin secretion. Nutritional guidelines by the American Diabetes Association emphasize maintenance of optimal plasma glucose and lipid levels. Estimation of basal

energy requirements and activity level requirements plus additional adjustments for growing children, pregnancy, lactation, infection, illness, and surgery are necessary. Low-calorie diets (800–1500 kcal) and very low calorie diets (<800 kcal) with limits on cholesterol raising fats and added sugars are used to reduce body fat and decrease insulin resistance and to normalize plasma glucose, lipids, and lipoproteins.

Oral Antidiabetic Agents

The four major classes of oral agents are the secretagogues (sulfonylureas, meglitinides), which increase insulin availability; biguanides (metformin), which suppress excessive hepatic glucose release; thiazolidinediones or glitazones (rosiglitazone, pioglitazone), which improve insulin sensitivity; and α-glucosidase inhibitors (acarbose, miglitol), which delay gastrointestinal glucose absorption (**Fig. 16-3**). These agents, either as monotherapy or in various combinations, are used to maintain glucose control (fasting glucose, 90–130 mg/dL; peak postprandial glucose, <180 mg/dL; Hb A_{1c} <7%) in the initial stages of the disease.

Insulin secretagogues stimulate insulin secretion from pancreatic beta cells. They can also enhance insulin-stimulated peripheral tissue utilization of glucose. They work by closing adenosine triphosphate–dependent potassium channels and opening calcium channels leading to exocytosis of insulin-containing secretory granules. The sulfonylureas are usually the initial pharmacologic treatment for type 2 diabetes (**Table 16-3**). The second-generation agents (glyburide, glipizide, glimepiride) are more potent and have fewer side effects than their predecessors. Unfortunately, due to the natural history of type 2 diabetes with decreasing beta-cell function, these agents are not effective indefinitely. Hypoglycemia is the most common side effect. The demonstration of harmful cardiac effects from sulfonylureas is controversial, with some studies attributing an increase in in-hospital mortality to their use. Potassium adenosine triphosphate channels in the myocardium mediate ischemic preconditioning, which appears critical for myocardial protection and limitation of infarction size. Sulfonylureas may inhibit this protective response and potentially delay contractile recovery and result in larger myocardial infarctions.

The biguanides decrease hepatic gluconeogenesis and, to a lesser degree, enhance utilization of glucose by skeletal muscle and adipose tissue by increasing glucose transport across cell membranes. In addition to lowering glucose levels, they decrease plasma triglycerides and low-density lipoprotein cholesterol levels and reduce postprandial hyperlipemia and plasma free fatty acid levels and their oxidation. If ineffective alone, metformin is usually combined with a sulfonylurea. The risk of hypoglycemia is less than that with the sulfonylureas, and the risk of lactic acidosis is much less with metformin than its predecessor phenformin.

The thiazolidinediones or glitazones are insulin sensitizers that decrease insulin resistance by binding to peroxisome proliferator–activated receptors γ located in skeletal muscle, liver, and adipose tissue. These receptors are important regulators of insulin action and the expression and release of mediators of

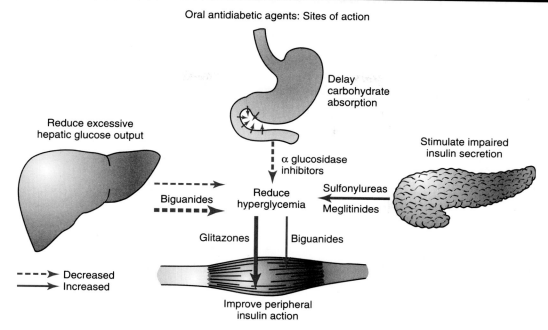

Oral antidiabetic agents: Sites of action

Figure 16-3 • Oral antidiabetic agents: sites of action. *(Adapted from Inzucchi S [ed]: The Diabetes Mellitus Manual: A Primary Companion to Ellenberg and Rifkin's Sixth Edition. New York, McGraw-Hill, 2005, p 168.)*

insulin resistance, lipid homeostasis, and adipocyte differentiation. These drugs influence genetic expression for encoding proteins for glucose and lipid metabolism, endothelial function, and atherogenesis and as a result may influence diabetic dyslipidemia in addition to hyperglycemia.

The α-glucosidase inhibitors inhibit α-glucosidase enzymes in the brush border of enterocytes in the proximal small intestine. They are administered before a main meal to ensure their presence at the site of action and result in a delay in the intraluminal production and subsequent absorption of glucose.

In most patients, oral agent therapy is initiated with a sulfonylurea or biguanide and titrated to achieve fasting and peak postprandial glucose American Diabetes Association recommendations (**Fig. 16-4**). Monotherapy studies usually demonstrate eventual failure, and a treat-to-failure strategy is used until combination therapy becomes necessary. Combination therapy with oral agents directed at more than one mechanism is effective. A sulfonylurea plus biguanide is the most widely studied combination. Triple oral therapy using a sulfonylurea, metformin, and a glitazone or acarbose is also used in clinical practice. If combination oral therapy is ineffective, the addition of a bedtime dose of intermediate-acting insulin is initiated

since hepatic glucose overproduction is typically most abnormal at night. If oral agents plus single-dose insulin therapy is ineffective, type 2 diabetics are switched to insulin exclusively. A combination of intermediate and regular insulin twice daily is commonly used for optimal control, although some patients require three or more injections. If increasing doses of insulin fail to achieve adequate control, reinstituting oral agents (metformin, a glitazone, acarbose) may be effective. Even in selected patients, discontinuing insulin and reinstituting oral therapy may work. Type 2 diabetics with excessive hyperglycemia (>300 mg/dL) associated with ketonuria or ketonemia, pregnancy, an acute myocardial infarction, or other acute situations need insulin immediately. Tight control of type 2 diabetes provides significant benefits in prevention and progression of microvascular disease and possibly macrovascular disease. In addition to treating hyperglycemia, all abnormalities of insulin resistance (the metabolic syndrome) must be managed with goals of therapy including Hb A_{1c} less than 7%, low-density lipoprotein less than 100 mg/dL, high-density lipoprotein greater than 40 mg/dL in men and greater than 50 mg/dL in women, triglycerides less than 200 mg/dL, and blood pressure less than 130/80.

TABLE 16-3 Sulfonylureas				
Drug	Initial Dose (mg/day)	Daily Dose Range (mg/day)	Duration (hr)	Doses/Day
Second Generation				
Glyburide	1.25–2.5	1.25–20	18–24	1–2
Glipizide	2.5–5.0	2.5–40	12–18	1–2
Glimepiride	1–2	4–8	24	1

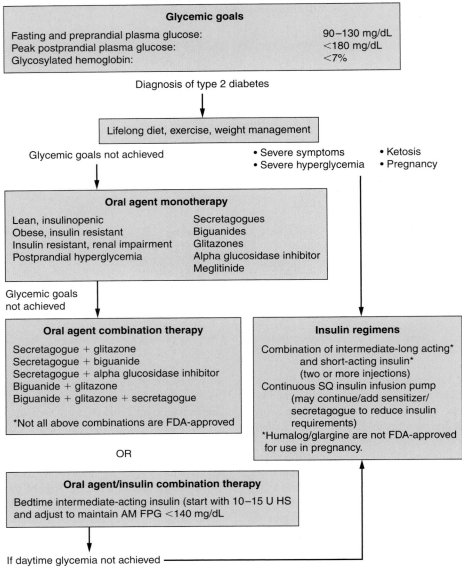

Glycemic goals

Fasting and preprandial plasma glucose:	90–130 mg/dL
Peak postprandial plasma glucose:	<180 mg/dL
Glycosylated hemoglobin:	<7%

Diagnosis of type 2 diabetes

Lifelong diet, exercise, weight management

Glycemic goals not achieved

• Severe symptoms
• Severe hyperglycemia

• Ketosis
• Pregnancy

Oral agent monotherapy

Lean, insulinopenic	Secretagogues
Obese, insulin resistant	Biguanides
Insulin resistant, renal impairment	Glitazones
Postprandial hyperglycemia	Alpha glucosidase inhibitor
	Meglitinide

Glycemic goals not achieved

Oral agent combination therapy

Secretagogue + glitazone
Secretagogue + biguanide
Secretagogue + alpha glucosidase inhibitor
Biguanide + glitazone
Biguanide + glitazone + secretagogue

*Not all above combinations are FDA-approved

Insulin regimens

Combination of intermediate-long acting*
and short-acting insulin*
(two or more injections)
Continuous SQ insulin infusion pump
(may continue/add sensitizer/
secretagogue to reduce insulin
requirements)
*Humalog/glargine are not FDA-approved
for use in pregnancy.

OR

Oral agent/insulin combination therapy

Bedtime intermediate-acting insulin (start with 10–15 U HS
and adjust to maintain AM FPG <140 mg/dL

If daytime glycemia not achieved

Figure 16-4 • Algorithm for treatment of type 2 diabetes. *(Adapted from Inzucchi S [ed]: The Diabetes Mellitus Manual: A Primary Companion to Ellenberg and Rifkin's Sixth Edition. New York, McGraw-Hill, 2005, p 193.)*

Insulin

Insulin is necessary to manage all type 1 diabetics and many type 2 diabetics (**Table 16-4**). In the United States, 30% of type 2 diabetics are treated with insulin. Conventional insulin therapy uses twice-daily injections. Intensive insulin therapy uses three or more daily injections or a continuous infusion.

The various forms of insulin include basal insulins, which are intermediate acting (NPH, lente, lispro protamine, aspart protamine) and administered twice daily or long acting (ultralente and glargine) and administered once daily, and insulins that are short acting (regular) or rapid acting (lispro, aspart), which provide glycemic control at mealtimes (prandial insulin). Conventional insulin therapy usually requires twice-daily injections of combinations of intermediate-acting and short-/rapid-acting insulins such as Humulin 70/30 insulin (70% NPH, 30% regular), Novolog 70/30 (70% insulin aspart

protamine plus 30% insulin aspart) or Humalog 75/25 (75% insulin lispro protamine plus 25% insulin lispro) (**Fig. 16-5**). For Humulin 70/30, injections are given 30 minutes before breakfast and 30 minutes before dinner. For Novolog 70/30 and Humalog 75/25, injections are given 5 to 15 minutes before breakfast and 5 to 15 minutes before dinner. Twice-daily separate injections of NPH insulin and regular insulin or NPH insulin and rapid-acting insulin (lispro, aspart) are another conventional method of administration.

Intensive insulin therapy uses three or four daily injections or a continuous infusion with more frequent glucose monitoring. Three daily injections includes NPH plus short-acting (regular) or rapid-acting (lispro, aspart) insulin before breakfast, short-acting or rapid-acting insulin before dinner, and NPH insulin at bedtime (**Fig. 16-6**). Four daily injections can include a single injection of NPH, lente, or insulin glargine (Lantus) at

TABLE 16-4 Insulin

Insulins	Onset	Peak	Duration
Short Acting			
Human regular	30 min	2–4 hr	5–8 hr
Lispro (Humalog)	10–15 min	1–2 hr	3–6 hr
Aspart (Novolog)	10–15 min	1–2 hr	3–6 hr
Intermediate			
Human NPH	1–2 hr	6–10 hr	10–20 hr
Lente	1–2 hr	6–10 hr	10–20 hr
Long Acting			
Ultralente	4–6 hr	8–20 hr	24–48 hr
Glargine (Lantus)	1–2 hr	Peakless	~ 24 hr

bedtime plus short-acting or rapid-acting insulin before break-fast, lunch, and dinner (**Figs. 16-7** and **16-8**). A subcutaneous infusion pump uses regular or rapid-acting insulin with a usual range of 0.5 to 2.0 units per hour (**Fig. 16-9**). A typical total daily basal dose of insulin equals weight (kg) × 0.3, with the

hourly rate obtained by dividing by 24. Basal rates vary during a 24-hour period with lower rates required at bedtime, higher rates between 3 and 9 AM and intermediate rates during the day. Premeal boluses may also be used, and insulin rates must be adjusted for exercise. Ideal glycemic goals for type 1 diabetics include the following: before meals, 70 to 120 mg/dL; after meals, less than 150 mg/dL; at bedtime, 100 to 130 mg/dL; and at 3:00 AM more than 70 mg/dL.

For many type 2 diabetics, early and aggressive initiation of insulin therapy has demonstrated beneficial effects. Reports of remissions of type 2 diabetes with early intensive insulin treatment suggests that it should be prescribed early rather than as a treatment of last resort. Unlike oral agents, insulin has no upper dose limit and can be adjusted over time to achieve near-normal glucose levels. Many type 2 diabetics require 0.6 to 1.0 U/kg per day. The amount of insulin needed is not related to the degree of hyperglycemia but to body adiposity and other factors of insulin resistance. In most studies, obese type 2 diabetics require significant daily doses (100–200 units) to achieve near-normal glycemia. Fortunately, blood glucose levels for type 2 diabetics are much less labile than for type 1 diabetics and adjustment of the dose is less necessary. Insulin therapy is usually initiated with 10 to

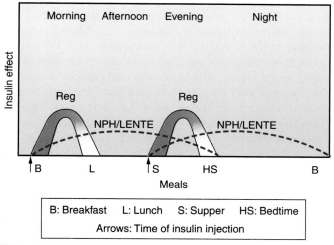

Figure 16-5 • Insulin effect from two daily doses of NPH + regular. (*Adapted from Hirsch IB, Farkas-Hirsch R, Skyler JS: Intensive insulin therapy for treatment of type I diabetes. Diabetes Care 1990;13.*)

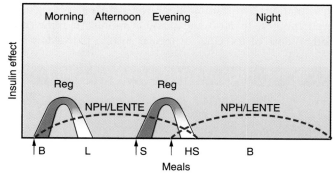

Figure 16-6 • Insulin effect of the three injections per day regimen (NPH + regular in morning, regular before supper, NPH at bedtime).

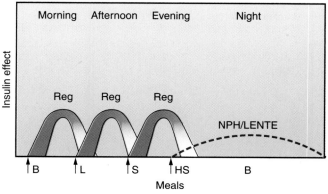

Figure 16-7 • Insulin effect of the four injections per day regimen of short-acting insulin before each meal and NPH at bedtime.

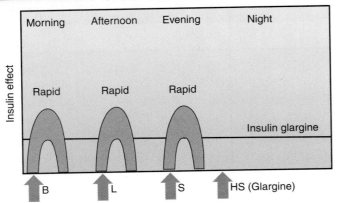

Figure 16-8 • Insulin effect of multiple-dose regimen: three premeal doses of rapid-acting insulin (lispro/aspart) + basal insulin (glargine). B, breakfast; HS, bedtime; L, lunch; S, supper.

15 units of intermediate-acting insulin at bedtime with the dose being adjusted until fasting levels are therapeutic, or, alternatively, administering long-acting insulin glargine in the evening. If glucose levels remain elevated during the day, intermediate-acting insulin is added in the morning with or without short- or rapid-acting insulin. Type 2 diabetics who benefit most from insulin therapy are those who demonstrate catabolism with ketonuria, persistently elevated glucose levels despite oral therapy, severe hypertriglyceridemia, uncontrolled weight loss or severe dehydration with hyperglycemia, or the desire to maintain near-normal glycemia or induce remission.

Hypoglycemia is the most frequent and dangerous complication of insulin therapy. Approximately 30% of type 1 diabetics experience one or more severe hypoglycemic attacks per year. The incidence is three times higher in the intensive therapy group than the conventional group. The hypoglycemic effect can be exacerbated by simultaneous administration of alcohol, sulfonylureas, biguanides, thiazolidinediones, angiotensin-converting enzyme (ACE) inhibitors, monoamine oxidase inhibitors, and nonselective β-blockers. β-Blockers may exacerbate hypoglycemia by inhibiting adipose tissue lipolysis, which serves as an alternate fuel when patients become hypoglycemic. Defective counterregulatory responses by glucagon and epinephrine to reduced plasma glucose levels contribute

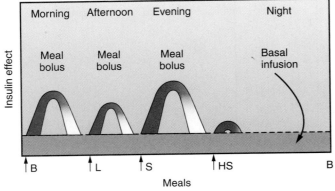

Figure 16-9 • Insulin effect of continuous subcutaneous infusion of short-/rapid-acting insulin before meals and snacks.

to this complication. Repetitive episodes of hypoglycemia, especially at night, results in hypoglycemia unawareness where the patient does not respond with the appropriate autonomic warning symptoms before neuroglycopenia. The diagnosis in adults requires a plasma glucose level less than 50 mg/dL. Symptoms are adrenergic (sweating, tachycardia, palpitations, restlessness, pallor) and neuroglycopenic (fatigue, confusion, headache, somnolence, convulsions, coma). Treatment, if conscious, includes the administration of sugar in the form of sugar cubes, glucose tablets or soft drinks, and, if unconscious, glucose 0.5 g/kg IV or glucagon 0.5 to 1.0 mg IV, IM, or SC.

Prognosis

Diabetic Ketoacidosis

Diabetic ketoacidosis (DKA) is a complication of decompensated diabetes mellitus. The signs and symptoms of DKA are primarily the result of abnormalities in carbohydrate and fat metabolism. Episodes of DKA occur more commonly in type 1 diabetics and are precipitated by infection or acute illness (cerebrovascular accident, myocardial infarction, acute pancreatitis) 30% to 40% of the time, insulin omission 15% to 20% of the time, and the new onset of diabetes mellitus in 15% to 20% of cases. High glucose levels exceed the threshold for renal tubular absorption creating a significant osmotic diuresis with marked hypovolemia. A tight metabolic coupling between hepatic gluconeogenesis and ketogenesis results in an overproduction of ketoacids by the liver. DKA results in an excess of glucose counterregulatory hormones with glucagon activating lipolysis with free fatty acids providing the substrate for ketogenesis. An increase in ketoacid (β-hydroxybutyrate, acetoacetate, acetone) production creates a metabolic acidosis (Table 16-5). An increased anion gap $(Na^+ - [Cl^- + HCO_3^-]$ normal: $8-14$ mEq/L) is present. Substantial deficits of water, potassium, and phosphorus exist, although laboratory values of these electrolytes appear normal or elevated. Hyponatremia results from the effect of hyperglycemia and hyperosmolarity on water distribution. The deficit of potassium is 3 to 5 mEq/kg and the deficit of phosphorus can lead to diaphragmatic and skeletal muscle dysfunction and impaired myocardial contractility.

The treatment of DKA consists of giving large amounts of normal saline, effective doses of insulin, and electrolyte supplementation. Rehydration alone will reduce plasma glucose levels by 30% to 50% and possibly more. An intravenous loading dose of 0.1 U/kg of regular insulin plus a low-dose

TABLE 16-5 Diagnostic Features of DKA	
Glucose (mg/dL)	≥300
pH	≤7.3
HCO₃⁻ (mEq/L)	≤18
SOsm (mOsm/L)	<320
Ketones	++-+++
DKA, diabetic ketoacidosis; SOsm, serum osmolarity.	

insulin infusion of 0.1 U/kg per hour is initiated. The effects of insulin are surprisingly limited and primarily due to inhibition of hepatic glucose production. The average decline in blood glucose is 75 to 100 mg/dL per hour with correction to target values ($\sim$ 250 mg/dL) occurring in 4 to 6 hours and correction to target values for acidosis and HCO_3^- levels in 8 to 12 hours. A normal pH is obtained in approximately 24 hours. Insulin administration is necessary until a normal acid base status is achieved. The insulin rate is reduced when hyperglycemia is controlled, the pH is greater than 7.3, and HCO_3^- greater than 18 mEq/L. Potassium and phosphate are replaced with KCl and K_2PO_4, respectively. Magnesium is replaced as needed. Sodium bicarbonate is administered for a pH less than 7.1. The infrequent but devastating development of cerebral edema results from correction of hyperglycemia without simultaneous elevation of plasma Na. The overall mortality rate for DKA is 5% to 10% and 15% to 28% for patients older than 65 years of age and may approach 45% in patients with coma.

Hyperglycemic Hyperosmolar Syndrome

Hyperglycemic hyperosmolar syndrome (HHS) is characterized by severe hyperglycemia, hyperosmolarity, and dehydration usually in elderly (older than 60 years) type 2 diabetics who live alone, are socially isolated, and experience an acute illness such as infection, myocardial infarction, cerebrovascular accident, pancreatitis, intestinal obstruction, endocrinopathy, renal failure, or a burn. The entire syndrome evolves over days to weeks with a persistent glycosuric diuresis. As the glucose load exceeds the renal tubular maximum for glucose reabsorption, a massive solute diuresis occurs with total body water depletion. The patient presents with polyuria, polydipsia, hypovolemia, hypotension, tachycardia, and organ hypoperfusion. The early administration of large volumes of crystalloid fluids is necessary to prevent this syndrome. Hyperosmolarity (>340 mOsm/L) is responsible for an obtunded mental status or coma (**Table 16-6**). Patients may have some degree of metabolic acidosis but do not demonstrate a ketosis. Vascular occlusions secondary to mesenteric artery thrombosis, low-flow states, or diffuse intravascular coagulation are an important complication of HHS.

Treatment includes significant fluid resuscitation, insulin, and electrolyte supplementation. If the plasma osmolarity is greater than 320 mOsm/L, large volumes (1000–1500 mL/hr) of 0.45% normal saline should be administered until the osmolarity is less than 320 mOsm/L, at which time large volumes (1000–1500 mL/hr) of 0.9% normal saline is

TABLE 16-6 Diagnostic Feature of Hyperglycemic Hyperosmolar Syndrome	
Glucose (mg/dL)	≥600
pH	≥7.3
HCO_3^- (mEq/L)	≥15
SOsm (mOsm/L)	≥350
SOsm, serum osmolarity.	

administered. Insulin is initiated with an intravenous bolus of 15 units of regular insulin followed by a 0.1-U/kg per hour infusion. The insulin infusion is decreased to 2 to 3 U/hr when the glucose decreases to 250 to 300 mg/dL. The rate of glucose decrease is predictable at 75 to 150 mg/dL per hour, and the amount of insulin required is comparable to DKA. Significant hyperglycemia persists only if renal blood flow and glomerular filtration rate remain reduced. A normally perfused kidney will not permit extreme hyperglycemia. Electrolyte deficits are significant but usually less severe than in DKA. The mortality rate of HHS is 10% to 15%.

Glycemic Control

Controlled clinical trials and epidemiologic studies have analyzed the relationship between the degree of glycemic control and the incidence of microvascular and macrovascular complications. Randomized, controlled clinical trials have unequivocally established that strict control of glycemia can decrease the risk of microangiopathic (nephropathy, peripheral neuropathy, retinopathy) complications of diabetes. Microvascular dysfunction is unique to diabetics and is characterized by nonocclusive, microcirculatory impairment with vascular permeability and impaired autoregulation of blood flow and vascular tone.

Hyperglycemia is essential for the development of these changes and intensive glycemic control (near normal range) delays the onset and slows progression of microvascular effects, demonstrating significant improvements in all outcomes for all microvascular complications. The major morbidity and mortality from type 2 diabetes, however, is secondary to accelerated atherosclerosis, a multifactorial disease process not solely due to hyperglycemia. As a result, treatment must be directed at multiple risk factors in addition to hyperglycemia such as hypertension, hyperlipidemia, and smoking. A growing number of epidemiologic studies have demonstrated an association between the degree of glycemia and macrovascular (cardiovascular, cerebrovascular, and peripheral vascular disease) complications, but large randomized clinical trials have not convincingly shown that macrovascular disease is affected by glycemic control. The macrovascular pathology is morphologically and functionally similar to nondiabetics and is characterized by atherosclerotic lesions of the coronary and peripheral arterial circulations.

Microvascular Complications

Nephropathy Approximately 30% to 40% of type 1 diabetics and 5% to 10% of type 2 diabetics develop end-stage renal disease. The kidneys demonstrate glomerulosclerosis with glomerular basement membrane thickening, arteriosclerosis, and tubulointerstitial disease. The clinical course is characterized by hypertension, albuminuria, peripheral edema, and a progressive decrease in glomerular filtration rate. Basement membrane thickening develops within 2 to 3 years of the diagnosis of diabetes. Renal function remains normal on laboratory testing for approximately 15 years, at which time proteinuria develops, indicating advanced glomerulosclerosis. Proteinuria is the earliest laboratory manifestation of diabetic renal disease. Within 5 years of proteinuria, the blood urea nitrogen and creatinine increase and a significant percentage of these patients progress to renal failure in 3 to 5 years. When the glomerular filtration rate decreases to less than 15 to 20 mL/min, the ability of the kidneys to excrete potassium and acids is impaired and patients become hyperkalemic and metabolically acidotic. Hypertension, hyperglycemia, hypercholesterolemia, and microalbuminuria accelerate the decrease in the glomerular filtration rate. Hypertension is a most important factor responsible for the progression of diabetic renal disease. Treatment of hypertension can markedly slow progression. Hypertension is managed with a low-sodium diet, low doses of diuretics, and one or several antihypertensive agents including a β_1-antagonist, ACE inhibitor, angiotensin II receptor blocker, calcium channel blocker, and/or an α_1-blocker. Even though β-blockers can cause hypoglycemia by inhibiting hepatic glucose production, impairing the counterregulatory hormone response to hypoglycemia, and masking the clinical signs of hypoglycemia, they are still highly effective. ACE inhibitors provide an added benefit in diabetics by retarding the progression of proteinuria and the decrease in the glomerular filtration rate. The initiation of tight control after the onset of proteinuria has unfortunately been ineffective in stopping the progression to renal failure. Treatment of a dyslipidemia and keeping the patient on a low-protein diet are also important. If end-stage renal disease develops, there are four options: hemodialysis, peritoneal dialysis, continuous ambulatory peritoneal dialysis, and transplantation. In fact, every third patient started on dialysis in the United States has diabetes mellitus. For hemodialysis, vascular access is established when the serum creatinine reaches 4 to 5 mg/dL and dialysis is initiated at a level of 6 to 8 mg/dL. Patients receiving a kidney transplant, especially if the organ is from a living/human HLA-identical donor, demonstrate a longer survival than those on dialysis. A combined kidney/pancreas transplant results in lower mortality than dialysis or renal transplantation alone and may prevent recurrence of diabetic nephropathy in the transplanted kidney.

Peripheral Neuropathy More than 50% of patients who have had diabetes for more than 25 years will develop a peripheral neuropathy. Glycemic control is the only effective treatment. There are two stages of a diabetic peripheral neuropathy: subclinical and clinical. The subclinical stage demonstrates laboratory evidence of slowed sensory and motor nerve conduction and elevated sensory perception thresholds in the absence of clinical signs and symptoms. The clinical stage demonstrates symptoms and/or neurologic deficits. Quantitative sensory tests measuring vibratory and temperature thresholds, electrodiagnostic studies of nerve conduction, and electromyography define the degree of dysfunction. A distal symmetrical diffuse sensorimotor polyneuropathy is the most common form. Sensory deficits usually overshadow motor findings and appear in the toes or feet and progress proximally toward the chest in a "stocking glove" distribution. Loss of large sensory and motor fibers produces a loss of light touch and proprioception, and muscle weakness. Loss of small fibers decreases the perception of pain and temperature and produces dysesthesias, paresthesias, and neuropathic pain. Foot ulcers develop from mechanical and traumatic events to distal extremities compromised by a loss of cutaneous sensitivity to pain and temperature and impaired perfusion from the microcirculatory defect and autonomic dysfunction. Significant morbidity results from recurrent infections, foot fractures (Charcot's joint), and subsequent amputations. The treatment of a peripheral neuropathy includes optimal glucose control, and nonsteroidal anti-inflammatory agents, antidepressants, and anticonvulsants for pain control.

Retinopathy Diabetic retinopathy results from a variety of microvascular changes including occlusion, dilation, increased permeability, and microaneurysm formation resulting in hemorrhages, exudates, and growth of abnormal vessels and fibrous tissue. Visual impairment can range from minor changes in color vision to total blindness. Strict glycemic control and blood pressure control can reduce the risk of development and progression of retinopathy.

Macrovascular Complications

Cardiovascular disease is a major cause of morbidity and the leading cause of mortality in diabetics. It commonly presents as angina, a myocardial infarction, congestive heart failure, or sudden death and results from atherosclerotic coronary artery disease and hypertension. A dyslipidemia is the major contributor to the initiation and development of atherosclerotic lesions. The hallmark of diabetic dyslipidemia is hypertriglyceridemia with poorly controlled type 1 and 2 diabetics demonstrating elevated triglycerides, low levels of high-density lipoprotein cholesterol, and an abnormally small, dense, more atherogenic low-density lipoprotein cholesterol. This dyslipidemia is caused by the lack of appropriate insulin signaling and is exacerbated by poor glucose control. As a result, statin therapy (3-hydroxy-3-methylglutaryl coenzyme A reductase inhibitors) should be considered for all diabetics. Increased oxidative stress and vascular inflammation are other mechanisms of atherosclerosis and increase the tendency for thrombosis. Prevention of coronary artery disease in diabetics includes aggressive management of elevated lipids, elevated glucose, and hypertension, as well as aspirin for thrombolysis. Medical management of symptomatic coronary artery disease includes β_1-blockers, ACE inhibitors, nitrates, calcium channel blockers, statins, fibrates, antiplatelet drugs, and possibly thrombolysis, stent placements, or, in severe cases, coronary artery bypass. Between 20% and 30% of patients presenting to a hospital with a myocardial infarction have diabetes and benefit from all the above as well as rigid glucose control. Congestive heart failure with diastolic dysfunction and decreased left ventricular compliance is initially treated with ACE inhibitors, diuretics, and digoxin and, after stabilization, benefits from β-blockers and calcium channel blockers. Hypertension is present in greater than 70% of diabetics and is treated with weight loss, exercise, a low-sodium diet, cessation of smoking, and the use of antihypertensive medications. A low dose of a diuretic in combination with an ACE inhibitor and/or an angiotensin II receptor blocker are commonly initiated, with a calcium channel blocker, β-blocker, or α-blocker added, if necessary.

Diabetic autonomic neuropathy (DAN) can affect any part of the autonomic nervous system. Autonomic disturbances can be subclinical or clinical, with the former demonstrating abnormalities on quantitative function tests and the latter presenting with clinical signs and symptoms. Subclinical DAN can occur within a year or two after diagnosis, while clinical DAN does not develop for many years and depends on the duration of diabetes and the degree of metabolic control. Symptomatic autonomic neuropathy, excluding impotence, is rare and present in less than 5% of diabetics. The pathogenesis is not completely understood and may involve metabolic, microvascular, and/or autonomic etiologies. Intensive glycemic control is critical in preventing its onset and slowing its progression. Cardiovascular autonomic neuropathy is a common type of DAN and is characterized by abnormalities in heart rate control and central/peripheral vascular dynamics. A resting tachycardia and a loss of heart rate variability during deep breathing are early signs. A heart rate that fails to respond to exercise is indicative of significant cardiac denervation. Limited exercise tolerance results from impaired sympathetic and parasympathetic responses responsible for cardiac output and peripheral blood flow. The heart may demonstrate systolic and diastolic dysfunction with a reduced ejection fraction. Dysrhythmias may be responsible for an episode of sudden death. Patients with coronary artery disease may be asymptomatic during ischemic events. In its mildest form, patients demonstrate a resting tachycardia, and in the advance stages, severe orthostatic hypotension (>30 mm Hg with standing) is present. These changes result from damaged vasoconstrictor fibers, impaired baroreceptor function, and ineffective cardiovascular reactivity. The presence of cardiovascular autonomic neuropathy is demonstrated by testing cardiovascular reflexes and measuring a patient's resting heart rate, heart rate variability, response to a Valsalva maneuver, orthostatic changes in heart rate and systolic pressure, diastolic blood pressure response to sustained exercise, and the QT interval. In addition to cardiovascular effects, patients with DAN may demonstrate impaired respiratory reflexes and impaired ventilatory responses to hypoxia and hypercapnia.

Diabetic autonomic neuropathy can also affect every part of the gastrointestinal tract and may impair gastric secretion and gastric motility, causing gastroparesis diabeticorum in 25% of diabetics. Although clinically silent in many cases, symptomatic patients will have nausea, vomiting, early satiety, bloating, and epigastric pain. Treatment of gastroparesis includes strict blood glucose control, multiple small meals, reduced fat content in meals, and prokinetic agents such as metoclopramide. Diarrhea and constipation are also common among diabetics and may be related to DAN.

Awareness of hypoglycemia is particularly important for patients on intensive treatment programs with insulin. In most diabetics, low glucose levels stimulate catecholamine release, which produces hypoglycemic symptoms (diaphoresis, tremulousness), alerting the patient to treat. In DAN, the counterregulatory hormone responses are impaired and the warning signs eliminated, creating a dangerous situation of hypoglycemia unawareness.

Management of Anesthesia

The goals of anesthetic management of the diabetic patient include a thorough preoperative evaluation, an in-depth understanding of the pathophysiology of diabetes and the metabolic stress response, a significant knowledge and understanding of insulin, and possibly collaboration with the patient's internist/endocrinologist.

The stress response of surgery creates the classic hyperglycemic challenge. Activation of the sympathetic nervous system and release of catecholamines, cortisol, and growth hormone may be sufficient to convert a well-controlled diabetic to one with significant hyperglycemia and even ketoacidosis. In addition, surgery is associated with a reduction in insulin sensitivity (insulin resistance of surgery) in the periphery. A poorly controlled diabetic who is already in a catabolic state will experience profound metabolic effects from surgery and anesthesia. The magnitude of surgery is very important, with major surgery creating significant metabolic derangements and minor surgery demonstrating less risk. The effects of chronic hyperglycemia (coronary artery disease, myocardial infarction, congestive heart failure, peripheral vascular disease, hypertension, cerebrovascular accident, chronic renal failure, infection, neuropathy) are frequently present on preoperative evaluation and should be medically optimized before proceeding, but the effects of acute hyperglycemia are also dangerous and must be managed. Acute and chronic hyperglycemia appear to increase the risk of ischemic myocardial injury by decreasing coronary collateral blood flow and coronary vasodilator reserve, impairing coronary microcirculation, and causing endothelial dysfunction. Acute hyperglycemia causes dehydration, impaired wound healing, an increased rate of infection, worsening central nervous system/spinal cord injury with ischemia, and hyperviscosity with thrombogenesis. The possibility of infection (especially skin and soft tissue) and delay in wound healing result from a reduction in neutrophil number and function, impaired chemotaxis/phagocytosis, a reduction in capillary volume, a decrease in tensile wound strength, a decrease in fibroblast and collagen synthesis, and an increase in edema. Tight control of serum glucose in the perioperative period is important in managing the consequences of acute and chronic hyperglycemia.

Preoperative Evaluation

The preoperative evaluation should emphasize the cardiovascular, renal, neurologic, and musculoskeletal systems. A high index of suspicion should exist for myocardial ischemia and infarction. Silent ischemia is possible if an autonomic neuropathy is present. Stress testing should be considered if a patient exhibits two or more cardiac risk factors and is undergoing major surgery (see American Heart Association/American College of Cardiologists guidelines for specifics).

β_1-Antagonists should be used if coronary artery disease is present to decrease morbidity and mortality perioperatively. For renal disease, control of hypertension is a major priority, using ACE inhibitors. Meticulous attention to hydration status, avoiding nephrotoxins, and preserving renal blood flow are also essential. The presence of an autonomic neuropathy predisposes the patient to perioperative dysrhythmias and intraoperative hypotension, gastroparesis with possible aspiration, and hypoglycemia unawareness. The loss of compensatory sympathetic responses interferes with the detection and treatment of hemodynamic insults. Preoperative evaluation of the musculoskeletal system should focus on limited joint mobility of the neck from nonenzymatic glycosylation of proteins and abnormal cross-linking of collagen. Firm, woody, nonpitting edema of the posterior neck and upper back (scleredema of diabetes) coupled with impaired joint mobility limits complete range of motion of the neck and may render endotracheal intubation difficult.

Management of insulin in the preoperative period depends on the type of insulin that the patient takes and the timing of dosing (**Table 16-7**). If a patient takes subcutaneous insulin each night at bedtime, two thirds of this dose (NPH and regular) should be administered the night before surgery and one half of the usual morning NPH dose should be given on the day of surgery. The daily morning dose of regular insulin should be held. A 5% dextrose with 0.45% normal saline (D^5 ½ NS) intravenous infusion at 100 mL/hr should be initiated preoperatively. If the patient uses an insulin pump, the overnight rate should be decreased by 30% so that the patient receives 70% of the basal rate. On the morning of surgery, the pump can be kept infusing at the basal rate or discontinued and replaced with a continuous insulin infusion at the same rate, or the patient can be given subcutaneous glargine and the pump discontinued in 60 to 90 minutes. If the patient uses glargine and lispro or aspart for daily glycemic control, the patient should take two thirds of the glargine dose and the entire lispro or aspart dose the night before surgery and hold all morning dosing. Oral hypoglycemics should be discontinued 24 to 48 hours preoperatively. The sulfonylureas should also be avoided during the entire perioperative period since they block myocardial potassium adenosine triphosphate channels, which are responsible for ischemia- and anesthetic-induced preconditioning. Well-controlled type 2 diabetics do not require insulin for minor surgery. Poorly controlled type 2 diabetics and all type 1 diabetics having minor surgery and all diabetics having major surgery need insulin. For major surgery, if the serum glucose is greater than 270 mg/dL preoperatively, the surgery should be delayed while rapid control is achieved with intravenous insulin. If the serum glucose is greater than 400 mg/dL, the surgery should be postponed and the metabolic state restabilized.

Intraoperative Management

Aggressive glycemic control is important intraoperatively. Two major goals are to minimize hyperglycemia and avoid hypoglycemia. Ideally, a continuous infusion of insulin should be initiated at least 2 hours before surgery. A sliding scale with short-acting, subcutaneous insulin for glucose greater than 200 to 250 mg/dL is ineffective and should not be used. Intraoperative serum glucose levels should be maintained between 120 and 180 mg/dL. Levels above 200 mg/dL are likely to be detrimental in the perioperative period, causing glycosuria and dehydration and inhibiting phagocyte function and wound healing. Typically, one unit of insulin lowers glucose approximately 25 to 30 mg/dL. The initial hourly rate for a continuous insulin infusion is determined by dividing the total daily insulin requirement by 24. A typical rate is 0.02 U/kg per hour or 1.4 U/hr in a 70-kg patient. An insulin infusion can be prepared by mixing 100 units of regular insulin in 100 mL NS (1 U/mL). Insulin infusion requirements are higher for coronary artery bypass graft surgery (0.06 U/kg per hour), patients receiving steroids (0.04 U/kg per hour), patients with severe infection (0.04 U/kg per hour), and patients receiving hyperalimentation or vasopressor infusions. Insulin infusions should be accompanied by an infusion of D^5 ½ NS with 20 mEq KCl at 100 to 150 mL/hr to provide carbohydrate (at least 150 g/day) to inhibit hepatic glucose production and protein catabolism. Serum glucose should be monitored every hour and every 30 minutes for coronary artery bypass graft surgery or for patients with higher insulin requirements. Spot urine glucose monitoring is not reliable, although the urine can be tested for ketones if the glucose increases to more than 250 mg/dL. For serum glucose values less than 100 mg/dL, the D5 1/2 NS infusion rate should be 150 mL/hr; for 100 to 150 mg/dL, it should be 75 mL/hr; for 151 to 200 mg/dL, it should be 50 mL/hr, and for more than 200 mg/dL, a keep vein open (KVO) rate should be used.

Avoidance of hypoglycemia intraoperatively and postoperatively is especially critical since its recognition may be delayed by anesthetics, sedatives, analgesics, β-blockers, sympatholytics, and an autonomic neuropathy. Hypoglycemia is defined as a serum glucose less than 50 mg/dL in adults and 40 mg/dL in children. Treatment consists of 50 mL of 50% dextrose (i.e., D50), which increases the glucose 100 mg/dL or 2 mg/dL/mL.

Emergency Surgery

Emergency surgery places diabetics at risk of developing DKA or HHS. Surgery should be delayed for 4 to 6 hours to optimize the patient's metabolic status. DKA is more likely to develop in type 1 diabetics and is usually precipitated by infection, gastrointestinal obstruction, or trauma in the surgical patient. Patients present with hyperglycemia, hyperosmolarity, significant dehydration, ketosis, and acidosis. Severe dehydration is secondary to an osmotic diuresis, vomiting, hyperventilation, and reduced oral intake and can cause significant hypotension, circulatory shock, and acute tubular necrosis. Total body deficits of sodium and potassium are present, and frequently phosphate and magnesium deficits exist. Treatment includes large volumes of normal saline and insulin. An insulin bolus of 0.1 U/kg followed by an infusion of 0.1 U/kg

TABLE 16-7 Inpatient Insulin Algorithm

Goal BG: _____mg/dL
Standard Drip: Regular insulin 100 units/100 mL 0.9% NaCl via infusion device
Initiating the infusion
   Bolus dose: Regular insulin 0.1 unit/kg = _____units
   Algorithm 1: Start here for most patients.
   Algorithm 2: Start here if w/p CABG, s/p solid organ transplant or islet cell transplant, receiving glucocorticoids, vasopressors or diabetics receiving > 80 units/day of insulin as an outpatient

ALGORITHM 1		ALGORITHM 2		ALGORITHM 3		ALGORITHM 4	
BG	**Units/hr**	**BG**	**Units/hr**	**BG**	**Units/hr**	**BG**	**Units/hr**
< 60 = Hypoglycemia (See below for treatment)							
< 70	Off	< 70	Off	< 70	Off	< 70	Off
70–109	0.2	70–109	0.5	70–109	1	70–109	1.5
110–119	0.5	110–119	1	110–119	2	110–119	3
120–149	1	120–149	1.5	120–149	3	120–149	-5
150–179	1.5	150–179	2	150–179	4	150–179	7
180–209	2	180–209	3	180–209	5	180–209	9
210–239	2	210–239	4	210–239	6	210–239	12
240–269	3	240–269	5	240–269	8	240–269	16
270–299	3	270–299	6	270–299	10	270–299	20
300–329	4	300–329	7	300–329	12	300–329	24
330–359	4	330–359	8	330–359	14	> 330	28
> 360	6	> 360	12	> 360	16		

Moving from Algorithm to Algorithm
Moving up: An algorithm failure is defined as BG outside the goal range for 2 hours (see above goal), and the level does not change by at least 60 mg/dL within 1 hour.
Moving down: When BG is < 70 mg/dL for two checks **OR** if BG decreases by > 100 mg/dL in an hour.
Tube feeds or TPN: Decrease infusion by 50% if nutrition (tube feeds or TPN) is discontinued or significantly reduced. Reinstitute hourly BG checks every 4 hours.
Patient Monitoring
Check capillary BG every hour until it is within goal range for 4 hours, then decrease to every 2 hours for 4 hours, and if it remains at goal, may decrease to every 4 hours.
Treatment of Hypoglycemia (BG < 60 mg/dL)
Discontinue insulin drip
 and
Give D$_{50}$W IV
Patient conscious: 25 mL (½ amp)
Patient unconscious: 50 mL (1 amp)
Recheck BG every 20 minutes and repeat 25 minutes of D$_{50}$W IV if < 60 mg/dL. Restart drip once BG is > 70 mg/dL for two checks.
Restart drip with lower algorithm (see moving down)
Intravenous Fluids
 Most patients will need 5–10 g of glucose per hour (D$_5$W or D^5 ½ NS at 100–200 mL/hr or equivalent [TPN, enteral feeds])

BG, blood glucose; CABG, coronary artery bypass graft; TPN, total parenteral nutrition.

per hour is the initial prescription. Serum glucose is monitored hourly, and electrolytes are monitored every 2 hours. Potassium, magnesium, and phosphate deficits are replaced when urine production is documented. When serum glucose decreases to less than 250 mg/dL, intravenous fluids should include dextrose. Insulin is continued until acidosis resolves.

Sodium bicarbonate is not routinely given and is reserved for cases where the pH is less than 7.10.

HHS usually occurs in elderly, debilitated type 2 diabetics. These patients present with greater metabolic derangements than those with DKA and are severely dehydrated (~7–10 L), hyperosmolar (>320 mOsm/L), and hyperglycemic

(> 800–1000 mg/dL). They may present with confusion, focal central nervous system deficits, seizures, or coma. Surprisingly, electrolyte deficits (K^+, $PO4-$, Mg^{2+}) are less severe than in DKA. Treatment consists of larger volumes of normal saline and similar doses of insulin compared to patients with DKA. These patients are at significant risk of developing of cerebral edema and therefore correction of serum glucose and osmolarity should proceed gradually over a 12- to 24-hour period.

Postoperative Care

Aggressive insulin therapy in the intensive care unit (ICU) has demonstrated significant benefit in morbidity and mortality. Patients receiving conventional insulin therapy (serum glucose, 180–200 mg/dL) demonstrate significantly higher rates of ICU mortality, in-hospital mortality and morbidity including sepsis, renal failure, and anemia than patients who were tightly controlled (80–110 mg/dL). Possible reasons for improved outcome in the latter include better neutrophil and macrophage function, beneficial changes to mucosal/skin barriers, enhanced erythropoiesis, reduced cholestasis, improved respiratory muscle function, and decreased axonal degeneration.

The postoperative management of diabetics requires meticulous monitoring of insulin requirements. The predischarge 24-hour inpatient insulin requirement should be compared to the preoperative outpatient insulin dose. To determine the discharge dose, the total insulin (long, intermediate, short, rapid acting) dose for the most recent 24-hour period is calculated, and 50% of the discharge dose is prescribed as long- or intermediate-acting insulin and 50% as short- or rapid-acting insulin. If glargine is prescribed, it is usually given once at bedtime. If the patient takes intermediate-acting insulin twice daily, then two thirds of the dose should be taken in the morning and one third at bedtime.

Future Strategies for Treating Diabetes

At present, there are no established therapies to prevent or delay the onset of type 1 diabetes. The long prediabetic period gives hope that clinical disease might be delayed through therapies. Future strategies for managing type 1 diabetes include identifying patients at risk by genetic testing and altering risk factors, documenting and following patients prospectively in the prediabetic phase by identifying circulating autoantibodies and preventing the development or delaying progression of the disease or suppressing beta-cell destruction, and implementing biological approaches for patients with clinical disease such as islet cell transplantation, regeneration of beta cells, use of engineered beta cells, and insulin gene therapy. Future treatment options presently under investigation include noninjectable routes of insulin administration (inhaled, oral, nasal, transdermal), new injectable insulin formulations, an implantable artificial pancreas, implantable insulin pumps, and noninvasive continuous glucose sensors.

Future goals for the prevention of type 2 diabetes include identifying the responsible genes and understanding the mechanism of action to alter insulin secretion and action, and eliminating obesity. Emphasis on earlier diagnosis and treatment appears necessary, and resetting diagnostic criteria and treatment goals appears likely. Aggressive therapy with combinations of new oral agents to stimulate insulin action, overcome insulin resistance, and stimulate insulin secretion will be used.

INSULINOMA

Insulinomas are insulin-secreting tumors of pancreatic beta cells manifested clinically as fasting hypoglycemia. A failure of the plasma insulin concentration to decrease as the blood glucose concentration decreases is suggestive of the presence of an insulinoma. Diagnosis of inappropriate secretion of insulin by an islet cell tumor is difficult in the obese patient since obesity results in insulin resistance and in the need for increased circulating concentrations of this hormone. Approximately 10% of these tumors are malignant, metastasizing to the liver. Streptozotocin has activity against pancreatic beta cells and is used as palliative therapy for inoperable metastatic disease.

The principal challenge during anesthesia for surgical excision of an insulinoma is the maintenance of a normal blood glucose concentration. Profound hypoglycemia can occur, particularly during manipulation of the tumor, whereas marked hyperglycemia can follow successful surgical removal of the tumor. Nevertheless, a hyperglycemic response is both variable and unpredictable, making this observation an unreliable clinical indicator of the completeness of surgical removal of the tumor. An artificial pancreas that continuously analyzes the blood glucose concentration and automatically infuses insulin or glucose has been used for the intraoperative management of these patients. A blood glucose meter is necessary to permit frequent (every 15 minutes) measurement of the blood glucose concentration. Since evidence of hypoglycemia (hypertension, tachycardia, diaphoresis) may be masked during anesthesia, it is probably wise to include glucose in the intravenous fluids administered intraoperatively. The known ability of volatile anesthetics to inhibit insulin release is a theoretical advantage for the maintenance of anesthesia during surgical resection of an insulinoma, remembering that the efficacy of this effect is unproven in these patients. The minimum glucose level needed to maintain glucose transport across the blood-brain barrier and into brain cells is undefined. Some patients adapt to blood glucose concentrations as low as 40 mg/dL, whereas others could experience a hypoglycemic reaction when the blood glucose level is abruptly decreased from 300 mg/dL to 100 mg/dL.

THYROID DISEASE

The function of the thyroid gland is to secrete sufficient quantities of thyroid hormones to regulate cellular metabolism throughout the body. Patients may seek medical care for hyperfunctioning (hyperthyroidism) or hypofunctioning (hypothyroidism) of the thyroid gland. In addition, thyroid enlargement may accompany either condition or exist in the absence of any functional abnormality. To manage these patients effectively, the anesthesiologist should understand the anatomy and physiology of the thyroid gland and how to interpret thyroid function tests. He or she should have a thorough familiarity with the clinical presentation, diagnosis, treatment, and anesthetic implications of hyperthyroidism and thyroid storm and hypothyroidism and myxedema coma.

Anatomy and Physiology of the Thyroid Gland

The thyroid gland weighs approximately 20 g and is composed of two lobes joined by an isthmus. The gland is closely affixed to the anterior and lateral aspects of the trachea with the upper border of the isthmus located just below the cricoid cartilage. A pair of parathyroid glands is located on the posterior aspect of each lobe. A rich capillary network permeates the entire gland. The gland is innervated by the adrenergic and cholinergic nervous systems. A network of adrenergic fibers is associated with each thyroid cell, and adrenergic receptors are located in the cell membranes. The recurrent laryngeal nerve and external motor branch of the superior laryngeal nerve are in intimate proximity to the gland. Histologically, the thyroid is composed of numerous follicles filled with proteinaceous colloid. The major constituent of colloid is thyroglobulin, an iodinated glycoprotein, that serves as the substrate for thyroid hormone synthesis. The wall of each follicle is composed of cuboidal cells that become columnar with glandular stimulation. Twenty to 40 follicles form a lobule, and lobules are separated by connective tissue. The thyroid gland also contains parafollicular C cells, which produce calcitonin.

Normal quantities of thyroid hormones depend on exogenous iodine. The diet is the primary source of iodine, and in most areas of the United States, 500 μg is the average daily intake. The thyroid contains approximately 90% (i.e., 8000 μg) of the total iodine content in the body. Iodine is reduced to iodide in the gastrointestinal tract and rapidly absorbed into the blood (**Fig. 16-10**). Active transport of iodide from the plasma into the thyroid follicular cell is known as iodide trapping. Within the cell, iodide is converted to an oxidized form of iodine that is capable of combining with tyrosine residues of thyroglobulin. Peroxidase and hydrogen peroxide provide a potent oxidizing environment for this reaction. Each molecule of thyroglobulin contains approximately 140 tyrosine residues. Binding of iodine to thyroglobulin (i.e., organification) is catalyzed by an iodinase enzyme. Inactive monoiodotyrosine (MIT) and diiodotyrosine (DIT) are formed. Approximately 25% of the MIT and DIT undergo coupling (i.e., MIT + DIT = T_3 [3,5,3′-triiodothyronine {triiodothyronine}], DIT + DIT = T_4 [3,5,3′,5′-tetraiodothyronine {thyroxine}]) via thyroid peroxidase to form the active compounds T_3 and T_4. The remaining 75% never becomes hormones, and eventually the iodine is cleaved and recycled. T_3 and T_4 remain attached to thyroglobulin and are stored as colloid until they are released from thyroglobulin by hydrolysis by thyroid proteases and peptidases. Active hormones are released into the circulation, while unused iodotyrosines in the colloid undergo deiodination to yield free iodide for reuse. Since the thyroid contains a large store of hormones and has a low turnover rate, there is protection against depletion if synthesis is impaired or discontinued.

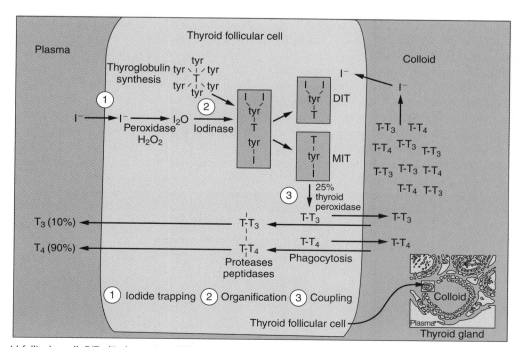

Figure 16-10 • Thyroid follicular cell. DIT, diiodotyrosine; MIT, monoiodotyrosine; T, thyroglobulin; T_3, 3,5,3′-triiodothyronine (triiodothyronine); T_4, 3,5,3′, 5′-tetraiodothyronine (thyroxine); tyr, tyrosine.

The T_4/T_3 ratio of secreted hormones is 10/1. Daily secretion of T_4 is approximately 80 to 100 µg. Upon entering the blood, T_4 and T_3 bind reversibly to three major proteins: thyroxine binding globulin (80% of binding), prealbumin (10%–15%), and albumin (5%–10%). Only the small amount of free fraction of hormone, however, is biologically active. The remainder serves as a metabolically inert reservoir. The elimination half-life ($T_{1/2}$) of T_4 is 7 to 8 days and the $T_{1/2}$ of T_3 is 3 days. Although only 10% of thyroid hormone secretion is T_3, T_3 is three to four times more active than T_4 per unit of weight and may be the only active thyroid hormone in peripheral tissues. The majority of T_3 (75%) is derived from monodeiodination of T_4 in the periphery. Ninety percent of thyroid hormone bound intracellularly is T_3 and 10% is T_4. Reverse T_3 is also formed in the peripheral tissues by monodeiodination but is metabolically inactive.

In the periphery, T_3 traverses cell membranes and binds to receptors in the cell nucleus, stimulating mRNA synthesis, which controls protein synthesis. Also, binding with mitochondria stimulates oxidative phosphorylation with adenosine triphosphate formation. At the plasma membrane level, T_3 influences transcellular flux of substrates and cations. Thyroid hormones stimulate virtually all metabolic processes, synthetic and catabolic. They influence growth and maturation of tissues, enhance tissue function, and stimulate protein synthesis and carbohydrate and lipid metabolism. Deiodinated pathways account for approximately 70% of the metabolism of T_3 and T_4. T_3 and T_4 are also conjugated in the liver with glucuronic acid and excreted into the bile.

Thyroid hormone acts directly on cardiac myocytes and vascular smooth muscle cells. In the heart, T_3 is transported via specific proteins across the myocyte cell membrane and enters the nucleus, binding to nuclear receptors, which bind to specific target genes. T_3-responsive genes code for structural and regulatory proteins (myosin, β-receptors, Ca^{2+} activated adenosine triphosphatase, phospholamban, and Ca^{2+}, Na^+, and K^+ channels) in the heart, which are important for systolic contractile function and diastolic relaxation. Thyroid hormone increases myocardial contractility directly, decreases systemic vascular resistance via direct vasodilation, and increases intravascular volume (**Table 16-8**). Ongoing research continues to evaluate the interaction of thyroid hormone with the autonomic nervous system. Most recent studies emphasize the direct effects of T_3 on the heart and vascular smooth muscle as responsible for the exaggerated hemodynamic effects of hyperthyroidism as opposed to a hyperactive sympathetic nervous system. Even though hyperthyroid patients appear to have increased numbers of β-receptors, these receptors demonstrate little or no increased sensitivity to adrenergic stimulation and surprisingly these patients have normal or low serum concentrations of catecholamines.

Regulation of thyroid function is controlled by the hypothalamus, pituitary, and thyroid glands, participating in a classic feedback control system. Thyrotropin-releasing hormone (TRH) is secreted from the hypothalamus, traverses the pituitary stalk, and promotes release of thyrotropin-stimulating hormone (TSH) from the anterior pituitary. TSH binds to specific receptors on the thyroid cell membrane and enhances all processes of synthesis and secretion of T_4 and T_3. TSH is the major regulator of thyroid structure and function. A decrease in TSH causes a reduction in synthesis and secretion of T_4 and T_3, a decrease in follicular cell size, and a decrease in the gland's vascularity. An increase in TSH yields an increase in hormone production and release and an increase in gland cellularity and vascularity. In addition to TRH, TSH secretion is influenced by plasma levels of T_4 and T_3. An increase in thyroid hormone release creates negative feedback within the thyrotropic cell in the pituitary, reducing TSH secretion. A decrease in thyroid hormone release promotes TSH secretion. In addition to the feedback system, the thyroid gland has an autoregulatory mechanism to maintain a consistent level of hormone stores. High organic iodine (i.e., bound to thyroglobulin) levels decrease iodide transport into the gland and low levels increase transport.

Diagnosis

Normal thyroid hormone levels do not exclude thyroid disease, and abnormal levels are not always indicative of disease. The laboratory tests most commonly used to evaluate thyroid function are serum free T_4 (F T_4) and serum TSH (**Table 16-9**). F T_4 is only approximately 0.02% of the total T_4. T_4 is a measurement of protein-bound and -unbound T_4. It is elevated in 90% of patients with hyperthyroidism and is low in 85% of patients with hypothyroidism. The T_3 resin uptake test (R T_3U), an indirect measure of the unbound fraction of T_4, is also used less frequently since an accurate test for F T_4 has been developed. The R T_3U test quantitates the degree of saturation of thyroxine-binding globulin sites by

TABLE 16-8 Cardiovascular Function and Thyroid Disease			
	Normal	**Hyperthyroidism**	**Hypothyroidism**
SVR (dyn-sec-cm^{-5})	1500–1700	700–1200	2100–2700
HR (bpm)	72–84	88–130	60–80
EF (%)	50–60	>60	<60
CO (L/min)	4.0–6.0	>7.0	<4.5
Blood volume (% of normal)	100	105.5	84.5

CO, cardiac output; EF, ejection fraction; HR, heart rate; SVR, systemic vascular resistance.
Adapted from Klein I, Ojamma K: Thyroid hormone and the cardiovascular system. N Engl J Med 2001;344:502.

TABLE 16-9 Thyroid Function Tests

Thyrotropin-stimulating hormone	0.4–5.0 mU/L
3,5,3′,5′-Tetraiodothyronine (thyroxine)	
Total	5.0–12.0 µg/dL
Freel	0.9–2.4 ng/dL
3,5,3′-Triiodothyronine (triiodothyronine)	70–195 ng/dL
Free thyroxine index	1.2–4.9
3,5,3′-Triiodothyronine uptake	24%–39%

T_4 and T_3. The resin uptake of radioactive T_3 is directly proportional to the fraction of F T_4 and inversely related to the thyroxine-binding globulin binding sites. Multiplying T_4 by the R T_3U gives the F T_4 index. The F T_4 index and free T_3 (F T_3) index are proportional to the F T_4 and F T_3. F T_3, total T_3, and F T_3 index are rarely used clinically.

The third generation of the TSH assay is now the single best test of thyroid hormone action at the cellular level. Small changes in thyroid function cause significant changes in TSH secretion. It is arguably the most significant advance in diagnosis and management of thyroid disease in the past decade. The normal level of TSH is 0.4 to 5.0 mU/L. A TSH level of 0.1 to 0.4 with normal levels of F T_3 and F T_4 is diagnostic of subclinical hyperthyroidism. A TSH level less than 0.03 mU/L with elevated T_3 and T_4 is diagnostic of overt hyperthyroidism. Thyroid storm may demonstrate TSH less than 0.01 mU/L. A TSH level of 5.0 to 10 mU/L with normal levels of F T_3 and F T_4 is diagnostic of subclinical hypothyroidism. A TSH level of more than 20 mU/L (may be as high as 200 or even 400 mU/L) with reduced levels of T_3 and T_4 is diagnostic of overt hypothyroidism.

Radioactive iodine uptake using ^{123}I, ^{131}I, or technetium-99 varies directly with the functional state of the thyroid. The percentage of tracer taken up by the thyroid in 24 hours is measured (normal range = 10%–25%). This test is usually used to confirm hyperthyroidism. The TRH stimulation test assesses the functional state of the TSH-secreting mechanism in response to TRH and is used to test pituitary function. Other tests that may be helpful include detection of serum antimicrosomal antibodies, antithyroglobulin antibodies, long-acting thyroid stimulator (LATS), thyroid-stimulating immunoglobulins, and thyroglobulin. Thyroid scans using ^{123}I or technetium-99m evaluate nodules as "warm" or normal, "hot" or hyperfunctioning, or "cold" or hypofunctioning. Ultrasonography is 90% to 95% accurate for determining whether a lesion is cystic, solid, or mixed.

Hyperthyroidism

Signs and Symptoms

Hyperthyroidism refers to hyperfunctioning of the thyroid gland with excessive secretion of active thyroid hormones. The majority of cases (i.e., 99%) of hyperthyroidism result from one of three pathologic processes: Graves' disease, toxic multinodular goiter, or a toxic adenoma. Regardless of the etiology, the signs and symptoms of hyperthyroidism are those of a hypermetabolic state. The patient is anxious, restless, and hyperkinetic and may be emotionally unstable. The skin is warm and moist, the face is flushed, the hair is fine, and the nails are soft and fragile. The eyes exhibit a wide-eyed stare with retraction of the upper eyelids. The patient may demonstrate increased sweating and complain of heat intolerance. Wasting, weakness, and fatigue of the proximal limb muscles is common. The patient usually complains of extreme fatigue but an inability to sleep. Increased bone turnover and osteoporosis may occur. A fine tremor of the hands and hyperactive tendon reflexes are common. Weight loss despite an increased appetite occurs secondary to increased calorigenesis. Bowel movements are frequent and diarrhea is not uncommon. The cardiovascular system is most threatened with hypermetabolism of peripheral tissues, increased cardiac work with tachycardia, arrhythmias (commonly atrial) and palpitations, a hyperdynamic circulation, increased myocardial contractility and cardiac output, and cardiomegaly. The etiology of cardiac responses is due to the direct effects of T_3 on the myocardium and the peripheral vasculature (see Table 16-8). Although cardiac failure rarely occurs, a thyrotoxic cardiomyopathy has been described with a lymphocytic and eosinophilic infiltration of the myocardium with fibrotic and fatty changes. Elderly patients with unexplained cardiac failure or rhythm disturbances, especially atrial in origin, should be evaluated for thyrotoxicosis.

Patients with subclinical hyperthyroidism are usually detected on routine laboratory screening. Most patients present with few if any signs or symptoms, although some may present with an elevated heart rate. Thyroid function tests reveal a normal T_3 and T_4 but a reduced TSH. Whether these patients should be treated is controversial. Benefits of treatment are not clearly established. If the TSH is between 0.1 and 0.5 mU/L, many clinicians will not treat. When the TSH drops below 0.1 mU/L, most patients receive treatment. Patients with subclinical hyperthyroidism are potentially at future risk of cardiac (atrial fibrillation) and central nervous system (emboli, cerebrovascular accident) complications.

Graves' disease or toxic diffuse goiter occurs in 0.4% of the United States population and is the leading cause of hyperthyroidism. The disease typically occurs in females (female-to-male ratio is 7:1) between the ages of 20 and 40 years. Although the etiology is unknown, Graves' disease appears to be a systemic autoimmune disease with thyroid-stimulating antibodies (long-acting thyroid stimulator, thyroid-stimulating immunoglobulins), binding to TSH receptors in the thyroid, activating adenyl cyclase and stimulating thyroid growth, vascularity, and hypersecretion of T_4 and T_3. The manifestations of the disease vary in intensity with the severity of the thyrotoxicosis, the age of the patient, the duration of the illness, and the involvement of other organ systems, especially cardiovascular. The disease is characterized by a classic triad of hyperthyroidism, exophthalmos, and dermopathy. The thyroid is usually diffusely enlarged, becoming two to three times normal size. Some glands secrete T_4 and T_3 at five to 15 times the normal amount. An ophthalmopathy occurs in

30% of cases and may include upper lid retraction, a wide-eyed stare, muscle weakness, proptosis, and an increase in intraocular pressure. Proptosis and muscle weakness are secondary to immunologic changes of extraocular muscles and retro-orbital tissues (i.e., edema, inflammation). When severe, the condition is termed malignant exophthalmos. Steroids, bilateral tarsorrhaphies, external radiation, or surgical decompression may be necessary in these cases. Fortunately, most cases are mild and follow a benign course and remit spontaneously. The dermopathy is characterized by edematous skin (pretibial myxedema) over the dorsum of the legs and feet and occurs in only 10% to 15% of cases.

Diagnosis

The diagnosis of Graves' disease is confirmed by elevated F T_4, T_3, F T_4 index, and R T_3U and an elevated radioactive iodine uptake. The TSH level is often low, and thyroid-stimulating antibodies are increased. In severe hyperthyroidism, the basal metabolic rate is markedly increased (30%–60%).

Toxic multinodular goiters usually arise from long-standing simple goiters and therefore occur mostly in patients older than 50 years of age. They may produce the most extreme thyroid enlargements, with some weighing more than 2000 g. They may cause dysphagia from esophageal compression, and a choking sensation and possibly inspiratory stridor from tracheal compression, especially with extension of the mass into the thoracic inlet behind the sternum. In severe cases, superior vena cava obstruction syndrome may also occur. However, hypermetabolism is usually less severe than with Graves' disease. There is no associated opthalmopathy or dermopathy. The diagnosis is confirmed by a thyroid scan demonstrating "hot" patchy foci throughout the gland or one or two "hot" nodules. Radioactive iodine uptake and serum T_4 and T_3 may only be slightly elevated. The goiter must be differentiated from a neoplasm, and a computed tomography (CT) scan and biopsy may be necessary.

A solitary toxic nodule (toxic adenoma) usually occurs in patients 30 to 40 years of age and may cause hyperthyroidism if the lesion exceeds 3 cm in diameter. The same diagnostic tests used for multinodular goiters are used for toxic adenomas.

An unusual presentation of thyrotoxicosis that may occur in association with Graves' disease, multinodular goiter, or toxic adenoma is T_3 toxicosis. In these patients, the serum T_4 and F T_4 are normal or low, while T_3 is increased. These patients may be more likely to have a long-term remission after withdrawal of antithyroid drug therapy than patients with the usual form of thyrotoxicosis in whom production of both T_4 and T_3 is increased.

Treatment

The first line of treatment for hyperthyroidism is the antithyroid drug propylthiouracil (PTU) or methimazole (Tapazole). Methimazole is currently more popular because of its faster response time and its ability to be administered as a single daily dose. These agents interfere with the synthesis of thyroid hormones by inhibiting organification and coupling. PTU has the added advantage of inhibiting the peripheral conversion of T_4 to T_3. PTU is prescribed for adults as 200 to 300 mg orally every 8 to 12 hours and methimazole as 10 to 20 mg orally every 12 hours. A euthyroid state can almost always be achieved in 6 to 8 weeks with either drug if a sufficient dose is given. The delay in effect is secondary to the large store of hormones existing in the gland prior to initiating therapy. Once euthyroidism is achieved, the dose is reduced and continued for 6 to 12 months and in some cases for 24 months. After euthyroidism has been achieved, a natural remission of the disease will often occur, but only less than 40% of patients remain well indefinitely after discontinuation of medication. Side effects occur in 3% to 12% of patients, with agranulocytosis being the most serious.

Iodide in high concentration inhibits release of hormones from the hyperfunctioning gland. Its effects occur immediately but last for only several weeks. Therefore, iodide is usually reserved for preparing hyperthyroid patients for surgery, managing patients with actual or impending thyroid storm, or treating patients with severe thyrocardiac disease. There is no need to delay surgery in an otherwise well-controlled thyrotoxic patient to initiate iodide therapy. High concentrations of iodide decrease all phases of thyroid synthesis and release and result in reduced gland size and possibly a decrease in vascularity. Iodide is administered orally as an SSKI (saturated solution of potassium iodide) solution, three drops orally every 8 hours for 10 to 14 days. Antithyroid drug therapy should precede the initiation of iodide because iodide alone will increase thyroid hormone stores and exacerbate the thyrotoxic state. Although parenteral NaI has been withdrawn from clinical use, oral iodide is equally efficacious. The radiographic contrast dye ipodate or iopanoic acid (0.5–3.0 g every day) contains iodide and demonstrates beneficial effects similar to those of inorganic iodide. In addition, ipodate inhibits the peripheral conversion of T_4 to T_3 and may also antagonize thyroid hormone binding to receptors. It is especially useful in the preoperative preparation of the thyrotoxic patient, reducing T_3 levels by 50% to 75% in 6 to 12 hours. Lithium carbonate 300 mg orally every 6 hours may be given in place of potassium iodide or ipodate if the patient is allergic to iodide.

β-Adrenergic antagonists do not affect the underlying thyroid pathology but may relieve signs and symptoms of increased adrenergic activity such as anxiety, sweating, heat intolerance, tremors, and tachycardia. Propranolol 40 to 80 mg orally every 6 to 8 hours, esmolol, metoprolol, and atenolol are effective. Propranolol has added features of impairing the peripheral conversion of T_4 to T_3 and reducing metabolic rate. For emergency use, intravenous propranolol in 0.2- to 1.0-mg boluses followed by an infusion or an intravenous esmolol 0.5 mg/kg bolus followed by an infusion is titrated to restore a normal heart rate.

Ablative therapy with radioactive ^{131}I or surgery is recommended for patients with Graves' disease in whom antithyroid drugs were ineffective or toxic or in whom a relapse occurred after 1 to 2 years of drug treatment and for patients with toxic multinodular goiter or a toxic adenoma. Also, patients who fail to follow medical regimens or fail to return for periodic examinations are candidates.

Radioactive ^{131}I therapy is the treatment of choice for hyperthyroidism in many large series because it is simple, effective, and economical. Standard doses deliver approximately 8500 rad to the thyroid and destroy the follicular cells. The remission rate is 80% to 98%. A major disadvantage of therapy is that 40% to 70% of treated patients become hypothyroid within 10 years. Patients are usually made euthyroid by antithyroid drugs prior to radioactive iodine therapy to avoid possible thyrotoxicosis from a radiation-induced thyroiditis. Radioactive iodine therapy has replaced subtotal thyroidectomy as the standard form of therapy for patients with Graves' disease requiring ablative therapy.

Surgery (i.e., subtotal thyroidectomy or possibly total thyroidectomy) results in prompt control of disease and a lower incidence of hypothyroidism (10%–30%) than radioactive iodine. Subtotal thyroidectomy corrects thyrotoxicosis in more than 95% of patients with a mortality rate of less than 0.1%. Complications from surgery are a major disadvantage of this form of therapy and include, in addition to hypothyroidism, hemorrhage with tracheal compression, unilateral or bilateral damage to the recurrent laryngeal nerve(s), damage to the motor branch of the superior laryngeal nerve, and damage to or inadvertent removal of the parathyroid glands.

Preparation of the hyperthyroid patient for surgery is extremely important. For elective surgery, all patients should be made euthyroid with a course of an antithyroid drug (PTU or methimazole) for 6 to 8 weeks preoperatively. A low TSH value should not be a contraindication to surgery. TSH values remain suppressed from prolonged hyperthyroidism in patients who have normalized T_3 and T_4 values. In addition, potassium iodide (SSKI solution) should be given for 7 to 14 days prior to surgery to reduce the gland's vascularity and hormonal release. β-Adrenergic blockers may be added in the preoperative period to control heart rate. Optimal patient response should dictate the timing of surgery.

For emergency surgery, an antithyroid drug (PTU or methimazole) should be administered even though it has a limited effect if taken for less than 2 weeks. No intravenous preparation is available, so the drug must be taken orally, via a nasogastric tube, or rectally. The antithyroid drug should precede iodide by 2 to 3 hours. Sodium iopanoate 500 mg orally twice daily and an intravenous β-blocker, preferably propranol, are essential for effective management. Glucocorticoids (dexamethasone 2 mg IV every 6 hours) should be administered to decrease hormone release and reduce the peripheral conversion of T_4 to T_3. This combination of medications is effective for any thyrotoxic patient presenting for thyroid or nonthyroid surgery. Euthyroidism can be achieved surprisingly quickly in approximately 5 to 7 days.

The treatment of hyperthyroidism during pregnancy includes low doses of antithyroid drugs. However, these drugs do cross the placenta and can cause fetal hypothyroidism. If the mother remains euthyroid on small doses of an antithyroid drug, the occurrence of fetal hypothyroidism is rare. Radioactive iodine treatment is contraindicated during pregnancy, and oral iodide therapy causes fetal goiter and hypothyroidism and is therefore contraindicated. The long-term use of propranolol is controversial since intrauterine growth retardation has been attributed to its use. Fortunately, pregnancy appears to attenuate the severity of hyperthyroidism and doses of antithyroid drugs can be kept low (i.e., PTU < 200 mg/day). If doses greater than 300 mg/day of PTU are needed during the first trimester, a subtotal thyroidectomy should be performed in the second trimester. Thyroid storm occurring in pregnancy is managed the same as in the nonpregnant patient.

Management of Anesthesia

In managing hyperthyroid patients for surgery, euthyroidism should definitely be established preoperatively. In elective cases, this may mean waiting a substantial time (6–8 weeks) for antithyroid drugs to become effective. In emergency cases, the use of an intravenous β-blocker, ipodate, cortisol, or dexamethasone and PTU is usually necessary. The anesthesiologist should be prepared to manage thyroid storm, especially in patients with uncontrolled or poorly controlled disease who present for emergency surgery. Premedication may include the use of a barbiturate, benzodiazepine, and/or a narcotic. Anticholinergic drugs (i.e., atropine) should be avoided since they may precipitate tachycardia and alter heat-regulating mechanisms. Intraoperatively, the need for invasive monitoring is determined on an individual basis and depends on the type of surgery to be performed and the medical condition of the patient. Controlled studies in hyperthyroid animals demonstrate no clinically significant increase in anesthetic requirements (i.e., minimum alveolar concentration, [MAC]). Establishing adequate anesthetic depth is extremely important to avoid exaggerated sympathetic nervous system (SNS) responses. Drugs that stimulate the SNS should be avoided (i.e., ketamine, pancuronium, atropine, ephedrine, epinephrine). No controlled patient studies have demonstrated one preferred anesthetic technique or anesthetic agent(s). For induction, thiopental, secondary to its thiourylene nucleus, decreases the peripheral conversion of T_4 to T_3 and may have a slight advantage over other induction agents. Succinylcholine and the nondepolarizing muscle relaxants with limited hemodynamic effects (e.g., vecuronium, rocuronium) have been used safely for intubation. Eye protection (eyedrops, lubricant, eye pads) is important, especially for patients with proptosis. For maintenance of anesthesia, any of the potent inhalation agents may be used. A concern in hyperthyroid patients is organ toxicity secondary to an increase in drug metabolism. Although animal studies demonstrate an increase in hepatotoxicity in hyperthyroid rats following exposure to isoflurane, no alterations in liver function have been demonstrated postoperatively in hyperthyroid patients rendered euthyroid preoperatively and administered this agent for surgery. Nitrous oxide and opioids are safe and effective in hyperthyroid patients. Muscle relaxants should be chosen based on their interaction with the SNS and their hemodynamic effects. Also, hyperthyroid patients may have co-existing muscle disease (e.g., myasthenia gravis) with reduced requirements for the nondepolarizing muscle relaxants necessitating careful titration to effect. Reversal of muscle relaxants should include glycopyrrolate instead of atropine in combination with an acetylcholinesterase inhibitor. For the treatment of intraoperative hypotension, a direct-acting vasopressor (phenylephrine) is preferred. Ephedrine, epinephrine, norepinephrine, and dopamine are avoided or administered in extremely low doses to prevent exaggerated hemodynamic responses. Regional anesthesia can be safely performed and in fact may be a preferred technique. Epinephrine containing local anesthetic solutions should be avoided. Fluids and phenylephrine are used to treat hypotension secondary to SNS blockade.

Removal of the thyrotoxic gland does not mean immediate resolution of thyrotoxicosis. The $T_{1/2}$ of T_4 is 7 to 8 days; therefore, β-blocker therapy may need to be continued in the postoperative period. Antithyroid drug therapy can be discontinued.

Thyroid storm and malignant hyperthermia can present with similar intraoperative and postoperative signs and symptoms (i.e., hyperpyrexia, tachycardia, hypermetabolism). Differentiation between the two may be extremely difficult. The preoperative detection of thyrotoxicosis (tremors, diaphoresis, fatigue, tachypnea, tachycardia, fever, an enlarged thyroid) is very important. Although thyrotoxicosis is an uncommon adult endocrine disorder, it is very rare in children. Regardless, thyrotoxicosis should be considered in the differential diagnosis of malignant hyperthermia in any age group.

Thyroid Storm

Thyroid storm is a life-threatening exacerbation of hyperthyroidism precipitated by trauma, infection, medical illness, or surgery. It is a clinical diagnosis. Thyroid function tests may not help in differentiating thyroid storm from symptomatic hyperthyroidism. Surprisingly, thyroid hormone levels may not be significantly higher than uncomplicated hyperthyroidism. It may be the acute, rapid increase in the plasma level that triggers the event. It most often occurs in the postoperative period in untreated or inadequately treated patients for emergency surgery. Patients present with extreme anxiety, fever, tachycardia, cardiovascular instability, and altered consciousness. The etiology is probably a shift from protein-bound thyroid hormone to free hormone secondary to circulating inhibitors to binding. Treatment includes rapid alleviation of thyrotoxicosis and general supportive care. Dehydration is managed with intravenous glucose containing crystalloid solutions, and cooling measures (e.g., cooling blanket, ice packs, cool humidified oxygen) are used to counter the fever. Necessary medications include propranolol, labetalol, or esmolol titrated to decrease heart rate to less than 90 bpm, and dexamethasone 2 mg every 6 hours or cortisol 100 to 200 mg every 8 hours. Antithyroid drugs (PTU 200–400 mg every 8 hours) may be administered through

a nasogastric tube, orally, or rectally. If circulatory shock is present, an intravenous direct vasopressor (phenylephrine) is indicated. A β-adrenergic blocker or digitalis is recommended for atrial fibrillation accompanied by a fast ventricular response. Serum thyroid hormone levels generally return to normal within 24 to 48 hours and recovery occurs within 1 week. Unfortunately, the mortality rate for thyroid storm remains surprisingly high at approximately 20%.

Hypothyroidism
Signs and Symptoms

Hypothyroidism or myxedema is a relatively common disease affecting 0.5% to 0.8% of the adult population. Primary hypothyroidism results in a decreased production of thyroid hormones despite adequate or increased levels of TSH and accounts for 95% of all cases of hypothyroidism. The most common cause in the United States is ablation of the gland by radioactive iodine or surgery. The second leading cause is idiopathic and probably autoimmune in origin, with autoantibodies blocking TSH receptors in the thyroid. Unlike Graves' disease, this immune response destroys receptors instead of stimulating them. Hashimoto's thyroiditis is autoimmune in origin and is characterized by goitrous enlargement and hypothyroidism in middle-aged women. Secondary hypothyroidism due to hypothalamic or pituitary disease accounts for 5% of cases of hypothyroidism.

In adults, hypothyroidism has a slow, insidious, progressive course. There is progressive slowing of mental and physical activity. In mild cases, patients tire easily and experience weight gain. In moderate to severe cases, patients develop fatigue, lethargy, apathy, and listlessness. Their speech becomes slow and their intellect becomes dull. With time, they experience cold intolerance, decreased sweating, constipation, menorrhagia, and slowing of motor function secondary to muscle stiffness and cramping. They gain weight despite a decrease in appetite. Physically, they demonstrate dry thickened skin, coarse facial features, dry brittle hair, a large tongue, a deep hoarse voice, and periorbital and peripheral edema. Accumulation of hydrophilic mucopolysaccharides in the dermis and other tissues is responsible for the immobile, nonpitting edema. Physiologically, cardiac output is decreased secondary to reductions in stroke volume and heart rate. Ventricular dysrhythmias may occur. Peripheral vascular resistance is increased and blood volume is reduced resulting in pale, cool skin (see Table 16-8). In advanced cases, myocardial contractility becomes reduced secondary to systolic and diastolic dysfunction, and the heart becomes enlarged and dilated (hypothyroid cardiomyopathy). Pericardial effusions are common. Baroreceptor function is also impaired. Hypothyroid patients usually have hypercholesterolemia and hypertriglyceridemia and may have coronary artery disease. The electrocardiogram in patients with overt hypothyroidism shows flattened or inverted T waves, low-amplitude P waves and QRS complexes, and sinus bradycardia. Hyponatremia and impairment of free water excretion are also common. Maximum breathing capacity and diffusion capacity are decreased, and ventilatory responsiveness to hypoxia and hypercarbia is depressed. Pleural effusions may result in dyspnea. Gastrointestinal function is slow, and an adynamic ileus may occur. Deep tendon reflexes demonstrate a prolonged relaxation phase.

Diagnosis

Diagnosis of primary hypothyroidism is confirmed by reduced levels of F T_4, T_4, T_3, R T_3U, and F T_4 index and an elevated TSH level. Subclinical hypothyroidism is more common than subclinical hyperthyroidism. Twenty percent of women older than 60 years of age have subclinical hypothyroidism. Like subclinical hyperthyroidism, it is associated with long-term cardiovascular consequences. Thyroid function tests demonstrate a normal T_4 and an elevated TSH from 5.0 to 10.0 mU/L (normal = 0.4–5.0 mU/L). Although most patients have few if any signs or symptoms, changes in myocardial structure and contractibility can occur secondary to systolic and diastolic dysfunction. Even though these changes are reversible with L-thyroxine, use of thyroid replacement remains controversial for subclinical disease. In mild hypothyroidism, patients have minor, nonspecific symptoms with a low or normal T_4 and a mean TSH of 18.0 mU/L. Overt hypothyroidism demonstrates obvious clinical signs and symptoms, a markedly low T_4, and a mean TSH of 90.0 mU/L. Basal metabolic rate may be decreased by 30% to 50%. Secondary hypothyroidism is diagnosed by reduced levels of F T_4, TSH, T_4, T_3, and R T_3U. A TRH stimulation test can confirm pituitary pathology as the cause. This test measures the responsiveness of the pituitary gland to intravenously administered TRH, the hypothalamic stimulator of TSH. In primary hypothyroidism, basal levels of TSH are elevated, and following TRH administration, the elevation is exaggerated. With pituitary dysfunction, there is a blunted or absent response to TRH.

Treatment

L-Thyroxine (levothyroxine sodium) is usually administered for the treatment of hypothyroidism. It has consistent potency, reliably restores levels of T_4 and T_3 to normal, and has a prolonged duration of action. L-Thyroxine has a gradual onset (6–12 hours), a peak effect in 10 to 12 days, and a $T_{1/2}$ of 7.5 days. L-Thyroxine 50 µg/day is the recommended starting dose with an increase to 100 µg/day within several weeks. A dose of 150 to 200 µg/day is sufficient to maintain a clinically euthyroid state. For the elderly or patients with coronary artery disease, 25 µg/day increasing monthly by 25-µg increments is recommended until euthyroidism is achieved. Patients with hypothyroid cardiomyopathy notice improvement in myocardial function in 2 to 4 months on 100 µg/day of L-thyroxine. A dose of 150 µg/day can reverse myocardial impairment and pericardial effusions. The first evidence of a therapeutic response to thyroid hormone is sodium and water diuresis and a reduction in the TSH level. Other alternative preparations include thyroid extract USP, L-triiodothyronine (liothyronine sodium), and liotrix, a combination

of T_4 and T_3 in a 4:1 ratio. Thyroid extract 60 mg is equivalent to 100 µg L-thyroxine, which is equivalent to 25 µg L-triiodothyronine. The optimal daily dose for each is based on clinical response and TSH or T_3 and T_4 levels. Although the combination of T_4 and T_3 has no advantages over T_4 alone in patients with primary hypothyroidism, a combination of T_4 and slow-release T_3 may yield better plasma levels and is recommended by some experts, although more studies are needed. This combination may more physiologically mimic normal thyroid gland secretion.

Management of Anesthesia

No studies have analyzed anesthetic requirements of hypothyroid patients, although by clinical observation, they appear to have an increased sensitivity to anesthetic drugs. The effect of thyroid activity on the MAC of potent inhalation agents is considered not to be clinically significant. Increased sensitivity is probably secondary to reduced cardiac output, decreased blood volume, abnormal baroreceptor function, decreased hepatic metabolism, and decreased renal excretion.

Hypothyroid patients may be at an increased risk when receiving either general or regional anesthesia for a number of reasons. Airway compromise secondary to a swollen oral cavity, edematous vocal cords, or goitrous enlargement may be present. Decreased gastric emptying increases the risk of regurgitation and aspiration. A hypodynamic cardiovascular system characterized by decreased cardiac output, stroke volume, heart rate, baroreceptor reflexes, and intravascular volume may be compromised by surgical stress and cardiac depressant anesthetic agents. Decreased ventilatory responsiveness to hypoxia and hypercarbia are enhanced by anesthetic agents. Hypothermia occurs quickly and is difficult to prevent and difficult to treat. Hematologic abnormalities such as anemia (25%–50% of patients) and platelet and coagulation factor (especially VIII) dysfunction, electrolyte imbalances (hyponatremia), and hypoglycemia are common and require close monitoring intraoperatively. Decreased neuromuscular excitability is enhanced by anesthetic drugs.

Despite these potential risks, patients with subclinical hypothyroidism usually present no anesthetic problems. Elective surgery can proceed without special preparation. Patients with mild to moderate disease should probably receive daily L-thyroxine (100–200 µg/day) in the preoperative period. If they do not receive preoperative thyroid supplementation, it is debatable as to whether they are at increased risk. Patients with overt disease are definitely at increased risk. Elective surgery is contraindicated until these patients are euthyroid. Decreased myocardial function and ventilatory drive return to normal within 3 to 6 months on L-thyroxine 150 µg/day. If emergency surgery is necessary, the potential for severe cardiovascular instability intraoperatively and myxedema coma in the postoperative period is high. If emergency surgery can be delayed for 24 to 48 hours, intravenous thyroid replacement therapy will be more effective. Although intravenous L-thyroxine takes 10 to 12 days to yield a peak basal metabolic rate, intravenous triiodothyronine is effective in 6 hours with a peak basal metabolic rate seen in 36 to 72 hours. L-Thyroxine 300 to 500 μg or L-triiodothyronine 25 to 50 μg intravenously are acceptable initial doses. Steroid coverage with hydrocortisone or dexamethasone is necessary since decreased adrenal cortical function often accompanies hypothyroidism. Phosphodiesterase inhibitors such as Milrinone may be effective in the treatment of reduced myocardial contractility since its mechanism of action does not depend on β-receptors, whose number and sensitivity may be reduced with hypothyroidism.

When managing hypothyroid patients for elective surgery, preoperative sedation should be avoided. These patients can be extremely sensitive to narcotics and sedatives and may even be lethargic secondary to their disease. Regional anesthesia is recommended if there are no contraindications (e.g., coagulation abnormalities) and the nature of the surgery permits it. Invasive monitoring is determined on an individual basis and depends on the type of surgery and the medical condition of the patient. Patients with a hypodynamic cardiovascular system frequently require intra-arterial blood pressure monitoring and a central venous pressure or pulmonary artery (Swan-Ganz) catheter or transesophageal echo to monitor intravascular volume and cardiac status. Dextrose in normal saline is the recommended intravenous fluid to avoid hypoglycemia and minimize hyponatremia secondary to impaired free water clearance. General anesthesia should be administered through an endotracheal tube following either a rapid sequence induction or an awake intubation if a difficult airway is present. Ketamine is the preferred induction agent since it will support blood pressure and heart rate if SNS activity is not impaired. Nitrous oxide may also be an effective induction agent. Barbiturates or benzodiazepines may be used; however, central nervous system and cardiovascular system depression is unpredictable and may be significant. Succinylcholine or the intermediate-acting nondepolarizing muscle relaxants can be used for intubation. For maintenance, nitrous oxide 70% with small doses of a short-acting opioid or benzodiazepine or ketamine, and an intermediate-acting nondepolarizing muscle relaxant (vecuronium, rocuronium) may offer an advantage. Hypothyroid patients are very sensitive to the myocardial depressant effects of the potent inhalation agents. Vasodilation in the presence of possible hypovolemia and impaired baroreceptor activity can produce significant hypotension. From a cardiovascular standpoint, pancuronium is a preferred muscle relaxant; however, reduced skeletal muscle activity in these patients coupled with a reduction in hepatic metabolism necessitates cautious dosing and close monitoring. Reversal of muscle relaxants is accomplished in the usual fashion with an acetylcholinesterase inhibitor and an anticholinergic agent. Controlled ventilation is recommended during all cases since these patients tend to hypoventilate if allowed to breathe spontaneously. Also, overventilation must be guarded against since metabolism is decreased and carbon dioxide production is reduced. Postoperative ventilatory support should be anticipated to manage possible delayed emergence. Pharmacologic support of intraoperative hypotension is best treated with ephedrine, dopamine, or epinephrine and not a pure α-adrenergic agonist (phenylephrine). Unresponsive hypotension may require supplemental steroid administration. Postoperative analgesia is best managed with regional techniques or small doses of opioids and/or ketorolac.

Patients with hypothyroidism and angina or other symptoms of coronary artery insufficiency present a unique circumstance. Historically, deliberate induction of hypothyroidism was a recognized therapy for some patients with incapacitating angina and relief was gained at the expense of symptomatic hypothyroidism. Although angina is uncommon in hypothyroidism, it can appear or worsen during treatment of the hypothyroid state with thyroid hormone. Medical management of such patients is particularly difficult. Therefore, patients presenting with both should have angiographic evaluation of the coronary arteries before hormone replacement is attempted. If surgically remediable disease is demonstrated, coronary artery bypass graft surgery can be successfully accomplished despite hypothyroidism. Coronary revascularization can permit the necessary thyroid hormone replacement and reinstitution of the euthyroid state.

Myxedema Coma

Myxedema coma is a rare severe form of hypothyroidism characterized by delirium or unconsciousness, hypoventilation, hypothermia (80% of patients), bradycardia, hypotension, and a severe dilutional hyponatremia. It occurs most commonly in elderly women with a long history of hypothyroidism. Ironically, most patients are not comatose. Hypothermia (as low as 80°F) is a cardinal feature and results from impaired thermoregulation from defective hypothalamic function (a target tissue of thyroid hormone). It is a medical emergency with a mortality rate greater than 50% and requires immediate aggressive treatment. Infection, trauma, cold, and central nervous system depressants predispose hypothyroid patients to myxedema coma. This is the one indication for intravenous thyroxine. L-Thyroxine in a 300- to 500-μg loading dose followed by a maintenance dose of 50 to 200 μg/day or L-triiodothyronine in a 25- to 50-μg loading dose followed by a maintenance infusion is recommended. L-Triiodothyronine has a more rapid onset and may be preferred. Administration of at least 65 μg/day in the initial days of therapy is associated with lower mortality. Combinations of T_4 and T_3 can also be used. Intravenous hydration with glucose-containing saline solutions, temperature regulation, correction of electrolyte imbalances, and stabilizing the cardiac and pulmonary systems are necessary. Mechanical ventilation is frequently necessary. Heart rate, blood pressure, and temperature usually improve within 24 hours, and a relative euthyroid state is achieved in 3 to 5 days. Intravenous hydrocortisone 100 to 300 mg/day is also prescribed to treat possible adrenal insufficiency (AI), a common sequela of hypothyroidism.

Euthyroid sick syndrome occurs in critically ill patients with significant nonthyroidal illness who demonstrate abnormal thyroid function tests. These tests demonstrate low levels of T_3 and T_4 and a normal TSH. As illness increases in severity, the T_3 and T_4 levels decrease further. The etiology of this response is not understood. Euthyroid sick syndrome may be a physiologic response to stress, and it can be induced by surgery. No treatment for thyroid function is necessary. Differentiating hypothyroidism from euthyroid sick syndrome is necessary and can be extremely difficult. A serum TSH level is the best aid. Levels greater than 10 mU/L indicate hypothyroidism, while levels less than 5.0 mU/L indicate euthyroidism. Values between 5 to 10 mU/L may represent mild hypothyroidism. Hypothyroidism is diagnosed by clinical signs and symptoms (dry skin, depressed deep tendon reflexes, bradycardia, hypothermia), reduced T_3 and T_4 levels, and an elevated TSH. Once diagnosed, hypothyroid patients should receive L-thyroxine.

Changes in thyroid function tests have also been documented following uncomplicated acute myocardial infarctions, congestive heart failure, and cardiopulmonary bypass. Significant depression of T_3 levels occurs, but the administration of T_3 does not appear efficacious. In addition, the use of T_3 as an inotrope has not demonstrated any significant or substantial improvement in cardiac performance.

Cretinism is extreme hypothyroidism that occurs during fetal life, infancy, and early childhood resulting in growth failure and mental retardation. The diagnosis must be made and treatment administered within a few weeks after birth to prevent organ damage.

Goiter

A goiter results from compensatory hypertrophy and hyperplasia of follicular epithelium secondary to a reduction in thyroid hormone output. The etiology may be a deficient intake of iodine, a dietary (i.e., cassava) or pharmacologic (i.e., phenylbutazone, lithium) goitrogen, or a defect in the hormonal biosynthetic pathway. The size of the goiter is determined by the level and duration of hormone insufficiency. In most cases, a goiter is associated with a euthyroid state with the increased mass and cellular activity eventually overcoming the impairment in hormone synthesis. However, hypothyroidism or hyperthyroidism occurs in some cases. Patients with simple, nontoxic goiter are euthyroid. Simple, nontoxic goiter is a forerunner of toxic multinodular goiter. In the United States, most cases of simple nontoxic goiter are of unknown etiology and are treated with L-thyroxine 100 μg/day, increasing to 150 to 200 μg/day with disappearance of the goiter in 3 to 6 months. Surgery is indicated only if medical therapy is ineffective and the goiter is compromising the airway or is cosmetically unacceptable.

Thyroid Tumors

Surgical resection of benign nodules or carcinomas rarely creates problems for the anesthesiologist. In the majority of these cases, the patient is euthyroid and the mass is relatively small. However, in some cases, the thyroid may be dangerously large and compromise the patients' airway. Hashimoto's thyroiditis

can be associated with a very large gland that may compress the trachea and esophagus, thereby creating difficulty with breathing and swallowing. Long-standing large multinodular goiters can present with airway compression and symptoms of respiratory compromise. A cervical goiter with substernal extension, although rare, frequently presents with life-threatening respiratory obstruction. Anaplastic carcinomas of the thyroid may be so invasive that removing tumor from the trachea or establishing a tracheostomy is all that can be done to relieve respiratory embarrassment.

The anesthetic management of a patient for surgical removal of a large thyroid mass that compromises the airway presents a major challenge. Examination of a CT scan of the neck will demonstrate anatomic abnormalities. Sedatives and narcotics should be avoided or used with great caution prior to and during endotracheal tube placement. Awake intubation with an armored (anode) tube using fiberoptic bronchoscopy is probably the safest method to assess the degree of obstruction and establish the airway. Surgical removal of the mass may reveal underlying tracheomalacia and a collapsible airway. Tracheal extubation should be performed with as much caution and concern as intubation.

If the mass extends into the substernal regional (i.e., anterior mediastinal mass), superior vena cava obstruction, major airway obstruction, and/or cardiac compression may occur. The latter two may become apparent only upon induction of general anesthesia. The etiology of airway obstruction appears to result from changes in lung and chest wall mechanics that occur with changes in patient position or with the onset of muscle paralysis. During spontaneous respiration, the larger airways are supported by negative intrathoracic pressure and the effects of extrinsic compression may be apparent in only the most severe cases. With cessation of spontaneous respiration, compensatory mechanisms are removed and airway obstruction may occur. In addition, positive pressure ventilation may demonstrate total airway occlusion. A preoperative history of dyspnea in the upright or supine position is predictive of possible airway obstruction during general anesthesia. A CT scan must be examined to assess the extent of the tumor. Flow volume loops in the upright and supine positions will demonstrate the site of obstruction and the degree of obstruction to airflow in the upper airway and trachea. Limitations in the inspiratory limb of the loop indicate extrathoracic airway obstruction, and delayed flow in the expiratory limb indicates intrathoracic obstruction. Echocardiography in the upright and supine positions will assess the degree of cardiac compression. If practical, local anesthesia is recommended in patients requiring surgery. If general anesthesia is necessary, preoperative shrinkage of the tumor by radiation or chemotherapy is recommended unless, in the case of a biopsy for diagnosis, the altered histologic appearance would prevent an accurate diagnosis. Unfortunately, goiters are not sensitive to radiation therapy. To manage such cases, an awake intubation with fiberoptic bronchoscopy using an anode tube is recommended. The patient is placed in the semi-Fowler's position and administered a volatile anesthetic with nitrous oxide and oxygen using spontaneous ventilation. Muscle relaxants are avoided. The ability to change the patient's position must be possible. Following tumor resection, the airway should be examined by fiberoptic bronchoscopy to detect tracheomalacia and determine whether and when tracheal extubation is appropriate. A rigid bronchoscope should be available to reestablish the airway if collapse occurs. Cardiopulmonary bypass should be on standby during the case.

Complications of Thyroid Surgery

Morbidity from thyroid surgery approaches 13%. Recurrent laryngeal nerve injury may be unilateral or bilateral and temporary or permanent. The injury may result from excess trauma to the nerve(s) (abductor and/or adductor fibers of the recurrent laryngeal nerve), inadvertent ligation, or transection. Paralysis of the abductor muscles to the vocal cords results in the involved cord assuming a median or paramedian position. If secondary to trauma and unilateral, the patient experiences hoarseness but no airway obstruction. Function usually returns in 3 to 6 months and invariably in 9 to 12 months. Ligation or transection results in permanent hoarseness. Bilateral involvement is more serious since the patient usually experiences airway obstruction and problems with coughing and respiratory toilet. A temporary or permanent tracheostomy, depending on the degree of damage, is usually necessary. Injury to the adductor fibers of the recurrent laryngeal nerve(s) (less common than injury to the abductor fibers) results in paralysis of the adductor muscle(s), and pulmonary aspiration is likely. The anesthesiologist must know whether injury to the recurrent laryngeal nerve(s) has occurred or is suspected in order to plan appropriately for emergence from anesthesia. Also, injury to the motor branch of the superior laryngeal nerve, which innervates the inferior pharyngeal constrictor and cricothyroid muscles, can occur during thyroid dissection. This injury limits the force of projection of one's voice and the ability to create high tones.

The most common etiology for hypoparathyroidism from thyroid surgery is damage to the blood supply of the parathyroid glands and not inadvertent removal. One functioning parathyroid gland with an adequate blood supply is all that is necessary to avoid hypoparathyroidism. The signs and symptoms of hypocalcium occur in the first 24 to 48 hours postoperatively. Anxiety, circumoral numbness, tingling of the fingertips, muscle cramping, and a positive Chvostek's sign and Trousseau's sign are indicative of hypocalcemia. Stridor can occur and can proceed to laryngospasm. Immediate treatment with intravenous calcium gluconate (1 g, 10 mL of a 10% solution) or calcium chloride (1 g, 10 mL of a 10% solution) is necessary. A continuous infusion of calcium for several days is also recommended. For long-term management, oral calcium and vitamin D_3 are prescribed or autotransplantation of parathyroid tissue may be performed.

Tracheal compression from an expanding hematoma may cause respiratory compromise in the immediate postoperative period. If bleeding occurs, it is usually from branches of the inferior thyroid or superior thyroid artery. If the rate of bleeding is such that surgical drains do not afford protection, swelling of the neck and bulging of the wound occurs demanding immediate attention. If untreated, respiratory compromise occurs. If time permits, the patient should be returned to the operating room for treatment. If necessary, the wound should be opened, clots evacuated, and bleeding vessels secured restoring a free airway at the bedside. Attempts at tracheal intubation are very difficult and time-consuming because of tracheal deviation and compression, and a frantic, hypoxic patient. Therefore, hematoma evacuation is the first line of treatment. A thyroid tray, including a tracheostomy set, should always be available at the bedside during the postoperative period to remove sutures/clips and open a wound emergently. Tracheostomy is not required, and in fact contraindicated, if the wound is decompressed early.

PHEOCHROMOCYTOMA

Pheochromocytomas are catecholamine-secreting tumors that arise from chromaffin cells of the sympathoadrenal system. Pheochromocytomas account for less than 0.1% of all cases of hypertension in adults. Although they are an uncommon cause of hypertension, their detection is imperative since they have lethal potential and are one of the few truly curable forms of hypertension. Uncontrolled catecholamine release can result in malignant hypertension, cerebrovascular accidents, and myocardial infarctions. They present a great challenge to anesthesiologists both in the operating room and in the ICU. Before diagnostic urine screening tests became available and prior to the institution of preoperative α-adrenergic blockade (i.e., early to mid 1960s), 25% to 50% of hospital deaths in patients with a pheochromocytoma occurred during the induction of anesthesia or during surgical procedures for unrelated disorders.

The precise etiology of a pheochromocytoma is unknown. Pheochromocytomas are usually (90%) an isolated finding. Ten percent of pheochromocytomas are inherited (familial) as an autosomal dominant trait. Both sexes are equally affected, and the tumor can present at any age with the peak incidence occurring in the third to fifth decades of life. Ten percent of pheochromocytomas occur in children. Variable clinical presentations are responsible for difficulties in diagnosis. Familial pheochromocytomas usually occur as bilateral adrenal tumors or as extra-adrenal tumors that appear in the same anatomic site over successive generations. Recent advances in genetic testing allow for early identification of patients with a familial pheochromocytoma before signs and symptoms occur. Familial pheochromocytomas can also be part of the multiple endocrine neoplastic syndromes and can occur in association with several neuroectodermal dysplasias. Patients with multiple endocrine neoplastic 2a syndrome have a pheochromocytoma, medullary carcinoma of the thyroid, and hyperparathyroidism. Patients with multiple endocrine neoplastic 2b syndrome have a pheochromocytoma, medullary carcinoma of the thyroid, alimentary tract ganglioneuromatosis, thickened corneal nerves, and a marfanoid habitus. In multiple endocrine neoplastic 2a and 2b syndromes, pheochromocytomas are usually located bilaterally in the adrenal glands and are seldom malignant. Almost 100% of patients with the multiple endocrine neoplastic 2 syndromes have or will develop bilateral benign adrenal medullary pheochromocytomas. Of the neuroectodermal dysplasias, 10% to 25% of patients with von Hippel-Lindau syndrome (i.e., hemangioblastoma of the cerebellum and a retinal angioma) may have a pheochromocytoma, less than 1% of patients with von Recklinghausen's disease (i.e., neurofibromatosis) have a pheochromocytoma, and patients with tuberous sclerosis and Sturge-Weber syndrome can have a pheochromocytoma.

Malignant spread usually proceeds via venous and lymphatic channels with a predilection for liver and bone, although spinal cord, lung, brain, and lymph nodes may also be affected. Metastatic spread from apparently benign primaries is well recognized. The incidence of malignancy is 10%, although improved diagnostic methods (i.e., ^{131}I-metaiodobenzylguanidine [MIBG] scintigraphy) may yield a higher rate in the future. The 5-year survival rate for patients with malignancy is 44%. Following resection of benign disease, 5% to 10% of patients have a benign recurrence.

Eighty percent of pheochromocytomas are located in the adrenal medulla. The right gland is involved more often than the left. Twenty percent of pheochromocytomas are extra-adrenal in location, with the majority being located in the abdomen in association with the sympathetic ganglia. The organ of Zuckerkandl near the aortic bifurcation is the most common extra-adrenal site. Two percent of extra-adrenal pheochromocytomas occur in the neck and thorax. Failure of involution of chromaffin tissue in childhood is the best explanation for the development of extra-adrenal pheochromocytomas. Contrary to previous beliefs, most extra-adrenal pheochromocytomas follow a benign course. Adult pheochromocytomas are solid, highly vascular tumors usually 3 to 5 cm in diameter and average 100 g in weight (range, 1.0–4000 g). The average-size adult pheochromocytoma contains 100 to 800 mg of norepinephrine.

Pheochromocytomas are tumors of the SNS. The SNS remains intact and active in the presence of these tumors. The manifestations of a pheochromocytoma are the result of the hormones released by the tumor. Most pheochromocytomas secrete norepinephrine either alone or more commonly combined with a smaller amount of epinephrine in a ratio of 85:15, the inverse of the ratio secreted by the normal adrenal gland. Approximately 15% of tumors secrete predominantly epinephrine. Some dopamine-secreting pheochromocytomas have been described. Most pheochromocytomas are not under neurogenic control and secrete catecholamines autonomously.

Signs and Symptoms

Hypertension, continuous or paroxysmal, is the most frequent manifestation of the disease. Headache, sweating, pallor, and palpitations are other classic signs and symptoms. Most patients are symptomatic, and attacks range from infrequent (i.e., once a month or less) to numerous (i.e., many times per day) and may last from less than a minute to several hours. They may occur spontaneously or be precipitated by physical stimuli, psychic stimuli, or medications. Hypertension is present in more than 80% of adult patients. Paroxysmal hypertension associated with a normal blood pressure between crises occurs in 50% of patients. Thirty percent of patients will have sustained hypertension. Twenty-four–hour ambulatory blood pressure monitoring has shown that many crises are asymptomatic. Orthostatic hypotension is also a common finding and considered to be secondary to hypovolemia and impaired venous and arterial vasoconstrictor reflex responses. Hemodynamic signs depend on the predominant catecholamine secreted. With norepinephrine, α-adrenergic effects predominate, and patients usually have systolic and diastolic hypertension and a reflex bradycardia. With epinephrine, β-adrenergic effects predominate, and patients usually have systolic hypertension, diastolic hypotension, and tachycardia. Some patients remain normotensive in spite of high levels of circulating norepinephrine. The regulation of blood pressure in pheochromocytoma patients appears more complex than traditional views suggest. The extent of increases in arterial blood pressure appears to have little relation to the prevailing levels of circulating catecholamines. An imbalance between endogenous vasodilators (i.e., dopamine, serotonin, enkephalins, and vasoactive intestinal peptide) and circulating catecholamines may account for this. Despite the 10-fold higher levels of circulating catecholamines, the hemodynamics are not greatly different between patients with pheochromocytomas and patients with essential hypertension. Both groups have an increased systemic vascular resistance, usually a normal cardiac output, and a slightly decreased plasma volume. Long-term exposure to high levels of catecholamines does not appear to produce hemodynamic responses characteristic of acute administration. A desensitization of the cardiovascular system or a down-regulation of adrenergic receptors may explain this finding. The sensitivity of smooth muscle cells is decreased secondary to a decrease in the number of receptors or an alteration in receptor-effector coupling. The hypertensive crises do, however, mimic the hemodynamic responses of acute catecholamine administration. Blood vessels of pheochromocytoma patients usually require extremely high concentrations of catecholamines to constrict and produce hypertension.

A catecholamine-induced cardiomyopathy may also occur. The true incidence of clinically significant cardiomyopathies is unclear. A global reduction in myocardial pump function results from the net reduction in viable myofibrils and the down-regulation of β-receptors. The etiology appears multifactorial and includes catecholamine-induced permeability changes of the sarcolemmal membranes leading to excess calcium influx, toxicity from oxidized products of catecholamines, and damage by free radicals. In addition, high catecholamine levels affect the heart via coronary vasoconstriction through α-adrenergic pathways reducing coronary blood flow and potentially creating ischemia. Both dilated and hypertrophic cardiomyopathies, as well as left ventricular outflow tract obstruction, have been demonstrated echocardiographically. Echocardiographic findings are usually normal in patients without cardiac symptoms (dyspnea, chest pain) or other clinical evidence of cardiac involvement. Electrocardiogram abnormalities may include elevation or depression of the ST segment, flattening or inversion of T waves, prolongation of the QT interval, high or peaked P waves, left axis deviation, and arrhythmias. These changes are usually transient, diffuse, variable, and normalize with α- and/or β-blockade. The cardiomyopathy appears reversible if catecholamine stimulation is removed early before fibrosis has occurred. Distinct from a cardiomyopathy, pheochromocytoma patients may develop cardiac hypertrophy with congestive heart failure secondary to sustained hypertension.

Since pheochromocytomas are notoriously variable in their secretory activity, they have been called "great mimics," and their presentation may be confused with thyrotoxicosis, malignant hypertension, diabetes mellitus, malignant carcinoid syndrome, or gram-negative septicemia. Although pheochromocytoma patients rarely have frank diabetes, most have an elevated blood glucose level secondary to catecholamine stimulation of glycogenolysis and an inhibition of insulin release.

Diagnosis

When a pheochromocytoma is clinically suspected, excess catecholamine secretion must be demonstrated. Various diagnostic tests have been suggested, but none is ideal. Regardless of which test is chosen, the clinical circumstances must be strictly controlled (i.e., for posture, exercise, emotion, medications) to yield reliable results. Concomitant medical conditions (i.e., alcoholism, hypothyroidism, hypovolemia) may yield misleading results.

The most sensitive test for high-risk patients (familial pheochromocytoma or classic symptoms) is plasma-free metanephrines. Catecholamines are metabolized to free metanephrines within tumor cells, and these metabolites are continuously released into the circulation. Plasma free normetanephrine greater than 400 pg/mL and/or metanephrine greater than 220 pg/mL is diagnostic of a pheochromocytoma. If normetanephrine is 112 to 400 pg/mL or metanephrine is 61 to 220 pg/mL, the diagnosis is equivocal. A pheochromocytoma is excluded if normetanephrine is less than 112 pg/mL and metanephrine is less than 61 pg/mL.

The determination of elevated urinary free catecholamine levels and their metabolites (i.e., metanephrine, normetanephrine, vanillylmandelic acid) is a frequently used diagnostic test. It is easy to perform and readily available; however, 24-hour collections can be inconvenient and unreliable. Measurement of vanillylmandelic acid is the oldest and least expensive test, but it is nonspecific. The determination of elevated metanephrines is the single best urine screening test. For patients with a low probability of having a pheochromocytoma, a 24-hour urine for metanephrines and catecholamines is sufficient.

Precisely executed measurement of plasma catecholamines is a favored initial test by many experts. The majority of patients have a significant elevation of norepinephrine, epinephrine, or both, although some patients with a pheochromocytoma have normal levels at rest. Plasma concentrations of total catecholamines greater than 2000 pg/mL are diagnostic of a pheochromocytoma. Values between 500 and 2000 pg/mL are equivocal, and 500 pg/mL or less rules out the diagnosis. In the majority of cases, the demonstration of increased levels of either plasma catecholamines or urinary free catecholamines and their metabolites should suffice to make the diagnosis. Results are equivocal in 5% to 10% of patients, and in these cases, the clonidine suppression test may be used. Clonidine is an α₂-agonist that acts on the central nervous system to diminish efferent sympathetic outflow. In patients with a pheochromocytoma, increased plasma catecholamines result from tumor release, bypassing normal storage and release mechanisms. Clonidine acts to lower plasma catecholamines in patients without a pheochromocytoma while having no effect on catecholamine levels in pheochromocytoma patients.

In the past, provocative testing with histamine and tyramine was used to elicit excess catecholamine release from the tumor. However, the incidence of morbidity was considered too high, and these tests have been abandoned. A glucagon stimulation test is now considered to be the safest and most specific provocative test. Glucagon acts directly on the tumor to release catecholamines. This test is limited to patients with a diastolic blood pressure of less than 100 mm Hg. A positive test yields a plasma catecholamine increase of at least three times the baseline values or more than 2000 pg/mL within 1 to 3 minutes of glucagon administration. At present, most centers diagnose a pheochromocytoma by urine testing for free catecholamines and their metabolites and/or measuring plasma catecholamines and add the clonidine suppression test and/or the glucagon stimulation test in equivocal cases. Of these tests, which is the single most reliable one remains controversial.

Tumor location can be predicted by the pattern of catecholamine production (**Table 16-10**). Specific radiographic tests can pinpoint the location. CT and MRI are the optimal noninvasive anatomic adrenal imaging studies. CT detects more than 95% of adrenal masses greater than 1.0 cm in diameter.

TABLE 16-10	Pattern of Catecholamine Production and Tumor Site		
	Adrenal	**Extra-adrenal**	**Adrenal + Extra-adrenal**
Norepinephrine	61%	31%	8%
Epinephrine	100%	—	—
Norepinephrine + epinephrine	95%	—	5%
Adapted from Kaser H: Clinical and diagnostic findings in patients with chromaffin tumors: Pheochromocytomas, pheochromoblastomas. Recent Results Cancer Res 1990;118:97–105.			

MRI offers advantages over CT that include better differentiation of small adrenal lesions, better differentiation among different types of adrenal lesions, no intravenous contrast is needed, and no radiation exposure occurs. With certain MRI sequences, pheochromocytomas have high signal intensity and light up brightly. In contrast to CT and MRI, which provide primarily anatomic information,[131]I-MIBG and ^{123}I-MIBG provide functional information. MIBG is an analogue of guanethidine, similar in structure to norepinephrine, and taken up by adrenergic neurons and concentrated in catecholamine-secreting tumors. MIBG is detected by scintigraphy. This is a physiologic test that localizes based on pharmacologic activity. It is especially useful in detecting extra-adrenal pheochromocytomas, metastatic deposits, and confirming that an adrenal mass is a functional pheochromocytoma. MIBG can screen the entire body with exquisite contrast and is the initial localizing procedure of choice at many institutions. CT, MRI, and ^{131}I-MIBG scintigraphy are complementary studies in localizing pheochromocytomas. A positron emission scan and selective venous catheterization with sampling of catecholamines from the adrenal vein and other sites are other useful tests.

Management of Anesthesia
Preoperative Management

There are no controlled, randomized, prospective clinical studies on the value of adrenergic blockade for pheochromocytoma patients in the perioperative period. However, following the introduction of α-adrenergic blockers during the preoperative period, the mortality from excision of a pheochromocytoma decreased from 40% to 60% in 1951 to 0% to 6% in 1967. Some authors attribute this result more to advances in anesthetic techniques, monitoring techniques, and the availability of fast-acting medications than to the use of α-blockers. Since most pheochromocytomas secrete predominantly norepinephrine, medical therapy has depended on α-blockade to lower blood pressure, increase intravascular volume, prevent paroxysmal hypertensive episodes, allow resensitization of adrenergic receptors, and decrease myocardial dysfunction. Although a significantly reduced intravascular volume may accompany a pheochromocytoma, the majority of patients have a normal or only slightly decreased intravascular volume. α-Blockade appears to protect myocardial performance and tissue oxygenation from adverse catecholamine effects.

Phenoxybenzamine is the most frequently prescribed α-blocker for preoperative use. It is a noncompetitive α_1-antagonist with some α_2-blocking properties. As a noncompetitive blocker, it is difficult for excess catecholamines to overcome the blockade. Its long duration of action permits oral dosing only twice daily. The usual starting regimen is 10 to 20 mg twice daily, with most patients requiring 60 to 250 mg/day. The goal of therapy is normotension, a resolution of symptoms, elimination of ST-T changes on the electrocardiogram, and elimination of arrhythmias. Overtreatment can result in severe orthostatic hypotension. The optimal duration of α-blockade therapy is undetermined and may range from 3 days to 2 weeks or longer. Because of its prolonged effect on α-receptors, it has been recommended to discontinue it 24 to 48 hours before surgery to avoid vascular unresponsiveness immediately following removal of the tumor. Some anesthesiologists administer only one half to two thirds of the morning dose preceding surgery to address similar concerns. Some surgeons request its discontinuation 48 hours preoperatively to allow them to use hypertensive episodes intraoperatively as cues to localize areas of metastasis. However, regardless of the completeness of α-blockade preoperatively, significant hypertension usually occurs with manipulation of the tumor. Unfortunately, being an $\alpha_{1,2}$-blocker, phenoxybenzamine may enhance catecholamine secretion through α_2-blockade, which will result in tachycardia.

Prazocin, a pure α_1-competitive blocker, can be used instead of phenoxybenzamine. It is shorter acting, causes less tachycardia, and is easier to titrate to a desired end point than phenoxybenzamine. Initial doses of 1.0 mg three times daily may be increased to 8 to 12 mg/day to obtain the desired effect. It has been criticized for its failure to prevent hypertensive episodes adequately in the preoperative period, although it has strong advocates. Other α_1-blockers include doxazosin and terazosin. Doxazosin at doses of 2 to 6 mg/day may be as effective in controlling hypertension as phenoxybenzamine and causes fewer side effects before (tachycardia) and after (hypotension) surgical removal.

If tachycardia (i.e., heart rates > 120 bpm) or other arrhythmias result following α_2-blockade from phenoxybenzamine, a β-adrenergic blocker is prescribed. A nonselective β-blocker should never be administered prior to α-blockade because blockade of vasodilatory β_2-receptors results in unopposed α-agonism, resulting in vasoconstriction and hypertensive crises. Propranolol, a nonselective $\beta_{1,2}$-blocker with a half-life greater than 4 hours, is most frequently used. Most patients require 80 to 120 mg/day. In some patients with epinephrine-secreting pheochromocytomas, doses up to 480 mg/day may be needed. β-Blockers must be used cautiously since a small but significant number of patients have an underlying cardiomyopathy and congestive heart failure may be precipitated. Atenolol, metoprolol, and labetalol have been used successfully, although experience is limited and complications have been reported with the latter. The degree of α- and β-blockade provided by labetalol (i.e., β effects exceed α effects) may not be appropriate for certain pheochromocytoma patients. In very rare circumstances, β-blockade has been selected before α-blockade. A patient with a solely epinephrine-secreting pheochromocytoma and coronary artery disease may benefit greatly from the β_1-selective agent esmolol. Esmolol has a fast onset and short elimination half-life and can be administered intravenously in the immediate preoperative period.

α-Methylparatyrosine (metyrosine) inhibits the rate-limiting enzyme tyrosine hydroxylase of the catecholamine synthetic pathway and may decrease catecholamine production by 50% to 80%. Usual doses range from 250 mg twice daily to 3 to 4 g/day. It is especially useful for malignant and inoperable tumors. Side effects including extrapyramidal reactions and crystalluria have limited its use. In combination with phenoxybenzamine during the preoperative period, it has been shown to facilitate intraoperative hemodynamic management.

The calcium channel blockers and the ACE inhibitors may be used to control hypertension. Calcium is a trigger for catecholamine release from the tumor and excess calcium entry into myocardial cells contributes to the catecholamine mediated cardiomyopathy. Nifedipine, diltiazem, and verapamil have all been used to control preoperative hypertension as has captopril, the ACE inhibitor. An α_1-blocker plus a calcium channel blocker (verapamil 120–240 mg every day or nifedipine 30–90 mg every day) is an effective combination for resistant cases.

Intraoperative Management

Elective surgery is recommended whenever possible. Optimal preparation with α-adrenergic blockade $\pm$ β-blockade $\pm$ α-methylparatyrosine and correction of possible hypovolemia are essential. Intraoperative goals include avoiding drugs or maneuvers that may provoke catecholamine release or potentiate catecholamine actions and maintaining cardiovascular stability, preferably with short-acting drugs. The periods of greatest danger occur secondary to hypertension and/or arrhythmias during anesthetic induction, intubation, surgical incision, abdominal exploration and particularly during tumor manipulation, and secondary to hypotension following ligation of the tumor's venous drainage. Intraoperative monitoring should include standard monitoring devices plus an arterial catheter, a central venous pressure or pulmonary arterial catheter, and a urinary catheter. If available, transesophageal echocardiography provides additional valuable information on myocardial function. An arterial catheter enables monitoring of blood pressure on a beat-to-beat basis in addition to drawing arterial blood for necessary laboratory tests (e.g., hematocrit/hemoglobin, arterial blood gases, glucose). A central venous pressure catheter is usually sufficient for patients without cardiac symptoms or other clinical evidence of cardiac involvement. A pulmonary artery catheter may be necessary to manage the large fluid requirements, major volume shifts, and possible underlying myocardial dysfunction in patients with very active tumors. Significant fluid requirements needed to prevent hypotension after tumor removal may indicate altered pressure-volume relationships induced by sudden catecholamine withdrawal. A large positive fluid balance is usually required to keep intravascular volumes within a normal range.

Intraoperative ultrasonography can be used to localize small, functional tumors and to perform adrenal-sparing procedures or partial adrenalectomies. Adrenal-sparing procedures are particularly valuable when removing bilateral adrenal pheochromocytomas. Laparoscopy can be used for tumors less than 4 to 5 cm in size. Hypertension frequently occurs during pneumoperitoneum as well as during adrenal manipulation.

Virtually every anesthetic technique for pheochromocytoma resection has been advocated or discredited based on anecdotal reports. Both general $\pm$ regional anesthesia have been successfully administered. Medications can cause a hypertensive response via (1) direct stimulation of tumor cells, (2) stimulation of the SNS, (3) release of accumulated catecholamine stores in nerve endings, (4) interfering with neuronal uptake of catecholamines, and (5) inducing hypersensitivity of catecholamine receptors or potentiating the effect of catecholamines on arterioles. Although all anesthetic drugs have been used with some degree of success, certain drugs should theoretically be avoided to prevent possible adverse hemodynamic responses. Morphine and atracurium can cause histamine release, which may provoke release of catecholamines from the tumor. Atropine, pancuronium, and succinylcholine are examples of vagolytic or sympathomimetic drugs that may stimulate the SNS. Although halothane in high concentrations is effective in attenuating hemodynamic responses (i.e., hypertension, tachycardia) to anesthetic and surgical stimuli, it sensitizes the myocardium to catecholamines and should probably be avoided. Droperidol, chlorpromazine, metoclopramide, and ephedrine have all created significant hypertensive responses. Anesthetic drugs that appear safe include thiopental, etomidate, benzodiazepines, fentanyl, sufentanil, alfentanil, enflurane, isoflurane, nitrous oxide, vecuronium, and rocuronium. Despite these recommendations, the choice of anesthetic is not as crucial as the understanding with which the agents are used. Factors that stimulate catecholamine release such as fear, stress, pain, shivering, hypoxia, and hypercarbia must be minimized or avoided in the perioperative period.

Virtually all patients exhibit increases in systolic arterial pressure in excess of 200 mm Hg for periods of time intraoperatively irrespective of preoperative α-blockade. A number of antihypertensive drugs must be prepared and ready for immediate administration. Sodium nitroprusside, a direct vasodilator, is the agent of choice because of its potency, immediate onset of action, and short duration of action. Phentolamine, a competitive α-adrenergic blocker and a direct vasodilator, is effective, although tachyphylaxis and tachycardia are associated with its use. Nitroglycerin is effective but is required in large doses to control significant hypertensive episodes and may also cause tachycardia. Labetalol, with more β- than α-blocking properties, is preferred for predominantly epinephrine-secreting tumors. Magnesium sulfate inhibits release of catecholamines from the adrenal medulla and peripheral nerve terminals, reduces sensitivity of α-receptors to catechols, is a direct vasodilator, and is an antiarrhythmic. However, like all antihypertensive medications, it is suboptimal in controlling hypertension during tumor manipulation. Mixtures of antihypertensive drugs such as nitroprusside, esmolol, diltiazem, and phentolamine have been recommended to control refractory hypertension. Increasing the depth of anesthesia is also an option, although this approach may accentuate the hypotension accompanying tumor vein ligation.

Arrhythmias are usually ventricular in origin and managed with either lidocaine or β-blockers. Lidocaine is short acting and has minimal negative inotropic action. Although propranolol has been widely used, esmolol, a selective β_1-blocker, offers several advantages. Esmolol has a rapid onset and is short acting (i.e., elimination half-life of 9 minutes), allowing adequate control of heart rate, and may also provide protection against catecholamine-induced cardiomyopathy and ischemia and the development of postoperative hypoglycemia. Amiodarone, an antiarrhythmic agent that prolongs the duration of the action potential of atrial and ventricular muscle, has been used as an alternative to β-blockers (metoprolol) to treat supraventricular tachycardia associated with hypercatecholaminemia.

Hypotension following tumor vein ligation is usually significant and occurs secondary to a combination of factors including an immediate decrease in plasma catecholamines (i.e., half-lives of norepinephrine and epinephrine are approximately 1–2 minutes), vasodilation from residual α-blockade with phenoxybenzamine, intraoperative fluid and blood loss, and increased anesthetic depth. Hypotension with systolic pressures in the 70s is not infrequent. To prevent precipitous hypotension, volume expansion to a pulmonary capillary wedge pressure of 16 to 18 mm Hg should be attained prior to tumor vein ligation. Lactated Ringer's solution or physiologic saline are the recommended fluids for use prior to tumor removal and a dextrose-containing solution should be added after tumor removal. A decrease in anesthetic depth will also aid in controlling hypotension. With a decrease in plasma catecholamines immediately following resection, insulin levels increase and hypoglycemia may occur. Fortunately, significant blood loss is unusual during resection of most intra-abdominal pheochromocytomas. Intraoperative blood salvage resulting in post-resection hypertension secondary to catecholamine-laden blood has been reported. Vasopressors (e.g., phenylephrine, norepinephrine) and inotropes (e.g., dopamine) should be ready for administration if hypotension is slow to respond to fluid resuscitation. Adequate fluid therapy is essential and is the major factor responsible for the reduction (i.e., < 2%) in operative mortality. Vasopressors and inotropes should be viewed as a secondary treatment modality. Residual α-adrenergic blockade and down-regulation of receptors make some patients much less responsive to vasopressors. Glucocorticoid therapy should be administered if a bilateral adrenalectomy is performed or if hypoadrenalism is a possibility.

Postoperative Management

The majority of patients become normotensive following complete tumor resection. Plasma catecholamine levels do not return to normal until 7 to 10 days after surgery due to a slow release of stored catecholamines from peripheral nerves. Fifty percent of patients are hypertensive for several days following surgery, and 25% to 30% of patients remain hypertensive indefinitely. This hypertension is sustained rather than paroxysmal, lower than before surgery, and not accompanied by the classic features of hypercatecholaminemia. The differential diagnosis for persistent hypertension includes a missed pheochromocytoma, surgical complications with subsequent renal ischemia, and underlying essential hypertension.

Hypotension is the most frequent cause of death in the immediate postoperative period. Large volumes of fluid are necessary since the peripheral vasculature is unresponsive to the reduced levels of catechols. In addition to the reduction in plasma catecholamines and third-space fluid losses, the residual effects of phenoxybenzamine and α-methylparatyrosine, secondary to long half-lives, are present for up to 36 hours. Vasopressor therapy may be necessary but is a secondary consideration. Steroid supplementation is necessary for patients who had bilateral adrenalectomies or if hypoadrenalism is suspected.

Hypoglycemia may occur because of excess insulin release and inadequate lipolysis and glycogenolysis. Nonselective β-blockers (e.g., propranolol) may aggravate hypoglycemia by decreasing sympathetic tone and masking signs of hypoglycemia. Dextrose-containing solutions should be included as part of the fluid therapy, and plasma glucose levels should be monitored for 24 hours.

Patients usually remain in the ICU for at least 24 hours. Adequate pain control is essential, although somnolence and an increased sensitivity to narcotic analgesics have been observed. The need for controlled ventilation is dictated by the extent of surgery, the site of surgery, and the patient's medical condition.

Pediatrics

Ten percent of pheochromocytomas occur in the pediatric population. Multiple (30%), extra-adrenal (30%), and bilateral (20%) pheochromocytomas are more common in children than adults.

Conclusion

The perioperative morbidity rate associated with removal of a pheochromocytoma is approximately 24% and the mortality rate is 2.4%. An in-depth knowledge and understanding of the pathophysiology of the tumor are the most important elements in designing an anesthetic plan. Recent advances in diagnostic and localization methods and potential future development of more effective antihypertensive medications will aid in providing better care to this patient population. Thorough preoperative patient preparation; good communication among the medical internist/endocrinologist, surgeon, and anesthesiologist; meticulous intraoperative preparation; and expert anesthetic management intraoperatively and postoperatively are necessary in managing these patients.

ADRENAL GLAND DYSFUNCTION

The adrenal glands consist of the adrenal cortex and the adrenal medulla. The body's adjustments to the upright posture and responses to stress, as produced by hemorrhage, sepsis, anesthesia, and surgery, are dependent on normal function of the adrenal glands. The adrenal cortex is responsible for the synthesis of three groups of hormones classified as glucocorticoids (cortisol essential for life), mineralocorticoids (aldosterone), and androgens. Corticotropin (ACTH) is secreted by the anterior pituitary gland in response to corticotropin-releasing hormone (CRH), which is synthesized in the hypothalamus and carried to the anterior pituitary in the portal blood. ACTH stimulates the adrenal cortex to produce cortisol. Maintenance of systemic blood pressure by cortisol reflects the importance of this hormone in facilitating conversion of norepinephrine to epinephrine in the adrenal medulla. Hyperglycemia in response to cortisol secretion reflects gluconeogenesis and inhibition of the peripheral use of glucose by cells. Retention of sodium and excretion of potassium are facilitated by cortisol. The anti-inflammatory effects of cortisol and other glucocorticoids (cortisone, prednisone, methylprednisolone, dexamethasone, triamcinolone) are particularly apparent in the presence of high serum concentrations of these hormones. Aldosterone secretion is regulated by the renin-angiotensin system and the serum concentrations of potassium. Aldosterone regulates the extracellular fluid volume by promoting resorption of sodium by the renal tubules. In addition, aldosterone promotes renal tubular excretion of potassium. The adrenal medulla is a specialized part of the sympathetic nervous system that is capable of synthesizing norepinephrine and epinephrine. The only important disease process associated with the adrenal medulla is pheochromocytoma. Adrenal medulla insufficiency is not known to occur.

Hypercortisolism (Cushing's Syndrome)

Cushing's syndrome is categorized as ACTH-dependent Cushing's syndrome (inappropriately high plasma ACTH concentrations stimulate the adrenal cortex to produce excessive amounts of cortisol) and ACTH-independent Cushing's syndrome (excessive production of cortisol by abnormal adrenocortical tissues causes the syndrome and suppresses secretion of CRH and ACTH). The term Cushing's disease is reserved for Cushing's syndrome caused by excessive secretion of ACTH by pituitary ACTH tumors (microadenomas). These microadenomas account for nearly 70% of patients with ACTH-dependent Cushing's syndrome. Acute ectopic ACTH syndrome (rapid onset of systemic hypertension, edema, hypokalemia, glucose intolerance) is another form of ACTH-dependent Cushing's syndrome that is most often associated with small-cell lung carcinoma. Benign or malignant adrenocortical tumors are the most common cause of ACTH-independent Cushing's syndrome.

Diagnosis

There are no pathognomonic signs or symptoms that confirm the diagnosis of Cushing's syndrome. The most common symptom is the relatively sudden onset of weight gain, which is usually central and often accompanied by thickening of the facial fat, which rounds the facial contour (moon facies), and a florid complexion due to telangiectasias. Systemic hypertension, glucose intolerance, oligomenorrhea, or amenorrhea in premenopausal women, decreased libido in men, and spontaneous ecchymoses are frequent concomitant findings. Skeletal muscle wasting and weakness manifest as difficulty climbing stairs. Depression and insomnia are often present. The diagnosis of Cushing's syndrome is confirmed by demonstrating cortisol hypersecretion based on 24-hour urinary secretion of cortisol. Determining whether a patient's hypercortisolism is ACTH dependent or ACTH independent requires reliable measurements of plasma ACTH using immunoradiometric assays. Because most patients with ACTH-dependent Cushing's syndrome have Cushing's disease, the goal is to identify the patients who have the less common ectopic ACTH syndrome. The high-dose dexamethasone suppression test distinguishes Cushing's disease from the ectopic ACTH syndrome (complete resistance present). Imaging procedures provide no information about adrenal cortex function and are useful only for determining the location of a tumor.

Treatment

The treatment of choice for patients with Cushing's disease is transsphenoidal microadenomectomy if a clearly circumscribed microadenoma can be identified and resected. Alternatively, patients may undergo 85% to 90% resection of the anterior pituitary. Pituitary radiation and bilateral total adrenalectomy are necessary in some patients. Surgical removal of the adrenal gland is the treatment for adrenal adenoma or carcinoma.

Management of Anesthesia

Management of anesthesia for patients with hypercortisolism must consider the physiologic effects of excessive cortisol secretion (**Table 16-11**). Preoperative evaluation of systemic blood pressure, electrolyte balance, and the blood glucose concentration are especially important. Osteoporosis is a consideration when positioning patients for the operative procedure.

The choice of drugs for preoperative medication, induction of anesthesia, and maintenance of anesthesia is not influenced by the presence of hypercortisolism. Etomidate may transiently decrease the synthesis and release of cortisol by the adrenal cortex. Surgical stimulation predictably increases the release of cortisol from the adrenal cortex. It seems unlikely that this stress-induced release would produce a different effect from that in normal patients. Furthermore, attempts to decrease adrenal cortex activity with opioids, barbiturates, or volatile anesthetics are probably futile, as any drug-induced inhibition is likely overridden by surgical stimulation.

TABLE 16-11 Physiologic Effects of Excess Cortisol Secretion
Systemic hypertension
Hyperglycemia
Skeletal muscle weakness
Osteoporosis
Obesity
Menstrual disturbances
Poor wound healing
Susceptibility to infection

Even regional anesthesia may not be effective in preventing increased cortisol secretion during surgery. Doses of muscle relaxants should probably be decreased initially in view of skeletal muscle weakness, which frequently accompanies hypercortisolism. In addition, the presence of hypokalemia could influence responses to nondepolarizing muscle relaxants. Mechanical ventilation of the patient's lungs during surgery is recommended, as skeletal muscle weakness, with or without co-existing hypokalemia, may decrease strength in the muscles of breathing. Regional anesthesia is acceptable, but the likely presence of osteoporosis, with possible vertebral body collapse, is a consideration.

Plasma cortisol concentrations decrease promptly after microadenomectomy or bilateral adrenalectomy, for which replacement therapy is recommended. In this regard, a continuous infusion of cortisol (100 mg/day IV) may be initiated intraoperatively. Likewise, patients with metastatic disease involving the adrenal glands may show development of acute AI, suggesting the need to institute supplemental therapy. Transient diabetes insipidus and meningitis may occur after microadenomectomy.

Primary Hyperaldosteronism (Conn's Syndrome)

Primary hyperaldosteronism (Conn's syndrome) is present when there is excess secretion of aldosterone from a functional tumor (aldosteronoma) independent of a physiologic stimulus. Aldosteronomas occur more often in women than in men and only rarely in children. Occasionally, primary aldosteronism is associated with pheochromocytoma, primary hyperparathyroidism, or acromegaly. Secondary hyperaldosteronism is present when increased circulating serum concentrations of renin, as associated with renovascular hypertension, stimulate the release of aldosterone. Aldosteronism associated with Bartter syndrome is not accompanied by systemic hypertension. The prevalence of primary aldosteronism in patients with essential hypertension appears to be less than 1%.

Signs and Symptoms

Clinical signs and symptoms of primary aldosteronism are nonspecific, and some patients are completely asymptomatic. Symptoms may reflect systemic hypertension (headache) or hypokalemia (polyuria, nocturia, skeletal muscle cramps, skeletal muscle weakness). Systemic hypertension (diastolic blood pressure often 100–125 mm Hg) reflects aldosterone-induced sodium retention and the resulting increased extracellular fluid volume. This hypertension may be resistant to treatment. Aldosterone promotes renal excretion of potassium resulting in hypokalemic metabolic alkalosis. Increased urinary excretion of potassium (more than 30 mEq/day) in the presence of hypokalemia suggests primary aldosteronism. Hypokalemic nephropathy can result in polyuria and an inability to concentrate urine optimally. Skeletal muscle weakness is presumed to reflect hypokalemia. Hypomagnesemia and abnormal glucose tolerance may be present.

Diagnosis

Spontaneous hypokalemia in patients with systemic hypertension is highly suggestive of aldosteronism. Plasma renin activity is suppressed in almost all patients with untreated primary aldosteronism and in many with essential hypertension; with secondary aldosteronism, however, the plasma renin activity is high. A plasma aldosterone concentration less than 9.5 ng/dL at the end of a saline infusion rules out primary aldosteronism. A syndrome exhibiting all the features of hyperaldosteronism (systemic hypertension, hypokalemia, suppression of the renin-angiotensin system) may result from chronic ingestion of licorice.

Treatment

Initial treatment of hyperaldosteronism consists of supplemental potassium and administration of a competitive aldosterone antagonist, such as spironolactone. Skeletal muscle weakness due to hypokalemia may require treatment with potassium administered intravenously. Systemic hypertension may require treatment with antihypertensive drugs. Accentuation of hypokalemia due to drug-induced diuresis is decreased by using a potassium-sparing diuretic such as triamterene. Definitive treatment for an aldosterone-secreting tumor is surgical excision. Bilateral adrenalectomy may be necessary if multiple aldosterone-secreting tumors are found.

Management of Anesthesia

Management of anesthesia for the treatment of hyperaldosteronism is facilitated by preoperative correction of hypokalemia and treatment of systemic hypertension. Persistence of hypokalemia may modify responses to nondepolarizing muscle relaxants. Furthermore, it must be appreciated that intraoperative hyperventilation of the patient's lungs can decrease the plasma potassium concentration. Inhaled or injected drugs are acceptable for maintenance of anesthesia. The use of sevoflurane is questionable, however, if hypokalemic nephropathy and polyuria are present preoperatively. Measurement of cardiac filling pressures via a right atrial or pulmonary artery catheter may be useful during surgery for adequate evaluation of the intravascular fluid volume and the response to intravenous infusion of fluids. Indeed, aggressive preoperative preparation can convert the excessive intravascular fluid volume status of these patients to unexpected hypovolemia, manifesting as hypotension in response to vasodilating anesthetic drugs, positive pressure ventilation of the lungs, body position changes, or sudden surgical blood loss. The existence of orthostatic hypotension detected during the preoperative evaluation is a clue to the presence of unexpected hypovolemia in these patients. Acid base status and plasma electrolyte concentrations should be measured frequently during the perioperative period. Supplementation with exogenous cortisol is probably unnecessary for surgical excision of a solitary adenoma in the adrenal cortex. Bilateral mobilization of the adrenal glands to excise multiple functional tumors, however, may introduce the need for exogenous administration of cortisol. A continuous intravenous infusion of cortisol, 100 mg every 24 hours, may be initiated on an empirical basis if transient hypocortisolism due to surgical manipulation is a consideration.

Hypoaldosteronism

Hyperkalemia in the absence of renal insufficiency suggests the presence of hypoaldosteronism. Heart block secondary to hyperkalemia and orthostatic hypotension and hyponatremia may be present. Hyperkalemia is sometimes abruptly enhanced by hyperglycemia. Hyperchloremic metabolic acidosis is a predictable finding in the presence of hypoaldosteronism.

Isolated deficiency of aldosterone secretion may reflect congenital deficiency of aldosterone synthetase or hyporeninemia due to defects in the juxtaglomerular apparatus or treatment with ACE inhibitors that leads to loss of angiotensin stimulation. Hyporeninemic hypoaldosteronism typically occurs in patients older than 45 years of age with chronic renal disease and/or diabetes mellitus. Indomethacin-induced prostaglandin deficiency is a reversible cause of this syndrome. Treatment of hypoaldosteronism includes liberal sodium intake and daily administration of fludrocortisone.

Adrenal Insufficiency
Signs and Symptoms

There are two types of AI: primary and secondary. In primary disease (Addison's disease), the adrenal glands are unable to elaborate sufficient quantities of glucocorticoid, mineralocorticoid, and androgen hormones. The most common etiology for this rare endocrinopathy is bilateral adrenal destruction from autoimmune disease. More than 90% of the glands must be involved before signs of AI appear. The insidious onset of Addison's disease is characterized by fatigue, weakness, anorexia, nausea and vomiting, cutaneous and mucosal hyperpigmentation, cardiopenia secondary to chronic hypotension, hypovolemia, hyponatremia, and hyperkalemia. In secondary AI, a failure in elaboration of CRH or ACTH occurs secondary to hypothalamic/pituitary disease or suppression of the hypothalamic-pituitary axis. Unlike Addison's disease, there is only a glucocorticoid deficiency with secondary disease. The most common cause is iatrogenic and includes pituitary surgery, pituitary irradiation, or most commonly the use of synthetic glucocorticoids. These patients lack cutaneous hyperpigmentation and may demonstrate only mild electrolyte abnormalities. Cortisol is one of the few hormones essential for life. It participates in carbohydrate and protein metabolism, fatty acid mobilization, electrolyte and water balance, and the anti-inflammatory response. It facilitates catecholamine synthesis and action, modulates β-receptor synthesis, regulation, coupling, and responsiveness and contributes to normal vascular permeability and tone and cardiac contractility. Cortisol accounts for 95% of the adrenal gland's glucocorticoid activity, with corticosterone and cortisone contributing some activity. Estimates of daily cortisol secretion are less than previously reported and are the equivalent of 15 to 25 mg/day of hydrocortisone or 5 to 7 mg/day of prednisone.

Surgery is one of the most potent and best studied activators of the hypothalamic-pituitary-adrenal (HPA) axis. The degree of activation of the axis depends on the magnitude and duration of surgery and the type and depth of anesthesia. During surgery in patients with an intact normally functioning HPA axis, CRH, ACTH, and cortisol levels all increase significantly. Deep general anesthesia or regional anesthesia postpones the usual intraoperative glucocorticoid surge until the postoperative period. Increases in ACTH begin with surgical incision and remain elevated during surgery with the peak level occurring with pharmacologic reversal of muscle relaxants and extubation of the patient at the end of the procedure and continuing into the immediate postoperative period. During major surgery, cortisol release may increase from a preoperative level of 15 to 25 mg/day to 75 to 150 mg/day, yielding a plasma cortisol level of 30 to 50 μg/dL. An uncomplicated cholecystectomy in an otherwise normal patient will yield a plasma cortisol level of 27 to 34 μg/dL 30 minutes after incision and 46 to 49 μg/dL 5 hours after surgery. Patients in the ICU may demonstrate plasma cortisol levels greater than 60 μg/dL. A low normal plasma cortisol level in response to stress is 25 μg/dL.

Diagnosis

Critically ill patients with cortisol levels less than 20 μg/dL have AI. The classic definition of AI includes a baseline plasma cortisol less than 20 μg/dL and a cortisol level less than 20 μg/dL following an ACTH stimulation test. The short 250-μg ACTH stimulation test is a reliable test of the integrity of the entire HPA axis. All steroids, except dexamethasone, must be discontinued for 24 hours before testing. Cortisol levels are measured at 30 and 60 minutes following the administration of ACTH. A normal ACTH stimulation test yields a plasma cortisol level greater than 25 μg/dL. A positive test demonstrates a poor response to ACTH and indicates an impairment of the adrenal cortex. Absolute AI is characterized by a low baseline cortisol level and a positive ACTH stimulation test. Relative AI has a higher baseline cortisol level but a positive ACTH stimulation test.

Treatment

The most common cause of AI is exogenous steroids (Table 16-12). In 2001, 34 million prescriptions were written for steroids. Patients take steroid preparations to treat a number of illnesses including arthritis, bronchial asthma, malignancies, allergies, collagen vascular diseases, and inflammatory ailments of the cardiovascular system, brain, kidney, liver, eye, skin, and gastrointestinal tract. Those who take steroids long term may exhibit signs and symptoms of AI during the stressful perioperative period. This presentation may be secondary to prolonged hypothalamic/pituitary suppression and/or inadequate exogenous steroid replacement. In addition, if steroids are abruptly withdrawn in the perioperative period, the manifestations of AI may appear within 24 to 36 hours. For patients with a history of long-term steroid use, it may take 6 to 12 months from the time of discontinuation

TABLE 16-12 Glucocorticoid Preparations

Steroid	POTENCY		Equivalent Dose (Oral or IV, mg)
	Anti-inflammatory (Glucocorticoid)	Na⁺ Retention (Mineralocorticoid)	
Short Acting			
Cortisol	1	1	20
Cortisone	0.8	0.8	25
Intermediate Acting			
Prednisone	4	0.8	5
Prednisolone	4	0.8	5
Methylprednisolone	5	0.5	4
Triamcinolone	5	0	4
Long Acting			
Dexamethasone	30–40	0	0.75

Adapted from Stoelting RK, Dierdorf SF: Endocrine disease. In Stoelting RK (ed): Anesthesia and Co-Existing Disease. New York, Churchhill Livingstone, 1993, p 358.

of the steroids for the adrenal glands to recover full function. Hypothalamic-pituitary function returns before adrenocortical function. A normal response to the ACTH test indicates normal HPA axis function. Recovery from short courses of steroids may take several days. For example, oral prednisone 25 mg twice daily for 5 days results in a reduced response to exogenous ACTH for 5 days.

Preoperative glucocorticoid coverage should be provided for patients with a positive ACTH stimulation test, Cushing's syndrome, and AI or are at risk of HPA axis suppression or AI based on prior glucocorticoid therapy. Adrenal suppression is much more common than AI and is of concern because overt AI, although uncommon, may occur under the stressful conditions of surgery and anesthesia.

Patients taking prednisone less than 5 mg/day (morning dose) for any length of time, even years, do not demonstrate clinically significant HPA axis suppression and do not require perioperative supplementation, although they need to receive their normal daily steroid dose. The timing of dosing is significant because normal cortisol secretion is diurnal with maximal release in the early morning, and negative feedback is greater with bedtime doses. Any patient who has received a glucocorticoid in doses equivalent to more than 20 mg/day of prednisone for more than 3 weeks within the past year is considered to have adrenal suppression and is at risk of AI and needs perioperative supplementation. Doses of steroids between these two extremes (> 5 mg/day but < 20 mg/day for > 3 weeks within the past year) may have HPA axis suppression and should probably receive supplementation. Patients receiving more than 2 g/day of topical steroids or more than 0.8 mg/day of inhaled steroids on a long-term basis may have adrenal suppression and should probably receive supplementation. Interestingly, patients receiving 7.5 mg/day of prednisone for several months all demonstrated an abnormal ACTH test

but no difference in perioperative outcome (hypotension, tachycardia) minus perioperative supplementation.

Patients with known or suspected adrenal suppression or AI should receive their baseline therapy plus supplementation in the perioperative period. Supplementation is individualized based on the surgery (**Table 16-13**). No benefit has been determined from excessive dosing and/or prolonged duration of supplementation therapy. When administering more than 100 mg/day of hydrocortisone, the clinician should also consider substituting methylprednisolone with its lower mineralocorticoid effects to avoid the attendant fluid retention, edema, and hypokalemia.

Management of Anesthesia

Acute AI may present in patients at risk of either primary or secondary AI. As anesthesiologists, we most likely will see the latter. However, ICU patients suffering from Addison's disease from autoimmune deficiency syndrome, meningococcemia, tuberculosis, sepsis, or shock may require our care. The clinical presentation is characterized by severe nausea and vomiting,

TABLE 16-13 Steroid (Hydrocortisone) Supplementation

Superficial surgery Dental, biopsies	None
Minor surgery Inguinal hernia, colonoscopy	25 mg IV
Moderate surgery Cholecystectomy, colon	50–75 mg IV, taper 1–2 days
Severe surgery Cardiovascular, liver, Whipple	100–150 mg IV, taper 1–2 days
Intensive care unit Sepsis, shock	50–100 mg q 6–8 hr for 2 days to 1 wk, taper

abdominal pain, lethargy, weakness, hypovolemia, hypotension, and possibly shock. Therapy includes treatment of the etiology, repletion of circulating glucocorticoids, and replacement of water and sodium deficits. Glucocorticoid replacement may include intravenous hydrocortisone, methylprednisolone, or dexamethasone. If ACTH stimulation testing will be required to assist in establishing a diagnosis of primary or secondary disease, dexamethasone is preferred because it does not alter cortisol levels. A bolus of 100 mg of hydrocortisone followed by a continuous infusion at 10 mg/hr is a recommended prescription. A 100-mg bolus of hydrocortisone every 6 hours is also an acceptable option. The continuous infusion has the advantage of maintaining the plasma cortisol at stress levels greater than 830 nmol/L (30 µg/dL). When the patient's condition stabilizes, the steroid dose is reduced with eventual conversion to an oral preparation. For primary disease, the mineralocorticoid fludrocortisone is not necessary acutely because isotonic saline replaces sodium loss, and in the case of high doses of hydrocortisone, mineralocorticoid properties exist. With tapering of steroids, fludrocortisone (100 µg/day) may be necessary in managing primary disease. Volume deficits may be substantial (2–3 L), and 5% glucose in normal saline is the fluid of choice. Hemodynamic support with vasopressors such as dopamine may be necessary. Metabolic acidosis and hyperkalemia usually resolve with fluids and steroids.

Fortunately, few cases of adrenal crisis have been reported in the operating room. Acute AI should be considered in the differential diagnosis of hemodynamic instability only after more common etiologies have been treated or ruled out, such as hypovolemia, anesthetic overdose, cardiopulmonary disorders, or surgical mechanical problems. Patients in circulatory shock and unresponsive to the usual therapeutic interventions of volume, vasopressors, and inotropes may have AI and require immediate glucocorticoids.

No specific anesthetic agent(s) and/or technique(s) are recommended in managing patients with or at risk of AI. Etomidate inhibits the synthesis of cortisol transiently in normal patients and should be avoided in this patient population. Patients with untreated AI presenting for emergency surgery should be managed aggressively with invasive monitoring including an arterial catheter and a central venous or pulmonary artery catheter, intravenous corticosteroids, and fluid and electrolyte resuscitation. Minimal doses of anesthetic agents and drugs are recommended since myocardial depression and skeletal muscle weakness are frequently part of the clinical presentation.

Intensive Care Unit Management

AI is a common and underdiagnosed entity among critically ill patients. Patients at risk have infection and systemic inflammation from tuberculosis, meningococcemia, human immunodeficiency virus, sepsis, and/or diffuse intravascular coagulation. The incidence of AI in high-risk, critically ill patients with hypotension, shock, and sepsis is approximately 30% to 40%. Approximately 33% of human immunodeficiency virus–infected patients admitted to the ICU have AI most likely caused by high levels of cytokines (interleukin-1,

interleukin-6, interferon alfa) and inflammatory peptides that impair the response of pituitary cells and inhibit the HPA axis. Cytokines also cause glucocorticoid resistance by impairing glucocorticoid receptor binding affinity. Hypotension is a common presentation, and hydrocortisone is required for vascular tone, endothelial cell integrity, normal vascular permeability, β-receptor function, and catecholamine synthesis and action. Acute AI has variable presentations with the systemic vascular resistance, cardiac output, and pulmonary capillary wedge pressure being low, normal, or high, while chronic AI is characterized by low systemic vascular resistance and depressed myocardial contractility. Patients at risk of AI who present with hypotension refractory to fluids and vasopressors may have adrenal dysfunction. Laboratory values reveal hyponatremia, hypoglycemia, and hyperkalemia. All patients suspected of having AI should be tested for serum cortisol and have an ACTH stimulation test, especially if the stress level in uncertain. Free serum cortisol, not total, will offer a better reflection of the HPA axis in critically ill patients with hypoproteinemia. Studies have shown that 39% of ICU patients with severe hypoproteinemia had lower-than-expected serum total cortisol, but serum free cortisol was consistently elevated, suggesting a significant increase in secretion. The ability to measure free cortisol levels may prevent the unnecessary treatment of many critically ill patients with normal adrenal function. With the exception of patients with vasopressor-dependent shock, significant doses of glucocorticoids should be reserved for patients with proven AI. The definitive Corticus study is currently under way testing the effectiveness of hydrocortisone therapy for patients with septic shock and positive ACTH stimulation tests.

Prior to 1989, large doses of steroids (300–1000 mg/day hydrocortisone) with tapers lasting days, even weeks, were given to treat sepsis with no beneficial effect and possibly harmful immunosuppressive effects associated with increased mortality. In addition, the deleterious effects of excess glucocorticoids include hyperglycemia, hypertension, hypervolemia, and induced psychosis. Since 1997, steroids have been given as replacement therapy for sepsis-induced AI. Lower, more physiologic doses of glucocorticoids reverse shock and confer a survival advantage. Physiologic doses during a stressful state are equal to 300 mg/day of cortisol. Therefore, for sepsis, 200 to 300 mg/day of hydrocortisone for a minimum of 5 to 7 days followed by tapering for 5 to 7 days results in overall improvement in shock reversal and survival in patients with vasopressor-dependent septic shock. Additional studies are needed to determine whether physiologic doses are beneficial to septic patients without shock or patients with shock but not vasopressor dependence. The treatment for critically ill patients with AI includes fluids, electrolytes, hydrocortisone, antibiotics if indicated, and organ support.

PARATHYROID GLAND DYSFUNCTION

The four parathyroid glands are located behind the upper and lower poles of the thyroid gland and produce parathormone, a polypeptide hormone. Parathormone is released into the systemic circulation by a negative feedback mechanism that depends on the plasma calcium concentration. Hypocalcemia stimulates the release of parathormone, whereas hypercalcemia suppresses both the synthesis and release of this hormone. Parathormone maintains normal plasma calcium concentrations (4.5–5.5 mEq/L) by promoting the movement of calcium across three interfaces represented by the gastrointestinal tract, renal tubules, and bone.

Hyperparathyroidism

Hyperparathyroidism is present when the secretion of parathormone is increased. Serum calcium concentrations may be increased, decreased, or unchanged. Hyperparathyroidism is classified as primary, secondary, or ectopic.

Primary Hyperparathyroidism

Primary hyperparathyroidism results from excessive secretion of parathormone due to a benign parathyroid adenoma, carcinoma of a parathyroid gland, or hyperplasia of the parathyroid glands. A benign parathyroid adenoma is responsible for primary hyperparathyroidism in approximately 90% of patients; carcinoma of a parathyroid gland is responsible for less than 5% of affected patients. Hyperplasia usually involves all four parathyroid glands, although not all glands may be enlarged to the same degree. Hyperparathyroidism due to an adenoma or hyperplasia is the most common presenting symptom of multiple endocrine neoplasia 1 syndrome.

Diagnosis Hypercalcemia (serum calcium concentration > 5.5 mEq/L and ionized calcium concentration > 2.5 mEq/L) is the hallmark of primary hyperparathyroidism. Primary hyperparathyroidism is the most common cause of hypercalcemia in the general population, whereas cancer is the most common cause in hospitalized patients. Modest increases in plasma calcium concentrations discovered incidentally in otherwise asymptomatic patients are most likely due to parathyroid adenomas, whereas marked hypercalcemia (> 7.5 mEq/L) is more likely due to cancer. Use of automated methods to measure serum calcium concentrations has detected primary hyperparathyroidism in a surprisingly large number of individuals, especially postmenopausal women. Patients in surgical ICUs for prolonged periods of time may develop hypercalcemia, which may reflect increased secretion of parathormone in response to repeated episodes of hypocalcemia due to sepsis, shock, and blood transfusions. Urinary excretion of cyclic adenosine monophosphate is increased in patients with primary hyperparathyroidism. Measurement of serum parathormone concentrations is not always sufficiently reliable to confirm the diagnosis of primary hyperparathyroidism

Signs and Symptoms Hypercalcemia is responsible for the broad spectrum of signs and symptoms that accompany primary hyperparathyroidism and that affect multiple organ systems (**Table 16-14**). Symptoms due to hypercalcemia reflect changes in ionized calcium concentrations, which is the physiologically active form of calcium and represents approximately 45% of the total serum calcium concentration.

TABLE 16-14 Signs and Symptoms of Hypercalcemia Due to Hyperparathyroidism

Organ System	Signs and Symptoms
Neuromuscular	Skeletal muscle weakness
Renal	Polyuria and polydipsia
	Decreased glomerular filtration rate
	Kidney stones
Hematopoietic	Anemia
Cardiac	Prolonged PR interval
	Short QT interval
	Systemic hypertension
Gastrointestinal	Vomiting
	Abdominal pain
	Peptic ulcer
	Pancreatitis
Skeletal	Skeletal demineralization
	Collapse of vertebral bodies
	Pathologic fractures
Nervous system	Somnolence
	Decreased pain sensation
	Psychosis
Ocular	Calcifications (band keratopathy)
	Conjunctivitis

Ionized serum calcium concentrations are dependent on arterial pH and the plasma albumin concentration. For this reason, it is preferable to measure ionized calcium concentrations directly using an ion-specific electrode.

Early signs and symptoms of primary hyperparathyroidism and associated hypercalcemia include sedation and vomiting. Skeletal muscle weakness and hypotonia are frequent complaints and may be so severe as to suggest the presence of myasthenia gravis. Loss of skeletal muscle strength and mass is most notable in the proximal musculature of the lower extremities. This skeletal muscle weakness is a neuropathy (muscle biopsies resemble amyotrophic lateral sclerosis) and not a myopathy. The cause of the neuropathy is unclear, but it is not related to hypercalcemia; it is reversible, as skeletal muscle strength often improves following surgical removal of the excess parathormone-producing tissues.

Persistent increases in plasma calcium concentrations can interfere with urine concentrating ability, and polyuria results. Oliguric renal failure can occur in advanced cases of hypercalcemia. Renal stones, especially in the presence of polyuria and polydipsia, must arouse suspicion of primary hyperparathyroidism. Increased serum chloride concentrations (>102 mEq/L) are most likely due to the influence of parathormone on renal excretion of bicarbonate, producing a mild metabolic acidosis. Anemia, even in the absence of renal dysfunction, is a consequence of primary hyperparathyroidism. Peptic ulcer disease is frequent and may reflect potentiation of gastric acid secretion by calcium. Acute and chronic pancreatitis is associated with primary hyperparathyroidism. Even in the absence of peptic ulcer disease or pancreatitis, abdominal pain that often accompanies hypercalcemia can mimic an acute surgical abdomen.

Systemic hypertension is common, and the electrocardiogram may reveal prolonged PR intervals, whereas QT intervals are often shortened. When serum calcium concentrations exceed 8 mEq/L, cardiac conduction disturbances are likely. The classic skeletal consequence of primary hyperparathyroidism is osteitis fibrosa cystica. Radiographic evidence of skeletal involvement includes generalized osteopenia, subcortical bone resorption in the phalanges and distal ends of the clavicles, and the appearance of bone cysts. Bone pain and pathologic fractures may be present. There may be deficits of memory and cerebration, with or without personality changes or mood disturbances, including hallucinations. Loss of sensation for pain and vibration may occur.

Treatment Primary hyperparathyroidism and the associated hypercalcemia are treated initially by medical means followed by definitive surgical removal of the diseased or abnormal portions of the parathyroid glands.

Medical Management Saline infusion (150 mL/hr) is the basic treatment for all patients with symptomatic hypercalcemia. Intravascular fluid volume may be depleted by vomiting, polyuria, and urinary loss of sodium. The calcium-lowering effect of saline hydration alone is limited, and it is often necessary to add loop diuretics (furosemide 40–80 mg IV every 2–4 hours) to the therapeutic regimen but only after the intravascular fluid volume has been optimized. Central venous pressure monitoring may be useful for guiding fluid replacement in these patients. Loop diuretics inhibit sodium (and therefore calcium) reabsorption in the proximal loop of Henle. The goal is a daily urine output of 3 to 5 L. Addition of loop diuretics to saline hydration increases calcium excretion only if the saline infusion is adequate to restore the intravascular fluid volume necessary for delivery of calcium to the renal tubules. Thiazide diuretics are not administered for treatment of hypercalcemia, as these drugs may enhance renal tubular reabsorption of calcium.

Bisphosphonates such as disodium etidronate administered intravenously are the drugs of choice for the treatment of life-threatening hypercalcemia. These drugs bind to hydroxyapatite in bone and act as potent inhibitors of osteoclastic bone resorption. The effectiveness of bisphosphonates allows surgery to be performed under elective conditions rather than as an emergency in unstable hypercalcemic patients. Hemodialysis can also be used to lower serum calcium concentrations promptly, as can calcitonin, but the effects of this hormone are transient. Mithramycin inhibits the osteoclastic activity of parathormone, producing prompt lowering of serum calcium concentrations. The toxic effects (thrombocytopenia, hepatotoxicity, nephrotoxicity) of mithramycin, however, limits its use.

Surgical Management Definitive treatment of primary hyperparathyroidism is surgical removal of the diseased or abnormal portions of the parathyroid glands. Successful surgical treatment is reflected by normalization of serum calcium concentrations within 3 to 4 days and a decrease in the urinary excretion of cyclic adenosine monophosphate. Postoperatively, the first potential complication is hypocalcemic tetany. The hypomagnesemia that occurs postoperatively aggravates the hypocalcemia and renders it refractory to treatment. Acute arthritis may occur following parathyroidectomy. Hyperchloremic metabolic acidosis, in association with deterioration of renal function, may occur transiently after parathyroidectomy.

Management of Anesthesia There is no evidence that any specific anesthetic drugs or techniques are necessary in patients with primary hyperparathyroidism undergoing elective surgical treatment of the disease. Maintenance of hydration and urine output is important during perioperative management of hypercalcemia. The existence of somnolence before induction of anesthesia introduces the possibility that intraoperative anesthetic requirements could be decreased. Ketamine is an unlikely selection in patients with co-existing personality changes attributed to chronic hypercalcemia. The possibility of co-existing renal dysfunction is a consideration when selecting sevoflurane, as impaired urine concentrating ability associated with polyuria and hypercalcemia could be confused with anesthetic-induced fluoride nephrotoxicity. Co-existing skeletal muscle weakness suggests the possibility of decreased requirements for muscle relaxants, whereas hypercalcemia might be expected to antagonize the effects of nondepolarizing muscle relaxants. Increased sensitivity to succinylcholine and resistance to atracurium have been described in a patient with hyperparathyroidism. In view of the unpredictable response to muscle relaxants, it is probably important to decrease the initial dose of these drugs and to monitor the response produced at the neuromuscular junction using a peripheral nerve stimulator. Monitoring the electrocardiogram for manifestations of adverse cardiac effects of hypercalcemia is often recommended, although there is evidence that the QT interval may not be a reliable index of changes in serum calcium concentrations during anesthesia. Theoretically, hyperventilation of the lungs in undesirable, as respiratory alkalosis lowers serum potassium concentrations and leaves the actions of calcium unopposed. Nevertheless, by lowering ionized fractions of calcium, alkalosis could also be beneficial. Careful positioning of hyperparathyroid patients is necessary because of the likely presence of osteoporosis and the associated vulnerability to pathologic fractures.

Secondary Hyperparathyroidism

Secondary hyperparathyroidism reflects an appropriate compensatory response of the parathyroid glands to secrete more parathormone to counteract a disease process that produces hypocalcemia. For example, chronic renal disease impairs elimination of phosphorous and decreases hydroxylation of vitamin D, resulting in hypocalcemia and compensatory hyperplasia of the parathyroid glands with increased release of parathormone. Because secondary hyperparathyroidism is adaptive rather than autonomous, it seldom produces hypercalcemia. Treatment of secondary hyperparathyroidism is best directed at controlling the underlying disease, as is achieved by normalizing serum phosphate concentrations in patients with renal disease by administering an oral phosphate binder.

On occasion, transient hypercalcemia may follow otherwise successful renal transplantation. This response reflects the inability of previously hyperactive parathyroid glands to adapt quickly to normal renal excretion of calcium and phosphorous and to hydroxylation of vitamin D. The parathyroid glands usually return to normal size and function with time, although parathyroidectomy is occasionally necessary.

Ectopic Hyperparathyroidism

Ectopic hyperparathyroidism (humoral hypercalcemia of malignancy, pseudohyperparathyroidism) is due to secretion of parathormone (or a substance with similar endocrine effects) by tissues other than the parathyroid glands. Carcinoma of the lung, breast, pancreas, or kidney and lymphoproliferative disease are the most likely ectopic sites for parathormone secretion. Ectopic hyperparathyroidism is more likely than primary hyperparathyroidism to be associated with anemia and increased plasma alkaline phosphatase concentrations. A role for prostaglandins in the production of hypercalcemia in these patients is suggested by the calcium-lowering effects produced by indomethacin, which is an inhibitor of prostaglandin synthesis.

Hypoparathyroidism

Hypoparathyroidism is present when secretion of parathormone is absent or deficient or peripheral tissues are resistant to the effects of the hormone (**Table 16-15**). Absence or deficiency of parathormone is almost always iatrogenic, reflecting inadvertent removal of the parathyroid glands, as during thyroidectomy. Pseudohypoparathyroidism is a congenital disorder in which the release of parathormone is intact but the kidneys are unable to respond to the hormone. Affected patients manifest mental retardation, calcification of

TABLE 16-15 Etiology of Hypoparathyroidism
Decreased or Absent Parathormone
Accidental removal of parathyroid glands during thyroidectomy
Parathyroidectomy to treat hyperplasia
Idiopathic (DiGeorge syndrome)
Resistance of Peripheral Tissues to Effects of Parathormone
Congenital
Pseudohypoparathyroidism
Acquired
Hypomagnesemia
Chronic renal failure
Malabsorption
Anticonvulsive therapy (phenytoin)
Unknown
Osteoblastic metastases
Acute pancreatitis

the basal ganglia, obesity, short stature, and short metacarpals and metatarsals.

Diagnosis Measurement of serum calcium concentrations and the ionized fractions of calcium is the most valuable diagnostic indicator for hypoparathyroidism. In this regard, a serum calcium concentration less than 4.5 mEq/L and an ionized calcium concentration lower than 2.0 mEq/L are indicative of hypoparathyroidism.

Signs and Symptoms Signs and symptoms of hypoparathyroidism depend on the rapidity of the onset of hypocalcemia.

Acute hypocalcemia can occur after accidental removal of the parathyroid glands during thyroidectomy and is likely to manifest as perioral paresthesias, restlessness, and neuromuscular irritability, as evidenced by a positive Chvostek's sign or Trousseau's sign. A positive Chvostek's sign consists of facial muscle twitching produced by manual tapping over the area of the facial nerve at the angle of the mandible. The Chvostek's sign is positive in the absence of hypocalcemia in 10% to 15% of patients. A positive Trousseau's sign is carpopedal spasm produced by 3 minutes of limb ischemia produced by a tourniquet. Inspiratory stridor reflects neuromuscular irritability of the intrinsic laryngeal musculature.

Chronic hypocalcemia is associated with complaints of fatigue and skeletal muscle cramps that may be associated with a prolonged QT interval on the electrocardiogram. The QRS complex, PR interval, and cardiac rhythm usually remain normal. Neurologic changes include lethargy, cerebration deficits, and personality changes reminiscent of hyperparathyroidism. Chronic hypocalcemia is associated with formation of cataracts, calcification involving the subcutaneous tissues and basal ganglia, and thickening of the skull. Chronic renal failure is the most common cause of chronic hypocalcemia.

Treatment Treatment of acute hypocalcemia consists of an infusion of calcium (10 mL of 10% calcium gluconate IV) until signs of neuromuscular irritability disappear. Correction of any co-existing respiratory or metabolic alkalosis is indicated. For treatment of hypoparathyroidism not complicated by symptomatic hypocalcemia, the approach is administration of oral calcium and vitamin D. An exogenous parathyroid hormone replacement preparation is not yet practical for clinical use. Thiazide diuretics may be useful, as these drugs cause sodium depletion without proportional potassium excretion, thereby tending to increase serum calcium concentrations.

Management of Anesthesia Management of anesthesia in the presence of hypocalcemia is designed to prevent any further decreases in the serum calcium concentrations and to treat the adverse effects of hypocalcemia, particularly those on the heart. In this regard, it is important to avoid iatrogenic hyperventilation as it will further aggravate the clinical picture. Administration of whole blood containing citrate usually does not decrease serum calcium concentrations because calcium is rapidly mobilized from body stores. The ionized calcium concentration can be decreased, however, with rapid infusions of blood (500 mL every 5–10 minutes, as during cardiopulmonary bypass or liver transplantation) or

TABLE 16-16 Hypothalamic and Related Pituitary Hormones

Hypothalamic Hormone	Action	Pituitary Hormone or Organ Affected	Action
Corticotropin-releasing hormone	Stimulatory	Corticotropin	Stimulates secretion of cortisol and androgens
Thyrotropin-releasing hormone	Stimulatory	Thyrotropin	Stimulates secretion of thyroxine and triiodothyronine
Gonadotropin-releasing hormone	Stimulatory	Follicle-stimulating hormone	Stimulates secretion of estradiol*
		Luteinizing hormone	Stimulates secretion of progesterone,* stimulates ovulation,* stimulates secretion of testosterone,† stimulates spermatogenesis†
Growth hormone–releasing hormone	Stimulatory	Growth hormone	Stimulates production of insulin-like growth factor
Dopamine	Inhibitory	Prolactin	Stimulates lactation*
Somatostatin	Inhibitory	Growth hormone	
Vasopressin (antidiuretic hormone)	Stimulatory	Kidneys	Stimulates free-water reabsorption
Oxytocin	Stimulatory	Uterus	Stimulates uterine contractions*
		Breasts	Stimulates milk ejection*

*Actions in females.
†Actions in males.
Adapted from Vance ML: Hypopituitarism. N Engl J Med 1994;330:1651–1662.

when metabolism or elimination of citrate is impaired by hypothermia, cirrhosis of the liver, or renal dysfunction.

PITUITARY GLAND DYSFUNCTION

The pituitary gland, located in the sella turcica at the base of the brain, consists of the anterior pituitary and posterior pituitary. The anterior pituitary secretes six hormones under control of the hypothalamus (**Table 16-16**). In this regard, the hypothalamus controls the function of the anterior pituitary by means of vascular connections (hormones travel via the hypophyseal portal veins to reach the anterior pituitary). The hypothalamic-anterior pituitary–target organ axis is composed of tightly coordinated systems in which hormonal signals from the hypothalamus stimulate or inhibit secretion of anterior pituitary hormones, which in turn act on target organs and modulate hypothalamic and anterior pituitary activity (closed loop or negative feedback system). The posterior pituitary is composed of terminal neuron endings that originate in the hypothalamus. Vasopressin (antidiuretic hormone [ADH]) and oxytocin are synthesized in the hypothalamus and are subsequently transported along the hypothalamic neuronal axons for storage in the posterior pituitary. Stimulus for the release of these hormones from the posterior pituitary arises from osmoreceptors in the hypothalamus that sense plasma osmolarity.

Overproduction of anterior pituitary hormones is most often reflected by hypersecretion of ACTH (Cushing's syndrome) by anterior pituitary adenomas. Hypersecretion of other tropic hormones rarely occurs. Underproduction of a single anterior pituitary hormone is less common than generalized pituitary hypofunction (panhypopituitarism). The anterior pituitary gland is the only endocrine gland in which a tumor, most often a chromophobe adenoma, causes destruction by compressing the gland against the bony confines of the sella turcica. Metastatic tumor, most often from the breast or lung, also occasionally produces pituitary hypofunction. Endocrine features of panhypopituitarism are highly variable and depend on the rate at which the deficiency develops and the patient's age. For example, gonadotropin deficiency (amenorrhea, impotence) is typically the first manifestation of global pituitary dysfunction. Hypocortisolism occurs 4 to 14 days after hypophysectomy, whereas hypothyroidism is not likely to manifest before 4 weeks. CT and MRI are useful for radiographic assessment of the pituitary gland.

Acromegaly

Acromegaly is due to excessive secretion of growth hormone in adults, most often by an adenoma in the anterior pituitary gland. Failure of plasma growth hormone concentrations to decrease 1 to 2 hours after ingestion of 75 to 100 g of glucose is presumptive evidence of acromegaly, as are growth hormone concentrations higher than 3 ng/mL. A skull radiograph and CT are useful for detecting enlargement of the sella turcica, which is characteristic of anterior pituitary adenomas.

Signs and Symptoms

Manifestations of acromegaly reflect parasellar extension of the anterior pituitary adenoma and peripheral effects produced by the presence of excess growth hormone (**Table 16-17**). Headache and papilledema reflect increased intracranial pressure due to expansion of the anterior pituitary adenoma. Visual disturbances are due to compression of the optic chiasm by the expanding overgrowth of surrounding tissues. Overgrowth of soft tissues of the upper airway (enlargement of the tongue and epiglottis) and increased length of the mandible may make upper airway management difficult. Polypoid masses reflect overgrowth of pharyngeal tissues, making the patient's upper airway susceptible to obstruction. Hoarseness and abnormal movement of the vocal cords or paralysis of a recurrent laryngeal nerve may be due to stretching by overgrowth of the cartilaginous structures. In addition, involvement of the cricoarytenoid joints can result in alterations in the patient's voice due to impaired movement of the vocal cords. The subglottic diameter may be decreased in acromegalic patients. Stridor or a history of dyspnea is suggestive of acromegalic involvement of the upper airway.

Peripheral neuropathy is common and likely reflects trapping of nerves by skeletal, connective, and soft-tissue overgrowth. Flow through the ulnar artery may be compromised in patients exhibiting symptoms of carpal tunnel syndrome. Even in the absence of such symptoms, approximately one half of patients with acromegaly have inadequate collateral blood flow through the ulnar artery in one or both hands. Glucose intolerance and, on occasion, diabetes mellitus requiring treatment with insulin reflects the effects of growth hormone on carbohydrate metabolism. The incidence of systemic hypertension, ischemic heart disease, osteoarthritis, and osteoporosis seems to be increased. Lung volumes are increased, and ventilation-to-perfusion mismatching may be increased. The patient's skin becomes thick and oily, skeletal muscle weakness may be prominent, and complaints of fatigue are common.

TABLE 16-17 Manifestations of Acromegaly

Parasellar
Enlarged sella turcica
Headache
Visual field defects
Rhinorrhea

Excess Growth Hormone
Skeletal overgrowth (prognathism)
Soft-tissue overgrowth (lips, tongue, epiglottis, vocal cords)
Connective tissue overgrowth (recurrent laryngeal nerve paralysis)
Peripheral neuropathy (carpal tunnel syndrome)
Visceromegaly
Glucose tolerance
Osteoarthritis
Osteoporosis
Hyperhydrosis
Skeletal muscle weakness

Treatment

Transsphenoidal surgical excision of pituitary adenomas is the preferred initial therapy. When adenomas have extended beyond the sella turcica, surgery or radiation is no longer feasible; medical treatment with suppressant drugs (bromocriptine) may be an option.

Management of Anesthesia

Management of anesthesia for patients with acromegaly is complicated by changes induced by excessive secretion of growth hormone. Particularly important are changes in the upper airway. Distorted facial anatomy may interfere with placing an anesthesia face mask. Enlargement of the tongue and epiglottis predisposes to upper airway obstruction and interferes with visualization of the vocal cords by direct laryngoscopy. The distance between the lips and vocal cords is increased by overgrowth of the mandible. The glottic opening may be narrowed, owing to enlargement of the vocal cords, which combined with subglottic narrowing may necessitate use of a smaller internal diameter tracheal tube than would have been predicted based on the patient's age and size. Nasal turbinate enlargement may preclude the passage of nasopharyngeal or nasotracheal airways. The preoperative history of dyspnea on exertion or the presence of hoarseness or stridor suggests involvement of the larynx by acromegaly. In this instance, indirect laryngoscopy may be indicated to quantitate the extent of vocal cord dysfunction. When difficulty placing a tracheal tube is anticipated, it may be prudent to consider an awake fiberoptic tracheal intubation. Indeed, the incidence of difficult laryngoscopy and tracheal intubation has been reported to be increased in acromegalic patients. Anticipation of the possible need to insert a smaller diameter tracheal tube and minimizing the mechanical trauma to the upper airway and vocal cords are important considerations, as additional edema can result in airway obstruction after the tracheal tube is removed.

When placing a catheter in the radial artery, it is important to consider the possibility of inadequate collateral circulation at the wrist. Monitoring blood glucose concentrations is useful if diabetes mellitus or glucose intolerance accompanies acromegaly. Doses of nondepolarizing muscle relaxants are guided by the use of a peripheral nerve stimulator, particularly if skeletal muscle weakness exists before anesthesia induction. Skeletal changes that accompany acromegaly may make performance of regional anesthesia technically difficult or unreliable. There is no evidence that hemodynamic instability or alterations in pulmonary gas exchange accompany anesthesia in acromegalic patients.

Diabetes Insipidus

Diabetes insipidus reflects the absence of vasopressin (ADH) owing to destruction of the posterior pituitary (neurogenic diabetes insipidus) or failure of renal tubules to respond to ADH (nephrogenic diabetes insipidus). Neurogenic and nephrogenic diabetes insipidus are differentiated based on the response to desmopressin, which concentrates urine in the presence of neurogenic, but not nephrogenic, diabetes insipidus. Classic manifestations of diabetes insipidus are polydipsia and a high output of poorly concentrated urine despite increased serum osmolarity. Diabetes insipidus that develops during or immediately after pituitary gland surgery is generally due to reversible trauma to the posterior pituitary and is therefore transient.

Initial treatment of diabetes insipidus consists of intravenous infusion of electrolyte solutions if oral intake cannot offset polyuria. Chlorpropamide, an oral hypoglycemic drug, potentiates the effects of ADH on renal tubules and may be useful for treating nephrogenic diabetes insipidus. Treatment of neurogenic diabetes insipidus is with ADH administered intramuscularly every 2 to 4 days or by intranasal administration of DDAVP.

Management of anesthesia for patients with diabetes insipidus includes monitoring the urine output and serum electrolyte concentrations during the perioperative period.

Inappropriate Secretion of Antidiuretic Hormone

Inappropriate secretion of ADH can occur in the presence of diverse pathologic processes, including intracranial tumors, hypothyroidism, porphyria, and carcinoma of the lung,

particularly undifferentiated small-cell carcinoma. Inappropriate secretion of ADH is alleged to occur in most patients following major surgery. Inappropriately increased urinary sodium concentrations and osmolarity in the presence of hyponatremia and decreased serum osmolarity are highly suggestive of inappropriate ADH secretion. Hyponatremia is due to dilution, reflecting expansion of the intravascular fluid volume secondary to hormone-induced resorption of water by renal tubules. Abrupt decreases in serum sodium concentrations, especially less than 110 mEq/L, can result in cerebral edema and seizures.

Treatment of inappropriate secretion of ADH consists of restricted oral fluid intake (approximately 500 mL/day), antagonism of the effects of ADH on the renal tubules by administration of demeclocycline, and intravenous infusions of sodium chloride. Often restriction of oral fluid intake is sufficient treatment for inappropriate secretion of ADH not associated with symptoms secondary to hyponatremia. Restriction of oral fluid intake and administration of demeclocycline, however, are not immediately effective in the management of patients manifesting acute neurologic symptoms due to hyponatremia. In these patients, intravenous infusions of hypertonic saline sufficient to increase serum sodium concentrations 0.5 mEq/L/hr are recommended. Overly rapid correction of chronic hyponatremia has been associated with central pontine myelinolysis.

KEY POINTS

- Diabetes mellitus results from an inadequate supply of insulin and an inadequate tissue response to insulin, yielding increased circulating glucose levels with eventual microvascular and macrovascular complications.

- The effects of chronic hyperglycemia (coronary artery disease, myocardial infarction, congestive heart failure, peripheral vascular disease, hypertension, cerebrovascular accident, chronic renal failure, diabetic autonomic neuropathy) and acute hyperglycemia ($\downarrow$volume [i.e., hypovolemia], delayed wound healing, infection) are common and dangerous in diabetics presenting for surgery. Aggressive insulin therapy in the perioperative period has demonstrated significant benefit in reducing morbidity and mortality.

- The direct effects of T_3 on the heart and vascular smooth muscle are responsible for the exaggerated hemodynamic effects of hyperthyroidism as opposed to a hyperactive sympathetic nervous system.

- The third generation TSH assay is the single best test of thyroid hormone action at the cellular level.

- Every effort should be made to render hyperthyroid patients euthyroid preoperatively.

- When caring for surgical patients with hyperthyroidism or hypothyroidism, the clinician must be prepared to manage the decompensated sequelae (thyroid storm or

myxedema coma, respectively) of each during the perioperative period.

- Since most pheochromocytomas secrete predominantly norepinephrine, preoperative α-blockade is necessary to lower blood pressure, increase intravascular volume, prevent paroxysmal hypertensive episodes, allow resensitization of adrenergic receptors, and decrease myocardial dysfunction.

- The intraoperative periods associated with greatest danger in a patient with a pheochromocytoma occur secondary to hypertension and/or dysrhythmias, which may occur during anesthetic induction, intubation, surgical incision, abdominal exploration, and particularly during tumor manipulation. In addition, hypotension, which occurs following ligation of the tumor's venous drainage, is also of significant concern.

- Increases in CRH, ACTH, and cortisol begin with surgical incision and remain elevated during surgery with the peak level occurring with pharmacologic reversal of muscle relaxants and extubation of the patient and continuing into the immediate postoperative period.

- The most common cause of AI is exogenous steroids.

- Any patient who has received a glucocorticoid in doses equivalent to more than 20 mg/day of prednisone for more than 3 weeks (within the past year) is considered to have adrenal suppression and is at increased risk of AI and will need perioperative supplementation.

- Hydrocortisone 200 to 300 mg/day for a minimum of 5 to 7 days followed by tapering for 5 to 7 days results in overall improvement in shock reversal and survival in patients with vasopressor-dependent septic shock.

- Primary hyperparathyroidism is the most common cause of hypercalcemia in the general population. A benign parathyroid adenoma is most commonly responsible, and the associated hypercalcemia is treated medically (saline, furosemide, bisphosphonates) followed by surgical removal of the tumor.

- Overproduction of anterior pituitary hormones is most often reflected by hypersecretion of ACTH (Cushing's syndrome) by an anterior pituitary adenoma.

- Diabetes insipidus that develops during or immediately after pituitary gland surgery is generally due to reversible trauma to the posterior pituitary and is transient.

- Inappropriate secretion of ADH is alleged to occur in most patients following major surgery, although the exact clinical significance is quite variable.

REFERENCES

Al-Mohaya S, Naguib M, Abdelaif M, et al: Abnormal responses to muscle relaxants in a patient with primary hyperparathyroidism. Anesthesiology 1986;65:554–556.

American Diabetes Association: Clinical practice recommendations. Diabetes Care 2002;25(Suppl 1):S33.

Annane D, Sebille V, Charpentier C, et al: Effect of treatment with low doses of hydrocortisone and fludrocortisone on mortality in patients with septic shock. JAMA 2002;288:862–871.

Axelrod L: Perioperative management of patients treated with glucocorticoids. Endocrinol Metab Clin N Am 200;32:367–383.

Boutros AR, Bravo EL, Zanettin G: Perioperative management of 63 patients with pheochromocytoma. Cleve Clin J Med 1990;57:613–617.

Bravo E, Fouad-Tarazi F, Rossi G, et al: A reevaluation of the hemodynamics of pheochromocytoma. Hypertension 1990;15(suppl I): I128–I131.

Bravo EL: Evolving concepts in the pathophysiology, diagnosis, and treatment of pheochromocytoma. Endocrine Rev 1994;15:356–368.

Bravo EL: Pheochromocytoma: An approach to antihypertensive management. Ann N Y Acad Sci 2002;970:1–10.

Bravo EL, Gifford RW: Pheochromocytoma. Endrocrinol Metab Clin North Am 1993;22:329.

Bravo EL, Tagle R: Pheochromocytoma: State-of-the-art and future prospects. Endocr Rev 2003;24:539–553.

Burch HB, Wartofsky L: Life-threatening thyrotoxicosis: thyroid storm. Endocrinol Metab Clin North Am 1993;22:263–277.

Burman KD, Wartofsky L: Thyroid function in the intensive care unit Setting. Crit Care Clin 2001;17:43–55.

Col NF, Surks MI, Daniels GH: Subclinical thyroid disease: Clinical applications. JAMA 2004;291:239–243.

Compkin TV: Radial artery cannulation, potential hazard in patients with acromegaly. Anaesthesia 1980;35:1008–1009.

Cooper DS: Hyperthyroidism. Lancet 2003;362:459–468.

Cooper MS, Stewart PM: Corticosteroid insufficiency in acutely ill patients. N Engl J Med 2003;348:727–734.

Coursin DB, Connery LE, Ketzler JT: Perioperative diabetic and hyperglycemic management issues. Crit Care Med 2004; 32(Suppl):S116–S125.

Coursin DB, Wood KE: Corticosteroid supplementation for adrenal insufficiency. JAMA 2002;287:236.

DeWitt DE, Hirsch IB: Outpatient insulin therapy in type 1 and type 2 diabetes mellitus. JAMA 2003;289:2254–2264.

Drop LJ, Cullen DJ: Comparative effects of calcium chloride and calcium gluceptate. Br J Anaesth 1980;52:501–505.

Executive summary of the third report of the National Cholesterol Education Program (NCEP) Expert Panel on Detection, Evaluation, and Treatment of High Blood Cholesterol in Adults (Adult Treatment Panel III). JAMA 2001;285:2486–2497.

Finney SJ, Zekvaeld C, Elia A, et al: Glucose control and mortality in critically ill patients. JAMA 2003;290:2041–2047.

Furnary AP, Gao G, Grunkemeier GL, et al: Continuous insulin infusion reduces mortality in patients with diabetes undergoing coronary artery bypass grafting. J Thorac Cardiovasc Surg 2003;125:1007–1018.

Gangat Y, Triner L, Baer L, et al: Primary aldosteronism with uncommon complications. Anesthesiology 1976;45:542–544.

Ganguly A: Primary aldosteronism. N Engl J Med 1998;339:1828–1834.

Gifford RW, Manger WM, Bravo EL: Pheochromocytoma. Endocrinol Metab Clin North Am 1994;23:387.

Goldstein DS, Eisenhofer G, Flynn JA, et al: Diagnosis and localization of pheochromocytoma. Hypertension 2004;43:907–910.

Gu W, Pagel PS, Warltier DC, et al: Modifying cardiovascular risk in diabetes mellitus. Anesthesiology 2003;98:774–779.

Hassan SZ, Matz G, Lawrence AM, Collins PA: Laryngeal stenosis in acromegaly. Anesth Analg 1976;55:57–60.

Heath DA: Hypercalcemia in malignancy: Fluids and bisphosphonate are best when life is threatened. BMJ 1989;298:1468–1469.

Hirsch IB, Farkas-Hirsch R, Skyler JS: Intensive insulin therapy for treatment of type I diabetes. Diabetes Care 1990;13:1265.

Hirsch IB, McGill JB, Cryer PE: Perioperative management of surgical patients with diabetes mellitus. Anesthesiology 1991;74:346–359.

Holland OB: Hypoaldosteronism-disease or normal response. N Engl J Med 1991;324:488–489.

Inzucchi S (ed): The Diabetes Mellitus Manual: A Primary Care Companion to Ellenberg and Rifkin's Sixth Edition. New York, McGraw-Hill, 2005.

Kitahata LM: Airway difficulties associated with anaesthesia in acromegaly. Br J Anaesth 1971;43:1187–1190.

Klein I, Ojamma K: Thyroid hormone and the cardiovascular system. N Engl J Med 2001;344:501–509.

Langley RW, Burch HB: Perioperative management of the thyrotoxic patient. Endocrinol Metab Clin North Am 2003;32:519–534.

Lazar HL, Chipkin SR, Fitzgerald CA, et al: Tight glycemic control in diabetic coronary artery bypass graft patients improves perioperative outcomes and decreases recurrent ischemic events. Circulation 2004;109:1497–1502.

Lenders J, Pacak K, Walther M, et al: Biochemical diagnosis of pheochromocytoma: Which is best? JAMA 2002;287:1427–1434.

Luce JM: Physicians should administer low-dose corticosteroids selectively to septic patients until an ongoing trial is completed. Ann Intern Med 2004;141:70–72.

Melmed S: Acromegaly. N Engl J Med 1990;322:966–975.

Mihai R, Farndon JR: Parathyroid disease and calcium metabolism. Br J Anaesth 2000;85:29–43.

Minneci PC, Deans KJ, Banks SM, et al: Meta-analysis: The effect of steroids on survival and shock during sepsis depends on the dose. Ann Intern Med 2004;141:47–56.

Muier JJ, Endres SM, Offord K, et al: Glucose management in patients undergoing operation for insulinoma removal. Anesthesiology 1983;59:371–375.

Orth DN: Cushing's syndrome. N Engl J Med 1995;332:791–803.

Pacak K, Linehan WM, Eisenhofer G, et al: Recent advances in genetics, localization, and treatment of pheochromocytoma. Ann Intern Med 2001;134:315–329.

Panzer C, Beazley R, Braverman L: Rapid preoperative preparation for severe hyperthyroid Graves' disease. J Clin Endocrinol Metab 2004;89:2142–2144.

Porte D Jr: B-cells in type II diabetes mellitus. Diabetes 1991;40:166–180.

Pulver JJ, Cullen BF, Miller DR, Valenta LJ: Use of the artificial beta cell during anesthesia for surgical removal of an insulinoma. Anesth Analg 1980;59:950–952.

Ringel MD: Management of hypothyroidism and hyperthyroidism in the intensive care unit. Crit Care Clin 2001;17:59.

Roberts CG, Ladenson PW: Hypothyroidism. Lancet 2004; 363:793–803.

Roland EJL, Wierda JMKH, Turin BY, et al: Pharmacodynamic behavior of vecuronium in primary hyperparathyroidism. Can J Anaesth 1994;41:694–698.

Schmitt H, Buchfelder M, Radespiel-Troger M, et al: Difficult intubation in acromegalic patients: Incidence and predictability. Anesthesiology 2000;93:110–114.

Seidman PA, Kofke WA, Policare R, et al: Anaesthetic complications of acromegaly. Br J Anaesth 2000;84:179–182.

Southwick JP, Katz J: Unusual airway difficulty in the acromegalic patient—indications for tracheostomy. Anesthesiology 1979;51:72-73.

Stathatos N, Wartofsky L: Perioperative management of patients with hypothyroidism. Endocrinol Met Clin North Am 2003;32:503–518.

Sterns RH, Riggs JE, Schochet SS: Osmotic demyelination syndrome following correction of hyponatremia. N Engl J Med 1986;314:1535–1542.

Surks MI, Ortiz E, Daniels GH, et al: Subclinical thyroid disease: Scientific review and guidelines for diagnosis and management. JAMA 2004;291:228–238.

The Diabetes Control and Complications Trial (DCCT) Research Group: The effect of intensive treatment of diabetes on the development and progression of long-term complications in insulin-dependent diabetes mellitus. N Engl J Med 1993;329: 977–986.

United Kingdom Prospective Diabetes Study (UKPDS) Group: Intensive blood-glucose control with sulphonylureas or insulin compared with conventional treatment and risk of complications in patients with type 2 diabetes. Lancet 1998;352:837.

Vance ML: Hypopituitarism. N Engl J Med 1994;330:1651–1662.

Van den Berghe G, Wouters P, Weekers F, et al: Intensive insulin therapy in critically ill patients. N Engl J Med 2001;345:1359–1367.

Van den Berghe G, Wouters PJ, Bouillon R, et al: Outcome benefit of intensive insulin therapy in the critically ill: Insulin dose versus glycemic control. Crit Care Med 2003;31:359–366.

VanHeerden JA, Edis AJ, Service FJ: The surgical aspect of insulinomas. Ann Surg 1979;189:677–682.

Wartofsky L: Combined levotriiodothyronine and levothyroxine therapy for hypothyroidism: Are we a step closer to the magic formula? Thyroid 2004;14:247–248.

Weatherill D, Spence AA: Anaesthesia and disorders of the adrenal cortex. Br J Anaesth 1984;56:741–747.

CHAPTER 17

Hematologic Disorders

Christine S. Rinder

ERYTHROCYTE DISORDERS

Disease states may be related to abnormal concentrations (anemia, polycythemia) or structures of hemoglobin (Hb). Oxygen-carrying capacity and adequacy of tissue oxygen delivery are often the most important clinical manifestations of these derangements.

Physiology of Anemia

Anemia, like fever, is a sign of disease manifesting clinically as a numeric deficiency of erythrocytes (red blood cells [RBCs]). There is no single laboratory value that defines anemia. Indeed, the hematocrit may be unchanged despite acute blood loss, whereas in parturients, decreased hematocrit values reflect increases in plasma volume and not anemia.

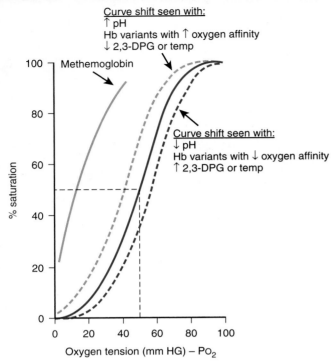

Figure 17-1 • Normal oxyhemoglobin dissociation curve and factors that result in displacement of O_2 dissociation. 2,3-DPG, 2,3-diphosphoglycerate; Hb, hemoglobin.

Nevertheless, in adults, anemia is usually defined as Hb concentrations less than 11.5 g/dL (hematocrit, 36%) for women and less than 12.5 g/dL (hematocrit, 40%) for men. Decreases in hematocrit that exceed 1% every 24 hours can only be explained by acute blood loss or intravascular hemolysis.

The most important adverse effects of anemia are decreased tissue oxygen delivery owing to associated decreases in arterial content of oxygen (CaO_2). For example, decreases in Hb concentrations from 15 g/dL to 10 g/dL result in a 33% decrease in CaO_2. Compensation for decreased CaO_2 is accomplished by a rightward shift of the oxyhemoglobin dissociation curve (facilitates release of oxygen from Hb to tissues) and increased cardiac output as a reflection of decreased blood viscosity (**Fig. 17-1**). Furthermore, when oxygen delivery to tissues is inadequate, the kidneys release erythropoietin, which subsequently stimulates erythroid precursors in the bone marrow to produce additional RBCs. Fatigue and decreased exercise tolerance reflect the inability of the cardiac output to increase further and maintain tissue oxygenation, especially in anemic patients who become physically active. There are many causes and forms of anemia, with the most common causes of chronic anemia being iron deficiency, the presence of chronic diseases, thalassemia, and anemia due to acute blood loss.

Anesthetic Considerations for Anemia Minimum acceptable Hb concentrations that should be present before proceeding with elective surgery in patients with chronic anemia

cannot be recommended. Although Hb concentrations of 10 g/dL are commonly cited as a reference point, there is no evidence that Hb values below this level mandates the need for perioperative RBC transfusions. Ultimately, the decision to administer RBCs during the perioperative period is influenced by the risks of anemia (decreased oxygen-carrying capacity) and the risks of transfusions (transmissible diseases, hemolytic and nonhemolytic transfusion reactions, immunosuppression). The risks of anemia in addition to decreased tissue oxygen delivery vary among individuals, depending on co-existing medical diseases, age, and the magnitude of the blood loss. In this regard, decisions to transfuse patients to specific preoperative Hb concentrations must be individualized, taking into consideration several factors.

Although guidelines for perioperative management of anemia and the need for RBC transfusions have been developed, it is important to recognize that no controlled studies have documented the Hb concentrations at which RBC transfusions prevent myocardial ischemia or infarction and improve clinical outcome. Furthermore, there is no evidence that postoperative morbidity (wound healing, infection) is adversely affected when surgery is performed in the presence of mild to moderate anemia. Overall there is little evidence to support the efficacy of RBC transfusions, including transfusions in patients with cardiovascular disease. The American College of Surgeons recommends RBC transfusions to normovolemic patients with anemia only if symptoms are present. An Hb level of 8 g/dL was suggested as a "transfusion trigger" by the Transfusion Practice Committee of the American Association of Blood Banks, whereas a threshold of 7 g/dL was suggested by the National Institutes of Health Consensus Conference on Perioperative Blood Transfusion. Nevertheless, there is some concern that liberalization of transfusion guidelines and increased acceptance of acute intraoperative decreases in Hb concentrations may predispose certain patients to complications such as ischemic optic neuropathy.

Increased 2,3-DPG concentrations in RBCs are principally responsible for maintaining oxygen-carrying capacity in the presence of chronic anemia. In this regard, cardiac output does not increase in chronically anemic patients until Hb concentrations decrease to approximately 7 g/dL. In vitro data suggest that peak oxygen-carrying capacity occurs at a hematocrit of 30%. Below this hematocrit level, oxygen-carrying capacity decreases, whereas above this level, the oxygen-carrying capacity may decrease as a result of decreased tissue blood flow owing to increased blood viscosity. Preoperative transfusions of packed RBCs can be administered to increase Hb concentrations, recognizing that a period of approximately 24 hours is needed to restore intravascular fluid volume. Compared with similar volumes of whole blood, packed RBCs produce approximately twice the increase in Hb concentrations.

If elective surgery is performed in the presence of chronic anemia, it seems prudent to minimize the likelihood of significant changes that could further interfere with oxygen delivery to tissues. For example, drug-induced decreases in cardiac output or a leftward shift of the oxyhemoglobin dissociation curve owing to respiratory alkalosis from iatrogenic hyperventilation of the patient's lungs could interfere with tissue oxygen delivery. Decreased body temperature also shifts the oxyhemoglobin dissociation curves to the left. Decreased tissue oxygen requirements may accompany depressant effects of anesthetic drugs and hypothermia, offsetting the decreases in tissue oxygen delivery associated with anemia to unpredictable degrees. Nevertheless, signs and symptoms of inadequate tissue oxygen delivery due to anemia during anesthesia are difficult to appreciate. Efforts to offset the impact of surgical blood loss by such measures as normovolemic hemodilution and intraoperative blood salvage are considerations in selected patients. Effects of anesthesia on the sympathetic nervous system and cardiovascular responses may blunt the usual increase in cardiac output associated with acute normovolemic anemia.

Volatile anesthetics may be less soluble in the plasma of anemic patients, reflecting a decrease in the concentration of lipid-rich RBCs. As a result, establishment of arterial partial pressures of volatile anesthetics in the plasma of anemic patients might be accelerated. Nevertheless, effects of decreased solubility of volatile anesthetics owing to anemia is probably offset by the impact of increased cardiac output. Therefore, it seems unlikely that clinically detectable differences in the rate of induction of anesthesia or vulnerability to an anesthetic overdose would be present in anemic patients any more than in normal patients. Although supporting evidence is not available, it is likely that a decision to replace intraoperative blood loss with whole blood or packed RBCs will be made when Hb concentrations decrease acutely to less than 7 g/dL, especially if there is co-existing anemia or cardiovascular or cerebrovascular disease.

Disorders Affecting the Red Cell Structure

The oxygen required by tissues for aerobic metabolism is supplied by the circulating mass of mature erythrocytes (RBCs). The circulating RBC population is continually renewed by the erythroid precursor cells in the marrow, under the control of both humoral and cellular growth factors. This cycle of normal erythropoiesis is a carefully regulated process. Oxygen sensors within the kidney detect minute changes in the amount of oxygen available to tissue and by releasing erythropoietin are able to adjust erythropoiesis to match tissue requirements.

The mature RBC at rest takes the shape of a biconcave disk with a mean diameter of 8 μm, a thickness of 2 μm, and a volume of 90 fL. It lacks a nucleus and mitochondria, and 33% of its contents are made up of a single protein, Hb. Intracellular energy requirements are largely supplied by glucose metabolism, which is targeted at maintaining Hb in a soluble, reduced state, providing appropriate amounts of 2,3-diphosphoglycerate (2,3-DPG), and generating adenosine triphosphate to support membrane function. Without a nucleus or protein metabolic pathway, the cell has a limited life span of 100 to 120 days. However, the unique structure of the adult RBC provides maximum flexibility as the cell travels through the microvasculature.

Hereditary Spherocytosis

Abnormalities in membrane protein composition can result in lifelong hemolytic anemia. Hereditary spherocytosis (HS) is inherited in an autosomal dominant pattern in more than 60% of patients, with sporadic mutations in another 20%, and the remaining cases classified as recessive. HS is the most common inherited hemolytic anemia in Europe and the United States, with a frequency of 1 in 5000 individuals. The principal defect in HS is a deficiency in membrane skeletal proteins, usually spectrin and ankyrin. These cells show abnormal osmotic fragility and shortened circulation half-life. Patients with HS can be clinically silent, and approximately one third have a very mild hemolytic anemia and rarely show spherocytes on their peripheral smear. Some patients, however, can have a more severe degree of hemolysis and resulting anemia, with less than 5% of patients developing life-threatening anemia. HS patients often have splenomegaly and experience symptoms of easy fatigability in proportion to their chronic anemia. HS patients are at risk of episodes of hemolytic crisis, often precipitated by viral or bacterial infection. These crises will worsen the chronic anemia and may be associated with jaundice. Infection with parvovirus B19 infection, however, can produce a profound, albeit transient (10–14 days) aplastic crisis. The risk of pigment gallstones is high in HS patients and should be considered in patients complaining of biliary colic. The anesthetic risk of these patients is largely dictated by the severity of their anemia, whether their hemolysis is steady state or they are currently experiencing an exacerbation of that hemolysis due to concurrent infection.

Anesthetic Considerations Episodic anemia, often triggered by viral or bacterial infection and cholelithiasis, must be taken into consideration.

Hereditary Elliptocytosis

Hereditary elliptocytosis is produced by an abnormality in one of the membrane proteins, spectrin or glycophorin, that make the erythrocyte less pliable. Hereditary elliptocytosis is inherited as an autosomal dominant disorder and is prevalent in regions where malaria is endemic, reaching a frequency of as much as 3 in 100. The diagnosis of hereditary elliptocytosis is most often an incidental finding, where the majority of cells demonstrate an elliptical and even a rodlike appearance. The majority of hereditary elliptocytosis patients are heterozygous and only rarely experience hemolysis. In contrast, homozygosity (<10%) or compound heterozygous defects may demonstrate greater degrees of hemolysis and, accordingly, more severe anemia

Anesthetic Considerations See discussion of anemia.

Acanthocytosis

Acanthocytosis is another defect in membrane structure found in patients with a congenital lack of lipoprotein-β (abetalipoproteinemia) and infrequently with severe cirrhosis or pancreatitis. It results from cholesterol or sphingomyelin accumulation on the outer membrane of the erythrocyte. This accretion gives the membrane a spiculated appearance that signals the splenic macrophages of the reticuloendothelial system to cull it from the circulation, producing hemolysis.

Anesthetic Considerations See previous discussion of anemia.

Paroxysmal Nocturnal Hemoglobinuria

Paroxysmal nocturnal hemoglobinuria is a clonal disorder that may arise in hematopoietic cells anywhere from the second to the eighth decade of life. A number of different mutations have been identified, but all result in abnormalities in or reductions of a membrane protein known as glycosyl-phosphatidyl glycan. This protein is found in all hematopoietic cells and serves to anchor specific secondary proteins to the membrane, so-called glycosylphosphatidyl glycan–linked proteins. Patients often present with hemolytic anemia and are at increased risk of venous thrombosis due to activation of coagulation by the dysregulated complement activation. Alternatively, absence of protectin, a critical glycosyl phosphatidyl glycan-linked protein, may be associated with a dysplastic or aplastic marrow, suggestive of damage to all hematopoietic precursor cells. Paroxysmal nocturnal hemoglobinuria tends to be a chronic disorder, with hemolytic anemia and deficiencies in other marrow constituents. Median life expectancy after diagnosis is 8 to 10 years.

Anesthetic Considerations See previous discussion of anemia and hypercoagulability discussion at the end of the chapter.

Disorders Affecting the Red Cell Metabolism

Lacking a nucleus and having a limited (120 days) life expectancy, the erythrocyte can maintain a very narrow spectrum of activities necessary to carry out its oxygen transport functions. The stability of the RBC membrane and the solubility of intracellular Hb depend on four glucose-supported metabolic pathways. These four pathways are illustrated in **Figure 17-2**. The most clinically relevant pathways are described below.

Embden-Meyerhoff Pathway

The Embden-Meyerhoff pathway (nonoxidative or anaerobic pathway) is responsible for generation of the adenosine triphosphate necessary for membrane function and the maintenance of cell shape and pliability. Defects in anaerobic glycolysis are associated with increased cell rigidity and decreased survival, which produces a hemolytic anemia. Unlike deficiencies in the phosphogluconate pathway, described later, deficiencies of the glycolytic pathway do not have any typical morphologic red cell changes that herald their presence, nor are they subject to hemolytic crisis after exposure to oxidants. The severity of their hemolysis is highly variable and largely unpredictable from patient to patient.

Phosphogluconate Pathway

In a similar fashion, the phosphogluconate pathway couples oxidative metabolism with nicotinamide adenine dinucleotide phosphate and glutathione reduction. It counteracts environmental oxidants and prevents globin denaturation. When

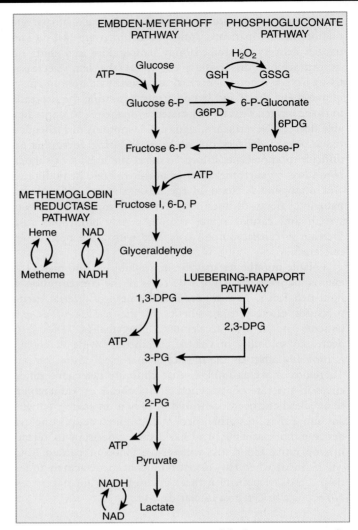

Figure 17-2 • Diagrammatic representation of the four most common disorders affecting the red cell metabolism. 6PDG, 6-phosphogluconate dehydrogenase; ATP, adenosine triphosphate; G6PD, glucose-6-phosphate dehydrogenase; GSH, glutathione reductase; GSSG, oxidized glutathione; NAD, nicotinamide adenine dinucleotide; NADH, reduced form of nicotinamide adenine dinucleotide.

patients lack either of the two key enzymes, glucose-6-phosphate dehydrogenase (G6PD) or glutathione reductase, denatured Hb precipitates on the inner surface of the RBC membrane, resulting in membrane damage and hemolysis.

Glucose-6-Phosphate Dehydrogenase Deficiency

Erythrocytes contain higher levels of glutathione reductase than any other cell in the body. Indeed, precious resources are continually tapped to maintain high reserves of this antioxidant critical to protecting the red cell from the toxicity of the very oxygen it is transporting.

G6PD deficiency is one of the most prevalent disease-causing mutations, affecting hundreds of millions of people worldwide, with regional variants predominating in Mediterranean, Southeast Asia, and Chinese territories. Encoded on the X chromosome, it is subject to dose compensation by

X chromosome inactivation. The remaining enzymes of the glutathione pathway are on autosomal chromosomes, and deficiencies of these are very rare, but generally manifest symptoms resembling G6PD deficiency. G6PD activity is highest in young red cells and declines with age, with half-life of approximately 60 days. The clinical manifestations of G6PD deficiency can be divided into three categories: a chronic hemolytic anemia; an acute, episodic hemolytic anemia; and no apparent risk of hemolysis. Acute insults that either precipitate new or aggravate pre-existing hemolytic anemias are most commonly infections, drugs, or fava bean ingestion. Methylene blue is a particular concern, as it may be administered therapeutically for methemoglobinemia (discussed later). If a patient manifesting methemoglobinemia with already compromised oxygen delivery is also G6PD deficient, methylene blue administration may be life threatening.

Anesthetic Considerations Anesthetic risk is largely a function of the severity and acuity of the anemia, as discussed previously. Drugs known to precipitate hemolytic crisis must, of course, be avoided, and perioperative infections may be of special concern.

Pyruvate Kinase Deficiency

Pyruvate kinase deficiency is the most common erythrocyte enzyme defect causing congenital hemolytic anemia. Although less prevalent than glucose-6-phosphate dehydrogenase deficiency (see previous section), pyruvate kinase deficiencies are considerably more likely to manifest a chronic hemolytic anemia. Accumulations of 2,3-DPG in the RBCs causes a shift of the oxyhemoglobin dissociation curve to the right to facilitate oxygen release from Hb to the peripheral tissues. Splenectomy does not totally prevent hemolysis but does decrease the rate of RBC destruction. The severity of the clinical presentation ranges from a mild, fully compensated process without anemia to a life-threatening, transfusion-requiring hemolytic anemia present at birth. Severely affected individuals may be chronically jaundiced, develop pigmented gallstones, and manifest splenomegaly. Splenectomy frequently improves the chronic hemolysis and may even eliminate the need for transfusions. An autosomal recessive mutation, pyruvate kinase deficiency is found worldwide, but shows a higher prevalence among people of northern European extraction and from some regions of China. In these populations, the frequency of heterozygosity may reach as high as 1%.

Anesthetic Considerations Anesthetic risk is largely a function of the severity and acuity of the anemia, as discussed previously.

Methemoglobin Reductase Pathway

The methemoglobin reductase pathway uses the pyridine nucleotide–reduced nicotinamide adenine dinucleotide generated from anaerobic glycolysis to maintain heme iron in its ferrous state. An inherited mutation of the methemoglobin reductase enzyme (also referred to as reduced nicotinamide adenine dinucleotide–diaphorase or cytochrome b_5 reductase) results in an inability to counteract oxidation of Hb to methemoglobin, the ferric form of Hb that will not transport oxygen. Patients with type I reduced nicotinamide adenine dinucleotide-diaphorase deficiency accumulate small amounts of methemoglobin in circulating red cells, whereas type II patients have severe cyanosis and mental retardation. Methemoglobinemia is discussed in detail in the section entitled "Hemoglobins with Decreased Oxygen Affinity."

Luebering-Rapaport Pathway

Finally, the Luebering-Rapaport pathway is responsible for the production of 2,3-DPG (also known as 2,3-bisphosphoglycerate). A single enzyme, bisphospheroglyceromutase, mediates both the synthase activity, resulting in 2,3-DPG formation, and the phosphatase activity that then converts 2,3-DPG to 3-phosphoglycerate, returning it to the glycolytic pathway. The balance of formation versus metabolism of 2,3-DPG is pH sensitive, with alkalosis favoring the synthetase activity and acidosis the phosphatase activity. The 2,3-DPG response is also influenced by the supply of phosphate to the cell. Severe phosphate depletion in patients with diabetic ketoacidosis or nutritional deficiency can result in a reduced 2,3-DPG production response.

The Hemoglobin Molecule

The RBC is basically a container for Hb, each containing an active heme group and overall representing approximately 90% of the dry weight of the red cell. Each heme group is capable of binding to an oxygen molecule. The respiratory motion of Hb, that is, the uptake and release of oxygen to tissues, involves a specific change in molecular structure. As Hb shuttles from its deoxyhemoglobin to its oxyhemoglobin form, CO_2 and 2,3-DPG are expelled from their position between the β-globin chains, opening the molecule to receive oxygen. Furthermore, oxygen binding by one of the heme groups increases the affinity of the other groups to oxygen loading. This interaction is responsible for the sigmoid shape of the oxygen dissociation curve.

Inherited defects in Hb structure can interfere with this respiratory motion. Most defects are substitutions of a single amino acid in either the α- or β-globin chains. Some interfere with molecular movement, restricting the molecule to either a low- or high-affinity state, whereas others either change the valency of heme iron from ferrous to ferric or reduce the solubility of the Hb molecule. Hb S (sickle cell disease) is an example of a single amino acid substitution that results in reduced solubility, typically causing precipitation of the abnormal Hb.

Disorders of Hemoglobin Resulting in Hemolysis

Sickle S Hemoglobin

Sickle cell disease is a disorder caused by the substitution of a valine for glutamic acid in the β-globin subunit. In the deoxygenated state, this Hb S undergoes conformational changes exposing a hydrophobic region of the molecule. In extreme states of deoxygenation, causing a high percentage of the resident Hb within the erythrocyte to undergo these states, the hydrophobic regions aggregate, resulting in distortion of the erythrocyte membrane, oxidative damage to the membrane, impaired deformability, and a shortened life span. Sickle cell anemia, the homozygous form of Hb S disease, presents early in life with a severe hemolytic anemia and vaso-occlusive disease involving the marrow, spleen, kidney, and central nervous system. Patients experience episodic painful crises characterized as bone and joint pain that may or may not be associated with concurrent illness. The severity and progression of the disease are remarkably varied. Organ damage can start early in childhood, with recurrent splenic infarction culminating in loss of splenic function in the first decade of life. The renal medulla is another prime target, with loss of concentrating ability an early feature of the disease progressing to chronic renal failure usually in the third or fourth decade' of life. Pulmonary and neurologic complications are the leading causes of morbidity and mortality. Lung damage results from chronic progressive lung damage due to persistent inflammatory reactions punctuated by acute chest syndrome, a pneumonia-like complication characterized by a new pulmonary infiltrate involving at least one complete lung segment and at least one of the following: chest pain, fever higher than 38.5°C, tachypnea, wheezing, or cough. Neurologic complications may include stroke, usually infarctive in adolescence and hemorrhagic later in adult life.

Anesthetic Considerations The sickle cell trait does not cause an increase in perioperative morbidity or mortality: by contrast, sickle cell disease patients have a high incidence of perioperative complications. Risk factors for such complications include age, frequency of hospitalizations and/or transfusions for episodes of crisis, evidence of organ damage such as low baseline oxygen saturation, elevated creatinine, cardiac dysfunction, history of central nervous system events, and concurrent infection. The risk intrinsic to the type of surgery is an important consideration, with minor procedures such as inguinal hernia repair and extremity surgery considered low risk, intra-abdominal operations such as cholecystectomy considered more intermediate risk, and intracranial and intrathoracic procedures classified as high risk. Among orthopedic procedures, however, hip surgery and hip replacement in particular are associated with a considerable risk of complications, including excessive blood loss in more than 70% of patients and sickle cell events in 19% of patients.

The goals of preoperative transfusion management have changed in recent years. Studies examining the effects of aggressive transfusion strategies aimed at increasing the ratio of normal Hb to sickle Hb have found no benefit compared to more the more conservative goal of achieving a preoperative hematocrit of 30%. Indeed, the aggressive strategy necessitated significantly more transfusions, and the complications of those transfusions outweighed their benefit. Accordingly, low-risk procedures rarely require any preoperative transfusions, and patients undergoing moderate- to high-risk operations need only have any preoperative anemia corrected to a target hematocrit of 30%. Choice of anesthetic technique does not appear to significantly affect the risk of complications stemming from sickle cell disease. The usual secondary goals of avoiding dehydration, acidosis, and hypothermia during anesthesia theoretically should also reduce the risk of perioperative sickling events. Occlusive orthopedic tourniquets are not contraindicated in sickle cell disease, although as mentioned above, the incidence of perioperative complications is increased. Postoperative pain requires aggressive management, as pain at the operative site and pain due to vaso-occlusive events can exacerbate complications of this disease. Patients may have a degree of tolerance to opioids, and while a subset of patients may have drug addition, this consideration should not lead clinicians to undertreat this patient population.

The complication known as *acute chest syndrome* may develop typically 2 to 3 days into the postoperative period and demands aggressive focus on oxygenation, adequate analgesia, and frequently blood transfusion to correct anemia and improve oxygenation. Inhaled nitric oxide to reduce pulmonary hypertension and improve blood oxygenation has shown promise, but at present is not widely available.

Sickle C Hemoglobin

Hb C is prevalent at approximately one fourth the frequency of Hb S. Hb C causes the erythrocyte to lose water via enhanced activity of the potassium-chloride cotransport system, resulting in cellular dehydration that in the homozygous (CC) state may produce a mild-to-moderate hemolytic anemia. Ironically, the presence of both Hb S and Hb C (Hb SC), traits that in isolation produce no symptoms, together produces a tendency toward sickling and the associated complications approaching that of Hb SS disease. It appears that the dehydration produced by Hb C increases the concentration of Hb S within the erythrocyte, exacerbating its insolubility and tendency to polymerize.

Anesthetic Considerations The anesthetic risks of Hb SC are not as well studied as with Hb SS, but one investigation suggested that perioperative transfusions considerably reduce the incidence of sickle complications in this subset.

Hemoglobin Sickle–β-Thalassemia

Among African Americans, the gene frequency of β-thalassemia is one tenth that of Hb S. The clinical presentation of this compound heterozygous state is largely determined by whether it is associated with reduced amounts of Hb A present (sickle cell-β+ thalassemia) or no Hb A whatsoever (sickle cell-β_{zero} thalassemia). In the absence of any Hb A, patients experience acute vaso-occlusive crises, acute chest syndrome, and other sickling complications at rates approaching those of Hb SS.

Anesthetic Considerations They are the same as those for homozygous sickle S Hb.

Unstable Hemoglobins

Hbs are made unstable by structural changes that reduce their solubility or make them more susceptible to oxidation of amino acids within the globin chains. More than 100 unique unstable Hb variants have been documented, most associated with only minimal clinical manifestations. The mutations typically impair globin folding or heme-globin binding that stabilizes the heme moiety within the hydrophobic globin pocket. Once freed from its cleft, the heme binds nonspecifically to other regions of the globin chains, causing them to form a precipitate containing globin chains and chain fragments and heme, called the Heinz body. Heinz bodies interact with the red cell membrane, reducing its deformability and favoring its removal by splenic macrophages. Unstable Hbs vary in their propensity to form Heinz bodies, and, accordingly, the severity of the associated anemia. Hemolysis may be aggravated by the development of additional oxidant stresses, such as infections or the ingestion of oxidant agents. Anesthetic management of these patients is largely dictated by the degree of hemolysis occurring in an individual patient, with transfusion during bouts of severe hemolysis and avoidance of oxidizing agents. Patients with recurring bouts of severe hemolysis or morbidity because of chronic anemia may be considered for splenectomy, which is usually effective in reducing and even eliminating symptoms.

Anesthetic Considerations These patients may have severe anemia and hemoglobin-induced renal injury. Care must be taken to avoid use of oxidizing agents.

Disorders of Hemoglobin Resulting in Reduced or Ineffective Erythropoiesis: Macrocytic/ Megaloblastic Anemia

Disruption of the erythroid precursor maturation sequence can result from deficiencies in vitamins such as folic acid and vitamin B_{12}, exposure to chemotherapeutic agents, or a preleukemic state. Since these are all defects in nuclear maturation, patients present with macrocytic anemias and megaloblastic bone marrow morphology.

Folate and B_{12} Deficiency Anemias

Folic acid and vitamin B_{12} deficiencies are primary causes of macrocytic anemia in adults. Both vitamins are essential for normal DNA synthesis, and high turnover tissues such as marrow are the first to become affected when these vitamins are in short supply. In deficiency states, the marrow precursors appear much larger than normal and are unable to complete cell division. Accordingly, the marrow becomes megaloblastic, and macrocytic red cells are released into the circulation. Prevalence of deficiencies of these vitamins varies considerably in different parts of the world. In developed countries, alcoholism is a frequent source of folate deficiency, both because of the poor dietary habits of the alcoholic and alcohol's interference with folate metabolism. In developing countries where tropical and nontropical sprue is more widespread, malabsorption may increase the frequency of B_{12} deficiencies.

Sustained exposure to nitrous oxide can produce an impairment of vitamin B_{12} activity. Nitrous oxide can oxidize the cobalt atom of the vitamin, reducing its cofactor activity and causing impairment in synthesis of both methionine and S-adenosylmethionine synthesis. This action requires long exposure to high concentrations of nitrous oxide and only pertains to situations where scavenging systems are inadequate, as might be found in dental offices or with recreational use of the gas.

A full-blown macrocytic anemia due to folate or vitamin B_{12} deficiency may result in Hb levels less than 8 to 10 g/dL, a mean cell volume of 110 to 140 fL (normal = 90 fL), a normal reticulocyte count, and increased levels of lactate dehydrogenase and bilirubin. In addition to megaloblastic anemia, vitamin B_{12} deficiency is associated with bilateral peripheral neuropathy due to degeneration of the lateral and posterior columns of the spinal cord. There are symmetrical paresthesias with loss of proprioceptive and vibratory sensations, especially in the lower extremities. Gait is unsteady, and deep tendon reflexes are diminished. Memory impairment and mental depression may be prominent. These neurologic deficits are progressive unless parenteral vitamin B_{12} is provided. Nonmedical abuse of nitrous oxide may be associated with neurologic findings similar to those that accompany vitamin B_{12} deficiency and pernicious anemia.

Treatment of folate and vitamin B_{12} deficiencies can be corrected by parenteral vitamin preparations, which in cases of intestinal malabsorption becomes the preferred route. Emergency correction, either in preparation for imminent surgery or life-threatening anemia, takes the form of red cell transfusions.

Anesthetic Considerations Management of anesthesia in patients with megaloblastic anemia due to vitamin B_{12} deficiency is influenced by the need to maintain delivery of oxygenated arterial blood to peripheral tissues. The presence of neurologic changes may detract from selection of regional anesthetic techniques or the use of peripheral nerve blocks. The use of nitrous oxide is questionable, as this drug has been shown to inhibit activity of methionine synthetase by oxidizing the cobalt atom of vitamin B_{12} from an active to an inactive state. Even relatively short exposures to nitrous oxide may produce megaloblastic changes.

Disorders of Hemoglobin Resulting in Reduced or Ineffective Erythropoiesis: Microcytic Anemia

Defects in hemoglobinization, including severe iron deficiency and inherited defects in globin chain synthesis, the thalassemias, produce microcytic, hypochromic anemia and markedly ineffective erythropoiesis.

Iron Deficiency Anemia

Nutritional deficiency of iron is a cause of anemia only in infants and small children. In adults, iron deficiency anemia can only reflect depletion of iron stores owing to chronic blood loss, most likely from the gastrointestinal tract or from the female genital tract (menstruation). Parturients are susceptible to the development of iron deficiency anemia because of increased RBC mass during gestation and the needs of the fetus for iron. Symptoms of iron deficiency anemia depend on the actual Hb concentrations.

Diagnosis Patients experiencing chronic blood loss may not be able to absorb sufficient iron from the gastrointestinal tract to form Hb as rapidly as RBCs are lost. As a result, RBCs are often produced with too little Hb, resulting in microcytic hypochromic anemia. Nevertheless, most cases of iron deficiency anemia in the United States are mild, exhibiting Hb concentrations of 9 to 12 g/dL. The absence of stainable iron in bone marrow aspirates is confirmatory for iron deficiency anemia. Demonstrations of decreased serum ferritin concentrations serve as cost-effective alternative tests to bone marrow examinations for the diagnosis of iron deficiency anemia.

Treatment Treatment of iron deficiency anemia is with ferrous iron salts, such as ferrous sulfate administered orally. Iron stores are replenished slowly. Therapy should be continued for at least 1 year after the source of blood loss that caused the iron deficiency anemia is corrected. Favorable responses to iron therapy are characterized by increases in Hb concentrations of approximately 2 g/dL in 3 weeks or return of Hb concentrations to normal levels in 6 weeks. Continued bleeding is reflected by reticulocytosis and failure of Hb concentrations to increase in response to iron therapy. Recombinant human erythropoietin may be used to treat drug-induced anemia or to improve Hb concentrations before elective surgery.

Defective Production of Globin Chains: The Thalassemias

Globin chains are assembled by cytoplasmic ribosomes under the control of two clusters of closely linked genes on chromosomes 11 and 16. The final globin molecule is a tetramer of two α-globin and two non–α-globin chains. In the adult, 96% to 97% of the Hb is made up of two α-globin and two β-globin chains (Hb A) with minor components of Hb F and A_2.

An inherited defect in globin chain synthesis, known as thalassemia, is one of the leading causes of microcytic anemia in children and adults. This disorder shows a strong geographic influence, with β-thalassemia predominating in Africa and the Mediterranean area, and α-thalassemia and Hb E dominant in Southeast Asia.

Thalassemia Minor

Most individuals with thalassemia are thalassemia minor patients who are heterozygotes for either an α-globin (α-thalassemia trait) or β-globin (β-thalassemia trait) gene mutation. While the mutation may decrease synthesis of the affected globin chain by up to 50% of normal, producing hypochromic and microcytic RBCs, the anemia is usually modest (Hb 10–14 g/dL at worst), and relatively little accumulation of the unaffected globin occurs. Accordingly, the morbidity associated with chronic hemolysis and ineffective erythropoiesis is rarely encountered.

Thalassemia Intermedia

Thalassemia intermedia patients present with more severe anemia and prominent microcytosis and hypochromia. They have symptoms attributable both to their anemia and also may have hepatosplenomegaly, cardiomegaly, and skeletal changes secondary to marrow expansion. These patients have either a milder form of homozygous β-thalassemia, a combined α- and β-thalassemia defect, or β-thalassemia with high levels of Hb F.

Thalassemia Major

Thalassemia major patients develop severe, life-threatening anemia during their first few years of life. To survive childhood, they require long-term transfusion therapy to correct their anemia and suppress their high level of ineffective erythropoiesis. Otherwise, they either die during childhood or have marked changes due to their disease and the complications of therapy. The severity of thalassemia is remarkably variable, even among patients with seemingly identical genetic mutations. In its most severe forms, patients exhibit three defects that markedly depress their oxygen-carrying capacity: (1) ineffective erythropoiesis, (2) hemolytic anemia, and (3) hypochromia with microcytosis. The deficit in oxygen-carrying capacity produces maximum erythropoietin release, and marrow erythroblasts respond by increasing their unbalanced globin synthesis. The accumulating unpaired globins aggregate and precipitate, forming inclusion bodies that cause membrane damage to the RBCs. Some of these defective RBCs are destroyed within the marrow, resulting in ineffective erythropoiesis. Some abnormal erythrocytes escape into the circulation, where their altered morphology can cause accelerated clearance (hemolytic anemia) or, at best, reduced capacity to transport oxygen due to their lowered Hb content (hypochromia with microcytosis). Other features of severe thalassemia include those attributable to massive marrow hyperplasia (frontal bossing, maxillary overgrowth, stunted growth, osteoporosis), and extramedullary hematopoiesis (hepatomegaly). Hemolytic anemia may produce splenomegaly together with extreme dyspnea and orthopnea, over time resulting in congestive heart failure and mental retardation. Transfusion therapy will ameliorate many of these changes, but complications due to iron overload such as cirrhosis, right-sided heart failure, and endocrinopathy frequently require chelation therapy. Some patients demonstrate reduced transfusion requirements after splenectomy, and laparoscopic splenectomy has dramatically shortened recovery times. However, the greater risk of postsplenectomy sepsis in younger patients argues for deferment of surgery until after 5 years of age whenever possible, and for well-transfused and well-chelated patients, splenectomy may not be indicated. Bone marrow transplantation was first performed for thalassemia major in 1982 and is a therapeutic option for younger patients with HLA-identical siblings.

Anesthetic Considerations The severity of the thalassemia is a critical determinant of the degree of organ damage and the anesthetic risks. In its mildest forms, a chronic, compensated anemia is the major concern. With more aggressive forms of the disorder, the anemia is more severe, and associated features may include spleno- and hepatomegaly, skeletal malformations, congestive heart failure, mental retardation, and complications of iron overload such as cirrhosis, right-sided heart failure, and endocrinopathies.

Hemoglobins with Increased Oxygen Affinity
Hemoglobin Chesapeake, J-Capetown, Kemsey, Creteil

Hb mutations increasing the oxygen binding avidity of the heme moiety cause the oxygen dissociation curve to shift to the left, reducing the Po_{50} (the partial pressure of oxygen at which the Hb is 50% saturated with oxygen). Many types of mutations can increase oxygen affinity, even those causing loss of 2,3-DPG binding. These Hbs bind oxygen more readily than normal and retain more oxygen at lower Po_2 levels. Accordingly, they deliver less oxygen to tissues at normal capillary Po_2 levels, and blood returns to the lungs still saturated with oxygen. Since these variant Hbs cannot acquire more oxygen in the lungs, despite their higher affinity, the net result is that at normal hematocrits, a mild tissue hypoxia results, triggering increased erythropoietin production leading to polycythemia. Patients with only mild erythrocytosis do not require intervention. Patients exhibiting high hematocrits (>55%–60%), whose blood viscosity may further compromise oxygen delivery, may require preoperative exchange transfusion and careful avoidance of hemoconcentration both pre- and intraoperatively. Hemodilution and blood loss, however, resulting in a modest anemia, may cause critical decreases the tissue oxygen delivery, even for hematocrits normally tolerated by patients with normal Hbs.

Anesthetic Considerations Tissue oxygen delivery at baseline may be barely adequate, making even modest decreases in hematocrit potentially dangerous. By the same token, very high hematocrits (>55%–60%) may compromise tissue perfusion and induce hypercoagulability.

Hemoglobins with Decreased Oxygen Affinity
Methemoglobinemias

Methemoglobin is formed when the iron moiety in the Hb is oxidized from the ferrous (Fe^{2+}) state to the ferric (Fe^{3+}) state. The normal Hb, upon binding oxygen, partially transfers an electron from the iron to the oxygen, moving the iron close to its ferric state and the oxygen resembles superoxide (O_2^-). Deoxygenation ordinarily returns the electron to the iron, but methemoglobin forms if the electron is not returned. The normal erythrocyte maintains methemoglobin levels at 1% or less by the methemoglobin reductase enzyme system consisting of nicotinamide adenine dinucleotide–dehydratase, antidiuretic hormone–diaphorase, and erythrocyte cytochrome b_3. Methemoglobin is a markedly left-shifted Hb that, due to its higher oxygen affinity, delivers little oxygen to the tissues. At levels below 30% of the total Hb content, methemoglobin causes no compromise in tissue oxygenation. Between 30% and 50%, however, patients begin to exhibit symptoms of oxygen deprivation, and above 50%, coma and death can ensue.

Methemoglobinemias of clinical importance can arise from three mechanisms: globin chain mutations favoring formation of methemoglobin (M Hbs), mutations impairing efficacy of the methemoglobin reductase system, and toxic exposure to substances that oxidize normal Hb iron at a rate that exceeds the capacity of normal reducing mechanisms.

M Hbs arise from mutations that stabilize the heme iron in the ferric (Fe^{3+}) state, making it relatively resistant to reduction by the methemoglobin reductase system. The methemoglobin has a brownish-blue color that does not change to red on exposure to oxygen, giving patients a cyanotic appearance independent of their Pao_2. Patients with M Hbs are usually asymptomatic, as their methemoglobin levels rarely exceed 30% of their total Hb, the level at which clinical symptoms develop.

Mutations impairing the methemoglobin reductase system rarely result in methemoglobinemia levels greater than 25%. Like their Hb M counterparts, affected patients may exhibit a slate-gray pseudocyanosis despite normal Pao_2 levels. Exposure to chemical agents that directly oxidize Hb or produce reactive oxygen intermediates that oxidize Hb may produce an acquired methemoglobinemia that is virtually the only situation in which life-threatening amounts of methemoglobin accumulate. Very young infants have lower levels of methemoglobin reductase in their erythrocytes and may accordingly manifest greater susceptibility to these oxidizing agents.

Emergency treatment of toxic methemoglobinemia begins with 1 to 2 mg/kg of intravenous methylene blue as a 1% solution in saline infused over 3 to 5 minutes. This treatment is usually effective, but may be repeated after 30 minutes. Methylene blue acts through the reduced nicotinamide adenine dinucleotide phosphate reductase system and accordingly requires the activity of G6PD. Patients who are G6PD deficient and patients severely affected may require exchange transfusions. Mild cases of methemoglobin intoxication do not require treatment, and identification of the source of the oxidizing agent is all that is needed.

Anesthetic Considerations Avoidance of oxidizing agents critical for patients with congenital mutations favoring development of methemoglobin, measurement of blood pH and occasionally methemoglobin levels may be required for the rare patient at risk of developing severe degrees of methemoglobinemia (>30%).

Disorders of Red Cell Production
Hypoproliferation

Constitutional Aplastic Anemia (Fanconi Anemia) Fanconi anemia is an autosomal recessive disorder that presents with severe pancytopenia usually in the first two decades of life and often progresses to acute leukemia. The gene frequency in Western societies is approximately 1 in 200 persons, and in white South Africans may be as high as 1 in 80. When fully expressed (1 per 100,000 live births), the disorder is associated with progressive marrow failure, multiple physical defects, chromosomal abnormalities, and cancer predisposition. However, patients may present without the classic

TABLE 17-1 Classes of Drugs Associated with Marrow Damage

Antibiotics (chloramphenicol, penicillin, cephalosporins, sulfonamides, amphotericin B, streptomycin)
Antidepressants (lithium, tricyclics)
Antiepileptics (dilantin, carbamazepine, valproic acid, phenobarbital)
Anti-inflammatory drugs (phenylbutazone, nonsteroidals, salicylates, gold salts)
Antiarrhythmics (lidocaine, quinidine, procainamide)
Antithyroidal drugs (propylthiouracil)
Diuretics (thiazides, pyrimethamine, furosemide)
Antihypertensives (captopril)
Antiuricemics (allopurinol, colchicine)
Antimalarials (quinacrine, chloroquine)
Hypoglycemics (tolbutamide)
Platelet inhibitors (ticlopidine)
Tranquilizers (prochlorperazine, meprobamate)

physical defects, and the diagnosis should be considered in children and young adults with acute myelogenous leukemia.

Drug and Radiation-associated Marrow Damage Anemia Marrow damage anemia is a predictable side effect of chemotherapy, and the anemia that develops is usually mild except in cases of high-dose, multidrug chemotherapy that can produce pancytopenia. As long as the drug does not irreversibly damage the marrow, recovery is usually full, provided there is a sufficient infection-free period. High-energy radiation can also produce a marrow damage anemia, the degree of which is usually predictable depending on the type of radiation, the dose, and the extent of marrow exposure. Long-term exposure to low levels of external radiation or ingested radioisotopes can also produce aplastic anemia, although the dose relationship is considerably less predictable.

Several drugs have been associated with the development of severe, often irreversible, aplastic anemia. **Table 17-1** shows classes of drugs that have been associated with marrow damage; some, such as chloramphenicol, can produce severe, irreversible aplastic anemia after only a few doses of the drug, while most, such as phenylbutazone, propylthiouracil, and tricyclic antidepressants, are associated with more gradual onset of pancytopenia that is reversible if the drug is immediately withdrawn.

Infection-associated Marrow Damage Anemia Marrow damage can result from direct invasion of the marrow itself by an infectious agent, miliary tuberculosis being perhaps the best example, or by immunosuppression of stem cell growth. Aplastic anemia is seen following viral illnesses such as viral hepatitis, Epstein-Barr virus infection, human immunodeficiency virus, and rubella. Parvovirus B19 infection can cause an acute, reversible pure red cell aplasia in patients with congenital hemolytic anemias (sickle cell anemia, hereditary spherocytosis, etc., and in human immunodeficiency virus patients who cannot clear the virus). Although most of these anemias are spontaneously reversible, some, especially after viral (non-A, non-B, non-C) hepatitis, can produce fatal aplastic anemia.

Anemia Due to Hematologic or Other Marrow-Involving Malignancy Anemias may be caused by any leukemia that reduces the number of erythroid precursors, whether by diverting the stem cells away from the erythroid pathway or crowding them out of the marrow by virtue of shear numbers. Solid tumors such as breast, lung, and prostate cancers may metastasize to the marrow, producing a similar hypoproliferative anemia. In addition to leukemias, clonal expansion of other marrow constituents, as in myelodysplastic syndromes and myeloproliferative disorders, frequently are also capable of crowding out RBC precursors resulting in anemia. By contrast, clonal expansion of erythroid cells in the marrow, or erythrocytosis, may produce the disorder known as polycythemia vera (PV), discussed in the next section.

Anesthetic Considerations Patients may present for surgery with anemia and thrombocytopenia to a degree that transfusions are necessary. The severity of the immunocompromise will affect the need for and choice of antibiotic coverage.

Polycythemia

Sustained hypoxia usually results in a compensatory rise in the RBC mass and hematocrit. Although this increases the oxygen-carrying capacity of blood, it also increases blood viscosity. Tissue oxygen delivery is maximal at a hematocrit of 33% to 36% (Hb of 11–12 g/dL), assuming no changes in cardiac output or regional blood flow. Above this level, an increase in viscosity will tend to slow blood flow and decrease oxygen delivery. This effect is relatively minor until the hematocrit exceeds 50%, at which time blood flow to key organs such as the brain can be significantly reduced.

Physiology of Polycythemia Polycythemia or erythrocytosis are terms to describe an abnormally elevated hematocrit. Even modest increases in the hematocrit level can have a major impact on whole blood viscosity. An increase in hematocrit can result from a reduction in plasma volume (relative polycythemia) without a true increase in red cell mass. In addition, acute decreases in plasma volume, as may be seen with preoperative fasting, can convert an asymptomatic polycythemia into one where hyperviscosity may threaten tissue perfusion. When the hematocrit rises to levels much above 50% to 55%, whole blood viscosity increases exponentially, especially in small vessels with low flow/shear rates, such as capillaries. The cerebral circulation in particular appears vulnerable to reductions in flow with increased viscosity.

The clinical signs and symptoms of an elevated hematocrit vary depending on the underlying disease process and the rate of onset. Patients with modest chronic polycythemia, as is seen with chronic lung disease, will complain of very few symptoms until the hematocrit rises above 55% to 60%, when headaches and easy fatigability become commonplace. Hematocrit levels greater than 60% can be life threatening, as the increase in viscosity threatens organ perfusion. Patients with hematocrits in this range are also at risk of venous and arterial thrombosis, with 40% of patients experiencing at lease one thrombotic event during the course of their illness.

Primary Polycythemia Primary polycythemia, also known as polycythemia vera or PV, is a stem cell disorder giving rise to proliferation of a clone of hematopoietic precursors, nearly 100% of which arise from a mutation in the *JAK-2* gene. This clonal expansion most commonly produces an excess of erythrocytes, but platelets and leukocytes may also be increased. The criteria for a diagnosis of PV include an elevated hematocrit or RBC mass, normal arterial oxygenation, and splenomegaly not attributable to another cause. PV may appear at any age, but most patients develop the disease in their sixth or seventh decade. Thrombosis, especially cerebral thrombosis, is often the presenting symptom, and patients generally require aggressive, regular phlebotomy to a hematocrit of 45% for men and 38% to 40% for women. Patients may also require myelosuppressive drugs such as hydroxyurea to control their hematocrit. Long term, approximately 30% of patients will die of thrombotic complications and another 30% will succumb to cancer, with half of these developing myelofibrosis and acute leukemia.

PV patients requiring surgery are at increased risk of perioperative thrombosis and, paradoxically, hemorrhage. The increased risk of thrombosis is the predictable combination of the PV patient's baseline hypercoagulability augmented by the approximately 100-fold increase associated with surgery. The etiology of the bleeding diathesis associated with PV is often attributable to an acquired von Willebrand's disease (vWD) caused by abnormally low amounts of the ultra-large von Willebrand's factor (vWF) multimers essential to normal platelet adhesion (see section entitled "von Willenbrand Disease"). The hyperviscosity associated with a high hematocrit favors the conformational change in vWF that renders it vulnerable to enzymatic cleavage. Accordingly, the most hemostatically effective larger multimers become depleted, creating a risk of bleeding. Thus, aggressive phlebotomy and avoidance of extreme dehydration lower the risk of both thrombosis and hemorrhage in the PV patient in the perioperative period.

Anesthetic Considerations Preoperative phlebotomy when indicated, perioperative hypercoagulability *and* potential for bleeding diathesis.

Secondary Polycythemia Due to Hypoxia An increase in the RBC mass without evidence of changes in other hematopoietic cell lines is a normal physiologic response to hypoxia, regardless of cause. Thus, individuals living at high altitudes up to 7000 feet experience a compensatory polycythemia that is physiologically effective and not associated with clinical abnormalities. At higher altitudes, humans are at risk of both acute and chronic mountain sickness, manifest by severe headaches, nausea, vomiting, and disorientation due to cerebral edema.

Significant cardiopulmonary disease can also result in sufficient tissue hypoxia to induce polycythemia, the most dramatic example being congenital heart disease with a severe right-to-left shunt and associated cyanosis. Extremely low cardiac output, whether congenital or acquired, may cause renal release of erythropoietin and an associated increased hematocrit.

Pulmonary disease can also result in a hypoxic polycythemia, the classic case being the very obese patient who develops hypoventilation (Pickwickian syndrome). Inherited defects in Hb, such as high-affinity Hb and defects in 2,3-DPG amount or function, may cause polycythemia despite apparently preserved oxygen saturation of erythrocytes due to reduced tissue oxygen delivery (leftward shift in the oxyhemoglobin dissociation curve, discussed in the section on abnormal Hbs). Defects/drugs producing significant methemoglobinemia (also discussed with abnormal Hbs), where the Hb is stabilized in the oxidized or ferric state, increasing the Hb affinity for oxygen and also resulting in a leftward shift of the oxyhemoglobin dissociation curve and a compensatory polycythemia. Disorders producing methemoglobinemia are distinguished for their pseudocyanotic appearance resulting from the brownish appearance of the ferric Hb due to its inability to reflect red light upon oxygenation. (Please see "Hemoglobins with Decreased Oxygen Affinity" for detailed discussion of the anesthetic implications of these latter disorders.)

Anesthetic Considerations Oxygen therapy, preoperative phlebotomy when indicated, perioperative hypercoagulability *and* potential for bleeding diathesis.

Secondary Polycythemia Due to Increased Erythropoietin Production Renal disease and several erythropoietin-secreting tumors have been associated with secondary polycythemia. Hydronephrosis, polycystic renal disease, renal cysts, and both benign and malignant renal tumors can result in increased erythropoietin production. Uterine myomas, hepatomas, and cerebellar hemangiomas also have been shown capable of secreting erythropoietin. Patients after renal transplantation can develop erythrocytosis that is unrelated to erythropoietin production, possibly due to the red cell growth–promoting effects of angiotensin II, as angiotensin-converting enzyme inhibitors will reverse the polycythemia. In addition, surreptitious use of recombinant erythropoietin by high-performance athletes may produce the finding of polycythemia in an otherwise healthy individual.

Management of patients with secondary polycythemia will vary depending on the specific cause. Patients with mild hypoxic polycythemia should be left alone, as the improved tissue oxygen delivery more than compensates for the modest increased viscosity. In patients with very high hematocrits, where treatment of the underlying disorder is not an option, phlebotomy may be indicated to reduce the thrombotic and hemorrhagic complications of the disorder, much as it would be for primary polycythemia (PV).

Anesthetic Considerations Preoperative phlebotomy when indicated, perioperative hypercoagulability *and* potential for bleeding diathesis.

DISORDERS OF HEMOSTASIS

Normal Hemostasis

Any disruption of vascular endothelium is a potent stimulus to clot formation. As a localized process, clotting acts to seal the break in vascular continuity, limit blood loss, and begin the process of wound healing. Prevention of an exuberant response that would result in pathologic thrombosis involves several counterbalancing mechanisms, including anticoagulant properties of intact endothelial cells, circulating inhibitors of activated coagulation factors, and localized fibrinolytic enzymes. Most abnormalities in hemostasis involve a defect in one or more of the integrated steps in this coagulation process. It is important, therefore, to understand the physiology of hemostasis.

Fifty years ago, two groups simultaneously described the "waterfall" or "cascade" model of soluble coagulation. The cascade model dovetailed well with the clotting assays that were developed at that time to guide warfarin and heparin dosing, and these tests came to be the gold standard for measuring soluble coagulation. Although this cascade model continues to be useful for interpretation of laboratory clotting tests, it does not accurately represent in vivo clotting.

In vivo coagulation follows exposure of the blood to a source of tissue factor (TF), typically on subendothelial cells following damage to a blood vessel. The intrinsic, or contact, pathway of coagulation has *no role* in these earliest clotting events. TF-initiated coagulation has two phases, one an *initiation* phase and a second, the *propagation* phase. The initiation phase begins as exposed TF binds to factor VIIa, picomolar amounts of which are present in the circulation. This VIIa-TF complex catalyzes the conversion of small amounts of factor X to Xa, which in turn generates similarly small amounts of thrombin.

The seemingly trivial amount of thrombin formed during the initiation phase triggers the propagation phase, which fosters explosive thrombin generation in abundance. Thrombin ramps up its own formation by activating platelets and factors (FV, FVIII), setting the stage for formation of the FVIIIa–IXa complex, a pivotal point in the propagation phase. Formation of this FVIIIa–IXa complex allows FXa generation to switch from a TF-VIIa complex–catalyzed reaction to one produced by the intrinsic Xase pathway. This switch is of enormous kinetic advantage, with the intrinsic Xase complex exhibiting 50-fold higher efficiency at Xa generation. The bleeding diathesis associated with hemophilia, with its intact initiation phase and absent propagation phase, is testament to the hemostatic importance of the propagation phase.

The commonly used laboratory tests of soluble coagulation only measure the kinetics of the initiation phase. The prothrombin time (PT) and activated partial thromboplastin time (aPTT) both have as endpoints the first appearance of fibrin gel, which occurs after completion of less than 5% of the total reaction. These tests are sensitive at detecting severe deficiencies in clotting factors, for example, hemophilia, and in guiding warfarin/heparin therapy; however, they do not model the sequence of events necessary for hemostasis and do not necessarily predict the risk of intraoperative bleeding.

In the venous circulation, the kinetic advantage of coagulation cascade assembly on the platelet surface is readily apparent; however, relatively small numbers of platelets are needed

to fulfill this function. To increase the risk of venous bleeding, the platelet count must decrease to very low levels, that is, less than 10,000/μL. This contrasts sharply with the arterial circulation, in which the minimum platelet count needed to ensure hemostasis for operative procedures is at least five times that number (see "Arterial Coagulation" below).

Hemostatic Disorders Affecting Coagulation Factors of the Initiation Phase

Table 17-2 lists both inherited and acquired hemostatic disorders.

Factor VII Deficiency

Hereditary deficiency of factor VII is a rare autosomal recessive disease with highly variable clinical severity. Only homozygous deficient patients have factor VII levels generally low enough (<15%) to have symptomatic bleeding. These patients are easily recognized from their unique laboratory pattern of a prolonged prothrombin time (PT) but normal partial thromboplastin time (PTT).

Anesthetic Considerations The treatment of a single-factor deficiency state depends on the severity of the deficiency. Most patients with mild to moderate factor VII deficiency can be treated with infusions of fresh frozen plasma (FFP). Patients with factor VII levels less than 1% generally require treatment with a more concentrated source of factor VII. The preferred product for prophylaxis of patients with factor VII deficiency

TABLE 17-2 Categorization of Coagulation Disorders
Hereditary
Hemophilia A
Hemophilia B
Von Willebrand's disease
Afibrinogenemia
Factor V deficiency
Factor VIII deficiency
Hereditary hemorrhagic telangiectasia
Protein C deficiency
Antithrombin III deficiency
Acquired
Disseminated intravascular coagulation
Perioperative anticoagulation
Intraoperative coagulopathies
Dilutional thrombocytopenia
Dilution of procoagulants
Massive blood transfusions
Type of surgery (cardiopulmonary bypass, brain trauma, orthopedic surgery, urologic surgery, obstetric delivery)
Drug-induced hemorrhage
Drug-induced platelet dysfunction
Idiopathic thrombocytopenic purpura
Thrombotic thrombocytopenic purpura
Catheter-induced thrombocytopenia
Vitamin K deficiency

is Proplex T (factor IX complex) because of its high level of factor VII. Treatment of factor VII deficiency with active bleeding is either Proplex T or the activated form, recombinant factor VIIa (NovoSeven), usually beginning with a dose of 20 to 30 μg/kg, with redosing according to prothrombin time results (see "Acquired Factor VIII or IX Inhibition" for comprehensive discussion of recombinant factor VIIa).

Congenital Deficiencies in Factors X, V, and Prothrombin (II)

Congenital deficiencies in factors X, V, and prothrombin are also inherited as autosomal recessive traits and severe deficiencies are quite rare, on the order of one in one million live births. Patients with severe deficiencies in any of these factors demonstrate prolongations of both the PT and PTT. Patients with congenital factor V deficiency may also have a prolonged bleeding time because of the relationship between factor V and platelet function in supporting clot formation.

Anesthetic Considerations Deficiencies in factors X, V, and prothrombin are can be corrected with FFP. The concentration of the vitamin K–dependent factors in FFP is approximately the same as that of normal plasma in vivo. Therefore, to obtain a significant increase in the level of any factor, a considerable volume of FFP must be infused. As a rule of thumb, at least four to six units of FFP are needed to attain a 20% to 30% increase in any missing factor level. This level represents a considerable volume of plasma (800–1200 mL) and may present a significant cardiovascular challenge to the patient. Moreover, the duration of effectiveness of this replacement therapy depends on the turnover time of each factor, which then dictates how often repeated infusions of FFP will be needed to maintain a factor level. Factor V is stored in platelet granules, and, particularly in a bleeding patient, platelet transfusion is an ideal alternative way to express deliver the missing factor V to the site of bleeding.

For a severe deficiency in a patient facing surgery with a significant risk of blood loss, several prothrombin complex concentrates (PCCs) are commercially available. The advantage of these products is that factor levels of 50% or higher can be achieved without the risk of volume overload. The disadvantages of PCCs are the risk induction of widespread thrombosis, thromboembolism, and disseminated intravascular coagulation (DIC). It is also important to recognize the variation in factor levels in the different products. Konyne-HT and Bebulin VH (factor IX complex) contain factors X and prothrombin in roughly equivalent amounts, while the prothrombin levels in Pronine-HT are more than twice the levels of factor X.

Hemostatic Disorders Affecting Coagulation Factors of the Propagation Phase

Defects in the propagation phase of coagulation convey a significant bleeding tendency. Some of these propagation phase defects are associated with an isolated prolongation of the activated partial thromboplastin time (aPTT). The X-linked recessive disorders hemophilia A and B are the principal examples of this type of abnormality. A marked reduction in either factor VIII or IX is associated with spontaneous and excessive hemorrhage, especially hemarthroses and muscle hematomas. A deficiency in factor XI, which is encoded by a gene on chromosome 4, also prolongs the aPTT but typically results in a less severe bleeding tendency. Not all deficiencies causing prolongation of the aPTT are associated with bleeding, however. The initial activation stimulus for this laboratory test is surface contact activation of factor XII (Hageman factor) to produce XIIa. This reaction is facilitated by the presence of high molecular weight kininogen and the conversion of pre-kallikrein to the active protease kallikrein, and deficiency in any of these three factors causes prolongation of the aPTT. However, as described in the Normal Hemostasis section these contact activation factors play *no role* in either the initiation phase or the propagation phase of clotting in vivo; thus, deficiencies of factor XII, high molecular weight kininogen, and prekallikrein are not associated with clinical bleeding. Patient with deficiencies in these particular factors require no special management except alteration of their coagulation testing to allow accurate measurement of physiologic factors critical to in vivo hemostasis.

Congenital Factor VIII Deficiency: Hemophilia A

The factor VIII gene is a very large, 186-kb gene on the X chromosome. The most severe hemophiliacs generally have an inversion or deletion of major portions of the X chromosome genome or a missense mutation, resulting in factor VIII activity of less than 1% of normal. Other mutations, including point mutations and minor deletions, generally result in milder disease with factor VIII levels greater than 1%. In some patients, a functionally abnormal protein is produced, which causes a discrepancy between the immunologic measurement of factor VIII antigen (protein) and the coagulation assay of factor VIII activity.

As a rule of thumb, clinical severity of hemophilia A is best correlated with the factor VIII activity level. Severe hemophiliacs have factor VIII activity levels less than 1% of normal (<0.01 U/mL) and are usually diagnosed during childhood because of frequent, spontaneous hemorrhages into joints, muscles, and vital organs. They require frequent treatment with factor VIII replacement and even then are at risk of developing a progressive, deforming arthropathy.

Factor VIII levels as low as 1% to 5% of normal are enough to reduce the severity of the disease. These patients are at increased risk of hemorrhage with surgery or trauma but have much less difficulty with spontaneous hemarthroses or hematomas. Patients with factor levels between 6% and 30% are only mildly affected and may go undiagnosed well into adult life. They are at risk, however, for excessive bleeding with a major surgical procedure. Female carriers of hemophilia A can also be at risk with surgery. Lyonization of the X chromosome is not purely random, so that 10% of female carriers can have factor VIII activity less than 30%.

Severe hemophilia A patients have a significantly prolonged PTT, whereas with milder disease, the PTT may be only a few seconds longer than normal. Since the tissue factor VII–dependent (extrinsic) pathway of laboratory clotting is intact, the PT is normal.

Anesthetic Considerations Whenever major surgery is necessary in a patient with hemophilia A, the factor VIII level must be brought to near normal (100%) for the procedure. This requires an initial infusion of 50 to 60 U/kg (3500–4000 units in a 70-kg patient). Since the half-life of factor VIII is approximately 12 hours in adults, repeated infusions of 25 to 30 U/kg every 8 to 12 hours will be needed to keep the plasma factor VIII level above 50%. When lower doses (20–30 U/kg) are used, mean postinfusion plasma levels will peak at approximately 30% to 50% (for each unit per kilogram infused, the plasma VIII level will increase ~2%). In children, the half-life of factor VIII may be as short as 6 hours, necessitating more frequent infusions and laboratory assays to confirm efficacy. Peak and trough factor VIII levels should be measured to confirm the appropriate dosing level and dosing interval. Therapy must be continued for up to 2 weeks to avoid postoperative bleeding that disrupts wound healing. Longer periods of therapy may be required in patients who undergo bone or joint surgery. In this situation, 4 to 6 weeks of replacement therapy may be needed.

Up to 30% of severe hemophilia A patients exposed to factor VIII concentrate or recombinant product will eventually develop inhibitor antibodies, some within 10 to 12 days of first exposure. Newer recombinant preparations have not resulted in a reduction in the incidence of inhibitor formation. (See "Acquired Factor VIII or IX Inhibitors" for a complete discussion of patients with this complication.)

Congenital Factor IX Deficiency: Hemophilia B

Hemophilia B patients have a similar clinical spectrum of disease as is found with hemophilia A. Factor IX levels of less than 1% are associated with severe bleeding, whereas more moderate disease is seen in patients with levels of 1% to 5%. Patients with factor IX levels of between 5% and 40% generally have very mild disease. Milder hemophiliacs (>5% factor IX activity) may not be detected until surgery is performed or the patient has a dental extraction. Similar to the laboratory findings with hemophilia A, hemophilia B patients have a prolonged PTT and a normal PT.

Anesthetic Considerations General guidelines for managing hemophilia B patients do not differ significantly from those for hemophilia A patients. Recombinant/purified product or factor IX–PCC are used to treat mild bleeding episodes or as prophylaxis with minor procedures. However, a note of caution is needed when using factor IX–PCC preparations, which can contain activated clotting factors, at higher doses. When given in amounts sufficient to increase factor IX levels to 50% or greater, there is an increased risk of thromboembolic complications, especially in patients undergoing orthopedic procedures. Therefore, it is essential to use only recombinant IX in treating patients undergoing major orthopedic surgery and those with severe traumatic injuries or liver disease.

As for factor VIII replacement, purified factor IX concentrates or recombinant IX are used over several days to treat bleeding in hemophilia B. Because of absorption to collagen sites in the vasculature, recovery of factor IX is approximately half that of factor VIII, making dosing approximately double that for factor VIII concentrates. Therefore, in order to achieve a 100% plasma level in a severe hemophilia B patient, a dose of 100 U/kg (7000 units in a 70-kg patient) needs to be administered. At the same time, factor IX has a half-life of 18 to 24 hours, so repeated infusions at 50% of the original dose every 12 to 24 hours are usually sufficient to keep the factor IX plasma level above 50%. Like factor VIII recommendations, doses of 30 to 50 U/kg will generally give mean factor IX levels of 20% to 40%, which is adequate for less severe bleeds.

Acquired Factor VIII or IX Inhibitors

Hemophilia A patients are at significant risk of developing circulating inhibitors to factor VIII, with an incidence of 30% to 40% in patients severely deficient in factor VIII. Hemophilia B patients are less likely to develop an inhibitor to factor IX; only 3% to 5% of patients will become affected during their lifetime. A severe hemophilia-like syndrome can occur in genetically normal individuals secondary to the appearance of an acquired autoantibody to either factor VIII or, very rarely, to factor IX. These patients are usually middle-aged or older with no personal or family history of abnormal bleeding who present with the sudden onset of severe, spontaneous hemorrhage.

A test known as a *mixing study* is required to detect the presence of an inhibitor. This study is performed by mixing *patient* plasma and *normal* plasma in a 1:1 ratio to determine whether the prolonged PTT shortens. The mixing study of a classic hemophilia A patient with a deficiency in factor VIII activity but no circulating VIII inhibitor will usually show a shortening of the PTT to within 4 seconds or less of the normal PTT control. In contrast, a patient with a factor VIII inhibitor will not correct the PTT to that extent, if at all. It is also important to quantitate the factor VIII activity level and, using a modification of the PTT called the Bethesda assay method to measure the inhibitor titer (Bethesda units of inhibitor/milliliters of plasma). In general, factor VIII inhibitor patients fall into one of two groups according to the level of inhibitor. High responders (>10 U/mL) demonstrate a marked inhibitor response after any factor infusion, such that levels cannot be neutralized by high-dose replacement therapy. The response is typical of induction of an alloantibody, and the patient is constantly at risk of an anamnestic response when re-exposed to factor antigen. In contrast, low responders develop and maintain relatively low levels of inhibitor that are constant despite repeated exposure to factor VIII replacement.

Anesthetic Considerations Management of the hemophilia A patient with an inhibitor will vary according to whether the patient is a high or low responder. Low responders have titers less than 5 to 10 Bethesda U/mL and do not show anamnestic responses to factor VIII concentrates, whereas the high responders can have titers of several thousand Bethesda units and dramatic anamnestic responses to therapy. Patients in the low-responder category can usually be managed with factor VIII concentrates. Larger initial and maintenance doses of factor VIII are required and frequent assays of factor VIII levels are essential to guide therapy. When the titer of the factor VIII inhibitor exceeds 5 to 10 U/mL (high responder category), treatment with factor VIII concentrates is not feasible. Major life-threatening bleeds can be treated with bypass products such as activated PCCs (Autoplex T, FEIBA), or recombinant factor VIIa (NovoSeven). Treatment with activated PCCs runs the risk of initiating DIC or widespread thromboembolism, so recombinant factor VIIa is becoming the treatment of choice for acquired inhibitors. As discussed in the Normal Hemostasis section, although hemophiliacs can generate Xa via factor VIIa binding to tissue factor in the initiation phase, in the propagation phase, they are unable to generate Xa and the subsequent thrombin burst on the platelet surface in the absence of factor VIII or IX. Recombinant factor VIIa in high concentrations appears to essentially replace the VIIIa/IXa Xase complex requirement by binding to the platelet surface and increasing both Xa generation and the thrombin burst, unaffected by factor VIII or IX inhibitors. For active bleeding of patients with inhibitors, a dose of 90 to 120 μg/kg intravenously is recommended every 2 to 3 hours until hemostasis is achieved. Continuous infusions of factor VIIa have also been used to manage patients undergoing surgery. Laboratory monitoring will demonstrate a shortening of the PT, but this may not correlate with the clinical control of hemostasis. Although the thrombin formed via VIIa is not as strong as that seen with factor VIII therapy, recombinant VIIa therapy is successful in controlling bleeding in more than 80% of inhibitor patients. The risk of serious side effects, including widespread or local thrombosis, appears to be acceptable.

Severe hemophilia B patients are also at risk of developing a factor IX inhibitor, but the incidence is far less than in hemophilia A. A modified Bethesda assay is similarly used to quantitate the inhibitor level. Usually, factor IX inhibitor patients can be managed acutely using recombinant VIIa or the PCC products noted above.

Patients who develop an autoantibody to factor VIII or IX without a history of hemophilia can present with life-threatening hemorrhage and may exhibit very high inhibitor levels in excess of several thousand Bethesda units. Treatment with recombinant factor VIIa or an activated prothrombin concentrate is required; factor VIII or IX alone will not be effective.

Factor XI Deficiency

The only other defect causing an isolated prolongation of the PTT and a bleeding tendency is factor XI deficiency (Rosenthal's disease). It is inherited as an autosomal recessive trait and, therefore, affects males and females equally. It is much rarer than either hemophilia A or B, but it affects up to 5% of Jews of Ashkenazi descent from Eastern Europe. Generally, the bleeding tendency, if present at all, is quite mild and may only be apparent following a surgical procedure. Hematomas and hemarthroses are very unusual, even in those patients with factor XI levels of less than 5%. Patients homozygous for the type II mutation (Glu117Stop) have very low levels of factor XI and can develop a factor XI inhibitor when exposed to plasma therapy.

Anesthetic Considerations The treatment of factor XI deficiency depends on the severity of the deficiency and bleeding history. Most patients' factor XI deficiency can be treated with infusions of FFP. Treatment of factor XI deficiency with active bleeding is either PCCs or recombinant factor VIIa (NovoSeven), usually beginning with a dose of 20 to 30 μg/kg, with redosing according to prothrombin time results. Management of factor XI inhibitors is comparable to that of hemophilia A and B inhibitors and is discussed under "Acquired Factor VIII or IX Inhibitors."

Congenital Abnormalities in Fibrinogen

Congenital abnormalities in fibrinogen production will obviously interfere with the final step in the generation of a fibrin clot. Decreased levels of fibrinogen, either hypofibrinogenemia or afibrinogenemia, are relatively rare conditions inherited as autosomal recessive traits. Patients with afibrinogenemia have a severe bleeding diathesis with both spontaneous and posttraumatic bleeding. Since the bleeding can begin during the first few days of life, this condition may be initially confused with hemophilia. Hypofibrinogenemic patients usually do not have spontaneous bleeding but may have difficulty with surgery. Severe bleeding can be anticipated in patients with plasma fibrinogen levels below 50 to 100 mg/dL.

Dysfibrinogenemia

A more common defect is the production of an abnormal fibrinogen. Fibrinogen is synthesized in the liver under the control of three genes on chromosome 4. More than 300 different mutations producing dysfunctional and, at times, reduced amounts of fibrinogen have been reported, resulting in a dysfibrinogenemia. Many of these mutations are inherited as autosomal dominant traits. The clinical presentation of dysfibrinogenemia is highly variable. Patients who demonstrate both a reduced amount and a dysfunctional fibrinogen (hypodysfibrinogenemia) usually exhibit excessive bleeding. This is also true for a few families who are homozygous for dysfibrinogenemia. Most dysfibrinogenemic patients, however, appear to be heterozygous for the trait, and, although they have abnormal coagulation tests, most do not have a bleeding tendency. Overall, approximately 60% of dysfibrinogenemias are clinically silent, whereas the remainder can present with either a bleeding diathesis or a paradoxically thrombotic tendency, in equal measure. A small number of dysfibrinogenemias have been associated with spontaneous abortion and poor wound healing.

Laboratory evaluation of fibrinogen involves measurements of both fibrinogen concentration and function. The most accurate quantitative measurement of total fibrinogen protein is provided by immunoassay or a protein precipitation technique. Other screening tests for fibrinogen dysfunction include the thrombin time (TT) and clotting time using a venom enzyme such as reptilase. Both are sensitive to fibrinogen dysfunction. Definitive diagnosis and subclassification of dysfibrinogenemia require fibrinopeptide chain analysis by sodium dodecyl sulfate–polyacrylamide gel electrophoresis and amino acid sequencing.

Anesthetic Considerations Most patients with dysfibrinogenemia have no clinical disease and, therefore, do not require therapy. For those who are symptomatic or are at risk of bleeding with surgery, cryoprecipitate therapy is warranted. To increase the fibrinogen level by at least 100 mg/dL in the average-size adult, 10 to 12 units of cryoprecipitate should be infused, followed by two to three units each day (fibrinogen is catabolized at a rate of 25% per day). By contrast, dysfibrinogenemia patients with a thrombotic tendency will require long-term anticoagulation.

Factor XIII Deficiency

Stability of the fibrin clot is hemostatically important. Factor XIII (fibrin-stabilizing factor) deficiency is a rare autosomal recessive disorder with an estimated prevalence of one in five million. Patients present at birth with persistent umbilical or circumcision bleeding. Adult patients demonstrate a severe bleeding diathesis, characterized by recurrent soft-tissue bleeding, poor wound healing, and a high incidence of intracranial hemorrhage. Typically, the bleeding is somewhat delayed based on the role of factor XIII in stabilizing the fibrin clot. Blood clots form but are weak and unable to maintain hemostasis. Fetal loss in women with factor XIII deficiency can approach 100%, suggesting a critical role for this factor in maintaining pregnancy.

Factor XIII deficiency should be considered in a patient with a severe bleeding diathesis who has otherwise normal coagulation screening tests, including PT, PTT, fibrinogen level, platelet count, and bleeding time. Clot dissolution in 5M urea can be used as a screen. Definitive diagnosis after an abnormal screen can be accomplished by enzyme-linked immunosorbent assay. Patients at risk of severe hemorrhage have factor XIII levels of 1% of normal. Heterozygotes (factor XIII levels of approximately 50%) usually exhibit no bleeding tendency.

Anesthetic Considerations Factor XIII–deficient patients can be treated with FFP, cryoprecipitate, or a plasma-derived factor XIII concentrate, Fibrogammin P. Preoperative prophylaxis is possible using intravenous injections of 10 to 20 U/kg at 4- to 6-week intervals depending on the patient's preinfusion plasma factor XIII level. Acute hemorrhage should be treated with an infusion of 50 to 75 U/kg body weight. Factor XIII has a long circulating half-life of 7 to 12 days, and adequate hemostasis is achieved with even very low plasma concentrations (1%–3%).

ARTERIAL COAGULATION

Disorders Affecting Platelet Number

The normal circulating platelet count is maintained within relatively narrow limits (150,000–450,000 platelets/μL in Northern Europeans and 90,000–300,000 platelets/μL in people of Mediterranean descent). The platelet volume is inversely related to the platelet count, so the mass of circulating platelets is the same for these two populations. Approximately one third of platelets are sequestered in the spleen at any one time. Since a platelet has a life span of approximately 9 to 10 days, some 15,000 to 45,000 platelets/μL must be produced each day to maintain a steady state.

Anesthetic Considerations: General Concepts for Thrombocytopenia Regardless of the cause of thrombocytopenia, platelet transfusions are appropriate if the patient is experiencing a life-threatening hemorrhage, is bleeding into a closed space such as an intracranial hemorrhage, or requires life-saving surgery. Long-term management usually requires other therapeutic maneuvers to either improve platelet production or decrease high levels of platelet destruction.

Platelet transfusion therapy must be tailored to the severity of the thrombocytopenia, the presence of bleeding complications, and the patient's underlying disorder. For relatively minor procedures such as catheter insertions, biopsies, or lumbar puncture, the platelet count should be greater than 20,000 to 30,000/μL. If major surgery is required, the platelet count should, if possible, be increased to 50,000 to 100,000/μL to control bleeding. Each unit of apheresis platelets or six units of random donor platelets (six pack) should increase the platelet count in a normal size (70 kg) adult by approximately 50,000/μL. This condition assumes, of course, no problems with alloimmunization and no increased rate of platelet destruction. With increased platelet consumption, platelet counts within 1 hour after transfusion and at frequent intervals are important in planning for further platelet transfusion needs.

One unit of single-donor apheresis platelets is equivalent to a random donor pool of four to eight units. For patients who become alloimmunized to random donor platelets, blood banks can provide HLA-matched, single-donor platelets. Random and single-donor platelets do not need to be ABO compatible. However, in Rh-negative patients, particularly women of child-bearing age, sufficient RBCs are transfused in the platelet pool to increase the risk of sensitizing the recipient. Therefore, such patients should receive platelets from Rh-negative donors or be treated with RhoGAM following transfusion of Rh-positive product.

There are no specific symptoms or unique clinical features that definitely point to the presence of thrombocytopenia. Patients with very low platelet counts, usually less than 15,000/μL, demonstrate significant bleeding from multiple sites including the nose, mucous membranes, gastrointestinal tract, skin, and vessel puncture sites. One sign that strongly suggests thrombocytopenia is the appearance of a petechial rash involving the skin or mucous membranes. This condition is usually most pronounced over the lower extremities (increased hydrostatic pressure). The diagnosis of thrombocytopenia is best organized according to the normal physiology of (1) platelet production, (2) distribution in circulation, and (3) destruction. This protocol provides an overall classification that helps guide the differential diagnosis of specific disease states.

Disorders Resulting in Platelet Production Defects: Congenital

Production disorders may be caused by megakaryocyte aplasia or hypoplasia in the bone marrow.

Congenital hypoplastic thrombocytopenia with absent radii (TAR syndrome) is usually inherited in an autosomal recessive manner. Thrombocytopenia develops in the third trimester or early after birth, often initially severe ($<30,000/\mu L$), but slowly improves over time nearing the normal range by age 2. Patients often have obvious bilateral radial anomalies, and abnormalities of other bones may also occur.

Fanconi Syndrome

The hematologic manifestations of Fanconi anemia do not usually appear until approximately 7 years of age, although thrombocytopenia has been reported in neonates. The bone marrow shows reduced cellularity and reduced numbers of megakaryocytes. Treatment is rarely necessary in the neonatal period, and stem cell transplantation is curative in the majority of children once severe bone marrow failure has developed.

May-Hegglin Anomaly

The patient with May-Hegglin anomaly typically has giant platelets in circulation and Döhle bodies (basophilic inclusions) in white blood cells. Platelet production is variably ineffective; one third of patients are significantly thrombocytopenic and at risk of bleeding.

Wiskott-Aldrich Syndrome

Wiskott-Aldrich syndrome is an X-linked disorder that presents with a combination of eczema, immunodeficiency, and thrombocytopenia. Circulating platelets are smaller than normal, function poorly because of granule defects, and have a reduced survival. The latter, however, is not enough to explain the severity of the thrombocytopenia; ineffective thrombopoiesis is the principal abnormality.

Autosomal Dominant Thrombocytopenia

Patients with autosomal dominant thrombocytopenia generally show increased megakaryocyte mass with ineffective production and in some cases, the release of macrocytic platelets into circulation. Many of these patients have nerve deafness and nephritis (Alport's syndrome).

Disorders Resulting in Platelet Production Defects: Acquired

A failure in platelet production can result from marrow damage where all aspects of normal hematopoiesis are depressed even to the point of marrow aplasia (aplastic anemia). Reductions in marrow megakaryocyte mass are seen in patients receiving radiation therapy or cancer chemotherapy, as a result of exposure to toxic chemicals such as benzene and insecticides, to common drugs such as thiazide diuretics, alcohol, and estrogens, or as a complication of viral hepatitis. Infiltration of marrow by a malignant process will also disrupt thrombopoiesis. Hematopoietic malignancies including multiple myeloma, the acute leukemias, lymphoma, and myeloproliferative disorders frequently produce a platelet production defect; metastatic carcinoma and Gaucher's disease are rarer causes.

Ineffective thrombopoiesis is also seen in patients with vitamin B_{12} or folate deficiency, including patients with alcoholism and defective folate metabolism. The defect is identical to the maturation defect seen in the RBC and white blood cell lines. Marrow megakaryocyte mass is increased, but effective platelet production is reduced. This failure in platelet production is rapidly reversed by appropriate vitamin therapy.

Anesthetic Considerations Platelet transfusions are a mainstay in the management of patients with platelet production disorders. See "Anesthetic Considerations: General Concepts for Thrombocytopenia" for a discussion of platelet transfusions. Patients with ineffective thrombopoiesis secondary to an intrinsic abnormality of megakaryocytes may be treated similarly to those with a production disorder when there is need for urgent surgery of a bleeding episode. Ineffective thrombopoiesis associated with either vitamin B_{12} or folate deficiency should be immediately treated with appropriate vitamin therapy. Recovery of the platelet count to normal occurs within a matter of days, making platelet transfusion unnecessary in all but the most acute situations.

Platelet Destruction Disorders: Nonimmune Destruction

Platelet consumption as a part of intravascular coagulation is seen in several clinical settings. When the entire coagulation pathway is activated, the process is referred to as DIC. DIC can be dramatic, with severe thrombocytopenia and marked prolongations of coagulation factor assays leading to bleeding, or it can be low grade, with little or no thrombocytopenia and less tendency for bleeding. Platelet consumption can also occur as an isolated process (so-called platelet DIC). Viral infections, bacteremia, malignancy, high-dose chemotherapy, and vasculitis can result in sufficient endothelial cell damage to dramatically increase the rate of platelet clearance without full activation of the coagulation pathway. Basically, this is an accentuation of the normal vessel repair process, where platelets adhere to exposed subendothelial surfaces and then aggregate with fibrinogen binding. With marked endothelial disruption, enough platelets will be consumed to result in thrombocytopenia. Vessel occlusion by formation of platelet thrombi is rare but can occasionally occur with severe vasculitis. Acquired immunodeficiency syndrome patients can develop a consumptive thrombocytopenia with organ damage secondary to arterial thrombosis.

Thrombotic thrombocytopenic purpura (TTP), hemolytic uremic syndrome (HUS), and HELLP syndrome are the most important examples of nonimmune destruction of platelets. Although the underlying pathophysiologies are distinctly different, these entities can lead to thrombus formation and organ damage.

Thrombotic Thrombocytopenic Purpura

TTP may present as a symptom complex that includes fever; thrombocytopenia with an otherwise negative DIC screen (normal PT, PTT, and fibrinogen levels); multiple small vessel occlusions (platelet thrombi) involving the kidney, central nervous system, and, on occasion, skin and distal extremities; and a microangiopathic hemolytic anemia with schistocytosis (mechanical fragmentation of RBCs flowing past intra-arteriolar platelet thrombi). However, the triad of schistocytosis, thrombocytopenia, and elevated lactate dehydrogenase (evidence of a hemolysis) is more common and considered sufficient for diagnosis. TTP can occur as a familial disease, a sporadic illness without apparent cause (idiopathic), a chronic relapsing condition, or a complication of marrow transplantation or drug therapy (quinine, ticlopidine, mitomycin C, interferon-α, pentostatin, gemcitabine, tacrolimus, or cyclosporine). Preeclamptic women with HELLP syndrome can also evolve to full-blown TTP peri- or postpartum.

TTP is perhaps the purest example of increased platelet destruction secondary to activation, aggregation, and thrombus formation resulting in organ damage. The underlying mechanism with familial or cyclic disease involves a deficiency of vWF-cleaving protease activity (ADAMTS13 deficiency) secondary to an inherited mutation of the *ADAMTS13* gene resulting in persistent circulation of ultra-large (UL) vWF multimers. Plasma exchange is effective at both removing some of the ULvWF multimers and restoring the von Willebrand factor-cleaving protease activity.

Hemolytic-Uremic Syndrome

HUS is most often seen in children who present with bloody diarrhea secondary to *Escherichia coli* 0157:H7 or related bacteria that produce Shiga-like toxin. Acute renal failure dominates the presentation; thrombocytopenia and anemia are less pronounced than seen with TTP and neurologic signs are absent. With the exception of the rare infant with severe HUS, these patients do not need plasmapheresis or FFP therapy. Most children spontaneously recover with hemodialysis support, and the mortality rate is less than 5%. In contrast, adults infected with *E. coli* 0157:H7 can present with a combination of features of both HUS or TTP, usually with less renal involvement. Since the mortality in older children and adults is higher, they should be treated with both plasma exchange and hemodialysis, regardless of the pattern of illness.

HELLP Syndrome

Thrombocytopenia is a frequent complication of pregnancy. Mild thrombocytopenia (platelet counts between 70,000 and 150,000/μL) is seen in 6% to 7% of women nearing gestation and represents a physiologic change, similar to the dilutional anemia of pregnancy. Thrombocytopenia in association with hypertension is observed in 1% to 2% of pregnancies, and as many as 50% of preeclamptic mothers will develop a DIC-like picture with severe thrombocytopenia, platelet counts of 20,000 to 40,000/μL, at the time of delivery. This is referred to as HELLP syndrome when the combination of red cell hemolysis (H), elevated liver enzymes (EL), and low platelet count (LP) is present. Physiologically, HELLP syndrome very much resembles TTP. Control of the patient's hypertension and completion of the delivery is usually enough to bring this process to a halt. However, a few patients will go on to full-blown TTP-HUS following delivery. Postpartum TTP is a life-threatening illness with a poor prognosis. Treatment with both plasma exchange and intravenous immunoglobulin has yielded variable results.

Anesthetic Considerations Proper management of patients with platelet destruction disorders depends on the diagnosis. In those individuals who have nonimmune destruction as a part of DIC, platelet and plasma transfusions are supportive: the only truly effective therapy is the treatment of the underlying cause of the DIC. If the primary condition can be corrected, coagulation factors and platelet count will recover. Patients with TTP or HUS should only receive platelet transfusions for life-threatening bleeding. With TTP or HUS, potential harm from platelet transfusions is of even greater concern; they may lead to increased thrombosis and organ damage (including sudden cardiac death) secondary to marked platelet aggregation and activation. Surgery should be delayed whenever possible until the underlying disorder is brought under control.

HUS and HELLP syndrome present a somewhat different therapeutic challenge. HUS in children can usually be managed without plasmapheresis, although dialysis may be necessary when renal failure is severe. HELLP syndrome, like preeclampsia, usually resolves with delivery of the fetus. However, a small number of women will convert to a TTP-like syndrome postpartum. They should be aggressively pheresed with plasma exchange. Response is generally poor once there is organ damage.

Platelet Destruction Disorders: Autoimmune Destruction

Thrombocytopenia is a common manifestation of autoimmune disease. The severity of the thrombocytopenia is highly variable. With some conditions, the platelet count falls to as low as 1000 to 2000/μL. In other patients, the ability of the megakaryocytes to increase platelet production results in a compensated state with platelet counts ranging from 20,000/μL to near normal levels.

Diagnosis of immune destruction can usually be made from the clinical presentation, an increase in the reticulated (RNA-containing) platelets in blood, and demonstration of an increase in marrow megakaryocyte number and ploidy. Expansion of the megakaryocyte mass is taken as prima facie evidence that a high rate of platelet production is trying to compensate for a shortened survival of platelets in circulation.

Thrombocytopenic Purpura in Adults

The differential diagnosis of autoimmune thrombocytopenia in the adult begins with a careful history to identify any exposure to drugs, blood products, or viral infections. Adults can develop posttransfusion purpura following exposure to a blood product, most often RBCs or platelets. Although multiparous PL^{A-1}-negative women are at greatest risk, posttransfusion purpura has been reported in both men and women. Usually, a potent alloantibody with PL^{A-1} specificity is readily detected in the patient's plasma.

Drug-induced Autoimmune Thrombocytopenic Purpura Several drugs can produce immune thrombocytopenia. Quinine, quinidine, and sedormid are the best known and have been studied extensively. Clinically, patients present with severe thrombocytopenia, with platelet counts less than 20,000/µL. These drugs act as haptens to trigger antibody formation and then serve as obligate molecules for antibody binding to the platelet surface. Thrombocytopenia can also occur within hours of the first exposure to a drug because of preformed antibodies. This has been reported with varying frequency (0%–13%) with abciximab (ReoPro) and other glycosylphosphatidyl glycan Ib/IIIa inhibitors. Other drugs, such as α-methyldopa, sulfonamides, and gold salts, also stimulate autoantibodies. They are not, however, obligate haptens in the resultant platelet destruction.

Heparin-induced Thrombocytopenia The association of heparin with thrombocytopenia deserves special discussion. Heparin-induced thrombocytopenia (HIT) can take one of several forms. A modest decrease in the platelet count, HIT type I (nonimmune HIT) may be observed in a majority of patients within the first day of full-dose unfractionated heparin (UH) therapy. This relates to passive heparin binding to platelets, resulting in a modest shortening of platelet life span. It is transient and clinically insignificant.

A second form of HIT, HIT type II or immune-mediated HIT, demands more attention. In patients receiving heparin for more than 5 days, antibodies to the heparin-platelet factor 4 complex can form, which are capable of binding to platelet Fc receptors and inducing platelet activation and aggregation. Platelet activation results in further release of heparin-platelet factor 4 and the appearance of platelet microparticles in circulation, both of which magnify the procoagulant state. Furthermore, heparin-platelet factor 4 complex binding to endothelial cells stimulates thrombin production. In vivo, this leads to both an increased clearance of platelets with resultant thrombocytopenia and venous and/or arterial thrombus formation, with the potential for severe organ damage (loss of limbs, stroke, myocardial infarction) as well as unusual sites of thrombosis (adrenal, portal vein, skin).

The incidence of HIT type II varies with the type and dose of heparin used and the duration of therapy. While 10% to 15% of patients receiving bovine UH develop an antibody, less than 6% of patients receiving porcine heparin will do so. The risk of heparin-induced thrombosis is lower than the incidence of antibody formation. Less than 10% of those who develop an antibody to the heparin–heparin-platelet factor 4 complex will exhibit a thrombotic event. However, the risk varies considerably with the clinical situation and can reach 40% or more in the postoperative setting when high circulating levels of both activated platelets and thrombin are present, for example, following orthopedic surgery. Several studies have also suggested that the HIT antibody has a negative impact on clinical outcome even in the absence of overt thrombosis. HIT antibody–positive patients undergoing coronary artery bypass surgery or heparin therapy for unstable angina have been reported to have a significant increase in adverse events, including prolonged hospitalization, stroke, myocardial infarction, and even death.

The association of heparin with significant thrombocytopenia should not be taken lightly. Patients placed on full-dose UH for more than 5 days or who have previously received heparin should be routinely monitored with every other day platelet counts. A greater than 50% decrease in platelet count, even if the absolute platelet count is within the normal range, can signal the appearance of an HIT type II antibody and, therefore, mandates stopping the heparin and substituting a direct thrombin inhibitor, such as lepirudin or argatroban. If heparin is continued, and this includes even low-dose subcutaneous heparin or low molecular weight heparin (LMWH), there is a significant risk of a major thromboembolic event depending on the clinical situation.

An acute form of HIT type II can occur in patients restarted on heparin within 20 days of a previous exposure. When an HIT antibody is already present, a patient restarted on heparin can exhibit an acute drug reaction with a sudden onset of severe dyspnea, shaking chills, diaphoresis, hypertension, and tachycardia. Such patients are at extreme risk of a fatal thromboembolism if heparin is continued.

Anesthetic Considerations for Drug-Induced Thrombocytopenia As always, platelet transfusions are appropriate if the patient is experiencing a life-threatening hemorrhage or is bleeding into a closed space such as an intracranial hemorrhage. Platelet transfusion therapy must be tailored to the severity of the thrombocytopenia, the presence of bleeding complications, and the patient's underlying disorder. In patients with autoimmune thrombocytopenia secondary to drug ingestion, the most important management step is to discontinue the drug. Corticosteroid therapy may speed recovery in patients with an idiopathic thrombocytopenic purpura (ITP)–like picture, such as may be seen in patients reacting to sulfamethoxazole. The rate of recovery will then depend on both the clearance rate of the drug and the ability of marrow megakaryocytes to proliferate and increase platelet production. Even when the platelet count is very low, bleeding is unlikely and patients can be allowed to recover on their own.

Human immunodeficiency virus–infected thrombocytopenic patients who require urgent surgery should also be given platelet transfusions as appropriate. For more elective operations planned for patients who develop thrombocytopenia early in their disease, consideration may be given to treatment with zidovudine well before scheduling surgery. Approximately 60% of patients will show a response, and up to 50% will have a long-lasting improvement in their platelet counts. The effect is not immediate; it can take up to 1 to 2 months before the platelet count improves. In those patients who do not respond, splenectomy can help in more than 85% of the cases if done early in the course of disease. Corticosteroids, intravenous immunoglobulin, and intravenous anti-D (WinRho) have also been used in patients with acquired immunodeficiency syndrome. With disease progression, human immunodeficiency virus–infected patients develop a platelet production defect that only responds to platelet transfusion therapy.

The management of HIT is a different matter. To prevent a life-threatening thromboembolic event in patients with HIT, all heparin forms, including the small amounts used in line maintenance, must be stopped immediately. Any delay, such as waiting for an assay result or a further decrease in the platelet count, puts the patient at increased risk of thrombosis. Substitution of LMWH is not an option inasmuch as there is significant antibody cross-reactivity. In the setting of a thrombotic event or when continued anticoagulation is required, HIT patients should be started on a direct thrombin inhibitor, such as lepirudin or argatroban. After a baseline PTT, lepirudin is given as an intravenous bolus of 0.4 mg/kg, followed by a continuous infusion at a rate of approximately 0.15 mg/kg per hour, adjusted to keep the PTT between 1.5 and 2.5 times normal. Argatroban is given as an infusion of approximately 2.0 μg/kg per minute, titrated to keep the PTT between 1.5 and 3 times normal. Oral anticoagulants should never be started until there is continuous and successful coverage with a direct thrombin inhibitor. The immediate reduction in protein C levels with the initiation of warfarin therapy can lead to worsening thrombosis, including massive skin necrosis and venous limb gangrene. Since factor VII levels may mirror the decrease in protein C, venous limb gangrene can be associated with a rapid increase in the international normalized ratio (INR) after initiating warfarin. If this occurs, warfarin should be discontinued, and vitamin K given to reverse the effect.

Idiopathic Thrombocytopenic Purpura Thrombocytopenia unrelated to a drug, infection, or autoimmune disease is generally classified as (autoimmune) ITP. This diagnosis can only be made by excluding all other causes of nonimmune and immune destruction. Similar to immune thrombocytopenia in children, it can be an acute disease in adults. However, most adult cases proceed to a chronic form of ITP where a continued high level of marrow platelet production is required to maintain a chronically low to near-normal platelet count in the face of a shortened platelet life span. Typically, thrombocytopenia must be severe before bleeding becomes a problem. This condition reflects the fact that the high level of platelet destruction that occurs in these patients is balanced by a high marrow production of platelets that demonstrate greater than normal function. The latter provides some protection for the patient; ITP patients with platelet counts even as low as 2000/μL are usually not at great risk of a major organ or intracerebral bleed. Patients with chronic ITP generally show less severe thrombocytopenia, with platelet counts of 20,000 to 100,000/μL.

Platelet survival in the most severely affected patients can be measured in hours rather than days, with destruction mainly in the spleen. Transfused platelet life span is also shortened. Some patients demonstrate only modest shortening in platelet survival, suggesting a subnormal rate of platelet production. Although most ITP patients receiving platelet transfusions rapidly destroy the infused platelets, up to 30% of patients demonstrate near-normal posttransfusion platelet increments and survival.

Anesthetic Considerations Severe autoimmune thrombocytopenia (ITP) with bleeding manifestations in adults should be treated as a medical emergency with high-dose corticosteroids for the first 3 days. If there is need for emergency surgery or clinical evidence of intracranial hemorrhage, the patient should also be given intravenous immunoglobulin and platelet transfusions at least every 8 to 12 hours, regardless of the effect on the platelet count. Some patients who receive platelet transfusions will show a relatively normal posttransfusion increment and reasonable survival. However, even when there is no posttransfusion increment, sufficient numbers of the transfused platelets may survive to improve hemostasis.

Some adults do not respond to corticosteroids and go on to develop chronic ITP. If ITP persists for more than 3 to 4 months, it is extremely unlikely that the patient will spontaneously recover. In this case, splenectomy should be considered if the platelet count is below 10,000 to 20,000/μL. Approximately 50% of patients will achieve a permanent remission after splenectomy. If splenectomy is recommended for a patient with chronic ITP, it is extremely important to immunize with pneumococcal, meningococcal, and *Haemophilus influenzae* vaccines prior to surgery to reduce the risk of postsplenectomy sepsis. In children younger than 5 years of age, postsplenectomy prophylactic antibiotic therapy may also be advisable.

Management of chronic ITP in pregnancy deserves special attention. Most women can be managed throughout their pregnancy with no medication, modest amounts of prednisone, or intermittent use of intravenous immunoglobulin. In those cases where the thrombocytopenia is severe, higher dose steroid therapy, 0.5 to 1 mg/kg prednisone per day together with weekly intravenous immunoglobulin, during the last 2 to 3 weeks of pregnancy, may be needed to prevent maternal bleeding. Even with severe ITP in the mother, most children are born with normal platelet counts. Less than 4% will have a platelet count below 20,000/μL and less than 1% will exhibit a bleeding complication. Neonatal platelet counts may continue to decrease for 7 or more days following delivery. Therefore, children at risk should have their platelet counts checked every 2 to 3 days until the count increases.

Despite the low incidence of bleeding complications in children born to ITP mothers, prophylactic cesarean section is still recommended by some obstetricians to decrease the chance of intracranial hemorrhage. There is no good evidence that cesarean section is significantly better at protecting the child. Moreover, this approach actually increases the risk of serious maternal bleeding and often requires platelet transfusion support. Although the risk of the fetus reflects the severity of the mother's ITP, this relationship is not a hard-and-fast rule. A child with severe thrombocytopenia and bleeding complications may be born to a mother with apparently mild disease.

Qualitative Platelet Disorders

Abnormalities in platelet function are often first appreciated as a complication of an acute illness or surgery, and multiple aggravating factors may play a role in determining the severity of the bleeding tendency. Consequently, this is not a time when an accurate diagnosis is easily made, and treatment should address as many potential contributing factors as possible. This list includes discontinuing drugs that inhibit platelet function, empirically replacing vWF or treating with desmopressin (DDAVP) and, according to the severity of the patient's bleeding, transfusing normal platelets. Although this approach lacks precision, it is effective.

As a general principle, the nature of the functional abnormality will guide the choice of therapy. For example, the vWD patient who lacks normal amounts of vWF will respond to agents that increase plasma vWF levels. In this situation, the platelets will function normally once the vWF abnormality is corrected. In contrast, patients with congenital defects of platelet receptor expression, granule content, or platelet metabolism will require platelet transfusion. As for the acquired abnormalities of platelet function, the best approach to therapy lies somewhere in between. There is clinical evidence that patients with acquired defects secondary to drug ingestion, uremia, and liver disease will respond to vWF replacement, DDAVP, or both. DDAVP is a synthetic analogue of the antidiuretic hormone vasopressin, which, when given intravenously, stimulates a release of vWF from endothelial cells to produce an immediate increase in plasma vWF and factor VIII activity. This enhances platelet function and shortens the bleeding time and is discussed in greater depth in "von Willebrand's Disease."

Congenital Disorders Affecting Platelet Function

vWD is the most common inherited abnormality affecting platelet *function*. All other disorders, including Bernard-Soulier syndrome, Glanzmann thrombasthenia, dense and α-granule deficiencies, and disorders of secretory and procoagulant activities, directly affect platelets and are quite rare. These defects can be grouped according to the in vitro functional defect. Bernard-Soulier syndrome is a disorder of adhesion, whereas Glanzmann thrombasthenia is characterized by defective aggregation. The other defects are classified as disorders of granule secretion and platelet metabolism.

von Willebrand's Disease

vWD is inherited as either an autosomal dominant or recessive trait with an estimated prevalence ranging from 1 in 100 to 3 in 100,000 individuals. However, severe vWD

with a history of life-threatening bleeding is seen in fewer than five individuals per million in Western countries. In the case of type 1 vWD, 40% of involved family members carry the allele for vWD but have normal or only slightly reduced vWF levels, both functional and antigenic. Even though autosomal dominant parents transmit the abnormal gene to 50% of their children, symptomatic disease is seen in only 30% to 40% of offspring. Patients with a single recessive gene are typically asymptomatic but can show abnormal vWF antigen and activity levels. Double heterozygote offspring, born to parents who each carry one defective gene, can exhibit severe disease (type 3 vWD). Rarely, acquired type 2 vWD, secondary to autoantibodies directed at vWF, can be seen in patients with lymphomyeloproliferative disorders or immunologic disease states.

As with the other platelet functional defects, symptomatic vWD patients usually present with mucocutaneous bleeding, especially epistaxis, easy bruising, menorrhagia, and gingival and gastrointestinal bleeding. As vWF also serves as a carrier protein for factor VIII, increasing its plasma half-life, some vWD patients may also have a prolonged PTT. Of note, patients with very low factor VIII levels can exhibit hemarthroses and deep tissue bleeds. From a population perspective, however, the number of patients with slight to moderate reductions in vWF activity far exceeds the number with overt clinical bleeding. This can lead to a gross overdiagnosis of vWD, if the vWF level is the sole criteria for diagnosis. Therefore, the diagnosis of "clinically important" vWD, especially type 1 vWD, should be limited to those patients who demonstrate abnormal bleeding, typically in association with an aggravating factor such as drugs, trauma, and surgery. If vWD is considered to be a contributing factor to a patient's bleeding, it should be empirically treated and the laboratory evaluation postponed until the patient is clinically stable and has not received either blood products or drugs for several weeks.

Screening laboratory evaluation for vWD should include measurements of bleeding time, platelet count, PT, and aPTT. Patients with mild type 1 vWD will generally have near-normal studies. With more severe disease, the bleeding time is markedly prolonged, ranging from 15 to more than 30 minutes, whereas the platelet count is normal. Patients with severe deficiencies of vWF or defective binding of factor VIII to vWF will have a prolonged PTT secondary to low levels of factor VIII in plasma. Specific assays of vWF levels and function are then necessary to confirm the diagnosis.

Full evaluation of vWD patients requires measurements of factor VIII coagulant activity, vWF antigen, vWF activity (ristocetin cofactor or collagen binding activity), and vWF multimer distribution by agarose gel electrophoresis. These studies are of diagnostic importance in the classification of vWD, which, in turn, is important in planning clinical management.

Type 1 Disease Type 1 vWD is the most common variant, accounting for 80% of observed cases. It represents a quantitative defect in plasma vWF levels. Clinical severity of the disease is quite variable, but generally correlates with the overall reduction in the plasma levels of vWF and factor VIII. In patients and families with histories of repeated and severe bleeding episodes, vWF antigen and vWF activity are usually reduced less than 15% to 25% of normal. These patients can be said to truly have type 1 vWD. They should be treated aggressively for any bleeding episode and given prophylaxis treatment for even minor surgical procedures. At the same time, a moderately low vWF level (<50%), by itself, does not make the diagnosis. The majority of such individuals will not suffer from an increased bleeding tendency and, therefore, should not be labeled as having vWD.

Type 1 vWD appears to result from a defect in vWF release from the Weibel-Palade bodies of endothelial cells; platelet and endothelial stores of vWF are normal in most patients. This is supported clinically by the observation that type 1 vWD patients demonstrate a release of vWF from endothelial cells with administration of DDAVP. Furthermore, vWF behaves as an acute phase reactant. Pregnancy, estrogen use, and inflammatory states can increase vWF levels, even to the point of masking the diagnosis of mild type 1 vWD.

Type 2 Disease Type 2 vWD is characterized by a qualitative defect in plasma vWF. This can involve a reduction in the larger vWF multimers (types 2A and 2B vWD) or variable changes in vWF antigen and factor VIII binding (types 2M and 2N vWD). The absence of the larger multimers results in a disproportionate decrease in the vWF activity (ristocetin cofactor activity) when compared with vWF antigen. Factor VIII activity is less likely to be reduced in types 2A, 2B, and 2M vWD but is severely affected with type 2N disease. Type 2 disease is further divided into 2A, 2B 2M, and 2D variants. While each has specific genetic derangements in vWF, clinically the differences are not significant.

Type 3 Disease Type 3 vWD is characterized by a virtual absence of circulating vWF antigen and very low levels of both vWF activity and factor VIII (3%–10% of normal). These patients experience severe bleeding with mucosal hemorrhage, hemarthroses, and muscle hematomas reminiscent of hemophilia A or B. However, unlike classic hemophilia, their bleeding times are very prolonged.

Anesthetic Considerations As is clear from the previous discussion, the type of vWD and its severity, and the nature, urgency, and location of the surgical procedure all factor into the therapeutic management of a patient with vWF. The major agents useful in this disorder include DDAVP, an agent that optimizes plasma levels of endogenous vWF, and blood products that contain vWF in high concentrations.

As discussed above, DDAVP is a synthetic analogue of the antidiuretic hormone vasopressin, which when given intravenously, stimulates release of vWF from endothelial cells to produce an immediate rise in plasma vWF and factor VIII activity. This enhances platelet function and shortens the bleeding time. It can be very effective in correcting the bleeding defect in vWD. Because of its impact on factor VIII levels, DDAVP has also been used to manage patients with mild hemophilia A who are undergoing minor surgery. Platelet functional abnormalities due to

aspirin, glycosylphosphatidyl glycan Ib/IIIa inhibitors, uremia, or liver disease are partially corrected by DDAVP's release of very large vWF multimers. However, more efficient dialysis and erythropoietin therapy in uremic patients have significantly decreased their bleeding tendency, obviating the need for long-term DDAVP therapy.

Success in treating vWD patients with DDAVP depends on the disease type. Patients with type 1 vWD show the best response, with a shortening of the bleeding time and an increase in vWF and factor VIII levels. However, when a full biologic response is defined as a reduction in bleeding time to less than 12 minutes, together with at least a threefold increase in vWF and factor VIII to levels greater than 30 IU/dL, less than a third of DDAVP-treated type 1 vWD patients meet the full criteria. The value of treatment with DDAVP in type 2 patients is even less certain. Type 2A or 2M vWD patients show poor, if any, biologic response. In addition, type 3 vWD patients will not respond to the drug since these patients lack endothelial stores of vWF. Both vWF and factor VIII must be provided to reliably treat bleeding in type 3 vWD.

DDAVP formulations include both intravenous and intranasal preparations. DDAVP is administered intravenously in a dose of 0.3 μg/kg. It should be diluted in 30 to 50 mL of saline and infused over 10 to 20 minutes to minimize side effects, especially the tachycardia and hypotension. Like its parent compound, DDAVP will cause headache, lightheadedness, nausea, and facial flushing in patients, especially when given rapidly. The drug also has a mild antidiuretic effect that can lead to water intoxication if the patient receives multiple treatments and large volumes of parenteral fluids. A highly concentrated nasal spray can be self-administered in women with type 1 vWD for the management of menorrhagia. It can also be effective in controlling the bleeding associated with tooth extractions or minor surgery in vWD and mild hemophilia A patients. A 300-μg dose of intranasal DDAVP (Stimate nasal spray), administered by the application of 100 μL of a 1.5-mg/mL solution to each nostril, will increase the vWF level three- to fivefold.

DDAVP therapy is most effective in treating mild bleeding episodes or in preventing bleeding during minor surgery. Patients with baseline vWF and factor VIII levels of greater than 10 to 20 IU/dL also seem to do the best, demonstrating three- to fivefold increases in vWF levels. However, even when the patient's response is suboptimal (fails to meet the full biologic response criteria, see previously), bleeding may be partially contained, or, in the case of surgical prophylaxis, blood loss and the need for transfusion are reduced. A drawback of DDAVP is the short-lived nature of its effect. The improvement in the bleeding time and vWF level is limited to 12 to 24 hours. The response to repeated doses can decrease because of the development of tachyphylaxis. In those situations where control of the patient's bleeding tendency is critical, such as following major surgery, DDAVP alone will be inadequate and vWF replacement is recommended.

vWF replacement is considered the more reliable therapy for severe bleeding and surgical prophylaxis and can be achieved by the transfusion of cryoprecipitate or purified concentrates containing the vWF–factor VIII complex. Cryoprecipitate is a readily available and effective blood product that contains concentrated fibrinogen, vWF, and factors VIII and XIII. Similar to DDAVP therapy, it results in an immediate shortening of the bleeding time, which correlates with the infusion of the larger vWF multimers. The dose schedule for cryoprecipitate is highly empirical. Patients with severe type 1 or 3 disease are managed like a severe hemophilia A patient, by increasing factor VIII levels to 50% to 70% for major surgery and 30% to 50% for minor surgery or less severe bleeding.

Because there is still a risk of transfusion-transmitted infection with cryoprecipitate, purified commercial preparations of factor VIII–vWF concentrate are now recommended. Not all purified factor VIII preparations used in the treatment of hemophilia A are suitable for the treatment of vWD. The concentrate must contain the larger vWF multimers to be effective. One preparation rich in vWF and approved for use in the United States is Humate P. The recommended doses (expressed in IU of both vWF and factor VIII) for bleeding management and surgical prophylaxis are an initial loading dose of 40 to 75 IU/kg IV, followed by repeat doses of 40 to 60 IU/kg at 8- to 12-hour intervals. Once bleeding is controlled, a single daily dose of concentrate is sufficient since the half-life of the factor VIII–vWF complex in vWD patients is 24 to 26 hours.

Acquired Abnormalities of Platelet Function

Acquired platelet dysfunction is seen in association with hematopoietic disease, as part of a systemic illness, or as a result of drug therapy. Often, the relationship is so strong that the mere presence of a specific drug or clinical condition is enough to make the diagnosis.

Myeloproliferative Disease Patients with myeloproliferative disorders (i.e., PV, myeloid metaplasia, idiopathic myelofibrosis, essential thrombocythemia, and chronic myelogenous leukemia) frequently exhibit abnormal platelet function. Some of these patients have very high platelet counts and demonstrate either abnormal bleeding or a tendency for arterial or venous thrombosis, or even both. In patients with PV, expansion of the total blood volume and an increase in blood viscosity may also contribute to the thrombotic risk. Other laboratory findings can be quite variable. The bleeding time may be prolonged, but is a poor predictor of abnormal bleeding. Perhaps the most consistent laboratory abnormalities in bleeding patients are defects in epinephrine-induced aggregation and dense and α-granule function. Bleeding due to an acquired form of vWD may also be observed in these disorders, secondary to a loss of higher molecular weight vWF multimers.

Dysproteinemia Abnormal platelet function, including defects in adhesion, aggregation, and procoagulant activity, are observed in patients with dysproteinemias. Almost one third of patients with Waldenström macroglobulinemia or IgA myeloma will have a demonstrable defect; immunoglobulin G multiple myeloma patients are less commonly affected. The level (concentration) of the monoclonal protein spike appears to correlate with the abnormalities in platelet function. Fibrinogen

breakdown fragments can also interfere with platelet function. This condition is illustrated by the functional defect that appears in patients with DIC and fibrin/fibrinogen breakdown. Fibrin fragments impair both fibrin polymerization and platelet aggregation. Of course, failure of platelet thrombus formation in the DIC patient is usually multifactorial, with thrombocytopenia, hypofibrinogenemia, and a loss of dense and α-granule function secondary to platelet activation all playing a role.

Uremia Untreated uremic patients consistently show a defect in platelet function that correlates with the severity of the uremia and anemia. It appears that the uncleared metabolic product guanidinosuccinic acid acts as an inhibitor of platelet function by inducing endothelial cell nitric oxide release. Platelet adhesion, activation, and aggregation are abnormal, and thromboxane A_2 generation is decreased.

Most patients with severe uremia have a prolonged bleeding time in excess of 30 minutes. This condition is corrected by hemodialysis. It may also relate to the patient's anemia since the bleeding time shortens with either transfusion or erythropoietin therapy. For acute bleeding episodes, DDAVP therapy can improve platelet function transiently. Infusion of conjugated estrogens (0.6 mg/kg per day) for 5 days will also shorten the bleeding time. This improvement takes several days to appear and can last for up to 2 weeks. The mechanism of the conjugated estrogen effect appears to be the normalization of plasma levels of nitric oxide metabolites.

Liver Disease In general, the most likely cause of hemorrhage in a liver disease patient is a discrete defect, such as bleeding varices or a gastric/duodenal ulcer. If, however, the patient has widespread bleeding, including ecchymoses and oozing from intravenous sites, a coagulopathy should be considered. Patients with liver disease have a multifaceted defect in coagulation. Thrombocytopenia related to hypersplenism and a failed thrombopoietin response is common. Platelet dysfunction, secondary to high levels of circulating fibrin degradation products, further increases the bleeding tendency. In addition, reduced production of factor VII (the principal cause of the prolonged PT in liver disease patients) and low-grade, chronic DIC with increased fibrinolysis add to the coagulopathy.

Inhibition by Drugs Several classes of drugs also affect platelet function (**Table 17-3**). Aspirin and the nonsteroidal anti-inflammatory drugs have a well-recognized impact on platelet function. Aspirin is a powerful inhibitor of platelet thromboxane A_2 synthesis through its irreversible inhibition of cyclo-oxygenase function. Nonsteroidal anti-inflammatory drugs (e.g., indomethacin, ibuprofen, sulfinpyrazone) also inhibit platelet cyclo-oxygenase, but the effect is reversible and lasts only as long as the drug is in circulation. From the clinical viewpoint, these agents are weak inhibitors of platelet function and are usually not associated with severe clinical bleeding. However, they will contribute to bleeding when other aggravating factors, such as other anticoagulants, a gastrointestinal disorder, or surgery, are present. Certain foods and food additives (vitamins C and E, omega-3 fatty acids, Chinese black tree fungus) can also reversibly inhibit platelet function through the cyclo-oxygenase pathway.

TABLE 17-3 Drugs That Inhibit Platelet Function

Strong Association
Aspirin (and aspirin-containing medications)
Clopidogrel/ticlopidine
Abciximab (ReoPro)
Nonsteroidal anti-inflammatory drugs: Naproxen, ibuprofen, indomethacin, phenylbutazone, piroxicam, ketorolac
Mild to Moderate Association
Antibiotics, usually only in high doses
  Penicillin, also carbenicillin, penicillin G, ampicillin, ticarcillin, nafcillin, mezlocillin
  Cephalosporins
  Nitrofurantoin
Volume expanders: dextran, hydroxyethyl starch
Heparin
Fibrinolytic agents: EACA, aprotinin
Weak Association
Oncologic drugs: daunorubicin, mithramycin
Cardiovascular drugs: β-blockers, calcium channel blockers, nitroglycerin, nitroprusside, quinidine
Alcohol

EACA, epsilon aminocaproic acid.

The impact of antibiotics on platelet function can be a major contributor to hemorrhage in critically ill patients. The penicillins, including carbenicillin, penicillin G, ticarcillin, ampicillin, nafcillin, and to a lesser extent mezlocillin, interfere with both platelet adhesion and platelet activation/aggregation. These drugs bind to the platelet membrane and interfere with vWF binding and the response of platelets to agonists such as adenosine diphosphate and epinephrine. Significant clinical bleeding can occur in the critically ill patient receiving one of these antibiotics in very high doses. The presence of aggravating factors of the critical illness is important since abnormal bleeding is rarely seen when antibiotics are used in generally healthy patients. Platelet dysfunction has also been reported with selected cephalosporins, including moxalactam and cefotaxime. Most other antibiotics in this class do not produce a defect.

Volume expanders, such as the neutral polysaccharide dextran, can interfere with platelet aggregation and procoagulant activity when infused in large amounts. This result can be a significant disadvantage in the trauma or surgical setting when a dextran solution is being used for volume support. At the same time, dextran is occasionally used in the vascular surgery setting to prevent platelet thrombosis. Hydroxyethyl starch, a more popular volume expander, is less likely to interfere with platelet function but will cause a detectable defect if given in doses in excess of 2 L of the 6% solution. Many other drugs have been reported to cause platelet dysfunction occasionally. This list includes several cardiovascular drugs, alcohol, and several of the oncologic drugs. The mechanisms involved have not been clearly defined.

Anesthetic Considerations for Qualitative Platelet Disorders Unlike the case for disorders resulting in thrombocytopenia, the therapeutic goal in qualitative platelet disorders is

less exact and may require frequent reassessment. Because the platelets are dysfunctional, the absolute platelet number does not predict bleeding risk. Treatment with DDAVP may "overcome" a mild to moderate platelet defect, as described for anesthetic considerations with vWD, especially if the risk of bleeding is relatively minor. For procedures where the bleeding risk is more substantial, platelet transfusions may be required. Normalization of the bleeding time, the platelet function analyzer, or the thromboelastogram may be used as end points, but will not guarantee adequacy of platelet function for the challenge of surgery. As a general rule, sufficient transfusions to increase the percentage of "normal functioning platelets" into the 10% to 20% range will be sufficient to correct platelet-related therapy.

Platelets become quite dysfunctional in the setting of hypothermia (<35°C) and acidosis (pH <7.3), and platelets transfused into a patient with either or both of these conditions will rapidly become dysfunctional as well.

HYPERCOAGULABLE DISORDERS

Sources of hypercoagulability can be divided into two major classes: a congenital predisposition caused by one or more genetic abnormalities, often referred to as thrombophilia, and acquired or environmental hypercoagulability.

Heritable Causes of Hypercoagulability
Hereditary conditions predisposing to venous thromboembolism (VTE) can conceptually be divided into conditions that either decrease endogenous antithrombotic proteins, or increase prothrombotic proteins (**Table 17-4**).

Thrombophilia Due to Decreased Antithrombotic Proteins
Hereditary Antithrombin Deficiency Antithrombin (AT, also called AT III) is the most important of the body's defenses against clot formation in healthy vessels or at the perimeter of

TABLE 17-4 Major Hereditary Conditions Linked to Hypercoagulability

	Prevalence in Healthy Controls	Prevalence in Patients with First DVT(%)	DVT Likelihood by Age 60(%)
Antithrombin deficiency*	0.2	1.1	62
Protein C deficiency*	0.8	3	48
Protein S deficiency*	1.3	1.1	33
Factor V$_{Leiden}$*	3.5	20	6
Prothrombin 20210A*	2.3	18	<5

*All numbers pertain to heterozygous state.
DVT, deep venous thrombosis.

a site of active bleeding. AT III deficiency is inherited as an autosomal dominant trait, with an estimated frequency of 1 per 1000 to 5000 individuals. Homozygous AT deficiency is generally not compatible with life or even fetal survival to term. Typically, a heterozygote patient has an AT III level between 40% and 70% of normal. Individuals who are heterozygous for AT deficiency are roughly 20 times more likely than nondeficient individuals to develop VTE at some point in their lives (see Table 17-4), usually in association with some triggering event that further increases their hypercoagulability. In one study of 18 AT-deficient individuals, more than 40% of the VTE that developed did so in association with either surgery or pregnancy. Only 11% of the VTEs were spontaneous, that is, they had no known precipitating factors.

Hereditary Protein C and Protein S Deficiency Hereditary deficiencies in protein C (PC) and protein S (PS) have adversely affect thrombin regulation. However, instead of limiting the activity of thrombin already formed, congenital deficiencies in PC and PS hamper the affected individual's ability to limit rates of thrombin generation. With heterozygous deficiencies, the relative surplus of factors Va and VIIIa that results from defective inactivation ensures that both the tenase and prothrombinase complexes are able to act with enhanced kinetics, generating an overabundance of thrombin and setting the stage for risk of the same order of magnitude as antithrombin deficiency. Moreover, synthesis of PC and PS are both vitamin K dependent, with PC having the shorter half-life. Accordingly, individuals who are PC deficient are at particular risk of thrombosis if warfarin therapy is initiated in the absence of protective *previous* anticoagulation by heparin. Specifically, during the first days of warfarin treatment, before inhibition of vitamin K has decreased factors VII, IX, and XI sufficiently to provide the intended *anti*coagulation, modest suppression of PC synthesis may compound the already subnormal PC levels, resulting in paradoxically heightened *hyper*coagulability.

Thrombophilia Due to Increased Prothrombotic Proteins

Factor V_{Leiden} Dahlback first described activated protein C (APC) resistance in a single family in 1993 and subsequently found that among other VTE patients, their plasma often exhibited resistance to the normal anticoagulant effect of APC. Specifically, addition of exogenous APC to their plasma did not prolong the aPTT of these VTE patients when compared with the prolongation found by APC treatment of plasma from non-VTE controls. The gene responsible for this effect, the factor V_{Leiden} gene, differs from the normal gene by a single nucleotide, producing an amino acid substitution at one of the sites where APC normally cleaves factor Va, thereby rendering it refractory to inactivation. Accordingly, factor Va_{Leiden} stays active in the circulation longer than normal, fostering increased thrombin generation.

As the sole source of hypercoagulability, factor V_{Leiden} is viewed as having low to intermediate procoagulant risk. Patients who are heterozygous for factor V_{Leiden} have a five- to

sevenfold increased risk of VTE, while the risk of homozygous carriers is increased up to 80-fold. Factor V_{Leiden} occurs at a high frequency in the general population; its prevalence varies considerably in different ethnic populations, present in approximately 5% of people of northern European descent but rarely in patients of African or Asian descent. Accordingly, depending on the ethnic makeup of the community, up to one in 20 patients presenting for routine surgery can be expected to have a degree of heightened risk attributable to this gene.

Prothrombin G20210A Gene Mutation Another thrombophilia that operates via an increase in prothrombotic proteins is known as the prothrombin gene mutation (G20210A). This gene was described by Poor and colleagues in 1996, noting that 18% of VTE patients and about 1% of healthy controls had a mutation in the gene for prothrombin at base 20210. This particular location is in the 3′ region of the gene that is not translated. Instead, the mutation renders the "end" cleavage signal of the gene inefficient, causing additional amounts of mRNA to be transcribed. Accordingly, the levels of the inactive zymogen, prothrombin, are considerably higher in affected individuals than in the general population. When this mutation is the only thrombophilic risk factor, the VTE risk is relatively low (see Table 17-4); most carriers of this gene will not have had an episode of VTE before age 50. The importance of this thrombophilia, as for FV_{Leiden}, resides in the frequency of the gene, rather than its potency. Also similar to FV_{Leiden}, ethnicity plays a significant role in the prevalence of this gene, occurring in about 4% of individuals of European descent but rarely in patients of African or Asian descent.

Acquired Causes of Hypercoagulability
Myeloproliferative Disorders

Myeloproliferative disorders, especially PV, essential thrombocytosis, and paroxysmal nocturnal hemoglobinuria, are associated with an increased incidence of thrombophlebitis, pulmonary embolism (PE), and arterial occlusions. Patients with these conditions are also at risk of thrombosis of splenic, hepatic, portal, and mesenteric vessels. The pathogenesis of the thrombosis in these patients is not clear. Both the thrombocytosis and an abnormality in platelet function may play a role. Increased activation and aggregation of platelets has been postulated as a cause for the hypercoagulable state.

Malignancies

Patients with certain malignancies demonstrate a marked thrombotic tendency. Adenocarcinomas of the pancreas, colon, stomach, and ovaries are the leading tumors associated with thromboembolic events. In fact, these malignancies can first present with a single or multiple episodes of deep venous thrombosis or migratory superficial thrombophlebitis. Overall, patients who present with primary thrombophlebitis show a 25% to 30% incidence of recurrence, and 20% of these will turn out to have cancer. The pathogenesis of the thrombotic tendency appears to relate to a combination of release of procoagulant factor(s) by the tumor, which can directly activate factor X, endothelial damage by tumor invasion, and blood stasis. Laboratory testing may show no abnormalities or some combination of thrombocytosis, elevation of the fibrinogen level, and low-grade DIC. In the latter case, it is assumed that the tumor must be a thromboplastic stimulus to coagulation.

Pregnancy and Oral Contraceptive Use

Pregnancy and oral contraceptive use have been reported to increase the risk of thrombosis. The overall incidence of thrombosis is approximately 1 in 1500 pregnancies (a five- to sixfold increase in relative risk), but is higher in women with an inherited hypercoagulable state, a history of deep venous thrombosis or PE, a positive family history of thromboembolic disease, or are obese, kept at bedrest for a prolonged period, or require cesarean section. The risk of PE is highest during the third trimester and immediate postpartum period and is a leading cause of maternal death. Of the inherited hypercoagulable states, Antithrombin III–deficient women are at the greatest risk and deserve to be anticoagulated throughout pregnancy. Factor V Leiden and the prothrombin G20201A mutation are associated with much less risk. Women with one of these inherited traits do not need to be anticoagulated unless they have a history of a PE or recurrent deep venous thromboses.

The association of oral contraceptives with thrombosis and thromboembolism also appears to be multifactorial. Since low-dose estrogen contraceptive pills have been introduced, the incidence has decreased significantly. However, women who also smoke, have a history of migraine headaches, or carry an inherited hypercoagulable defect are at increased risk (30-fold) of venous thrombosis, PE, and cerebrovascular thrombosis. At the same time, there appears to be less of a relationship between the use of estrogen at the time of menopause and the occurrence of thrombosis.

Nephrotic Syndrome Patients

Nephrotic syndrome patients are at risk of thromboembolic disease including renal vein thrombosis. The explanation for this is unclear. It has been attributed to lower than normal levels of antithrombin III or PC secondary to renal loss of the coagulation protein, factor XII deficiency, platelet hyperactivity, abnormal fibrinolytic activity, and higher than normal levels of other coagulation factors. Hyperlipidemia and hypoalbuminemia have also been proposed as possible etiologic factors.

Antiphospholipid Antibodies

An increased tendency for both venous and arterial thrombosis is seen in patients who develop a circulating lupus anticoagulant (antiphospholipid/anticardiolipin antibodies) in association with systemic lupus erythematosus or, more often, as the only manifestation of autoimmune disease. The term anticoagulant is, therefore, a clinical misnomer. Antiphospholipid antibodies are a mix of several immunoglobulin G, immunoglobulin M, and, less commonly, immunoglobulin A antibodies directed at phospholipid-associated proteins, particularly prothrombin and β_2-glycoprotein I. They are clinically defined by the method of detection. Lupus anticoagulant antibodies are detected by their prolongation of the PTT and, in some cases, the PT, while anticardiolipin antibodies are measured directly by immunoassay. Anticardiolipin antibody is defined by its reactivity to cardiolipin, β_2-glycoprotein I, or other anionic phospholipids. While the two forms of antibody are closely related, the risk of thrombosis appears to be greater with lupus anticoagulants or anticardiolipin antibodies with activity specifically directed at β_2-glycoprotein I.

The exact mechanism of action has yet to be defined; it has been suggested that the antibodies somehow activate endothelial cells to increase the expression of vascular adhesion molecule-1 and E-selectin. This may then increase the binding of white blood cells and platelets to the endothelial surface, leading to thrombus formation. Other suggested mechanisms of action include interference with PC activation, reduction in PS levels, and the development of a HIT-like platelet defect.

Clinical studies of patients with lupus anticoagulants have shown an increased propensity for thrombosis, with 30% to 60% of patients experiencing one or more thrombotic events during their lifetime. Isolated venous thrombosis or thromboembolism make up two thirds of the cases; cerebral thrombosis accounts for the other third. Coronary, renal, retinal, subclavian, and pedal artery occlusions are less common. Up to 20% of patients presenting with a VTE not associated with other disease, surgery, or trauma will demonstrate antiphospholipid antibodies. Therefore, along with factor V_{Leiden} and the prothrombin gene mutation, the presence of an antiphospholipid antibody must be considered as one of the top causes of thromboembolic disease in younger individuals. Patients can also present with catastrophic antiphospholipid syndrome characterized by multiorgan failure secondary to widespread small vessel thrombosis, thrombocytopenia, acute respiratory distress syndrome, DIC, and, on occasion, an autoimmune hemolytic anemia. This clinical picture is indistinguishable from that of TTP. Bacterial infections often appear to be triggering events for this syndrome.

Anesthetic Considerations for Venous Hypercoagulability
Current antithrombotic strategies range from simple management approaches like early ambulation to the combination of subcutaneous heparin with elastic stockings followed by conversion to outpatient warfarin with associated laboratory monitoring. Surgical patients may present with a host of VTE risk factors, all of which must be considered when balancing the degree of thrombotic risk and the costs (monetary and bleeding risk) of aggressive perioperative anticoagulation. A number of professional societies have synthesized a four-tiered approach to risk stratification of surgery patients that permits the intensity of prophylaxis to be adjusted to an individual patient's VTE risk.

Prophylaxis strategies may take the form of pharmacologic or physical methods. Drugs that have proven to be suitable for VTE prophylaxis include UH, LMWH, the oral anticoagulant warfarin, direct thrombin inhibitors such as hirudin, and factor Xa inhibitors such as fondaparinux. Large trials suggest that subcutaneous administration of UH or LMWH confers a 60% to 70% risk reduction over placebo, depending on the type of surgery. By contrast, aspirin provides relatively weak prophylaxis, with a risk reduction of only 20% compared to placebo. Physical methods of prophylaxis such as graded compression elastic stockings have a 40% to 45% risk reduction, while intermittent pneumatic compression shows a risk reduction that approaches that of UH when used as the only prophylactic method. The management of patients presenting for surgery who are already on oral anticoagulants is discussed in a separate section to follow.

A number of investigations published in the late 1970s and early 1980s presented convincing evidence that regional anesthesia, usually consisting of neuraxial blockade, resulted in a decreased incidence of postoperative VTE. This finding was particularly true for lower extremity joint replacement surgery. With as many as 9% of hip arthroplasty patients developing symptomatic VTE and with asymptomatic VTE in the range of 45% to 65%, regional anesthesia became the preferred anesthetic technique for this surgery and other procedures with high VTE risk. However, even when neuraxial anesthesia was combined with techniques such as early ambulation and intraoperative antiembolism stockings, the VTE risk was still unacceptably high. As a result, postoperative prophylactic anticoagulation with drugs like warfarin and subcutaneous heparin became the standard of care for these high-risk operations.

With the advent of routine antithrombotic prophylaxis, however, the advantages of regional over general anesthesia are now less clear, raising the question whether, for patients receiving pharmacologic perioperative thromboprophylaxis, neuraxial anesthesia still reduces the risks of VTE. A meta-analysis of anesthesia for hip fracture surgery by the Cochrane Database of Systematic Reviews found that regional and general anesthesia appeared to produce comparable results for most outcomes studied. Seventeen trials were included, and only four included some form of pharmacologic or mechanical antithrombotic prophylaxis. Accordingly, although there was a slight reduction in VTE incidence associated with regional anesthesia, it was largely a function of older studies lacking in pharmacologic prophylaxis, and this did not translate into a significant difference in mortality. The recent U.S. Food and Drug Administration advisory prohibiting neuraxial anesthesia in patients receiving LMWH due to increased epidural hematoma risk may further limit the extension of regional anesthesia into the postoperative period. Furthermore, there is no evidence that the VTE risk reduction provided by regional anesthesia obviates the need for postoperative pharmacologic prophylaxis. In conclusion, no particular anesthetic technique is mandated for antithrombotic prophylaxis, and, except in special circumstances, effective antithrombotic drugs such as LMWH should probably not be withheld in the postoperative period to allow continued use of an epidural.

In patients who have an absolute contraindication to anticoagulation or have a major bleeding complication, the placement of a vena caval filter can be used to prevent recurrent pulmonary emboli. Available filters include the Greenfield filter, the bird's nest filter, the Simon nitinol filter, the Vena Tech filter, and the Gunther Tulip Retrievable Vena Caval Filter. The latter can be removed in 7 to 10 days if bleeding is controlled and anticoagulation reinstituted. The filters compare well in terms of efficacy, reducing the incidence of PE to less than 4% (median follow-up in most study series was 12–18 months), but are not more effective than long-term anticoagulation. In cancer patients who have failed anticoagulation, a vena caval filter combined with continued anticoagulation may provide greater protection. Complications include insertion site (20%–40%) and inferior vena caval thrombosis, tilting or migration of the filter, damage to the wall of the inferior vena cava, and filter fracture.

Anesthetic Considerations for Patients on Long-Term Anticoagulation

Perioperative management of patients receiving long-term anticoagulation requires special consideration of the risks of bleeding and thrombosis (**Table 17-5**). The risk of thrombosis when the preoperative patient is not effectively anticoagulated must be weighed against the risk of bleeding during and after surgery if anticoagulation is continued perioperatively. Details of the thrombosis that warranted anticoagulation, that is, the "inciting thrombus," are of primary importance. The risks associated with recurrence of thrombosis are greatest if the inciting thrombus was arterial, especially if associated with atrial fibrillation where recurrent embolism carries a 40% mortality; in contrast, recurrent lower-extremity VTE has a risk of associated sudden death of 6%. In addition, the time elapsed since the inciting thrombus is also critical, as the risk of recurrence decreases over time for both arterial and venous thrombi.

Most anticoagulated patients are managed on warfarin, an anticoagulation that gradually abates after stopping the drug.

TABLE 17-5	Recommendations for Preoperative and Postoperative Anticoagulation in Patients Being Treated with Oral Anticoagulants	
Indication	Before Surgery	After Surgery
Acute venous thromboembolism		
First 30 days	Heparin IV	Heparin IV
After 30 days	No change	Heparin IV
Recurrent venous thromboembolism	No change	Heparin SC
Acute arterial thromboembolism (first 30 days)	Heparin IV	Heparin IV
Mechanical heart valve	No change	Heparin SC
Nonvalvular atrial fibrillation	No change	Heparin SC

After discontinuing warfarin, the INR does not start to fall for approximately 29 hours, and then decreases with a half-life of approximately 22 hours. If a patient is considered to be at high risk without anticoagulation, bridging therapy in the form of therapeutic doses of UH or LMWH should be considered approximately 60 hours after the last dose of warfarin. In the case of intravenous UH, a window of 6 drug-free hours should be allowed prior to surgery. For LMWH, which may be given subcutaneously as an outpatient, doses should be given once or twice daily for 3 days before surgery, with the last dose no less than 18 hours preoperatively for a twice-daily dose (i.e., ~100 U/kg of LMWH) and 30 hours for a once-daily regimen (i.e., ~150–200 U/kg of LMWH). An additional 6-hour drug-free interval should be allowed if neuraxial anesthesia is planned.

Postoperative resumption of anticoagulation requires an evaluation of the risk of recurrent thrombosis and consideration of the degree to which surgery itself increases the patient's hypercoagulability (e.g., minor surgery versus major orthopedic surgery). This must be weighed against the bleeding risk associated with resumption of anticoagulation. Since there is a delay of approximately 24 hours after warfarin administration before the INR increases, warfarin should generally be resumed as soon as possible after surgery except in patients at high bleeding risk; consideration can be given to bridging therapy with intravenous or subcutaneous anticoagulation until the INR becomes therapeutic.

Acquired Hypercoagulability of the Arterial Vasculature

Atrial Fibrillation

Patients with atrial fibrillation, particularly atrial fibrillation with valvular disease, a dilated atrium, and evidence of heart failure or a previous embolus generally require moderate-dose warfarin therapy indefinitely. Patients with acute anterior wall infarctions who, because of a wall motion abnormality, are likely to form a mural thrombus need to receive warfarin for 2 to 3 months, after which there is little risk of embolism.

Antiphospholipid Antibodies

Patients with antiphospholipid antibodies (lupus anticoagulants) and thromboembolic disease can represent a major therapeutic challenge. These patients are at significant risk of both arterial and venous thromboses, and their management is discussed in "Acquired Causes of Hypercoagulability."

In summary, hypercoagulability, a state of exaggerated coagulation activation, plays a major role in the pathogenesis of VTE, a process that affects some two million Americans annually with an estimated mortality of 150,000 from PE. New heritable causes of hypercoagulability are being identified, and some genetic predisposition to thrombosis can be identified in more than 50% of deep venous thrombosis patients. Accordingly, anesthesiologists are being asked to care for an increasing number of patients carrying the diagnosis of hypercoagulability, many of whom receive long-term anticoagulation therapy. The perioperative period represents a time of high risk of VTE, with selected surgeries associated with a greater than 100-fold increased risk of thrombosis. Our knowledge of the optimum operative management of these patients inevitably lags behind the identification of their pathophysiology, making it incumbent on anesthesiologists to understand the mechanisms behind hypercoagulability and thereby make educated choices. Hypercoagulability plays a less clearly defined role in the pathophysiology of arterial thrombotic events, but the high morbidity and mortality associated with arterial occlusive events in the operative patient makes staying abreast of these developments important patient care.

KEY POINTS

- The erythrocyte and its major protein constituent Hb are highly specialized such that oxygen delivery can be rapidly adjusted to meet local tissue needs. Disorders affecting the formation, structure, metabolism, and turnover of these elements can impair their ability to perform this vital task in the operative patient.

- Preoperative management of sickle cell disease patients no longer mandates exchange transfusions to decrease the ratio of sickle Hb to normal Hb, but instead only requires whatever transfusions (if any) are needed to achieve a preoperative hematocrit of 30%.

- Recent advances in cell-based coagulation models have changed our fundamental understanding of in vivo clotting. This improved understanding has translated into a better appreciation of how specific defects in coagulation components affect the balance of hemostasis and what therapeutic interventions offer the best risk/benefit ratio.

- Sources of hypercoagulability can be divided into two major classes: a congenital predisposition that is usually lifelong and an acquired or environmental hypercoagulability such as surgery. In patients presenting with a first-time VTE, some congenital predisposition can be identified in up to 50% of cases. However, in almost all cases of VTE, some acquired or environmental hypercoagulability serves as a triggering event.

- Most disorders producing a state of venous hypercoagulability affect the generation or disposition of thrombin, whereas in the arterial circulation, platelet and endothelial function and regulation also critically affect the prothrombotic tendency.

REFERENCES

Bouchard BA, Butenas S, Mann KG, et al: Interaction between platelets and the coagulation system. In Michelson AD (ed): Platelets, Vol. 1. Amsterdam, Academic Press, 2002, pp 229–253.

Butenas S, Branda RF, van't Veer C, et al: Platelets and phospholipids in tissue factor-initiated thrombin generation. Thromb Haemost 2001;86:660–667.

Caprini JA, Arcelus JI, Reyna JJ: Effective risk stratification of surgical and nonsurgical patients for venous thromboembolic disease. Semin Hematol 2001;38(Suppl 5):12–19.

Crowther MA, Kelton JG: Congenital thrombophilic states associated with venous thrombosis: A qualitative overview and proposed classification system. Ann Intern Med 2003;138:128–134.

Firth PG, Head CA: Sickle cell disease and anesthesia. Anesthesiology 2004;101:766–785.

Greinacher A, Farner B, Kroll H, et al: Clinical features of heparin-induced thrombocytopenia including risk factors for thrombosis. Thromb Haemost 2005;94:132–135.

Gutt CN, Oniu T, Wolkener F, et al: Prophylaxis and treatment of deep vein thrombosis in general surgery. Am J Surg 2004; 189:14–22.

Hillman RS, Ault KA, Rinder HM: Hematology in Clinical Practice. New York, McGraw-Hill, 2005.

Mann KG, Brummel K, Butenas S: What is all that thrombin for? J Thromb Haemost 2003;1:1504–1515.

Marks PW, Glader B: Approach to anemia in the adult and child. In Hoffman R, Benz EL Jr, Shattil S, et al (eds): Hematology: Basic Principles and Practice. Philadelphia, Elsevier, 2005.

Practice guidelines for perioperative blood transfusion and adjuvant therapies. Anesthesiology 2006;105:198–208.

Savage B, Ruggeri ZM: Platelet thrombus formation in flowing whole blood. In Michelson AD (ed): Platelets, Vol. I. Philadelphia, Elsevier, 2007, pp 359–376.

Schafer A, Levine M, Konkle B, et al: Thrombotic disorders: Diagnosis and treatment. Hematology 2003;520–539.

Steinberg MH, Benz EL Jr: Pathobiology of the human erythrocyte and its hemoglobins. In Hoffman R, Benz EL Jr, Shattil S, et al (eds): Hematology: Basic Principles and Practice, Philadelphia, Elsevier, 2005.

Tefferi A: Polycythemia vera: A comprehensive review and clinical recommendations. Mayo Clin Proc 2003;78:174–194.

Turpie AGG, Chin BSP, Lip GLH: Venous thromboembolism: pathophysiology, clinical features, and prevention. The ABCs of antithrombotic therapy. BMJ 2002;325:887–890.

CHAPTER 18

Skin and Musculoskeletal Diseases

Jeffrey J. Schwartz

Myasthenia Gravis
- Classification
- Signs and Symptoms
- Treatment
- Management of Anesthesia

Myasthenic Syndrome

Rheumatoid Arthritic
- Signs and Symptoms
- Treatment
- Management of Anesthesia

Spondyloarthropathies
- Ankylosing Spondylitis
- Reactive Arthritis
- Juvenile Chronic Polyarthropathy
- Enteropathic Arthritis

Osteoarthritis

Paget's Disease

Marfan Syndrome
- Cardiovascular System
- Management of Anesthesia

Kyphoscoliosis
- Signs and Symptoms
- Management

Dwarfism
- Achondroplasia
- Russell-Silver Syndrome

Back Pain
- Acute Low Back Pain
- Lumbar Spinal Stenosis

Other Musculoskeletal Syndromes
- Rotator Cuff Tear
- Floppy Infant Syndrome
- Tracheomegaly
- Alcoholic Myopathy
- Prader-Willi Syndrome
- Prune-Belly Syndrome
- Mitochondrial Myopathies
- Multicore Myopathy
- Centronuclear Myopathy
- Meige Syndrome
- Spasmodic Dysphonia
- Juvenile Hyaline Fibromatosis
- Chondrodysplasia Calcificans Punctata
- Erythromelalgia
- Farber's Lipogranulomatosis
- McCune-Albright Syndrome
- Klippel-Feil Syndrome
- Osteogenesis Imperfecta
- Fibrodysplasia Ossificans
- Deformities of the Sternum
- Macroglossia

Diseases of the skin and musculoskeletal system manifest with obvious clinical signs since both of these systems are readily visible. However, less visible systemic effects of many of these disorders are also important.

EPIDERMOLYSIS BULLOSA

Epidermolysis bullosa is a group of genetic diseases of mucous membranes and skin, particularly the oropharynx and esophagus. Epidermis bullosa can be categorized as simplex, junctional, and dystrophic. In the simplex type, epidermal cells are fragile and mutations of genes encoding keratin intermediate filament proteins underlie the fragility. In the dystrophic types (incidence approximately one in every 300,000 births), the genetic mutation appears to be in the gene encoding the type of collagen that is the major component of anchoring fibrils.

Signs and Symptoms

Epidermolysis bullosa is characterized by bulla formation (blistering) due to separation within the epidermis followed by fluid accumulation. Bulla formation is typically initiated when lateral shearing forces are applied to the skin. Pressure applied perpendicular to the skin is not as great a hazard. Bulla formation can occur with even minimal trauma or can occur spontaneously.

The simplex form of epidermolysis bullosa is characterized by a benign course and normal development. By contrast, patients with the junctional form of epidermolysis bullosa rarely survive beyond early childhood. Most die of sepsis. Features that distinguish junctional epidermolysis bullosa from other forms are generalized blistering beginning at birth, absence of scar formation, and generalized mucosal involvement (gastrointestinal, genitourinary, respiratory). Manifestations of epidermolysis bullosa dystrophica include severe scarring with fusion of the digits (pseudosyndactyly), constriction of the oral aperture (microstomia) and esophageal stricture. The teeth are often dysplastic. Malnutrition, anemia, electrolyte derangements, and hypoalbuminemia are common, most likely reflecting chronic infection, debilitation, and renal dysfunction. Survival beyond the second decade is unusual. Diseases associated with epidermolysis bullosa include porphyria, amyloidosis, multiple myeloma, diabetes mellitus, and hypercoagulable states. Mitral valve prolapse may also accompany this disorder.

Treatment

Treatment of epidermolysis bullosa is symptomatic and supportive. Many of these patients are receiving corticosteroids. Infection of bullae with *Staphylococcus aureus* or with β-hemolytic streptococci is common.

Management of Anesthesia

Supplemental corticosteroids may be indicated during the perioperative period if patients have been on long-term treatment with these drugs. The main anesthetic concerns in patients with epidermolysis bullosa center on the serious complications that can occur if proper precautions are not taken during instrumentation. Avoidance of trauma to the skin and mucous membranes is crucial. Bulla formation can be caused by trauma from tape, blood pressure cuffs, tourniquets, adhesive electrodes, and rubbing the skin with alcohol wipes. Blood pressure cuffs should be padded with a loose cotton dressing. Electrodes should have the adhesive portion removed. Petroleum jelly gauze can help hold them in place. Anything that touches a patient should be well padded. Intravenous and intra-arterial catheters should be sutured or held in place with gauze wraps rather than tape. A nonadhesive pulse oximetry sensor should be used. A soft foam, sheepskin, or gel pad should be placed under the patient. All creases should be removed from the linen.

Trauma from the anesthetic face mask must be minimized by gentle application against the face. Lubrication of the face and mask with cortisol ointment, or indeed any lubricant, can be helpful. Upper airway instrumentation should be minimized because the squamous epithelium lining the oropharynx and esophagus is very susceptible to trauma. Frictional trauma to the oropharynx, such as that produced by an oral airway, can result in formation of large intraoral bullae and/or extensive hemorrhage from denuded mucosa. Nasal airways are equally hazardous. Esophageal stethoscopes should be avoided. Hemorrhage from ruptured oral bullae has been treated successfully with epinephrine-soaked gauze applied directly to the bullae.

Interestingly, endotracheal intubation has not been associated with laryngeal or tracheal complications in patients with epidermolysis bullosa dystrophica. Indeed, laryngeal involvement with this form of the disease is rare, and tracheal bullae have not been reported. This finding is consistent with the greater resistance of columnar epithelium to disruption compared to fragile squamous epithelium. Generous lubrication of the laryngoscope blade with cortisol ointment and/or petroleum jelly and selection of a smaller endotracheal tube than usual are recommended. Chronic scarring of the oral cavity can result in a narrow oral aperture and immobility of the tongue making tracheal intubation difficult. After intubation, the tube must be carefully immobilized with soft cloth bandages to prevent movement in the oropharynx, and the tube must be positioned so that it does not exert lateral forces at the corners of the mouth. Tape is not used to hold the endotracheal tube in place. It must be remembered that oropharyngeal suctioning can lead to life-threatening bulla formation. The risk of pulmonary aspiration may be increased in the presence of esophageal stricture.

Porphyria cutanea tarda has been reported to occur with increased frequency in patients with epidermolysis bullosa. This type of porphyria does not have the same implications for management of anesthesia, as does acute intermittent porphyria.

Propofol and ketamine are useful for avoiding airway manipulation when the operative procedure does not require controlled ventilation or skeletal muscle relaxation. Despite the presence of dystrophic skeletal muscle, there is no evidence that these patients are at increased risk of a hyperkalemic response when treated with succinylcholine. There are no known contraindications to the use of volatile anesthetics in these patients. As alternatives to general anesthesia, regional anesthetic techniques (spinal, epidural, brachial plexus block) have been recommended.

PEMPHIGUS

Pemphigus refers to a group of chronic autoimmune blistering (vesiculobullous) diseases that may involve extensive areas of the skin and mucous membranes. Cutaneous pemphigus is characterized by bullae of the skin and mucous membranes (mouth, upper airway, genitalia). Two histopathologically and clinically different types of pemphigus have been recognized: pemphigus vulgaris and pemphigus foliaceus. Cutaneous pemphigus closely resembles the oral manifestations of epidermolysis bullosa dystrophica. Involvement of the oropharynx is present in approximately 50% of patients with pemphigus. Extensive oropharyngeal involvement makes eating painful, and patients may decrease oral intake to the point that severe malnutrition develops. Denuding of skin and bulla formation can result in significant fluid and protein losses. The risk of secondary infection is substantial.

Pemphigus is an autoimmune disorder in which circulating antibodies attack antigenic sites on the surface of epidermal cells, resulting in destruction of these cells. Pemphigus may be associated with underlying malignancy, especially lymphoreticular cancer. As with epidermolysis bullosa, there may be an absence of intercellular bridges that normally prevent the separation of epidermal cells. Therefore, frictional trauma can result in bulla formation. Occasionally, infection or drug sensitivity is the inciting event for bulla formation. Pemphigus vulgaris is the most common form of pemphigus and is also the most significant because of its high incidence of oropharyngeal lesions.

Treatment

Treatment of pemphigus with corticosteroids has decreased the mortality associated with this disease from 70% to 5%. Biologic and immunosuppressive therapy with mycophenolate mofetil, rituximab, azathioprine, methotrexate, and cyclophosphamide has also been used successfully for early treatment of pemphigus. Immune globulin has replaced high-dose corticosteroids as a rescue therapy.

Management of Anesthesia

Management of anesthesia in patients with pemphigus and epidermolysis bullosa is similar. Preoperative evaluation must consider current drug therapy. Supplementation with corticosteroids may be necessary. Electrolyte derangements may be present due to chronic fluid losses through bullous skin lesions. Dehydration and hypokalemia are not uncommon.

Airway management may be difficult because of bullae in the oropharynx. Airway manipulation including direct laryngoscopy and endotracheal intubation can result in acute bulla formation, upper airway obstruction, and bleeding. Regional anesthesia, although controversial, has been successfully administered to these patients. Skin infection at the site selected for regional anesthesia is possible. Infiltration with a local anesthetic solution is usually avoided because of the risk of skin sloughing and bulla formation at the injection site. Propofol and ketamine are useful for general anesthesia in selected patients.

PSORIASIS

Psoriasis is a common chronic dermatologic disorder affecting 1% to 3% of the world's population. It is characterized by accelerated epidermal growth resulting in inflammatory erythematous papules covered with loosely adherent scales (chronic plaque psoriasis). Skin lesions are remitting and relapsing. Onset may occur during adolescence and young adulthood or at an older age. Synthesis of deoxyribonucleic acid in the epidermis of these patients is four times greater than in normal epidermis. Symmetrically distributed skin lesions typically involve the elbows, knees, hairline, and presacral region. An asymmetrical arthropathy occurs in approximately 5% to 8% of patients. This usually involves the small joints of the hands and feet, the large joints of the legs, or some combination of both. High output heart failure has been observed. Generalized pustular psoriasis is a rare form of the disease that may be complicated by hypoalbuminemia, sepsis, and renal failure.

Treatment

Treatment of psoriasis is directed at slowing the rapid proliferation of epidermal cells. Coal tar is effective because of its antimitotic action and its ability to inhibit enzymes. Although preparations containing coal tar can cause plaques to clear when used alone, they are usually used in combination with ultraviolet phototherapy. The use of coal tar is limited by its unpleasant odor and its potential to irritate normal skin. Coal tar is frequently used in shampoo preparations to prevent psoriatic scaling of the scalp. In rare cases, skin cancer has been associated with the therapeutic use of coal tar. Ointments containing salicylic acid are the most widely used keratolytic agents. They can be used alone or in combination with coal tar or topical corticosteroids. Topical corticosteroids are effective, but the disease promptly recurs when treatment is discontinued. Application of corticosteroids under occlusive dressings can result in significant systemic absorption and suppression of the pituitary-adrenal axis. Calcipotriene ointment (a vitamin D analogue) and tazarotene (a topical retinoid) can be used. Systemic therapy with methotrexate or cyclosporine and

biologic therapy with etanercept (a tumor necrosis factor inhibitor), infliximab (a monoclonal antibody to tumor necrosis factor), alefacept (an immunomodulatory fusion protein), or efalizumab (a monoclonal antibody to CD11a) may be required for severe cases. Toxic effects of these drugs include cirrhosis, renal failure, hypertension, and pneumonitis.

Management of Anesthesia

Management of anesthesia must include evaluation of the drugs being used for the treatment of psoriasis including topical corticosteroids and chemotherapeutic drugs. Skin trauma from venipuncture or the surgical incision can accentuate psoriasis in some patients. Patients with psoriasis often have a marked increase in skin blood flow that can contribute to altered thermoregulation.

MASTOCYTOSIS

Mastocytosis is a rare disorder of mast cell proliferation that can occur in a cutaneous form (urticaria pigmentosa) or in a systemic form. Urticaria pigmentosa is usually benign and asymptomatic. Children are most often affected. In nearly half of affected children, the small red-brown macules that are present on the trunk and extremities disappear by adulthood. In the systemic form of mastocytosis, mast cells proliferate in all organs (especially bone, liver, spleen) but not the central nervous system. Degranulation of mast cells with release of histamine, heparin, prostaglandins, and numerous enzymes (tryptases, hydrolases) may occur spontaneously or be triggered by nonimmune factors, including physical or psychologic stimuli, alcohol, and drugs known to release histamine. A rare form of systemic mastocytosis, known as malignant aggressive systemic mastocytosis, is characterized by diffuse mast cell proliferation in parenchymal organs, thrombocytopenia, and hemorrhage. These patients often require splenectomy.

Signs and Symptoms

Classic signs and symptoms of mastocytosis reflect degranulation of mast cells with anaphylactoid responses characterized by pruritus, urticaria, and flushing. These changes may be accompanied by hypotension and tachycardia. Hypotension may be so severe as to be life threatening. Although symptoms are usually attributed to histamine release from mast cells, H_1- and H_2-receptor antagonists are not always protective, and the incidence of bronchospasm is low. This suggests that vasoactive substances other than histamine (such as prostaglandins) may be involved. Bleeding is unusual in these patients even though mast cells contain heparin.

Management of Anesthesia

Management of anesthesia is influenced by the possibility of intraoperative mast cell degranulation and anaphylactoid reaction. Although the intraoperative period is usually uneventful in these patients, there are reports of life-threatening anaphylactoid reactions with even minor surgical procedures, emphasizing the need to have resuscitation drugs such as epinephrine immediately available when anesthetizing these patients. Preoperative administration of H_1- and H_2-receptor antagonists may be considered to decrease the clinical response to histamine release. However, these drugs do not interfere with the actual release of histamine from mast cells. Cromolyn sodium does inhibit mast cell degranulation and may decrease the risk of bronchospasm.

Some recommend preoperative skin testing of anesthesia-related drugs to help define which anesthetics would evoke mast cell degranulation. Fentanyl, propofol, and vecuronium have been administered to these patients without evoking mast cell degranulation as have succinylcholine and meperidine. Volatile anesthetics also appear to be acceptable to these patients. Monitoring serum tryptase concentration during the perioperative period may be useful for detecting the occurrence of mast cell degranulation.

Episodes of profound hypotension have been observed with administration of radiocontrast media to patients with mastocytosis. Therefore, it is prudent to pretreat these patients with H_1- and H_2-histamine receptor antagonists and a glucocorticoid before a procedure involving a dye contrast study.

ATOPIC DERMATITIS

Atopic dermatitis is the cutaneous manifestation of the atopic state. It is characterized by dry, scaly, eczematous, pruritic patches on the face, neck, and flexor surfaces of the arms and legs. Pruritus is the primary symptom. Systemic antihistamines are effective in decreasing pruritus, and corticosteroids may be indicated for short-term treatment of severe cases. Pulmonary manifestations of the atopic state, such as asthma, hay fever, otitis media, and sinusitis, may influence anesthetic management.

URTICARIA

Urticaria may be characterized as acute urticaria, chronic urticaria, or physical urticaria. Acute urticaria (hives) and angioedema affects 10% to 20% of the U.S. population at one time or another. In most people, the cause cannot be determined and the lesions resolve spontaneously or after administration of antihistamines. Only a minority of patients have lesions for a long period of time. With physical urticaria, physically stimulating the skin causes the formation of local wheals, itching, and in some cases angioedema. Cold urticaria accounts for 3% to 5% of all physical urticarias (**Table 18-1**). Urticarial vasculitis may be a presenting symptom of systemic lupus erythematosus and Sjögren's syndrome.

Chronic Urticaria

Chronic urticaria is characterized by circumscribed wheals and localized areas of edema produced by extravasation of fluid through blood vessel walls. The wheals are smooth, pink to red

TABLE 18-1 Features of Common Types of Chronic Urticaria

Type of Urticaria	Age Range (yr)	Clinical Features	Angioedema	Diagnostic Test
Chronic idiopathic	20–50	Pink or pale edematous papules or wheals, wheals often annular, pruritus	Yes	
Symptomatic dermatographism	20–50	Linear wheals with a surrounding bright-red flare at sites of stimulation, pruritus	No	Light stroking of skin causes wheal
Physical urticarias				
Cold	10–40	Pale or red swelling at sites of contact with cold surfaces or fluids, pruritus	Yes	Application of ice pack causes a wheal within 5 min of removing the ice (cold stimulation test)
Pressure	20–50	Swelling at sites of pressure (soles, palms, waist) lasting ≥ 2–24 hr, painful, pruritus	No	Application of pressure perpendicular to skin produces persistent red swelling after a latent period of 1–4 hr
Solar	20–50	Pale or red swelling at site of exposure to ultraviolet or visible light, pruritus	Yes	Radiation by a solar simulator for 30–120 sec causes wheals in 30 min
Cholinergic	10–50	Monomorphic pale or pink wheals on trunk, neck, and limbs, pruritus	Yes	Exercise or hot shower elicits wheals

Adapted from Greaves MW: Chronic urticaria. N Engl J Med 1995;332:1767–1772.

and surrounded by a bright red flare; they are usually intensely pruritic, can be found anywhere on hairless or hairy skin, and last less than 24 hours. Wheals lasting longer than 24 hours raise the possibility of other diagnoses including urticarial vasculitis. Chronic urticaria affects approximately twice as many women as men and often follows a remitting and relapsing course, with symptoms typically increasing at night. Angioedema describes urticaria involving the mucous membranes, particularly those of the mouth, pharynx, and larynx. Mast cells and basophils regulate urticarial reactions. When stimulated by certain nonimmunologic events or by immunologic factors (drugs, inhaled allergens), storage granules in these cells release histamine and other vasoactive substances such as bradykinin. These substances result in the localized vasodilation and transudation of fluid characteristic of urticarial lesions.

Except for patients with chronic urticaria for whom avoidable causes can be identified (for example, food additives), treatment is symptomatic. A tepid shower temporarily alleviates pruritus. Antihistamines (H_1-receptor antagonists) are the principal treatment for mild cases of recurring chronic urticaria. Terfenadine has a low potential for sedation and is a common treatment for mild cases of chronic urticaria. High doses of this drug have been associated with cardiac dysrhythmias. Doxepin is a tricyclic antidepressant drug with significant H_1-antagonist actions that is particularly useful when severe urticaria is associated with depression. The combination of H_1- and H_2-receptor antagonists may be more efficacious than use of H_1-receptor antagonists alone. If antihistamines do not control chronic urticaria, a course of systemic corticosteroids may be considered. The course of this treatment is usually limited to 21 days because prolonged use of corticosteroids is invariably associated with a decreased efficacy and an increase in side effects. A 2% topical spray of ephedrine is useful for treating oropharyngeal edema. Swelling involving the tongue may require urgent treatment with epinephrine.

All patients with chronic urticaria should be advised to avoid angiotensin-converting enzyme inhibitors, aspirin, and other nonsteroidal anti-inflammatory drugs (NSAIDs).

Cold Urticaria

Cold urticaria is characterized by development of urticaria and angioedema following exposure to cold. The most common triggering factors are cold air currents, rain, aquatic activities, snow, cold foods and beverages, and contact with cold objects. Severe cold urticaria may be life threatening with laryngeal edema, bronchospasm, and hypotension. The diagnosis is based on skin stimulation at a temperature of $0°$ to $4°C$ for 1 to 5 minutes (cold stimulation test). Immunologic mechanisms may be associated with the development of cold urticaria. Immunoglobulin E concentrations may be increased. Cutaneous mast cells rather than basophils in the bloodstream are the target cells for degranulation, although basophil degranulation is possible with profound hypothermia. Tryptase is an important marker of mast cell degranulation.

The primary objective of treatment of cold urticaria is to prevent systemic reactions caused by known triggers. Antihistamines may decrease the incidence of recurrence and prolong the time that a cold stimulus is tolerated before a reaction occurs.

Management of anesthesia includes avoidance of drugs that are likely to evoke histamine release. Drugs requiring cold storage should be avoided or warmed before injection. Other prophylactic measures include warming intravenous fluids and increasing the ambient temperature of the operating room. Preoperative administration of H_1- and H_2-receptor antagonists and corticosteroids has been recommended, especially when intraoperative hypothermia is unavoidable as may be the case during surgery requiring cardiopulmonary bypass.

ERYTHEMA MULTIFORME

Erythema multiforme is a recurrent disease of the skin and mucous membranes characterized by lesions ranging from edematous macules and papules to vesicular or bullous lesions that may ulcerate. Attacks are associated with viral infection (especially herpes simplex), infection with hemolytic streptococci, cancer, collagen vascular disease, and drug-induced hypersensitivity.

Stevens-Johnson syndrome (erythema multiforme major) is a severe manifestation associated with multisystem dysfunction. High fever, tachycardia, and tachypnea may occur. Drugs associated with the onset of this syndrome include antibiotics, analgesics, and certain over-the-counter medications. Corticosteroids are used in the management of severe cases.

The hazards of administering anesthesia to patients with Stevens-Johnson syndrome are similar to those encountered in anesthetizing patients with epidermolysis bullosa. For example, involvement of the upper respiratory tract can make management of the airway and tracheal intubation difficult. The presence of pulmonary blebs makes these patients vulnerable to pneumothorax, particularly with positive pressure ventilation. Pulmonary blebs also prohibit the use of nitrous oxide. Patients with particularly severe Stevens-Johnson syndrome should be treated in a burn unit.

SCLERODERMA

Scleroderma (systemic sclerosis) is characterized by inflammation, vascular sclerosis, and fibrosis of the skin and viscera. Microvascular changes produce tissue fibrosis and organ sclerosis. Injury to vascular endothelial cells results in vascular obliteration and leakage of serum proteins into the interstitial space. These proteins produce tissue edema, lymphatic obstruction, and ultimately fibrosis. In some patients, the disease evolves into the CREST syndrome (*C*alcinoses, *R*aynaud's phenomenon, *E*sophageal hypomotility, *S*clerodactyly, *T*elangiectasia). The prognosis is poor and is related to the extent of visceral involvement. No drugs or treatments have proved safe and effective in altering the underlying disease process in scleroderma.

The etiology of scleroderma is unknown but the disease process has the characteristics of both a collagen vascular disease and an autoimmune disease. The typical onset is at 20 to 40 years of age, and women are most often affected. Pregnancy accelerates the progression of scleroderma in approximately half of patients. The incidence of spontaneous abortion, premature labor, and perinatal mortality is high.

Signs and Symptoms

Manifestations of scleroderma occur in the skin and musculoskeletal system, nervous system, cardiovascular system, lungs, kidneys, and gastrointestinal tract.

Skin and Musculoskeletal Systems

Skin exhibits mild thickening and diffuse nonpitting edema. As scleroderma progresses, the skin becomes taut, leading to limited mobility and flexion contractures, especially of the fingers. Skeletal muscles may develop myopathy, manifesting as weakness, particularly of proximal skeletal muscle groups. Plasma creatine kinase concentration is typically increased. Mild inflammatory arthritis can occur, but most limitation in joint movement is due to the thickened, taut skin. Avascular necrosis of the femoral head may occur.

Nervous System

Peripheral or cranial nerve neuropathy has been attributed to nerve compression by thickened connective tissue surrounding the nerve sheath. Facial pain suggestive of trigeminal neuralgia may occur as a result of this thickening. Keratoconjunctivitis sicca (dry eyes) exists in some patients and may predispose to corneal abrasions.

Cardiovascular System

Changes in the myocardium reflect sclerosis of small coronary arteries and the conduction system, replacement of cardiac muscle with fibrous tissue, and the indirect effects of systemic and pulmonary hypertension. These changes result in cardiac dysrhythmias, cardiac conduction abnormalities, and congestive heart failure. Intimal fibrosis of pulmonary arteries is associated with a high incidence of pulmonary hypertension, which may progress to cor pulmonale. Pulmonary hypertension is often present, even in asymptomatic patients. Pericarditis and pericardial effusion with or without cardiac tamponade are not infrequent. Changes in the peripheral portion of the vascular tree are common and typically involve intermittent vasospasm in the small arteries of the digits. Raynaud's phenomenon occurs in most cases and may be the initial manifestation of scleroderma. Oral or nasal telangiectasias may be present.

Lungs

The effects of scleroderma on the lungs are a major cause of morbidity and mortality. Diffuse interstitial pulmonary fibrosis may occur independent of the vascular changes that lead to pulmonary hypertension. Arterial hypoxemia resulting from decreased diffusion capacity is not unusual in these patients, even at rest. Although dermal sclerosis does not decrease chest wall compliance, pulmonary compliance is diminished by fibrosis.

Kidneys

Renal artery stenosis as a result of arteriolar intimal proliferation leads to decreased renal blood flow and systemic hypertension. Development of malignant hypertension and irreversible renal failure was the most common cause of death in patients with scleroderma, but now scleroderma renal crisis is relatively rare. Angiotensin-converting enzyme inhibitors are effective in controlling hypertension and in improving the impaired renal function that accompanies hypertension. Corticosteroids can precipitate a renal crisis in patients with scleroderma.

Gastrointestinal Tract

Involvement of the gastrointestinal tract by scleroderma may manifest as dryness of the oral mucosa (xerostomia). Progressive fibrosis of the gastrointestinal tract causes hypomotility of the lower esophagus and small intestine. Dysphagia is a common complaint and is due to hypomotility of the esophagus. Lower esophageal sphincter tone is decreased, and reflux of gastric fluid into the esophagus is common. Symptoms resulting from this esophagitis can be treated with antacids. Bacterial overgrowth due to intestinal hypomotility can produce a malabsorption syndrome. Coagulation disorders reflecting malabsorption of vitamin K may be present. Broad-spectrum antibiotics are effective in the treatment of this type of malabsorption syndrome. Intestinal hypomotility can also manifest as intestinal pseudo-obstruction. Somatostatin analogues such as octreotide may improve intestinal motility. Prokinetic drugs such as metoclopramide are not effective.

Management of Anesthesia

Preoperative evaluation of patients with scleroderma must focus attention on the organ systems likely to be involved by this disease. Decreased mandibular motion and narrowing of the oral aperture due to taut skin must be appreciated before induction of anesthesia. Fiberoptic laryngoscopy may be necessary to facilitate endotracheal intubation through a small oral aperture. Oral or nasal telangiectasias may bleed profusely if traumatized during tracheal intubation. Intravenous access may be impeded by dermal thickening. Intra-arterial catheterization for blood pressure monitoring introduces the same concerns as in patients with Raynaud's phenomenon. Cardiac evaluation may provide evidence of pulmonary hypertension. Because of chronic systemic hypertension and vasomotor instability, patients with scleroderma may have a contracted intravascular volume. This may become manifest as hypotension during induction of anesthesia when anesthetic drugs with vasodilating properties exert their effects. Hypotonia of the lower esophageal sphincter puts patients at risk of regurgitation and pulmonary aspiration. Efforts to increase gastric fluid pH with antacids or H_2-receptor antagonists before induction of anesthesia are recommended.

443

Intraoperatively, decreased pulmonary compliance may require higher airway pressures to ensure adequate ventilation. Supplemental oxygen is indicated in view of the impaired diffusion capacity and vulnerability to the development of arterial hypoxemia. Events known to increase pulmonary vascular resistance, such as respiratory acidosis and arterial hypoxemia, must be prevented. These patients may be particularly sensitive to the respiratory depressant effects of opioids, and a period of postoperative ventilatory support may be required in patients with severe pulmonary disease.

The degree of renal dysfunction must be considered when selecting anesthetic drugs dependent on renal elimination. Regional anesthesia may be technically difficult because of the skin and joint changes that accompany scleroderma. Attractive features of regional anesthesia include peripheral vasodilation and postoperative analgesia. Measures to minimize peripheral vasoconstriction include maintenance of the operating room temperature above 21°C and administration of warmed intravenous fluids. The eyes should be protected to prevent corneal abrasions.

PSEUDOXANTHOMA ELASTICUM

Pseudoxanthoma elasticum is a rare hereditary disorder of elastic tissue. Elastic fibers degenerate and calcify with time. The most striking feature of this condition, and often the basis for the diagnosis, is the appearance of angioid streaks in the retina. Substantial loss of visual acuity may result from these ocular changes. Additional visual impairment may occur when vascular changes predispose to vitreous hemorrhage. Skin changes, consisting of yellowish, rectangular, elevated xanthoma-like lesions, primarily in the neck, axilla, and inguinal regions, are among the earliest clinical features. Interestingly, some tissues rich in elastic fibers, such as the lungs, aorta, palms, and soles, are not affected by this disease process.

Gastrointestinal hemorrhage is a frequent occurrence. Degenerative changes in the arteries supplying the gastrointestinal tract are thought to prevent vasoconstriction of these blood vessels in response to mucosal injury. The incidence of hypertension and ischemic heart disease is increased in these patients. Endocardial calcification can involve the conduction system and predispose to cardiac dysrhythmias and sudden death. Involvement of cardiac valves is frequent. Calcification of peripheral arteries, particularly the radial and ulnar arteries, is common. Psychiatric disturbances often accompany this disease.

Management of anesthesia in the presence of pseudoxanthoma elasticum is based on an appreciation of the abnormalities associated with this disease. Cardiovascular derangements are probably the most important considerations. The increased incidence of ischemic heart disease is considered when establishing limits for acceptable changes in blood pressure and heart rate. Electrocardiographic monitoring is particularly important in view of the potential for

cardiac dysrhythmias. Noninvasive blood pressure monitoring devices are usually selected. Trauma to the mucosa of the upper gastrointestinal tract, as may be produced by a gastric tube or esophageal stethoscope, should be minimized. There are no specific recommendations regarding the choice of anesthetic drugs or techniques.

EHLERS-DANLOS SYNDROME

Ehlers-Danlos syndrome consists of a group of inherited connective tissue disorders (at least nine distinct types have been described) due to abnormal production of procollagen and collagen. It is estimated that 1 in 5000 people is affected by this syndrome. The only form of Ehlers-Danlos syndrome associated with an increased risk of death is the type IV (vascular) syndrome. This form may be complicated by rupture of large blood vessels or disruption of the bowel. (See Chapter 8, "Vascular Diseases.")

Signs and Symptoms

All forms of Ehlers-Danlos syndrome cause signs and symptoms of joint hypermobility, skin fragility or hyperelasticity, bruising and scarring, musculoskeletal discomfort, and susceptibility to osteoarthritis. The gastrointestinal tract, uterus, and vasculature are particularly well endowed with type III collagen, accounting for complications such as spontaneous rupture of the bowel, uterus, or major arteries. Premature labor and excessive bleeding at the time of delivery are common obstetric problems. Dilation of the trachea is often present, and the incidence of pneumothorax is increased. Mitral regurgitation and cardiac conduction abnormalities are occasionally seen. Patients may exhibit extensive ecchymoses with even minimal trauma though a specific coagulation defect has not been identified.

Management of Anesthesia

Management of anesthesia in patients with Ehlers-Danlos syndrome must consider the cardiovascular manifestations of this disease and the propensity for these patients to bleed excessively. Avoidance of intramuscular injections or instrumentation of the nose or esophagus is important in view of the bleeding tendency. Trauma during direct laryngoscopy must be minimized. Placement of an arterial or central venous catheter must be tempered by the realization that hematoma formation may be extensive. Extravasation of intravenous fluids due to a displaced venous cannula may go unnoticed because of the extreme laxity of the skin. Maintenance of low airway pressure during assisted or controlled mechanical ventilation seems prudent in view of the increased incidence of pneumothorax. There are no specific recommendations for the selection of drugs to provide anesthesia. Regional anesthesia is not recommended because of the tendency of these patients to bleed and form extensive hematomas. Surgical complications may include hemorrhage and postoperative wound dehiscence.

POLYMYOSITIS AND DERMATOMYOSITIS

Polymyositis and dermatomyositis are multisystem diseases of unknown etiology, manifesting as inflammatory myopathies. Dermatomyositis has characteristic skin changes in addition to muscle weakness. These cutaneous changes include discoloration of the upper eyelids, periorbital edema, a scaly erythematous malar rash, and symmetrical erythematous atrophic changes over the extensor surfaces of joints. Abnormal immune responses may be responsible for the slowly progressive skeletal muscle damage of dermatomyositis and polymyositis. The concept that altered cellular immunity causes polymyositis is supported by the fact that 10% to 20% of these patients have occult neoplasms.

Signs and Symptoms

Muscle weakness involves proximal skeletal muscle groups, especially the flexors of the neck, shoulders, and hips. Patients may have difficulty climbing stairs. Dysphagia, pulmonary aspiration, and pneumonia can result from paresis of pharyngeal and respiratory muscles. Diaphragmatic and intercostal muscle weakness may contribute to ventilatory insufficiency. Increased serum creatine kinase concentrations parallel the extent and rapidity of skeletal muscle destruction. These diseases do not affect the neuromuscular junction.

Heart block secondary to myocardial fibrosis or atrophy of the conduction system, left ventricular dysfunction, and myocarditis can occur. Polymyositis can also be associated with systemic lupus erythematosus, scleroderma, and rheumatoid arthritis. A widespread necrotizing vasculitis may be present with childhood forms of this disease.

Diagnosis

The diagnosis of polymyositis or dermatomyositis is considered when proximal skeletal muscle weakness, an increased serum creatine kinase concentration, and a characteristic skin rash are present. Electromyography may demonstrate the triad of spontaneous fibrillation potentials, decreased amplitude of voluntary contraction potentials, and repetitive potentials on needle insertion. Skeletal muscle biopsy supports the clinical diagnosis. Muscular dystrophy and myasthenia gravis can mimic polymyositis.

Treatment

Corticosteroids are the usual treatment for polymyositis. Immunosuppressive therapy with methotrexate, azathioprine, cyclophosphamide, mycophenolate, or cyclosporine may be effective when the response to corticosteroids is inadequate. Intravenous immunoglobulin may be useful in refractory cases.

Management of Anesthesia

Management of anesthesia must consider the vulnerability of patients with polymyositis to pulmonary aspiration. In view of the skeletal muscle weakness, there has been concern that these patients could display abnormal responses to muscle relaxants. However, responses to nondepolarizing muscle relaxants and succinylcholine are normal in patients with polymyositis.

SYSTEMIC LUPUS ERYTHEMATOSUS

Systemic lupus erythematosus (SLE) is a multisystem chronic inflammatory disease characterized by antinuclear antibody production. However, these antinuclear antibodies have not been documented to be directly involved in the pathogenesis of this disease. SLE typically occurs in young women and may affect as many as 1 in 1000 women. Stresses such as infection, pregnancy, or surgery may exacerbate SLE. The onset of SLE can also be drug induced with procainamide, hydralazine, isoniazid, D-penicillamine, and α-methyldopa being the most frequently associated drugs. Susceptibility to the development of SLE with hydralazine or procainamide is related to acetylator phenotype. The disease is more likely to develop in those who metabolize these drugs slowly (slow acetylators). The clinical presentation of drug-induced SLE is similar to the naturally occurring form of the disease, but the progression is usually slower and the symptoms are usually mild and consist of arthralgias, a maculopapular rash, fever, anemia, and leukopenia. The natural history of SLE is highly variable. The presence of nephritis and hypertension is associated with a worse prognosis. Pregnancy in patients with SLE, especially those with nephritis or hypertension, is associated with a substantial risk of disease exacerbation and poor fetal outcome.

Signs and Symptoms

Clinical manifestations of SLE can be categorized as articular or systemic. Polyarthritis and dermatitis are the most common signs and symptoms. Many of the clinical manifestations of SLE are the result of tissue damage from a vasculopathy mediated by immune complexes. Others, such as thrombocytopenia and the antiphospholipid syndrome, are the direct result of antibodies to cell surface molecules or serum components.

Diagnosis

Detection of antinuclear antibodies is a sensitive screening test for SLE. These antibodies occur in more than 95% of patients. The diagnosis of SLE is very likely if patients have three of four typical manifestations: antinuclear antibodies, characteristic rash, thrombocytopenia, serositis, or nephritis. However, presentation may not always be so clear and features such as arthralgias, vague central nervous system symptoms, rash, Raynaud's phenomenon, and/or a weakly positive antinuclear antibody test may make the diagnosis more difficult.

Articular Manifestations

Symmetrical arthritis involving the hands, wrists, elbows, knees, and ankles is common and occurs in 90% of patients. This arthritis is characteristically episodic and migratory, with pain that is out of proportion to the apparent degree of synovitis present. Lupus arthritis does not involve the spine. Another form of skeletal involvement is avascular necrosis, which most often involves the head or condyle of the femur.

Systemic Manifestations

Systemic manifestations of SLE appear in the central nervous system, heart, lungs, kidneys, liver, neuromuscular system, and skin.

Neurologic complications can affect any part of the central nervous system. Cognitive dysfunction occurs in approximately one third of individuals. Psychological changes ranging from depression and anxiety to psychosomatic complaints to signs of organic psychosis with deterioration of intellectual capacity are seen in more than half of patients. Most serious central nervous system manifestations appear to be the result of vasculitis. Fluid and electrolyte disturbances, fever, hypertension, uremia, infection, and drug-induced effects may contribute to central nervous system dysfunction. Atypical migraine headaches are common and may be accompanied by cortical visual disturbances.

Pericarditis resulting in chest pain, a friction rub, electrocardiographic changes, and pericardial effusion is the most common cardiac manifestation of SLE. Myocarditis may result in abnormalities of cardiac conduction. Congestive heart failure can develop with extensive cardiac involvement. Valvular abnormalities can be identified by echocardiography. These include verrucous endocarditis (Libman-Sacks endocarditis) that can involve the aortic and/or mitral valves.

Pulmonary involvement can manifest as lupus pneumonia characterized by diffuse pulmonary infiltrates, pleural effusion, dry cough, dyspnea, and arterial hypoxemia. Pulmonary function tests in these patients show restrictive pulmonary disease. Recurrent atelectasis can result in the "shrinking" or "vanishing" lung syndrome. This may be a result of diaphragmatic weakness or elevation due to phrenic neuropathy. Pulmonary angiitis with lung hemorrhage may complicate severe SLE. Pulmonary hypertension is present in some patients.

The most common renal abnormality is glomerulonephritis with proteinuria that can result in hypoalbuminemia. Hematuria is a frequent finding. The glomerular filtration rate can decrease dramatically and result in oliguric renal failure.

Liver function tests are abnormal in approximately 30% of patients. Severe liver disease is most likely due to infection or to undiagnosed autoimmune hepatitis or primary biliary cirrhosis.

Neuromuscular manifestations include myopathy with proximal skeletal muscle weakness and increased serum creatine kinase concentration. Tendinitis is common and can result in tendon rupture.

Hematologic abnormalities may be present. Thromboembolism associated with antiphospholipid antibodies can be an important cause of central nervous system dysfunction. Leukopenia, granulocyte dysfunction, decreased complement levels, and functional asplenia have been implicated in an increased risk of infection. Thrombocytopenia and hemolytic anemia are present in some patients. The presence of circulating anticoagulants is reflected in a prolonged activated partial thromboplastin time. Patients with circulating anticoagulants often manifest a false-positive test for syphilis.

Some patients with lupus have cutaneous manifestations. The classic butterfly-shaped malar rash occurs in approximately half of patients. This rash can be transient and is often exacerbated by sunlight. Discoid lesions on the face, scalp, and upper trunk develop in approximately 25% of patients with SLE but may occur in the absence of any other features of SLE. Alopecia is common.

Treatment

Treatment is determined by individual disease manifestations. Arthritis and serositis can often be controlled with aspirin or NSAIDs. Antimalarial drugs such as hydroxychloroquine and quinacrine are also effective in treating the dermatologic and arthritic manifestations of SLE. Patients should use sunscreens and avoid intense sun exposure. Thrombocytopenia and hemolytic anemia usually respond to corticosteroid therapy. Danazol, vincristine, cyclophosphamide, or splenectomy can be used if thrombocytopenia does not respond to glucocorticoid administration. In view of the increased susceptibility to infection, the risk/benefit ratio of splenectomy must be carefully considered.

Corticosteroids are the principal treatment for severe manifestations of SLE. Corticosteroids effectively suppress glomerulonephritis and cardiovascular abnormalities. However, corticosteroid therapy can be a major cause of morbidity in patients with SLE. Death during the course of SLE may be due to coronary atherosclerosis. The development and progression of coronary atherosclerosis is accelerated by treatment with corticosteroids. Immunosuppressive treatment with alternative drugs such as cyclophosphamide, azathioprine, or mycophenolate mofetil may be preferable to prolonged treatment with high-dose corticosteroids.

Management of Anesthesia

Management of anesthesia is influenced by the magnitude of organ system dysfunction and the drugs used to treat SLE. Laryngeal involvement, including mucosal ulceration, cricoarytenoid arthritis, and recurrent laryngeal nerve palsy, may be present in as many as one third of patients.

TUMORAL CALCINOSIS

Tumoral calcinosis is a rare genetic disorder that presents as metastatic calcifications adjacent to large joints. Joint motion is unaffected, but the masses may enlarge and interfere with skeletal muscle function. Treatment consists of complete excision of the masses. The principal anesthetic consideration is the rare involvement of the hyoid bone, hypothyroid ligament, or cervical intervertebral joints by this disease process, leading to difficult exposure of the glottic opening during direct laryngoscopy.

MUSCULAR DYSTROPHY

Muscular dystrophy is a group of hereditary diseases characterized by painless degeneration and atrophy of skeletal muscles. There are progressive, symmetrical skeletal muscle weakness and wasting but no evidence of skeletal muscle denervation; that is, sensation and reflexes are intact. Increased permeability of skeletal muscle membranes precedes clinical evidence of muscular dystrophy. In order of decreasing frequency, muscular dystrophy can be categorized as pseudohypertrophic (Duchenne's muscular dystrophy), limb-girdle, facioscapulohumeral (Landouzy-Dejerine), nemaline rod myopathy, and oculopharyngeal dystrophy.

Pseudohypertrophic Muscular Dystrophy (Duchenne's Muscular Dystrophy)

Pseudohypertrophic muscular dystrophy is the most common (3 per 10,000 births) and most severe form of childhood progressive muscular dystrophy. The disease is caused by an X-linked recessive gene and becomes apparent in 2- to 5-year-old boys. Initial symptoms include a waddling gait, frequent falling, and difficulty climbing stairs, and these reflect involvement of the proximal skeletal muscle groups of the pelvic girdle. Affected muscles become larger as a result of fatty infiltration, and this accounts for the designation of this disorder as pseudohypertrophic. There is progressive deterioration in skeletal muscle strength, and typically these boys are confined to a wheelchair by age 8 to 10. Kyphoscoliosis can develop. Skeletal muscle atrophy can predispose to long bone fractures. Mental retardation is often present. Serum creatine kinase concentrations are 20 to 100 times normal, even early in the disease, reflecting increased permeability of skeletal muscle membranes and skeletal muscle necrosis. Approximately 70% of the female carriers of this disease also exhibit increased serum creatine kinase concentrations. Skeletal muscle biopsy early in the course of the disease may demonstrate necrosis and phagocytosis of muscle fibers. Death usually occurs at 15 to 25 years of age due to congestive heart failure and/or pneumonia.

Cardiopulmonary Dysfunction

Degeneration of cardiac muscle invariably accompanies this muscular dystrophy. Characteristically, the electrocardiogram reveals tall R waves in V_1, deep Q waves in the limb leads, a short PR interval, and sinus tachycardia. Mitral regurgitation may occur due to papillary muscle dysfunction or decreased myocardial contractility.

Chronic weakness of the respiratory muscles and a decreased ability to cough result in loss of pulmonary reserve and accumulation of secretions. These abnormalities predispose to recurrent pneumonia. Respiratory insufficiency often remains covert because overall activity is so limited. As the disease progresses, kyphoscoliosis contributes to further restrictive lung disease. Sleep apnea may occur and may contribute to development of pulmonary hypertension. Approximately 30% of deaths among individuals with pseudohypertrophic muscular dystrophy are due to respiratory causes.

Management of Anesthesia

Children with pseudohypertrophic muscular dystrophy may require anesthesia for muscle biopsy or correction of orthopedic deformities. Preparation for anesthesia must take into consideration the implications of increased skeletal muscle membrane permeability and decreased cardiopulmonary reserve. Hypomotility of the gastrointestinal tract may delay gastric emptying and, in the presence of weak laryngeal reflexes, can increase the risk of pulmonary aspiration. Succinylcholine is contraindicated because of the risk of rhabdomyolysis, hyperkalemia, and/or cardiac arrest. Cardiac arrest may be due to hyperkalemia or to ventricular fibrillation. Indeed, ventricular fibrillation during induction of anesthesia that included succinylcholine has been observed in patients later discovered to have this form of muscular dystrophy. The response to nondepolarizing muscle relaxants is normal.

Rhabdomyolysis, with or without cardiac arrest, has been observed in association with administration of volatile anesthetics to these patients even in the absence of succinylcholine administration. Dantrolene should be available because there is an increased incidence of malignant hyperthermia in these patients. Malignant hyperthermia has been observed after even brief periods of halothane administration, although most cases have been triggered by succinylcholine or prolonged inhalation of halothane. Regional anesthesia avoids the unique risks of general anesthesia in these patients. During the postoperative period, neuraxial analgesia may facilitate chest physiotherapy.

Monitoring is directed at early detection of malignant hyperthermia (capnography, temperature) and cardiac depression. Postoperative pulmonary dysfunction must be anticipated and attempts made to facilitate clearance of secretions. Delayed pulmonary insufficiency may occur up to 36 hours postoperatively even though skeletal muscle strength has apparently returned to its preoperative levels.

Limb-Girdle Muscular Dystrophy

Limb-girdle muscular dystrophy is a slowly progressive but relatively benign disease. Onset occurs from the second to the fifth decade. Shoulder girdle or hip girdle muscles may be the only skeletal muscles involved.

Facioscapulohumeral Muscular Dystrophy

Facioscapulohumeral muscular dystrophy is characterized by a slowly progressive wasting of facial, pectoral, and shoulder girdle muscles that begins during adolescence. Eventually the lower limbs are also involved. Early symptoms include difficulty raising the arms above the head or difficulty smiling. There is no involvement of cardiac muscle, and serum creatine kinase concentration is seldom increased. Recovery from atracurium-induced neuromuscular blockade may be faster than normal. The progression of this muscular dystrophy is slow and a long life is likely.

Nemaline Rod Muscular Dystrophy

Nemaline rod muscular dystrophy is an autosomal dominant disease characterized by slowly progressive or nonprogressive symmetrical dystrophy of skeletal and smooth muscle.

The diagnosis is confirmed by skeletal muscle biopsy. Histologic examination will demonstrate the presence of rods between normal myofibrils.

Affected individuals experience delayed motor development, generalized skeletal muscle weakness, a decrease in muscle mass, hypotonia, and loss of deep tendon reflexes. There are typical dysmorphic features and an abnormal gait, but intelligence is usually normal. Affected infants may present with hypotonia, dysphagia, respiratory distress, and cyanosis. Micrognathia and dental malocclusion are common. Other skeletal deformities include kyphoscoliosis and pectus excavatum. Restrictive lung disease may result from the myopathy and/or scoliosis. Cardiac failure due to dilated cardiomyopathy has been described.

Tracheal intubation may be difficult due to anatomic abnormalities such as micrognathia and a high-arched palate. Awake fiberoptic endotracheal intubation may be prudent. The respiratory depressant effects of drugs may be exaggerated in these patients due to respiratory muscle weakness and chest wall abnormalities. Ventilation-perfusion mismatching is increased, and the ventilatory response to carbon dioxide may be blunted. Bulbar palsy associated with regurgitation and aspiration may further complicate anesthetic management.

The response to succinylcholine and nondepolarizing neuromuscular blockers is unpredictable. There is no conclusive evidence that administration of succinylcholine evokes excessive potassium release. Indeed, resistance to succinylcholine has been described in some patients. Malignant hyperthermia has not been reported in patients with nemaline rod myopathy. Myocardial depression may accompany administration of volatile anesthetics if the disease process involves the myocardium. Plans for regional anesthesia must consider the possible respiratory compromise that could accompany a high motor block. In addition, the exaggerated lumbar lordosis and/or kyphoscoliosis may make neuraxial anesthesia technically difficult.

Oculopharyngeal Dystrophy

Oculopharyngeal dystrophy is a rare variant of muscular dystrophy characterized by progressive dysphagia and ptosis. Although experience is limited, these patients may be at risk of aspiration during the perioperative period and their sensitivity to muscle relaxants may be increased.

Emery-Dreifuss Muscular Dystrophy

Emery-Dreifuss muscular dystrophy is an X-linked recessive disorder characterized by development of skeletal muscle contractures that precede the onset of skeletal muscle weakness. These contractures are typically in a humeroperoneal distribution. Mental retardation is not present, and respiratory function is maintained. Cardiac involvement may be life threatening and present as congestive heart failure, thromboembolism, or bradycardia. In contrast to other muscular dystrophies, female carriers of this disorder may experience cardiac impairment.

MYOTONIC DYSTROPHY

Myotonic dystrophy designates a group of hereditary degenerative diseases of skeletal muscle characterized by persistent contracture (myotonia) after voluntary contraction of a muscle or following electrical stimulation (**Table 18-2**). Peripheral nerves and the neuromuscular junction are not affected. Electromyographic findings are diagnostic and are characterized by prolonged discharges of repetitive muscle action potentials. This inability of skeletal muscle to relax after voluntary contraction or stimulation results from abnormal calcium metabolism. Intracellular adenosine triphosphatase fails to return calcium to the sarcoplasmic reticulum so unsequestered calcium remains available to produce sustained skeletal muscle contraction. Interestingly, general anesthesia, regional anesthesia, and neuromuscular blockers are not able to prevent or relieve this skeletal muscle contraction. Infiltration of contracted skeletal muscles with local anesthetic may induce relaxation. Quinine (300–600 mg IV) has also been reported to be effective in some cases. Increasing the ambient temperature of the operating room decreases the severity of myotonia and the incidence of postoperative shivering, which can precipitate contraction of skeletal muscles. Most myotonic patients survive to adulthood with little impairment, and it is common for them to conceal their symptoms so they may present for surgery without the underlying myotonia being appreciated.

Myotonia Dystrophica

Myotonia dystrophica is the most common (2.4–5.5 per 100,000 population) and most serious form of myotonic dystrophy affecting adults. It is inherited as an autosomal dominant trait, with the onset of symptoms during the second or third decade. Unlike other myotonic syndromes, myotonia dystrophica is a multisystem disease, although skeletal muscles are affected most. Death from pneumonia or heart failure often occurs by the sixth decade of life. This reflects progressive involvement of skeletal muscle, cardiac muscle, and smooth muscle. Perioperative morbidity and mortality rates are high due principally to cardiopulmonary complications.

Treatment is symptomatic and may include use of phenytoin. Quinine and procainamide also have antimyotonic properties but can worsen cardiac conduction abnormalities. These three drugs depress sodium influx into skeletal muscle cells and delay the return of membrane excitability.

TABLE 18-2 Classification of Myotonic Dystrophies
Myotonic dystrophy (myotonia atrophica, Steinert's disease)
Myotonia congenita (Thomsen's disease)
Paramyotonia congenita
Hyperkalemic periodic paralysis
Acid-maltase deficiency (Pompe's disease)
Schwartz-Jampel syndrome (chondrodystrophic myotonia)

Signs and Symptoms

Myotonia dystrophica usually manifests as facial weakness (expressionless facies), wasting and weakness of the sternocleidomastoid muscles, ptosis, dysarthria, dysphagia, and inability to relax the handgrip (myotonia). Other characteristic features include the triad of mental retardation, frontal baldness, and cataracts. Endocrine gland involvement may be indicated by gonadal atrophy, diabetes mellitus, hypothyroidism, and adrenal insufficiency. Delayed gastric emptying and intestinal pseudo-obstruction may be present. Central sleep apnea may occur and may account for the frequent presence of hypersomnolence. There is an increased incidence of cholelithiasis, especially in men. Exacerbation of symptoms during pregnancy is common, and uterine atony and retained placenta often complicate vaginal delivery.

Cardiac dysrhythmias and conduction abnormalities presumably reflect myocardial involvement by the myotonic process. First-degree atrioventricular heart block is common and is often present before the clinical onset of the disease. Up to 20% of patients have mitral valve prolapse, but systemic complications from this are rare. Reports of sudden death may reflect development of complete heart block. Pharyngeal and thoracic muscle weakness makes these patients vulnerable to pulmonary aspiration.

Management of Anesthesia

Preoperative evaluation and management of anesthesia in patients with myotonia dystrophica must consider the likelihood of cardiomyopathy, respiratory muscle weakness, and the potential for abnormal responses to anesthetic drugs. Even asymptomatic patients have some degree of cardiomyopathy and so the myocardial depression produced by volatile anesthetics may be exaggerated. Cardiac dysrhythmias may need treatment. Anesthesia and surgery could aggravate cardiac conduction problems by increasing vagal tone.

Succinylcholine should not be administered because prolonged skeletal muscle contraction can result. However, the response to nondepolarizing neuromuscular blocking drugs is normal. Theoretically, reversal of neuromuscular blockade could precipitate skeletal muscle contraction, but adverse responses do not predictably occur with neostigmine use. Careful titration of neuromuscular blockade and administration of short-acting nondepolarizing muscle relaxants may obviate the need for reversal of neuromuscular blockade.

Patients with myotonia dystrophica are sensitive to the respiratory depressant effects of barbiturates, opioids, benzodiazepines, and propofol. This is most likely due to drug-induced central respiratory depression acting in tandem with weak and/or atrophic respiratory muscles. In addition, hypersomnolence and central sleep apnea contribute to the increased sensitivity to respiratory depressant drugs.

Myotonic contraction during surgical manipulation and/or the use of electrocautery may interfere with surgical access. Drugs such as phenytoin and procainamide, which stabilize skeletal muscle membranes, may be helpful in this situation. High concentrations of volatile anesthetics can also abolish myotonic contractions but at the expense of myocardial depression. Maintenance of normothermia and avoidance of shivering are very important since cold may induce myotonia.

Myotonia Congenita

Myotonia congenita is transmitted as an autosomal dominant trait and becomes manifest at birth or during early childhood. Skeletal muscle involvement is widespread, but there is not usually involvement of other organ systems. Muscle hypertrophy and myotonia are present. The disease does not progress nor does it result in a decreased life expectancy. Patients with myotonia congenita respond to phenytoin, mexiletine, or quinine therapy. The response to succinylcholine administration is abnormal.

Paramyotonia Congenita

Paramyotonia congenita is a rare autosomal dominant disorder characterized by generalized myotonia that is recognized during early childhood; as with myotonia congenita, generalized muscle hypertrophy may occur. This myotonia is unusual because, in contrast to other myotonias, the skeletal muscle stiffness in paramyotonia is often exacerbated by exercise. In other myotonias sustained exercise improves myotonia, the so-called warm-up phenomenon. Cold markedly aggravates the myotonia and flaccid paralysis may be present after the muscles are warmed. Some patients develop muscle paralysis independent of myotonia. This could be related to the serum potassium concentration and may be the reason that there is some doubt whether paramyotonia congenita and hyperkalemic periodic paralysis are separate entities. The electromyogram may be normal at room temperature, but typical myotonic discharges become evident as muscles are cooled. Treatment is similar to that of myotonia congenita.

Schwartz-Jampel Syndrome

Schwartz-Jampel syndrome is a rare childhood disorder of progressive skeletal muscle stiffness, myotonia, and ocular, facial, and skeletal abnormalities including micrognathia. Tracheal intubation is predictably difficult. There is blepharospasm and tense puckering of the mouth. These children may be susceptible to malignant hyperthermia.

PERIODIC PARALYSIS

Periodic paralysis is a spectrum of diseases characterized by intermittent acute attacks of skeletal muscle weakness or paralysis (sparing only a few muscles such as the muscles of respiration) and associated with hypokalemia or hyperkalemia (**Table 18-3**). The hyperkalemic form is much rarer than the hypokalemic form. Attacks generally last for a few hours but may persist for days. Muscle strength is normal between attacks.

Causes

The exact defect with familial periodic paralysis is unknown, although mutations in calcium and sodium channels are associated with hypokalemic and hyperkalemic periodic

TABLE 18-3 Clinical Features of Familial Periodic Paralysis

Type	Serum Potassium Concentration during Symptoms (mEq/L)	Precipitating Factors	Other Features
Hypokalemic	< 3.0	Large carbohydrate meal, strenuous exercise Glucose infusion, stress, menstruation, pregnancy, anesthesia, hypothermia	Cardiac dysrhythmias Electrocardiographic signs of hypokalemia
Hyperkalemic	> 5.5	Exercise, potassium infusion, metabolic acidosis, hypothermia	Skeletal muscle weakness may be localized to tongue and eyelids

paralysis, respectively. It is recognized that the mechanism of this disease is not related to any abnormality at the neuromuscular junction but rather to loss of muscle membrane excitability. Skeletal muscle weakness provoked by a glucose-insulin infusion confirms the presence of *hypokalemic* familial periodic paralysis, and skeletal muscle weakness after oral administration of potassium confirms the presence of *hyperkalemic* familial periodic paralysis. Acetazolamide is recommended for the treatment of both forms of familial periodic paralysis. Acetazolamide produces a nonanion gap acidosis, which protects against hypokalemia, and promotes renal potassium excretion, and thus protects against hyperkalemia as well.

Management of Anesthesia

A principal goal of anesthesia is avoidance of any events that can precipitate skeletal muscle weakness. Hypothermia must be avoided in patients with periodic paralysis, regardless of the nature of the potassium sensitivity. In patients undergoing cardiac surgery, it may be necessary to maintain normothermia during cardiopulmonary bypass. Nondepolarizing muscle relaxants can be safely administered to patients with periodic paralysis.

Hypokalemic Periodic Paralysis

Preoperative considerations include carbohydrate balance, correction of electrolyte abnormalities, and avoidance of events known to trigger hypokalemic attacks (psychological stress, cold, carbohydrate loads). Large carbohydrate meals can trigger hypokalemic episodes and should be avoided during the 24 hours preceding surgery. Glucose-containing solutions and drugs known to cause intracellular shifts of potassium such as β-adrenergic agonists must also be avoided. Mannitol can be administered in lieu of a potassium-wasting diuretic should the operative procedure require diuresis. Frequent perioperative monitoring (every 30–60 minutes) of serum potassium concentration is useful, and aggressive intervention (potassium chloride infused at a rate of up to 40 mEq/hr) to increase the serum potassium concentration may occasionally be needed. Hypokalemia may precede the onset of muscle weakness by several hours, so timely potassium supplementation may help avoid muscle weakness. Shorter acting neuromuscular blockers are preferable if skeletal muscle relaxation is required for the surgery.

Succinylcholine with its ability to increase serum potassium concentration transiently is acceptable in these patients. Regional anesthesia has been safely used.

Hyperkalemic Periodic Paralysis

Management of anesthesia in patients with hyperkalemic periodic paralysis includes preoperative potassium depletion with diuretics, prevention of carbohydrate depletion by administration of glucose-containing solutions, and avoidance of potassium-containing solutions and potassium-releasing drugs such as succinylcholine. Frequent monitoring of serum potassium concentration is indicated as is the availability of calcium for intravenous administration should signs of hyperkalemia appear on the electrocardiogram.

MYASTHENIA GRAVIS

Myasthenia gravis is a chronic autoimmune disorder caused by a decrease in functional acetylcholine receptors at the neuromuscular junction due to their destruction or inactivation by circulating antibodies (**Fig. 18-1**). Seventy percent to 80% of functional acetylcholine receptors can be lost, and this accounts for the weakness and easy fatigability of these patients and their marked sensitivity to nondepolarizing muscle relaxants. Indeed, the hallmarks of the disease are weakness and rapid exhaustion of voluntary muscles with repetitive use followed by partial recovery with rest. Skeletal muscles innervated by cranial nerves (ocular, pharyngeal, and laryngeal muscles) are especially vulnerable, as reflected by the appearance of ptosis, diplopia, and dysphagia, which are often the initial symptoms of the disease. Myasthenia gravis is not a rare disease. It has a prevalence of 1 in 7500. Women 20 to 30 years of age are most often affected, whereas men are often older than 60 years of age when their disease presents. Receptor-binding antibodies are present in more than 80% of patients with myasthenia gravis. The origin of these antibodies is unknown, but a relationship to the thymus gland is suggested by the association of myasthenia gravis with thymus gland abnormalities. For example, thymic hyperplasia is present in more than 70% of patients with myasthenia gravis, and 10% to 15% of these patients have thymomas. Other conditions that cause weakness of the cranial and somatic musculature must be considered in the differential diagnosis of myasthenia gravis (**Table 18-4**).

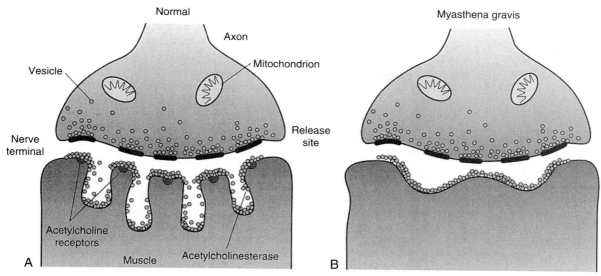

Figure 18-1 • Normal (**A**) and myasthenic (**B**) neuromuscular junctions. Compared with normal neuromuscular junctions, myasthenic neuromuscular junctions have fewer acetylcholine receptors, simplified synaptic folds, and widened synaptic spaces. *(From Drachman DB: Myasthenia gravis. N Engl J Med 1994;330:1797–1810. Copyright © 1994 Massachusetts Medical Society. All rights reserved.)*

Classification

Myasthenia gravis is classified based on the skeletal muscles involved and the severity of symptoms. Type I is limited to involvement of the extraocular muscles. Approximately 10% of patients show signs and symptoms confined to the extraocular muscles and are considered to have ocular myasthenia gravis. Patients in whom the disease has been confined to the ocular muscles for more than 3 years are unlikely to experience any progression in their disease. Type IIA is a slowly progressive, mild form of skeletal muscle weakness that spares the muscles of respiration. The response to anticholinesterase drugs and corticosteroids is good in these patients. Type IIB is a more rapidly progressive, severe form of skeletal muscle weakness. The response to drug therapy is not as good, and the muscles of respiration may be involved. Type III is characterized by acute onset and rapid deterioration of skeletal muscle strength within 6 months. It is associated with a high mortality

TABLE 18-4 Differential Diagnosis of Myasthenia Gravis		
Condition	**Symptoms and Characteristics**	**Comments**
Congenital myasthenic syndromes	Rare, early onset, not autoimmune	Electrophysiologic and immunocytochemical tests required for diagnosis
Drug-induced myasthenia gravis Penicillamine Nondepolarizing muscle relaxants Aminoglycosides Procainamide	Triggers autoimmune myasthenia gravis Increased sensitivity	Recovery within weeks of discontinuing the drug Recovery after drug discontinuation
Eaton-Lambert syndrome	Small cell lung cancer, fatigue	Incremental response on repetitive nerve stimulation, antibodies to calcium channels
Hyperthyroidism	Exacerbation of myasthenia gravis	Thyroid function abnormal
Graves' disease	Diplopia, exophthalmos	Thyroid-stimulating immunoglobulin present
Botulism	Generalized weakness, ophthalmoplegia	Incremental response on repetitive nerve stimulation, mydriasis
Progressive external ophthalmoplegia	Ptosis, diplopia, generalized weakness in some cases	Mitochondrial abnormalities
Intracranial mass compressing cranial nerves	Ophthalmoplegia cranial nerve weakness	Abnormalities on computed tomography or magnetic resonance imaging

Adapted from Drachman DB: Myasthenia gravis. N Engl J Med 1994;330:1797–1810. Copyright © 1994 Massachusetts Medical Society. All rights reserved.

rate. Type IV is a severe form of skeletal muscle weakness that results from progression of type I or II myasthenia.

Signs and Symptoms

The clinical course of myasthenia gravis is marked by periods of exacerbation and remission. Muscle strength may be normal in well-rested patients, but weakness occurs promptly with exercise. Ptosis and diplopia resulting from extraocular muscle weakness are the most common initial complaints. Weakness of pharyngeal and laryngeal muscles results in dysphagia, dysarthria, and difficulty handling saliva. Patients with myasthenia gravis are at high risk of pulmonary aspiration of gastric contents. Arm, leg, or trunk weakness can occur in any combination and is usually asymmetrical. Muscle atrophy does not occur. Myocarditis can result in atrial fibrillation, heart block, or cardiomyopathy. Other autoimmune diseases may occur in association with myasthenia gravis. For example, hyperthyroidism is present in approximately 10% of patients with myasthenia gravis. Rheumatoid arthritis, SLE, and pernicious anemia occur more commonly in patients with myasthenia than in those without myasthenia. Approximately 15% of neonates born to mothers with myasthenia gravis demonstrate transient (2–4 weeks) skeletal muscle weakness. Infection, electrolyte abnormalities, pregnancy, emotional stress, and surgery may precipitate or exacerbate muscle weakness. Antibiotics, especially the aminoglycosides, can aggravate the muscle weakness. Isolated respiratory failure may occasionally be the presenting manifestation of myasthenia gravis.

Treatment

Treatment modalities for myasthenia gravis include enhancing neuromuscular transmission with anticholinesterase drugs, thymectomy, immunosuppression, and short-term immunotherapy, including plasmapheresis and administration of immunoglobulin.

Anticholinesterase Drugs

Anticholinesterase drugs are the first line of treatment for myasthenia gravis. These drugs are effective because they inhibit the enzyme responsible for the hydrolysis of acetylcholine and thus increase the amount of neurotransmitter available at the neuromuscular junction. Pyridostigmine is the most widely used anticholinesterase drug for this purpose. The onset of effect occurs in 30 minutes, and peak effect is achieved in approximately 2 hours. Oral pyridostigmine lasts longer (3–6 hours) and produces fewer side effects than neostigmine. Pyridostigmine dosing is tailored to response, but the maximal useful dose of pyridostigmine rarely exceeds 120 mg every 3 hours. Higher doses may actually induce more muscle weakness, the so-called cholinergic crisis. The presence of significant muscarinic side effects (salivation, miosis, bradycardia) plus accentuated muscle weakness after administration of edrophonium (1–2 mg IV) confirms the diagnosis of a cholinergic crisis. Although anticholinesterase drugs benefit most patients, the improvements may be incomplete and may wane after weeks or months of treatment.

Thymectomy

Thymectomy is intended to induce remission or at least allow for the doses of immunosuppressive medications to be reduced. Patients with generalized myasthenia gravis are candidates for thymectomy. Preoperative preparation should optimize strength and respiratory function. Immunosuppressive drugs should be avoided if possible because they can increase the risk of perioperative infection. If the vital capacity is less than 2 L, plasmapheresis can be performed before surgery to improve the likelihood of adequate spontaneous respiration during the postoperative period. A surgical approach via median sternotomy optimizes visualization and removal of all thymic tissue. Alternatively, mediastinoscopy through a cervical incision has been advocated because it is associated with a smaller incision and less postoperative pain. The use of neuraxial analgesia minimizes postoperative pain and thus improves postoperative ventilation. The need for anticholinesterase medication may be decreased for a few days postoperatively, but the full benefit of thymectomy is often delayed for months after surgery. The mechanism by which thymectomy produces improvement is uncertain, although acetylcholine receptor antibody levels usually decrease following thymectomy.

Immunosuppressive Therapy

Immunosuppressive therapy (corticosteroids, azathioprine, cyclosporine, mycophenolate) is indicated when skeletal muscle weakness is not adequately controlled by anticholinesterase drugs. Corticosteroids are the most commonly used and most consistently effective immunosuppressive drugs for the treatment of myasthenia gravis. They are also associated with the greatest likelihood of adverse effects.

Short-Term Immunotherapy

Plasmapheresis removes antibodies from the circulation and produces short-term clinical improvement in patients with myasthenia gravis who are experiencing myasthenic crises or are being prepared for thymectomy. The beneficial effects of plasmapheresis are transient, and repeated treatment introduces the risk of infection, hypotension, and pulmonary embolism. The indications for administration of immunoglobulin are the same as for plasmapheresis. The effect is temporary, and this treatment has no effect on circulating concentrations of acetylcholine receptor antibodies.

Management of Anesthesia
Preoperative Preparation

Patients with myasthenia gravis often require ventilatory support after surgery. Therefore, it is important to advise these patients during the preoperative interview that they may be intubated and ventilated when they awaken. Criteria that correlate with the need for mechanical ventilation during the postoperative period following transsternal thymectomy include disease duration of longer than 6 years, the presence of chronic obstructive pulmonary disease unrelated to myasthenia gravis, a daily dose of pyridostigmine higher than

750 mg, and a vital capacity less than 2.9 L. These criteria are less predictive of the need for ventilatory support following transcervical thymectomy, indicating that this less invasive surgical approach produces less respiratory depression.

Muscle Relaxants

The acetylcholine receptor-binding antibodies of myasthenia gravis decrease the number of functional acetylcholine receptors, and this results in an increased sensitivity to non-depolarizing muscle relaxants. The balance between active and nonfunctional acetylcholine receptors modulates the sensitivity to nondepolarizing muscle relaxants. The initial muscle relaxant dose should be titrated according to response at the neuromuscular junction as monitored with a peripheral nerve stimulator. Monitoring these responses at the orbicularis oculi muscle may *overestimate* the degree of neuromuscular blockade but may help to avoid unrecognized persistent neuromuscular blockade in these patients.

It is possible that drugs used to treat myasthenia gravis can influence the response to muscle relaxants independent of the disease process. For example, anticholinesterase drugs inhibit not only true cholinesterase but also impair plasma pseudo-cholinesterase activity, introducing the possibility of a prolonged response to succinylcholine. They could also antagonize the effects of nondepolarizing muscle relaxants. However, neither of these effects is seen clinically. Corticosteroid therapy does not alter the dose requirements for succinylcholine but has been reported to produce resistance to the neuromuscular blocking effects of steroidal muscle relaxants such as vecuronium.

Measurement of neuromuscular function in patients with myasthenia gravis treated with pyridostigmine demonstrates *resistance* to the effects of succinylcholine. The ED_{95} is approximately 2.6 times normal (**Fig. 18-2**). Because the dose of succinylcholine commonly administered to normal patients (1.0–1.5 mg/kg) represents three to five times the ED_{95}, it is

likely that adequate intubating conditions can be achieved in patients with myasthenia gravis using these doses. The mechanism for the resistance to succinylcholine is unknown, but the decreased number of acetylcholine receptors at the post-synaptic neuromuscular junction may play a role.

In contrast to the resistance to succinylcholine, patients with myasthenia gravis exhibit marked sensitivity to nondepolarizing muscle relaxants. Even the small doses of nondepolarizing muscle relaxant intended to block succinylcholine-induced fasciculations can produce profound skeletal muscle weakness in some patients with myasthenia gravis. In patients with mild to moderate myasthenia gravis, the potency of atracurium and vecuronium is increased twofold compared to the response in normal patients (**Fig. 18-3**). Despite the increase in potency, the duration of action of intermediate-acting muscle relaxants is short enough that skeletal muscle paralysis can be achieved as the surgery requires yet these drugs can be predictably reversed at the conclusion of surgery.

Induction of Anesthesia

Induction of anesthesia with a short-acting intravenous anesthetic is acceptable for patients with myasthenia gravis. However, the respiratory depressant effects of these drugs may be accentuated. Tracheal intubation can often be accomplished without neuromuscular blockers because of intrinsic muscle weakness and the relaxant effect of volatile anesthetics on skeletal muscle.

Maintenance of Anesthesia

Maintenance of anesthesia is often provided with a volatile anesthetic with or without nitrous oxide. Volatile anesthetics can decrease the dose or even eliminate the need for muscle relaxants. Should administration of a nondepolarizing neuromuscular blocker be necessary, the initial dose should be decreased by one half to two thirds and the response monitored with a peripheral nerve stimulator. The relatively short

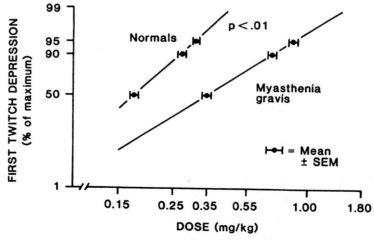

Figure 18-2 • Dose-response curves for succinylcholine in patients with myasthenia gravis are shifted to the right of curves for normal patients indicating that myasthenic patients are resistant to the neuromuscular blocking effects of this muscle relaxant. (*From Eisenkraft JB, Book WJ, Mann SM, et al: Resistance to succinylcholine in myasthenia gravis: A dose-response study. Anesthesiology 1988;69:760–763, with permission.*)

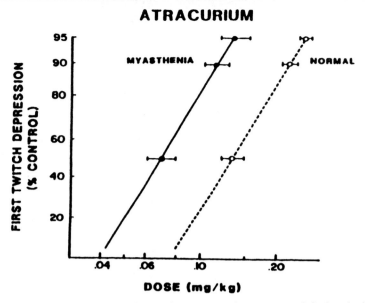

ATRACURIUM

Figure 18-3 • Dose-response curves for atracurium in patients with myasthenia gravis. The curves are shifted to the left of the curves for normal patients, indicating that myasthenic patients are sensitive to the neuromuscular blocking effects of this muscle relaxant and presumably other nondepolarizing muscle relaxants as well. *(From Smith CE, Donati F, Bevan DR: Cumulative dose-response curves for atracurium in patients with myasthenia gravis. Can J Anaesth 1989;36:402–406, with permission.)*

duration of action of short- and intermediate-acting muscle relaxants is a desirable characteristic in this patient group. The respiratory effects of opioids, which can linger into the post-operative period, detract from their use for maintenance of anesthesia.

Postoperative Care

At the conclusion of surgery, it is important to leave the endotracheal tube in place until clear evidence of the ability to maintain respiration is present. Skeletal muscle strength often seems adequate during the early postoperative period but may deteriorate a few hours later. The need for mechanical ventilation during the postoperative period should be anticipated in those patients meeting the criteria known to correlate with inadequate ventilation after surgery (see "Preoperative Preparation").

MYASTHENIC SYNDROME

Myasthenic syndrome (Eaton-Lambert syndrome) is a disorder of neuromuscular transmission that resembles myasthenia gravis (**Table 18-5**). This syndrome of skeletal muscle weakness, originally described in patients with small-cell carcinoma of the lung, has subsequently been described in patients without cancer. Myasthenic syndrome is an acquired autoimmune disease with immunoglobulin G antibodies to voltage-sensitive calcium channels that produces a deficiency of these channels at the motor nerve terminal. This deficiency restricts calcium entry when the terminal is depolarized. Anticholinesterase drugs effective in the treatment of myasthenia gravis do *not* produce an improvement in patients with myasthenic syndrome.

TABLE 18-5	Comparison of Myasthenic Syndrome and Myasthenia Gravis	
Parameter	**Myasthenic Syndrome**	**Myasthenia Gravis**
Manifestations	Proximal limb weakness (legs more than arms), exercise improves strength, muscle pain common, reflexes absent or decreased	Extraocular, bulbar, and facial muscle weakness, fatigue with exercise; muscle pain uncommon; reflexes normal
Gender	Males more often than females	Females more often than males
Co-existing pathology	Small-cell lung cancer	Thymoma
Response to muscle relaxants	Sensitive to succinylcholine and nondepolarizing muscle relaxants Poor response to anticholinesterases	Resistant to succinylcholine, sensitive to nondepolarizing muscle relaxants Good response to anticholinesterases

Patients with myasthenic syndrome are sensitive to the effects of both succinylcholine and nondepolarizing muscle relaxants. Antagonism of neuromuscular blockade with anticholinesterase drugs may be inadequate. The potential presence of myasthenic syndrome and the need to decrease the doses of muscle relaxants should be considered in patients undergoing bronchoscopy, mediastinoscopy, or exploratory thoracotomy for suspected lung cancer.

RHEUMATOID ARTHRITIS

Rheumatoid arthritis, the most common chronic inflammatory arthritis, affects approximately 1% of adults. The incidence is two to three times higher in women than in men. The etiology of rheumatoid arthritis is unknown, but it is suspected to be a complex interaction between genetic and environmental factors and the immune system. The disease is characterized by symmetrical polyarthropathy and significant systemic involvement (**Table 18-6**). Involvement of the proximal interphalangeal and metacarpophalangeal joints of the hands and feet helps distinguish rheumatoid arthritis from osteoarthritis, which typically affects weight-bearing joints and distal interphalangeal joints. The course of the disease is characterized by exacerbations and remissions. Rheumatoid nodules are typically present at pressure points, particularly below the elbows. Rheumatoid factor is an immunoglobulin G antibody that is present in the serum of up to 90% of patients with rheumatoid arthritis but is not present with osteoarthritis. However, the presence of rheumatoid factor is not specific to rheumatoid arthritis. It is also present in patients with viral hepatitis, SLE, bacterial endocarditis, sarcoidosis, and Sjögren's syndrome.

Signs and Symptoms

The onset of rheumatoid arthritis in adults may be acute, involving single or multiple joints, or insidious with symptoms such as fatigue, anorexia, and weakness preceding overt arthritis. In some patients, the onset of rheumatoid arthritis coincides with trauma, a surgical procedure, childbirth, or exposure to extremes of temperature.

Joint Involvement

Morning stiffness is a hallmark of rheumatoid arthritis. Several joints, often the hands, wrists, knees, and feet, are affected in a symmetrical distribution. Fusiform swelling is typical when there is involvement of the proximal interphalangeal joints. These joints are swollen and painful and remain stiff for several hours after the start of daily activity. Synovitis of the temporomandibular joint can produce marked limitation of mandibular motion. When the disease is progressive and unremitting, nearly every joint is affected except for the thoracic and lumbosacral spine.

Cervical spine involvement is frequent and may result in pain and neurologic complications. The most significant abnormality of the cervical spine is atlantoaxial subluxation and consequent separation of the atlanto-odontoid articulation. This deformity is best seen on a lateral radiograph of the neck. With the neck flexed, the separation of the anterior margin of the odontoid process from the posterior margin of the anterior arch of the atlas can exceed 3 mm. When this separation is severe, the odontoid process could protrude into the foramen magnum and exert pressure on the spinal cord or impair blood flow through the vertebral arteries. Since the odontoid process is often eroded, complications on the spinal cord may be minimized. Subluxation of other cervical vertebrae can also occur. Magnetic resonance imaging has confirmed the frequency of cervical spine involvement in rheumatoid arthritis.

Cricoarytenoid arthritis is common in patients with generalized rheumatoid arthritis. With acute cricoarytenoid arthritis, hoarseness, pain on swallowing, dyspnea, and stridor may accompany tenderness over the larynx. Redness and swelling of the arytenoids can be seen on direct laryngoscopy. With chronic cricoarytenoid arthritis, patients may be asymptomatic or manifest variable degrees of hoarseness,

TABLE 18-6 Comparison of Rheumatoid Arthritis and Ankylosing Spondylitis		
Parameter	**Rheumatoid Arthritis**	**Ankylosing Spondylitis**
Family history	Rare	Common
Gender	Female (30–50 years old)	Male (20–30 years old)
Joint involvement	Symmetrical polyarthropathy	Asymmetrical oligoarthropathy
Sacroiliac involvement	No	Yes
Vertebral involvement	Cervical	Total (ascending)
Cardiac changes	Pericardial effusion, aortic regurgitation, cardiac conduction abnormalities, cardiac valve fibrosis, coronary artery arteritis	Cardiomegaly, aortic regurgitation, cardiac conduction abnormalities
Pulmonary changes	Pulmonary fibrosis, pleural effusion	Pulmonary fibrosis
Eyes	Keratoconjunctivitis sicca	Conjunctivitis, uveitis
Rheumatoid factor	Positive	Negative
HLA-B27	Negative	Positive

dyspnea, and upper airway obstruction. Cricoarytenoid arthritis may make endotracheal intubation difficult.

Osteoporosis is ubiquitous in patients with rheumatoid arthritis.

Systemic Involvement

Many of the systemic manifestations of rheumatoid arthritis are a result of small and medium-sized artery vasculitis due to deposition of immune complexes. Systemic involvement is usually most obvious in patients with severe articular disease.

In the cardiovascular system, rheumatoid arthritis may manifest as pericarditis, myocarditis, coronary artery arteritis, accelerated coronary atherosclerosis, cardiac valve fibrosis, and formation of rheumatoid nodules in the cardiac conduction system. Aortitis with dilation of the aortic root may result in aortic regurgitation. Pericardial thickening or effusion is present in approximately one third of patients.

Vasculitis in small synovial blood vessels is an early finding in patients with rheumatoid arthritis, but more widespread vascular inflammation may occur, especially in older men. Patients may demonstrate a neuropathy (mononeuritis multiplex), skin ulcerations, and purpura. Neuropathy is presumed to be caused by deposition of immune complexes in the vasa nervorum. Manifestations of visceral ischemia, including bowel perforation, myocardial infarction, and cerebral infarction, are possible.

The most common pulmonary manifestation of rheumatoid arthritis is pleural effusion. Many of these effusions are small and asymptomatic. Rheumatoid nodules can develop in the pulmonary parenchyma and on pleural surfaces and may mimic tuberculosis or cancer on chest radiography. Progressive pulmonary fibrosis, associated with cough, dyspnea, and diffuse honeycomb changes on chest radiography, is rare. Costochondral involvement may affect chest wall motion and produce restrictive lung changes with decreased lung volumes and vital capacity. This may result in ventilation-perfusion mismatch and decreased arterial oxygenation.

Neuromuscular involvement can be seen with loss of strength in skeletal muscles adjacent to joints with active synovitis. Peripheral neuropathies due to nerve compression, carpal tunnel syndrome, and tarsal tunnel syndrome are common. Cervical nerve root compression is unlikely to accompany involvement of the cervical vertebrae by rheumatoid arthritis.

The most common hematologic abnormality in patients with rheumatoid arthritis is anemia of chronic disease, the severity of which usually parallels the severity of the rheumatoid arthritis. Felty's syndrome is rheumatoid arthritis with splenomegaly and leukopenia. Keratoconjunctivitis sicca (dry eyes) occurs in approximately 10% of patients with rheumatoid arthritis. The cause is lack of tear formation due to impaired lacrimal gland function. A similar process may involve the salivary glands, resulting in xerostomia (dry mouth). These are both manifestations of Sjögren's syndrome.

Mild abnormalities of liver function are common in patients with rheumatoid arthritis. Renal dysfunction may be secondary to amyloidosis or vasculitis or drug therapy.

Treatment

Treatment of rheumatoid arthritis includes efforts to relieve pain, preserve joint function and strength, prevent deformities, and attenuate systemic complications. These objectives may be met by a combination of drugs, physical therapy, occupational therapy, and orthopedic surgery.

Drug Therapy

Drug therapy is used to provide analgesia, control inflammation, and produce immunosuppression.

Nonsteroidal Anti-inflammatory Drugs NSAIDs are important for symptomatic relief of rheumatoid arthritis but have little role in changing the underlying disease process. They should not be used without the concomitant use of disease-modifying antirheumatic drugs (DMARDs). Aspirin remains an important drug for the initial treatment of rheumatoid arthritis, but its use has decreased because of the availability of newer NSAIDs. These drugs decrease swelling in affected joints and relieve stiffness, but associated gastrointestinal irritation and inhibition of platelet cyclooxygenase (COX) may necessitate discontinuation of these drugs. Selective COX-2 inhibitors are as effective as COX-1 inhibitors in producing analgesia and reducing inflammation, but they evoke fewer gastrointestinal side effects and do not interfere with platelet function. It appears, however, that some COX-2 inhibitors increase the risk of cardiac ischemic events. Both COX-1 and COX-2 drugs can adversely affect renal blood flow and glomerular filtration rate.

Corticosteroids Corticosteroids are potent anti-inflammatory drugs that decrease joint swelling, pain, and morning stiffness in patients with rheumatoid arthritis. However, the doses of systemic corticosteroids necessary to maintain desirable effects are often associated with significant long-term side effects including osteoporosis, osteonecrosis, increased susceptibility to infection, myopathy, hyperglycemia, and poor wound healing. Intra-articular corticosteroids produce beneficial effects lasting on average approximately 3 months, but repeated injections may result in cartilage destruction and osteonecrosis.

Corticosteroids are indicated as "bridge therapy," that is, to decrease inflammation rapidly while DMARDs are starting to work in controlling the disease process. Prednisone doses greater than 10 mg/day are rarely indicated for joint disease, but higher doses may be needed to treat other manifestations of rheumatoid arthritis, especially vasculitis

Disease-Modifying Antirheumatic Drugs DMARDs are a group of drugs that have the potential to modify or change the course of rheumatoid arthritis. They can slow or halt the progression of the disease. Included in this group are methotrexate, sulfasalazine, leflunomide, antimalarials, D-penicillamine, azathioprine, and minocycline. These drugs generally take 2 to 6 months to achieve their effects. Patients who fail to respond to one drug may respond to another.

Methotrexate is the preferred DMARD in the treatment of rheumatoid arthritis. It is given in a once-a-week dosing regimen. Methotrexate is primarily anti-inflammatory. Monitoring hematologic parameters and liver function tests are necessary in individuals being treated with methotrexate because of the risks of bone marrow suppression and cirrhosis. Daily folic acid therapy can decrease methotrexate toxicities.

It appears that cytokines, especially tumor necrosis factor α and interleukin-1, play a central role in the pathogenesis of rheumatoid arthritis. Interference with the function of tumor necrosis factor either by drug-induced receptor blockade or by monoclonal antibodies is effective in treating rheumatoid arthritis. Drugs such as infliximab (Remicade) and etanercept (Enbrel), tumor necrosis factor inhibitors, are quite effective in treating rheumatoid arthritis and act more rapidly than other DMARDs. Long-term toxicities such as infection (tuberculosis) and demyelinating syndromes are a concern. Anakinra, an interleukin-1 receptor antagonist, is effective against the signs and symptoms of rheumatoid arthritis, but its onset of action is slower and its overall effect is less than that of the tumor necrosis factor α inhibitors.

Gold, the oldest DMARD, is extremely effective therapy for some patients with rheumatoid arthritis, but it is not commonly used because of its frequent toxicities.

Surgery

Indications for surgery in patients with rheumatoid arthritis include intractable pain, impairment of joint function, and the need for joint stabilization. Eroded cartilage, ruptured ligaments, and progressive bone destruction can lead to impairment that is amenable only to surgical treatment. Arthroscopic surgery is used to remove cartilaginous fragments and to perform partial synovectomy. When joints are destroyed by the disease process, total replacement of large and small joints can be considered.

Management of Anesthesia

The multiorgan involvement and side effects of drugs used to treat rheumatoid arthritis must be appreciated when planning anesthetic management. Preoperatively, patients should be evaluated for airway involvement by this disease process. Compromise of the airway may occur at the cervical spine, temporomandibular joints, and cricoarytenoid joints. Flexion deformity of the cervical spine may make it difficult if not impossible to straighten the neck. Atlantoaxial subluxation may be present. Radiographic demonstration that the distance from the anterior arch of the atlas to the odontoid process exceeds 3 mm confirms the presence of atlantoaxial subluxation. This abnormality is important because the displaced odontoid process can compress the cervical spinal cord or medulla or occlude the vertebral arteries. When atlantoaxial subluxation is present, care must be taken to minimize movement of the head and neck during direct laryngoscopy to avoid further displacement of the odontoid process and damage to the spinal cord. It is helpful to evaluate preoperatively whether there is interference with vertebral artery blood flow during flexion, extension, or rotation of the head and cervical spine. This can be accomplished by having the awake patient demonstrate head movement or positioning that can be tolerated without discomfort or other symptoms.

Limitation of temporomandibular joint movement must be recognized before induction of anesthesia. The combination of limited mobility of these joints plus cervical spine stiffness may make visualizing the glottic opening by direct laryngoscopy difficult or impossible. Awake, sedated endotracheal intubation by fiberoptic laryngoscopy may be indicated if preoperative evaluation suggests that direct visualization of the glottic opening will be difficult. Involvement of the cricoarytenoid joints by arthritic changes is suggested by the preoperative presence of hoarseness or stridor or by the observation of erythema or edema of the vocal cords during direct laryngoscopy. Diminished movement of these joints can result in narrowing of the glottic opening and interference with translaryngeal passage of the tracheal tube or an increased risk of cricoarytenoid joint dislocation.

Preoperative pulmonary function studies plus measurement of arterial blood gases may be indicated if severe rheumatoid lung disease is suspected. Postoperative ventilatory support might be needed in this subset of patients. The effect of aspirin or NSAIDs on platelet function must be considered. Corticosteroid supplementation may be indicated in patients being treated long term with these drugs. Postextubation laryngeal obstruction may occur in patients with cricoarytenoid arthritis.

SPONDYLOARTHROPATHIES

Spondyloarthropathies are a group of nonrheumatic arthropathies that include ankylosing spondylitis, reactive arthritis (Reiter syndrome), juvenile chronic polyarthropathy, psoriatic arthritis, and enteropathic arthritis. These diseases are characterized by involvement of the spine, especially the sacroiliac joints, asymmetrical peripheral arthritis and synovitis, and absence of rheumatoid nodules or detectable circulating rheumatoid factor (see Table 18-6). There is a shared predilection for new bone formation at sites of chronic inflammation, and joint ankylosis often results. There is also a predilection for ocular inflammation. Causes of these seronegative spondyloarthropathies are unknown, but there is a strong association with HLA allele B27 (HLA-B27).

Ankylosing Spondylitis

Ankylosing spondylitis is a chronic, usually progressive, inflammatory disease involving the articulations of the spine and adjacent soft tissues. Spinal disease begins in the sacroiliac joints and moves cranially. The degree of spinal disease can range from just sacroiliac involvement to complete ankylosis of the spine. Hip involvement occurs in approximately one third of patients. Back pain characterized by morning stiffness that improves with activity and exercise plus radiographic evidence of sacroiliitis is highly suggestive of this diagnosis. The disease occurs predominantly in men and often begins in young adulthood. The strong familial incidence is supported by the finding that 90% of patients with ankylosing spondylitis are HLA-B27 positive compared to only 6% of the general population. Ankylosing spondylitis is often erroneously diagnosed as back pain due to lumbar disc degeneration.

Examination of the spine may demonstrate skeletal muscle spasm, loss of lordosis, and decreased mobility of the vertebral column.

Systemic involvement manifests as weight loss, fatigue, and low-grade fever. Conjunctivitis and uveitis occur in approximately 40% of patients. The uveitis is usually unilateral and manifests as visual impairment, photophobia, and eye pain. Distinctive pulmonary abnormalities associated with ankylosing spondylitis include apical cavitary lesions with fibrosis and pleural thickening that mimic tuberculosis. Arthritic involvement of the thoracic spine and costovertebral articulations can result in a decrease in chest wall compliance and, consequently, a decrease in vital capacity.

Treatment

Treatment of ankylosing spondylitis consists of exercises designed to maintain joint mobility and posture plus anti-inflammatory drugs. NSAIDs (indomethacin and diclofenac) are commonly used. Infliximab and etanercept may cause profound improvement in this disease, but patients often relapse when treatment is discontinued. For uveitis, topical corticosteroid eyedrops are an integral part of management.

Management of Anesthesia

Management of anesthesia in patients with ankylosing spondylitis is influenced by the magnitude of spinal involvement. The spinal column can be stiff and deformed and prevent appropriate cervical spine motion for endotracheal intubation. Awake fiberoptic tracheal intubation may be needed. Restrictive lung disease from costochondral rigidity and flexion deformity of the thoracic spine must be appreciated. Sudden or excessive increases in systemic vascular resistance are poorly tolerated if significant aortic regurgitation is present. Neurologic monitoring is a consideration for patients undergoing corrective spinal surgery. Epidural or spinal anesthesia is an acceptable alternative to general anesthesia for perineal or lower limb surgery. Regional anesthesia may be technically difficult due to limited joint mobility and closed interspinous spaces, but ossification of the ligamentum flavum is uncommon.

Reactive Arthritis

Reactive arthritis is an aseptic arthritis that occurs after an extra-articular infection, especially infection with *Chlamydia, Salmonella,* and *Shigella* species. When reactive arthritis is accompanied by extra-articular features such as urethritis, uveitis or conjunctivitis, and skin lesions, the term Reiter syndrome is often used. Predisposing factors include genetic makeup (HLA-B27 positive). Most of the signs of Reiter syndrome persist for only a few days, but arthritis progresses to sacroiliitis and spondylitis in approximately 20% of patients. Cricoarytenoid arthritis can also occur. Hyperkeratotic skin lesions cannot be distinguished from psoriasis, and the two diseases frequently overlap. Management consists of antibiotic treatment for the initial infection and NSAIDs or sulfasalazine for symptomatic relief of the arthritis.

Juvenile Chronic Polyarthropathy

The pathology of chronic juvenile polyarthropathy is similar to that of adult rheumatoid arthritis. Growth abnormalities may occur if arthritis appears before puberty. Hepatic dysfunction may be present, but cardiac involvement is unusual. An acute form of polyarthritis, which presents as fever, rash, lymphadenopathy, and splenomegaly in young children who are negative for rheumatoid factor and HLA-B27, is designated Still's disease. Aspirin is commonly used to treat this disorder. Corticosteroids can effectively control this disease, but their use is limited because of concerns about drug-induced growth retardation in these young patients.

Enteropathic Arthritis

Approximately 10% to 20% of patients with Crohn's disease and 2% to 7% of patients with ulcerative colitis have an inflammatory polyarthritis, most often involving the large joints of the lower extremities. In general, the arthritis activity parallels the activity of the gastrointestinal inflammation and measures that control the gut disease usually control the joint disease concomitantly. This arthritis is not linked to HLA-B27.

Inflammatory bowel disease can also be associated with sacroiliitis and spondylitis, which follow a pattern in which the joint inflammation waxes and wanes independently of the gastrointestinal inflammation. HLA-B27 is found in 50% of these patients. This arthritis is usually chronic and may become ankylosing spondylitis. Treatment is as described for ankylosing spondylitis.

OSTEOARTHRITIS

Osteoarthritis is by far the most common joint disease, one of the leading chronic diseases of the elderly, and a major cause of disability. Osteoarthritis is a degenerative process that affects articular cartilage. This process is different from rheumatoid arthritis because there is minimal inflammatory reaction in the joints. The pathogenesis is likely related to joint trauma from biomechanical stresses, joint injury, or abnormal joint loading due to neuropathy, ligamentous injury, or muscle atrophy. Pain is usually present on motion but is relieved by rest. Stiffness tends to disappear rapidly with joint motion, in contrast to the morning stiffness associated with rheumatoid arthritis, which can last for several hours.

One or several joints can be affected by osteoarthritis. The knees and hips are common sites of involvement. Bony enlargements, referred to as Heberden's nodes, are seen at the distal interphalangeal joints of the fingers. There may be degenerative disease of the vertebral bodies and intervertebral discs, which can be complicated by protrusion of the nucleus pulposus and compression of nerve roots. Degenerative changes are most significant in the mid to lower cervical spine and in the lower lumbar area. Radiographic findings include narrowing of the intervertebral disc spaces and osteophyte formation.

Although often overlooked, physical therapy and exercise programs can provide benefits for patients with osteoarthritis.

Maintaining muscle function is important for both cartilage integrity and pain reduction. Pain relief can also be achieved by application of heat, simple analgesics such as acetaminophen, and anti-inflammatory drugs. Symptomatic improvement with application of heat may be due to an increased pain threshold in warm tissues compared to that in cold tissues. Transcutaneous nerve stimulation and acupuncture can be effective in some patients. Systemic corticosteroids have no place in the treatment of osteoarthritis. Joint replacement surgery may be recommended when pain due to osteoarthritis is persistent and disabling or significant limitation of joint function is present.

PAGET'S DISEASE

Paget's disease of bone is characterized by excessive osteoblastic and osteoclastic activity, resulting in abnormally thick but weak bones. The cause is unknown but may reflect an excess of parathyroid hormone or a deficiency of calcitonin. A familial tendency is present, with white men older than 40 years of age affected most often. Bone pain is the most common symptom. Complications of Paget's disease involve bones (fractures and neoplastic degeneration), joints (arthritis), and the nervous system (nerve compression, paraplegia). Hypercalcemia and renal calculi may also occur. The most characteristic radiographic feature of Paget's disease is localized bone enlargement. Lytic and sclerotic bone changes may involve the skull. If the skull is affected, it may be grossly enlarged and irreversible hearing loss may occur. A radionuclide bone scan is the most reliable test to identify lesions due to Paget's disease. Serum alkaline phosphatase concentration (reflecting bone formation) and urinary hydroxyproline excretion (reflecting bone resorption) are usually increased.

Treatment of Paget's disease is designed to alleviate bone pain and to minimize or prevent progression of the disease. Calcitonin is a hormone secreted by the thyroid gland that inhibits osteoclastic activity and decreases bone resorption. Treatment with calcitonin decreases pain and the biochemical and radiographic abnormalities associated with Paget's disease. It may also stabilize the hearing loss due to Paget's disease. Bisphosphonates can induce marked and prolonged inhibition of bone resorption by decreasing osteoclastic activity. In contrast to the short-lived effects of calcitonin, disease activity remains low for many months, sometimes years, after treatment with bisphosphonates is stopped. Radiographically confirmed repair of osteolytic lesions may occur in response to treatment with bisphosphonates.

Conservative treatment of fractures in patients with Paget's disease is associated with a high risk of delayed union. Patients with Paget's disease who have severe arthritis of the hips or knees often benefit from joint replacement. Rarely osteotomy must be performed to correct bowing deformities of long bones. Patients with evidence of peripheral nerve compression, radiculopathy, or spinal cord compression require decompressive surgery.

MARFAN SYNDROME

Marfan syndrome, a connective tissue disorder, is inherited as an autosomal dominant trait. The incidence is 4 to 6 per 100,000 live births and the mean age of survival is 32 years. Characteristically, these patients have long tubular bones, giving them a tall stature and an "Abe Lincoln" appearance. Additional skeletal abnormalities include a high-arched palate, pectus excavatum, kyphoscoliosis, and hyperextensibility of the joints. Early development of pulmonary emphysema is characteristic and may further accentuate the impact of lung disease related to kyphoscoliosis. There is a high incidence of spontaneous pneumothorax. Ocular changes such as lens dislocation, myopia, and retinal detachment occur in more than half of patients with Marfan syndrome.

Cardiovascular System

Cardiovascular abnormalities are responsible for nearly all premature deaths in patients with Marfan syndrome. Defective connective tissue in the aorta and heart valves can lead to aortic dilation, dissection, or rupture and to prolapse of the cardiac valves, especially the mitral valve. Mitral regurgitation due to mitral valve prolapse is a common abnormality. The risk of bacterial endocarditis is increased in the presence of this valvular heart disease. Cardiac conduction abnormalities, especially bundle branch block, are common. Echocardiography is useful for detecting cardiac abnormalities in asymptomatic individuals. Prophylactic β-adrenergic blocker therapy is recommended for patients with a dilated thoracic aorta. Surgical replacement of the aortic valve and ascending aorta is indicated when the diameter of the ascending aorta exceeds 6 cm and substantial aortic regurgitation is present. Pregnancy poses a unique risk of rupture or dissection of the aorta in women with Marfan syndrome.

Management of Anesthesia

Preoperative evaluation of patients with Marfan syndrome should concentrate on cardiopulmonary abnormalities. In most patients, skeletal abnormalities have little impact on the airway. Care should be exercised, however, to avoid temporomandibular joint dislocation to which these patients are susceptible. In view of the risk of aortic dissection, it is prudent to avoid any sustained increase in systemic blood pressure, as can occur during direct laryngoscopy or in response to painful surgical stimulation. Invasive monitoring including transesophageal echocardiography may be a consideration in selected patients. A high index of suspicion must be maintained for the development of pneumothorax.

KYPHOSCOLIOSIS

Kyphoscoliosis is a spinal deformity characterized by anterior flexion (kyphosis) and lateral curvature (scoliosis) of the vertebral column. Idiopathic kyphoscoliosis, which accounts for 80% of cases, commonly begins during late childhood and may progress in severity during periods of rapid skeletal growth. The incidence of idiopathic kyphoscoliosis is approximately 4 per 1000 population. There may be a familial predisposition to this disease, and females are affec-ted four times more often than males. Diseases of the neuromuscular system, such as poliomyelitis, cerebral palsy, and muscular dystrophy, may also be associated with kyphoscoliosis.

Signs and Symptoms

Spinal curvature of more than 40 degrees is considered severe and is likely to be associated with physiologic derangements in cardiac and pulmonary function. Restrictive lung disease and pulmonary hypertension progressing to cor pulmonale are the principal causes of death in patients with kyphoscoliosis. As the scoliosis curve worsens, more lung tissue is compressed, resulting in a decrease in vital capacity and dyspnea on exertion. The work of breathing is increased because of the abnormal mechanical properties of the distorted thorax and by the increased airway resistance that results from small lung volumes. The alveolar-arterial oxygen difference is increased. Pulmonary hypertension is the result of increased pulmonary vascular resistance due to compression of lung vasculature and the response to arterial hypoxemia. The Pa_{CO_2} is usually maintained at normal levels, but an insult such as bacterial or viral upper respiratory tract infection can result in hypercapnia and acute respiratory failure. A poor cough contributes to frequent pulmonary infection.

Management of Anesthesia

Preoperatively, it is important to assess the severity of the physiologic derangements produced by this skeletal deformity. Pulmonary function tests reflect the magnitude of restrictive lung disease. Arterial blood gases are helpful for detecting unrecognized hypoxemia or acidosis that could be contributing to pulmonary hypertension. These patients may have preoperative pulmonary infection due to chronic aspiration. Certainly, any reversible component of pulmonary dysfunction, such as infection or bronchospasm, should be corrected prior to elective surgery.

Although no specific drug or drug combination can be recommended as optimal for patients with kyphoscoliosis, it should be remembered that nitrous oxide may increase pulmonary vascular resistance. This could be particularly problematic in patients with pulmonary hypertension. Monitoring central venous pressure may provide warning of an increase in pulmonary vascular resistance.

If surgery is undertaken to correct the spinal curvature, special anesthetic considerations concerning blood loss and recognition of surgically induced spinal cord damage are required. Controlled hypotension with a combination of volatile anesthetic and/or vasodilator may be selected to help minimize intraoperative blood loss. At the time that the spinal curvature is straightened/distracted, excessive traction on the spinal cord can result in spinal cord ischemia, which could produce paralysis. There are several maneuvers designed to detect spinal cord ischemia. One is the "wake-up test," which entails determining that no significant neuromuscular blockade is present by discontinuing the anesthetic until the patient is sufficiently awake to move both legs on command, thus confirming that spinal cord motor pathways are intact. Anesthesia is then reestablished and the operation completed. Another method to confirm an intact spinal cord is to monitor somatosensory and/or motor evoked potentials. The advantage of this monitoring is that patients need not be awakened intraoperatively. However, many anesthetic drugs, especially volatile anesthetics and nitrous oxide, interfere with the monitoring of evoked potentials and neuromuscular blockers cannot be used if motor evoked potentials are being monitored. Therefore, total intravenous anesthesia with an opioid and propofol or an opioid/propofol/low-dose (0.33 MAC) volatile anesthetic combination are usually chosen to provide general anesthesia. These techniques make it easier to interpret changes in amplitude and latency due to spinal cord ischemia. A wake-up test may still be necessary if abnormalities persist. At the conclusion of surgery, the principal concern is restoration of adequate ventilation. Postoperative mechanical ventilation may be necessary in some patients with severe kyphoscoliosis.

DWARFISM

Dwarfism can occur in two forms: *proportionate* dwarfism in which the limbs, trunk, and head size are in the same relative proportions as a normal adult and *disproportionate* dwarfism in which the limbs, trunk, and head size are not in the usual proportions of a normal adult.

Achondroplasia

Achondroplasia is the most common cause of disproportionate dwarfism. It occurs predominantly in females with an incidence of 1.5 per 10,000 births. Transmission is by an autosomal dominant gene, although an estimated 80% of cases represent spontaneous mutations. The basic defect is a decrease in the rate of endochondral ossification that, when coupled with normal periosteal bone formation, produces short tubular bones. The anticipated height of achondroplastic males is 132 cm (52 inches) and of females is 122 cm (48 inches). Kyphoscoliosis and genu varum are common. Premature fusion of the bones at the base of the skull can result in a shortened skull base and a stenotic foramen magnum. In addition, there may be functional fusion of the atlanto-occipital joint with odontoid hypoplasia, atlantoaxial instability, bulging discs, and severe cervical kyphosis. These changes may result in hydrocephalus or damage to the cervical spinal cord. Central sleep apnea in achondroplastic dwarfs may be a result of brainstem compression due to foramen magnum stenosis. Pulmonary hypertension leading to cor pulmonale is the most common cardiovascular disturbance that develops in dwarfs. Mental and skeletal muscle development are normal as is life expectancy for those who survive the first year of life.

Management of Anesthesia

Pituitary dwarfism is associated with proportionately smaller airways without anatomic abnormalities. A short laryngoscope handle, a range of blades, and oral or nasal airways appropriate for pediatric patients should be available for patients with pituitary dwarfism. In adult patients with pituitary dwarfism, the size of an endotracheal tube is more similar to that of pediatric patients than to normal-size adult patients.

Management of anesthesia in achondroplastic dwarfs is influenced by potential airway difficulties, cervical spine instability, and the potential for spinal cord trauma with neck extension (**Table 18-7**).

Achondroplastic dwarfs may undergo a number of specific operations, including suboccipital craniectomy for foramen magnum stenosis, laminectomy for spinal column stenosis or nerve root compression, and ventriculoperitoneal shunts. A history of obstructive sleep apnea may predispose to development of upper airway obstruction after sedation or induction of anesthesia. Abnormal bone growth can result in several potential anesthetic problems. Facial features including a large protruding forehead, short maxilla, large mandible, flat nose, and large tongue may result in difficulty attaining a good fit with the anesthesia face mask and in maintenance of a patent upper airway. Despite these anatomic characteristics, clinical experience has not confirmed difficulty with upper airway patency or endotracheal intubation in most of these patients.

In dwarfs with cervical kyphosis, tracheal intubation may be difficult because of an inability to align the axes of the airway. Hyperextension of the neck during direct laryngoscopy should be avoided because of the likely presence of foramen magnum stenosis. Fiberoptic-guided tracheal intubation may be a consideration in selected patients. Weight rather than age is the best guide for selecting the proper-size endotracheal tube.

Excess skin and subcutaneous tissue may make peripheral venous access technically difficult. Achondroplastic dwarfs undergoing suboccipital craniectomy, especially in the sitting position, are at risk of venous air embolism. A right atrial catheter is desirable should an air embolism occur but placing such a catheter may be technically difficult because of a short neck and the difficulty of identifying landmarks that may be obscured by excess soft tissue. Evoked potential monitoring is useful during surgery that may be associated with brainstem or spinal cord injury. Achondroplastic dwarfs respond normally to anesthetic drugs and neuromuscular blockers. Anesthetic techniques that permit rapid awakening may be desirable for prompt evaluation of neurologic function.

Cesarean section is necessary because a small, contracted pelvis combined with a near-normal birth weight infant produces cephalopelvic disproportion. Regional anesthesia might be considered, but technical difficulties may occur due to kyphoscoliosis and a narrow epidural space and spinal canal. The small epidural space may make it difficult to introduce an epidural catheter. Osteophytes, prolapsed intervertebral discs, or deformed vertebral bodies can also contribute to difficulties with neuraxial blockade. There are no data confirming appropriate doses of local anesthetics for epidural or spinal anesthesia in these patients. Epidural anesthesia may be preferable to spinal anesthesia because it permits titration of the local anesthetic drug to achieve the desired level of sensory blockade.

Russell-Silver Syndrome

Russell-Silver syndrome is a form of dwarfism characterized by intrauterine growth retardation with subsequent severe postnatal growth impairment, dysmorphic facial features (including mandibular and facial hypoplasia), limb asymmetry, congenital heart defects, and a constellation of endocrine abnormalities including hypoglycemia, adrenocortical insufficiency, and hypogonadism. Developmental and hormonal abnormalities tend to normalize with age, and individuals with this syndrome can achieve adult heights near 150 cm (~60 inches). Rapid depletion of limited hepatic glycogen stores, especially in small-for-gestational-age neonates, may predispose to hypoglycemia. The risk of hypoglycemia diminishes as the child grows and is usually absent after approximately 4 years of age.

Preoperative evaluation should consider the serum glucose concentration, especially in neonates at risk of hypoglycemia. Intravenous infusions containing glucose may be indicated preoperatively. Facial manifestations of this syndrome (similar to those in Goldenhar's and Treacher-Collins syndromes) may make direct laryngoscopy and exposure of the glottic opening difficult. An endotracheal tube smaller than the predicted size may be needed. Obtaining a good mask fit may also be difficult due to facial asymmetry. Administration of some drugs, such as muscle relaxants, based on body weight rather than body surface area may result in relative underdosing. Infants with Russell-Silver syndrome may be especially prone to intraoperative hypothermia because of their large surface-to-volume ratio. Unexplained tachycardia, diaphoresis, or somnolence after emergence from anesthesia may indicate hypoglycemia.

BACK PAIN

Low back pain is the most common musculoskeletal complaint requiring medical attention (**Table 18-8**). Risk factors

---

TABLE 18-7 Characteristics of Achondroplastic Dwarfs That May Influence Management of Anesthesia

Difficult exposure of the glottic opening
Foramen magnum stenosis
Odontoid hypoplasia with cervical instability
Kyphoscoliosis
Restrictive lung disease
Obstructive sleep apnea
Central sleep apnea
Pulmonary hypertension
Cor pulmonale
Hydrocephalus

for low back pain include male gender, frequent lifting of heavy objects, and smoking. In many patients, the cause of the back pain cannot be determined with certainty and is usually attributed to muscular or ligamentous strain, facet joint arthritis, or disc pressure on the annulus fibrosus, vertebral endplate, or nerve roots.

Acute Low Back Pain

Back pain improves within 30 days in 90% of patients. Continuing ordinary activities within the limits permitted by the pain leads to more rapid recovery than bed rest or back-mobilizing exercises. NSAIDs are often effective for analgesia for acute back pain. Pain arising from inflammation initiated by mechanical or chemical insult to a nerve root may be responsive to epidural administration of corticosteroids, but few patients experience symptomatic relief from epidural corticosteroids if radicular pain has been present for more than 6 months or if laminectomy has been performed. A herniated disc should be considered in patients with radiculopathy that is suggested by pain radiating down a leg or by symptoms reproduced by straight leg raising. Most lumbar disc herniations producing sciatica occur at the L4-5 and L5-S1 levels. Magnetic resonance imaging can confirm a herniated disc, but findings should be interpreted with caution because many asymptomatic people also have disc abnormalities. Surgical intervention is indicated in patients with persistent radiculopathy/neurologic deficits. Patients with persistent back pain after 30 days of conservative treatment (NSAIDs) should be evaluated for systemic illness.

Lumbar Spinal Stenosis

Lumbar spinal stenosis is narrowing of the spinal canal or its lateral recesses. It typically results from hypertrophic degenerative changes in spinal structures (extensive degenerative disc disease and/or osteophyte formation) and occurs most often in elderly patients with chronic back pain and sciatica. Symptoms include pain, numbness, and weakness in the buttocks that can extend down one or both legs. Symptoms often worsen with standing or walking and improve with the flexed or supine position. The diagnosis of lumbar spinal stenosis is confirmed by magnetic resonance imaging or myelography. Conservative measures may be helpful in some patients, but surgical decompression and fusion are needed for those with progressive functional deterioration.

OTHER MUSCULOSKELETAL SYNDROMES

Rotator Cuff Tear

Rotator cuff tear is the most common pathologic entity involving the shoulders. The prevalence of partial- or full-thickness rotator cuff tears is 5% to 40% as determined at postmortem examinations of adults older than age 40. The incidence of rotator cuff tears increases with age. As many as half of individuals older than 55 years of age have arthrographically

TABLE 18-8 Causes of Low Back Pain

Mechanical Low Back or Leg Pain (97%)
Idiopathic low back pain (lumbar sprain or strain) (70%)
Degenerative processes of discs and facets (age-related) (10%)
Herniated disc (4%)
Spinal stenosis (3%)
Osteoporotic compression fractures (4%)
Spondylolisthesis (2%)
Traumatic fracture (<1%)
Congenital disease (<1%)
  Severe kyphosis
  Severe scoliosis
Spondylolysis

Nonmechanical Spinal Conditions (1%)
Cancer (0.7%)
  Multiple myeloma
  Metastatic cancer
  Lymphoma and leukemia
  Spinal cord tumors
  Retroperitoneal tumors
  Primary vertebral tumors
Infection (0.01%)
  Osteomyelitis
  Paraspinal abscess
  Epidural abscess
Inflammatory arthritis
  Ankylosing spondylitis
  Psoriatic spondylitis
  Reiter syndrome
  Inflammatory bowel disease

Visceral Disease (2%)
Disease of pelvic organs
  Prostatitis
  Endometriosis
  Pelvic inflammatory disease
Renal disease
  Nephrolithiasis
  Pyelonephritis
  Perinephric abscess
Aortic aneurysm
Gastrointestinal disease
  Pancreatitis
  Cholecystitis
  Penetrating ulcer

Percentages indicate the estimated incidence of these conditions in adult patients.
Adapted from Deyo RO, Weinstein JN: Low back pain. N Engl J Med 2001;344:363–370.

detectable rotator cuff tears. Other shoulder pathology is less common. Adhesive capsulitis (frozen shoulder) occurs in approximately 2% of the adult population and in 11% of the adult diabetic population. The incidence of calcific tendinitis ranges from 3% to 7%. Shoulder pain ranks just behind back and neck pain as a cause of disability in workers.

Corticosteroid injection into the subacromial space may provide symptomatic relief in patients with impingement syndromes with or without rotator cuff tears, adhesive capsulitis, or supraspinatus tendinitis. Arthroscopic release or manipulation under anesthesia may be used in an attempt to restore shoulder motion. Total shoulder replacement (replacement of humeral and glenoid articular surfaces) reduces shoulder pain in most patients.

Brachial plexus anesthesia via the interscalene approach with continuous infusion of local anesthetic can provide anesthesia for shoulder surgery and postoperative analgesia. Ipsilateral hemidiaphragmatic paralysis virtually always occurs with an interscalene block. For this reason, interscalene block may be problematic and is best avoided in patients with severe chronic obstructive pulmonary disease or with neuromuscular diseases associated with weakness of the respiratory muscles. Wound infiltration or lavage with solutions containing a long-acting local anesthetic such as bupivacaine or ropivacaine can also provide postoperative analgesia following major shoulder surgery.

Floppy Infant Syndrome

Floppy infant syndrome is a term used to describe infants who have weak, hypotonic skeletal muscles. A diminished cough reflex and difficulty swallowing predisposed to aspiration and recurrent pneumonia is common. Progressive weakness and atrophy of skeletal muscles leads to contractures and kyphoscoliosis.

Anesthesia, such as for skeletal muscle biopsy to confirm the diagnosis, may be associated with increased sensitivity to nondepolarizing muscle relaxants and hyperkalemia and cardiac arrest after administration of succinylcholine. These infants are also susceptible to malignant hyperthermia. Ketamine can be useful for anesthesia because it does not cause significant respiratory depression.

Tracheomegaly

Tracheomegaly is characterized by marked dilation of the trachea and bronchi due to a congenital defect in elastin and smooth muscle fibers in the tracheobronchial tree or to their destruction after radiotherapy. The diagnosis is confirmed by measuring a tracheal diameter of more than 30 mm on chest radiography. Symptoms include a chronic productive cough and frequent pulmonary infection, perhaps related to chronic aspiration. The tracheal and bronchial walls are abnormally flaccid and may collapse during vigorous coughing. Aspiration during general anesthesia is possible, especially if maximal inflation of the endotracheal tube cuff does not produce an airtight seal.

Alcoholic Myopathy

Acute and chronic forms of proximal skeletal muscle weakness occur frequently in alcoholic patients. Distinguishing alcoholic myopathy from alcoholic neuropathy is based on proximal, rather than distal, skeletal muscle involvement, an increased serum creatine kinase concentration, myoglobinuria in acute cases, and rapid recovery after cessation of alcohol consumption.

Prader-Willi Syndrome

Prader-Willi syndrome manifests at birth as hypotonia, which may be associated with a weak cough, swallowing difficulties, and upper airway obstruction. Nasogastric feeding may be necessary during infancy. The syndrome progresses during childhood and is characterized by hyperphagia leading to obesity plus endocrine abnormalities including hypogonadism and diabetes mellitus. The pickwickian syndrome may develop in some patients. There is little growth in height and patients remain short. Mental retardation is often severe. There is a deletion in chromosome 15 in this syndrome, and an autosomal recessive mode of inheritance has been proposed.

Micrognathia, a high-arched palate, strabismus, a straight ulnar border, and congenital dislocation of the hip may be present. Dental caries are common and may be related to chronic regurgitation of gastric contents. Seizures are associated with this syndrome, but cardiac dysfunction does not accompany the Prader-Willi syndrome.

The principal anesthetic concerns in these patients center on hypotonia and altered metabolism of carbohydrates and fat. Weak skeletal musculature is associated with a poor cough and an increased incidence of pneumonia. Intraoperative monitoring of blood glucose concentration is necessary, and exogenous glucose administration may be needed because these patients use circulating glucose to manufacture fat rather than to meet basal energy needs. When calculating drug doses, one should consider the decreased skeletal muscle mass and increased fat content in these patients. Muscle relaxant requirements might be decreased in the presence of hypotonia. Succinylcholine has been administered without incident to these patients.

Disturbances in thermoregulation, often characterized by intraoperative hyperthermia and metabolic acidosis, have been observed, but a relationship to malignant hyperthermia has not been established. There is an increased incidence of perioperative aspiration pneumonitis.

Prune-Belly Syndrome

Prune-belly syndrome is characterized by congenital agenesis of the lower central abdominal musculature and the presence of urinary tract anomalies including gross ureteral dilatation, hypotonic bladder, prostatic hypoplasia, and bilateral undescended testes. The full syndrome appears only in males, and an incomplete syndrome may include up to 3% females. Recurrent respiratory tract infection reflects an impaired ability to cough effectively. It is unlikely that muscle relaxants are necessary during the management of anesthesia in these patients.

Mitochondrial Myopathies

Mitochondrial myopathies are a heterogeneous group of disorders of skeletal muscle energy metabolism. Mitochondria produce the energy requirements of skeletal muscle cells through the redox reactions of the electron transfer chain and oxidative phosphorylation, thereby producing adenosine triphosphate. Defects in this process result in abnormal fatigability with sustained exercise, skeletal muscle pain, and progressive weakness. The morphologic hallmark is large sub-sarcolemmal accumulations of abnormal mitochondria that appear as red-staining granules (ragged-red fibers). Disorders of mitochondrial metabolism may also involve other organ systems with high energy demands, such as the brain, heart, liver, and kidneys.

Kearns-Sayre Syndrome

Kearns-Sayre syndrome is a rare mitochondrial myopathy accompanied by progressive external ophthalmoplegia, retinitis pigmentosa, heart block, hearing loss, short stature, peripheral neuropathy, and impaired ventilatory drive. Dilated cardiomyopathy and congestive heart failure may be present.

General anesthesia for these patients must consider the risk of drug-induced myocardial depression, development of cardiac conduction defects, and hypoventilation during the early postoperative period

Multicore Myopathy

Multicore myopathy is a heterogeneous group of diseases characterized by proximal skeletal muscle weakness, a decrease in muscle mass, and musculoskeletal abnormalities such as scoliosis and high-arched palate. Recurrent pulmonary infection is common and may be related to the severity of the associated kyphoscoliosis. Cardiomyopathy may accompany this myopathy. Unlike other myopathies, serum creatine kinase concentration is usually normal in these individuals. Intelligence is normal, and the myopathy may have a benign course.

Preoperative assessment of respiratory function is necessary in the presence of kyphoscoliosis and recurrent lung infection. Difficulty swallowing and an inability to clear secretions may reflect pharyngeal and laryngeal muscle involvement. Postoperative aspiration may be associated with impaired upper airway reflexes and the lingering effects of drugs administered during anesthesia. It is important to recognize the potential relationship between multicore myopathy and malignant hyperthermia.

Centronuclear Myopathy

Centronuclear myopathy is a rare congenital myopathy characterized by progressive muscle weakness of extraocular, facial, neck, and limb muscles. The defect is a mutation in a gene important for muscle cell growth and differentiation. There are severe neonatal forms of this disease as well as slowly progressive forms that can begin anytime from birth to adulthood. Development of scoliosis with restrictive lung disease is an important manifestation of disease severity. Serum creatine kinase concentration is usually normal. The association of ptosis and strabismus with this myopathy increases the likelihood that these children will undergo surgery.

Management of anesthesia is influenced by the degree of skeletal muscle weakness, the presence of restrictive lung disease, and gastroesophageal reflux. Muscle relaxants are often avoided, and a nontriggering general anesthetic technique used.

Meige Syndrome

Meige syndrome is an idiopathic dystonic disorder that manifests as blepharospasm and oromandibular dystonia. It most often affects middle-aged to elderly women. Facial muscle spasms are characterized by symmetrical dystonic contractions of the facial muscles. Dystonia is aggravated by stress and disappears during sleep. The pathophysiology of this disease is unknown but may be related to dopamine hyperactivity or dysfunction of the basal ganglia. Drug therapy (antidopaminergics, anticholinergics, acetylcholine agonists, γ-aminobutyric acid agonists) may have some effect, and facial nerve block has been reported to provide sustained relief.

Spasmodic Dysphonia

Spasmodic dysphonia is a laryngeal disorder characterized by adductor or abductor dystonic spasms of the vocal cords. This syndrome typically manifests as abnormal phonation but on rare occasions is associated with respiratory distress. Stress can exacerbate it, and associated neurologic symptoms (tremors, weakness, dystonia of other skeletal muscle groups) are present in most patients. Botulinum toxin, which blocks neuromuscular transmission, may be effective for treating the spasms of torticollis, blepharospasm, and spasmodic dysphonia.

Preoperative fiberoptic or direct laryngoscopy may be necessary to define anatomic abnormalities and to estimate airway dimensions. The presence of laryngeal stenosis may necessitate the use of smaller-than-usual tracheal tubes. The risk of pulmonary aspiration may be increased by vocal cord dysfunction caused by therapeutic interventions such as botulinum toxin injection or recurrent laryngeal nerve interruption. Continued monitoring during the postoperative period is important, as these patients may experience respiratory difficulties.

Juvenile Hyaline Fibromatosis

Juvenile hyaline fibromatosis is a rare syndrome characterized by the presence of numerous dermal and subcutaneous nodules. Patients may have hypertrophic gingivae, osteolytic bone lesions, and stunted growth with normal mental development. Resistance to the effects of succinylcholine has been described in patients with juvenile hyaline fibromatosis.

Chondrodysplasia Calcificans Punctata

Chondrodysplasia calcificans punctata is a rare congenital syndrome caused by dysfunctional peroxisomes. It manifests as erratic cartilage calcification resulting in bone and skin lesions, cataracts, and cardiac malformations. In surviving children, abnormal growth leads to dwarfism, kyphoscoliosis, and subluxation of the hips. There is no available treatment. Orthopedic procedures are often necessary to offset functional limitations of the disease and to stabilize spine and limb malformations. Tracheal cartilage may be involved by the disease process, resulting in tracheal stenosis, which may complicate perioperative airway management.

Erythromelalgia

Erythromelalgia literally means red, painful extremities. Erythema, intense, burning pain, and increased temperature of the involved extremities are hallmarks of the disease. The feet, especially the soles, are most often involved, and males are affected twice as often as females. Primary erythromelalgia occurs more frequently than secondary erythromelalgia, which is associated with myeloproliferative disorders such as polycythemia vera. Intravascular platelet aggregation may be prominent. Aspirin is the most effective treatment for secondary erythromelalgia due to myeloproliferative diseases. Patients may seek relief by exposing the affected extremity to a cooler environment, such as immersing the afflicted extremity in cold water. Neuraxial opioids and local anesthetics may provide some pain relief.

Farber's Lipogranulomatosis

Farber's lipogranulomatosis is an inherited disorder due to a deficiency of ceramidase that results in accumulation of ceramide in tissues (pleura, pericardium, synovial lining of joints, liver, spleen, lymph nodes). Progressive arthropathy, psychomotor retardation, and nutritional failure are present, and most affected individuals die by 2 years of age as a result of airway and respiratory problems. Acute renal and hepatic failure may reflect accumulation of ceramide in these organs. Difficult airway management is a common problem because of granuloma formation in the pharynx or larynx. Tracheal intubation is best avoided in patients with upper airway involvement because laryngeal edema or bleeding from laryngeal granulomas is possible.

McCune-Albright Syndrome

McCune-Albright syndrome consists of a triad of physical signs: osseous lesions (polyostotic fibrous dysplasia), melanotic cutaneous macules (café au lait spots), and sexual precocity (autonomous ovarian steroid secretion). Conductive and neural deafness occur when osseous lesions involve the temporal bone and impinge on the cochlea. Bony fractures are likely during childhood. Some patients show other endocrine dysfunction, especially hyperthyroidism, acromegaly, and hypophosphatemia.

An important anesthetic implication of McCune-Albright syndrome is the presence of endocrine abnormalities, especially hyperthyroidism. Perioperative steroid supplementation may be a consideration when adrenal hyperactivity is present because these patients may exhibit an altered cortisol response to stress. Vascular fragility may make venous access difficult. These patients may have fragile bones, and particular care is needed during intraoperative positioning. Tracheal intubation may be difficult because of airway distortion associated with acromegaly or hypertrophy of soft tissue in the upper airway.

Klippel-Feil Syndrome

Klippel-Feil syndrome is characterized by a short neck resulting from a reduced number of cervical vertebrae or fusion of several vertebrae. Movement of the neck is limited and associated skeletal abnormalities include spinal stenosis and kyphoscoliosis. Mandibular malformations and micrognathia may be present. There is an increased incidence of cardiac and genitourinary anomalies. Management of anesthesia must consider the risk of neurologic damage during direct laryngoscopy due to cervical spine instability. Preoperative lateral neck radiographs help evaluate the stability of the cervical spine.

Osteogenesis Imperfecta

Osteogenesis imperfecta is a rare, autosomal dominant, inherited disease of connective tissue that affects bones, the sclera, and the inner ear. Bones are extremely brittle because of defective collagen production. The incidence of osteogenesis imperfecta is higher in females. Osteogenesis imperfecta can manifest in two forms: osteogenesis imperfecta congenita and osteogenesis imperfecta tarda. With the congenital form fractures occur in utero and death often occurs during the perinatal period. The tarda form typically manifests during childhood or early adolescence with the presence of blue sclerae fractures after minor trauma, kyphoscoliosis, bowing of the femur and tibia, and gradual onset of otosclerosis and deafness. Impaired platelet function may produce a mild bleeding tendency. Hyperthermia with hyperhidrosis can occur in patients with osteogenesis imperfecta. An increased serum thyroxine concentration associated with an increase in oxygen consumption occurs in at least 50% of patients with this disease.

Management of anesthesia is influenced by the co-existing orthopedic deformities and the potential for additional fractures during the perioperative period. Patients with osteogenesis imperfecta often have a decreased range of motion of the cervical spine due to remodeling of bone. Tracheal intubation must be accomplished with as little manipulation and trauma as possible because cervical and mandibular fractures may occur. Awake fiberoptic intubation is prudent if orthopedic deformities suggest that it will be difficult to visualize the glottic opening with direct laryngoscopy. Dentition is often defective, and teeth are vulnerable to damage during direct laryngoscopy. Succinylcholine-induced fasciculations may produce fractures. Kyphoscoliosis and pectus excavatum decrease vital capacity and chest wall compliance and can result in arterial hypoxemia due to ventilation-perfusion mismatching. Automated blood pressure cuffs may be hazardous since inflation can result in fractures. Regional anesthesia is acceptable in selected patients because it avoids the need for endotracheal intubation, but it may be technically difficult because of kyphoscoliosis. The coagulation status should be evaluated before selecting a regional anesthetic technique because osteogenesis imperfecta may be associated with a prolonged bleeding time despite a normal platelet count. Desmopressin may be effective in normalizing platelet function. These patients may have mild hyperthermia intraoperatively but it is not a forerunner of malignant hyperthermia.

Fibrodysplasia Ossificans

Fibrodysplasia ossificans is a rare inherited autosomal dominant disease, usually presenting before 6 years of age and characterized by myositis and proliferation of connective tissue. The term myositis ossificans is also applied to this disease, but fibrodysplasia ossificans may be a more correct term because this is principally a disease of connective tissue rather than of skeletal muscle. Connective tissue undergoes cartilaginous and osteoid transformation, eventually leading to displacement of skeletal muscles by ectopic bone formation. Body parts become rigid. Ectopic bone formation typically affects the muscles of the elbows, hips, and knees, leading to serious limitations of joint movement. Cervical spine involvement is common. There may be varying degrees of cervical fusion and the possibility of atlantoaxial subluxation. There may also be temporomandibular joint involvement. Muscles of the face, larynx, eyes, anterior abdominal wall, diaphragm, and heart usually escape involvement.

During the early stages of the disease, fever may occur at the same time as localized lumps appear in affected skeletal muscles. Alkaline phosphatase activity is increased during active phases of the disease. A restrictive breathing pattern can result from limitation of rib movement, but progression to respiratory failure is rare. Pneumonia, however, is a common complication. Abnormalities on the electrocardiogram include ST-segment changes and right bundle branch block. Deafness may occur, but mental retardation is unlikely. There is no effective therapy.

Deformities of the Sternum

Pectus carinatum (outward protuberance of the sternum) and pectus excavatum (inward concavity of the sternum) produce cosmetic problems, but functional impairment is unusual. Considerable narrowing of the distance between the posterior sternum and the anterior border of the vertebral bodies can be tolerated with little effect on cardiopulmonary function. Rarely is pectus excavatum associated with increased cardiac filling pressures or dysrhythmias. Obstructive sleep apnea may be more common in young children with pectus excavatum, perhaps due to greater inward movement of the sternum and the pliable costochondral apparatus.

Macroglossia

Macroglossia is an infrequent but potentially lethal postoperative complication that is most often associated with posterior fossa craniotomy performed in the sitting position. Possible causes of macroglossia include arterial compression, venous compression due to excessive neck flexion or a head-down position, or mechanical compression of the tongue by the teeth, an oral airway, or an endotracheal tube. It might also have a neurogenic origin. When the onset of macroglossia is immediate, it is easily recognized and airway obstruction does not occur because tracheal extubation is delayed. In some patients, however, obstruction to venous outflow from the tongue leads to development of regional ischemia from compression of the lingual arteries. This is followed by a reperfusion injury that does not occur until the venous outflow obstruction is relieved. As a result, the development of macroglossia may be delayed for 30 minutes or longer. There is then the risk of complete airway obstruction occurring at an unexpected time during the postoperative period.

KEY POINTS

- Epidermolysis bullosa and pemphigus are characterized by bulla formation (blistering) that can involve extensive areas of skin and mucous membranes. Even minor frictional trauma can result in bulla formation. Airway management may be difficult because of bullae in the oropharynx. Airway manipulation including direct laryngoscopy and endotracheal intubation can result in acute bulla formation, upper airway obstruction, and bleeding.

- Patients with scleroderma can present several anesthetic problems. Decreased mandibular motion and narrowing of the oral aperture due to taut skin may make efforts at endotracheal intubation difficult. Oral or nasal telangiectasias may bleed profusely if traumatized. Intravenous access may be impeded by dermal thickening. Systemic or pulmonary hypertension may be present. Hypotonia of the lower esophageal sphincter puts patients at risk of regurgitation and aspiration.

- Muscular dystrophy is characterized by progressive, symmetrical skeletal muscle weakness and wasting but no evidence of skeletal muscle denervation; that is, sensation and reflexes are intact. Increased permeability of skeletal muscle membranes precedes clinical evidence of muscular dystrophy. Patients with muscular dystrophy are malignant-hyperthermia susceptible.

- Myotonic dystrophy designates a group of hereditary degenerative diseases of skeletal muscle characterized by persistent contracture (myotonia) after voluntary contraction of a muscle or following electrical stimulation of the muscle. Peripheral nerves and the neuromuscular junction are not affected. This inability of skeletal muscle to relax after voluntary contraction or stimulation results from abnormal calcium metabolism.

- The clinical course of myasthenia gravis is marked by periods of exacerbation and remission. Muscle strength may be normal in well-rested patients, but weakness occurs promptly with exercise. Ptosis and diplopia resulting from extraocular muscle weakness are the most common initial signs. Weakness of pharyngeal and laryngeal muscles results in dysphagia, dysarthria, and difficulty handling saliva. Patients with myasthenia gravis are at high risk of pulmonary aspiration of gastric contents.

- The acetylcholine receptor–binding antibodies of myasthenia gravis decrease the number of functional acetylcholine receptors, and this results in an increased

KEY POINTS—cont'd

sensitivity to nondepolarizing muscle relaxants. However, patients with myasthenia gravis demonstrate *resistance* to the effects of succinylcholine.

- Myasthenic syndrome (Eaton-Lambert syndrome) is a disorder of neuromuscular transmission that resembles myasthenia gravis. Myasthenic syndrome is an acquired autoimmune disease with immunoglobulin G antibodies to voltage-sensitive calcium channels that produces a deficiency of these channels at the motor nerve terminal. Anticholinesterase drugs effective in the treatment of myasthenia gravis do *not* produce an improvement in patients with myasthenic syndrome.

- Cervical spine involvement is frequent in rheumatoid arthritis and may result in pain and neurologic complications. The most significant abnormality of the cervical spine is atlantoaxial subluxation and consequent separation of the atlanto-odontoid articulation. When this separation is severe, the odontoid process could protrude into the foramen magnum and exert pressure on the spinal cord or impair blood flow through the vertebral arteries.

- Involvement of the cricoarytenoid joints by rheumatoid arthritis is suggested by the presence of hoarseness or stridor or by the observation of erythema or edema of the vocal cords during direct laryngoscopy. Diminished movement of these joints can result in narrowing of the glottic opening and interference with translaryngeal passage of the endotracheal tube or an increased risk of cricoarytenoid joint dislocation.

- The spondyloarthropathies are a group of nonrheumatic arthropathies characterized by involvement of the spine, especially the sacroiliac joints, asymmetrical peripheral arthritis, and synovitis and absence of rheumatic nodules or detectable circulating rheumatoid factor. These diseases have a shared predilection for new bone formation at sites of chronic inflammation, and joint ankylosis often results. There is also a predilection for ocular inflammation.

- Osteoarthritis is by far the most common joint disease, one of the leading chronic diseases of the elderly and a major cause of disability. Osteoarthritis is a degenerative process that affects articular cartilage. This process is different from rheumatoid arthritis because there is minimal inflammatory reaction in the joints. The pathogenesis is likely related to joint trauma from biomechanical stresses, joint injury, or abnormal joint loading due to neuropathy, ligamentous injury, or muscle atrophy. Pain is usually present on motion but is relieved by rest.

- Kyphoscoliosis is a spinal deformity characterized by anterior flexion (kyphosis) and lateral curvature (scoliosis) of the vertebral column. Spinal curvature of more than 40 degrees is considered severe and is likely to be associated with physiologic derangements in cardiac and pulmonary function. Restrictive lung disease and pulmonary hypertension progressing to cor pulmonale are the principal causes of death in patients with kyphoscoliosis.

REFERENCES

Almahroos M, Kurban AK: Management of mastocytosis. Clin Dermatol 2003;21:274–277.

Ames WA, Mayou BJ, Williams KN: Anaesthetic management of epidermolysis bullosa. Br J Anaesth 1999;82:746–751.

D'Cruz DP: Systemic lupus erythematosus. BMJ 2006;332:890–894.

Dalakas MC, Hohlfeld R: Polymyositis and dermatomyositis. Lancet 2003;362:971–982.

Dedhia HV, DiBartolomeo A: Rheumatoid arthritis. Crit Care Clin 2002;18:841–854.

Dillon FX: Anesthesia issues in the perioperative management of myasthenia gravis. Semin Neurol 2004;24:83–94.

Kuczkowski KM: Labor analgesia for the parturient with an uncommon disorder: A common dilemma in the delivery suite. Obstet Gynecol Surv 2003;58:800–803.

O'Neill GN: Acquired disorders of the neuromuscular junction. Int Anesthesiol Clin 2006;44:107–121.

Pai S, Marinkovich MP: Epidermolyis bullosa: New and emerging trends. Am J Clin Dermatol 2002;3:371–380.

Wattendorf DJ, Muenke M: Prader-Willi syndrome. Am Fam Physician 2005;72:827–830.

White RJ, Bass SP: Myotonic dystrophy and paediatric anaesthesia. Paediatr Anaesth 2003;13:94–102.

Infectious Diseases

Michael S. Avidan

On December 4, 1967, Dr. William H. Stewart, the U.S. Surgeon General, informed a meeting of state and territorial health officials that infectious diseases were now conquered. He extolled the findings of the Centers for Disease Control and Prevention (CDC) a year earlier. Epidemic diseases such as smallpox, bubonic plague, and malaria were declared things of the past. Typhoid, polio, and diphtheria were ostensibly heading in the same direction. While syphilis, gonorrhea, and tuberculosis (TB) were not quite so readily defeated, it was suggested to be only a matter of time before every plague that had ever struck fear into the heart of decent Americans would be a distant memory. With the wisdom of hindsight, the irony in these proclamations is evident and the premature declaration of "mission accomplished" appears naive and even foolhardy. The grim reality is that we have probably experienced only a temporary reprieve from the devastation of plagues and infectious diseases. The 21st century will see their resurgence.

Infectious diseases are different from other co-existing diseases from the anesthesiologist's perspective in several respects. Patients may have co-existing infectious diseases that affect perioperative care when they present for surgery. These infections may be manifest or occult. Such diseases may be the reason behind the surgery or may alter the risks associated with surgery. Every patient undergoing surgery is also at risk of acquiring an infectious disease in the perioperative period. People undergoing surgery are vulnerable to infections both at the surgical site and where natural defenses are breached, such as the respiratory tract, the urinary tract, and the bloodstream. Additionally, apart from being contracted by patients, infectious diseases can be passed on to other patients and health professionals in the perioperative period. Anesthesiologists have a major responsibility to implement practices that are proven to decrease the acquisition and passage of infection as well as to prevent and treat complications associated with co-existing infections.

ANTIBIOTIC RESISTANCE

Before modern times humans had little understanding about infection and were subject to multiple devastating pandemics, such as the Black Death of the 14th century. **Box 19-1** presents some of the milestones that have advanced our ability to combat infection over the past millennia.

Since the discovery of penicillin in 1928, bacteria have undergone more mutations than have humans since we split millions of years ago from our ancestor in common with apes. In the past 40 years, there have been only two new antibiotic chemical classes: oxazolidinones (linezolid) and lipopeptides (daptomycin). Most classes of antibiotic were discovered in the 1940s and 1950s and are directed at a few specific aspects of bacterial physiology: biosynthesis of the cell wall and of DNA and proteins.[1] Pharmaceutical companies have generally retreated from antibacterial drugs, concentrating on chronic diseases in the interests of maximum profits. One of the reasons for widespread drug resistance among bacterial pathogens is the limited choice of

---

BOX 19-1 Important Events in Infectious Disease

Date	Event
1675	Antony van Leeuwenhoek discovered bacteria.
1796	Edward Jenner laid the foundation for vaccines.
1848	Ignaz Semmelweis discovered hand washing could prevent infection or contagion.
1857	Louis Pasteur introduced the germ theory of disease.
1867	Joseph Lister pioneered antiseptics during surgery.
1876	Robert Koch, by studying anthrax, showed the role of bacteria in disease.
1892	Dmitri Ivanovski discovered viruses.
1928	Alexander Fleming discovered penicillin.
1955	Jonas Salk developed polio vaccine.
1983	Luc Montagnier and Robert Gallo identified the virus that causes acquired immunodeficiency syndrome.

---

antibiotics that exploit a relatively narrow range of mechanisms.[1] It is encouraging that there are some new developments in the offing, such as the discovery of a small molecule, platensimycin, derived from *Streptomyces platensis*, that targets a seldom-exploited weakness in bacteria: fatty-acid biosynthesis. Such discoveries offer some consolation in the battle with resistant and emerging infections.[1] Perhaps this discovery will be translated into the development of new antimicrobial agents.

In recent decades, many new infections have either been discovered or have "emerged." Examples of emerging infectious diseases are:

Bacteria
Bartonella henselae: cat-scratch disease
Borrelia burgdorferi: Lyme disease
Ehrlichia chaffeensis: Ehrlichiosis (a form of "tick-bite fever")
Helicobacter pylori: peptic ulcer disease

Viruses
Ebola viruses: hemorrhagic fever
Hantaviruses: hemorrhagic fever
Hepatitis C virus: chronic hepatitis, cirrhosis
Hepatitis E virus: acute hepatitis
Human herpesvirus 6: roseola, infection in the immunocompromised
Human herpesvirus 8: Kaposi's sarcoma
Human immunodeficiency virus: acquired immunodeficiency syndrome (AIDS)
Nipah virus: encephalitis
Parvovirus B19: fifth disease, arthritis, anemia
Severe acute respiratory syndrome (SARS) coronavirus: severe acute respiratory syndrome
H5N1 influenza A: severe influenza

Parasites
Babesia protozoa: babesiosis (redwater fever, a form of tick-bite fever)

BOX 19-2 Antibiotic Resistance

New infections are emerging at an alarming rate.

Old infections, such as tuberculosis, are re-emerging with resistance to treatment.

Increasing numbers of gram-negative bacteria are resistant to all antibiotics.

Resistance becomes more dangerous when virulent organisms acquire antimicrobial resistance.

Resistance among virulent gram-positive organisms, such as *Streptococcus pneumoniae* and *Staphylococcus aureus*, is increasing.

No new drugs are being developed to target resistant gram-negative organisms.

What is perhaps even more concerning is that infectious diseases that appeared to be vanquished, such as tuberculosis (TB) and malaria, are having an alarming resurgence. Some reemerging pathogens, such as multidrug-resistant tuberculosis and extensively drug-resistant tuberculosis, have evolved resistance to previously successful antimicrobial therapy. Such trends are a cause for concern for the World Health Organization.

Multidrug-resistant organisms cause an increasing number of bacterial infections in hospitals. Bacteria are emerging with resistance to all available antibiotics. Examples include *Pseudomonas aeruginosa*, *Burkholderia cepacia*, *Acinetobacter baumanii*, *Stenotrophomonas maltophilia*, *Enterobacter cloacae*, *Serratia marcescens*, and *Klebsiella pneumoniae*.[2]

Much of the attention is presently focused on resistant gram-positive organisms, such as methicillin-resistant *Staphylococcus aureus*. But even if vancomycin fails, there are new drugs for gram-positive organisms such as linezolid and perhaps platensimycin in the future. Disturbingly, there is a near-total lack of developmental antibiotics active against the resistant gram-negative pathogens referred to previously.[3]

Box 19-2 summarizes concerns about the increasing resistance to antibiotics.

SURGICAL SITE INFECTIONS

In the days before Semmelweis and Lister, antiseptic techniques were unknown and postoperative surgical site infection (SSI) occurred more than 50% of the time. Semmelweis noticed that three times as many women were dying at the hands of medical students than midwifery students from puerperal fever or "the black death of the childbed." He proposed a connection between medical students' autopsies and the "examining finger, which introduces the cadaveric particles." In May 1847, he required medical students to wash hands with chlorine and the death rate plummeted. Lister applied Pasteur's germ theory to surgery seeking to achieve a sterile operating field, and in 1869 Lister's carbolic spray was first used. The application of antisepsis to surgery resulted in a

dramatic decline in surgical mortality. Despite major advances over the next 150 years, SSIs continued to occur at a rate of 2% to 5% for extra-abdominal surgeries and up to 20% for intra-abdominal surgeries. The CDC's National Nosocomial Infections Surveillance system, established in 1970, monitors reported trends in nosocomial infections in U.S. acute-care hospitals. SSIs are among the top three causes of nosocomial infection, accounting for 14% to 16% of all nosocomial infections among hospitalized patients.[4] SSIs render patients 60% more likely to spend time in ICU, five times more likely to need hospital readmission, and twice as likely to die. A recent resurgence in SSIs may be attributable to bacterial resistance, the increased implantation of prosthetic and foreign material, as well as the poor immune status of many patients undergoing surgery. The universal adoption of simple measures including frequent hand decontamination with alcohol and appropriate administration of prophylactic antibiotics would dramatically decrease the incidence of SSIs.[5]

SSIs are divided into superficial (involving skin and subcutaneous tissues), deep (fascial and muscle layers), and organ or tissue spaces (any area opened, manipulated during surgery) (**Fig. 19-1**).[6] *S. aureus*, including methicillin-resistant *S. aureus* is the predominant cause. Other causative organisms are coagulase-negative staphylococci, enterococci, coliforms, and *Clostridium perfringens*. Organ or tissue space infection after gastrointestinal surgery presents as peritonitis or intra-abdominal abscess. Common causative organisms are coliforms, *P. aeruginosa*, *Candida* spp., and *Bacteroides fragilis*. From 1991 to 1995, the incidence of fungal SSIs among patients at National Nosocomial Infections Surveillance hospitals increased.[7] The increased proportion of SSIs caused by resistant pathogens and *Candida* spp. may reflect increasing numbers of severely ill and immunocompromised surgical patients and the impact of widespread use of broad-spectrum antimicrobial agents.[4]

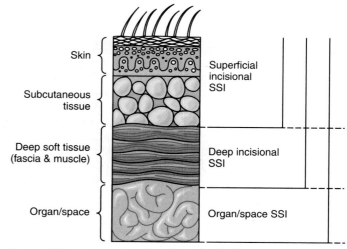

Figure 19-1 • Cross-section of abdominal wall depicting the Centers of Disease Control and Prevention classification of surgical site infection (SSI). (*Adapted from Horan TC, et al: CDC definitions of nosocomial surgical site infections, 1992: A modification of CDC definitions of surgical wound infections. Infect Control Hosp Epidemiol 1992;13:606–608.*)

Who Is at Risk?

The risk of SSI can be conceptualized according to the following relationship[4]:

Patient-related Factors

Illness, extremes of age, or immunocompromise including diabetes mellitus and corticosteroid therapy are associated with an increased risk of developing an SSI. The American Society of Anesthesiologists' score of 3 or more when combined with the type and duration of surgery has been shown to be predictive of the rate of SSIs.

Microbial Factors

Enzyme production (*S. aureus*), possession of polysaccharide capsule (*B. fragilis*), and the ability to bind to fibronectin in blood clots (*S. aureus* and *Staphylococcus epidermidis*) are mechanisms by which microorganisms exploit weakened host defenses and initiate infection. Biofilm formation, exemplified by *S. epidermidis*, is particularly important in the etiology of prosthetic material infections, for example, prosthetic joint infection. Coagulase-negative staphylococci produce glycocalyx and an associated component called "slime," which physically shields bacteria from phagocytes or inhibits the binding or penetration of antimicrobial agents.[8]

Wound-related Factors

Devitalized tissue, dead space, and hematoma formation are factors associated with the development of SSI. Historically, wounds have been described as clean, contaminated, and dirty according to the expected number of bacteria entering the surgical site. The presence of a foreign body (such as sutures) reduces the burden of organisms required to induce SSI.[4] Risk factors for SSI are summarized in **Table 19-1**.

Signs and Symptoms

SSIs typically present within 30 days of surgery with inflammation of the surgical site and evidence of poor healing.

Systemic features of infection, such as fever and malaise, may occur.

Diagnosis

There may be nonspecific evidence of infection, such as elevated white blood count, poor blood sugar control, and elevation of inflammatory markers, such as C-reactive protein and procalcitonin. But surgery itself is a great confounder leading to inflammation, thus rendering surrogate markers of infection unreliable. Pus at the wound sight is suggestive, but not invariable. The best way to document infection is by growing organisms from an aseptically obtained culture. Approximately one third of organisms cultured are staphylococci (*S. aureus* and *S. epidermidis*), *Enterococcus* spp. makes up more than 10%, and *Enterobacteriaceae* (*Escherichia coli*, *P. aeruginosa*, *Enterobacter* spp., *Proteus mirabilis*, and *K. pneumoniae*) make up the bulk of the remaining culprits.[9]

Table 19-2 reflects the criteria for diagnosing SSIs.

Management of Anesthesia

Preoperative

Active infections should be treated aggressively prior to surgery and, where possible, surgery should be postponed until infection has resolved. Several studies have shown that smoking may increase not only the incidence of respiratory infection, but also that of SSI.[10] Preoperative cessation of smoking for 4 to 8 weeks prior to orthopedic surgery decreases the incidence of wound-related complications. Preoperative alcohol consumption may result in immunocompromise. One month of preoperative abstinence reduces postoperative morbidity in alcohol abusers.[11]

Diabetes is an independent risk factor for infection, and optimization of preoperative diabetes treatment may decrease perioperative infection.[12] Malnutrition, whether manifesting as cachexia or obesity, is associated with increased perioperative infection.[13] Appropriate diet and weight loss may be beneficial prior to major surgery.

S. aureus is the most common organism implicated in SSIs, and carriage of *S. aureus* in the anterior nares has been identified as a risk factor for these infections. Topical mupirocin applied to the anterior nares has been successful in eliminating *S. aureus* and decreasing infections.[14] However, this intervention is not without its detractors as the net result may be the promotion of mupirocin-resistant *S. aureus*. Hair clipping is acceptable, but shaving increases the risks of SSI, probably owing to microcuts serving as portals for organisms. Preoperative skin cleaning with chlorhexidine may reduce the incidence of SSIs. There was a well-designed, randomized, prospective study in patients undergoing sternotomy for cardiac surgery. The application of 0.12% chlorhexidine gluconate solution as an oral rinse and as a nasal gel four times daily from the time of hospital admission until the time of removal of the nasogastric tube decreased the incidence of nosocomial infection by 6.4% (number needed to treat equals 16 to prevent one infection).[15] Active surveillance programs to eliminate nasal colonization in hospital surgical personnel have controlled outbreaks of *S. aureus* SSIs.

TABLE 19-1	Risk Factors for SSI	
Patient-related Factors	**Microbial Factors**	**Wound-related Factors**
Age	Enzyme production	Devitalized tissue
Nutritional status	Polysaccharide capsule	Dead space
ASA score > 2	Bind to fibronectin	Hematoma
Diabetes	Biofilm and slime	Contaminated
Smoking		Foreign material
Obesity		
Co-existing infections		
Colonization		
Immunocompromised		
Length of preoperative stay		

ASA, American Society of Anesthesiologists.

TABLE 19-2 Diagnosis of Surgical Site Infections

Type of SSI	Time Course	Criteria (at Least One)
Superficial incisional SSI	Within 30 days of surgery	Superficial pus drainage Organisms from superficial tissue or fluid Signs and symptoms (pain, redness, swelling, heat) Diagnosis by surgeon
Deep incisional SSI	Within 30 days of surgery or within 1 yr if prosthetic implant	Deep pus drainage Dehiscence or wound opened by surgeon (for fever > 38°C, pain, tenderness) Abscess (e.g., radiographically diagnosed) Diagnosis by surgeon or attending physician
Organ/space SSI	Within 30 days of surgery or within 1 yr if prosthetic implant	Pus from a drain in the organ/space Organisms from aseptically obtained culture of fluid or tissue in the organ/space Abscess involving the organ/space Diagnosis by a surgeon or attending physician

SSI, surgical site infection.

Intraoperative

Prophylactic Antibiotics It was recognized many years ago that prophylactic antimicrobial drugs prevent postoperative wound infections.[16] This is particularly true where the inoculum of bacteria is high, such as in colonic or vaginal surgery, or where there is insertion of an artificial device, for example, a hip prosthesis or heart valve. The organisms that are implicated in SSIs are usually those that are carried as colonizers, for example, in the nose or on the skin, by the patient at the time of surgery. Unless the patient has been in the hospital for some time prior to surgery, these are usually community organisms that have not developed multiple drug resistance. Gram-positive organisms are typical. Antibiotic prophylaxis (within 2 hours) prior to surgical incision is important; these organisms are introduced into the bloodstream with incision. Ideally, antibiotics should be given within 30 minutes of surgical incision. Currently, this recommendation is not being met, and there is tremendous variation in the timing of prophylactic antibiotics.[5] For most procedures, a single dose is adequate. Prolonged surgery (3 hours) may necessitate a second dose. Prophylaxis should usually be discontinued within 24 hours of the procedure. For cardiac surgery, the Joint Commission on Accreditation of Healthcare Organizations has recommended that the duration of prophylaxis be increased to 48 hours. Other surgeries may follow. A first-generation cephalosporin such as cefazolin is effective for many types of surgery. In general, the antibacterial spectrum, low incidence of side effects, and tolerability of cephalosporins have made them the ideal choice for prophylaxis.

For high-risk patients and procedures, the choice of appropriate antibiotics may be important in decreasing the incidence of SSIs. The increasing prevalence of both methicillin-resistant *S. aureus*, against which cephalosporins are ineffective and *Clostridium difficile*–associated diarrhea, a disorder associated with cephalosporin use, may result in the substitution of other agents, such as vancomycin, in the future. The recent alarming emergence of community-acquired methicillin-resistant *S. aureus* has seen the convergence of resistance, virulence, and high prevalence. From 2001 through 2002, there were 1647 cases of community-acquired methicillin-resistant *S. aureus* infection reported in Baltimore, MD, Atlanta, GA, and Minnesota communities, representing between 8% and 20% of all methicillin-resistant *S. aureus* isolates.[17]

When the small bowel is entered, coverage of gram-negative organisms is important, and for the large bowel and the female genital tract, the addition of anaerobic coverage is appropriate. Broadly speaking, infections associated with clean surgery are caused by staphylococcal species, and infections of contaminated surgery are polymicrobial in origin and comprise the flora of the viscus entered (e.g., *E. coli* and *B. fragilis* in colonic surgery). In a controversial study, it was demonstrated that ertapenem, a long-acting carbapenem, may be superior to cefotetan as antibiotic prophylaxis for the prevention of SSI following elective colorectal surgery.[18] The approach taken in this study is counterintuitive. Carbapenems as a class are last-line antimicrobials; they may be the only antibiotics effective against multidrug resistant gram-negative organisms, such as those with extended spectrum β-lactamase enzymes. The use of such drugs for prophylaxis, with the attendant risk of promoting resistance among gram-negative organisms to the carbapenem class, goes against fundamental principles of antibiotic prophylaxis. For high-risk patients, such as those with prosthetic devices or risk factors for infective endocarditis, broader spectrum prophylaxis is appropriate. The main risk factors for infective endocarditis are rheumatic heart disease, prosthetic heart valves, congenital heart disease, mitral valve prolapse with regurgitation, a previous episode of infective endocarditis, and hypertrophic

---

BOX 19-3 Antibiotic Prophylaxis

Administer within 30 minutes before incision.

Increase dose for larger patients.

Repeat dose when surgery exceeds 3 hours.

Use drugs appropriate to type of surgery.

Use drug appropriate for local resistance patterns.

Stop prophylaxis at 24 hours (or 48 hours for cardiac surgery).

Follow American Heart Association guidelines for patients at risk for endocarditis.

---

cardiomyopathy. Guidelines for antimicrobial prophylaxis for those considered at risk of infective endocarditis are published by the American Heart Association.[19] Additional considerations are listed in **Box 19-3**.

Physical and Physiologic Preventive Measures Several simple physical measures have been studied in relation to the incidence of postoperative infection. Much of the work has focused on the oxygen tension at the wound site. Destruction by oxidation, or oxidative killing, is the most important defense against surgical pathogens and depends on the partial pressure of oxygen in contaminated tissue. In patients with normal peripheral perfusion, the subcutaneous oxygen tension is linearly related to the arterial oxygen tension. An inverse correlation has been demonstrated between subcutaneous tissue oxygen tension and the rate of wound infections Tissue hypoxia appears to increase the vulnerability to infection.

Hypothermia has been shown to increase the incidence of SSI. In a study where patients were randomized to hypothermia and normothermia groups, SSI was present in 19% of patients in the hypothermia group, but in only 6% in the normothermia group.[20] Radiant heating at 38°C increases subcutaneous oxygen tension. This may be one of the mechanisms of decreased infection risk with increased temperature. In addition production of oxidative intermediates is related to core temperature, decreasing nearly fourfold over a 4°C range. Impaired neutrophil oxidative killing may contribute to the hypothermia-induced reduction in resistance to infection. Even for some neurosurgical procedures where mild hypothermia has previously been used routinely, hypothermia is associated with an increased risk of infection with no measurable improvement in neurologic function.[21]

Oxygen An easy method of improving oxygen tension is to increase the concentration of inspired oxygen. In a study of 500 patients undergoing colorectal resection, patients were randomized to receive 30% or 80% inspired oxygen during the operation and for 2 hours afterward. There was an absolute risk reduction of SSI of 6% (95% confidence interval = 1.2%–10.8%) in the group that received 80% oxygen.[22] This is an astonishing result. Unfortunately, a subsequent smaller study in a more heterogeneous patient population did not replicate these impressive results and suggested that 80% oxygen increases the risk of SSI.[23] This study had serious design flaws. In a recent Spanish multicenter study of 300 patients

undergoing colorectal resection, patients were randomized to receive 30% or 80% inspired oxygen during the operation and for 6 hours afterward.[24] There was an absolute risk reduction of SSI of 14.5% in the group that received 80% oxygen.[24] Thus two well-conducted studies have now demonstrated that perioperative administration of 80% oxygen decreases the incidence of SSI in patients undergoing colorectal resection. It is unknown whether the perioperative administration of 80% oxygen decreases the incidence of SSI in other surgical settings. The universal adoption of this treatment remains controversial as high inspired oxygen tension may also have adverse effects, such as causing pulmonary damage.

Analgesia Superior treatment of surgical pain is associated with increased postoperative subcutaneous oxygen partial pressures at wound sites. Adequate analgesia may therefore be associated with decreased incidence of SSI. This provides further impetus for aggressive treatment of postoperative pain.

Carbon Dioxide Hypocapnia occurs frequently during anesthesia and is deleterious for many reasons, such as profound vasoconstriction and impaired perfusion to vital organs. Hypercapnia is known to cause vasodilatation and increased skin perfusion. Intriguing research has shown that mild intraoperative hypercapnia increases subcutaneous and colonic oxygen tension.[25] Such increases in tissue oxygen partial pressure may be associated with a reduction in SSI risk. Interestingly, CO_2 is itself bacteriostatic. As CO_2 does not support combustion, a CO_2 environment may also allow the application to the wound of antiseptic ethanol solutions, which are highly bacteriocidal. It is likely, therefore, that interest will increase in possible applications for CO_2 in preventing SSIs.

Fluids There has been speculation that fluid administration may have a positive impact on the incidence of wound infection. Research findings have, however, yielded conflicting results. Supplemental perioperative fluid administration has been shown to increase tissue perfusion and tissue oxygen partial pressure. But there may be a fine balance, as excess fluids may be associated with increased morbidity, especially pulmonary complications. Recent studies have not replicated early findings that supplemental fluid administration decreases the incidence of SSIs. Striving for normovolemia is recommended based on current evidence.[26]

Glucose For patients with and without underlying diabetes, tight control of blood sugar has been suggested to decrease the incidence of SSIs and other infections. In a landmark study, aggressive use of insulin to maintain blood sugar between 80 and 110 mg/dL was shown to decrease episodes of septicemia (by 46%) and mortality in critically ill patients, especially following cardiac surgery.[27] There is currently insufficient information on intraoperative blood sugar control to make firm recommendations about goal blood sugar ranges and about which patients would derive the most benefit from tight control. Recent evidence suggests that variability in blood sugar concentrations, not just tight control, is associated with increased mortality among critically ill patients.[28] Results of studies to date therefore suggest that in the perioperative period, the ideal blood sugar goal should be a narrow

BOX 19-4 Tips to Decrease Surgical Site Infection

Ensure hand hygiene with alcohol.

Observe strict asepsis.

Use appropriate antibiotics: timing, dose, and duration.

Keep glucose tight and consistent.

Maintain normothermia.

Promote adequate tissue oxygenation.

BOX 19-5 Most Common Pathogens Associated with Bloodstream Infections (1992–1999)[32]

Pathogen (% of total)

Coagulase-negative staphylococci (37%)

Staphylococcus aureus (13%)

Enterococcus (13%)

Gram-negative bacilli (14%)

   Escherichia coli (2%)

   Enterobacter spp. (5%)

   Pseudomonas aeruginosa (4%)

   Klebsiella pneumoniae (3%)

Candida spp. (8%)

National Nosocomial Infections Surveillance (NNIS) System report, data summary from January 1990 May 1999, issued June 1999. Am J Infect Control 1999 27: 520–532.

physiologic range with minimal variability over time. High blood sugar is thought to inhibit leukocyte function and to provide a favorable environment for bacterial growth. Interestingly, the therapy for hyperglycemia may itself have beneficial effects; the administration of glucose, insulin, and potassium stimulates lymphocytes to proliferate and attack pathogens. Glucose, insulin, and potassium may play an important role in restoring immunocompetence to patients with immunocompromise.[29]

Box 19-4 lists several key elements in decreasing SSI.

BLOODSTREAM INFECTION

Bloodstream infections (BSIs) are among the top three nosocomial infections. Anesthesiologists have an important role in the prevention and often the treatment of BSIs. Central venous catheters are the predominant cause of nosocomial bacteremia and fungemia.[30] A total of 250,000 cases of central venous catheter–associated BSIs have been estimated to occur annually in the United States with an attributable mortality rate estimated at 12% to 25% for each infection.[31] The CDC recommends that the rate of catheter-associated BSIs be expressed as the number of catheter-associated BSIs per 1000 central venous catheter days.[32] This parameter is more useful than the rate expressed as the number of catheter-associated infections per 100 catheters (or percentage of catheters studied) because it accounts for BSIs over time and therefore adjusts risk of the number of days that the catheter is in use.[31]

Signs and Symptoms

Patients typically have nonspecific signs of infection with no obvious candidate source, no cloudy urine, purulent sputum, pus drainage, wound inflammation, other than an indwelling infected catheter. Inflammation at the catheter insertion site is suggestive. A sudden change in a patient's condition should alert an astute clinician to the possibility of a BSI. Important signs include mental status changes, hemodynamic instability, altered tolerance for nutrition, and generalized malaise.

Diagnosis

Catheter-associated BSIs are defined as bacteremia/fungemia in a patient with an intravascular catheter with at least one positive blood culture obtained from a peripheral vein, clinical manifestations of infection, and no apparent source for the BSI except the catheter. Bloodstream infections are considered to be associated with a central line if the line was in use during the 48-hour period before the development of the BSI. If the time interval between the onset of infection and device use is greater than 48 hours, there should be compelling evidence that the infection is related to the central line. The diagnosis is more compelling if, when a catheter is removed, the same organisms that grow from blood grow abundantly from the catheter tip.

Box 19-5 lists some of the pathogens associated with BSI.

Treatment

The best treatment is prevention, with BSI often leading to severe sepsis, multiorgan failure, and death. The source of the infection, usually a central venous catheter, should be removed and broad-spectrum empirical antimicrobial therapy should be initiated pending the results of the cultures, at which point therapy should be appropriately narrowed and targeted. Resistance patterns (both general and in individual hospitals) may dictate initial therapy. Data from the United States are very concerning. Most coagulase-negative staphylococci and more than 50% of *S. aureus* from ICUs are oxacillin resistant.[32] More than 25% of enterococci isolates from ICUs are vancomycin resistant,[32] and this proportion is increasing.[33] As for the gram-negative ICU isolates, many of them produce extended-spectrum β-lactamases, particularly *K. pneumoniae*, rendering them resistant to most antibiotics including even fourth-generation cephalosporins and extended spectrum penicillins, such as piperacillin/tazobactam.[34] Half of the *Candida* BSIs are associated with non-*Albicans* species, such as *Candida glabrata*, *Candida tropicalis*, *Candida parapsilosis*, and *Candida krusei*, which are likely to be resistant to fluconazole and itraconazole.[35] Based on these resistance patterns, it is difficult to strike a compromise between appropriate initial empirical coverage and not exhausting the last-line antimicrobial agents with the first salvo. Clinical judgment should be based on the severity of the patient's condition, the known susceptibility patterns of organisms at a particular institution, and the organisms that are currently implicated in infection in a particular environment. In order to delay widespread resistance to all antimicrobial agents, therapy *must* be narrowed as soon as organisms are identified and susceptibility is known. The principles of management for patients with BSIs are as for other causes of sepsis.

Preoperative

Anesthesiologists have an essential role to play in the prevention of BSIs. Many central venous catheters are placed by anesthesiologists who may be unaware about BSIs that present days later. The subclavian route is preferable to the internal jugular, which carries less risk of infection than the femoral route. The decision about route has to be balanced against the higher risk of pneumothorax with a subclavian catheter. A recent interventional study targeted five evidence-based procedures recommended by the CDC and identified as having the greatest effect on the rate of catheter-related BSIs and the lowest barriers to implementation.[36] The interventions were hand washing, the use of full-barrier precautions during central venous catheter insertion, cleaning the skin with chlorhexidine, avoiding the femoral site if possible, and removing unnecessary catheters. This evidence-based interventional study resulted in a large and sustained reduction (up to 66%) in rates of catheter-related BSIs that was maintained throughout the 18-month study period.[37] During insertion, catheter contamination rates can be further reduced by rinsing gloved hands in a solution of chlorhexidine in alcohol prior to handling the catheter. Sterility must be maintained with frequent hand decontamination and cleaning catheter ports each time with alcohol prior to accessing them. The same high standards of sterility should be applied for regional anesthetic techniques. Central venous catheters may be coated or impregnated with antimicrobial or antiseptic agents, such as silver/platinum/carbon impregnation or chlorhexidine/silver sulfadiazine or rifampicin/minocycline coating.[30] Such catheters have been associated with a lower incidence of BSIs.[30] Concerns about widespread adoption are increased costs and promotion of further microbial resistance. Such catheters may be indicated for the most vulnerable patients, such as those with immunocompromise.

Intraoperative

Transfusion of blood and blood components increase postoperative infection through two mechanisms: direct transmission of organisms and immunosuppression.[38] Even autologous blood transfusion results in natural killer cell inhibition and is intrinsically immunosuppressive. The mechanisms of immunosuppression may be related to the infusion of allogeneic donor leukocytes, or their products, present in the cellular blood products used for the transfusion. Blood transfusion–associated immunosuppression may be decreased by leukodepletion. Nonetheless, numerous studies have shown that transfusion is associated with increased morbidity and mortality. Analysis of a database of 4892 ICU patients suggested that blood transfusion is an independent predictor of an increased incidence of BSIs.[39] Transfusion is not a benign intervention and should be avoided wherever possible.

Transfusion of cellular blood components has been implicated in transmission of viral, bacterial, and protozoan diseases. Over the past 20 years, reductions in the risk of viral infection via blood components have been achieved. Until recently, the tests for viral contamination of blood components were based on the presence of antibodies. During early viral infection with human immunodeficiency virus (HIV) and hepatitis C virus, there is a "window period" during which antibodies are not yet present and there is a significant viral count. Those infected are healthy but highly infective during this window period. Mini-pool nucleic acid–amplification testing detects virus during the window period and has prevented transmission of approximately five HIV-1 and 56 hepatitis C virus infections annually in the United States and has decreased the risk of HIV-1 and hepatitis C virus transmission to one in two million blood transfusions.[40]

As a result of this success, bacterial contamination of blood products has emerged as the greatest residual source of transfusion-transmitted disease.[41] Each year, approximately nine million platelet-unit concentrates are transfused in the United States; an estimated one in 1000 to 3000 platelet units are contaminated with bacteria.[42] Platelets, to maintain viability and function, must be stored at room temperature, which creates an excellent growth environment for bacteria. In some instances, contaminated units contain large numbers of endotoxins as well as potentially virulent bacteria, such as coagulase-negative staphylococci, *S. aureus*, *Bacillus cereus*, *S. marcescens*, streptococci, and *P. aeruginosa*.[43] Only organisms that grow at cold temperature, such as *Yersinia enterocolitica*, are able to grow in refrigerated blood. The prevalence of severe episodes of transfusion-associated sepsis is probably approximately 1 in 50,000 for platelet units and 1 in 500,000 for red blood cell units transfused. Implementation of bacterial detection methods could improve safety and extend the shelf-life of platelets.[44] The use of urine dipsticks has been proposed to detect rapidly possible bacterial contamination in platelet concentrates. Low glucose and pH are suggestive of possible bacterial contamination. The new College of American Pathologists Checklist, which became effective in December 2003, is a Phase 1 requirement that calls for inspected facilities to have a platelet bacteria detection method in place.[45] While transfusion is undoubtedly a lot safer than in past years, new infectious agents continue to enter the donor population, and there is an inherent time delay before the new pathogens are definitively identified and new tests implemented in order to maintain consistent safety of the blood supply. A recent example is variant Creutzfeldt-Jakob disease, (**Box 19-6**) the agent responsible for bovine spongiform encephalopathy or mad cow disease. It was previously thought the variant Creutzfeldt-Jakob disease could not be spread via transfusion.[46] This illusion has been shattered by the transmission of variant Creutzfeldt-Jakob disease to recipients of blood components.[46,47] With its long incubation period of up to 40 years, many asymptomatic blood donors may pass

Variant Creutzfeldt-Jakob disease (CJD) is a human transmissible spongiform encephalopathy. Patients may have behavioral and psychiatric disturbances, failure of muscular coordination, and memory impairment. The major cause of variant CJD is the consumption of bovine spongiform encephalopathy–infected meat. The infective agent is a prion, which is an infectious protein lacking nucleic acid. Young people are frequently affected, and death typically occurs within 2 years of the onset of symptoms, although there is a long (up to decades) incubation period. Until recently it was not thought that variant CJD could be transmitted through blood component transfusion. It is now known that it can be. Prions are resistant to destruction and may survive cleaning and perhaps even surgical sterilization. It is not known whether variant CJD may be transmitted by contaminated surgical instruments or anesthetic devices, such as reusable laryngeal mask airways. Variant CJD cannot at present be diagnosed from a blood specimen.

Bloodstream infections (BSIs) are among the top three nosocomial infections.

Central venous catheters are the predominant cause of BSIs.

Resistant organisms are commonly implicated in BSIs.

Asepsis during central line insertion decreases the likelihood of BSI.

Blood component transfusion causes immunosuppression.

Platelets are often contaminated with bacteria.

Avoid blood component transfusion if possible.

Remove suspected catheters.

Management principles are as for sepsis.

on this disease unless techniques emerge to detect variant Creutzfeldt-Jakob disease in asymptomatic carriers. The best way to avoid infectious complications of transfusion is to avoid transfusion.

Postoperative

Remove central lines and pulmonary artery catheters as soon as they are no longer needed. Avoid unnecessary parenteral nutrition and even dextrose-containing fluid as these may be associated with increased risk of BSI. Food and sugar can usually be withheld for a while or given into the gut rather than into a vein.

Box 19-7 reiterates the previous discussion about BSIs.

SEPSIS

Sepsis is an umbrella term encompassing conditions where there are pathogenic microorganisms in the body. Sepsis may result in life-threatening conditions precipitated by the organisms, their toxins, and the body's own defensive inflammatory response. Sepsis is a spectrum of disorders on a continuum with localized inflammation at one end and severe generalized inflammatory response with multiorgan failure at the other end (**Fig. 19-2**).[48] Surgery and anesthesia should ideally be postponed until sepsis is at least partially treated. However, sometimes the underlying cause of sepsis requires urgent surgical intervention. This may be termed source control. Examples include abscesses, infective endocarditis, bowel perforation or infarction, infected prosthetic device (e.g., intravenous catheter, intrauterine device, pacemaker), endometritis, and necrotizing fasciitis. Organisms frequently implicated in sepsis include *Streptococcus pyogenes*, *Streptococcus pneumoniae*, *S. aureus*, gram-negative bacilli (e.g., *Klebsiella* spp., *E. coli*, *P. aeruginosa*, *H. influenzae*), *Neisseria meningitides*, *C. albicans*, and *C. perfringens*.

Bacterial components such as endotoxin and lipoteichoic acid, through their action on neutrophils and macrophages, induce a wide range of proinflammatory factors, including

tumor necrosis factor α and interleukin-1 and interleukin-6, and counterregulatory host responses, interleukin-4 and interleukin-10, that turn off production of the proinflammatory cytokines.[49] Recently, the pivotal roles of Toll-like receptors on cell surfaces have been recognized in binding to bacterial components and in promoting cytokine production and cellular activation.[49] Normally there is a balance between

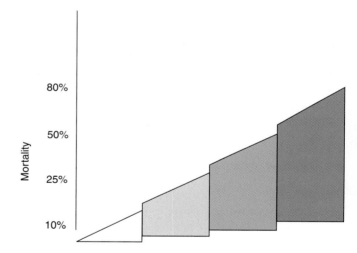

	Infection	Sepsis	Severe sepsis	Septic shock
Definition	Pathogens detected in blood or tissue	Infection plus systemic inflammatory response syndrome (SIRS)	Sepsis plus organ dysfunction: Lactic acidosis Oliguria Confusion Hepatic dysfunction	Severe sepsis plus hypotension (systolic BP < 90 mm Hg despite adequate fluid resuscitation)
Estimated mortality	0–10%	10%–25%	25%–50%	50%–80%

Figure 19-2 • Continuum of sepsis with definitions and approximate mortality rates. (*Adapted from Bone RC: Toward an epidemiology and natural history of systemic inflammatory response syndrome. JAMA 1992;268:3452–3455.*)

pro- and anti-inflammatory responses.[49,50] As a result of sepsis, the proinflammatory reaction (systemic inflammatory response syndrome) can cascade, out of control, with activation of complement, coagulation, widespread arterial vasodilatation, and altered capillary permeability. A range of abnormalities may result, leading to multiorgan dysfunction and death.[49] If there is a predominance of the compensatory anti-inflammatory response syndrome, which often occurs subsequently, patients become more vulnerable to infection, including opportunistic organisms.[50]

Signs and Symptoms

Signs and symptoms of sepsis are often nonspecific. Presentation varies according to the initial source of infection. The systemic inflammatory response syndrome (**Box 19-8**) is an important component of sepsis.[51]

Sepsis may result in multiple organ system failure. Features of infection, including fever, altered mental status, and encephalopathy, and deranged blood sugar may be present. Septic shock refers to hemodynamic instability that may accompany sepsis. Classically, there is hypotension, bounding pulses, and wide pulse pressure. These are characteristic signs of high-output cardiac failure and distributive shock, both of which may occur with sepsis.[50]

Diagnosis

A diagnosis of sepsis is surmised from history, signs, and symptoms. Confirmation is based on the isolation of specific causative pathogens. It is important to hone in on the culprit microbe to ensure that antimicrobial therapy is appropriate. Cultures should be sent from all sources where organism growth is suspected. Blood, urine, and sputum cultures are the default. Tissue samples, such as heart valves, bone marrow, and cerebrospinal fluid, are also important sources of organisms.

Treatment

The initial treatment of sepsis is with broad antimicrobial coverage coupled with supportive care of failing organ systems. Door-to-needle time has often been applied to thrombolytic medications, but the urgency of administering treatment is arguably even more pressing for life-threatening infections. The replication of virulent bacteria, such as *S. pyogenes*, is so rapid that every minute may be crucial. As soon as specific microbiologic information is available, therapy should be tailored according to the specific organism and its

---

BOX 19-8 Systemic Inflammatory Response Syndrome

Two or more of the following

White blood cell count > 11,000 or < 4000 ×10⁹/L or > 10% immature forms

Heart rate > 90 bpm

Temperature > 38°C or < 36°C

Respiratory rate > 20 breaths per minute or Paco₂ < 32 mm Hg

---

sensitivities. This is imperative for several reasons. Targeted therapy may decrease the likelihood of the emergence of multidrug-resistant organisms. Also, while some antimicrobials, such as penicillin, may have relatively narrow spectra of activity, they may be more effective at killing susceptible organisms than broad-spectrum alternatives. The choice of antimicrobial agent should not only be guided by in vitro susceptibility tests. Agents should also be chosen according to their ability to penetrate various tissues, including bone, cerebrospinal fluid, lung tissue, and abscess cavities.

Apart from targeted antimicrobial therapy, supportive treatment relating to organ system dysfunction is essential. Early goal-directed optimization targeting oxygen delivery and cardiac output might improve outcome in sepsis.[52] Parameters such as mixed venous or central venous saturation may be useful guides for therapeutic end points. Early fluid resuscitation is usually indicated. Appropriate use of inotropes and vasoconstrictors may be important. Apart from hemodynamic support, measures to bolster other failing organ systems should be taken[52,53] (**Table 19-3**).

Prognosis

Prognosis in sepsis depends on the virulence of the infecting pathogen(s), the stage at which appropriate treatment is initiated, the inflammatory response of the patient, the immune statues of the patient, and the extent of organ system dysfunction. It is impossible to predict the outcome for individual patients. General scoring systems for ICU and surgical patients, such as the APACHE II (Acute Physiology and Chronic Health Evaluation) and SAPS II scores provide useful epidemiological tools. The Organ Dysfunctions and/or Infection and Sepsis-Related Organ Failure Assessment scores were developed as epidemiological prognostication tools for patient populations with sepsis.

Management of Anesthesia
Preoperative

The most important questions for a patient with sepsis are whether the surgery may be postponed pending treatment of sepsis and whether, if surgery is urgent, the patient's condition may be improved prior to surgery. Septic patients may be extremely unstable and support of failing organ systems may occupy entirely the attention of the physician. Nonetheless, it is crucial to remember that the early and appropriate administration of antimicrobials may be the intervention that has the best chance to alter the course of the disease. The treatment algorithm (**Fig. 19-3**)[54] suggests goal-directed optimization of patients who present with sepsis.[52] Resuscitation should be targeted to achieve mean arterial pressure greater than 65 mm Hg, central venous pressure of 8 to 12 mm Hg, adequate urine output, a "normal" pH without a metabolic (lactic) acidosis, and a mixed venous or central venous saturation above 70%.[52]

Intraoperative

Intraoperative management of patients with sepsis is challenging. Patients with sepsis may have limited physiologic

TABLE 19-3 Organ System Dysfunction in Sepsis

Organ System	Manifestations of Dysfunction	Treatment and Support
Central nervous system	Encephalopathy, decreased Glasgow Coma Scale score	Consider airway protection (e.g., intubation), daily interruption of sedation to assess neurologic status
Cardiovascular	Vasodilatory shock, myocardial depression	Maintain mean arterial pressure > 65 mm Hg, central venous pressure of 8–12 cm H_2O, and central or mixed venous saturation > 70%; fluid resuscitation, vasoconstrictors (e.g., norepinephrine, vasopressin); inotropes (e.g., epinephrine)
Respiratory	Impaired oxygenation (decreased Pao_2/Fio_2), acute respiratory distress syndrome	Assisted ventilation with low tidal volumes (6–8 mL/kg ideal body mass) and target mean airway pressures < 30 cm H_2O
Renal	Renal failure (elevated creatinine)	Attempt to maintain urine output > 0.5 mL/kg/hr; renal replacement therapy such as continuous venovenous hemodialysis
Hematologic	Thrombocytopenia or disseminated intravascular coagulopathy	Target hemoglobin of 7–9 g/dL Treatment is controversial; consider heparin or recombinant activated protein C; anticoagulants are contraindicated at the time of surgery; platelet transfusion may be indicated for surgery
Gastrointestinal	Hepatic dysfunction (elevated bilirubin)	Treatment is supportive; fresh frozen plasma or vitamin K may be required to correct a deranged international normalized ratio at the time of surgery
Endocrine	Hyperglycemia, adrenal insufficiency	Insulin infusion to achieve blood sugars of 80–150 mg/dL; check random and stimulated adrenal function; consider empirical hydrocortisone (e.g., 50–100 mg IV for refractory hypotension)

reserve, rendering them vulnerable to hypotension and hypoxemia with induction of anesthesia. Invasive monitoring, such as invasive blood pressure and central venous access, is usually indicated. Sufficient intravenous access is essential to allow massive volume resuscitation as well as transfusion of blood and blood components. Antimicrobial prophylaxis appropriate for surgery is needed. Ideally, this could be combined with the treatment regimen for the pathogen thought to be responsible for the sepsis. Prophylactic antibiotics should ideally be administered within 30 minutes of skin incision. The same principles that apply in general to preventing infection following surgery apply to patients with sepsis undergoing surgery, such as stringent efforts to maintain normothermia and normoglycemia.[20,27] Infusions of inotropes (e.g., epinephrine) and vasoconstrictors (e.g., norepinephrine and vasopressin) should be available. Intravenous steroids may be indicated for refractory shock. The principles of management outlined in **Table 19-4** and Figure 19-3 apply.

Postoperative (If Applicable)

Patients with sepsis invariably merit ICU admission following surgery. In the ICU, the priorities are to support failing organ systems, to target antimicrobial therapy, and to try to minimize the likelihood of new infections (such as fungal infections and *C. difficile* or the emergence of resistant organisms). Another important postoperative priority is to continue antimicrobial therapy only for as long as it is indicated. The broad guidelines for the treatment of patients with sepsis in the ICU have been published in the "Surviving Sepsis" Consensus Guidelines[54] (see Fig. 19-3).

Box 19-9 summarizes the key points in approaching sepsis.

NECROTIZING SOFT-TISSUE INFECTION

This is a nonspecific blanket term that may encompass such diagnoses as gas gangrene, toxic shock syndromes, Fournier's gangrene, severe cellulitis, and flesh-eating infection. One of the most important aspects of these infections is that the severity may be underappreciated at the time of presentation. The organisms responsible are highly virulent, the clinical course is rampant, and mortality is high (up to 75%).[55] Fournier's gangrene was eponymously named for the French physician Jean Alfred Fournier, who described scrotal gangrene in five young men. He noted a sudden onset, rapid progression to gangrene, and an absence of a definite cause. Toxic shock syndrome was described in women and was attributed to staphylococcal infection. It was often associated with the presence of foreign bodies, such as tampons and indwelling contraceptive devices. Necrotizing soft-tissue infections are surgical emergencies and represent a subclass of severe sepsis with all the attendant complications.

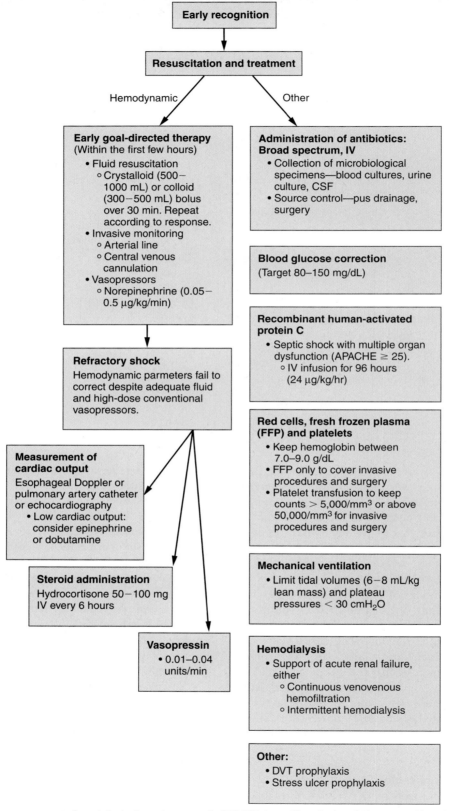

Figure 19-3 • Postoperative management of sepsis in the intensive care unit. APACHE, Acute Physiology and Chronic Health Evaluation II; CSF, cerebrospinal fluid; DVT, deep vein thrombosis; FFP, fresh frozen plasma.

TABLE 19-4 Clinical Pulmonary Infection Score Calculation

Parameter	Options	Score
Temperature (°C)	≥36.5 and ≤38.4 : 0	0
	≥38.5 and ≤38.9 : 1	1
	≥39 or ≤36 : 2	2
Blood leukocytes (mm³)	≥4000 and ≤11,000 : 0	0
	<4000 or >11000 : 1	1
	+ band forms ≥ 50%, add 1	Add 1
Tracheal secretions	Absence of tracheal secretions : 0	0
	Presence of non-purulent tracheal secretions : 1	1
	Presence of purulent tracheal secretions : 2	2
Oxygenation: Pao_2/Fio_2 (mm Hg)	>240 or ARDS : 0	0
	≤240 and no ARDS : 2	2
Pulmonary radiography	No infiltrate : 0	0
	Diffuse (or patchy) infiltrate 1	1
	Localized infiltrate : 2	2
Progression of pulmonary infiltrate	No radiographic progression : 0	0
	Radiographic progression (after cardiac failure and ARDS excluded) : 2	2
Culture of tracheal aspirate	Pathogenic bacteria cultured in rare or light quantity	0
	Pathogenic bacteria cultured in moderate or heavy quantity	1
	Same pathogenic bacteria seen on Gram stain	Add 1

ARDS, acute respiratory distress syndrome.
Reproduced from Luyt CE, Chastre J, Fagon JY: Value of the clinical pulmonary infection score for the identification and management of ventilator-associated pneumonia. Intensive Care Med 2004;30:844–852; with permission.

BOX 19-9 Sepsis

Sepsis may result in life-threatening conditions precipitated by organisms, their toxins, and the body's inflammatory response.

Normally there is a balance between pro- and anti-inflammatory responses.

Cultures should be sent from all sources where organism growth is suspected.

The initial treatment is with broad antimicrobial coverage coupled with supportive care of failing organ systems.

Early goal-directed optimization targeting oxygen delivery and cardiac output might improve outcome.

Broad guidelines for the treatment of patients with sepsis have been published in the Surviving Sepsis Consensus Guidelines.

Signs and Symptoms

Patients may presents with general features of infection, including malaise, fever, sweating, and altered mental status. Pain is invariable and may be out of proportion to physical signs. Specific features may include scrotal swelling and erythema, vaginal discharge, tissue inflammation, pus, or subcutaneous air (crepitus). The cutaneous signs are often surprisingly mild and are not reflective of the extent of tissue necrosis or the severity of the disease. This is because necrotizing skin infections begin in deep tissue planes.[56]

Hypotension is an ominous sign and may presage the progression to septic shock. The resolution of pain may also be ominous, as this may occur with the progression to gangrene.

Diagnosis

History is important in suggesting a diagnosis. Patients with a history of alcohol use, malnutrition, obesity, trauma, cancer, burns, older age, vascular disease, and diabetes are more susceptible. Patients who have underlying immunocompromise, such as those taking immunosuppressant therapy or those infected with HIV, are more frequently affected. There may be a high white blood cell count, thrombocytopenia, coagulopathy, electrolyte abnormalities, acidosis, hyperglycemia, elevated markers of inflammation such as C reactive protein, and radiographic evidence of extensive necrotic inflammation with subcutaneous air. Ultrasonography may be useful, and computed tomography or magnetic resonance imaging may delineate the extent of necrotic tissue. Blood, urine, and tissue cultures should be sent to the laboratory. Organisms most frequently grown from necrotic tissue include *S. pyogenes*, *S. aureus*, *S. epidermidis*, *Bacteroides* spp., *C. perfringens*, and gram-negative organisms, especially *E. coli*. Polymicrobial infection is common.[56] Multidrug-resistant organisms, such as enterococci, have been described.

Treatment

The definitive treatment is extensive surgical débridement of necrotic tissue coupled with appropriate antimicrobial therapy, which typically includes coverage of gram-positive, gram-negative, and anaerobic organisms. The principle of antimicrobial therapy is to start empirical broad coverage and to narrow the spectrum when specific organisms have been grown and their susceptibility has been tested. Antifungal agents may be added if fungal infection is strongly suspected. Clindamycin has been advocated as a useful agent for toxic shock syndrome as it is speculated to "turn off" staphylococcal and streptococcal toxin production. Topical therapy is beneficial. Natural unprocessed honey may be useful to digest necrotic tissue and to promote wound healing.[57] Hyperbaric oxygen therapy has been described and is of theoretical benefit.

Prognosis

There is a high mortality secondary to rampant sepsis caused by virulent organisms. If patients survive the initial insult, they may remain vulnerable to secondary infection. Patients may require repeated anesthesia for débridements, reconstructive surgery, and skin grafts.

Management of Anesthesia

Preoperative

The extent of the necrosis and the severity of the infection may not be immediately apparent. The anesthesiologist should treat such patients as having severe sepsis and try to resuscitate preoperatively. This may be best achieved in the ICU with goal-directed therapy, including intravenous fluids and improving global oxygen delivery, reflected by resolution of a lactic acidosis or an increase in central or mixed venous saturation. However, surgical débridement should not be postponed as delay is associated with increased mortality.

Intraoperative

Concern has been raised about the use of etomidate when patients have septic shock as they may already have adrenal insufficiency, which may be worsened theoretically even by a singly dose of etomidate.[58] Major fluid shifts, blood loss, and release of cytokines may occur intraoperatively. Good intravenous access is essential, and invasive arterial and central venous monitoring may provide valuable information. With the risk of bleeding, blood should be cross-matched and readily available. Patients are at risk of developing both hypovolemic and septic shock. The anesthesiologist should be prepared to treat both conditions.

Postoperative

As with sepsis in general, patients are at risk of developing multiorgan failure. Postoperative admission to an ICU is desirable. Antibiotic therapy should be continued in the postoperative period and should be targeted to the organisms that grow from tissue specimens.

Issues regarding necrotizing soft infections are reviewed in **Box 19-10**.

482

BOX 19-10 Necrotizing Soft-Tissue Infections

These are surgical emergencies with high mortality.

The cutaneous signs are not reflective of the extent of tissue necrosis.

Patients may be much sicker than they look.

Polymicrobial infection including aerobes and anaerobes is common.

The complications are as with sepsis, including multiorgan failure.

Goal-directed optimization and resuscitation might improve outcome.

TETANUS

Tetanus is caused by the gram-negative bacillus *Clostridium tetani*. Elaboration of the neurotoxin tetanospasmin by vegetative forms of these organisms is responsible for the clinical manifestations of tetanus. With the exception of botulinum toxin, tetanospasmin is the most powerful poison known to humans. Tetanospasmin, when elaborated into wounds, spreads centrally along motor nerves to the spinal cord or enters the systemic circulation to reach the central nervous system. This toxin affects the nervous system in several areas. In the spinal cord, tetanospasmin suppresses inhibitory internuncial neurons, resulting in generalized skeletal muscle contractions (spasms). In the brain, there is fixation of toxin by gangliosides. The fourth cerebral ventricle is believed to have selective permeability for tetanospasmin, resulting in early manifestations of trismus and neck rigidity. Sympathetic nervous system hyperactivity may manifest as the disease progresses.[59]

Signs and Symptoms

Trismus is the presenting symptom of tetanus in 75% of patients. The greater strength of the masseter muscles, compared with the opposing digastric and mylohyoid muscles, results in lockjaw. Indeed, these patients may initially seek dental attention. Rigidity of the facial muscles results in the characteristic appearance described as the "sardonic smile" (risus sardonicus). Spasm of laryngeal muscles can occur at any time. Intractable pharyngeal spasms following tracheal extubation has been described in patients with unrecognized tetanus.[60] Dysphagia may be due to spasm of the pharyngeal muscles. Spasm of the intercostal muscles and the diaphragm interferes with adequate ventilation. The rigidity of abdominal and lumbar muscles accounts for the opisthotonic posture. Skeletal muscle spasms are tonic and clonic in nature and are excruciatingly painful. Furthermore, the increased skeletal muscle work is associated with dramatic increases in oxygen consumption, and peripheral vasoconstriction can contribute to increased body temperature.

External stimulation, including sudden exposure to bright light, unexpected noise, or tracheal suction, can precipitate generalized skeletal muscle spasms, leading to inadequate ventilation and then death. Hypotension has been attributed to myocarditis. Isolated and unexplained tachycardia may be early manifestations of hyperactivity of the sympathetic nervous system. More often this hyperactivity manifests as transient systemic hypertension. Sympathetic nervous system responses to external stimuli are exaggerated, as demonstrated by cardiac tachydysrhythmias and labile systemic blood pressure. In addition, excessive sympathetic nervous system activity is associated with intense peripheral vasoconstriction, diaphoresis, and increased urinary excretion of catecholamines. Inappropriate secretion of antidiuretic hormone manifesting as hyponatremia as well as decreased plasma osmolarity may occur.

Treatment

Treatment of patients with tetanus is directed toward controlling the skeletal muscle spasms, preventing sympathetic nervous system hyperactivity, supporting ventilation, neutralizing circulating exotoxin, and surgically débriding the affected area to eliminate the source of the exotoxin. Diazepam (40–100 mg/day IV) is useful for controlling skeletal muscle spasms. If skeletal muscle spasms are not controlled by diazepam, administration of nondepolarizing muscle relaxants and mechanical ventilation of the patient's lungs via a tracheal tube are necessary. Indeed early, aggressive protection of the patient's upper airway is important, as laryngospasm may accompany generalized skeletal muscle spasms. Overactivity of the sympathetic nervous system is best managed with intravenous administration of β-antagonists such as propranolol and esmolol. Continuous epidural anesthesia has also been used to control tetanus-induced sympathetic nervous system hyperactivity.[61] The circulating exotoxin is neutralized with intramuscular human hyperimmunoglobulin. This neutralization does not alter the symptoms already present but does prevent additional exotoxin from reaching the central nervous system. Penicillin destroys the exotoxin-producing vegetative forms of *C. tetani*.

Management of Anesthesia

General anesthesia including tracheal intubation is a useful approach for surgical débridement. Such débridement is delayed until several hours after the patient has received antitoxin because tetanospasmin is mobilized into the systemic circulation during surgical resection. Monitoring often includes continuous recording of systemic blood pressure via an intra-arterial catheter and measuring the central venous pressure. Volatile anesthetics are useful for maintenance of anesthesia if excessive sympathetic nervous system activity is present. Drugs such as lidocaine, esmolol, metoprolol, magnesium, nicardipine, and nitroprusside should be readily available to treat excessive sympathetic nervous system activity during the perioperative period.

Box 19-11 reviews the key findings in tetanus.

PNEUMONIA

Combined with influenza, community-acquired pneumonia is one of the 10 leading causes of death in the United States.

> **BOX 19-11   Tetanus**
>
> The neurotoxin tetanospasmin expressed by *Clostridium tetani* is responsible for the clinical manifestations of tetanus.
>
> Tetanospasmin spreads centrally along motor nerves to the spinal cord or enters the systemic circulation to reach the central nervous system.
>
> Autonomic dysfunction with sympathetic nervous system hyperactivity is common.
>
> Generalized muscle spasm and lockjaw may occur.
>
> Treatment entails controlling muscle spasms, preventing sympathetic hyperactivity, supporting ventilation, neutralizing exotoxin, and débriding the affected area to eliminate the source of the exotoxin.

S. pneumoniae is by far the most frequent cause of bacterial pneumonia in adults. Other bacteria that cause pneumonia include *H. influenzae*, *Mycoplasma pneumoniae*, *S. aureus*, *Legionella pneumophilia*, *K. pneumoniae*, and *Chlamydia pneumoniae*. *S. pneumoniae* usually causes typical pneumonia. Influenzavirus, *M. pneumoniae*, chlamydia, legionella, adenovirus, and other microorganisms may cause atypical pneumonia.[62]

Diagnosis

An initial chill, followed by abrupt onset of fever, chest pain, dyspnea, fatigue, rigors, cough, and copious sputum production often characterize bacterial pneumonia, although symptoms vary. Nonproductive cough is a feature of atypical pneumonias. A detailed history may suggest possible causative organisms. Hotels and whirlpools are associated with Legionnaires' disease (*L. pneumoniae*) outbreaks. Fungal pneumonia may occur with cave exploration (*Histoplasma capsulatum*) and diving (*Scedosporium angiospermum*). *Chlamydia psittaci* pneumonia may follow contact with birds and Q fever (*Coxiella burnetti*) contact with sheep. Alcoholism may increase the risk of bacterial aspiration such as *K. pneumoniae*. Patients who are immunocompromised, such as those with AIDS, are at risk of fungal pneumonia, such as *Pneumocystis jiroveci* pneumonia (PCP).

Posteroanterior and lateral chest radiographs may be extremely helpful in diagnosing pneumonia.[63] Diffuse infiltrates are suggestive of an atypical pneumonia whereas a lobar radiographic opacification is suggestive of a typical pneumonia. Atypical pneumonia occurs more frequently in young adults. Radiography is useful for detecting pleural effusions and multilobar involvement. Polymorphonuclear leukocytosis is typical, and arterial hypoxemia may occur in severe cases of bacterial pneumonia. Arterial hypoxemia reflects intrapulmonary shunting of blood owing to perfusion of alveoli filled with inflammatory exudates.

Microscopic examination of sputum plus cultures and sensitivity testing may be helpful in suggesting the etiologic diagnosis of pneumonia and in guiding the selection of appropriate antibiotic treatment. *S. pneumoniae* and gram-negative organisms, such as *H. influenzae*, may be seen on sputum stain or culture. Unfortunately, sputum specimens are frequently inadequate and organisms do not invariably grow from sputum. Interpretation of sputum culture may be challenging, as there is frequent normal nasopharyngeal carriage of *S. pneumoniae*. If there is suspicion, sputum specimens should be sent for acid-fast bacilli (tuberculosis). Antigen detection in urine is a good test for *L. pneumophilia*. Blood antibody titers are helpful in diagnosing *M. pneumoniae*. Sputum polymerase chain reaction is useful for chlamydia.[62] Blood cultures are usually negative, but are important to rule our bacteremia. HIV is an important risk factor for pneumonia and should be tested for when pneumonia is suspected.

Treatment

For severe pneumonia, empirical therapy is typically a combination such as a cephalosporin (e.g., cefuroxime or ceftriaxone) plus a macrolide (e.g., azithromycin or clarithromycin) antibiotic. There may be an increasing role for newer quinolones such as moxifloxacin in the treatment of community-acquired pneumonia.[64] Therapy is advised for 10 days for *S. pneumoniae* and for 14 days for *M. pneumoniae* and *C. pneumoniae*. Therapy should be narrowed and targeted when the pathogen is identified. When symptoms resolve, therapy can be switched from intravenous to oral. The inappropriate prescription of antibiotics for nonbacterial respiratory tract infections is common and promotes antibiotic resistance. It has recently been demonstrated that even brief administration of macrolide antibiotics to healthy subjects promotes resistance of oral streptococcal flora that lasts for months.[65] Resistance of *S. pneumoniae* is becoming a major problem.

Prognosis

The Pneumonia Severity Index is a useful tool for aiding clinical judgment, guiding appropriate management, and suggesting prognosis.[66] Old age and co-existing organ dysfunction have a negative impact. Physical examination findings associated with worse outcome are

T temperature > 40°C or < 35°C

R respiratory rate > 30/min

A altered mental status

S systolic blood pressure < 90 mm Hg

H heart rate > 125/min

Laboratory findings and special investigations that are consistent with poorer prognosis include

H hypoxia (Po_2 < 60 mm Hg or saturation < 90% on room air)

E effusion

A anemia (hematocrit < 30%)

R renal: BUN (urea) > 64 mg/dL (23 mmol/L)

G glucose > 250 mg/dL (14 mmol/L)

A acidosis (pH < 7.35)

S sodium < 130 mmol/L

Aspiration Pneumonia

Most patients with depressed consciousness experience pharyngeal aspiration, which, in the presence of underlying diseases that impair host defense mechanisms and alterations in oropharyngeal flora, may manifest as aspiration pneumonia. Alcohol abuse, drug abuse, head trauma, seizures and other neurologic disorders, and administration of sedatives are most often responsible for the development of aspiration pneumonia. *K. pneumoniae* is frequently implicated in aspiration pneumonia associated with obtundation typical of alcoholic binges. Patients with abnormalities of deglutition or esophageal motility resulting from placement of nasogastric tubes, esophageal cancer, bowel obstruction, or repeated vomiting are prone to aspiration of gastric contents. Poor oral hygiene and periodontal disease predispose to aspiration pneumonia because of the presence of increased bacterial flora. Induction and recovery from anesthesia may place patients at increased risk of aspiration of gastric contents.

Clinical manifestations of pulmonary aspiration depend in large part on the nature and volume of aspirated material. Aspiration of large volumes of acidic gastric fluid (Mendelson's syndrome) produces fulminating pneumonia and arterial hypoxemia. Aspiration of particulate material may result in airway obstruction, and smaller particles may produce atelectasis. Radiographically, infiltrates are most common in dependent areas of the patient's lungs. Penicillin-sensitive anaerobes are the most likely cause of aspiration pneumonia. Clindamycin is an alternative to penicillin and may be superior for treating necrotizing aspiration pneumonia and lung abscess. Hospitalization or antibiotic therapy alters the usual oropharyngeal flora such that aspiration pneumonia in hospitalized patients often involves pathogens that are uncommon in community-acquired pneumonias. There are limited data to suggest that treatment of aspiration pneumonia with antibiotics improves outcome.

Management of Anesthesia

Anesthesia and surgery should ideally be deferred with acute infections. Patients with acute pneumonia are often dehydrated and may have renal insufficiency. However, overly aggressive volume resuscitation may worsen gas exchange and morbidity. Fluid management is therefore extremely challenging. Regional anesthesia may be superior. If general anesthesia is unavoidable, a protective ventilation strategy is appropriate with tidal volumes of 6 to 8 mL/kg ideal body mass and mean airway pressures less than 30 cm H_2O. The anesthesiologist should suction secretions, send distal sputum specimens for Gram stain and culture, and ensure that appropriate antibiotics are administered both for the pneumonia and to cover the surgery.

Postoperative Pneumonia

Postoperative pneumonia occurs in approximately 20% of patients undergoing major thoracic, esophageal, or major upper abdominal surgery but is rare in other procedures in previously fit patients. Chronic respiratory disease increases the incidence of postoperative pneumonia threefold. Other risk factors include obesity, age older than 70 years, and operations lasting more than 2 hours.[67]

Community-acquired pneumonia is one of the leading causes of death in the United States.

Streptococcus pneumoniae is the most frequent cause of bacterial pneumonia.

Empirical therapy for pneumonia is typically a combination such as a cephalosporin and a macrolide antibiotic.

Resistance of *S. pneumoniae* is becoming a major problem.

The Pneumonia Severity Index is a useful tool for aiding clinical judgment, guiding appropriate management, and suggesting prognosis.

Patients undergoing general anesthesia are at risk of aspiration pneumonia.

Patients undergoing major abdominal and thoracic surgery are at risk of postoperative pneumonia.

Lung Abscess

Lung abscess may develop after bacterial pneumonia. Alcohol abuse and poor dental hygiene are important risk factors. Septic pulmonary embolization, which is most common in intravenous drug abusers, may also result in formation of a lung abscess. A finding of an air-fluid level on the chest radiograph signifies rupture of the abscess into the bronchial tree, and foul-smelling sputum is characteristic. Antibiotics are the mainstay of treatment of a lung abscess. Surgery is indicated only when complications such as empyema occur. Thoracentesis is necessary to establish the diagnosis of empyema, and treatment requires chest tube drainage and antibiotics. Surgical drainage is necessary to treat chronic empyema.

Important considerations in the approach to pneumonia are listed in **Box 19-12**.

VENTILATOR-ASSOCIATED PNEUMONIA

Ventilator-associated pneumonia (VAP) is the most common nosocomial infection in the ICU and makes up one third of the total nosocomial infections.[68] Ten percent to 20% of patients with tracheal tubes and mechanical ventilation for more than 48 hours acquire VAP, with mortality rates of 15% to 50%.[69] Anesthesiologists and intensive care physicians have important roles to play in the prevention, diagnosis, and treatment of VAP. Several simple interventions may decrease the occurrence of VAP, including meticulous hand hygiene, oral care, limiting patient sedation, positioning patients semi-upright, aspiration of subglottic secretions, limiting intubation time, and considering the appropriateness of noninvasive ventilation support.[70]

Diagnosis

VAP is difficult to differentiate from other common causes of respiratory failure, such as acute respiratory distress syndrome and pulmonary edema. A tracheal tube or a tracheostomy tube provides a foreign surface that rapidly becomes colonized with upper airway flora. The mere presence of potentially pathogenic organisms in tracheal secretions is not diagnostic of VAP. A standardized diagnostic algorithm for VAP employing clinical and microbiologic data is used in the National Nosocomial Infections Surveillance System and the clinical pulmonary infection score to promote diagnostic consistency among clinicians and investigators. A clinical pulmonary infection score greater than 6 is consistent with a diagnosis of VAP (see Table 19-4).[71]

Both the National Nosocomial Infections Surveillance and the clinical pulmonary infection score are relatively sensitive for VAP (>80%) but nonspecific when applied to individual patients. In approximately half the patients suspected on clinical grounds of having VAP, the diagnosis is doubtful and distal airway cultures do not grow organisms. Arbitrary thresholds that have been proposed to suggest a diagnosis of VAP are 10^3 colony-forming units/mL (cfu/mL) of organisms grown from protected specimen brush, 10^4 cfu/mL of organisms grown from bronchoalveolar lavage, or 10^5 to 10^6 cfu/mL of organisms grown from tracheal aspirates.

Treatment and Prognosis

The treatment of VAP includes supportive care for respiratory failure plus therapy for the organisms most likely to be implicated. The most common pathogens are *P. aeruginosa* and *S. aureus*. Prognosis is improved if treatment is initiated early. Therefore, despite the high rate of false-positive diagnoses, broad-spectrum therapy should be initiated to cover resistant organisms such as methicillin-resistant *S. aureus* and *P. aeruginosa*. If known multidrug-resistant organisms, such as *A. baumanii* and extended-spectrum β-lactamase–producing organisms, a carbapenem antibiotic may be appropriate pending culture results. Treatment should be narrowed to target specific organisms according to cultures and sensitivities and should be stopped at 48 hours if cultures are negative. Eight days of therapy are usually sufficient, except for nonlactose fermenting gram-negative organisms, for which a 14-day course is recommended. **Figure 19-4** is an algorithm to guide treatment.[69]

Management of Anesthesia

Patients with VAP frequently require anesthesia for tracheostomy. Major surgery should be deferred until the pneumonia has resolved and respiratory function has improved. Tracheostomy is not an emergency procedure. It may be ill advised to proceed when patients have minimal pulmonary reserve, such as a requirement for more than 50% inspired oxygen or a positive end-expiratory pressure (PEEP) of 7.5 or higher. One of the major goals for the anesthesiologist is to ensure that patients with VAP do not experience a setback following anesthesia. Patients with respiratory failure may be PEEP dependent. When they are transported to the operating room, a PEEP valve should be used to decrease the likelihood of "derecruitment" of alveoli. In the operating room, protective mechanical ventilation should be used, with tidal volumes of 6 to 8 mL/kg of lean body mass. Ideally, the same ventilator

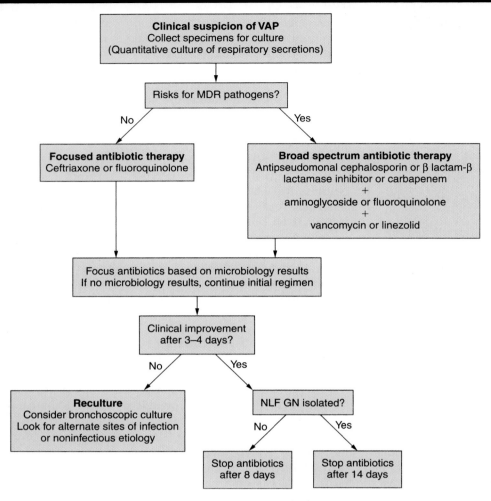

Figure 19-4 • Management of VAP. (*Adapted from Porzecanski I, Bowton DL: Diagnosis and treatment of ventilator-associated pneumonia. Chest 2006;130:597–604.*)

settings that were used in the ICU should be used, including mode of ventilation and PEEP. The lowest inspired oxygen should be administered to achieve adequate oxygen saturation (e.g., >95%). If the ventilator in the operating room is limited in its capabilities, consideration should be given to bringing an ICU ventilator into the operating room. If pneumonia is suspected and body fluids (e.g., pleural effusion, empyema, bronchial washing) are drained or suctioned, specimens should be sent to the laboratory for culture and identification of pathogens.

Important findings regarding VAP are listed in **Box 19-13**.

SEVERE ACUTE RESPIRATORY SYNDROME AND INFLUENZA

"There is no question that there will be another influenza pandemic someday. We simply don't know when it will occur or whether it will be caused by the H5N1 avian influenza virus. It would be prudent to develop robust plans for dealing with such a pandemic."[72]

Influenza A– and severe acute respiratory syndrome (SARS)–associated viruses are examples of respiratory viruses that may

---

BOX 19-13 Ventilator-associated Pneumonia

Several simple interventions may decrease the occurrence of VAP.

There is no gold standard for the diagnosis of VAP.

Early broad-spectrum antibiotic therapy decreases mortality with VAP.

When organisms are grown, therapy should be narrowed and targeted to the particular pathogen.

Eight days of therapy for VAP is sufficient, except for nonlactose fermenting gram-negative organisms, for which a 14-day course is recommended.

When no organisms grow from tracheal aspirates or bronchoalveolar lavage after 48 hours, antibiotics should generally be stopped.

If patients with VAP require anesthesia, a protective ventilation strategy should be adopted, similar to that in the ICU.

have rampant courses, high virulence, and high lethality. SARS struck like a bolt from the blue in 2002 to 2003 and was a grim reminder of our vulnerability to new infectious diseases. SARS affected mainly people in Asia, in the Pacific Rim, and in Canada. The causative agent is thought to be an RNA coronavirus that is passed on through contact and droplet spread. The virus is viable ex vivo for 24 to 48 hours. Many of the victims of the SARS outbreak were health workers, including anesthesiologists. The influenza pandemic of 1918 to 1919 was one of the major plagues to have affected humankind; it is estimated that Spanish flu left a trail of as many as 25 million corpses around the world in just 25 weeks. A new strain of avian influenza, the H5N1 strain, which is a subtype of influenza A, is now threatening humankind. Influenza is an RNA orthomyxovirus, which, like other RNA viruses, mutates at an alarming rate. The strain H5N1 is so named based on the capsular peptides, hemagglutinin, and neuraminidase. There are 16 known hemagglutinin subtypes and nine known neuraminidase subtypes of influenza A viruses. The Spanish flu was caused by an H1N1 strain of the virus, which continues to cause seasonal human influenza. According to the World Health Organization, pathogenic strains of H5N1 that infect humans may be fatal in approximately 66% of cases. Currently, H5N1 influenza A is passed from bird to human. The fear is that if there is recombination within a patient with concurrent H1N1 or H3N2 influenza A infection, the viruses may undergo recombination resulting in a lethal strain that can spread among humans (**Fig. 19-5**). Patients with acute respiratory viral infections may require care by anesthesiologists for such procedures as emergency intubation, tracheostomy, chest tube placement, mechanical ventilator support, or general ICU care.

Signs and Symptoms

Symptoms include nonspecific complaints of viral infection such as cough, sore throat, headache, diarrhea, arthralgia, and muscle pain. In more severe cases, patients may present with respiratory distress, confusion (encephalitis), and hemoptysis. Signs may include fever, tachycardia, sweating, conjunctivitis, rash, tachypnea, use of accessory respiratory muscles, cyanosis, and pulmonary features of pneumonia, pleural effusions, or pneumothorax. A chest radiograph may show patchy infiltrates, areas of opacification, pneumothoraces, and evidence of pleural effusions. Both H5N1 influenza A virus and SARS-coronavirus (CoV) may cause acute lung injury and acute respiratory distress syndrome. Complications include multiorgan failure and severe sepsis.

Diagnosis

In the context of an outbreak, history, symptoms, and presentation are usually sufficient to suggest a diagnosis. The incubation period for SARS-CoV and H5N1 influenza A is approximately a week. For influenza, the range described is between 2 and 17 days. A definitive diagnosis is made by detecting the virus in sputum. The problem with serology is that it may take 2 to 3 weeks for seroconversion (development of antibodies) after infection. Results of enzyme-linked

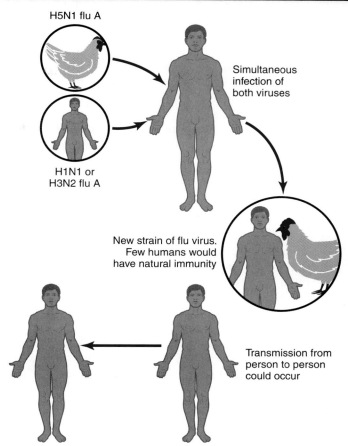

Figure 19-5 • How a pathogenic and contagious new strain of influenza could theoretically emerge.

immunosorbent assay and rapid influenza tests have been negative in patients infected with H5N1 influenza A. Rapid antigen detection kits have thus far yielded disappointing results for influenzaviruses.[73] Molecular methods, such as nucleic acid–based molecular techniques, show promise in providing mainstays for diagnosis in clinical laboratories. Reverse-transcriptase polymerase chain reaction kits are available and are useful for diagnosing both SARS-CoV and H5N1 influenza A. Influenzavirus may be missed in sputum and even nasopharyngeal specimens[74]; real-time polymerase chain reaction performed on tracheal aspirates and bronchoalveolar lavage fluid has yielded good diagnostic results.[72,74] A simple diagnostic DNA microarray that targeted only the matrix gene segment of influenza A has been developed that has a clinical sensitivity of 97% and a clinical specificity of 100% for influenza A strains H5N1 (avian), H1N1 (human) and H3N2 (human).[75] Electron microscopy may allow direct visualization of viral particles in patient samples,[76] but may not be practical for general diagnosis. Culture of this high-risk pathogen is restricted to certified containment level 3 facilities.[74] All specimens that test positive for influenza A (H5N1) must be confirmed by the National Microbiology Laboratory or its designate.[74]

Treatment

Vaccine development is a key component in the prevention of widespread viral infection and in the reduction of morbidity and mortality associated with many viral infections. Thus far, there is no vaccine for the SARS-CoV or for the H5N1 influenza A virus. In the case of influenza, neuraminidase inhibitors have been developed, including zanamivir and oseltamivir. These drugs may decrease the severity of infection, but there may be insufficient quantities in the event of a major outbreak. Other pharmacologic treatments for influenza include amantadine and rimantadine. Antiviral drugs are of modest benefit and help only if administered within the first 48 hours of symptoms.[77] There is no proven drug therapy that attenuates the course of SARS. Ribavirin has been used with questionable success. Vaccine development is difficult until the specific strain causing a pandemic is isolated, at which point there may be a delay of months during which the virus could wreak devastation. One of the interventions that may have yielded some success during the Spanish flu outbreak was the injection of blood from survivors into those with acute infections.

The mainstay of treatment for influenza and SARS is supportive care, which may include assisted ventilation as well as the array of supportive measures for sepsis. There may be benefit in draining pleural effusions and placing chest tubes for pneumothoraces. Antibiotics should be added for co-existing bacterial infections.

Prognosis

Prognosis depends on the pathogenicity of the infecting virus as well as the susceptibility of the infected person. Influenza and SARS may trigger a marked inflammatory response and a cytokine storm. A clinical picture indistinguishable from severe bacterial sepsis may result. Superinfection with bacteria is described and considerably worsens outcome.

Management of Anesthesia

Preoperative

The anesthesiologist should assess the patient with an appreciation of the potential lethality of the infection. Both patient and their family should be counseled about the high risks associated with SARS-CoV. These viruses are highly contagious and frequently lethal; strict isolation should be enforced and precautions to protect health workers must be taken. The same may apply to a potential (recombinant or newly evolved) influenza strain. Ideally, infected patients should be cared for in rooms with negative pressure to decrease aerosolized spread and contagion. Barrier precautions include the use of full-body disposable oversuits, double gloves, goggles, and powered air-purifying respirators with high-efficiency particulate air filters.[78,79] If these are not available, N95 masks (block 95% of particles) should be used rather than regular surgical masks. Filters should be placed in both limbs of breathing circuits to protect ventilators and anesthesia machines from contamination. All surfaces should be sterilized with alcohol and rooms should

---

> **BOX 19-14** | **Severe Acute Respiratory Syndrome and Influenza**
>
> Respiratory viruses may have rampant courses, high virulence, and high lethality.
>
> Both influenza and severe acute respiratory syndrome (SARS) may result in acute lung injury and acute respiratory distress syndrome.
>
> Complications of influenza and SARS include multiorgan failure and severe sepsis.
>
> Molecular methods, such as reverse-transcriptase polymerase chain reaction, allow diagnosis of SARS and influenza.
>
> The mainstay of treatment for influenza and SARS is supportive care.
>
> Barrier precautions are essential.
>
> Protective mechanical ventilation, as for acute respiratory distress syndrome, is indicated.

---

ideally not be used for other patients (if practical) for up to 48 hours after a person with SARS-CoV or H5N1 influenza A has been in the room. Even if it is not SARS or influenza, the same principles of infection control barrier precautions apply to any deadly contagious infection, whether occurring "naturally" or introduced by those with malevolent intent.

Intraoperative

Fears about contagion should not blind anesthesiologists to the high level of care required for these vulnerable patients. During the SARS outbreak in Hong Kong, fears about contagion may have affected patient management.[80] Experience from Canada has shown that when appropriate precautions are taken, spread of infection may be prevented. If mechanical ventilation is required, protective ventilation as for acute respiratory distress syndrome is indicated. Tidal volumes should be limited to 6 to 8 mL/kg lean body mass and mean airway pressure should be less than 30 cm H_2O. Sudden cardiorespiratory compromise could be reflective of an expanding pneumothorax. Draining of pleural effusions may improve ventilation and gas exchange. Care should be taken with bronchoscopy as this is a particularly high-risk procedure that results in aerosolization of viral particles.

Postoperative

Precautions to prevent spread of infection should be ongoing. The same treatment principles for acute respiratory distress syndrome and sepsis should apply.

Box 19-14 summarizes the previous discussion on SARS and influenza.

ACQUIRED IMMUNODEFICIENCY SYNDROME

AIDS was first described in 1981 in the United States. HIV and the AIDS pandemic pose a major threat to global health. It is estimated that more than 40 million people worldwide are infected with HIV, which is thought to have caused more than 25 million deaths to date.[81] The infection continues to spread apace, the most rapid increases being observed in Southern and Central Africa and in South Asia. The predominant mode of HIV transmission is heterosexual sex, and women represent a high proportion of new infections, including in developed countries.[82]

Increasing numbers of patients presenting for surgery are HIV seropositive or have AIDS. Anesthesiologists should be familiar with this disease and be aware of the impact of HIV on anesthesia.[83-85] An understanding of the pathogenesis of HIV and awareness of the possible drug interactions occurring with HIV therapy may help to guide the choice of anesthetic techniques. The possibility of nosocomial transmission of HIV highlights the need for anesthesiologists to enforce rigorous infection control policies to protect themselves, other health workers, and their patients. Antiretroviral therapy decreases the rate of disease progression, but there is no cure available nor is a vaccine likely in the foreseeable future.

HIV belongs to the family of Retroviridae and the genus Lentiviridae. Members of this genus are cytopathic (cell damaging), have long latent periods and run a chronic course. When cases of AIDS first appeared, its pathogenesis was frustratingly elusive because the disease does not appear immediately upon infection with HIV. There is a variable period during which the patient remains healthy but is viremic.

Signs and Symptoms

Acute seroconversion illness occurs with a high viral load soon after infection. After several months, there is a gradual decrease in the viremia as the immune response occurs. The viral load is often at a steady state as rate of viral production equals rate of destruction. Ninety-eight percent of T-helper lymphocytes (CD4 T cells) are located in lymph nodes, which are the major site of viral replication and T-cell destruction. There is a gradual involution of lymph nodes with a concomitant decrease in CD4 T cells and an increase in viral load as the inexorable onset of AIDS occurs (**Fig. 19-6**).

PCP (previously *Pneumocystis carinii*) does not usually occur until the CD4 count is less than 200 cells/mL. Breathlessness, night sweats, and weight loss are frequent complaints. Examination of the chest may be unremarkable. Complications include respiratory failure, pneumothorax, and chronic pulmonary disease. Cavitary lung disease can be due to

pyogenic bacterial lung abscess, pulmonary TB, fungal infections, and *Nocardia* spp. Kaposi's sarcoma and lymphoma can also affect the lung. Adenopathy can lead to tracheobronchial obstruction or compression of the great vessels. Endobronchial Kaposi's sarcoma may cause massive hemoptysis. HIV directly affects the lungs, causing a destructive pulmonary syndrome similar to emphysema.

Neurologic disease, ranging from AIDS dementia to infectious and neoplastic involvement, is common. Three diagnoses comprise the majority of predominantly focal cerebral diseases complicating AIDS: cerebral toxoplasmosis, primary central nervous system lymphoma, and progressive multifocal leukoencephalopathy. *Cryptococcus neoformans*, HIV, and TB can cause meningitis. Cardiac involvement in the course of HIV is common, but often clinically silent. Aggressive generalized vascular disease, including cardiac and cerebral, may occur as a complication of antiretroviral therapy. When patients exhibit unexplained hypotension, adrenal insufficiency should be considered as this may occur with advanced HIV infection.

Diagnosis

With the advent of highly active antiretroviral therapy (HAART), the prognosis for those infected with HIV is dramatically improved. It is important that the stigma attached to HIV infection is combated to enable routine testing. The standard test is an enzyme-linked immunosorbent assay, which usually becomes positive with the increase in antibodies to HIV 4 to 8 weeks after infection. During this initial window period, there is a high viral load and patients are more infectious. Confirmation of infection may be with a Western blot test or by measurement of HIV viral load in the blood.

With PCP, an AIDS-defining illness, the chest radiograph is normal in many instances. Typically, there is bilateral ground-glass shadowing. Pneumothoraces may be evident, and there may be multiple pneumatoceles. High-resolution computed tomography reveals a ground-glass appearance, even when the chest radiograph is normal. Lung-function tests show reduced lung volumes with decreased compliance and diminished diffusing capacity for carbon monoxide. Oxygen saturation measurements, or Pao_2, on exercise can be more helpful than lung function tests. If PCP is suspected, fiberoptic bronchoscopy and bronchoalveolar lavage should be performed. The advantage of an early

Figure 19-6 • The course of human immunodeficiency virus infection. AIDS, acquired immunodeficiency syndrome; HAART, highly active antiretroviral therapy.

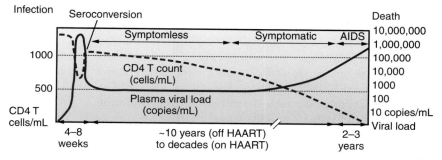

diagnosis compensates for a high frequency of negative examinations.

Disseminated TB is a potential cause of severe respiratory failure, and respiratory secretions should be examined routinely for acid-fast bacilli in AIDS patients with pulmonary infiltrates. Bacterial pneumonia (*S. pneumoniae, Moraxella catarrhalis, H. influenzae, S. aureus,* and *P. aeruginosa*) may also be the cause of severe acute respiratory failure; bacteria may be detected in sputum or bronchial washings.

Up to 50% of patients with HIV have abnormal echocardiographic findings at some point in their disease. Approximately 25% have pericardial effusions. Myocarditis, which is more common in advanced disease, may be caused by toxoplasmosis, disseminated cryptococcus, coxsackie B virus, cytomegalovirus, lymphoma, *Aspergillus* spp., and HIV itself. Ventricular dilatation and cardiac dysfunction may result.

With PI therapy, glucose intolerance and disorders of lipid metabolism are common. Random cortisol and tests of adrenal stimulation may reveal absolute and relative adrenal insufficiency.

Treatment

Three major classes of antiretroviral agents are currently in use:

1. Nucleoside analogue reverse-transcriptase inhibitors bind to the evolving viral DNA and prevent completion of reverse transcription.
2. Non-nucleoside analogue reverse-transcriptase inhibitors interfere with the transcriptional activity of this enzyme by binding to it directly, downstream of the active catalytic site.
3. Protease inhibitors (PIs) inhibit the HIV protease, which cleaves the polyprotein precursors that ultimately make up the core proteins of mature virions. PIs bind specifically to the active cleavage site.

Two new classes of antiretroviral agents have recently been developed. Integrase inhibitors act on the integrase enzyme, which the virus needs for incorporation of its proviral DNA into the infected cell's chromosomal DNA. If this enzyme is inhibited, HIV replication is thereby prevented. Raltegravir is the first FDA-approved integrase inhibitor. Chemokine receptor 5 (CCR5) antagonists prevent the binding of HIV to one of the co-receptors it uses to enter target cells. Integrase inhibitors and CCR5 antagonists, such as maraviroc, are effective in combination with other antiretroviral agents. Drugs from both classes are well tolerated and may be useful both as adjunctive therapy for resistant HIV strains and to delay the emergence of widespread viral resistance.

A typical antiretroviral regimen consists of three agents: a PI or non-nucleoside analogue reverse-transcriptase inhibitor combined with two nucleoside analogues. Such combination therapy has been termed HAART. In some circumstances, combinations of four or more drugs are used. The aim of therapy in treatment-naive patients is to achieve an undetectable viral load by 24 weeks of therapy and to improve and extend the length and quality of life. Numerous side effects and drug interactions complicate such

regimens and decrease compliance. Patients may acquire drug hypersensitivity reactions, resulting in fever, hypotension, and acute interstitial pneumonitis with respiratory failure. Concurrent use of zidovudine and corticosteroids may result in severe myopathy and respiratory muscle dysfunction. In addition, reports have documented several cases of respiratory failure related to HAART initiation and immune reconstitution resulting in a paradoxical worsening of *Pneumocystis* pneumonia. Distinguishing HAART-associated immune reconstitution with paradoxical worsening from *Pneumocystis* pneumonia treatment failure or a superimposed respiratory infection is often clinically challenging.[86] Of particular importance to anesthesiologists is that patients receiving HAART are subject to long-term metabolic complications, including lipid abnormalities and glucose intolerance, which may result in the development of diabetes, coronary artery, and cerebrovascular disease.[87]

A syndrome resembling acute gram-negative sepsis has been reported in patients taking nucleoside reverse-transcriptase inhibitors.[88,89] Lactic acidosis and hepatic steatosis are usually found. Patients develop high fever and can rapidly become confused and comatose. Nucleoside analogue drugs may cause inhibition of DNA polymerase gamma, the sole DNA polymerase required for the replication of mitochondrial DNA. This in turn causes mitochondrial dysfunction and impaired aerobic cellular respiration. Inhibition of oxidative phosphorylation and derangement of respiratory chain enzymes have been implicated.[88,89] Riboflavin has been suggested as a potential treatment. Unfortunately, most patients die despite ICU support.

PIs, particularly ritonavir, are inhibitors of cytochrome P-450. In contrast, drugs such as nevirapine are inducers of hepatic microsomal enzymes. These variable effects on liver enzymes complicate the dosing of drugs, including anesthetic and analgesic agents, many of which undergo hepatic metabolism (**Table 19-5**).

A combination of high-dose sulfamethoxazole (100 mg/kg per day) and trimethoprim (20 mg/kg per day) is the treatment of choice for PCP. Systemic steroid therapy, such as prednisolone (1 mg/kg per day), is advised for patients who have low oxygen saturation. Respiratory support and supplementary oxygen are invariably required. Continuous positive airway pressure has, in some instances, obviated the need for positive pressure ventilation.[90,91] The prognosis in patients who require mechanical ventilation despite adjunctive corticosteroid treatment is poor, and the use of PEEP can result in pneumothorax.

Empirical antibacterial treatment should be given when a bacterial pulmonary infection is suspected. Outbreaks of multidrug-resistant TB have occurred in patients with HIV infection and health care workers. Airborne transmission by inhalation of infective aerosols justifies appropriate isolation measures to protect medical staff and other patients from TB transmission.

Prognosis

Prior to 1995, the prospects for treatment of HIV had been rather gloomy. The situation changed dramatically as a result of four independent factors:

TABLE 19-5 Antiretroviral Drugs: Administration Tips and Side Effects

Drug Name	Administration	Common Side Effects
NRTIs		
Zidovudine (AZT/ZDV)	Oral/IV	Bone marrow suppression (neutropenia), GI upset, headache
Didanosine (DDI)	Empty stomach, oral	Peripheral neuropathy, pancreatitis, diarrhea
Zalcitabine (DDC)	Oral	Peripheral neuropathy, pancreatitis, oral ulcers
Stavudine (D4T)	Oral	Peripheral neuropathy
Lamivudine (3TC)	Oral	Anemia, GI upset
Abacavir	Oral	GI upset, potentially fatal acute hypersensitivity reactions
NNRTIs		
Nevirapine	Oral	Rash, hepatitis, liver enzyme (P-450) induction
Delavirdine	Oral	Rash, liver enzyme (P-450) induction
Efavirenz	Oral	Dizziness, rash, dysphoria, liver enzyme (P-450) induction
PIs		
Saquinavir	With fatty meal or up to 2 hr after meals	Diarrhea, increased transaminases, hyperlipidemia, P-450 inhibition
Indinavir	Empty stomach; 1.5 L water in 24 hr	Nephrolithiasis, hyperbilirubinemia, hyperlipidaemia, lipodystrophy, P-450 inhibition
Ritonavir	Refrigerate tablets	GI upset, circumoral parasthesia, hyperlipidaemia, lipodystrophy, P-450 inhibition
Nelfinavir	With food	Diarrhea, hyperlipidaemia, lipodystrophy, P-450 inhibition

GI, gastrointestinal; NNRTIs, non-nucleoside reverse transcriptase inhibitors; NRTIs, nucleoside reverse transcriptase inhibitors; PIs, protease inhibitors.

1. An improved understanding of the pathogenesis of HIV infection.
2. The availability of surrogate markers of immune function and plasma viral burden.
3. The development of new and more powerful drugs, such as the PIs and non-nucleoside reverse transcriptase inhibitors.
4. The completion of several large clinical end point trials that conclusively demonstrated that antiretroviral combinations significantly delayed the progression of HIV disease and improved survival.

Management of Anesthesia
Intraoperative

Universal precautions for the prevention of transmission of blood-borne viruses were recommended in 1987 by the CDC. These precautions recommend that every patient be regarded as potentially infected with a blood-borne virus. Following an accident with high-risk body fluid, such as a (hollow) needlestick injury, postexposure prophylaxis is recommended for health workers. This should commence as soon as possible after the injury, ideally within 1 to 2 hours, but can be considered up to 1 to 2 weeks after the injury. Very high risk exposures may be treated beyond this time with a view to modifying rather than preventing infection. A recommended postexposure prophylaxis regimen for a duration of 4 weeks is zidovudine 250 mg every 12 hours, lamivudine 150 mg every 12 hours, indinavir 800 mg every 8 hours. The high rate of toxicity and noncompliance may necessitate other regimens.

Focal neurologic lesions may increase intracerebral pressure precluding neuraxial anesthesia. Spinal cord involvement, peripheral neuropathy, and myopathy may occur with cytomegalovirus or HIV infection itself. Suxamethonium may be hazardous in this setting. HIV infection is associated with autonomic neuropathy, and this can manifest as hemodynamic instability during anesthesia or in the ICU. Invasive hemodynamic monitoring may be helpful for severe autonomic neuropathy. Steroid supplementation may decrease hemodynamic instability and should be considered for unexplained hypotension.

HIV infection does not increase the risk of postprocedural complications, including death, up to 30 days post-procedure. Thus, surgical intervention should not be limited because of HIV status and concern for subsequent complications. However, during anesthesia, tachycardia is more frequently seen in HIV-seropositive patients, and, postoperatively, high fever, anemia, and tachycardia are more frequent.

Several studies indicate that general anesthesia and opiates may have a negative effect on immune function. Although this immunosuppressive effect is probably of little clinical importance in healthy individuals, the implications for the HIV-infected patient are unknown. Immunosuppression resulting from general anesthetics occurs within 15 minutes of induction and may persist for as long as 3 to 11 days. Postoperative immunosuppression may last longer in inherently immunosuppressed patients and may predispose to the development of postoperative infections or facilitate tumor growth or metastasis.

There is little specific information concerning the overall risk of anesthesia and surgery in the HIV-seropositive patient.

The American Society of Anesthesiologists' physical status assessment and the inherent surgical risk probably provide a measure of global risk assessment. This information, when combined with the CDC stage of the HIV infection, the degree of immunosuppression, and the presence and severity of opportunistic infection or neoplasm, may offer the best predictor of global preoperative risk of the HIV-seropositive patient. With regard to anesthetic technique, regional anesthesia is the technique of choice except in certain cases of neuropathies.

HIV and AIDS are increasing in women of child-bearing age. In the ACTG-076 study, zidovudine monotherapy was shown dramatically to reduce the incidence of vertical transmission of HIV from 25.5% to 8.3%. However, zidovudine monotherapy has limited long-term benefit as HIV resistance develops rapidly. Therefore, in pregnancy, combination therapy is thought to be preferable. There are limited data on the use of PIs in pregnancy. A meta-analysis strongly suggested that cesarean section independently decreases the incidence of vertical transmission.[92] A combination of antiretroviral therapy and elective cesarean section reduces the rate of transmission to 2%. However, a cesarean section is a major surgical intervention that has well-reported complications. There is a higher incidence of morbidity after cesarean section compared with vaginal childbirth in healthy women. This includes more prolonged and intense pain, longer duration of bed rest, increased blood loss, and more frequent venous thrombosis and wound infection.[93] Many practitioners today do not recommend elective cesarean section to HIV-infected women who are compliant with antiretroviral therapy and have undetectable HIV viral loads. Unfortunately, the HIV-positive women (with low CD4 lymphocytes counts), whose infants theoretically will benefit most from caesarean delivery, are also the women who are most likely to experience postoperative complications.[93]

In studies of HIV seropositive parturients who were given regional anesthesia, there were no neurologic or infectious complications related to the anesthetic or obstetric course.[83,94] In the immediate postpartum period, the immune function measurements remained essentially unchanged, as did the severity of the disease. There have been fears that epidural and lumbar puncture in HIV-seropositive patients may allow entry of the virus into the central nervous system. The natural history of HIV includes central nervous system involvement early in the clinical course and expression of this infection varies widely. The safety of epidural blood patches for treatment of postdural puncture headache has been reported in HIV-seropositive patients, but, given the very small theoretical risk of introducing virus to the central nervous system, other analgesic strategies should be tried first.

Postoperative

APACHE II scoring significantly underestimates mortality risk in HIV-seropositive patients admitted to the ICU with a total lymphocyte count less than 200 cells/mL. This is

---

BOX 19-15 Human Immunodeficiency Virus and Acquired Immunodeficiency Syndrome

More than 25 million people have died of acquired immunodeficiency syndrome.

There is no cure in sight.

The initial enthusiasm that greeted highly active antiretroviral therapy has been tempered with the discovery of multidrug-resistant viral strains.

Anesthesiologists have contact with a broad range of patients, many of whom are human immunodeficiency virus seropositive without symptoms.

Rigorous infection control practice with universal precautions is imperative.

All clinicians should keep abreast of current knowledge about human immunodeficiency virus therapy in order that patients receive optimal treatment.

---

particularly true of patients admitted with pneumonia or sepsis. There is a diverse range of indications for critical care in patients with HIV infection. Historically, respiratory failure owing to *Pneumocystis* pneumonia has been the most common reason for admission to the ICU and accounted for 34% of cases. Mechanical ventilation for PCP and other pulmonary disorders is associated with a mortality rate exceeding 50%. In contrast, admission to the ICU and mechanical ventilation for nonpulmonary disorders is associated with a mortality rate of less than 25%. In patients with septic shock, HIV infection has been shown to be an independent predictor of poor outcome. In the era of HAART, fewer patients with HIV infection are admitted to the ICU with AIDS-defining illnesses, such as PCP. Many patients are now admitted with unrelated critical illness and are found coincidentally to be infected with HIV. Initiation of HAART in patients with PCP has been shown to improve outcome. However, this must be weighed against the problems associated with immune reconstitution, which may occur in septic patients when HAART is initiated.[86]

Box 19-15 lists key points in the approach to HIV/AIDS.

TUBERCULOSIS

Mycobacterium tuberculosis is an obligate aerobe responsible for TB.[95] This organism survives most successfully in tissues with high oxygen concentrations, which is consistent with the increased presentation of TB in the apices of the lungs.

In the past, most cases of TB in the United States were due to reactivation of an infection, especially in elderly individuals.[95] At present, most cases of TB occur in racial and ethnic minorities, foreign-born individuals from areas where TB is endemic (Asia and Africa), intravenous drug abusers, and those with HIV infection or AIDS. Any patient with TB should be tested for HIV. The appearance of multidrug-resistant strains of *M. tuberculosis* has contributed to the resurgence of TB worldwide. A concerning recent development has been the emergence within the context of the HIV epidemic of extensively drug-resistant TB in South Africa, which is not only more resistant to therapy but is also more virulent and frequently lethal.[96]

Almost all *M. tuberculosis* infections result from aerosol (droplet) inhalation. It has been estimated that up to 600,000 droplet nuclei are expelled with each cough and remain viable for several days. Although a single infectious unit is capable of causing infection in susceptible individuals, prolonged exposure in closed environments is optimal for transmission of infection. It is estimated that 90% of patients infected with *M. tuberculosis* never become symptomatic and are identified only by conversion of the tuberculin skin test. Often patients who acquire the infection early in life do not become symptomatic until much later. Patients who are HIV seropositive or immunocompromised are at much higher risk of becoming symptomatic.

Diagnosis

The diagnosis of TB is based on the presence of clinical symptoms, the epidemiologic likelihood of infection, and the results of diagnostic tests.[95] Symptoms of pulmonary TB often include persistent nonproductive cough, anorexia, weight loss, chest pain, hemoptysis, and night sweats. The most common test for TB is the tuberculin skin (Mantoux) test. The skin reaction is read in 48 to 72 hours, and a positive reading is generally defined as an induration of more than 10 mm. For patients with AIDS, a reaction of 5 mm or more is considered positive. The skin test is limited, and alternative screening and diagnostic tests are undergoing evaluation. The skin test is nonspecific and may be positive if people have received a bacille Calmette-Guérin vaccine or if they have been exposed to TB, or perhaps even other mycobacteria, even if there are no viable mycobacteria present at the time of the skin test.

Chest radiographs are important for the diagnosis of TB. Apical or subapical infiltrates are highly suggestive of infection. Bilateral upper lobe infiltration with the presence of cavitation is also common. Patients with AIDS may demonstrate a less classic picture on chest radiography, which may be further confounded by the presence of PCP. Tuberculous vertebral osteomyelitis (Pott's disease) is a common manifestation of extrapulmonary TB.[97]

Sputum smears and cultures are also used to diagnose TB. Smears are examined for the presence of acid-fast bacilli. This test is based on the ability of mycobacteria to take up and retain neutral red stains after an acid wash. It is estimated that 50% to 80% of individuals with active TB have positive sputum smears. Although the absence of acid-fast bacilli does not rule out TB, a positive sputum culture containing *M. tuberculosis* provides a definitive diagnosis.

Health care workers are at increased risk of occupational acquisition of TB.[95] For example, TB is twice as prevalent in physicians as in the general population. Persons involved with autopsies are uniquely at risk. Nosocomial outbreaks of TB have occurred especially among patients with AIDS. In 1994, CDC issued guidelines for the prevention of occupationally acquired TB among health care workers.[95,98] In the decade following these guidelines, there was a marked decrease in nosocomial TB and in multidrug-resistant TB outbreaks in the United States.[99] The guidelines were updated in 2005.[99]

Anesthesiologists are at increased risk of nosocomial TB by virtue of events surrounding the induction and maintenance of anesthesia that may induce coughing (tracheal intubation, tracheal suctioning, mechanical ventilation).[95] Bronchoscopy is a high-risk procedure associated with conversion of the tuberculin skin test in anesthesiologists. As a first step in preventing occupational acquisition of TB, anesthesia personnel should participate in annual tuberculin screening such that those who develop a positive skin test may be offered chemotherapy. The decision to take chemotherapy is not trivial as treatment for TB carries the serious toxicity. A baseline chest radiograph is indicated when a positive tuberculin skin test first manifests.

Treatment

Anti-TB chemotherapy has decreased mortality from TB by more than 90%.[95] With adequate treatment, more than 90% of patients who have susceptible strains of TB have bacteriologically negative sputum smears within 3 months. In the United States, vaccination with bacille Calmette-Guérin is not recommended, as it may not confer immunity and confounds the diagnosis of TB.

Some argue that, for protection of the community, people who have positive skin tests should receive chemotherapy with isoniazid. However, the flipside is that isoniazid is a toxic drug and treatment is only strictly indicated if there are radiographic features of pulmonary TB or if there are suggestive symptoms. The toxicity of isoniazid manifests in the peripheral nervous system, liver, and possibly the kidneys. Neurotoxicity may be prevented by daily administration of pyridoxine. Hepatotoxicity is most likely to be related to metabolism of isoniazid by hepatic acetylation. Depending on the genetically determined traits, patients may be characterized as slow or rapid acetylators. Hepatitis appears to be more common in rapid acetylators, consistent with the greater production of hydrazine, a potentially hepatotoxic metabolite of isoniazid. Persistent elevations of serum transaminase concentrations mandate that isoniazid be discontinued, but mild, transient increases do not.

Other drugs used to treat TB include pyrazinamide, rifampicin, and ethambutol. Adverse effects of rifampicin include thrombocytopenia, leukopenia, anemia, and renal failure. Hepatitis associated with increases in serum aminotransaminase concentrations occur in approximately 10% of patients being treated with rifampicin. In order to be curative, treatment for pulmonary TB is recommended for 6 months. Extrapulmonary TB usually requires a longer course. Noncompliance with therapy contributes to the emergence of resistant TB strains.

Management of Anesthesia

The preoperative assessment of patients considered to be at risk of TB includes a detailed history, including the presence of a persistent cough and the tuberculin status.[95] Elective surgical procedures should be postponed until patients are no longer considered infectious. Patients are considered non-infectious if they have received antituberculous chemotherapy, are improving clinically, and have had three consecutive negative sputum smears. If surgery cannot be delayed, it is important to limit the number of involved personnel, and high risk procedures (bronchoscopy, tracheal intubation, and suctioning) should be performed in a negative-pressure environment whenever possible. Patients should be transported to the operating room wearing a tight-fitting N-95 face mask to prevent casual exposure of others to airborne bacilli. Staff should also wear N-95 masks.

If patients have TB of the cervical spine, special precautions should be taken not to injure the spine during airway manipulation. A high efficiency particulate air filter should be placed in the anesthesia delivery circuit between the Y connector and the mask, laryngeal mask airway, or tracheal tube. Bacterial filters should be placed on the exhalation limb of the anesthesia delivery circuit to decrease the discharge of tubercle bacilli into the ambient air. Sterilization of anesthesia equipment (laryngoscope blades) is with standard methods using a disinfectant that destroys tubercle bacilli. Use of a dedicated anesthesia machine and ventilator is recommended.[95] Positive-pressure ventilation has been associated with massive hemoptysis in a patient with old pulmonary TB leading to the recommendation that maintenance of spontaneous breathing may be indicated in selected patients.[100] Postoperative care should, if possible, take place in an isolation room, preferably with negative pressure.

Box 19-16 lists important considerations in regard to tuberculosis.

CLOSTRIDIUM DIFFICILE

C. difficile is an anaerobic, gram-positive, spore-forming bacterium that is the major identifiable cause of antibiotic-associated diarrhea and pseudomembranous colitis.[101,102] Clindamycin was implicated in many cases of *C. difficile*, but it became apparent that many other antibiotics, such as penicillins, cephalosporins, and fluoroquinolones are similarly implicated. It is clear today that most antibiotics can alter bowel flora facilitating the growth of *C. difficile*. With the frequent use of broad-spectrum antibiotics, the incidence of *C. difficile* diarrhea has risen dramatically.[103] The prevalence of asymptomatic colonization in the hospital, especially in older people, is more than 20%. In approximately one third of those colonized, *C. difficile* produces toxins that cause diarrhea.[104] The two principal toxins are A and B toxins. Toxin B is approximately 1000 times more cytotoxic than toxin A. Toxin A activates macrophages and mast cells. Activation of these cells causes the production of inflammatory mediators, which leads to fluid secretion and increased mucosal permeability.[102] Toxin A is also an enterotoxin in that it loosens the tight junctions between the epithelial cells that line the colon, which helps toxin B enter into epithelial cells.

One systematic review identified several risk factors for *C. difficile*–associated diarrhea[105]:

Increasing age (excluding infancy)
Severe underlying disease
Nonsurgical gastrointestinal procedures
Presence of a nasogastric tube
Receiving antiulcer medications
Stay in the ICU
Long duration of hospital stay
Long duration of antibiotic course (risk doubles after 3 days)
Receiving multiple antibiotics
Immunosuppressive therapy
Recent surgical procedure
Sharing a hospital room with a *C. difficile*–infected patient

In recent years, *C. difficile* has been more frequent, more severe, more refractory to standard therapy and more likely to relapse. This may be attributable to a new strain of *C. difficile*, which produces large amounts of toxins.[106]

Signs and Symptoms

The most frequent symptoms are diarrhea and abdominal pain. Patients may be febrile with abdominal tenderness and distention. With perforation, patients may present with an acute abdomen.

Diagnosis

The diagnosis is made by detecting toxin in stool. Whenever a hospitalized patient has diarrhea, especially if they have received antibiotics, it is prudent to send stool for *C. difficile* detection. Diarrhea is not invariable, and an unexplained leukemoid reaction (increase in white cell count often greater than $30–50 \times 10^9/$L) should raise suspicion, especially if there are abdominal signs, such as an acute abdomen. An abdominal radiograph may show colonic dilatation. The most common confirmatory study is an enzyme immunoassay for *C. difficile* toxins A and B. The results are available in 2 to 4 hours. Specificity is high (up to 100%), but sensitivity ranges from 63% to 99%.[107] Therefore, it is advisable to send stool for *C. difficile* toxin detection over three sequential days in order to rule that *C. difficile* is unlikely.

A combination immunoassay tests for *C. difficile*–specific glutamate dehydrogenase, which has a high sensitivity for toxins A and B, with a high specificity. This test provides a high negative predictive value.[108] If doubt remains about the diagnosis, if response to therapy is poor, or if there is fulminant disease, sigmoidoscopy or computed tomography may provide a diagnosis and valuable prognostic information.[103]

Treatment

Therapy for patients with *C. difficile*–associated diarrhea comprises fluid and electrolyte replacement, withdrawal of current antibiotic therapy if possible, and targeted antibiotic treatment to eradicate *C. difficile*.[101] Treatment should be given orally, if possible. The first-line regimen is oral metronidazole 400 mg three times daily. An alternative is oral vancomycin 125 mg four times daily.[101] Vancomycin has a theoretical advantage over metronidazole as it is not well absorbed and may therefore better reach the site of infection. The major downside to vancomycin is that it may promote the growth of vancomycin-resistant enterococci. Vancomycin has been advocated as first-line treatment for patients in the ICU or for patients with low albumin levels.[109] Treatment is typically for at least 10 days, but should be continued until symptoms and diarrhea resolve. Probiotics such as *Saccharomyces boulardii* and *Lactobacillus rhamnosus* may be useful in restoring physiologic bowel flora and decreasing the recurrence of *C. difficile*. If there is an ileus, vancomycin enemas and intravenous metronidazole may be useful.

Prognosis

C. difficile infection accounts for considerable increases in the length of hospital stays and more than $1.1 billion in health care costs each year in the United States.[110] The condition is a common cause of significant morbidity and even death in elderly or debilitated patients. Twenty-five percent of patients have recurrent infection.[111]

Management of Anesthesia

Preoperative

It is generally the sickest patients with *C. difficile* colitis, including those who do not improve with conventional therapy, who present for surgery, such as subtotal colectomy and ileostomy. If they are hemodynamically unstable, major surgery may be deferred and an ileostomy, cecostomy, or colostomy may be done as a temporizing intervention.[112] Surgery carries a high mortality. Resuscitation and preoperative treatment metabolic derangements may be beneficial.

Intraoperative

Patients with fulminant *C. difficile* colitis are very ill, and hemodynamic instability is likely during anesthesia. Invasive monitoring may guide fluid administration and the use of inotropes and vasopressors. Dehydration, acid base, and electrolyte abnormalities may occur following episodes of diarrhea. Opiates decrease intestinal motility, which may exacerbate toxin-mediated disease.

Postoperative

One of the most important considerations is to prevent the spread of *C. difficile*. The spores are hardy and are not destroyed by alcohol. Strict contact and isolation precautions are essential, routine use of disposable gloves and gowns is important, and vigorous hand washing with soap and water may remove spores. Stethoscopes and ties are potential repositories for spores.

The previous discussion on *C. difficile* is summarized in **Box 19-17**.

BOX 19-17 *Clostridium difficile* Colitis

Clostridium difficile is the most common cause of diarrhea in hospitals.

Broad-spectrum antibiotics facilitate the growth of *C. difficile*.

Perioperative antibiotics should generally be stopped within 24 to 48 hours.

Clindamycin, cephalosporins, and fluoroquinolones have frequently been implicated.

There is an epidemic of virulent and refractory strain of *C. difficile*.

Oral vancomycin is the preferred treatment for seriously ill patients.

Isolation precautions and hand hygiene may decrease contagion.

KEY POINTS

- The 21st century will herald an increase in resistant infectious diseases and pandemics.

- There are no new antibiotics to treat resistant gram-negative organisms.

- Targeted preoperative, intraoperative, and postoperative interventions decrease the likelihood of SSI.

- Frequent hand decontamination with alcohol may be the single most effective intervention in decreasing infection.

- Use appropriate antibiotics at the right time, at the right dose, and for an appropriate duration.

- In order to delay widespread resistance to all antimicrobial agents, therapy *must* be narrowed as soon as organisms are identified and susceptibility is known.

- Cultures should be sent from all sources where organism growth is suspected.

- With necrotizing soft-tissue infections, the cutaneous signs are frequently not reflective of the extent of tissue necrosis.

- Ten percent to 20% of patients with tracheal tubes and mechanical ventilation for more than 48 hours acquire

KEY POINTS—cont'd

ventilator-associated pneumonia, with mortality rates of 15% to 50%.

- Respiratory viruses may have rampant courses, high virulence, and high lethality.

- HIV is a modern pandemic, which, owing to combination therapy, has become a chronic disease with morbidity associated with both the infection and its treatment.

- A concerning recent development has been the emergence within the context of the HIV epidemic of

extensively drug resistant TB, which is not only more resistant to therapy but is also more virulent and frequently lethal.

- There is a growing epidemic of virulent *C. difficile* associated diarrhea in hospitalized patients, which may be associated with the widespread use of broad-spectrum antibiotics.

REFERENCES

1. Wang J, Soisson SM, Young K, et al: Platensimycin is a selective FabF inhibitor with potent antibiotic properties. Nature 2006;441:358–361.

2. Nordmann P, Poirel L: Emerging carbapenemases in gram-negative aerobes. Clin Microbiol Infect 2002;8:321–331.

3. Livermore DM: The threat from the pink corner. Ann Med 2003;35:226–234.

4. ManGram AJ, Horan TC, Pearson ML, et al: Guideline for Prevention of Surgical Site Infection, 1999. Centers for Disease Control and Prevention (CDC) Hospital Infection Control Practices Advisory Committee. Am J Infect Control 1999;27:97–132; quiz 133–134; discussion 96.

5. Classen DC, Evans RS: The timing of prophylactic administration of antibiotics and the risk of surgical-wound infection. N Engl J Med 1992;326:281–286.

6. Horan TC, Gaynes RP, Martone WJ, et al: CDC definitions of nosocomial surgical site infections, 1992: A modification of CDC definitions of surgical wound infections. Infect Control Hosp Epidemiol 1992;13:606–608.

7. Jarvis WR: Epidemiology of nosocomial fungal infections, with emphasis on *Candida* species. Clin Infect Dis 1995;20:1526–1530.

8. Christensen GD, Baddour LM, Simpson WA: Phenotypic variation of *Staphylococcus epidermidis* slime production in vitro and in vivo. Infect Immun 1987;55:2870–2877.

9. National Nosocomial Infections Surveillance (NNIS) report, data summary from October 1986–April 1996, issued May 1996. A report from the National Nosocomial Infections Surveillance (NNIS) System. Am J Infect Control 1996;24:380–388.

10. Myles PS, Jacono GA, Hunt JO, et al: Risk of respiratory complications and wound infection in patients undergoing ambulatory surgery: Smokers versus nonsmokers. Anesthesiology 2002;97:842–847.

11. Tonnesen H, Rosenberg J, Nielsen HJ, et al: Effect of preoperative abstinence on poor postoperative outcome in alcohol misusers: Randomised controlled trial. BMJ 1999;318:1311–1316.

12. Malone DL, Genuit T, Tracy JK, et al: Surgical site infections: Reanalysis of risk factors. J Surg Res 2002;103:89–95.

13. Cantürk Z, Cantürk Z, Okay E, et al: Nosocomial infections and obesity in surgical patients. Obes Res 2003;11:769–775.

14. Perl TM, Cullen JP, Wenzel PP, et al: Intranasal mupirocin to prevent postoperative *Staphylococcus aureus* infections. N Engl J Med 2002;346:1871–1877.

15. Segers P, Speekenbrink RG, Ubbink DT, et al: Prevention of nosocomial infection in cardiac surgery by decontamination of the nasopharynx and oropharynx with chlorhexidine gluconate: A randomized controlled trial. JAMA 2006;296:2460–2466.

16. Feltis JM Jr, Hamit HF: Use of prophylactic antimicrobial drugs to prevent postoperative wound infections. Am J Surg 1967;114:867–870.

17. Fridkin SK, Hageman JC, Morrison M, et al: Methicillin-resistant *Staphylococcus aureus* disease in three communities. N Engl J Med 2005;352:1436–1444.

18. Itani KM, Wilson SE, Awad SS, et al: Ertapenem versus cefotetan prophylaxis in elective colorectal surgery. N Engl J Med 2006;355:2640–2651.

19. Bonow RO, Carabello DO, de Leon AC, et al: Guidelines for the management of patients with valvular heart disease: Executive summary. A report of the American College of Cardiology/American Heart Association Task Force on Practice Guidelines (Committee on Management of Patients with Valvular Heart Disease). Circulation 1998;98:1949–1984.

20. Kurz A, Sessler DI, Lenhardt R: Perioperative normothermia to reduce the incidence of surgical-wound infection and shorten hospitalization. Study of Wound Infection and Temperature Group. N Engl J Med 1996;334:1209–1215.

21. Todd MM, Hindman BJ, Clarke WR, et al: Mild intraoperative hypothermia during surgery for intracranial aneurysm. N Engl J Med 2005;352:135–145.

22. Greif R, Akça O, Horn FP, et al: Supplemental perioperative oxygen to reduce the incidence of surgical-wound infection. Outcomes Research Group. N Engl J Med 2000;342:161–167.

23. Pryor KO, Fahey TJ 3rd, Lien CA, Goldstein PA: Surgical site infection and the routine use of perioperative hyperoxia in a general surgical population: A randomized controlled trial. JAMA 2004;291:79–87.

24. Belda FJ, Aguilera L, Garcia de la Asuncion J, et al: Supplemental perioperative oxygen and the risk of surgical wound infection: A randomized controlled trial. JAMA 2005; 294:2035–2042.

25. Fleischmann E, Herbst F, Kugener A, et al: Mild hypercapnia increases subcutaneous and colonic oxygen tension in patients given 80% inspired oxygen during abdominal surgery. Anesthesiology 2006;104:944–949.

26. Mauermann WJ, Nemergut EC: The anesthesiologist's role in the prevention of surgical site infections. Anesthesiology 2006;105:413–421; quiz 439–440.

27. van den Berghe G, Wouters P, Weekers F, et al: Intensive insulin therapy in the critically ill patients. N Engl J Med 2001;345:1359–1367.

28. Egi M, Bellomo R, Stochowski E, et al: Variability of blood glucose concentration and short-term mortality in critically ill patients. Anesthesiology 2006;105:244–252.

29. Hill AF, Polvino WJ, Wilson DB: The significance of glucose, insulin and potassium for immunology and oncology: A new model of immunity. J Immune Based Ther Vaccines 2005;3:5.

30. Fraenkel D, Rickard C, Thomas P, et al: A prospective, randomized trial of rifampicin-minocycline-coated and silver-platinum-carbon-impregnated central venous catheters. Crit Care Med 2006;34:668–675.

31. O'Grady NP, Alexander H, Dellinger FP, et al: Guidelines for the prevention of intravascular catheter-related infections. Centers for Disease Control and Prevention. MMWR Recomm Rep 2002;51:1–29.

32. National Nosocomial Infections Surveillance (NNIS) System report, data summary from January 1990–May 1999, issued June 1999. Am J Infect Control 1999;27:520–532.

33. Fridkin SK, Edwards JR, Courval JM, et al: The effect of vancomycin and third-generation cephalosporins on prevalence of vancomycin-resistant enterococci in 126 U.S. adult intensive care units. Ann Intern Med 2001;135:175–183.

34. Fridkin SK, Gaynes RP: Antimicrobial resistance in intensive care units. Clin Chest Med 1999;20:303–316.

35. Pfaller MA, Jones RN, Messer A, et al: National surveillance of nosocomial blood stream infection due to species of *Candida* other than *Candida albicans*: frequency of occurrence and antifungal susceptibility in the SCOPE ProGram. SCOPE Participant Group. Surveillance and Control of Pathogens of Epidemiologic. Diagn Microbiol Infect Dis 1998;30:121–129.

36. Mermel LA: Prevention of intravascular catheter-related infections. Ann Intern Med 2000;132:391–402.

37. Pronovost P, Needham D, Berenholtz S, et al: An intervention to decrease catheter-related bloodstream infections in the ICU. N Engl J Med 2006;355:2725–2732.

38. Hill GE, Frawley WH, Griffith KE, et al: Allogeneic blood transfusion increases the risk of postoperative bacterial infection: A meta-analysis. J Trauma 2003;54:908–914.

39. Shorr AF, Jackson WL, Kelly KM, et al: Transfusion practice and blood stream infections in critically ill patients. Chest 2005;127:1722–1728.

40. Stramer SL, Glynn SA, Kleinman SH, et al: Detection of HIV-1 and HCV infections among antibody-negative blood donors by nucleic acid-amplification testing. N Engl J Med 2004;351:760–768.

41. Brecher ME, Hay SN: Bacterial contamination of blood components. Clin Microbiol Rev 2005;18:195–204.

42. Fatal bacterial infections associated with platelet transfusions—United States, 2004. MMWR Morb Mortal Wkly Rep 2005;54:168–170.

43. Yomtovian RA, Palavecino EL, Dykstra AH, et al: Evolution of surveillance methods for detection of bacterial contamination of platelets in a university hospital, 1991 through 2004. Transfusion 2006;46:719–730.

44. Brecher ME, Hay SN: Improving platelet safety: bacterial contamination of platelets. Curr Hematol Rep 2004;3:121–127.

45. Burns KH, Werch JB: Bacterial contamination of platelet units: A case report and literature survey with review of upcoming American Association of Blood Banks requirements. Arch Pathol Lab Med 2004;128:279–281.

46. Aguzzi A, Glatzel M: Prion infections, blood and transfusions. Nat Clin Pract Neurol 2006;2:321–329.

47. Llewelyn CA, Hewitt PE, Knight RS, et al: Possible transmission of variant Creutzfeldt-Jakob disease by blood transfusion. Lancet 2004;363:417–421.

48. Bone RC, Sprung CL, Sibbald WJ, Definitions for sepsis and organ failure and guidelines for the use of innovative therapies in sepsis. The ACCP/SCCM Consensus Conference Committee. American College of Chest Physicians/Society of Critical Care Medicine. Chest 1992;101:1644–1655.

49. Riedemann NC, Guo RF, Ward PA: Novel strategies for the treatment of sepsis. Nat Med 2003;9:517–524.

50. Hotchkiss RS, Karl IE: The pathophysiology and treatment of sepsis. N Engl J Med 2003;348:138–150.

51. Bone RC: Toward an epidemiology and natural history of SIRS (systemic inflammatory response syndrome). JAMA 1992;268:3452–3455.

52. Rivers E, Nguyen B, Havstad S, et al: Early goal-directed therapy in the treatment of severe sepsis and septic shock. N Engl J Med 2001;345:1368–1377.

53. Russell JA: Management of sepsis. N Engl J Med 2006;355: 1699–1713.

54. Dellinger RP, Carlet JM, Masur H, et al: Surviving Sepsis Campaign guidelines for management of severe sepsis and septic shock. Crit Care Med 2004;32:858–873.

55. McHenry CR, Piotrowski JJ, Petrinic D, Malangoni D: Determinants of mortality for necrotizing soft-tissue infections. Ann Surg 1995;221:558–563; discussion 563–565.

56. Headley AJ: Necrotizing soft tissue infections: A primary care review. Am Fam Physician 2003;68:323–328.

57. Efem SE: Recent advances in the management of Fournier's gangrene: preliminary observations. Surgery 1993;113:200–204.

58. Jackson WL Jr: Should we use etomidate as an induction agent for endotracheal intubation in patients with septic shock? A critical appraisal. Chest 2005;127:1031–1038.

59. Tsueda K, Oliver PB, Richter RW: Cardiovascular manifestations of tetanus. Anesthesiology 1974;40:588–592.

60. Baronia AK, Singh PK, Dhiman RK: Intractable pharyngeal spasm following tracheal extubation in a patient with undiagnosed tetanus. Anesthesiology 1991;75:1111.

61. Southorn PA, Blaise GA: Treatment of tetanus-induced autonomic nervous system dysfunction with continuous epidural blockade. Crit Care Med 1986;14:251–252.

62. Lutfiyya MN, Henley E, Chang LF, Reyburn SW: Diagnosis and treatment of community-acquired pneumonia. Am Fam Physician 2006;73:442–450.

63. Niederman MS, Mandell LA, Anzueto A, et al: Guidelines for the management of adults with community-acquired pneumonia. Diagnosis, assessment of severity, antimicrobial therapy, and prevention. Am J Respir Crit Care Med 2001; 163:1730–1754.

64. Guthrie R: Community-acquired lower respiratory tract infections: Etiology and treatment. Chest 2001;120:2021–2034.

65. Malhotra-Kumar S, Lammen C, Conen S, et al: Effect of azithromycin and clarithromycin therapy on pharyngeal carriage of macrolide-resistant streptococci in healthy volunteers: A randomised, double-blind, placebo-controlled study. Lancet 2007;369:482–490.

66. Fine MJ, Auble TE, Yealy DM, et al: A prediction rule to identify low-risk patients with community-acquired pneumonia. N Engl J Med 1997;336:243–250.

67. Start RD, Cross SS: ACP. Best practice no 155. Pathological investigation of deaths following surgery, anaesthesia, and medical procedures. J Clin Pathol 1999;52:640–652.

68. Rello J, Ollendorf DA, Oster G, et al: Epidemiology and outcomes of ventilator-associated pneumonia in a large US database. Chest 2002;122:2115–2121.

69. Porzecanski I, Bowton DL: Diagnosis and treatment of ventilator-associated pneumonia. Chest 2006;130:597–604.

70. Craven DE: Preventing ventilator-associated pneumonia in adults: sowing seeds of change. Chest 2006;130:251–260.

71. Luyt CE, Chastre J, Fagon JY: Value of the clinical pulmonary infection score for the identification and management of ventilator-associated pneumonia. Intensive Care Med 2004;30:844–852.

72. Webster RG, Govorkova EA: H5N1 influenza—continuing evolution and spread. N Engl J Med 2006;355:2174–2177.

73. Chan KH, Lam SY, Puthavathana P, et al: Comparative analytical sensitivities of six rapid influenza A antigen detection test kits for detection of influenza A subtypes H1N1, H3N2 and H5N1. J Clin Virol 2007;38:169–171.

74. Majury A, Ash J, Toye B, et al: Laboratory diagnosis of human infection with avian influenza. CMAJ 2006;175:1371.

75. Dawson ED, Moore CL, Dankbar DM, et al: Identification of A/H5N1 influenza viruses using a single gene diagnostic microarray. Anal Chem 2007;79:378–384.

76. Johnsen CK, Bottiger B, Blom J: Confirmation of electron microscopy results by direct testing of viruses adhered to grids using nucleic acid amplification techniques. J Virol Methods 2006;134:92–98.

77. Ebell MH: Diagnosing and treating patients with suspected influenza. Am Fam Physician 2005;72:1789–1792.

78. Kamming D, Gardam M, Chung F: Anaesthesia and SARS. Br J Anaesth 2003;90:715–718.

79. Peng PW, Wong DT, Bevon D, Gardam M: Infection control and anesthesia: lessons learned from the Toronto SARS outbreak. Can J Anaesth 2003;50:989–997.

80. Sihoe AD, Wong RH, Lee AT, et al: Severe acute respiratory syndrome complicated by spontaneous pneumothorax. Chest 2004;125:2345–2351.

81. The global HIV and AIDS epidemic, 2001. MMWR Morb Mortal Wkly Rep 2001;50:434–439.

82. Gayle H: An overview of the global HIV/AIDS epidemic, with a focus on the United States. AIDS 2000;14(Suppl 2):S8–S17.

83. Avidan MS, Groves P, Blott M, et al: Low complication rate associated with cesarean section under spinal anesthesia for HIV-1-infected women on antiretroviral therapy. Anesthesiology 2002;97:320–324.

84. Avidan MS, Jones N, Pozniak AL: The implications of HIV for the anaesthetist and the intensivist. Anaesthesia 2000; 55:344–354.

85. Hughes SC: HIV and anesthesia. Anesthesiol Clin North Am 2004;22:379–404.

86. Cinque P, Bossolasco S, Brambilla AM, et al: The effect of highly active antiretroviral therapy-induced immune reconstitution on development and outcome of progressive multifocal leukoencephalopathy: Study of 43 cases with review of the literature. J Neurovirol 2003;9(Suppl 1):73–80.

87. Haugaard SB: Toxic metabolic syndrome associated with HAART. Expert Opin Drug Metab Toxicol 2006;2:429–445.

88. Bonnet F, Balestre E, Bernardin E, et al: Risk factors for lactic acidosis in HIV-infected patients treated with nucleoside reverse-transcriptase inhibitors: A case-control study. Clin Infect Dis 2003;36:1324–1328.

89. Claessens YE, Chiche JD, Mira JP, Cariou A: Bench-to-bedside review: Severe lactic acidosis in HIV patients treated with nucleoside analogue reverse transcriptase inhibitors. Crit Care 2003;7:226–232.

90. Gregg RW, Friedman BC, Williams JF, et al: Continuous positive airway pressure by face mask in Pneumocystis carinii pneumonia. Crit Care Med 1990;18:21–24.

91. Kesten S, Rebuck AS: Nasal continuous positive airway pressure in Pneumocystis carinii pneumonia. Lancet 1988;2:1414–1415.

92. The mode of delivery and the risk of vertical transmission of human immunodeficiency virus type 1—a meta-analysis of 15 prospective cohort studies. The International Perinatal HIV Group. N Engl J Med 1999;340:977–987.

93. Grubert TA, Reindell D, Kästner R, et al: Complications after caesarean section in HIV-1-infected women not taking antiretroviral treatment. Lancet 1999;354:1612–1623.

94. Hughes SC, Dailey DA, Landers DA, et al: Parturients infected with human immunodeficiency virus and regional anesthesia. Clinical and immunologic response. Anesthesiology 1995;82:32–37.

95. Tait AR: Occupational transmission of tuberculosis: implications for anesthesiologists. Anesth Analg 1997;85:444–451.

96. Gandhi NR, Moll A, Sturm AW, et al: Extensively drug-resistant tuberculosis as a cause of death in patients co-infected with tuberculosis and HIV in a rural area of South Africa. Lancet 2006;368:1575–1580.

97. Pollard BA, El-Beheiry H: Pott's disease with unstable cervical spine, retropharyngeal cold abscess and progressive airway obstruction. Can J Anaesth 1999;46:772–775.

98. Guidelines for preventing the transmission of *Mycobacterium* tuberculosis in health-care facilities, 1994—CDC. Notice of final revisions to the "Guidelines for Preventing the Transmission of Mycobacterium Tuberculosis in Health-Care Facilities, 1994." Fed Regist 1994;59:54242–54303.

99. Jensen PA, Lambert LA, Iodemarco MF, Rizon R, et al: Guidelines for preventing the transmission of Mycobacterium tuberculosis in health-care settings, 2005. MMWR Recomm Rep 2005;54:1–141.

100. Wang YL, Hong CL, Chung HS, et al: Massive hemoptysis after the initiation of positive pressure ventilation in a patient with pulmonary tuberculosis. Anesthesiology 2000;92:1480–1482.

101. Starr J: *Clostridium difficile* associated diarrhoea: Diagnosis and treatment. BMJ 2005;331:498–501.

102. Hurley BW, Nguyen CC: The spectrum of pseudomembranous enterocolitis and antibiotic-associated diarrhea. Arch Intern Med 2002;162:2177–2184.

103. Dallal RM, Harbrecht DG, Boujoukas AJ, et al: Fulminant *Clostridium difficile*: An underappreciated and increasing cause of death and complications. Ann Surg 2002; 235:363–372.

104. McCoubrey J, Starr J, Martin H, Poxton JR, et al: *Clostridium difficile* in a geriatric unit: A prospective epidemiological study employing a novel S-layer typing method. J Med Microbiol 2003;52:573–578.

105. Bignardi GE: Risk factors for *Clostridium difficile* infection. J Hosp Infect 1998;40:1–15.

106. Bartlett JG: Narrative review: The new epidemic of *Clostridium difficile*-associated enteric disease. Ann Intern Med 2006;145:758–764.

107. Schroeder MS: *Clostridium difficile*–associated diarrhea. Am Fam Physician 2005;71:921–928.

108. Massey V, Gregson DB, Chagla AH, et al: Clinical usefulness of components of the Triage immunoassay, enzyme immunoassay for toxins A and B, and cytotoxin B tissue culture assay for the diagnosis of *Clostridium difficile* diarrhea. Am J Clin Pathol 2003;119:45–49.

109. Fernandez A, Anand G, Friedenberg F: Factors associated with failure of metronidazole in *Clostridium difficile*–associated disease. J Clin Gastroenterol 2004;38:414–418.

110. Kyne L, Hamel MB, Polavaram R, Kelly CP: Health care costs and mortality associated with nosocomial diarrhea due to *Clostridium difficile*. Clin Infect Dis 2002;34:346–353.

111. Bartlett JG: Clinical practice. Antibiotic-associated diarrhea. N Engl J Med 2002;346:334–339.

112. Viswanath YK, Griffiths CD: The role of surgery in pseudomembranous enterocolitis. Postgrad Med J 1998; 74:216–219.

Cancer

Nalini Vadivelu

Cancer is the second most frequent cause of death in the United States, exceeded only by heart disease. Cancer develops in one of every three Americans, and one of every five cancer victims dies of the effects of their disease. The number of deaths is increasing, reflecting the growing elderly population and a decrease in the number of deaths from heart disease.

MECHANISM

Cancer results from an accumulation of mutations in genes that regulate cellular proliferation. Genes are involved in carcinogenesis by virtue of inherited traits that predispose to cancer (altered metabolism of potentially carcinogenic components, decreased level of immune system function) or mutation of normal genes into oncogenes. The inheritance of a mutated allele is commonly followed by the loss of the second allele, leading to inactivation of a tumor suppressor gene and triggering malignant transformation. A critical gene related to cancer in humans is the tumor suppressor *p53*. This gene is not only essential for cell viability, but it is critical for monitoring damage to deoxyribonucleic acid (DNA). Inactivation of *p53* is an early step in the development of many types of cancer.

Stimulation of oncogene formation by carcinogens (tobacco, alcohol, sunlight) is estimated to be responsible for 80% of cancers in the United States. Tobacco use accounts for more cases of cancer than all other known carcinogens combined. The fundamental event that causes cells to become malignant is an alteration in the structure of DNA. The responsible mutations occur in cells of target tissues, with these cells becoming the ancestors of the entire future tumor cell population. Clonal evolution to even more undifferentiated cells reflects high mutation rates and contributes to the development of tumors that are resistant to drug, hormonal, and antibody therapy. Mutations have no effect on germ cells and are not transmitted genetically.

Cancer cells must evade the host's immune surveillance system, which is designed to seek out and destroy tumor cells. Most mutant cells stimulate the host's immune system to form antibodies (see "Immunology of Cancer Cells"). In support of a protective role of the immune system is the increased incidence of cancer in immunosuppressed patients, such as those with acquired immunodeficiency syndrome and those receiving organ transplants.

DIAGNOSIS

Cancer often becomes clinically evident when tumor bulk compromises the function of vital organs. The initial diagnosis of cancer is often by aspiration cytology or biopsy (needle, incisional, excisional). Monoclonal antibodies that recognize antigens for specific cancers (prostate, lung, breast, ovary) may aid in the diagnosis of cancer (see "Immunology of Cancer Cells"). A commonly used staging system for solid tumors is the TNM system based on tumor size (T), lymph node involvement (N), and distant metastasis (M). This system further groups patients into stages ranging from the best prognosis (stage I) to the poorest prognosis (stage IV). Tumor invasiveness is related to the release of various tumor mediators that modify the surrounding microenvironment in such a way as to permit cancer cells to spread along the lines of least resistance. Lymphatics lack a basement membrane so local spread of cancer is influenced by the anatomy of the regional lymphatics. For example, regional lymph node involvement occurs late in squamous cell cancer of the vocal cords because these structures have few lymphatics, whereas regional lymph node involvement is an early manifestation of supraglottic cancer because this region is rich in lymphatics. Imaging techniques including computed tomography and magnetic resonance imaging are used for further delineation of tumor presence and spread.

TREATMENT

Treatment of cancer includes chemotherapy, radiation, and surgery. Surgery is often necessary for the initial diagnosis of cancer (biopsy) and subsequent definitive treatment to remove the entire tumor or distant metastases or to decrease the tumor mass. Palliative and rehabilitative therapy may require surgery. Adequate relief of acute and chronic pain associated with cancer is a mandatory part of treatment.

Chemotherapy

Drugs administered for cancer chemotherapy may produce significant side effects (**Table 20-1**). These side effects may have important implications for the management of anesthesia during surgical procedures for cancer treatment as well as operations unrelated to the presence of cancer.

Angiogenesis Inhibitors

Cancer cells secrete proteins that facilitate angiogenesis (creation of new blood vessels) and tissue invasion, such as vascular endothelial growth factor, fibroblast growth factors, and matrix metalloproteinases. Signaling proteins have been identified, such as Flk-1 kinase, that are activated in endothelial cells after binding of angiogenic growth factors. Drugs that

TABLE 20-1	Principal Toxicities of Commonly Used Cancer Chemotherapeutic Drugs
Drug	**Effect**
Bleomycin (Blenoxane)	Interstitial pneumonitis/pulmonary fibrosis
Busulfan (Myleran)	Interstitial pneumonitis/pulmonary fibrosis
Cisplatin (Platinol)	Ototoxicity, peripheral neuropathy, renal failure
Cyclophosphamide (Cytoxan)	Plasma cholinesterase inhibition, hemorrhagic cystitis
Doxorubicin (Adriamycin)	Dose-dependent cardiomyopathy
L-Asparaginase (Elspar)	Hypersensitivity reactions/anaphylaxis, pancreatitis
Melphalan (Alkeran)	Development of secondary leukemias, sterility
Mitomycin	Hemolytic uremic syndrome
Paclitaxel (Taxol)	Hypersensitivity reactions, peripheral neuropathy
Vincristine (Oncovin)	Peripheral neuropathy, autonomic neuropathy

prevent angiogenesis, such as endostatin, may be useful in the treatment of cancer.

Acute and Chronic Pain

Cancer patients may experience acute pain associated with pathologic fractures, tumor invasion, surgery, radiation, and chemotherapy A frequent source of pain is related to metastatic spread of the cancer, especially to bone. Nerve compression or infiltration may be a cause of pain. Patients with cancer who experience frequent and significant pain exhibit signs of depression and anxiety.

Pathophysiology

Organic causes of cancer pain may be subdivided into nociceptive and neuropathic pain. Nociceptive pain includes somatic and visceral pain and refers to pain due to the peripheral stimulation of nociceptors in somatic or visceral structures. Somatic pain is related to tumor involvement of somatic structures such as bones or skeletal muscles and is often described as aching, stabbing, or throbbing. Visceral pain is related to lesions in a hollow or solid viscus and is described as diffuse, gnawing, or crampy if a hollow viscus is involved. It is more commonly described as aching or sharp if a solid viscus is involved. Nociceptive pain is typically responsive to both nonopioids and opioids. Neuropathic pain involves peripheral or central afferent neural pathways and is commonly described as burning or lancinating pain. Patients experiencing neuropathic pain often respond poorly to opioids. Pain can be controlled in cancer patients with drug therapy or by invasive procedures.

Trauma associated with surgery for removal of cancerous tissue may also be a cause of chronic pain. Scars and injury of soft tissue and of sensory afferents that innervate the surgical area may all contribute to the development of chronic pain. Chronic postmastectomy pain may impair the activities in a woman's life. Multimodal analgesia with local anesthetics and gabapentin may be effective in preventing both acute and chronic postmastectomy pain and reducing analgesic consumption after breast surgery. Recently gabapentin has been shown to reduce analgesic requirements for *acute* postoperative pain but does not significantly affect the development of *chronic* pain.

Drug Therapy

Drug therapy is the cornerstone of cancer pain management because of its efficacy, rapid onset of action, and relatively low cost. Mild to moderate cancer pain is initially treated with nonsteroidal anti-inflammatory drugs and acetaminophen. Nonsteroidal anti-inflammatory drugs are especially effective for managing bone pain, which is the most common cause of cancer pain. The next step in management of moderate to severe pain includes addition of codeine or one of its analogues. When cancer pain is severe, opioids are the major drugs used. Morphine is the most commonly selected opioid and can be administered orally. When the oral route of administration is inadequate, alternative routes (intravenous,

subcutaneous, epidural, intrathecal, transmucosal, transdermal) are considered. Fentanyl is available in transdermal and transmucosal delivery systems. There is no maximum safe dose of morphine and other μ-agonist opioids. Tolerance to opioids does occur but need not be a clinical problem. Unnecessary fear of addiction is a major reason opioids are underused despite the fact that addiction is rare when these drugs are correctly used to treat pain in cancer patients.

Tricyclic antidepressant drugs are recommended for those who remain depressed despite improved pain control. These drugs are also effective in the absence of depression and appear to have direct analgesic effects and cause potentiation of opioids. Anticonvulsants are useful for management of chronic neuropathic pain. Corticosteroids can decrease pain perception, have a sparing effect on opioid requirements, improve mood, increase appetite, and lead to weight gain.

Neuraxial Analgesia

Neuraxial analgesia is an effective way to control pain in cancer patients undergoing surgery and may play a role in providing preemptive analgesia. Neuraxial analgesia with local anesthetics provides immediate pain relief in patients whose pain cannot be relieved with oral or intravenous analgesics and is frequently used for the treatment of cancer pain. Neuraxial analgesia is not performed in patients with local infection, bacteremia, and systemic infection because of the increased risk of epidural abscess. However, in the presence of intractable cancer pain, there may be a role for the use of epidural analgesia despite meningeal infection. Morphine may be administered intrathecally or epidurally for management of acute and chronic cancer pain. Spinal opioids may be delivered for weeks to months via a long-term, subcutaneously tunneled, exteriorized catheter or an implanted drug delivery system. The implantable systems can be intrathecal or epidural and typically feature a drug reservoir and the capability for external reprogramming. Patients are typically considered for neuraxial opioid administration when systemic opioid administration has failed as a result of the onset of intolerable adverse (systemic) side effects or adequate analgesia cannot be achieved. Neuraxial administration of opioids is usually successful, but some patients require an additional low concentration of local anesthetic to achieve adequate pain control.

Neurolytic Procedures Neurolytic procedures intended to destroy sensory components of nerves cannot be used without also destroying motor and autonomic nervous system fibers. Important aspects of determining the suitability of destructive nerve blocks are the location and quality of the pain, the effectiveness of less destructive treatment modalities, life expectancy, the inherent risks associated with the block, and the availability of experienced anesthesiologists to perform the procedures. In general, constant pain is more amenable to destructive nerve blocks than is intermittent pain. Neurolytic celiac plexus block (alcohol, phenol) has been used to treat pain originating from abdominal viscera, for example, pancreatic cancer. The block is associated with significant side effects, but analgesia usually lasts 6 months or longer.

Neurosurgical procedures (neuroablative or neurostimulatory) for managing cancer pain are reserved for patients unresponsive to other less invasive procedures. Cordotomy involves interruption of the spinothalamic tract in the spinal cord and is considered for treatment of unilateral pain involving the lower extremity, thorax, or upper extremity. Dorsal rhizotomy involves interruption of sensory nerve roots and is used when pain is localized to specific dermatomal levels. Dorsal column stimulators or deep brain stimulators may be used in selected patients.

IMMUNOLOGY OF CANCER CELLS

Tumor cells are antigenically different from normal cells and may therefore elicit immune reactions similar to those that cause rejection of allografts. Antigens present in cancer cells but not in normal cells are designated *tumor-specific* antigens. Conversely, *tumor-associated* antigens (α-fetoprotein, prostate-specific antigen [PSA], carcinoembryonic antigen) are present in cancer cells and normal cells, but concentrations are higher in tumor cells. Because tumor-associated antigens may be present in normal tissues, measurements of these antigens may be less useful for the diagnosis of cancer than for monitoring patients with known malignant disorders.

Antibodies to tumor-associated antigens can be used for the immunodiagnosis of cancer. The use of monoclonal antibodies to detect proteins encoded by oncogenes or other types of tumor-associated antigens is a common method for identifying cancer. Monoclonal antibodies to various tumor-associated antigens can be labeled with radioisotopes and injected to monitor the spread of cancer or be used as carriers of immunotoxins or drugs. The enormous antigenic diversity of many forms of cancer makes the development of an effective vaccine a formidable task. Alternatively, attempts may be made to enhance a patient's overall level of immunity with nonspecific immunopotentiators such as bacille Calmette-Guérin and interferons. Most spontaneously occurring tumors appear to be weakly antigenic. Some can activate suppressor T cells to dampen the intensity of immune responses to tumor antigens.

PARANEOPLASTIC SYNDROMES

Paraneoplastic syndromes manifest as pathophysiologic disturbances that may accompany cancer (**Table 20-2**). Certain of these pathophysiologic disturbances (superior vena cava obstruction, increased intracranial pressure, pericardial tamponade, renal failure, hypercalcemia) may manifest as life-threatening medical emergencies.

Fever and Weight Loss

Fever may accompany any type of cancer but is particularly likely with metastases to the liver. Increased body temperature

TABLE 20-2	Pathophysiologic Manifestations of Paraneoplastic Syndromes

Fever
Anorexia
Weight loss
Anemia
Thrombocytopenia
Coagulopathy
Neuromuscular abnormalities
Ectopic hormone production
Hypercalcemia
Hyperuricemia
Tumor lysis syndrome
Adrenal insufficiency
Nephrotic syndrome
Ureteral obstruction
Pulmonary hypertrophic osteoarthropathy and digital clubbing
Pericardial effusion
Pericardial tamponade
Superior vena cava obstruction
Spinal cord compression

may accompany rapidly proliferating tumors, such as leukemias and lymphomas. Fever may reflect tumor necrosis, inflammation, the release of toxic products by cancer cells, or the production of endogenous pyrogens.

Anorexia and weight loss are frequent occurrences in patients with cancer, especially lung cancer. In addition to the psychological effects of cancer on appetite, cancer cells compete with normal tissues for nutrients and may eventually cause nutritive death of normal cells. Hyperalimentation is indicated for nutritional support when malnutrition is severe, especially if elective surgery is planned.

Hematologic Abnormalities

Anemia is usually a direct result of the effects of cancer, such as gastrointestinal bleeding or tumor replacement of bone marrow. Cancer chemotherapy is another common cause of bone marrow suppression and anemia. Acute hemolytic anemia may accompany lymphoproliferative diseases. Solid tumors, especially metastatic breast cancer, can lead to pancytopenia. In contrast, an increased amount of erythropoietin, as produced by a renal cell carcinoma or hepatoma, can produce polycythemia. Thrombocytopenia can be due to chemotherapy or to the presence of an unrecognized cancer. Disseminated intravascular coagulation may occur in patients with advanced cancer, especially when hepatic metastases are present. There is an association between venous thromboembolism and a subsequent diagnosis of cancer. Cancer diagnosed at the same time as or within 1 year after an episode of venous thromboembolism is often associated with an advanced stage of cancer and a poor prognosis. Recurrent venous thrombosis due to unknown mechanisms may be associated with pancreatic cancer.

Neuromuscular Abnormalities

Neuromuscular abnormalities occur in 5% to 10% of patients with cancer. The most common is the skeletal muscle weakness (myasthenic syndrome) associated with lung cancer. Potentiation of depolarizing and nondepolarizing muscle relaxants has been observed in patients with co-existing skeletal muscle weakness, particularly when such weakness is associated with undifferentiated small cell lung cancer.

Ectopic Hormone Production

Active hormones are produced by a number of tumors, resulting in predictable physiologic effects (**Table 20-3**).

Hypercalcemia

Cancer is the most common cause of hypercalcemia in hospitalized patients, reflecting local osteolytic activity from bone metastases especially breast cancer or the ectopic parathyroid hormonal activity associated with tumors that arise from the kidneys, lungs, pancreas, or ovaries. The rapid onset of hypercalcemia that occurs in patients with cancer may manifest as lethargy and coma. Polyuria and dehydration may accompany hypercalcemia, which is further exaggerated by bone pain and immobility. Opioids administered to relieve pain can result in further immobility, vomiting, or dehydration.

Tumor Lysis Syndrome

Tumor lysis syndrome is caused by sudden destruction of tumor cells by chemotherapy, leading to the release of uric acid, potassium, and phosphate. This syndrome occurs most often after treatment of hematologic neoplasms, such as acute lymphoblastic leukemia. Acute renal failure can accompany the hyperuricemia. Hyperkalemia and resulting cardiac dysrhythmia are more likely in the presence of renal dysfunction. Hyperphosphatemia can lead to secondary hypocalcemia, which increases the risk of cardiac dysrhythmias from hypokalemia and can cause neuromuscular symptoms such as tetany.

Adrenal Insufficiency

Adrenal insufficiency caused by complete replacement of the adrenal glands by metastatic tumor is rare. More often there is relative adrenal insufficiency owing to partial replacement of the adrenal cortex by tumor or suppression of adrenal cortical function by prolonged treatment with corticosteroids. Adrenal insufficiency is most often seen in patients with metastatic disease due to melanoma, retroperitoneal tumors, lung cancer, or breast cancer. The stress of the perioperative period may unmask adrenal insufficiency. Clinical manifestations include fatigue, dehydration, oliguria, and cardiovascular collapse. Treatment of acute adrenal insufficiency consists of bolus intravenous administration of cortisol repeated at 6- to 8-hour intervals or given by continuous infusion until oral replacement of a glucocorticoid and mineralocorticoid can be initiated.

Renal Dysfunction

Renal complications of cancer reflect invasion of the kidneys by tumor, damage from tumor products, or chemotherapy. Deposition of tumor antigen-antibody complexes on the glomerular membrane results in changes characteristic of the nephrotic syndrome. Extensive retroperitoneal cancer can lead to bilateral ureteral obstruction and uremia, especially in patients with cancer of the cervix, bladder, or prostate. Percutaneous nephrostomy is indicated if a ureter is totally obstructed. Chemotherapy can destroy large numbers of tumor cells. Acute hyperuricemic nephropathy due to precipitation of uric acid crystals in the renal tubules is prevented by administration of allopurinol in combination with hydration and alkalinization of the urine. Methotrexate and cisplatin are the chemotherapeutic drugs most often associated with nephrotoxicity.

TABLE 20-3 Ectopic Hormone Production		
Hormone	**Associated Cancer**	**Manifestations**
Corticotropin	Lung (small cell), thyroid (medullary), thymoma, carcinoid islet cell tumor	Cushing's syndrome
Antidiuretic hormone	Lung (small cell), pancreas, lymphoma	Water intoxication
Gonadotropin	Lung (large cell), ovary, adrenal	Gynecomastia, precocious puberty
Melanocyte-stimulating hormone Parathyroid hormone	Lung (small cell), renal lung (squamous cell), pancreas, ovary	Hyperpigmentation, hyperparathyroidism
Thyrotropin	Choriocarcinoma, testicular (embryonal)	Hyperthyroidism
Thyrocalcitonin	Thyroid (medullary)	Hypocalcemia
Insulin	Retroperitoneal tumors	Hypoglycemia

Acute hemorrhagic cystitis is a complication of cyclophosphamide therapy.

Acute Respiratory Complications

The acute onset of dyspnea may reflect extension of the tumor or the effects of chemotherapy. Bleomycin-induced interstitial pneumonitis and fibrosis are the most commonly encountered pulmonary complications of chemotherapy. Elderly patients and those with co-existing lung disease or previous radiation therapy receiving large dose of bleomycin are at greatest risk of pulmonary toxicity. Pulmonary toxicity rarely occurs when the total dose of bleomycin is less than 150 mg/m^2. The most common symptoms of interstitial pneumonitis are the insidious onset of nonproductive cough, dyspnea, tachypnea, and occasionally fever 4 to 10 weeks after initiation of bleomycin therapy. These symptoms appear in 3% to 6% of patients treated with bleomycin. Incipient toxicity can be detected by measuring carbon monoxide diffusing capacity. The alveolar-to-arterial oxygen difference is usually increased in affected patients. The appearance of radiographic changes, such as bilateral diffuse pulmonary infiltrates, probably portends irreversible pulmonary fibrosis. In the absence of a biopsy, the clinical and radiographic features of bleomycin-induced pneumonitis can be difficult to distinguish from pneumonia due to *Pneumocystis carinii*. Corticosteroids are the only treatment for the acute effects of drug-induced pneumonitis. However, once interstitial and alveolar fibrosis have occurred, they are irreversible.

Acute Cardiac Complications

Pericardial effusion caused by metastatic invasion of the pericardium can lead to cardiac tamponade. Lung cancer seems to be the most common cause of pericardial tamponade. Malignant pericardial effusion is the most common cause of electrical alternans on the electrocardiogram. Paroxysmal atrial fibrillation or flutter may be an early manifestation of malignant involvement of the pericardium or myocardium. Optimal treatment of malignant pericardial effusion consists of prompt removal of the fluid followed by surgical creation of a pericardial window

Cardiac toxicity manifesting as cardiomyopathy occurs in 1% to 5% of patients treated with doxorubicin or daunorubicin. Cardiotoxicity may manifest initially as symptoms suggestive of an upper respiratory tract infection (nonproductive cough) followed by rapidly progressive congestive heart failure that is often refractory to inotropic drugs or mechanical cardiac assistance. Cardiomegaly and/or pleural effusion may be evident on chest radiography. Patients who have undergone radiation therapy, particularly to the mediastinum, or patients who are on concurrent cyclophosphamide therapy seem to be more susceptible to the development of cardiomyopathy. In contrast to life-threatening cardiomyopathy, approximately 10% of treated patients show nonspecific, usually benign, changes on the electrocardiogram (nonspecific ST-T changes, low QRS voltage, atrial

or ventricular premature beats) that do not reflect an underlying cardiomyopathy.

Superior Vena Cava Obstruction

Obstruction of the superior vena cava is caused by spread of cancer into the mediastinum or directly into the caval wall, most often by lung cancer. Engorgement of veins above the level of the heart occurs, particularly the jugular veins and those in the arms. Dyspnea and airway obstruction may be present. Edema of the arms and face is usually prominent. Hoarseness may reflect edema of the vocal cords. Increased intracranial pressure manifests as nausea, seizures, and decreased levels of consciousness and is most likely due to the increase in cerebral venous pressures. Treatment consists of prompt radiation or chemotherapy, even without a cytologic diagnosis to decrease the size of the tumor and thus relieve venous and airway obstruction. Bronchoscopy and/or mediastinoscopy to obtain a tissue diagnosis can be very hazardous, especially in the presence of co-existing airway obstruction and increased pressure in the mediastinal veins.

Spinal Cord Compression

Spinal cord compression results from the presence of metastatic lesions in the epidural space, most often breast, lung, or prostate cancer or lymphoma. Symptoms include pain, skeletal muscle weakness, sensory loss, and autonomic nervous system dysfunction. Computed tomography and magnetic resonance imaging can visualize the limits of compression. Radiation therapy is a useful treatment when neurologic deficits are only partial or in development. Once total paralysis has developed, the results of surgical laminectomy or of radiation to decompress the spinal cord are usually poor. Corticosteroids are often administered to minimize the inflammation and edema that can result from radiation directed at tumors in the epidural space.

Increased Intracranial Pressure

Metastatic brain tumors, most often from lung and breast cancer, present initially as mental deterioration, focal neurologic deficits, or seizures. Treatment of an acute increase in intracranial pressure caused by a metastatic lesion includes corticosteroids, diuretics, and mannitol. Radiation therapy is the usual palliative treatment, but surgery can be considered for patients with only a single metastatic lesion. Intrathecal administration of chemotherapeutic drugs is necessary when the tumor involves the meninges.

MANAGEMENT OF ANESTHESIA

Preoperative evaluation of patients with cancer includes consideration of the pathophysiologic effects of the disease (see Tables 20-2 and 20-3) and recognition of the potential adverse effects of cancer chemotherapeutic drugs (see Table 20-1).

TABLE 20-4	Preoperative Tests in Patients with Cancer
Hematocrit	
Platelet count	
White blood cell count	
Prothrombin time	
Electrolytes	
Liver function tests	
Renal function tests	
Blood glucose concentrations	
Arterial blood gases	
Chest radiography	
Electrocardiography	

Preoperative tests to detect side effects of chemotherapy are listed in **Table 20-4.**

Side Effects of Chemotherapy

Pulmonary and Cardiac Toxicity

The possible presence of pulmonary or cardiac toxicity is a consideration in patients being treated with chemotherapeutic drugs known to be associated with these complications. A preoperative history of drug-induced pulmonary fibrosis (dyspnea, nonproductive cough) or congestive heart failure will influence the subsequent conduct of anesthesia. In patients treated with bleomycin, it may be helpful to monitor arterial blood gases in addition to oximetry and to carefully titrate intravascular fluid replacement, keeping in mind that these patients are at risk of development of interstitial pulmonary edema presumably because of impaired lymphatic drainage from the pulmonary fibrosis. Whether bleomycin increases the likelihood of oxygen toxicity in the presence of high inspired concentrations of oxygen is not certain, but it seems prudent to adjust the delivered oxygen concentration to the minimum that provides the desired Sp_{O_2}. Depressant effects of anesthetic drugs on myocardial contractility may be enhanced in patients with drug-induced cardiac toxicity.

Neurotoxicity

Anticancer chemotherapy can cause a number of neurotoxic side effects including peripheral neuropathy and encephalopathy

Peripheral Neuropathy Vinca alkaloids, particularly vincristine, affect the microtubules causing sensorimotor peripheral neuropathy. Virtually all patients treated with vincristine develop paresthesias in their digits. Autonomic nervous system neuropathy may accompany the paresthesias. These changes are reversible. Cisplatin causes dose-dependent large-fiber neuropathy by damaging dorsal root ganglia. Loss of proprioception in these patients may be sufficiently severe to interfere with ambulation. Performance of regional anesthesia in patients being treated with cisplatin chemotherapy may be influenced by the realization that subclinical neurotoxicity is present in a large percentage of patients and cisplatin neurotoxicity may extend several months beyond discontinuation of treatment. Administration of local anesthetics and epinephrine in this situation might produce a clinically significant injury. Severe diffuse brachial plexopathy has been described following an interscalene block in a patient receiving cisplatin chemotherapy. Paclitaxel causes dose-dependent ataxia that may be accompanied by paresthesias in the hands and feet and proximal skeletal muscle weakness. Corticosteroids (prednisone or its equivalent at 60–100 mg/day) may cause a myopathy characterized by weakness of the neck flexors and proximal weakness of the extremities. The first sign of corticosteroid-induced neuromuscular toxicity is difficulty rising from the sitting position. Respiratory muscles may also be affected. Corticosteroid-induced peripheral neuropathy usually resolves when the drug is discontinued.

Encephalopathy Many cancer chemotherapeutic drugs can cause encephalopathy. High-dose cyclophosphamide may be associated with acute delirium. High-dose cytarabine may cause acute delirium or cerebellar degeneration, both of which are usually reversible. Reversible acute encephalopathy may accompany the intravenous or intrathecal administration of methotrexate. Prolonged administration of methotrexate, especially in conjunction with radiation therapy, can lead to progressive irreversible dementia.

Preoperative Preparation

Correction of nutrient deficiencies, anemia, coagulopathy, and electrolyte abnormalities may be needed preoperatively. Nausea and vomiting are the most common and distressing side effects of chemotherapy and, to some extent, of radiation treatment. Serotonin antagonist drugs, such as ondansetron, droperidol, and metoclopramide may help control nausea in these patients. Tricyclic antidepressants are useful for potentiating the analgesic effects of opioids and producing some inherent analgesia. Opioids used to manage cancer pain may be responsible for preoperative sedation.

The presence of hepatic or renal dysfunction may influence the choice of anesthetic drugs and muscle relaxants. Although not a consistent observation, the possibility of a prolonged response to succinylcholine is a consideration in patients being treated with alkylating chemotherapeutic drugs such as cyclophosphamide. Attention to aseptic technique is important because immunosuppression occurs with most chemotherapeutic agents. Immunosuppression produced by anesthesia, surgical stimulation, or even blood transfusion during the perioperative period could exert effects on the patient's subsequent response to cancer. There is concern that, because of their suppression of the immune response, some anesthetic drugs may assist in tumor growth or enhance aggregation of some cancer proteins.

Cancer patients may have life-threatening airway difficulties and upper airway obstruction with head, neck, and chest tumors. Preoperative preparation is required to assess potential difficulties that may arise in securing the airway. Awake fiberoptic intubation is the gold standard for difficult airway management. In some patients, tracheostomy may be indicated.

Postoperative Considerations

Postoperative mechanical ventilation may be required, particularly following invasive or prolonged operations and in patients with drug-induced pulmonary fibrosis. Patients with drug-induced cardiac toxicity are more likely to experience postoperative cardiac complications.

COMMON CANCERS ENCOUNTERED IN CLINICAL PRACTICE

The most commonly encountered cancers in adults are lung cancer, breast cancer, colon cancer, and prostate cancer. Lung cancer is the second most common malignancy in men surpassed only by prostate cancer, whereas in women the incidence of lung cancer is increasing and is now exceeded only by breast cancer.

Lung Cancer

Lung cancer is the leading cause of cancer deaths among men and women and accounts for nearly one third of all cancer deaths in the United States. It is largely a preventable disease, since more than 90% of lung cancer deaths are related to cigarette smoking. The high mortality resulting from lung cancer (5-year survival rate of 15%) reflects its aggressive biology and advanced stage at the time of diagnosis.

Etiology

The strong association of cigarette smoking with lung cancer is well established. Smoking marijuana produces a greater carbon monoxide and tar burden than smoking a similar quantity of tobacco and thus may pose an additional risk factor for lung cancer in cigarette smokers. The mutagens and carcinogens present in cigarette smoke may cause chromosomal damage and over time may cause malignancy. Other carcinogens that cause lung cancer include ionizing radiation (by-product of coal and iron mining), asbestos (increases the incidence of lung cancer in nonsmokers and acts as a synergistic co-carcinogen with tobacco smoke), and naturally occurring radon gas. Adjuvant radiation therapy for breast cancer following mastectomy is associated with an increased risk of lung cancer.

There is a familial risk of lung cancer that is related to genetic and ecogenetic factors and to exposure to passive smoking. Inhalation of second-hand smoke increases the risk of lung cancer and contributes to the development of childhood respiratory infections and asthma. Cigarette smokers who develop emphysema are at increased risk of the development of lung cancer. Acquired immunodeficiency syndrome may be associated with an increased incidence of lung cancer. Cessation of cigarette smoking decreases the risk and incidence of lung cancer to that of nonsmokers after approximately 10 to 15 years have elapsed.

Signs and Symptoms

Patients with lung cancer present with features related to the extent of the disease, including local and regional manifestations, signs and symptoms of metastatic disease, and various paraneoplastic syndromes related indirectly to the cancer (see Table 20-2). Cough, hemoptysis, wheezing, stridor, dyspnea, or pneumonitis from airway obstruction may be presenting clinical signs. Mediastinal metastases may cause hoarseness (recurrent laryngeal nerve compression), superior vena cava syndrome, cardiac dysrhythmias, or congestive heart failure from pericardial effusion and tamponade. Pleural effusion results in increasing dyspnea and often chest pain. Generalized weakness, fatigue, anorexia, and weight loss are common.

Histologic Subtypes

Clinical manifestations of lung cancer vary with the histologic subtype (**Table 20-5**). Non-small cell lung cancer, which includes squamous cell carcinoma, adenocarcinoma, and large cell carcinoma, accounts for 75% to 80% of all new cases of lung cancer.

Squamous cell cancers arise in major bronchi or their primary divisions (central origin) and are usually detected by sputum cytology. These tumors tend to grow slowly and may reach a large size before they are finally detected because of hemoptysis and bronchial obstruction with associated atelectasis, dyspnea, and fever from pneumonia. Cavitation may be evident on chest radiography.

Adenocarcinomas most often originate in the lung periphery. These tumors commonly present as subpleural nodules

TABLE 20-5 Clinical and Pathologic Features of Lung Cancer

| Histologic Subtype | Incidence (%) | 5-YEAR SURVIVAL (%) | | Associated Symptoms |
		All Cases	Resectable Cases	
Squamous cell	25–40	11	40	Hypercalcemia
Adenocarcinoma	30–50	5	30	Hypercoagulability, osteoarthropathy
Large cell	10	4	30	Gynecomastia, galactorrhea
Small cell	15–24	2	5–10	Inappropriate antidiuretic hormone secretion, ectopic corticotropin secretion, Eaton-Lambert syndrome

Adapted from Skarin AT: Lung cancer. Sci Am Med 1997;1–20.

and have a tendency to invade the pleura and induce pleural effusions that contain malignant cells. Lung adenocarcinomas may be difficult to differentiate morphologically from malignant mesothelioma and adenocarcinoma that has metastasized from other sites (breast, gastrointestinal tract, pancreas).

Large cell carcinomas are usually peripheral in origin and present as large, bulky tumors. Like adenocarcinomas, these tumors metastasize early and preferentially to the central nervous system.

Small cell carcinomas are usually of central bronchial origin and have a high frequency of early lymphatic invasion especially to lymph nodes in the mediastinum and metastases to liver, bone, central nervous system, adrenal glands, and pancreas. Prominent mediastinal lymphadenopathy may lead to the erroneous diagnosis of malignant lymphoma. Superior vena cava syndrome may result from mediastinal compression. Small cell tumors have a marked propensity to produce polypeptides and ectopic hormones resulting in metabolic abnormalities. These patients do not usually present before the disease process is widespread.

Diagnosis

Cytologic analysis of sputum is often sufficient for the diagnosis of lung cancer, especially when the cancer arises in proximal endobronchial locations where shedding of cells is likely to occur. Peripheral lesions as small as 3.0 mm can be detected by high-resolution computed tomography. Lung cancer screening has been recommended for patients who are at highest risk, such as cigarette smokers with chronic obstructive lung disease. However, despite new diagnostic techniques, the overall 5-year survival rates remain approximately 15%, and most patients still present with advanced disease.

Flexible fiberoptic bronchoscopy, in combination with a biopsy, brushings, or washings, is a standard procedure for initial evaluation of lung cancer. Peripheral lung lesions can be diagnosed by percutaneous fine-needle aspiration guided by fluoroscopy, ultrasonography, or computed tomography. Video-assisted thoracoscopic surgery is useful for diagnosing peripheral lung lesions and pleura-based tumors. Computed tomography is sensitive for detecting pulmonary metastases. Brain magnetic resonance imaging and head computed tomography are useful for detecting metastases even in patients without neurologic abnormalities. Mediastinoscopy and video-assisted thoracoscopy provide the opportunity to biopsy lymph nodes and stage the tumor.

Treatment

Surgical resection (lobectomy, pneumonectomy) is the most effective treatment for lung cancer. In patients with impaired pulmonary function, wedge resection may be selected. *Resectability* refers to the extent of the disease and whether the tumor can be entirely removed. This is determined by staging procedures. *Operability* refers to the medical status of the patient and includes an assessment of the patient's overall surgical risk and the amount of functional lung tissue that will remain postoperatively. It is estimated that approximately 30% of patients with newly diagnosed non-small cell lung cancers have locally advanced nonresectable disease at the time of diagnosis, and another 40% have confirmed metastatic disease.. Surgery has little effect on survival when the disease has spread to unilateral mediastinal lymph nodes. Even among those considered surgically curable, recurrent metastatic disease develops in approximately half of these patients within 5 years. For these reasons, many patients with non-small cell lung cancers are candidates for chemotherapy alone or in combination with surgery or radiation therapy. Video-assisted thoracoscopy is the preferred surgical approach, especially for wedge resection and lobectomy. Standard thoracotomy is needed for more complex procedures or pneumonectomy.

The 5-year survival is unaffected by traditional adjuvant treatments, including radiation, chemotherapy, immunotherapy, and combinations of these treatments. Radiotherapy is effective in palliating symptoms from tumor invasion in most patients.

Management of Anesthesia

Management of anesthesia in patients with lung cancer includes preoperative consideration of tumor-induced effects such as malnutrition, pneumonia, pain, and ectopic endocrine effects such as hyponatremia (see Table 20-3). When resection of lung tissue is planned, it is important to evaluate underlying pulmonary and cardiac function, especially for the presence of pulmonary hypertension.

Hemorrhage and pneumothorax are the most frequently encountered complications of mediastinoscopy. The mediastinoscope can also exert pressure on the right innominate artery, causing loss of the distal pulse and an erroneous diagnosis of cardiac arrest. Likewise, unrecognized compression of the right innominate artery of which the right carotid artery is a branch may manifest as a postoperative neurologic deficit. Bradycardia during mediastinoscopy may be due to stretching of the vagus nerve or trachea compression by the mediastinoscope.

Colorectal Cancer

Colon cancer is second only to lung cancer as a cause of cancer death in the United States. The incidence and mortality from this cancer has not changed appreciably during the past several decades. Almost all colorectal cancers are adenocarcinomas, and the disease generally occurs in adults older than 50 years.

Etiology

Most colorectal cancers arise from premalignant adenomatous polyps. Large polyps, especially those larger than 1.5 cm in diameter, are more likely to contain invasive cancer. Although adenomatous polyps are common (present in more than 30% of patients older than 50 years), less than 1% of adenomatous polyps ever become malignant. It is thought that adenomatous polyps require at least 5 years of growth before they become clinically significant. The evolution of normal colonic mucosa to a benign adenomatous polyp that contains cancer and then to life-threatening invasive cancer is associated with a series of genetic events that involve the mutational activation of a proto-oncogene and the loss of several genes that normally suppress tumorigenesis.

Most colorectal cancers appear to be related to diet, with the disease occurring in the greatest incidence among individuals in upper socioeconomic classes living in urban areas. There is a direct correlation between calories consumed, dietary fat and oil, and meat protein. Available data indicate that a high intake of animal fat is the dietary element that is most strongly associated with the risk of colon cancer. As many as 25% of patients with colorectal cancer have a family history of the disease. Inflammatory bowel disease is associated with an increased incidence of colorectal cancer. Cigarette smoking for longer than 35 years appears to increase the risk of colorectal cancer.

Diagnosis

The rationale for colorectal cancer screening is that early detection and removal of localized superficial tumors and precancerous lesions in asymptomatic individuals increases the cure rate. Screening programs (digital rectal examination, examination of the stool for occult blood, colonoscopy) appear to be particularly useful for persons who have first-degree relatives with a history of the disease, especially if these relatives developed the colorectal cancer before 55 years of age. There is evidence that annual or biennial fecal occult blood testing is associated with a decreased incidence of colorectal cancer.

Signs and Symptoms

The presenting signs and symptoms of colorectal cancer reflect the anatomic location of the cancer. Because stool is relatively liquid as it passes into the right colon through the ileocecal valve, tumors in the cecum and ascending colon can become large and markedly narrow the bowel lumen without causing obstructive symptoms. Ascending colon cancers frequently ulcerate, leading to chronic blood loss in the stool. These patients experience symptoms related to anemia, including fatigue and, in some patients, angina pectoris.

Stool becomes more concentrated as it passes into the transverse colon. Transverse colon cancers cause abdominal cramping, occasional bowel obstruction, and even perforation. Abdominal radiographs reveals characteristic abnormalities in the colonic gas pattern, reflecting narrowing of the lumen ("napkin ring lesion"). Colon cancers developing in the rectosigmoid portion of the large intestine result in tenesmus and thinner stools. Anemia is unusual despite the passage of bright red blood from the rectum (often attributable to hemorrhoids).

Colorectal cancers initially spread to regional lymph nodes and then through the portal venous circulation to the liver, which represents the most common visceral site of metastases. Colorectal cancers rarely spread to lung, bone, or brain in the absence of liver metastases. A preoperative increase in the serum concentration of carcinoembryonic antigen suggests that the tumor will recur following surgical resection. Carcinoembryonic antigen is a glycoprotein that is also increased in the presence of other cancers (stomach, pancreas, breast, lung) and nonmalignant conditions (alcoholic liver disease, inflammatory bowel disease, cigarette smoking, pancreatitis).

Treatment

The prognosis for patients with adenocarcinoma of the colorectum depends on the depth of tumor penetration into the bowel wall and the presence or absence of regional lymph node involvement and distant metastases (liver, lung, bone). Radical surgical resection, which includes the blood vessels and lymph nodes draining the involved bowel, offers the best potential for cure. Surgical management of cancers that arise in the distal rectum may necessitate a permanent sigmoid colostomy (abdominoperineal resection). Because most recurrences occur within 3 to 4 years, the cure rate for colorectal cancer is often estimated by 5-year survival rates.

Radiation therapy is a consideration in patients with rectal tumors since the risk of recurrence following surgery is significant. Postoperative radiation therapy causes transient diarrhea and cystitis, but permanent damage to the small intestine and bladder is uncommon. Use of chemotherapy in patients with advanced colorectal cancers rarely results in a satisfactory response.

Management of Anesthesia

Management of anesthesia for surgical resection of colorectal cancers may be influenced by anemia and the effects of metastatic lesions in liver, lung, bone, or brain. Chronic large bowel obstruction probably does not increase the risk of aspiration during induction of anesthesia, although abdominal distention could interfere with adequate ventilation and oxygenation. Blood transfusion during surgical resection of colorectal cancers has been alleged to be associated with a decrease in the length of patient survival. This could reflect immunosuppression produced by transfused blood. For this reason, careful review of the risks and benefits of blood transfusions in these patients is prudent.

Prostate Cancer

Prostate cancer is the second leading cause of death among men who die of cancer. The reported number of cases of prostate cancer has increased dramatically, presumably reflecting the widespread use of PSA testing. The incidence of prostate cancer is highest in African Americans and lowest in Asians. The presence of the hereditary prostate cancer gene mutation (HPC-1) greatly increases the risk of developing prostate cancer. The possibility that vasectomy may be associated with an increased risk of prostate cancer has not been substantiated. Prostate cancer is almost always an adenocarcinoma.

Diagnosis

The use of PSA-based screening has changed the way prostate cancer is diagnosed. An increased serum PSA concentration may indicate the presence of prostate cancer in asymptomatic men and prompt a digital rectal examination. Detection of a discrete nodule or diffuse induration on digital rectal examination leads to suspicion of prostate cancer, especially in the presence of impotence or symptoms of urinary obstruction (frequency, nocturia, hesitancy, urgency). However, the rectal examination can evaluate only the posterior and lateral aspects of the prostate. If the rectal examination indicates the possible presence of cancer, transrectal ultrasonography and biopsy are needed regardless of the PSA concentration. There is a much greater likelihood of detecting cancer if the PSA level is higher than 10 ng/mL, regardless of the findings on rectal examination. Infrequently, patients present with symptoms of metastatic disease, such as bone pain and weight loss.

Treatment

Focal, well-differentiated prostate cancers are usually cured by transurethral resection. However, progressive disease may develop in up to 16% of these patients within 8 years. For this reason, more aggressive treatment such as radical prostatectomy or radiation may be indicated in subsets of these patients, especially those younger than 65 years of age. If lymph nodes are involved, radical prostatectomy or definitive radiation therapy may be recommended. Radical prostatectomy can be performed via a retropubic or perineal approach. The retropubic approach permits the surgeon to take lymph node samples for frozen section before beginning the prostatectomy. Radiation therapy can be delivered either by an external beam or by implantation of radioactive seeds. The decision to select surgery or radiation is based on the side effects of each treatment. Impotence and urinary incontinence are risks of radical prostatectomy. Preservation of the neurovascular bundles on each side of the prostate may decrease the risk of impotence following surgery. Radiation therapy produces impotence less often, but debilitating cystitis or proctitis may develop.

Hormone therapy is indicated for management of metastatic prostate cancer because these tumors are under the trophic influence of androgens. Androgen deprivation therapy dramatically reduces testosterone levels and causes tumor regression. Androgen deprivation can be obtained by surgical castration, administration of exogenous estrogens such as diethylstilbestrol, use of analogues of luteinizing hormone–releasing hormone that inhibit the release of pituitary gonadotropins, use of antiandrogens, such as flutamide that block the action of androgens at target tissues, and use of combination therapy, such as an antiandrogen in combination with a luteinizing hormone–releasing hormone agonist or bilateral orchiectomy.

When advanced prostate cancers become resistant to hormone therapy, incapacitating bone pain often develops. Systemic chemotherapy with mitoxantrone plus corticosteroids or estramustine plus a taxane may be effective in palliating pain. In the terminal phases of the disease, high doses of prednisone for short periods may produce subjective improvement.

Breast Cancer

Women in the United States have a 12.6% lifetime risk of developing breast cancer. The risk of death from breast cancer is approximately 4%. Most women in whom breast cancer is diagnosed do not die of the disease. It is estimated that more than 2 million women in the United States are now living with a history of breast cancer. Because of increased awareness and use of screening mammography, in situ cancers now account for approximately 20% of newly diagnosed cases of breast cancer.

Risk Factors

The principal risk factors for development of breast cancer are increasing age (75% of cases occur in patients older than 50 years of age) and family history (a first-degree relative diagnosed with breast cancer before age 50 increases the risk three- to fourfold). Reproductive risk factors that increase the risk of breast cancer include early menarche, late menopause, late first pregnancy, and nulliparity, which are all presumed to prolong exposure of the breasts to estrogen. Two breast cancer susceptibility genes (BRCA1, BRCA2) are mutations that are inherited as autosomal dominant traits.

Screening

Recommended screening strategies for breast cancer include the triad of breast self-examination, clinical breast examination by a professional, and screening mammography. Clinical breast examination by a professional and regular mammography appear to decrease mortality from breast cancer by approximately one third in women older than age 50. Annual screening mammography is recommended for all women older than age 40. A small percentage of breast cancers are not detected by mammography, so alternative screening methods such as ultrasonography and/or magnetic resonance imaging may be of value in selected patients.

Prognosis

Axillary lymph node invasion and tumor size are the two most important determinants of outcome in patients with early breast cancer. Other established prognostic factors include the estrogen and progesterone receptor content of the primary tumor and its histologic grade. The absence of estrogen and progesterone receptor expression is associated with a poorer prognosis. Most tumors that express receptors are responsive to endocrine therapy.

Treatment

Although radical mastectomy (removal of the involved breast, axillary contents, and underlying chest wall musculature) was the principal treatment for invasive breast cancer in the past, it is seldom used in current practice. Breast conservation therapy, including lumpectomy with radiation therapy, simple mastectomy, and modified radical mastectomy provide similar survival rates. Because the likelihood of distant micrometastases is highly correlated with the number of lymph nodes containing tumor invasion, axillary lymph node dissection provides prognostic information. Sentinel lymph node mapping involves injection of a radioactive tracer or isosulfan blue dye into the area around the primary breast tumor. The injected substance tracks rapidly to the dominant axillary lymph node (sentinel node). If the sentinel node is tumor free, the remaining lymph nodes are also likely to be tumor free, and further axillary surgery can be avoided. Administration of isosulfan blue dye causes a transient decrease in SpO_2, usually of approximately 3%. The morbidity associated with breast cancer surgery is now largely related to side effects of lymph node dissection such as lymphedema and restricted arm motion. Obesity, weight gain, and infection in the arm are additional risk factors for development of lymphedema. To minimize the risk of lymphedema, it is reasonable to protect the ipsilateral arm from venipuncture, compression, infection, and exposure to heat.

Radiation is an important component of breast conservation therapy since lumpectomy alone is associated with a high incidence of recurrence. Postmastectomy radiation is reserved for women with extensive local disease, such as skin and chest wall invasion and extensive lymph node involvement.

Systemic Treatment Many women with early-stage breast cancer already have distant micrometastases at the time of diagnosis. Systemic therapy is intended to prevent or delay recurrence of the disease. Tamoxifen therapy, chemotherapy, and ovarian ablation are the most commonly used modes of systemic therapy.

Tamoxifen Tamoxifen is a mixed estrogen agonist-antagonist that has become the most commonly prescribed antineoplastic drug. The principal beneficial effect of tamoxifen is related to its interaction with estrogen receptors. Five years of tamoxifen therapy in patients with estrogen receptor–positive tumors is associated with a significant reduction in the risk of recurrence. Benefits of tamoxifen therapy are similar for node-positive and node-negative patients. However, tamoxifen does not alter outcome in patients with minimal or no estrogen receptor expression in their tumors.

Tamoxifen can cause body temperature disturbances ("hot flashes"), vaginal discharge, and an increased risk of developing endometrial cancer. Megestrol (progestin) may be administered to decrease the severity of the hot flashes associated with tamoxifen treatment. Tamoxifen lowers the serum cholesterol and low-density lipoprotein concentrations, but the importance of these effects in reducing the risk of ischemic heart disease is unclear Tamoxifen preserves bone density in postmenopausal women by its proestrogenic effects and may decrease the incidence of osteoporosis-related fractures of the hip, spine, and radius. There is an increased risk of thromboembolic events, including deep venous thrombosis, pulmonary embolism, and stroke with tamoxifen therapy. Raloxifene, like tamoxifen, is a selective estrogen-receptor modulator.

Chemotherapy Combination chemotherapy decreases the rate of recurrence and mortality from breast cancer in both node-positive and node-negative patients. The maximum benefit seems to be in node-positive women younger than 50 years of age. A commonly used combination chemotherapy regimen includes cyclophosphamide, methotrexate, and 5-fluorouracil. Regimens including doxorubicin, paclitaxel, and docetaxel are also being used. The chemotherapy dose is an important determinant of cell kill. Conventional adjuvant chemotherapy usually begins within a few months of surgery. Chemotherapy or radiation before surgery may be used in selected patients in an attempt to decrease tumor size and improve breast conservation. In high-risk women with multiple positive lymph nodes, high-dose chemotherapy with alkylating drugs combined with autologous bone marrow transplantation may be considered.

Chemotherapy for breast cancer has adverse effects that typically resolve following treatment such as nausea and vomiting, hair loss, and bone marrow suppression. The most serious late sequelae of chemotherapy are leukemia and doxorubicin-induced cardiac impairment. Clinically significant congestive heart failure develops in 0.5% to 1.0% of women treated with standard anthracycline-based chemotherapy regimens. Patients with symptoms of cardiac disease or congestive heart failure should be evaluated with an electrocardiogram and echocardiography. Myelodysplastic syndromes or acute myeloid leukemia can arise after chemotherapy, but the incidence is low (0.2%–1.0%). High-dose radiation therapy may be associated with brachial plexopathy or nerve damage, pneumonitis, pulmonary fibrosis, and cardiac injury.

Supportive Treatment Palliation of symptoms and prevention of complications are primary goals when treating advanced breast cancer. The most common site of breast cancer metastases is bone. Regular administration of bisphosphonates (pamidronate, clodronate) in addition to hormone therapy or chemotherapy can decrease bone pain and lower the incidence of bone complications by inhibiting osteoclastic activity. Erythropoietin may be useful for diminishing symptoms of chemotherapy-related bone marrow suppression. The cardiotoxicity of doxorubicin may be decreased by the use of the cardioprotective drug dexrazoxane or liposomal preparations. Adequate pain control is usually achieved with sustained-release oral and/or transdermal opioid preparations.

Management of Anesthesia

Preoperative evaluation includes a review of potential side effects related to chemotherapy. Placement of intravenous catheters in the arm at risk of lymphedema is avoided because exacerbation of lymphedema and susceptibility to infection are considerations. It is also necessary to protect that arm from compression (as with a blood pressure cuff) and heat exposure. The presence of bone pain and pathologic fractures is noted when considering regional anesthesia and when positioning patients during surgery. Selection of anesthetic drugs, techniques, and special monitoring is influenced more by the planned surgical procedure than by the presence of breast cancer. If isosulfan blue dye is injected during the surgical procedure, it is likely that pulse oximetry will demonstrate a transient spurious decrease in the measured SpO_2 value (approximately a 3% decrease).

LESS COMMON CANCERS ENCOUNTERED IN CLINICAL PRACTICE

Less commonly encountered cancers include cardiac tumors, head and neck cancer, and cancers involving the endocrine glands, liver, gallbladder, genitourinary tract, and reproductive organs. Lymphomas and leukemias are examples of cancers involving the lymph glands and blood-forming elements.

Cardiac Tumors

Cardiac tumors may be primary or secondary, benign or malignant. Metastatic cardiac involvement usually from adjacent lung cancer occurs 20 to 40 times more often than a primary malignant cardiac tumor.

Cardiac Myxomas

Cardiac myxomas account for most benign cardiac tumors that occur in adults. Approximately 70% of cardiac myxomas occur in the left atrium, and the remaining 30% occur in the right atrium. Myxomas often demonstrate considerable movement within the cardiac chamber during the cardiac cycle.

Signs and Symptoms Signs and symptoms of cardiac myxomas reflect interference with filling and emptying of the involved cardiac chamber and release of emboli composed of myxomatous material or thrombi that have formed on the tumor (**Table 20-6**). Left atrial myxoma may mimic mitral valve disease with development of pulmonary edema. Right atrial myxoma mimics tricuspid disease and can be associated with impaired venous return and evidence of right heart failure. Right atrial myxoma may manifest as isolated tricuspid stenosis, dyspnea, and/or arterial hypoxemia. Embolism occurs in approximately one third of patients with cardiac myxomas. Because most myxomas are located in the left atrium, systemic embolism is particularly frequent and often involves the retinal and cerebral arteries. Cardiac myxomas may occur as part of a syndrome that includes cutaneous myxomas, myxoid fibroadenomas of the breast, pituitary adenomas, and adrenocortical hyperplasia with Cushing's syndrome.

TABLE 20-6 Signs and Symptoms of Cardiac Myxomas
Refractory congestive heart failure
Unexplained cardiac rhythm disturbances
Syncope related to changes in body position
Unexplained systemic or pulmonary emboli
Pulmonary hypertension of unknown cause

Diagnosis Echocardiography can determine the location, size, shape, attachment, and mobility of cardiac myxomas. There are reports of the incidental discovery of cardiac myxomas during intraoperative echocardiographic monitoring of patients undergoing emergency arterial embolectomy. Cardiac myxomas of at least 0.5 to 1.0 cm in diameter can also be identified by computed tomography and magnetic resonance imaging.

Treatment Surgical resection of cardiac myxomas is usually curative. After the diagnosis has been established, prompt surgery is indicated because of the possibility of embolic complications and sudden death. In most cases, cardiac myxomas can be easily removed because they are pedunculated. Intraoperative fragmentation of the tumor must be avoided. All chambers of the heart are examined to eliminate the presence of multifocal tumors. Mechanical damage to a heart valve or adhesion of the tumor to valve leaflets may necessitate valvuloplasty or valve replacement.

Management of Anesthesia Anesthetic considerations in patients with cardiac myxomas include the possibility of low cardiac output and arterial hypoxemia due to obstruction at the mitral or tricuspid valve. Symptoms of obstruction may be exacerbated by changes in body position. The presence of a right atrial myxoma prohibits placement of right atrial or pulmonary artery catheters. Supraventricular cardiac dysrhythmias may follow surgical removal of atrial myxomas. In some patients, permanent cardiac pacing may be required because of atrioventricular conduction disturbances.

Head and Neck Cancers

Head and neck cancers account for approximately 5% of all cancers in the United States, with a predominance in men older than 50 years of age. Most patients have a history of excessive alcohol use and cigarette smoking. The most common sites of metastases are lung, liver, and bone. Hypercalcemia may be associated with bone metastases, and altered liver function tests presumably reflect alcohol-induced disease. Preoperative nutritional therapy may be indicated before surgical resection of the tumor. The goal of chemotherapy, if selected, is to decrease the bulk of the primary tumor or known metastases, thereby enhancing the efficacy of subsequent surgery or radiation. A secondary goal is eradication of occult micrometastases.

Thyroid Cancer

Papillary and follicular thyroid cancers are among the most curable cancers. Thyroid cancers are more frequent in women. External radiation to the neck during childhood increases the risk of papillary thyroid cancer as does a family history of thyroid cancer. Medullary thyroid cancers may be associated with pheochromocytomas in an autosomal dominant disorder known as multiple endocrine neoplasia type 2. This type of thyroid cancer typically produces large amounts of thyrocalcitonin, providing a sensitive measure of the presence of the disease as well as its cure.

Subtotal and total thyroidectomy result in lower recurrence rates than more limited thyroidectomy. Even with total thyroidectomy some thyroid tissue remains, as detected by postoperative scanning with iodine 131. Risks of total thyroidectomy include recurrent laryngeal nerve injury (2%) and permanent (2%) hypoparathyroidism. Patients with papillary thyroid cancers require dissection of paratracheal and tracheoesophageal lymph nodes. The growth of papillary and follicular tumor cells is controlled by thyrotropin, and inhibition of thyrotropin secretion with thyroxine improves long-term survival. External beam radiation can be used for palliative treatment of obstruction and bony metastases.

Esophageal Cancer

Esophagectomy is often performed for carcinoma of the esophagus and is associated with significant morbidity and mortality. Excessive alcohol consumption and chronic cigarette smoking are independent risk factors for development of squamous cell carcinoma of the esophagus. The risk of adenocarcinoma is highest in people with Barrett's esophagus, a complication of gastroesophageal reflux disease. Dysphagia and weight loss are the initial symptoms of esophageal cancer in most patients. The dysphagia may be associated with malnutrition. Difficulty swallowing may result in regurgitation and increase the risk of aspiration. The disease has usually metastasized by the time clinical symptoms are present. However, in patients with Barrett's esophagus who undergo routine endoscopic surveillance for cancer, the disease can be diagnosed at a very early stage. The lack of a serosal layer around the esophagus and the presence of an extensive lymphatic system can result in rapid spread of tumor to adjacent lymph nodes.

The results of primary radiation therapy resemble those of radical surgery, with a 5-year survival rate of 20% to 30% in those with squamous cell cancer. Chemotherapy and radiation may be instituted prior to attempting surgical resection. Adenocarcinomas are radioinsensitive, but chemotherapy and surgery may improve survival. Palliation may include surgical placement of a feeding tube, bougienage, or endoscopic stent placement.

The likelihood of underlying alcohol-induced liver disease, chronic obstructive pulmonary disease from cigarette smoking, and cross-tolerance with anesthetic drugs in alcohol abusers are considerations during anesthetic management of patients with esophageal cancer. Extensive weight loss often parallels a decrease in intravascular fluid volume and manifests as hypotension during induction and maintenance of anesthesia.

Gastric Cancer

The incidence of gastric cancer has decreased dramatically since 1930 when it was the leading cause of cancer-related death among men in the United States. Achlorhydria (loss of gastric acidity), pernicious anemia, chronic gastritis, and *Helicobacter* infection contribute to the development of gastric cancer. The presenting features of gastric cancer (indigestion, epigastric distress, anorexia) are indistinguishable from those of benign peptic ulcer disease. Approximately 90% of gastric cancers are adenocarcinomas, and approximately half of them occur in the distal portion of the stomach. Gastric cancer is usually far advanced when signs such as weight loss, palpable epigastric mass, jaundice, or ascites appear.

Complete surgical eradication of gastric tumors with resection of adjacent lymph nodes is the only treatment that may be curative. Resection of the primary lesion can also offer the best palliation. Gastric cancer is relatively resistant to radiation therapy, but it is one of the few gastrointestinal tumors that may have some response to chemotherapy.

Liver Cancer

Liver cancer occurs most often in men with liver disease caused by hepatitis B or hepatitis C virus, alcohol consumption, and hemochromatosis. Initial manifestations are typically abdominal pain, a palpable abdominal mass and constitutional symptoms such as anorexia and weight loss. There may be compression of the inferior vena cava and/or portal vein, lower extremity edema, ascites, and jaundice. Laboratory studies reflect the abnormalities associated with the underlying chronic liver disease. Liver function tests are likely to be abnormal. Computed tomography and magnetic resonance imaging of the liver can determine the anatomic location of the tumor, although angiography may be more useful for distinguishing hepatocellular cancer (hypervascular) from hepatic metastases (hypovascular) and for determining whether a tumor is resectable. Radical surgical resection or liver transplantation offers the only hope for survival, but most patients with liver cancer are not surgical candidates because of extensive cirrhosis, impaired liver function, and the presence of extrahepatic disease. Chemotherapy and radiation therapy are of limited value.

Pancreatic Cancer

Pancreatic cancer, despite its low incidence, is the fourth most common cause of cancer-related death in men and women in the United States. There is no evidence linking this cancer to caffeine ingestion, cholelithiasis, or diabetes mellitus, but cigarette smoking, obesity, and chronic pancreatitis show a positive correlation. Approximately 95% of pancreatic cancers are ductal adenocarcinomas, with most occurring in the head of the pancreas. Abdominal pain, anorexia, and weight loss are the usual initial symptoms. Pain suggests retroperitoneal invasion and infiltration of splanchnic nerves. Jaundice reflects biliary obstruction in patients with tumor in the head of the pancreas. Diabetes mellitus is rare in patients who develop pancreatic cancer.

Pancreatic cancer may appear as a localized mass or as diffuse enlargement of the gland. Biopsy is needed to confirm the diagnosis. Complete surgical resection is the only effective treatment of ductal pancreatic cancer. Patients most likely to have resectable lesions are those with tumors in the head of the pancreas that cause painless jaundice. Extrapancreatic spread eliminates the possibility of surgical cure. The two most commonly employed surgical resection techniques are total pancreatectomy and pancreaticoduodenectomy (Whipple procedure). Total pancreatectomy is technically easier but has the disadvantage of producing diabetes mellitus and malabsorption. Only 10% of patients who undergo complete pancreatic resection survive 5 years. The median survival for patients with unresectable tumors is 5 months. Palliative procedures include radiation, chemotherapy, and surgical diversion of the biliary system to relieve obstruction. Celiac plexus block with alcohol or phenol is the most effective intervention for treating the pain associated with pancreatic cancer. A complication of celiac plexus block is hypotension due to sympathetic denervation in these often hypovolemic patients. Computed tomography guidance may be used to confirm proper needle placement before injecting any solution intended to act on the celiac plexus.

Renal Cell Cancer

Renal cell cancer most often manifests itself as hematuria, mild anemia, and flank pain. Risk factors include a family history of renal cancer and cigarette smoking. Renal ultrasonography can help identify renal cysts, and computed tomography and magnetic resonance imaging are useful for determining the presence and extent of renal cell cancers. Laboratory testing may reveal eosinophilia and liver function abnormalities. Paraneoplastic syndromes especially hypercalcemia due to ectopic parathyroid hormone secretion and erythrocytosis due to ectopic erythropoietin production are not uncommon. The only curative treatment for renal adenocarcinoma confined to the kidneys is radical nephrectomy with regional lymphadenectomy. Radical nephrectomy is not helpful in patients with distant metastases, but chemotherapy may show some efficacy. The 5-year survival rate in patients with metastatic disease is 3% to 10%.

Bladder Cancer

Bladder cancer occurs more often in men and is associated with cigarette smoking and chronic exposure to chemicals used in the dye, leather, and rubber industries. The most common presenting feature is hematuria, either gross or microscopic.

Treatment of noninvasive bladder cancer includes endoscopic resection and intravesical chemotherapy. Carcinoma in situ of the bladder often behaves aggressively and may require cystectomy to help prevent muscle invasion and metastatic spread. In men, radical cystectomy includes removal of the bladder, prostate, and proximal urethra. In women, a hysterectomy, oophorectomy, and partial vaginectomy are required. Urinary diversion is either by ureteroileostomy (ileal conduit) or creation of an artificial bladder (neobladder) from segments of small bowel. Traditional treatment for metastatic disease includes radiation and chemotherapy.

Testicular Cancer

Although testicular cancer is rare, it is the most common cancer in young men and represents a tumor that can be cured even when distant metastases are present. Orchipexy before 2 years of age is recommended for cryptorchidism to decrease the risk of testicular cancer. Testicular cancer usually presents as a painless testicular mass. When the diagnosis is suspected, an inguinal orchiectomy is performed and the diagnosis is histologically confirmed. A transscrotal biopsy is not performed because disruption of the scrotum may predispose to local recurrence and/or metastatic spread to inguinal lymphatics. Germ cell cancers, which account for 95% of testicular cancers, can be subdivided into seminomas and nonseminomas. Seminomas often metastasize through regional lymphatics to the retroperitoneum and mediastinum, and nonseminomas spread hematogenously to viscera, especially the lungs.

Patients with seminomas that do not extend beyond the retroperitoneal lymph nodes are treated with radiation. Chemotherapy is recommended when seminomas are large, present as several anatomic levels of nodal involvement, or have spread above the diaphragm. Nonseminomas are not radiation sensitive and are treated with retroperitoneal lymph node dissection and combination chemotherapy. Side effects of chemotherapy in these patients may include anemia, cardiac toxicity, pulmonary toxicity, nephrotoxicity, and peripheral neuropathy.

Uterine Cervix Cancer

Uterine cervix cancer is the most common gynecologic cancer in females aged 15 to 34 years. Human papillomavirus infection of the uterine cervix is the principal cause of cervical cancer. Carcinoma in situ as detected by a Papanicolaou smear is treated with a cone biopsy, whereas more extensive local disease or disease that has metastasized is treated with some combination of surgery, radiation therapy, and chemotherapy.

Uterine Cancer

Cancer involving the uterine endometrium occurs most frequently in women 50 to 70 years of age and may be associated with estrogen replacement therapy at menopause, more than 5 years of tamoxifen treatment for breast cancer, obesity, hypertension, and diabetes mellitus. Endometrial cancer is often diagnosed at an early stage because more than 90% of patients present with postmenopausal or irregular bleeding. The initial evaluation of these patients often includes fractional dilation and curettage. In the absence of metastatic disease, a total abdominal hysterectomy and bilateral salpingo-oophorectomy with or without radiation to the pelvic and periaortic lymph nodes is the treatment. Hormone therapy with progesterone may be useful for treating patients with metastatic disease. Metastatic endometrial cancer responds poorly to chemotherapy.

Ovarian Cancer

Ovarian cancer is the most deadly of the gynecologic malignancies. Ovarian cancer is most likely to develop in women who experience early menopause or who have a family history of ovarian cancer. Early ovarian cancer is usually asymptomatic, so advanced disease is usually present by the time the cancer is finally discovered. Widespread intra-abdominal metastases to lymph nodes, omentum, and peritoneum are often present. Surgery is the treatment of both early-stage and advanced ovarian cancer. Aggressive tumor debulking, even if all cancer cannot be removed, improves the length and quality of survival. Intraperitoneal chemotherapy is indicated postoperatively in most women and is usually well tolerated.

Cutaneous Melanoma

The incidence of cutaneous melanoma is increasing more rapidly than that of any other cancer. Sunlight (ultraviolet light) is an important environmental factor in the pathogenesis of melanoma. Melanoma is suspected when there is a change in the color, size, shape, or surface of a mole or the appearance of a new pigmented lesion. The initial treatment of a suspected lesion is wide and deep excisional biopsy often with sentinel node mapping. Melanoma can metastasize to virtually any organ. Treatment of metastatic melanoma is directed at palliation and can include resection of a solitary metastasis, simple or combination chemotherapy, and immunotherapy.

Bone Cancer

Bone cancers include multiple myeloma, osteosarcoma, Ewing's tumor, and chondrosarcoma.

Multiple Myeloma

Multiple myeloma (plasma cell myeloma, myelomatosis) is a malignant neoplasm characterized by poorly controlled growth of a single clone of plasma cells, which produce a monoclonal immunoglobulin. Multiple myeloma accounts for approximately 10% of hematologic cancers and 1% of all cancers in the United States. The disease is more common in elderly patients (median age at time of diagnosis is 65 years), and it occurs twice as often in African Americans as in whites. The cause of multiple myeloma is unknown. Its extent, complications, sensitivity to drugs, and clinical course vary greatly among patients.

Signs and Symptoms

The most frequent manifestations of multiple myeloma are bone pain (often from vertebral collapse), anemia, thrombocytopenia, neutropenia, hypercalcemia, renal failure, and recurrent bacterial infection reflecting bone marrow invasion by tumor cells. Extramedullary plasmacytomas can produce compression of the spinal cord. This occurs in approximately 10% of patients. Other extramedullary sites of tumor invasion include the liver, spleen, ribs and skull. Peripheral neuropathy is uncommon and is usually caused by amyloidosis. Inactivation of plasma procoagulants by myeloma proteins may interfere with coagulation. These proteins coat the platelets and interfere with platelet function. The presence of hypercalcemia from excessive bone destruction should be suspected in patients with myeloma who develop nausea, fatigue,

confusion, or polyuria. Renal insufficiency occurs in approximately 25% of patients with multiple myeloma either due to deposition of an abnormal protein (Bence-Jones protein) in renal tubules or the development of acute renal failure. Amyloidosis or immunoglobulin deposition disease can cause nephrotic syndrome or contribute to renal failure. Recurrent bacterial infection is a major cause of morbidity in patients with multiple myeloma and is most common in those with bone marrow suppression, impaired immune responses due to advanced disease, or granulocytopenia caused by chemotherapy. The combination of hypogammoglobulinemia, granulocytopenia, and depressed cell-mediated immunity increases the risk of infection. Development of fever in patients with multiple myeloma is an indication for antibiotic therapy. In an estimated 20% of patients, multiple myeloma is diagnosed by chance in the absence of symptoms when screening laboratory studies reveal increased serum protein concentrations.

Treatment Treatment of overt symptomatic multiple myeloma most often includes autologous stem cell transplantation and chemotherapy. Palliative radiation is limited to patients who have disabling pain and a well-defined focal process that has not responded to chemotherapy. The median duration of remission is approximately 2 years and the median survival approximately 3 years. Signs of spinal cord compression due to an extramedullary plasmacytoma require early confirmation and prompt radiation. Urgent decompressive laminectomy to avoid permanent paralysis may be needed if radiation is not effective. Chemotherapy reverses mild renal failure in many patients with multiple myeloma, but temporary hemodialysis may be necessary in the presence of renal failure to permit time for chemotherapy to become effective. Erythropoietin therapy may be indicated to treat anemia. Prevention of dehydration is important if hypercalcemia is present. Hypercalcemia requires prompt treatment with intravenous saline infusion and administration of furosemide. Bed rest is avoided because inactivity leads to further mobilization of calcium from bone and venous thrombosis due to venous stasis.

Management of Anesthesia The presence of compression fractures requires caution when positioning these patients during anesthesia and surgery. Fluid therapy will depend on the degree of renal insufficiency and/or hypercalcemia. Pathologic fractures of the ribs may impair ventilation and predispose to development of pneumonia.

Osteosarcoma

Osteosarcoma occurs most often in adolescents and typically involves the distal femur and proximal tibia. A genetic predisposition is suggested by the association of this tumor with retinoblastoma. Magnetic resonance imaging is used to assess the extent of the primary lesion and the existence of metastatic disease, especially in the lungs. Serum alkaline phosphatase concentrations are likely to be increased and the levels correlate with prognosis. Treatment consists of combination chemotherapy followed by surgical excision/amputation. Success of chemotherapy may permit limb salvage procedures in selected patients. Pulmonary resection may be indicated in patients with solitary metastatic lung lesions. Nonmetastatic disease has an 85% to 90% survival rate.

Ewing's Tumor

Ewing's tumor or sarcoma usually occurs in children and young adults and most often involves the pelvis, femur, and tibia. Ewing's sarcoma is highly malignant, and metastatic disease is often present at the time of diagnosis. Treatment consists of surgery, local radiation, and combination chemotherapy.

Chondrosarcoma

Chondrosarcoma usually involves the pelvis, ribs, or upper end of the femur or humerus in young or middle-aged adults. This tumor often grows slowly and can be treated by radical surgical excision of larger lesions and radiation of smaller lesions.

LYMPHOMAS AND LEUKEMIAS

Hodgkin's Disease

Hodgkin's disease is a lympho [...] tive (Epstein-Barr virus), gene [...] tions. Another factor that [...] development of lymphoma is [...] patients after organ transplar [...] human immunodeficiency vi [...] diagnostic test in patients [...] lymph node biopsy.

Hodgkin's disease is a lym[p...] presentation consists of lymph [...] tions. Cervical and anterior n [...] common. Pruritus can be gene [...] and unexplained weight loss [...] anemia is often present. Per [...] cord compression may occu [...] growth. Bone marrow and c [...] ment is unusual in Hodgkin's disease but not in other lymphomas.

[Handwritten note: Notes in PPT. file "Case studies Hematology"]

Staging of the disease is accomplished by computed tomography and positron emission tomography scanning of the chest, abdomen, and pelvis; biopsy of available nodes; and bone marrow biopsy. Precise definition of the extent of nodal and extranodal disease is necessary to select the proper treatment strategy. Radiation therapy is curative for localized early stage Hodgkin's disease. Bulkier or more advanced Hodgkin's disease is treated by combination chemotherapy. Cure can be achieved with 20-year survival rates of approximately 90%.

Leukemia

Leukemia is the uncontrolled production of leukocytes owing to cancerous mutation of lymphogenous cells or myelogenous cells. Lymphocytic leukemias begin in lymph nodes and are named according to the type of hematopoietic cells that are primarily involved. Myeloid leukemia begins as cancerous production of myelogenous cells in bone marrow with spread to extramedullary organs. The principal difference between normal hematopoietic stem cells and leukemia cells is the ability of the latter to continue to divide. The result is an expanding mass of cells that infiltrate the bone marrow, rendering patients functionally aplastic. Anemia may be profound. Eventually, bone marrow failure is the cause of fatal infections or hemorrhage due to thrombocytopenia. Leukemia cells may also infiltrate the liver, spleen, lymph nodes, and meninges, producing signs of dysfunction at these sites. Extensive use of nutrients by rapidly proliferating cancerous cells depletes amino acids, leading to patient fatigue and metabolic starvation of normal tissues.

Acute Lymphoblastic Leukemia

Acute lymphoblastic leukemia accounts for approximately 15% of all leukemias in adults. Central nervous system dysfunction is common. Affected patients are highly susceptible to life-threatening opportunistic infection, including that due to *Pneumocystis carinii* and cytomegalovirus. Chemotherapy [...] ly as 70% of children and 25% to 45% of

[...]phocytic Leukemia

[...]hocytic leukemia is one of the most common [...]lts, accounting for approximately 25% of all [...]ally in elderly patients. This form of leukemia [...] children. The diagnosis of chronic lympho[...] confirmed by the presence of lymphocytosis [...] infiltrates in bone marrow. Signs and symp[...] ariable, with the extent of bone marrow infil[...]ermining the clinical course. Autoimmune [...] a and hypersplenism that result in pancyto[...]ocytopenia may be prominent. Lymph node [...] obstruct the ureters. Corticosteroids may be [...] the hemolytic anemia, but splenectomy may [...]ecessary. Single or combination chemother- apy is the usual treatment, with radiation therapy reserved for treatment of localized nodal masses or an enlarged spleen.

Acute Myeloid Leukemia

Acute myeloid leukemia is characterized by an increase in the number of myeloid cells in bone marrow and arrest of their maturation, frequently resulting in hematopoietic insufficiency (granulocytopenia, thrombocytopenia, anemia). Clinical signs and symptoms of acute myeloid leukemia are diverse and nonspecific, but they are usually attributable to the leukemic infiltration of the bone marrow. Approximately one third of patients with AML will have significant or life-threatening infection when initially seen. Other patients will present with complaints of fatigue, bleeding gums or nose bleeds, pallor, and headache. Dyspnea on exertion is common. Leukemic infiltration of various organs (hepatomegaly, splenomegaly, lymphadenopathy), bones, gingiva, and the central nervous system can produce a variety of signs. Hyperleukocytosis (more than 100,000 cells/mm^3) can result in signs of leukostasis with ocular and cerebrovascular dysfunction or bleeding. Metabolic abnormalities may include hyperuricemia and hypocalcemia.

Chemotherapy is administered to induce remission. Complete and sustained remission can be achieved in 70% to 80% of patients who are younger than 60 years of age and in approximately 50% of patients older than 60 years of age. Bone marrow transplantation may be a consideration in patients who do not achieve an initial remission or who relapse after chemotherapy.

Chronic Myeloid Leukemia

Chronic myeloid leukemia manifests as myeloid leukocytosis with splenomegaly. Typically, leukocyte alkaline phosphatase is markedly decreased in these patients. High leukocyte counts may predispose to vascular occlusion. Hyperuricemia is common and is treated with allopurinol. Cytoreduction therapy with hydroxyurea, chemotherapy, leukopheresis, and splenectomy may be necessary. Allogenic stem cell transplantation is a potentially curative therapy with 10-year survival rates of 30% to 60%. However, transplant-related mortality may be significant.

Chemotherapy for Treatment of Leukemia

A kilogram of leukemia cells (approximately 10^{12} cells) appears to be a lethal mass. Symptoms leading to the diagnosis of leukemia are unlikely until the tumor load is approximately 10^9 cells. Chemotherapy is intended to decrease the number of tumor cells so organomegaly regresses and function of the bone marrow improves. Drugs used for chemotherapy are principally those that depress bone marrow activity. Therefore, hemorrhage and infection will determine the maximum doses of the chemotherapeutic drugs. Destruction of tumor cells by chemotherapy produces a uric acid load that may result in urate nephropathy and/or gouty arthritis. Nutritional support of patients undergoing chemotherapy may be necessary to prevent hypoalbuminemia and loss of immunocompetence.

Bone Marrow Transplantation for Treatment of Leukemia

Hematopoietic stem cell transplantation offers an opportunity for cure of several otherwise fatal diseases. Autologous bone marrow transplantation entails collection of the patient's own bone marrow for subsequent reinfusion, whereas allogeneic transplantation uses bone marrow or peripheral blood elements from an immunocompatible donor. Regardless of the type of bone marrow transplantation, recipients must undergo a preoperative regimen designed to achieve functional bone marrow ablation. This is produced by a combination of total body radiation and chemotherapy. Bone marrow is usually harvested by repeated aspirations from the posterior iliac crest. For allogeneic bone marrow transplantation with major AB incompatibility between donor and recipient, it is necessary to remove mature erythrocytes from the graft to avoid a hemolytic transfusion reaction. Removal of T cells from the allograft can decrease the risk of graft-versus-host disease.

Processing of the harvested bone marrow (eradicating malignant cells, removing incompatible erythrocytes) may take 2 to 12 hours. The condensed bone marrow volume (approximately 200 mL) is then infused into the recipient through a central venous catheter. From the systemic circulation, the bone marrow cells pass into the recipient's bone marrow, which provides the microenvironment necessary for maturation and differentiation of the cells. The time necessary for bone marrow engraftment is usually 10 to 28 days, during which time protective isolation of the patient may be required. While awaiting engraftment, it may be necessary to administer platelets to maintain the count above 20,000 cells/mm^3 and erythrocytes to maintain the hematocrit above 25%.

Anesthesia for Bone Marrow Transplantation

General or regional anesthesia is required during aspiration of bone marrow from the iliac crests. Nitrous oxide might be avoided in the donor because of potential bone marrow depression associated with this drug. However, there is no evidence that nitrous oxide administered during bone marrow harvesting adversely affects marrow engraftment and subsequent function. Substantial fluid losses may accompany this procedure. Blood replacement may be necessary, either with autologous blood transfusion or by reinfusion of separated erythrocytes obtained during the harvest. Perioperative complications are rare, although discomfort at bone puncture sites is predictable.

Complications of Bone Marrow Transplantation

In addition to prolonged myelosuppression, bone marrow transplantation is associated with several unusual complications.

Graft-Versus-Host Disease Graft-versus-host disease is a life-threatening complication of bone marrow transplantation manifesting as organ system dysfunction most often involving the skin, liver, and gastrointestinal tract (**Table 20-7**). Severe rash, even desquamation, jaundice, and diarrhea are usually seen. This response occurs when immunologically competent cells in the graft target antigens on the recipient's cells.

Graft-verus-host disease can be divided into two somewhat distinct clinical entities: acute disease, which occurs during the first 30 to 60 days after bone marrow transplantation, and chronic disease, which develops at least 100 days after transplantation. Patients undergoing allogeneic bone marrow transplantation typically undergo prophylactic treatment for acute graft-versus-host disease. Even with prophylaxis, however, most adult patients experience some degree of graft-versus-host disease after allogeneic bone marrow transplantation. The chronic form of graft-versus-host disease shares certain clinical characteristics with other immunologic disorders, such as scleroderma.

TABLE 20-7	Manifestations of Graft-Versus-Host Disease

Pancytopenia and immunodeficiency
Maculopapular rash, erythroderma, desquamation
Oral ulceration and mucositis
Esophageal ulceration
Diarrhea
Hepatitis with coagulopathy
Bronchiolitis obliterans
Interstitial pneumonitis
Pulmonary fibrosis
Renal failure

Graft Rejection Graft rejection occurs when immunologically competent cells of host origin destroy the cells of donor origin. This is rarely seen in well-matched related-donor transplants but can be seen in transplants from alternative donors.

Pulmonary Complications Pulmonary complications following allogeneic bone marrow transplantation include infection, adult respiratory distress syndrome, chemotherapy-induced lung damage, and interstitial pneumonia. When interstitial pneumonitis occurs 60 days or more after bone marrow transplantation, it is most likely due to cytomegalovirus or fungal infection.

Veno-occlusive Disease of the Liver Veno-occlusive disease of the liver may occur following allogeneic and autologous bone marrow transplantation. Primary symptoms of veno-occlusive disease include jaundice, tender hepatomegaly, ascites, and weight gain. Progressive hepatic failure and multiorgan failure can develop and the mortality is high.

The understanding of cancer and its symptoms and management is vital for our professional as well as personal well-being. Cancer has complex social ramifications and is a major health problem. More avenues for research and more facilities for recognition and treatment of cancer are opening up, and there is hope for better control of and even a cure for cancer.

KEY POINTS

- Stimulation of oncogene formation by carcinogens (tobacco, alcohol, sunlight) is estimated to be responsible for 80% of cancers in the United States. Tobacco use accounts for more cases of cancer than all other known carcinogens combined. The fundamental event that causes cells to become malignant is an alteration in the structure of DNA. The responsible mutations occur in cells of target tissues, with these cells becoming the ancestors of the entire future tumor cell population.

- A commonly used staging system for solid tumors is the TNM system based on tumor size (T), lymph node involvement (N), and distant metastasis (M). This system further groups patients into stages ranging from the best prognosis (stage I) to the poorest prognosis (stage IV).

- Drugs administered for cancer chemotherapy may produce significant side effects including interstitial pneumonitis, peripheral neuropathy, renal dysfunction, cardiomyopathy, and hypersensitivity reactions. These side effects may have important implications for the management of anesthesia during surgical procedures for cancer treatment as well as operations unrelated to the presence of cancer

- Cancer patients may experience acute pain associated with pathologic fractures, tumor invasion, surgery, radiation, and chemotherapy. A frequent source of pain is related to metastatic spread of the cancer, especially to bone. Nerve compression or infiltration may be a cause of pain.

Patients with cancer who experience frequent and significant pain exhibit signs of depression and anxiety.

- Drug therapy is the cornerstone of cancer pain management because of its efficacy, rapid onset of action, and relatively low cost. Mild to moderate cancer pain is initially treated with nonsteroidal anti-inflammatory drugs and acetaminophen, which are especially effective for managing bone pain, which is the most common cause of cancer pain. The next step in management of moderate to severe pain includes addition of codeine or one of its analogues. When cancer pain is severe, opioids are the major drugs used. There is no maximum dose of morphine or other μ-agonist opioids. Tolerance to opioids does occur but need not be a clinical problem.

- Spinal opioids may be delivered for weeks to months via a long-term, subcutaneously tunneled, exteriorized catheter or an implanted drug delivery system. The implantable systems can be intrathecal or epidural. Patients are typically considered for neuraxial opioid administration when systemic opioid administration has failed as a result of intolerable adverse (systemic) side effects or inadequate analgesia. Neuraxial administration of opioids is usually successful, but some patients require an additional low concentration of local anesthetic to achieve adequate pain control.

- Important aspects of determining the suitability of destructive nerve blocks are the location and quality of the pain, the effectiveness of less destructive treatment

Continued

KEY POINTS—cont'd

modalities, life expectancy, the inherent risks associated with the block, and the availability of experienced anesthesiologists to perform the procedures. In general, constant pain is more amenable to destructive nerve blocks than intermittent pain.

- Cancer is the most common cause of hypercalcemia is hospitalized patients, reflecting local osteolytic activity from bone metastases, especially breast cancer, or the ectopic parathyroid hormonal activity associated with tumors that arise from the kidneys, lungs, pancreas, or ovaries. The rapid onset of hypercalcemia that occurs in patients with cancer may manifest as lethargy or coma. Polyuria and dehydration may accompany hypercalcemia, which is further exaggerated by bone pain and immobility.

- Renal complications of cancer reflect invasion of the kidneys by tumor, damage from tumor products, or chemotherapy. Deposition of tumor antigen-antibody complexes on the glomerular membrane can result in nephrotic syndrome. Extensive retroperitoneal cancer can lead to bilateral ureteral obstruction and uremia, especially in patients with cancer of the cervix, bladder, or prostate. Chemotherapy can destroy large numbers of tumor cells and result in acute hyperuricemic nephropathy due to precipitation of uric acid crystals in the renal tubules. Methotrexate and cisplatin are the chemotherapeutic drugs most often associated with nephrotoxicity.

REFERENCES

Armitage JO: Bone marrow transplantation. N Engl J Med 1994;330:827–838.

Breivik H: The future role of the anaesthesiologist in pain management. Acta Anaesthesiol Scand 2005;49:922–926.

Burstein HJ, Winer EP: Primary care for survivors of breast cancer. N Engl J Med 2000;343:1086–1094.

Congedo E, Aceto P, Petrucci R, et al: Preoperative anesthetic evaluation and preparation in patients requiring esophageal surgery for cancer. Rays 2005;30:341–345.

Exner HJ, Peters J, Eikermann M: Epidural analgesia at the end of life: Facing empirical contraindications. Anesth Analg 2003;97:1740–1742.

Fassoulaki A, Triga A, Melemeni A, Sarantopoulos C: Multimodal analgesia with gabapentin and local anesthetics prevents acute and chronic pain after breast surgery for cancer. Anesth Analg 2005;101:1427–1432.

Homburger JA, Meiler SE: Anesthesia drugs, immunity and long-term outcome. Curr Opin Anaesthesiol 2006;19:423–428.

Kvolik S, Glavas-Obrovac L, Sakic K, et al: Anesthetic implications of anticancer chemotherapy. Eur J Anaesthesiol 2003;20:859–871.

Lavand'homme P, De Kock M, Waterloos H: Intraoperative epidural analgesia combined with ketamine provides effective preventive analgesia in patients undergoing major digestive surgery. Anesthesiology 2005;103:813–820.

Martin RF, Rossi RL: Multidisciplinary considerations for patients with cancer of the pancreas or biliary tract. Surg Clin N Am 2000;80:709–728.

Minai FN, Monem A: Paraneoplastic syndrome of renal cell carcinoma. J Coll Physicians Surg Pak 2006;16:81–82.

Reardon MJ, Walkes JC, Benjamin R: Therapy insight: Malignant primary cardiac tumors. Nat Clin Pract Cardiovasc Med 2006;3:548–553.

Reynen K: Cardiac myxomas. N Engl J Med 1995;333:1610–1617.

Sorensen HT, Mellemkjaer L, Olsen JH, Baron JA: Prognosis of cancers associated with venous thromboembolism. N Engl J Med 2000;343:1846–1850.

Stewart AF: Hypercalcemia associated with cancer. N Engl J Med 2005;352:373–379.

Testini M, Nacchiero M, Portincasa P, et al: Risk factors of morbidity in thyroid surgery: Analysis of the last 5 years of experience in a general surgery unit. Int Surg 2004;89:125–130.

Vokach-Brodsky L, Jeffrey SS, Lemmens HJ, Brock-Utne FG: Isosulfan blue affects pulse oximetry. Anesthesiology 2000;93:1002–1003

CHAPTER 21

Diseases Related to Immune System Dysfunction

Christine S. Rinder

Inadequate Innate Immunity
- Neutropenia
- Abnormalities of Phagocytosis
- Deficiencies in Components of the Complement System

Excessive Innate Immunity
- Neutrophilia
- Asthma

Misdirected Innate Immunity
- Angioedema

Inadequate Adaptive Immunity
- Defects of Antibody Production
- Combined Defects

- Defects of T Lymphocytes
- Allergic Reactions
- Anaphylaxis
- Drug Allergy
- Eosinophilia

Misdirected Adaptive Immunity
- Autoimmune Disorders

Anesthesia and Immunocompetence
- Resistance to Infection
- Resistance to Cancer

The human immune system can be divided into two pathways, one encompassing *innate* immunity and the other *adaptive* or *acquired* immunity. Innate immunity may be thought of as the rapid response team. It is always present, mounts the initial response to any infection, recognizes targets that are common to many pathogens, and has no specific memory. Its cellular elements are neutrophils, macrophages, monocytes, and natural killer cells and its noncellular elements include the complement system, acute-phase proteins, and proteins of the contact activation pathway. Adaptive immunity has a more delayed time course and may take days to activate when challenged by an unfamiliar antigen. However, adaptive immunity is capable of developing memory and is more rapidly induced by antigen when memory is present. Adaptive immunity consists of a humoral component that is mediated by B lymphocytes that produce antibodies and a cellular component dominated by T lymphocytes. Defects specific to each of these immune systems generally predispose to infection with a characteristic subset of pathogenic organisms (**Table 21-1**). Both innate and acquired immunity exhibit defects that can be divided into three categories: (1) injury caused by an inadequate immune response, (2) injury caused by an excessive immune response, (3) injury caused by a misdirection of the immune response.

TABLE 21-1	Pathogens Associated with Specific Immune Defects				
Organism	Phagocyte Defect	Complement Defect	B-Cell Defect and Antibody Deficiency	T-Cell Defect or Deficiency	Combined B-and T-Cell Deficiency
Bacteria	Staphylococci, *Pseudomonas*, enteric flora	*Neisseria*, pyogenic bacteria	Streptococci, staphylococci, *Haemophilus*, *Neisseria meningitidis*	Bacterial sepsis, especially *Salmonella typhi*	Similar to antibody deficiency, especially *N. meningitides*
Viruses			Enteroviruses	Cytomegalovirus, Epstein-Barr virus, varicella, chronic respiratory and intestinal viruses	All
Mycobacterium	Nontuberculous mycobacteria			Nontuberculous mycobacteria	
Fungi	*Candida, Nocardia, Aspergillus*		Severe intestinal giardiasis	*Candida, Pneumocystis, Histoplasma, Aspergillus*	Similar to T-cell defect, especially *Pneumocystis* and *Toxoplasma*
Special features			Recurrent sinopulmonary infections, sepsis, chronic meningitis	Aggressive disease with opportunistic pathogens, failure to clear infections	

INADEQUATE INNATE IMMUNITY

Neutropenia

Neutropenia is defined as an absolute granulocyte count less than 2000/μL in whites or 1500/μL in African Americans. It is not until the granulocyte count decreases to less than 500/μL, however, that a patient is at significant risk of infection of the skin, mouth (teeth and periodontal tissue), pharynx, and lung. If the count decreases to less than 100/μL, the chance of gram-positive or gram-negative sepsis or fungal infection increases dramatically.

Neutropenia in Pediatric Patients

Several neutropenic syndromes can be observed in newborns and young children. Neonatal sepsis is the most common cause of severe neutropenia within the first few days of life. A transient neutropenia can be observed in children born to mothers with autoimmune disease or as a result of maternal hypertension or drug ingestion. Persistent neutropenia can occur as a result of defects in neutrophil production, maturation, or survival.

The autosomal dominant disorder *cyclic neutropenia* is a particularly well-studied cause of childhood neutropenia. It is characterized by recurrent episodes of neutropenia that are not always associated with infection but that occur in regular cycles every 3 to 4 weeks. Each episode is characterized by 1 week of reduced granulocyte production, followed by a period of reactive monocytosis, and then spontaneous recovery of normal granulocyte production. The granulocytopenia can be severe enough to result in recurrent, severe bacterial infection that requires antibiotic therapy. As the child grows older, the cyclical nature of the neutrophil production can diminish and result in a chronic, persistent granulocytopenia. The postulated mechanism of cyclic neutropenia is a defect in a feedback mechanism that normally stimulates precursor cells to respond to growth factors such as granulocyte colony–stimulating factor (G-CSF).

Kostmann's syndrome is an autosomal recessive disorder of neutrophil maturation. Patients with Kostmann's syndrome appear to have a normal population of early progenitor cells that are somehow suppressed, inhibiting normal maturation. They are at risk of severe, life-threatening infection. Most respond to therapy with G-CSF.

Neutropenia in Adults

Acquired defects in the production of neutrophils in adults are very common. Typical causes include cancer chemotherapy and treatment of acquired immunodeficiency syndrome with zidovudine. Neutropenia usually reflects the impact of a particular drug on stem cell and early myelocytic progenitor proliferation. In most cases, the marrow recovers once the drug is withdrawn. Many drugs have been associated with neutropenia. Among the most prominent of these are the injectable gold salts, chloramphenicol, antithyroid medications (carbimazole and propylthiouracil), analgesics (indomethacin, acetaminophen, and phenacetin), tricyclic antidepressants, and phenothiazines. However, virtually any drug can, on occasion, produce severe, life-threatening neutropenia. Therefore, when neutropenia occurs in the course of medical treatment, the possibility that it is drug induced must be considered.

Autoimmune-related neutropenia is observed with collagen vascular or autoimmune diseases. The two most common associations are with systemic lupus erythematosus (where the neutropenia can occur alone or be accompanied by thrombocytopenia) and rheumatoid arthritis. *Felty's syndrome* is the triad of rheumatoid arthritis, splenomegaly, and neutropenia. Other causes of splenomegaly and neutropenia include lymphoma, myeloproliferative disease, and severe liver disease with portal hypertension. In these latter situations, it is often difficult to decide whether the granulocytopenia is caused simply by splenic sequestration or whether it also has an autoimmune component. Splenectomy in patients with Felty's syndrome or myelofibrosis has been reported to significantly improve neutrophil production.

Acute, life-threatening granulocytopenia can occur in patients with overwhelming sepsis. A decreasing white cell count in a patient with pneumococcal sepsis or peritonitis is a bad prognostic sign. It reflects a rate of granulocyte use that exceeds the marrows ability to produce new cells. Alcoholic patients are especially susceptible to infection-induced granulocytopenia. Both folic acid deficiency and direct toxic effects of alcohol on marrow precursor cells cripple the ability to produce new neutrophils in response to infection.

Some patients present with neutropenia without obvious cause. Usually, the reduction in the number of circulating granulocytes is relatively mild and therefore is not associated with life-threatening infection. When the granulocytopenia is accompanied by abnormalities of other blood elements (anemia and thrombocytopenia), it is likely that the patient is developing a myeloproliferative or myelodysplastic disorder. Lymphoproliferative disease, especially T- suppressor cell malignancies, can also present with granulocytopenia and an increased incidence of skin and mucous membrane infection. Human immunodeficiency virus infection is a common cause of T-cell dysfunction. In these patients, loss of the T-helper subset and overexpression of the T-suppressor subset is associated with abnormalities of neutrophil production and function.

Abnormalities of Phagocytosis

Chronic granulomatous disease is a genetic disorder in which granulocytes lack the ability to generate reactive oxygen species. The granulocytes can migrate to a site of infection and ingest organisms but are unable to kill them. Therefore, *Staphylococcus aureus* and certain gram-negative bacteria that are normally killed by phagocytosis and lysosomal digestion are responsible for most of the infections in these patients. The condition is usually diagnosed during childhood or early adult life when patients present with recurrent microabscesses and chronic granulomatous inflammation.

The primary substrate for the enzymatic generation of reactive oxygen species is the reduced form of nicotinamide adenine dinucleotide phosphate. Patients deficient in neutrophil glucose 6-phosphate dehydrogenase are unable to generate large amounts of the reduced form of nicotinamide adenine dinucleotide phosphate, thus limiting their ability to generate

the oxidase needed to kill ingested microorganisms. As with chronic granulomatous disease, neutrophil *glucose 6-phosphate dehydrogenase–deficient* patients are at lifelong risk of recurrent infection with catalase-positive microorganisms.

Leukocyte adhesion deficiency is a relatively rare deficiency of a subunit of the integrin family of leukocyte adhesion molecules. This subunit is critical for cellular adhesion and chemotaxis. Leukocyte adhesion deficiency patients are at high risk of recurrent bacterial infection associated with a lack of pus formation.

Chédiak-Higashi syndrome is a rare multisystem disease characterized by partial oculocutaneous albinism, frequent bacterial infection, a mild bleeding diathesis, progressive neuropathy, and cranial nerve defects. Many patients succumb to infection before age 20. The neutrophils of these patients contain giant granules that can cause neutrophils to be perceived as abnormal by immune surveillance cells. Many white blood cells are destroyed before leaving the bone marrow. Accordingly, many patients have moderate neutropenia. Chemotaxis, phagocytosis, and the ability to kill ingested bacteria are also abnormal.

Specific granule deficiency syndrome is another rare congenital disorder characterized by neutrophils that exhibit impaired chemotaxis and bactericidal activity. Patients are prone to recurrent bacterial and fungal infection and often deep-seated abscesses. Skin and pulmonary infections appear to predominate and most of these respond well to aggressive antibiotic therapy. Affected patients frequently survive into their adult years.

Management of Patients with Neutropenia or Abnormal Phagocytosis

Patients with neutropenia or a qualitative disorder of granulocyte function often benefit significantly from antibiotic therapy and use of recombinant G-CSF. Recombinant G-CSF significantly reduces the duration of absolute neutropenia in patients receiving ablative chemotherapy and autologous bone marrow transplantation, shortens the length of antibiotic therapy, and reduces the risk of life-threatening bacteremia and the incidence of fungal infection. G-CSF therapy has been approved for the reversal of the neutropenia associated with human immunodeficiency virus infection and the prevention of worsening neutropenia with human immunodeficiency virus therapy. Neutropenic patients undergoing elective surgery may benefit from a course of G-CSF therapy preoperatively to reduce the risk of perioperative infection. Patients with dysfunctional phagocytes may be candidates for bone marrow transplantation.

Deficiencies in Components of the Complement System

Deficiencies in virtually all the soluble complement components have been described. Defects in early components of the classic pathway of complement activation (C1q, C1r, C2, and C4) predispose to autoimmune inflammatory disorders resembling systemic lupus erythematosus. Deficiencies in the common pathway component C3 are usually fatal in utero. Deficiencies in the terminal complement components C5 through C8 are associated with recurrent infection and rheumatic diseases. Patients with deficiencies in C9 and components of the alternative pathway (factor D and properdin) are predisposed to neisserial infection. Factor H deficiency is associated with familial relapsing hemolytic uremic syndrome. Deficiency of the complement regulator C1 inhibitor does not cause immunodeficiency but rather hereditary angioedema.

EXCESSIVE INNATE IMMUNITY

Neutrophilia

The earliest response to an infection is the emigration of granulocytes out of the circulation and into the site of bacterial invasion. The rapidity and magnitude of the increase in the number of circulating granulocytes in response to infection are remarkable. Within hours of the onset of a severe infection, the granulocyte count increases two- to fourfold. This increase represents a change in the marginated and circulating pools of granulocytes and the delivery of new granulocytes from the bone marrow. *Neutrophilia* is defined as an absolute granulocyte count in excess of 7000 segmented granulocytes plus bands per microliter. Major causes of neutrophilia are listed in **Table 21-2**.

An increase in the granulocyte count does not produce specific symptoms or signs unless the count exceeds 100,000/μL. Such marked leukocytosis can produce leukostasis in the spleen that can result in splenic infarction and leukostasis in the lungs that is associated with a decrease in oxygen-diffusing capacity. Granulocytes can also accumulate in the skin to produce nontender, purplish nodules (chloromas). Unlike immature blasts, mature granulocytes do not invade brain tissue, so neurologic complications do not result from reactive granulocytosis.

The clinical features associated with moderate granulocytosis are those of the primary disease stimulating the outpouring of neutrophils. Major bacterial infection, especially deep-seated infection or peritonitis, is associated with granulocyte counts of 10,000 to 30,000/μL or more, together with an increase in the number of band forms. Reactive monocytosis is seen in patients with tuberculosis, subacute bacterial endocarditis, or severe granulocytopenia. Parasitic infestations are typically associated with an elevated eosinophil count, whereas basophilia is seen in patients with chronic myelogenous leukemia. As a general rule, sustained granulocyte counts of 50,000/μL or higher indicate a noninfectious, malignant disease process such as a myeloproliferative disorder. The appearance of very immature myelocytic cells in the circulation and accompanying changes in other cell lines (increased or decreased platelets or red blood cells) are also signs of hematologic malignancy.

Granulocytosis is an expected side effect of glucocorticoid therapy that interferes with the egress of granulocytes from the circulation into tissues. Patients receiving prednisone 60 to 100 mg/day often have white blood cell counts of 15,000 to 20,000/μL.

Asthma

Asthma is characterized by an exaggerated bronchoconstrictor response to certain stimuli (see Chapter 9, "Respiratory Diseases"). Triggers for this bronchospasm may be unrelated to the immune system such as exposure to cold, exercise, stress, or inhaled irritants. These triggers produce *intrinsic* asthma. Placement of an endotracheal tube and exposure to cold inhaled gases may also trigger this type of asthma. This response is considered part of innate immunity. By contrast, triggers that stimulate activation of the immune system and immunoglobulin (Ig) E release, such as inhaled allergens, produce *extrinsic* asthma and are part of adaptive immunity. Symptoms of extrinsic or allergic asthma are highly variable and can include cough, dyspnea, and wheezing. Treatment consists of administration of β-agonists, anticholinergic drugs, corticosteroids, and leukotriene inhibitors.

MISDIRECTED INNATE IMMUNITY

Angioedema

Angioedema may be hereditary or acquired and is characterized by episodic edema (due to increased vascular permeability) of the skin (face and extremities) and mucous membranes (gastrointestinal tract). The most common hereditary form of angioedema results from an autosomal dominant deficiency or dysfunction of *C1 esterase inhibitor*. This serine protease inhibitor (serpin) regulates the complement pathway and has activity against the antibody-independent complement pathway and the fibrinolytic pathway. Most importantly, however, is the

TABLE 21-2 Clinical Conditions Associated with Neutrophilia

Disorder	Mechanism
Infection/inflammation	Increased neutrophil production and marrow release of neutrophils
Stress/metabolic disorders (preeclampsia, diabetic ketoacidosis)	Increased neutrophil production
Steroid treatment	Demargination of neutrophils
Myeloproliferative disease	Increased marrow neutrophil release and demargination of neutrophils
Splenectomy	Decrease in splenic trapping of neutrophils

ability of this serpin to inhibit bradykinin and factor XII, enzymes of the contact activation pathway. The absence of this serpin leads to a release of vasoactive mediators that increase vascular permeability and produce edema. Patients deficient in this regulatory enzyme experience repeated bouts of facial and/or laryngeal edema lasting 24 to 72 hours. The onset of susceptibility to these attacks usually begin in the second decade of life and may be triggered by menses, trauma, infection, stress, or estrogen-containing oral contraceptives. Dental surgery can be an important trigger of laryngeal attacks. Abdominal attacks usually present with excruciating pain, nausea, vomiting, and/or diarrhea, and supportive care must address both pain and fluid losses.

C1 esterase inhibitor deficiency can be acquired by patients with lymphoproliferative disorders. These patients have antibodies to C1 inhibitor, and this gives rise to a syndrome that closely mimics hereditary angioedema. Angiotensin-converting enzyme inhibitors used for the treatment of hypertension and heart failure can also precipitate angioedema in 0.1% to 0.7% of patients. This drug-induced angioedema is thought to result from increased availability of bradykinin made possible by the angiotensin-converting enzyme inhibitor's blockade of bradykinin catabolism. The angioedema may develop unexpectedly after prolonged drug use and may affect the face, upper airway, or larynx.

Patients experiencing recurrent angioedema, whether hereditary or acquired, require prophylaxis before a stimulating procedure such as dental surgery or any surgery requiring endotracheal intubation. Androgens such as danazol and stanozolol have been the mainstay of prophylactic therapy, both long term and prior to surgery or dental manipulation. Antifibrinolytic therapy (ϵ-aminocaproic acid, tranexamic acid, or aprotinin) has also been used. Anabolic steroids (androgens) are believed to increase hepatic synthesis of C1 esterase inhibitor, whereas antifibrinolytics are believed to act by inhibiting plasmin activation. The preferred treatment for an acute attack of angioedema is C1 inhibitor concentrate (25 U/kg) or fresh frozen plasma (two to four units) to replace the deficient enzyme. It is important to note that androgens, catecholamines, antihistamines, and antifibrinolytics are not useful in the treatment of acute attacks of angioedema. Should upper airway obstruction develop during acute attacks of hereditary angioedema, tracheal intubation may be lifesaving until the edema subsides.

Management of Anesthesia

Pretreatment of patients with hereditary angioedema should be considered prior to elective surgery in which airway trauma (including placement of a laryngeal mask airway or endotracheal tube) is anticipated. It is prudent to ensure the ready availability of C1 inhibitor concentrates for intravenous infusion should an acute attack occur. Incidental trauma to the oropharynx, such as that produced by suctioning, should be minimized. Regional anesthetic techniques are well tolerated as are intramuscular injections.. The choice of drugs to produce general or regional anesthesia is not influenced by the presence of hereditary angioedema.

Emergency Airway Management

Management of the airway during an acute attack of laryngeal edema includes administration of supplemental oxygen and consideration of endotracheal intubation. When performing laryngoscopy, it is important to have personnel and equipment available to perform tracheostomy if needed, but airway swelling may become so severe that even tracheostomy may be ineffective in providing a patent airway. Swelling may extend into the airway to such an extent that death is possible unless C1 inhibitor replacement therapy is undertaken.

INADEQUATE ADAPTIVE IMMUNITY

Defects of Antibody Production

X-linked agammaglobulinemia is an inherited defect in the maturation of B cells. Mature B cells are missing or reduced in the circulation and lymphoid tissues have no plasma cells. Therefore, functional antibody is not produced. Affected boys have recurrent pyogenic infection during the latter half of their first year of life as maternal antibodies wane. Therapy with intravenous immunoglobulin every 3 to 4 months allows the majority of these children to survive into adulthood.

Combined Defects

Severe combined immunodeficiency syndromes are caused by a number of genetic mutations that affect T-, B-, or natural killer–cell function. The most common form of severe combined immunodeficiency syndrome is the *X-linked form of combined immunodeficiency*, with a prevalence of approximately 1 in 50,000 live births and accounting for approximately half of severe combined immunodeficiency syndrome cases in the United States. The disease is caused by a defect in a receptor that transduces lymphocyte responses to interleukins. B-lymphocyte numbers are usually normal, but immunoglobulin levels are low and specific antibody responses do not occur. The only treatment that substantially prolongs life expectancy is bone marrow or stem cell transplantation from an HLA-compatible donor.

Adenosine deaminase deficiency is another form of severe combined immunodeficiency syndrome, accounting for approximately 15% of all severe combined immunodeficiency syndromes. The adenosine deaminase enzyme is critical in purine metabolism. The adenosine deaminase enzyme is most abundant in lymphocytes and deficiency allows for accumulation of toxic levels of purine intermediates leading to T-cell death. There is profound lymphopenia together with skeletal abnormalities of the ribs and hips. Bone marrow or stem cell transplantation or enzyme replacement with bovine adenosine deaminase enzyme is of benefit in increasing life expectancy.

Ataxia-telangiectasia is a syndrome consisting of cerebellar ataxia, oculocutaneous telangiectasias, chronic sinopulmonary disease, and immunodeficiency. The genetic basis of this disorder is a gene mutation in the surveillance system that monitors DNA for double-strand breaks. With this syndrome, DNA damage that occurs during cell division is missed and defective cells are released into the circulation. One consequence of this defect is the production of dysfunctional lymphocytes. These patients also have a considerable predisposition to malignancy, especially leukemia and lymphoma. Ataxia-telangiectasia patients are so susceptible to radiation-induced injury that bone marrow transplantation is not possible. Supportive therapy includes intravenous immunoglobulin administration.

Defects of T Lymphocytes

DiGeorge syndrome (thymic hypoplasia) is a result of a gene deletion. Features include absent or diminished thymus development, hypoplasia of the thyroid and parathyroid glands, cardiac malformations, and facial dysmorphism. The degree of immunocompromise correlates with the amount of thymic tissue present. Complete absence of the thymus produces a severe combined immunodeficiency syndrome–like phenotype with bacterial, fungal, and parasitic infections all being problems. There are no T cells. Partial DiGeorge syndrome requires no therapy. Complete DiGeorge syndrome is treated by thymus transplantation or infusion of mature T cells.

EXCESSIVE ADAPTIVE IMMUNITY

Allergic Reactions

Immune-mediated allergic reactions are classified according to their mechanism. Type I allergic reactions are IgE mediated and involve mast cells and basophils. Anaphylaxis is an example of a type I reaction. Type II reactions mediate cytotoxicity with IgG, IgM, and complement. Type III reactions produce tissue damage via immune complex formation or deposition. Type IV reactions exhibit T lymphocyte–mediated delayed hypersensitivity. Anaphylactoid reactions appear to be caused by mediator release from mast cells and basophils through a nonimmune mechanism.

Anaphylaxis

Anaphylaxis is a life-threatening manifestation of antigen-antibody interaction. This type of allergic reaction can occur when previous exposure to antigens, e.g., from drugs or foods, has evoked production of antigen-specific IgE antibodies. Subsequent exposure to the same or a chemically similar antigen results in antigen-antibody interactions that initiate marked degranulation of mast cells and basophils. Initial manifestations usually occur within 5 to 10 minutes of exposure to the antigen. Vasoactive mediators released by degranulation of mast cells and basophils are responsible for the clinical manifestations of anaphylaxis (**Table 21-3**). Urticaria and pruritus are common. Primary vascular collapse occurs in approximately 25% of cases of fatal anaphylaxis. Extravasation of up to 50% of intravascular fluid into the extracellular fluid space reflects the marked increase in capillary permeability that accompanies anaphylaxis. Indeed, hypovolemia is a likely cause of hypotension in these patients, although negative inotropic actions of leukotrienes could also play a role.

TABLE 21-3 Vasoactive Mediators Released During Anaphylaxis

Mediator	Physiologic Effect
Histamine	Increased capillary permeability, peripheral vasodilation, bronchoconstriction
Leukotrienes	Increased capillary permeability, intense bronchoconstriction, negative inotropy, coronary artery vasoconstriction
Prostaglandins	Bronchoconstriction
Eosinophil chemotactic factor	Attraction of eosinophils
Neutrophil chemotactic factor	Attraction of neutrophils
Platelet-activating factor	Platelet aggregation and release of vasoactive amines

Laryngeal edema, bronchospasm, and arterial hypoxemia may accompany anaphylaxis. The incidence of anaphylaxis during anesthesia has been estimated to be between 1:3500 and 1:13,000.

Diagnosis

The diagnosis of anaphylaxis can be suggested by the often dramatic nature of the clinical manifestations in close temporal relationship to exposure to a particular antigen. When only a few symptoms are present, however, the response may mimic pulmonary embolism, acute myocardial infarction, aspiration, or a vasovagal reaction. Anesthetic drugs may alter vasoactive mediator release and delay early recognition of anaphylaxis. Hypotension and cardiovascular collapse may be the only manifestations of anaphylaxis in patients under general anesthesia.

Immunologic and biochemical proof of anaphylaxis can be provided by an increased plasma tryptase concentration within 1 to 2 hours of the suspected allergic drug reaction. Tryptase, a neutral protease stored in mast cells, is liberated into the systemic circulation during anaphylactic but not anaphylactoid reactions. Its presence verifies that mast-cell activation and mediator release have occurred, and thus it serves to distinguish immunologic from chemical reactions. The concentration of tryptase in plasma generally reflects the severity of the reaction. Plasma histamine concentration returns to baseline within 30 to 60 minutes of an anaphylactic reaction, so measurement of plasma histamine concentration must be done immediately after treatment of the reaction.

Identification of the offending antigen can be provided by a positive intradermal test (wheal and flare response), which confirms the presence of specific IgE antibodies. Skin testing should not be performed within 6 weeks of an anaphylactic reaction because mast-cell and basophil-mediator depletion can produce a false-negative result. Because of the risk of inducing a systemic reaction, testing must be done with a dilute, preservative-free solution of suspected antigen and only by trained personnel with appropriate resuscitative equipment immediately available.

The radioallergosorbent test and enzyme-linked immunosorbent assay are commercially available antigen preparations for in vitro testing of antibodies to a test antigen.

Treatment

The immediate goals of treatment of anaphylaxis are reversal of hypotension and hypoxemia, replacement of intravascular volume and inhibition of further cellular degranulation, and release of vasoactive mediators. Several liters of crystalloid and/or colloid solution must be infused to restore intravascular fluid volume and blood pressure. Epinephrine is indicated in doses of 10 to 100 μg IV. Early intervention with epinephrine is critical for reversing the life-threatening events characteristic of anaphylaxis. Epinephrine, by increasing intracellular concentrations of cyclic adenosine monophosphate, restores membrane permeability and decreases the release of vasoactive mediators. The β-agonist effects of epinephrine relax bronchial smooth muscle and reverse bronchospasm. The dose of epinephrine should be doubled and repeated every 1 to 2 minutes until a satisfactory blood pressure response has been obtained. If anaphylaxis is not life threatening, subcutaneous rather than intravenous epinephrine may be used in a dose of 0.3 to 0.5 mg.

Antihistamines such as diphenhydramine compete with membrane receptor sites normally occupied by histamine and might decrease some manifestations of anaphylaxis such as pruritus and bronchospasm. However, administration of an antihistamine is not effective in treating anaphylaxis once vasoactive mediators have been released. The negative inotropic effect and bronchospasm due to leukotrienes are not influenced by antihistamines. β_2-Agonists such as albuterol delivered by metered-dose inhaler or nebulization are useful for the treatment of bronchospasm associated with anaphylaxis.

Corticosteroids are often administered intravenously to patients experiencing life-threatening anaphylaxis. Although these drugs have no known effect on degranulation of mast cells or antigen-antibody interactions, the favorable effects of corticosteroids may reflect enhancement of the β-agonist effects of other drugs and inhibition of the release of arachidonic acid responsible for the production of leukotrienes and prostaglandins. Corticosteroids may be uniquely helpful in patients experiencing life-threatening allergic reactions due to activation of the complement system.

Drug Allergy

Epidemiology

In the general population, penicillin accounts for most fatal anaphylactic drug reactions. Drug sensitivity has been implicated in 3.4% to 4.3% of anesthesia-related deaths. The incidence of allergic drug reactions during anesthesia may be increasing, probably due to the frequent administration of several drugs to a patient and cross-sensitivity among the drugs. Allergic reactions to drugs may be due to anaphylaxis, anaphylactoid reactions, or activation of the complement system. More than one mechanism may be involved in the production of an allergic drug reaction in a particular patient. Regardless of the mechanism responsible for life-threatening allergic drug reactions, the manifestations and treatment are identical.

It is not possible to reliably predict which patients are likely to experience anaphylaxis after administration of drugs that are usually innocuous. However, patients with a history of allergy (asthma, food, drugs) have an increased incidence of anaphylaxis, possibly related to a genetic predisposition to form increased amounts of IgE antibodies. Patients allergic to penicillin have a three- to fourfold greater risk of experiencing an allergic reaction to *any* drug. A history of allergy to specific drugs elicited during the preoperative evaluation is helpful but previous uneventful exposure to a drug does not eliminate the possibility of anaphylaxis on subsequent exposure.

Allergic drug reactions must be distinguished from drug intolerance, idiosyncratic reactions, and drug toxicity (**Table 21-4**). The occurrence of undesirable pharmacologic effects at a low dose of drug reflects intolerance, whereas idiosyncratic reactions are undesirable responses to a drug independent of the dose administered. Evidence of histamine release along veins into which drugs are injected reflects localized and nonimmunologic release of histamine insufficient to evoke an anaphylactoid reaction. Patients manifesting this localized response should not be diagnosed as allergic to the drug.

Allergic Drug Reactions during the Perioperative Period

Allergic drug reactions have been reported with most drugs that may be administered during anesthesia (**Table 21-5**). The exceptions to this generalization are ketamine and benzodiazepines. Cardiovascular collapse is the predominant manifestation of a life-threatening allergic drug reaction in an anesthetized patient. Bronchospasm is present in fewer patients. It is important to consider the possible role of latex sensitivity when a presumed allergic reaction to a drug occurs. It may be that many allergic reactions attributed to drugs are, in fact, a result of latex allergy. It is estimated that as many as 15% of allergic reactions during anesthesia are due to latex.

Most drug-induced allergic reactions manifest within 5 to 10 minutes of exposure to the offending drug. An important exception is the allergic response to latex, which is typically delayed for as long as 30 minutes. An allergic reaction should be considered whenever there is an abrupt decrease in blood pressure. In one tenth of patients, the only manifestation of an intraoperative allergic reaction is hypotension. Extravasation of fluid into the extracellular space is a result of a marked increase in capillary permeability, and the resulting hypovolemia is the principal cause of hypotension during a drug-induced allergic reaction. Bronchospasm may be particularly

TABLE 21-4 | Characteristics of Drug Allergy Versus Drug Toxicity

Parameter	Drug Allergy	Drug Toxicity
Mechanism	Antigen-antibody interaction	Dependent on chemical properties of drug
Manifestations	Hypotension Bronchospasm Urticaria	Variable
Predictability	Poor	Good
Previous exposure	Required	Not required
Dose related	No	Yes
Onset	Usually within 5–10 min	Usually delayed
Incidence	Low	High if dose is sufficient

severe and difficult to treat in patients with obstructive pulmonary disease.

Muscle Relaxants

Muscle relaxants are responsible for more than 60% of drug-induced allergic reactions during the intraoperative period. Approximately half of patients who experience an allergic reaction to one muscle relaxant are also allergic to other muscle relaxants. Cross-sensitivity among muscle relaxants emphasizes the structural similarities of these drugs, especially the presence of one or more antigenic quaternary ammonium groups. Muscle relaxant-allergic patients may remain sensitized (positive radioallergosorbent test) for up to 30 years after first developing antibodies. IgE antibodies develop to quaternary or tertiary ammonium ions. Many over-the-counter drugs and cosmetics contain these ammonium ions and are capable of sensitizing an individual. Consequently, anaphylaxis may develop on the first exposure to a muscle relaxant in a patient sensitized by one of these products. Neostigmine and morphine contain ammonium ions that are also capable of cross-reacting with antibodies to muscle relaxants. A patient with a history of anaphylaxis to any muscle relaxant should be skin tested preoperatively for all drugs that are likely to be used in the upcoming anesthetic.

Nonimmune reactions to muscle relaxants include direct mast cell degranulation that causes release of histamine and other mediators. Benzylisoquinolinium compounds such as tubocurare, metocurine, atracurium, and mivacurium are more likely to cause direct mast cell degranulation than aminosteroid compounds like pancuronium, vecuronium, and rocuronium.

Induction Drugs

Allergic reactions after barbiturate administration for induction of anesthesia are rare but can be life threatening. Most reported cases are in patients with a history of food allergies, rhinitis, or asthma and previous uneventful exposure to a barbiturate during anesthesia.

Life-threatening allergic reactions have occurred after first or subsequent exposure to propofol. Patients with a history of allergy to other drugs seem to be more vulnerable to propofol allergy. Bronchospasm occurs more often in patients experiencing allergic reactions to propofol than with other anesthetic drugs.

Local Anesthetics

Local anesthetic-induced allergic reactions are rare despite the frequent use of these drugs and the common labeling of patients as allergic to drugs in this class. It is estimated that only 1% of all local anesthetic reactions are allergic reactions. The mechanism of an adverse response to a local anesthetic can often be determined by careful questioning and review of past medical records describing the event. For example, the occurrence of *hypotension* and seizures is characteristic of a systemic reaction due to toxic blood levels of a local anesthetic. This is most likely to occur with inadvertent intravascular injection during performance of regional anesthesia. These episodes of local anesthetic toxicity are often erroneously labeled as allergic reactions. Tachycardia and *hypertension* associated

TABLE 21-5 | Intraoperative Allergic Drug Reactions

Drug	Incidence (%)	Anaphylactic	Anaphylactoid	Nonspecific Mast Cell/Basophil Degranulation
Muscle relaxants	60	X		X
Latex	15	X		
Antibiotics	5–10	X		
Hypnotics	<5	X		
Opioids	<5	X		X
Radiocontrast media	<5		X	
Protamine	<5	X	X	

with injection of a local anesthetic most likely reflects systemic absorption of epinephrine from the local anesthetic solution. Urticaria, laryngeal edema, and bronchoconstriction are likely to indicate a true local anesthetic-induced allergic reaction.

Ester-type local anesthetics are metabolized to the highly antigenic compound para-aminobenzoic acid and are more likely than amide-type local anesthetics that are not metabolized to compound para-aminobenzoic acid to evoke an allergic reaction. Local anesthetic solutions may also contain methylparaben or propylparaben as preservatives with bacteriostatic and fungistatic properties. The structural similarity of these preservatives to compound para-aminobenzoic acid may render them antigenic. As a result, anaphylaxis may actually be due to stimulation of antibody production by the preservative and not by the local anesthetic.

It is not uncommon to have to consider the safety of administering a local anesthetic to a patient with a history of allergy to this class of drugs. It is generally agreed that cross-sensitivity does not exist between ester- and amide-based local anesthetics. It should, therefore, be acceptable to administer amide-based local anesthetics to patients with a history of allergy to ester-based local anesthetics and vice versa. It is also important to use only preservative-free local anesthetic solutions since preservatives may also be responsible for allergic reactions. It is reasonable to recommend intradermal testing with preservative-free local anesthetics in the occasional patient with a convincing allergic history in whom failure to document a safe local anesthetic drug would prevent the use of local or regional anesthesia.

Opioids

Anaphylaxis after administration of opioids is very rare, perhaps reflecting the similarity of these drugs to naturally occurring endorphins. Fentanyl has been associated with allergic reactions following systemic and neuraxial administration. Morphine, but not fentanyl or its related derivatives, may directly evoke the release of histamine from mast cells and basophils.

Volatile Anesthetics

Clinical manifestations of halothane-induced hepatitis suggest a drug-induced allergic reaction. These include eosinophilia, fever, rash, and previous exposure to halothane. The plasma of patients with a clinical diagnosis of halothane hepatitis may contain antibodies that react with halothane-induced liver antigens (neoantigens). These neoantigens are formed by the covalent interaction of reactive oxidative trifluoroacetyl halide metabolites of halothane with hepatic microsomal proteins. Acetylation of liver proteins, in effect, changes these proteins from self to nonself (neoantigens), resulting in the formation of antibodies against these now foreign proteins. It is postulated that subsequent antigen-antibody interactions are responsible for the liver injury associated with halothane hepatitis. Similar oxidative halide metabolites are produced after exposure to enflurane, isoflurane, and desflurane but not sevoflurane, indicating the possibility of cross-sensitivity to volatile

anesthetics in susceptible patients. Based on the degree of metabolism of these volatile anesthetics, it is predictable that the incidence of anesthetic-induced allergic hepatitis would be greatest after halothane, intermediate with enflurane, minimal with isoflurane, and remote with desflurane.

Protamine

Anaphylactic reactions following administration of protamine are more likely to occur in patients who are allergic to seafood (protamine is derived from salmon sperm) and in patients with diabetes mellitus who are being treated with protamine-containing insulin preparations. After vasectomy, men may also be at increased risk of allergic reactions to protamine since they develop circulating antibodies to spermatozoa. Protamine is capable of causing direct histamine release from cells. Protamine may also activate the complement pathway and cause release of thromboxane, leading to bronchoconstriction and pulmonary hypertension. Patients known to be allergic to protamine present a therapeutic dilemma when neutralization of heparin is required because no alternative drug to reverse the effects of heparin is available.

Antibiotics

The structural similarity between penicillin and cephalosporins (both contain β-lactam rings) suggests the possibility of cross-sensitivity. However, the incidence of life-threatening allergic reactions following administration of cephalosporins is low (0.02%), and the incidence of allergic reactions to cephalosporins is only minimally increased in patients with a history of penicillin allergy.

Blood and Plasma Volume Expanders

Allergic reactions to properly cross-matched blood occur in approximately 1% to 3% of patients. Synthetic colloid solutions (dextran, hydroxyethyl starch) have been implicated in anaphylactic and anaphylactoid reactions, with manifestations ranging from rash and modest hypotension to bronchospasm and shock. Low molecular weight dextran cannot induce antibody formation but may react with antibodies formed in response to previous exposure to polysaccharides of viral or bacterial origin. Dextran may also activate the complement system, producing signs of an allergic reaction.

Radiocontrast Media

Iodine in contrast media injected intravenously for radiographic studies evokes allergic reactions in approximately 5% of patients. The risk of an allergic reaction is increased in patients with a history of allergies to other drugs or foods. Many of the allergic reactions to contrast media seem to be anaphylactoid and can be modified by pretreatment with corticosteroids and histamine antagonists and limitation of the iodine dose.

Latex-Containing Medical Devices

Cardiovascular collapse during anesthesia and surgery may be attributable to anaphylaxis triggered by latex (natural rubber). A feature that distinguishes latex-induced allergic reactions from drug-induced allergic reactions is the delayed onset of the reaction, typically longer than 30 minutes after exposure to the latex. By contrast, most drug-induced allergic reactions occur within 5 to 10 minutes following drug administration. It may take time for the responsible antigen to be eluted from rubber gloves and absorbed across mucous membranes into the systemic circulation in amounts sufficient to cause an allergic reaction. Contact with latex at mucosal surfaces is probably the most significant route of latex exposure. However, inhalation of latex antigens is also a common route of exposure and sensitization in health care workers. Cornstarch powder in gloves is not immunogenic but can act as an airborne vehicle for latex antigens that have been absorbed by the powder.

Sensitized patients develop IgE antibodies directed specifically against latex antigens. Skin testing can confirm latex hypersensitivity, but anaphylaxis has occurred during skin testing. The radioallergosorbent test and enzyme-linked immunosorbent assay are available for the in vitro detection of latex-specific IgE antibodies. These tests are equally sensitive and specific and avoid the risk of anaphylaxis associated with skin testing.

Questions about itching, conjunctivitis, rhinitis, rash, or wheezing after inflating toy balloons or wearing latex gloves or following dental or gynecologic examinations involving latex gloves may be helpful in identifying sensitized patients. Operating room personnel and patients with spina bifida have an increased incidence of latex allergy that is thought to reflect frequent exposure to latex devices such as bladder catheters and gloves. Latex sensitivity most often manifests as cutaneous sensitivity from direct contact with latex gloves or bronchospasm due to inhalation of latex antigens. Latex sensitivity is recognized as an occupational hazard for operating room personnel. The incidence of latex sensitivity in anesthesiologists may exceed 15%. Health care workers are at increased risk of development of severe latex allergic reactions should they themselves become patients and undergo surgery.

Management of Anesthesia

Patients at high risk of latex sensitivity (those with spina bifida, multiple previous operations, history of fruit allergies; health care workers; atopic individuals) should be questioned for symptoms related to exposure to natural rubber during their daily routine or previous surgical procedure. Intraoperative management is characterized by a latex-free environment. Nonlatex gloves (styrene, neoprene) are used by all personnel who may be in contact with a latex-sensitive patient. Medications should not be withdrawn from multidose bottles with latex caps or injected through latex ports on intravenous delivery tubing. Intravenous and bladder catheters, drains, anesthesia delivery tubing, ventilator bellows, endotracheal tubes, laryngeal mask airways, nasogastric tubes, blood pressure cuffs, pulse oximeter probes, electrocardiogram pads, and syringes must also be latex free.

Eosinophilia

Clinically significant eosinophilia is defined as a sustained absolute eosinophil count of greater than 1000 to 1500/μL. Moderate eosinophilia is commonly seen with a wide spectrum of disorders, including parasitic infestations, systemic allergic disorders, collagen vascular diseases, various forms of dermatitis, drug reactions, and tumors. Hodgkin's disease and both B- and T-cell non-Hodgkin's lymphomas can present with 2eosinophilia. Even when there is no obvious sign of an underlying lymphoma, up to 25% of patients with apparent idiopathic eosinophilia will have an expanded clone of aberrant T cells, which produce high levels of interleukin-5.

Hypereosinophilia (an eosinophil count > 5000/μL) is associated with tissue damage secondary to release of basic protein by the eosinophil. Irreversible endomyocardial fibrosis producing a restrictive cardiomyopathy is common in patients who maintain eosinophil counts greater than 5000/μL. In patients with eosinophilic leukemia, idiopathic hypereosinophilic syndrome or Löffler's syndrome, eosinophil counts can reach 20,000 to 100,000/μL. Widespread organ dysfunction and rapidly progressive heart disease are associated with these conditions. These patients need aggressive treatment with both corticosteroids and hydroxyurea. Leukopheresis can be used to acutely lower the eosinophil count.

MISDIRECTED ADAPTIVE IMMUNITY

Autoimmune Disorders

The challenge of adaptive immunity is the need for immune cells to be capable of responding efficiently to an enormous number of foreign antigens yet still be able to recognize and tolerate "self" antigens. There is growing evidence that major immunologic stimuli, such as infection, can activate some self-reactive lymphocytes. In the aftermath of such an immunologic challenge, part of the clean up of these primed lymphocytes is widespread apoptosis, that is, these self-reactive lymphocytes are signaled to self-destruct. Transient autoimmunity appears to be a relatively common by-product of a major immune response. The specific defects that cause autoimmunity to persist and become a chronic, self-destructive immune disorder are not well understood at the present time. Perhaps some genetic predisposition and/or a particular infection or other inciting event causes autoimmunity to persist and become problematic. **Table 21-6** lists some diseases with an autoimmune basis.

The anesthetic implications of autoimmune disorders can be partitioned into three categories. The first category is anesthetic considerations for certain vulnerable organs specific to the particular autoimmune disorder. Examples of this include cervical instability with rheumatoid arthritis, renal injury with systemic lupus erythematosus, and liver failure with chronic active hepatitis. The second category is the consequences of therapy being used to treat the disorder. The potential for addisonian crisis in patients being treated with corticosteroids is well recognized.

TABLE 21-6 Examples of Autoimmune Diseases

Rheumatic
Rheumatoid arthritis
Scleroderma
Sjögren's syndrome
Mixed connective tissue disease
Systemic lupus erythematosus

Gastrointestinal
Chronic active hepatitis
Ulcerative colitis
Crohn's disease

Endocrine
Type I diabetes mellitus
Hashimotos thyroiditis
Graves' disease

Neurologic
Myasthenia gravis
Multiple sclerosis

Hematologic
Idiopathic thrombocytopenic purpura

Renal
Goodpasture's syndrome

Some of the newer therapies inhibit particular facets of the immune response, such as the B cell–depleting monoclonal antibody rituximab, which is now in common use for treating forms of lymphoma. The third category, especially in patients with long-standing autoimmune disorders, is the risk of accelerated atherosclerosis and associated cardiovascular complications such as heart disease and stroke. Some studies suggest that the risk of cardiovascular morbidity and mortality is increased approximately 50-fold by autoimmune diseases. Some of this added risk may be due to the therapy for autoimmune diseases since chronic corticosteroid treatment is associated with both hypertension and diabetes mellitus. Even after controlling for these comorbidities, patients with autoimmune disorders have an eightfold increased risk of cardiovascular disease. Therefore, patients with long-standing autoimmune disease presenting for surgery need a thorough evaluation for the presence of cardiovascular disease that could increase their perioperative risk.

ANESTHESIA AND IMMUNOCOMPETENCE

Exposure to anesthesia and performance of surgery may affect immunocompetence and alter the incidence of perioperative infection or the response to cancer.

Resistance to Infection

It is conceivable that anesthesia-induced depression of the immune system can increase the risk of development of perioperative infection or augment the severity of co-existing infection. Local and inhaled anesthetics (nitrous oxide) may produce dose-dependent inhibition of mobilization and migration of polymorphonuclear leukocytes. However, the effects produced by these drugs are probably clinically insignificant, considering the usual duration of anesthesia and the total dose of drug administered. The incidence of postoperative infection seems to be more related to surgical trauma and to the release of cortisol and catecholamines that are known to inhibit phagocytosis. It appears that the effects of anesthetics on resistance to infection are transient, reversible, and of lesser importance compared with the prolonged immunosuppressive effects of cortisol and catecholamine release as part of the hormonal response to surgery. Mild perioperative hypothermia ($<36°C$) has been associated with an increased risk of postoperative infection.

If hormonal responses to surgical stimulation are undesirable in respect to infection risk, it could be reasoned that light anesthesia, which does not reliably attenuate sympathetic nervous system activity, is less desirable than deeper levels of general anesthesia. Regional anesthesia may decrease the hormonal response to surgical stimulation. However, to date, there is no convincing evidence that the incidence of perioperative infection can be altered by the depth of anesthesia or the technique selected to produce surgical anesthesia.

Resistance to Cancer

Immunocompetence is essential for the host to resist cancer. There is concern that some patients with a preoperative diagnosis of cancer might experience rapid tumor growth after anesthesia and surgery, perhaps due to enhancement of tumor cell replication and spread by decreasing host resistance. Despite these concerns, there is no evidence that the short-term effects of anesthetic drugs are of any significance in the resistance of a host to cancer.

KEY POINTS

- The immune system can be divided into two pathways, one encompassing *innate* immunity and the other *adaptive* or *acquired* immunity.

- Innate immunity mounts the initial response to any infection, recognizes targets that are common to many pathogens, and has no specific memory. Its cellular elements are neutrophils, macrophages, monocytes, and natural killer cells and its noncellular elements include the complement system, acute-phase proteins, and proteins of the contact activation pathway.

Continued

KEY POINTS—cont'd

- Adaptive immunity has a more delayed onset and may take days to activate when challenged by an unfamiliar antigen. However, adaptive immunity is capable of developing memory and is more rapidly induced by antigen when memory is present. Adaptive immunity consists of a humoral component that is mediated by B lymphocytes that produce antibodies and a cellular component dominated by T lymphocytes.

- Angioedema may be hereditary or acquired and is characterized by episodic edema (due to increased vascular permeability) of the skin (face and extremities) and mucous membranes (gastrointestinal tract). The most common hereditary form of angioedema results from an autosomal dominant deficiency of C1 esterase inhibitor.

- The treatment of an acute attack of angioedema is C1 inhibitor concentrate or fresh frozen plasma to replace the deficient enzyme. Androgens, catecholamines, antihistamines, and antifibrinolytics are *not* useful in the treatment of acute attacks of angioedema.

- Anaphylaxis is a life-threatening manifestation of antigen-antibody interaction.

- Initial manifestations occur within 5 to 10 minutes of exposure to the antigen. Vasoactive mediators released by degranulation of mast cells and basophils are responsible for the clinical manifestations of anaphylaxis.

- Treatment of anaphylaxis requires reversal of hypotension, replacement of intravascular volume and inhibition of further cellular degranulation, and release of vasoactive mediators. Early intervention with epinephrine is critical. Epinephrine, by increasing intracellular concentrations of cyclic adenosine monophosphate, restores membrane permeability and decreases the release of vasoactive mediators. The β-agonist effects of epinephrine relax bronchial smooth muscle and reverse bronchospasm.

- Muscle relaxants are responsible for more than 60% of drug-induced allergic reactions during the intraoperative period. Approximately half of patients who experience an allergic reaction to one muscle relaxant are also allergic to other muscle relaxants.

- Anaphylaxis triggered by latex (natural rubber) can cause cardiovascular collapse during anesthesia and surgery. A feature that distinguishes latex-induced allergic reactions from drug-induced allergic reactions is the delayed onset of the reaction, typically longer than 30 minutes after exposure to the latex.

- Latex sensitivity is recognized as an occupational hazard for operating room personnel. The incidence of latex sensitivity in anesthesiologists exceeds 15%.

- Patients with autoimmune disorders have an eightfold increased risk of cardiovascular disease. Therefore, patients with long-standing autoimmune disease presenting for surgery need a thorough evaluation for the presence of cardiovascular disease that could increase their perioperative risk.

REFERENCES

Bracho FA: Hereditary angioedema. Curr Opin Hematol 2005;12:493–498.

Cleary AM, Insel RA, Lewis DB: Disorders of lymphocyte function. In Hoffman R, Benz EJ, Shattil SJ (eds): Hematology: Basic Principles and Practice. Philadelphia, Elsevier Science, 2004.

Dinauer MC, Coates TD: Disorders of phagocyte function and number. In Hoffman R, Benz EJ, Shattil SJ (eds): Hematology: Basic Principles and Practice. Philadelphia, Elsevier Science, 2004.

Gompels MM, Lock RJ, Abinum M, et al: C1 inhibitor deficiency: Consensus document. Clin Exp Immunol 2005;139: 379–394.

Hepner DL, Castells MC: Latex allergy: An update. Anesth Analg 2003;96:1219–1229.

Hepner DL, Castells MC: Anaphylaxis during the perioperative period. Anesth Analg 2003;97:1381–1395.

Kay AB: Allergy and allergic diseases. N Engl J Med 2001;344:30–37, 109–113.

Kemp SF, Lockey RF: Anaphylaxis: A review of causes and mechanisms. J Allergy Clin Immunol 2002;110:341–348.

Mertes PM, Laxenaire MC: Allergic reactions occurring during anaesthesia. Eur J Anaesthesiol 2002;19:240–262.

Walport MJ: Complement. N Engl J Med 2001;344:1058–1066, 1140–1151.

CHAPTER 22

Psychiatric Disease/ Substance Abuse/ Drug Overdose

Roberta L. Hines
Katherine E. Marschall

Depression
- Diagnosis
- Treatment

Bipolar Disorder
- Treatment
- Management of Anesthesia

Schizophrenia
- Treatment
- Neuroleptic Malignant Syndrome

Anxiety Disorders

Substance Abuse
- Diagnosis
- Treatment
- Alcoholism
- Cocaine

- Opioids
- Barbiturates
- Benzodiazepines
- Amphetamines
- Hallucinogens
- Marijuana

Drug Overdose
- Cyclic Antidepressant Overdose
- Salicylic Acid Overdose
- Acetaminophen Overdose

Poisoning
- Methyl Alcohol Ingestion
- Ethylene Glycol Ingestion
- Organophosphate Overdose
- Carbon Monoxide Poisoning

The prevalence of psychiatric diseases is such that these entities will often co-exist in patients undergoing anesthesia and surgery. Effects of and potential drug interactions with psychotropic medications are important perioperative considerations. Substance abuse and drug dependence can be viewed as types of psychiatric disease. In addition, substance abuse and suicide represent significant occupational hazards for anesthesiologists.

DEPRESSION

Depression is the most common psychiatric disorder, affecting 2% to 4% of the population. It is distinguished from normal sadness and grief by the severity and duration of the mood disturbances. Patients with depression who have had a manic episode are classified as having manic-depressive disease or bipolar disorder. There is a familial pattern of major

TABLE 22-1 Characteristics of Severe Depression

Depressed mood
Markedly diminished interest or pleasure in almost all
  activities
Fluctuations in body weight and appetite
Insomnia or hypersomnia
Restlessness
Fatigue
Feelings of worthlessness or guilt
Decreased ability to concentrate
Suicidal ideation

TABLE 22-2 Commonly Used Antidepressant Medications

Drug Class	Generic Name	Trade Name
SSRI	Fluoxetine	Prozac
	Paroxetine	Paxil
	Sertraline	Zoloft
	Fluvoxamine	Luvox
	Citalopram	Celexa
Tricyclics	Amitriptyline	Elavil
	Imipramine	Tofranil
	Protriptyline	Vivactil
	Doxepin	Sinequan
MAOI	Phenylzine	Nardil
	Tranylcypromine	Parnate
Atypical	Bupropion	Wellbutrin
	Trazodone	Desyrel
	Nefazodone	Serzone
	Ventafaxine	Effexor

MAOI, monoamine oxidase inhibitor; SSRI, selective serotonin reuptake inhibitor.

depression, and females are affected more often than males. Approximately 15% of patients with major depression commit suicide. Pathophysiologic causes of major depression are unknown, although abnormalities of amine neurotransmitter pathways are the most likely etiologic factors.

Diagnosis

The diagnosis of major depression is based on the persistent presence of at least five of the symptoms noted in **Table 22-1**. Organic causes of irritability or mood changes and the normal reaction to the death of a loved one must be excluded. Alcoholism and major depression often co-exist, and it is presumed that toxic effects of alcohol on the brain are responsible. Depression and dementia may be difficult to distinguish in elderly patients. All patients with depression should be evaluated for the potential to commit suicide. Suicide is the eighth leading cause of death among Americans. Interestingly, physicians have moderately higher (men) to much higher (women) suicide rates than the general population. Most suicide victims have been under the care of a physician shortly before their death, emphasizing the importance of recognizing at-risk patients. Hopelessness is the most important aspect of depression associated with suicide.

Treatment

Depression can be treated with antidepressant medications, psychotherapy, and/or electroconvulsive therapy (ECT). An estimated 70% to 80% of patients respond to pharmacologic therapy, and at least 50% who do not respond to antidepressants do respond favorably to ECT. ECT is usually reserved for patients resistant to antidepressant drugs or those with medical contraindications to treatment with these drugs. Patients with depression plus psychotic symptoms (delusions, hallucinations, catatonia) require both antidepressant and antipsychotic drugs.

Approximately 50 years ago, neurochemical hypotheses regarding depression postulated that decreased availability of norepinephrine and serotonin at specific synapses in the brain are associated with depression and conversely that an increased concentration of these neurotransmitters is associated with mania. Subsequent studies have generally supported the hypotheses that catecholamine and serotonin metabolism are important in mood states, although the exact mechanisms remain to be elucidated. Almost all drugs with antidepressant properties affect catecholamine and/or serotonin availability in the central nervous system (**Table 22-2**).

The selective serotonin reuptake inhibitors (SSRIs) block reuptake of serotonin at presynaptic membranes with relatively little effect on adrenergic, cholinergic, histaminergic, or other neurochemical systems. As a result, they are associated with few side effects.

Tricyclic antidepressants are thought to affect depression by inhibiting synaptic reuptake of norepinephrine and serotonin. However, they also affect other neurochemical systems including histaminergic and cholinergic systems. Consequently, they have a large range of side effects including postural hypotension, cardiac dysrhythmias, and urinary retention.

Monoamine oxidase inhibitors (MAOIs) are inhibitors of both the A and B forms of brain monamine oxidase and as such change the concentration of neurotransmitters by preventing breakdown of catecholamines and serotonin.

Venlafaxine is a methylamine antidepressant that selectively inhibits reuptake of norepinephrine and serotonin without affecting other neurochemical systems. Other atypical antidepressants have more diverse effects including inhibition of reuptake of serotonin and dopamine, antagonism of specific serotonin receptors, dopamine receptor blockade, presynaptic α_2-blockade resulting in increases in norepinephrine and serotonin release, and histamine receptor blockade.

Selective Serotonin Reuptake Inhibitors

Serotonin is produced by hydroxylation and decarboxylation of L-tryptophan in presynaptic neurons, then stored in vesicles that are released and bound to postsynaptic receptors when needed for neurotransmission. A reuptake mechanism allows for return of serotonin to the presynaptic vesicles. Metabolism is by monoamine oxidase type A. Serotonin-specific reuptake inhibitors, as their name implies, inhibit the reuptake of serotonin from the neuronal synapse without significant effects on reuptake of norepinephrine and dopamine.

SSRIs comprise the most widely prescribed class of antidepressants and are the drugs of choice to treat mild to moderate depression. These drugs are also effective for treating panic disorders, posttraumatic stress disorder, bulimia, dysthymia, obsessive-compulsive disorder, and irritable bowel syndrome. Common side effects of SSRIs are insomnia, agitation, headache, nausea, diarrhea, and sexual dysfunction. Appetite suppression is associated with fluoxetine therapy. Abrupt cessation of SSRI use, especially with paroxetine and fluvoxamine, which have short half-lives and no active metabolites, can result in a discontinuation syndrome that can mimic serious illness and can be distressing and uncomfortable. Discontinuation symptoms typically begin 1 to 3 days after abrupt cessation of SSRI use and may include dizziness, irritability, mood swings, headache, nausea and vomiting, dystonia, tremor, lethargy, myalgias, and fatigue. Symptoms can be relieved within 24 hours of restarting SSRI therapy.

Among SSRIs, fluoxetine is a potent inhibitor of certain hepatic cytochrome P-450 enzymes. As a result, this drug may increase plasma concentrations of drugs that depend on hepatic metabolism for clearance. For example, the addition of fluoxetine to treatment with tricyclic antidepressant drugs may result in two- to fivefold increases in the plasma concentrations of tricyclic drugs. Some cardiac antidysrhythmic drugs and some β-adrenergic antagonists are also metabolized by this enzyme system, and fluoxetine inhibition of enzyme activity may result in potentiation of their effects.

Serotonin Syndrome

Serotonin syndrome is a potentially life-threatening adverse drug reaction that may occur with therapeutic drug use, overdose, or interaction between serotoninergic drugs. A large number of drugs have been associated with the serotonin syndrome. These include SSRIs, atypical and cyclic antidepressants, MAOIs, opiates, cough medicine, antibiotics, weight reduction drugs, antiemetic drugs, antimigraine drugs, drugs of abuse (especially "Ecstasy"), and herbal products (**Table 22-3**).

Typical symptoms of serotonin syndrome include agitation, delirium, autonomic hyperactivity, hyperreflexia, clonus, and hyperthermia (**Fig. 22-1**). Additional syndromes to consider in the differential diagnosis of serotonin syndrome are listed in **Table 22-4**. Treatment includes supportive measures and control of autonomic instability, excess muscle activity, and hyperthermia. Cyproheptadine, a 5-HT$_{2A}$ antagonist, can be used to bind serotonin receptors. It is only available for oral use.

TABLE 22-3	Drug and Drug Interactions Associated with Serotonin Syndrome

Drugs Associated with Serotonin Syndrome:
SSRIs
Atypical and cyclic antidepressants
Monoamine oxidase inhibitors
Anticonvulsant drugs: valproate
Analgesics: meperidine, fentanyl, tramadol, pentazocine
Antiemetic drugs: ondansetron, granisetron, metoclopramide
Antimigraine drugs: sumatriptan
Bariatric medications: sibutramine
Antibiotics: linezolide, ritonavir
Over-the-counter cough medicine: dextromethorphan
Drugs of abuse: ecstasy, LSD, foxy methoxy, Syrian rue
Dietary supplements: St. John's wort, ginseng
Other: lithium

Drug Interactions Associated with Severe Serotonin Syndrome:
Phenylzine and meperidine
Tranylcypromine and imipramine
Phenylzine and SSRIs
Paroxetine and buspirone
Linezolide and citalopram
Modobemide and SSRIs
Tramadol, venlafaxine, and mirtazapine

SSRIs, selective serotonin reuptake inhibitors.
Modified from Boyer EW, Shannon M: The serotonin syndrome. N Engl J Med 2005;352:1112–1120. Copyright 2005 Massachusetts Medical Society. All rights reserved.

Tricyclic Antidepressants

Before the availability of SSRIs, tricyclic antidepressants were the most commonly prescribed drugs for treating depression. Now they are used in selected patients with depression and as adjuvant therapy for patients with chronic pain syndromes. Side effects of antidepressant drugs influence drug choice because all these drugs are equally effective if administered in equivalent doses. In addition to causing sedative and

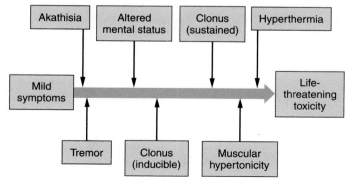

Figure 22-1 • Spectrum of clinical findings in serotonin syndrome. Manifestations range from mild to life threatening. The *vertical arrows* suggest the approximate point at which clinical findings initially appear in the spectrum of the disease. (*Adapted from Boyer EW, Shannon M: The serotonin syndrome. N Engl J Med 2005;352:1112–1120. Copyright 2005 Massachusetts Medical Society. All rights reserved.*)

TABLE 22-4 Drug-Induced Hyperthermic Syndromes

Syndrome	Time to Onset	Causative Drugs	Outstanding Features	Treatment
Malignant hyperthermia	Within minutes	Succinylcholine, inhalation anesthetics	Muscle rigidity, severe hypercarbia	Dantrolene, supportive care
Neuroleptic malignant syndrome	24–72 hr	Dopamine antagonist antipsychotic drugs	Muscle rigidity, stupor/coma, bradykinesia	Bromocriptine or dantrolene, supportive care
Serotonin syndrome	Up to 12 hr	Serotoninergic drugs including SSRIs, MAOIs, and atypical antidepressants	Clonus, hyperreflexia, agitation; may have muscle rigidity	Cyproheptadine, supportive care
Sympathomimetic syndrome	Up to 30 min	Cocaine, amphetamines	Agitation, hallucinations, myocardial ischemia, dysrhythmias, no rigidity	Vasodilators α- and β-blockers, supportive care
Anticholinergic poisoning	Up to 12 hr	Atropine, belladonna	Toxidrome of hot, red, dry skin, dilated pupils, delirium, no rigidity	Physostigmine, supportive care
Cyclic antidepressant overdose	Up to 6 hr	Cyclic antidepressants	Hypotension, stupor/coma, wide-complex dysrhythmias, no rigidity	Serum alkalinization, magnesium

MAOIs, monoamine oxidase inhibitors; SSRIs, selective serotonin reuptake inhibitors.

anticholinergic effects, tricyclic antidepressants can cause cardiovascular abnormalities, including orthostatic hypotension and cardiac dysrhythmias.

Patients being treated with tricyclic antidepressants may have altered responses to drugs administered during the perioperative period. Increased availability of neurotransmitters in the central nervous system can result in increased anesthetic requirements. Likewise, increased availability of norepinephrine at postsynaptic receptors in the sympathetic nervous system can be responsible for exaggerated blood pressure responses following administration of indirect-acting vasopressors, such as ephedrine. The potential for significant hypertension is greatest during acute treatment (first 14–21 days) with tricyclic antidepressants, whereas long-term treatment is associated with down-regulation of receptors.

Long-term treatment with tricyclic antidepressants may alter the response to pancuronium. Tachydysrhythmias have been observed following administration of pancuronium to patients who were also receiving imipramine. Presumably, there is an interaction between tricyclic antidepressants and the anticholinergic and sympathetic stimulating effects of pancuronium. Ketamine, meperidine, and epinephrine-containing local anesthetic solutions might produce adverse responses similar to those seen with pancuronium and are best avoided.

Monoamine Oxidase Inhibitors

Patients who do not respond to antidepressants may benefit from treatment with MAOIs. MAOIs inhibit norepinephrine and serotonin breakdown, so there is more norepinephrine and serotonin available for release. The principal clinical problem associated with use of these drugs is the occurrence of significant systemic hypertension if patients ingest foods containing tyramine (cheeses, wines) or receive sympathomimetic drugs. Both tyramine and sympathomimetic drugs are potent stimuli for norepinephrine release. Orthostatic hypotension is the most common side effect observed in patients being treated with MAOIs (**Table 22-5**). The mechanism for this hypotension is unknown, but it may reflect accumulation of false neurotransmitters such as octopamine, which are less potent than norepinephrine. This mechanism may also explain the antihypertensive effects observed with long-term use of MAOIs.

As noted earlier (see "Serotonin Syndrome"), adverse interactions between MAOIs and other serotoninergic drugs have been observed. In the anesthetic environment, the interaction with the opioid meperidine has been the most notable.

Management of Anesthesia Anesthesia can be safely conducted in patients being treated with MAOIs despite earlier recommendations that these drugs be discontinued 14 days prior to elective operations to permit time for regeneration of new enzyme. Proceeding with anesthesia and surgery in patients being treated with MAOIs influences the selection and doses of drugs to be administered. Benzodiazepines are

TABLE 22-5 Side Effects of Monoamine Oxidase Inhibitors

Sedation
Blurred vision
Orthostatic hypotension
Tyramine-induced hypertensive crisis
Excessive effects of sympathomimetic drugs
Potential for serotonin syndrome

acceptable for pharmacologic treatment of preoperative anxiety. Induction of anesthesia can be safely accomplished with most intravenous induction agents, keeping in mind that central nervous system effects and depression of ventilation may be exaggerated. Ketamine, a sympathetic stimulant, should be avoided. Serum cholinesterase activity may decrease in patients treated with phenelzine, so the dose of succinylcholine may need to be reduced. Nitrous oxide combined with a volatile anesthetic is acceptable for maintenance of anesthesia. Anesthetic requirements may be increased due to increased concentrations of norepinephrine in the central nervous system. Fentanyl has been administered intraoperatively to patients being treated with MAOIs without apparent adverse effects. The choice of nondepolarizing muscle relaxants is not influenced by treatment with MAOIs, with the possible exception of pancuronium. Spinal or epidural anesthesia is acceptable, although the potential of these anesthetic techniques to produce hypotension and the consequent need for vasopressors may mitigate in favor of general anesthesia. The addition of epinephrine to local anesthetic solutions should probably be avoided.

During anesthesia and surgery, it is important to avoid stimulating the sympathetic nervous system as, for example, by light anesthesia, topical cocaine spray, or injection of indirect-acting vasopressors to decrease the incidence of systemic hypertension. If hypotension occurs and vasopressors are needed, direct-acting drugs such as phenylephrine are recommended. The dose should probably be decreased to minimize the likelihood of an exaggerated hypertensive response.

Postoperative Care Provision of analgesia during the postoperative period is influenced by the potential adverse interactions between opioids, especially meperidine and MAOIs, resulting in severe serotonin syndrome (see Table 22-3). If opioids are needed for postoperative pain management, morphine is a preferred drug. Alternatives to opioid analgesia such as nonopioid analgesics, nonsteroidal anti-inflammatory drugs, and peripheral nerve blocks should be considered. Neuraxial opioids provide effective analgesia, but experience is too limited to permit recommendations regarding use of this approach in patients being treated with MAOIs.

Electroconvulsive Therapy

Despite many decades of use, the exact mechanism of the therapeutic effect of ECT remains unknown. Alterations in neurophysiologic, neuroendocrinologic, and neurochemical systems are thought to be involved but have not been clearly elucidated. What is clear is that electrically induced seizures of at least 25-second duration are necessary for a therapeutic effect. ECT is indicated for treating severe depression in patients who are unresponsive to drug therapy or who are suicidal. The electrical current may be administered to both hemispheres or only to the nondominant hemisphere, which may reduce memory impairment. The electrical stimulus produces a grand mal seizure consisting of a brief tonic phase followed by a more prolonged clonic phase.

TABLE 22-6	Side Effects of Electroconvulsive Therapy

Parasympathetic nervous system stimulation
    Bradycardia
    Hypotension
Sympathetic nervous system stimulation
    Tachycardia
    Hypertension
Dysrhythmias
Increased cerebral blood flow
Increased intracranial pressure
Increased intraocular pressure
Increased intragastric pressure

The electroencephalogram shows changes similar to those present during spontaneous grand mal seizures. Typically, patients undergo six to 12 "induction" treatments during hospitalization and then may continue weekly, biweekly, or monthly "maintenance" therapy. More than two thirds of ECT patients show significant improvement in their depressive symptoms.

In addition to the seizure and its neuropsychiatric effects, ECT produces significant cardiovascular and central nervous system effects (**Table 22-6**). The typical cardiovascular response to the ECT stimulus consists of 10 to 15 seconds of parasympathetic stimulation producing bradycardia, with a reduction in blood pressure followed by sympathetic nervous system activation, resulting in tachycardia and hypertension lasting several minutes. These changes may be undesirable in patients with ischemic heart disease. Indeed, the most common causes of death associated with ECT are myocardial infarction and cardiac dysrhythmias, although overall mortality rates are low, approximately 1 in 5000 treatments. Transient myocardial ischemia, however, is not an uncommon event. Other cardiovascular changes in response to ECT include decreased venous return caused by the increased intrathoracic pressure that accompanies the seizure and/or positive-pressure ventilation and ventricular premature beats that presumably reflect excess sympathetic nervous system activity. Patients with acute coronary syndromes, decompensated congestive heart failure, significant dysrhythmias, and severe valvular heart disease require cardiologic consultation prior to initiation of ECT.

Cerebrovascular responses to ECT include marked increases in cerebral blood flow (up to sevenfold) and blood flow velocity (more than double) compared to pretreatment values. Cerebral oxygen consumption increases as well. The rapid increase in systemic blood pressure may transiently overwhelm cerebral autoregulation and may result in a dramatic increase in intracranial pressure. Thus, the use of ECT is prohibited in patients with known space-occupying lesions or head injury. The cerebral hemodynamic changes are also associated with increased wall stress on cerebral aneurysms and intracranial aneurysm disease is another contraindication to ECT.

Increased intraocular pressure is an inevitable side effect of electrically induced seizures. Increased intragastric pressure also occurs during seizure activity. Transient apnea, postictal confusion or agitation, nausea and vomiting, and headache may follow the seizure. The most common long-term effect of ECT is memory impairment.

Management of Anesthesia Anesthesia for ECT must be brief, provide the ability to monitor and limit the physiologic effects of the seizure, and minimize any interference with seizure activity or duration. Patients are fasted. Administration of glycopyrrolate intravenously 1 to 2 minutes before induction of anesthesia and delivery of the electrical current may be useful in decreasing excess salivation and bradycardia. The magnitude of treatment-induced hypertension can be ameliorated by the use of nitroglycerin intravenously, sublingually, or transcutaneously. Likewise, esmolol 1 mg/kg IV administered just prior to induction of anesthesia can attenuate the tachycardia and hypertension associated with ECT, and it does so better than labetalol. Many other drugs including calcium channel blockers, ganglionic blockers, α_2-agonists and antagonists, and direct-acting vasodilators have been used to treat the sympathetic overactivity during ECT, but they do not appear to offer any specific advantages over esmolol or nitroglycerin therapy.

Methohexital (0.5–1.0 mg/kg IV) is the standard drug used for induction of anesthesia for ECT. It has a rapid onset and rapid recovery, short duration of action, and minimal anticonvulsant effects. Thiopental offers no advantage over methohexital and may be associated with longer recovery times. Propofol is an alternative to methohexital and is associated with a lower blood pressure and heart rate response to ECT. Recovery time is similar following administration of methohexital or propofol, but the anticonvulsant effect of propofol can be manifested by shortened seizure duration.

Intravenous injection of succinylcholine promptly after induction is intended to attenuate the potentially dangerous skeletal muscle contractions and bone fractures that can result from seizure activity. Doses of 0.3 to 0.5 mg/kg IV are sufficient to attenuate skeletal muscle contractions and still permit visual confirmation of seizure activity. The most reliable method to confirm electrically induced seizure activity is the electroencephalogram. Alternatively, tonic and clonic movements in an extremity that has been isolated from the circulation by applying a tourniquet before administration of succinylcholine are evidence that a seizure has occurred. Succinylcholine-induced myalgias are remarkably uncommon, occurring in approximately 2% of patients undergoing ECT. There is no evidence that succinylcholine-induced release of potassium is increased by ECT. Ventilatory support and oxygen supplementation are continued as necessary until there is complete recovery to pretreatment cardiopulmonary status. Because repeated anesthesia is necessary, it is possible to establish the dose of the anesthetic induction drug and succinylcholine that produces the most predictable and desirable effects in each patient.

Occasionally, ECT is necessary in a patient with a permanent cardiac pacemaker or cardioverter/defibrillator. Fortunately, most of these devices are shielded and are not adversely affected by the electrical currents necessary to produce seizures, but it is prudent to have an external magnet available to ensure the capability of converting pacemakers to asynchronous modes should malfunction occur in response to the externally delivered electrical current or myopotentials from the succinylcholine or the seizure. Monitoring the ECG, the plethysmographic waveform of the pulse oximeter, and palpation of peripheral arterial pulses documents the uninterrupted function of cardiac pacemakers. Implantable cardioverters/defibrillators should be turned off prior to ECT and reactivated when the treatment is finished.

Safe and successful use of ECT has been described in patients following cardiac transplantation. In such patients, the lack of vagal innervation to the heart eliminates the risk of bradydysrhythmias. However, the sympathetic responses still occur.

BIPOLAR DISORDER

Bipolar disorder, previously called manic-depressive disorder, is, characterized by marked mood swings from depressive episodes to manic episodes with normal behavior often seen in between these episodes. Eight percent to 10% of patients with bipolar disorder commit suicide. The manic phase of bipolar disorder is manifested clinically by sustained periods of expansive euphoric mood in which the patient is subject to grandiose ideas and plans. The mood disturbance is sufficiently severe to cause marked impairment in occupational functioning and in social activities and relationships so there is risk of harm to self and others. Irritability and hyperactivity are also present, and, in severe cases, psychotic delusions and hallucinations may appear (**Table 22-7**).

The genetic pattern in bipolar disorder suggests autosomal dominance with variable penetrance. Presumably, there are abnormalities in neuroendocrine pathways that result in aberrant regulation of one or more amine neurotransmitter systems. Thus, the pathophysiology of bipolar disorder, to the extent that it is known, is similar to that of major depressive illness. The evaluation of mania must exclude the effects of substance abuse drugs, medications, and concomitant medical conditions.

TABLE 22-7 Manifestations of Mania
Expansive, euphoric mood
Inflated self-esteem
Decreased need for sleep
Flight of ideas
More talkative than usual
Distractibility
Psychomotor agitation

Treatment

Mania necessitates prompt treatment, usually in a hospital setting to protect patients from potential harmful actions. Lithium remains a mainstay of treatment, but antiepileptic drugs such as carbamazepine and valproate are often used. Olanzapine is another treatment option. When manic symptoms are severe, lithium may be administered in combination with an antipsychotic drug until the acute symptoms abate.

Lithium

Lithium is an alkali metal, a monovalent cation, and is minimally protein bound. It does not undergo biotransformation and is renally excreted. Lithium is efficiently absorbed after oral administration. Its therapeutic serum concentration for acute mania is 0.8 to 1.2 mEq/L and for prophylaxis approximately 0.4 mEq/L. Because of its narrow therapeutic index, monitoring serum lithium concentration is necessary to prevent toxicity. The therapeutic effects of lithium are most likely related to actions on second messenger systems based on phosphatidylinositol turnover. Lithium also affects transmembrane ion pumps and has inhibitory effects on adenylate cyclase.

Common side effects of lithium therapy include cognitive dysfunction, weight gain, and tremor. Lithium inhibits release of thyroid hormone and results in hypothyroidism in approximately 5% of patients. Long-term administration of lithium may also result in polyuria due to a form of vasopressin-resistant diabetes insipidus. Cardiac problems may include sinus bradycardia, sinus node dysfunction, atrioventricular block, T-wave changes, and ventricular irritability. Leukocytosis in the range of 10,000 to 14,000 cells/mm^3 is common.

Toxicity occurs when the serum lithium concentration exceeds 2 mEq/L, with signs of skeletal muscle weakness, ataxia, sedation, and widening of the QRS complex. Atrioventricular heart block, hypotension, and seizures may accompany severe lithium toxicity. Hemodialysis may be necessary in this medical emergency.

Lithium is excreted entirely by the kidneys. Reabsorption of lithium occurs in the proximal tubule in exchange for sodium. Diuretic use can affect the serum lithium concentration. Thiazide diuretics trigger an increase in lithium reabsorption in the proximal tubule, whereas loop diuretics do not promote lithium reabsorption. Administration of sodium-containing solutions or osmotic diuretics enhances renal excretion of lithium and results in lower lithium levels. Concomitant administration of nonsteroidal anti-inflammatory drugs and/or angiotensin-converting enzyme inhibitors increases the risk of lithium toxicity.

Management of Anesthesia

Evidence of lithium toxicity is important to consider during the preoperative evaluation. Review of the most recent serum lithium concentration is necessary and inclusion of lithium in the measurements of the patient's serum electrolytes during the perioperative period is very useful. To prevent significant renal reabsorption of lithium, it is reasonable to administer sodium-containing intravenous solutions during the perioperative period. Stimulation of urine output with thiazide diuretics must be avoided. The electrocardiogram should be monitored for evidence of lithium-induced conduction problems or dysrhythmias. The association of sedation with lithium therapy suggests that anesthetic requirements may be decreased in these patients. Monitoring the effects of neuromuscular blockade is indicated because the duration of both depolarizing and nondepolarizing muscle relaxants may be prolonged in the presence of lithium.

SCHIZOPHRENIA

Schizophrenia (Greek "split mind") is the major psychotic mental disorder. It is characterized by abnormal reality testing or thought processes. The essential features of the illness include two broad categories of symptoms. Positive symptoms are those that reflect distortion or exaggeration of normal behavior and include delusions and hallucinations. Negative symptoms represent a loss or diminution in normal function and include flattened affect, apathy, social, or occupational dysfunction including withdrawal, and changes in appearance and hygiene. Subtypes of schizophrenia include the paranoid type, the disorganized type, the catatonic type, and the undifferentiated type. In some patients, the disorder is persistent, whereas in others, there are exacerbations and remissions.

Treatment

Hypotheses concerning the etiology of schizophrenia suggest that the disorder is the result of neurotransmitter dysfunction, specifically of the neurotransmitters dopamine and serotonin. Drugs that affect dopamingeric function by blocking dopamine receptors, especially D_2 and D_4 receptors, have demonstrated the ability to improve a variety of psychotic symptoms, especially positive symptoms. The older ("traditional") antipsychotic drugs have broad-spectrum dopamine receptor–blocking properties, affecting all dopamine receptor subtypes. As a result, these drugs have many motor side effects. These troubling side effects include tardive dyskinesia (choreoathetoid movements), akathisia (restlessness), acute dystonia (contraction of skeletal muscles of the neck, mouth and tongue), and parkinsonism. Some of these effects diminish over time, but some persist even after drug discontinuation. Concurrent administration of anticholinergic medication may lessen some of these motor abnormalities. Acute dystonia resolves with administration of diphenhydramine (25–50 mg IV).

Newer antipsychotic drugs, also called "atypical" antipsychotic drugs, have variable effects on dopamine receptor subtypes and on serotonin receptors, especially the 5-HT$_{2A}$ receptor. These newer drugs appear to be quite effective in relieving the negative symptoms of schizophrenia and have fewer extrapyramidal side effects than the classic drugs (Table 22-8).

For the anesthesiologist, important effects of antipsychotic medications include α-adrenergic blockade causing postural hypotension, prolongation of the QT interval potentially

TABLE 22-8 Commonly Used Antipsychotic Medications

Class	Generic Name	Trade Name	EPSEs	Special Side Effects
Traditional Drugs				
Phenothiazines	Chlorpromazine	Thorazine	Common	
	Perphenazine	Trilafon		
	Fluphenazine	Prolixin		
	Trifluoperazine	Stelazine		
	Thioridazine	Mellaril		
Butyrophenones	Haloperidol	Haldol	Common	Retinal pigmentation
Thioxanthines	Thiothixene	Navane	Common	
Atypical Drugs				
	Risperidone	Risperdal	Uncommon	
	Clozapine	Clozaril	Rare	Agranulocytosis
	Quetiapine	Seroquel	Uncommon	Cataracts
	Olanzapine	Zyprexa	Uncommon	Neutropenia
	Ziprasidone	Geodon	Uncommon	Prolonged QT interval

EPSEs, extrapyramidal side effects.

producing torsade de pointes, seizures, hepatic enzyme elevations, abnormal temperature regulation, and sedation. Drug-induced sedation may decrease anesthetic requirements.

Neuroleptic Malignant Syndrome

Neuroleptic malignant syndrome is a rare, potentially fatal complication of antipsychotic drug therapy that is presumed to reflect dopamine depletion in the central nervous system. This syndrome can occur anytime during the course of antipsychotic treatment but often is manifest during the first few weeks of treatment or following an increase in drug dose. Clinical manifestations usually develop over 24 to 72 hours and include hyperpyrexia, severe skeletal muscle rigidity, rhabdomyolysis, autonomic hyperactivity (tachycardia, hypertension, cardiac dysrhythmias), altered consciousness, and acidosis. Skeletal muscle spasm may be so severe that mechanical ventilation becomes necessary. Renal failure may occur due to myoglobinuria and dehydration.

Treatment of neuroleptic malignant syndrome requires immediate cessation of antipsychotic drug therapy and supportive therapy (ventilation, hydration, cooling). Bromocriptine (5 mg PO every 6 hours) or dantrolene (up to 6 mg/kg daily as a continuous infusion) may decrease skeletal muscle rigidity Mortality rates approach 20% in untreated patients, with death due to cardiac dysrhythmias, congestive heart failure, hypoventilation, or renal failure. Patients who have this syndrome are likely to experience a recurrence when treatment with antipsychotic drugs is resumed so a switch to a less potent antidopaminergic drug or to an atypical antipsychotic drug is usually made.

Because there are similarities between neuroleptic malignant syndrome and malignant hyperthermia, the possibility that patients with a history of neuroleptic malignant syndrome are vulnerable to developing malignant hyperthermia is an important issue to consider (see Table 22-4). At the present time, there is no evidence of a pathophysiologic link between the two syndromes, and there is no familial pattern or evidence of inheritance in neuroleptic malignant syndrome. However, until any association between neuroleptic malignant syndrome and malignant hyperthermia is clearly disproved, careful metabolic monitoring during general anesthesia is recommended. Note that succinylcholine has been used without problems for ECT in patients with a history of neuroleptic malignant syndrome.

ANXIETY DISORDERS

Anxiety disorders are associated with distressing symptoms such as nervousness, sleeplessness, hypochondriasis, and somatic complaints. It is useful clinically to consider anxiety disorders as occurring in two different patterns: (1) chronic generalized anxiety and (2) episodic, often situation-dependent, anxiety. Anxiety resulting from identifiable stresses is usually self-limited and rarely requires pharmacologic treatment. The presence of unrealistic or excessive worry and apprehension may be cause for drug therapy. Short-term and often dramatic relief is afforded by almost any benzodiazepine. Performance anxiety ("stage fright") is a type of situational anxiety that is often treated with β-blockers that do not produce sedation or allay anxiety but do eliminate the motor and autonomic manifestations of anxiety. Supplemental cognitive behavioral therapy, relaxation techniques, hypnosis, and psychotherapy are also very useful in treating anxiety disorders.

Panic disorders are qualitatively different from generalized anxiety. The patient typically experiences, *without provocation*, discrete periods of intense fear, apprehension, and a sense of impending doom. Dyspnea, tachycardia, diaphoresis, paresthesias, nausea, chest pain, and fear of dying may be present and may be confused with medical conditions such as angina pectoris and epilepsy. Several classes of medications are effective in reducing panic attacks and include SSRIs, benzodiazepines, cyclic antidepressants, and MAOIs. They have approximately comparable efficacy.

SUBSTANCE ABUSE

Substance abuse may be defined as self-administration of drugs that deviates from accepted medical or social use, which, if sustained, can lead to physical and psychological dependence. The incidence of substance abuse and drug-related deaths is high among physicians, especially during the first 5 years after medical school graduation. Dependence is diagnosed when patients manifest at least three of nine characteristic symptoms, with some of the symptoms having persisted for at least 1 month or occurred repeatedly (**Table 22-9**). Physical dependence develops when the presence of a drug in the body is necessary for normal physiologic function and prevention of withdrawal symptoms. Typically, the withdrawal syndrome consists of a rebound in the physiologic systems modified by the drug. Tolerance is a state in which tissues become accustomed to the presence of a drug such that increased doses of that drug become necessary to produce effects similar to those observed initially with smaller doses. Substance abusers can manifest cross-tolerance to drugs, making it difficult to predict analgesic or anesthetic requirements. Most often, *long-term* substance abuse results in increased analgesic and anesthetic requirements, whereas additive or even synergistic effects may occur in the presence of *acute* substance abuse. It is important to recognize the signs of drug withdrawal during the perioperative period. Certainly, acute drug withdrawal should not be attempted during the perioperative period.

Diagnosis

Substance abuse is often first suspected or recognized during the medical management of other conditions, such as

TABLE 22-9	Characteristic Symptoms of Psychoactive Drug Dependence

Drug taken in higher doses or for longer periods than intended

Unsuccessful attempts to reduce use of the drug

Increased time spent obtaining the drug

Frequent intoxication or withdrawal symptoms

Restricted social or work activities because of drug use

Continued drug use despite social or physical problems related to drug use

Evidence of tolerance to the effects of the drug

Characteristic withdrawal symptoms

Drug use to avoid withdrawal symptoms

hepatitis, acquired immune deficiency syndrome, and pregnancy. Patients almost always have a concomitant personality disorder and display antisocial traits. Sociopathic characteristics (school dropout, criminal record, multiple drug abuse) seem to predispose to, rather than result from, drug addiction. Approximately 50% of patients admitted to hospitals with factitious disorders are drug abusers, as are some chronic pain patients. Psychiatric consultation is recommended in all cases of substance abuse.

Drug overdose is the leading cause of unconsciousness observed in patients admitted to emergency departments. Often more than one class of drug as well as alcohol has been ingested. Conditions other than drug overdose may result in unconsciousness, emphasizing the importance of laboratory tests (electrolytes, blood glucose concentrations, arterial blood gases, renal and liver function tests) for confirming the diagnosis. The depth of central nervous system depression can be estimated based on the response to painful stimulation, activity of the gag reflex, presence or absence of hypotension, respiratory rate, and size and responsiveness of the pupils.

Treatment

Regardless of the drug or drugs ingested, the manifestations are similar; assessment and treatment proceed simultaneously. The first step is to secure the airway and support ventilation and circulation. Absence of a gag reflex is confirmatory evidence that protective laryngeal reflexes are dangerously depressed. In this situation, a cuffed endotracheal tube should be placed to protect the lungs from aspiration. Body temperature is monitored, as hypothermia frequently accompanies unconsciousness due to drug overdose. Decisions to attempt removal of ingested substances (gastric lavage, forced diuresis, hemodialysis) depend on the drug ingested, the time since ingestion, and the degree of central nervous system depression. Gastric lavage may be beneficial if less than 4 hours have elapsed since ingestion. Gastric lavage or pharmacologic stimulation of emesis is not recommended when the ingested substances are hydrocarbons or corrosive materials or when protective laryngeal reflexes are not intact. After gastric lavage or emesis, activated charcoal can be administered to absorb any drug remaining in the gastrointestinal tract. Hemodialysis may be considered when potentially fatal doses of drugs have been ingested, when there is progressive deterioration of cardiovascular function, or when normal routes of metabolism and renal excretion are impaired. Treatment with hemodialysis is of little value when the ingested drugs are highly protein bound or avidly stored in tissues because of their lipid solubility.

Alcoholism

Alcoholism is defined as a primary chronic disease with genetic, psychosocial, and environmental factors that influence its development and manifestations. Alcoholism affects at least 10 million Americans and is responsible for 200,000 deaths annually. Up to one third of adult patients have medical problems related to alcohol (**Table 22-10**). The diagnosis of alcoholism requires a high index of suspicion combined with nonspecific but suggestive symptoms (gastritis, tremor, history of falling, unexplained episodes of amnesia). The possibility of alcoholism is often overlooked in the elderly.

Male gender and family history of alcohol abuse are the two major risk factors for alcoholism. Adoption studies indicate that male children of alcoholic parents are more likely to become alcoholic, even when raised by nonalcoholic adoptive parents. Other forms of psychiatric disease such as depression or sociopathy are not increased in the children of alcoholic parents.

Although alcohol appears to produce widespread nonspecific effects on cell membranes, there is evidence that many of its neurologic effects are mediated by actions at receptors for the inhibitory neurotransmitter, γ-aminobutyric acid (GABA). When GABA binds to receptors, it causes chloride channels in the receptors to open, thereby hyperpolarizing the neurons and making the occurrence of depolarization less likely.

TABLE 22-10 Medical Problems Related to Alcoholism

Central Nervous System Effects
Psychiatric disorders (depression, antisocial behavior)
Nutritional disorders (Wernicke-Korsakoff)
Withdrawal syndrome
Cerebellar degeneration
Cerebral atrophy

Cardiovascular Effects
Cardiomyopathy
Cardiac dysrhythmias
Hypertension

Gastrointestinal and Hepatobiliary Effects
Esophagitis
Gastritis
Pancreatitis
Hepatic cirrhosis
Portal hypertension

Skin and Musculoskeletal Effects
Spider angiomata
Myopathy
Osteoporosis

Endocrine and Metabolic Effects
Decreased serum testosterone concentrations (impotence)
Decreased gluconeogenesis (hypoglycemia)
Ketoacidosis
Hypoalbuminemia
Hypomagnesemia

Hematologic Effects
Thrombocytopenia
Leukopenia
Anemia

Alcohol appears to increase GABA-mediated chloride ion conductance. A shared site of action for alcohol, benzodiazepines, and barbiturates would be consistent with the ability of these different classes of drugs to produce cross-tolerance and cross-dependence.

Treatment

Treatment of alcoholism mandates total abstinence from alcohol. Disulfiram may be administered as an adjunctive drug along with psychiatric counseling. The unpleasantness of symptoms (flushing, vertigo, diaphoresis, nausea, vomiting) that accompanies alcohol ingestion in the presence of disulfiram is intended to serve as a deterrent to the urge to drink. These symptoms reflect the accumulation of acetaldehyde from oxidation of alcohol, which cannot be further oxidized because of disulfiram-induced inhibition of aldehyde dehydrogenase activity. Compliance with long-term disulfiram therapy is often poor, and this drug has not been documented to have advantages over placebo for achieving total alcohol abstinence. Medical contraindications to disulfiram use include pregnancy, cardiac dysfunction, hepatic dysfunction, renal dysfunction, and peripheral neuropathy. Emergency treatment of an alcohol-disulfiram interaction includes intravenous infusion of crystalloids and, occasionally, transient maintenance of systemic blood pressure with vasopressors.

Overdose

The intoxicating effects of alcohol parallel its blood concentration. In patients who are not alcoholics, blood alcohol levels of 25 mg/dL are associated with impaired cognition and coordination. At blood alcohol concentrations higher than 100 mg/dL, signs of vestibular and cerebellar dysfunction (nystagmus, dysarthria, ataxia) increase. Autonomic nervous system dysfunction may result in hypotension, hypothermia, stupor, and, ultimately, coma. Intoxication with alcohol is often defined as a blood alcohol concentrations greater than 80 to 100 mg/dL, and levels above 500 mg/dL are usually fatal owing to depressed ventilation. Chronic tolerance from prolonged excessive alcohol ingestion may cause alcoholic patients to remain sober despite potentially fatal blood alcohol concentrations. The critical aspect of treating life-threatening alcohol overdose is maintenance of ventilation. Hypoglycemia may be profound if excessive alcohol consumption is associated with food deprivation. It must be appreciated that other central nervous system depressant drugs are often ingested simultaneously with alcohol.

Withdrawal Syndrome

Physiologic dependence on alcohol manifests as a withdrawal syndrome when the drug is discontinued or when there is decreased intake.

Early Manifestations The earliest and most common withdrawal syndrome is characterized by generalized tremors that may be accompanied by perceptual disturbances (nightmares, hallucinations), autonomic nervous system hyperactivity (tachycardia, hypertension, cardiac dysrhythmias), nausea, vomiting, insomnia, and mild confusional states with agitation. These symptoms usually begin within 6 to 8 hours after a substantial decrease in blood alcohol concentration and are typically most pronounced at 24 to 36 hours. These withdrawal symptoms can be suppressed by the resumption of alcohol ingestion or by administration of benzodiazepines, β-antagonists or α$_2$-agonists. In clinical situations, diazepam is usually administered to produce sedation; a β-antagonist is added if tachycardia is present. The ability of sympatholytic drugs to attenuate these symptoms suggests a role for autonomic nervous system hyperactivity in the etiology of alcohol withdrawal syndrome.

Delirium Tremens

Approximately 5% of patients experiencing alcohol withdrawal syndrome exhibit delirium tremens, a life-threatening medical emergency. Delirium tremens occurs 2 to 4 days after the cessation of alcohol ingestion, manifesting as hallucinations, combativeness, hyperthermia, tachycardia, hypertension or hypotension, and grand mal seizures.

Treatment of delirium tremens must be aggressive, with administration of diazepam (5–10 mg IV every 5 minutes) until the patient becomes sedated but remains awake. Administration of β-adrenergic antagonists such as propranolol and esmolol is useful to suppress manifestations of sympathetic nervous system hyperactivity. The goal of β-antagonist therapy is to decrease the heart rate to less than 100 bpm. Protection of the airway with a cuffed endotracheal tube is necessary in some patients. Correction of fluid, electrolyte (magnesium, potassium), and metabolic (thiamine) derangements is important. Lidocaine is usually effective when cardiac dysrhythmias occur despite correction of electrolyte abnormalities. Physical restraint may be necessary to decrease the risk of self-injury or injury to others. Despite aggressive treatment, mortality from delirium tremens is approximately 10%, principally due to hypotension, cardiac dysrhythmias, or seizures.

Wernicke-Korsakoff Syndrome

Wernicke-Korsakoff syndrome reflects a loss of neurons in the cerebellum (Wernicke's encephalopathy) and a loss of memory (Korsakoff's psychosis) due to the lack of thiamine (vitamin B$_1$), which is required for the intermediary metabolism of carbohydrates. This syndrome is not an alcohol withdrawal syndrome, but its occurrence establishes that a patient is, or has been, physically dependent on alcohol. In addition to ataxia and memory loss, many of the patients exhibit global confusion states, drowsiness, nystagmus, and orthostatic hypotension. An associated peripheral polyneuropathy is almost always present.

Treatment of Wernicke-Korsakoff syndrome consists of intravenous administration of thiamine, with normal dietary intake when possible. Because carbohydrate loads may precipitate this syndrome in thiamine-depleted patients, it may be useful to administer thiamine before initiation of glucose infusions to malnourished or alcoholic patients.

Alcohol and Pregnancy

Alcohol crosses the placenta and may result in decreased birth weight. High blood concentrations of alcohol (>150 mg/dL) may result in the fetal alcohol syndrome, characterized by craniofacial dysmorphology, growth retardation, and mental retardation. There is an increased incidence of cardiac malformations, including patent ductus arteriosus and septal defects.

Management of Anesthesia

Management of anesthesia in patients being treated with disulfiram should consider the potential presence of disulfiram-induced sedation and hepatotoxicity. Decreased drug requirements could reflect additive effects from co-existing sedation or the ability of disulfiram to inhibit metabolism of drugs other than alcohol. For example, disulfiram may potentiate the effects of benzodiazepines. Acute, unexplained hypotension during general anesthesia could reflect inadequate stores of norepinephrine due to disulfiram-induced inhibition of dopamine β-hydroxylase. This hypotension may respond to ephedrine, but direct-acting sympathomimetics such as phenylephrine may produce a more predictable response in the presence of norepinephrine depletion. Use of regional anesthesia may be influenced by the presence of disulfiram-induced polyneuropathy. Alcohol-containing solutions, as used for skin cleansing, probably should be avoided in disulfiram-treated patients.

Cocaine

Cocaine use for nonmedical purposes is a public health problem with important economic and social consequences. Myths associated with cocaine abuse are that it is sexually stimulating, nonaddictive, and physiologically benign. In fact, cocaine is highly addictive; casual use is not possible once addiction occurs, and life-threatening side effects accompany cocaine use. Cocaine produces sympathetic nervous system stimulation by blocking the presynaptic uptake of norepinephrine and dopamine, thereby increasing the postsynaptic concentrations of these neurotransmitters. Because of this blocking effect, dopamine is present in high concentrations in synapses, producing the characteristic "cocaine high."

Side Effects

Acute cocaine administration is known to cause coronary vasospasm, myocardial ischemia, myocardial infarction, and ventricular cardiac dysrhythmias, including ventricular fibrillation. Associated systemic hypertension and tachycardia further increase myocardial oxygen requirements at a time when coronary oxygen delivery is decreased by the effects of cocaine on coronary blood flow. Cocaine use can cause myocardial ischemia and hypotension that lasts as long as 6 weeks after discontinuing cocaine use. Excessive sensitivity of the coronary vasculature to catecholamines after long-term exposure to cocaine may be due in part to cocaine-induced depletion of dopamine stores. Lung damage and pulmonary edema have been observed in patients who smoke cocaine.

Cocaine-abusing parturients are at higher risk of spontaneous abortion, abruptio placenta, and fetal malformations. Cocaine causes a dose-dependent decrease in uterine blood flow and may produce hyperpyrexia, which can contribute to seizures. There is a temporal relationship between the recreational use of cocaine and cerebrovascular accidents. Long-term cocaine abuse is associated with nasal septal atrophy, agitated behavior, paranoid thinking, and heightened reflexes. Symptoms associated with cocaine withdrawal include fatigue, depression, and increased appetite. Death due to cocaine use has occurred with all routes of administration (intranasal, oral, intravenous, inhalation) and is usually due to apnea, seizures, or cardiac dysrhythmias. Persons with decreased plasma cholinesterase activity (elderly patients, parturients, those with severe liver disease) may be at risk of sudden death when using cocaine because this enzyme is essential for metabolizing the drug.

Cocaine overdose evokes overwhelming sympathetic nervous system stimulation of the cardiovascular system. Uncontrolled hypertension may result in pulmonary and cerebral edema, whereas the effects of increased circulating catecholamine concentrations may include coronary artery vasoconstriction, coronary vasospasm, and platelet aggregation.

Treatment

Treatment of cocaine overdose includes administration of nitroglycerin to manage myocardial ischemia. Although esmolol has been recommended for treating tachycardia due to cocaine overdose, there is evidence that β-adrenergic blockade accentuates cocaine-induced coronary artery vasospasm. α-Adrenergic blockade may be effective in the treatment of coronary vasoconstriction due to cocaine. Administration of intravenous benzodiazepines such as diazepam is effective in controlling seizures associated with cocaine toxicity. Active cooling may be necessary if hyperthermia accompanies cocaine overdose.

Management of Anesthesia

Management of anesthesia in patients acutely intoxicated with cocaine must consider the vulnerability of these patients to myocardial ischemia and cardiac dysrhythmias. Any event or drug likely to increase already enhanced sympathetic nervous system activity must be carefully considered before its selection. It seems prudent to have nitroglycerin readily available to treat signs of myocardial ischemia associated with tachycardia or hypertension. Unexpected agitation during the perioperative period may reflect the effects of cocaine ingestion. Increased anesthetic requirements may be present in acutely intoxicated patients, presumably reflecting increased concentrations of catecholamines in the central nervous system. Thrombocytopenia associated with cocaine abuse may influence the selection of regional anesthesia.

In the absence of acute intoxication, long-term abuse of cocaine has not been shown to be predictably associated with adverse anesthetic interactions, although the possibility of cardiac dysrhythmias remains a constant concern. The rapid metabolism of cocaine probably decreases the likelihood that an acutely intoxicated patient will present to the operating room.

Administration of topical cocaine plus epinephrine for medically indicated purposes followed by administration of a volatile anesthetic that sensitizes the myocardium may exaggerate the cardiac-stimulating effects of cocaine. Cocaine use for medically indicated purposes should be avoided in patients with hypertension or coronary artery disease and in patients receiving drugs that potentiate the effects of catecholamines such as MAOIs.

Opioids

Contrary to common speculation, opioid dependence rarely develops from the use of these drugs to treat acute postoperative pain. It is possible to become addicted to opioids in less than 14 days, however, if the drug is administered daily in ever-increasing doses. Opioids are abused orally, subcutaneously, or intravenously for their euphoric and analgesic effects. Numerous medical problems are encountered in opioid addicts, especially intravenous abusers (**Table 22-11**). Evidence of the presence of these medical problems in opioid addicts should be sought during the preoperative evaluation. Tolerance may develop to some of the effects of opioids (analgesia, sedation, emesis, euphoria, hypoventilation) but not to others (miosis, constipation). Fortunately, as tolerance increases, so does the lethal dose of the opioid. In general, there is a high degree of cross-tolerance among drugs with morphine-like actions, although tolerance wanes rapidly when opioids are withdrawn from addicts.

Overdose

The most obvious manifestation of opioid overdose (usually heroin) is a slow breathing rate with a normal to increased tidal volume. Pupils are usually miotic, although mydriasis may occur if hypoventilation results in severe hypoxemia. Central nervous system manifestations range from dysphoria to unconsciousness; seizures are unlikely. Pulmonary edema occurs in a large proportion of patients with heroin

TABLE 22-11 Medical Problems Associated with Chronic Opioid Abuse
Hepatitis
Cellulitis
Superficial skin abscesses
Septic thrombophlebitis
Endocarditis
Systemic septic emboli
Acquired immunodeficiency syndrome
Aspiration pneumonitis
Malnutrition
Tetanus
Transverse myelitis

overdose. The etiology of pulmonary edema is poorly understood, but hypoxemia, hypotension, neurogenic mechanisms, and drug-related pulmonary endothelial damage are considerations. Gastric atony is a predictable accompaniment of acute opioid overdose. Fatal opioid overdose is most often an outcome of fluctuations in the purity of street products or the combination of opioids with other central nervous system depressants. Naloxone is the specific opioid antagonist administered to maintain an acceptable respiratory rate, usually more than 12 breaths per minute.

Withdrawal Syndrome

Although withdrawal from opioids is rarely life threatening, it is unpleasant and may complicate management during the perioperative period. In this regard, it is useful to consider the time to onset, peak intensity, and duration of withdrawal after abrupt withdrawal of opioids (**Table 22-12**). Opioid withdrawal symptoms develop within seconds after intravenous administration of naloxone. Conversely, it is usually possible to abort the withdrawal syndrome by reinstituting administration of the abused opioid or by substituting methadone (2.5 mg equivalent to 10 mg of morphine). Clonidine may also attenuate opioid withdrawal symptoms presumably by replacing opioid-mediated inhibition with α_2-agonist-mediated inhibition of the sympathetic nervous system in the brain.

Opioid withdrawal symptoms often include manifestations of excess sympathetic nervous system activity (diaphoresis, mydriasis, hypertension, tachycardia). Craving for the drug and anxiety are followed by yawning, lacrimation, rhinorrhea, piloerection (origin of the term "cold turkey"), tremors, skeletal muscle and bone discomfort, and anorexia. Insomnia, abdominal cramps, diarrhea, and hyperthermia may develop. Skeletal muscle spasms and jerking of the legs (origin of the term "kicking the habit") follow, and cardiovascular collapse is possible. Seizures are rare, and their occurrence should raise suspicion about other etiologies of seizures, such as unrecognized barbiturate withdrawal or underlying epilepsy.

Rapid Opioid Detoxification

Rapid opioid detoxification using high doses of an opioid antagonist (nalmefene) administered during general anesthesia followed by naltrexone maintenance has been proposed as a cost-effective alternative to conventional detoxification approaches. There is evidence that opioid withdrawal, primarily involving the nucleus locus ceruleus, peaks and then recovers to near baseline within 4 to 6 hours after administering high doses of opioid antagonists. Subsequent administration of naloxone to patients who have undergone rapid detoxification under general anesthesia should produce no evidence of opioid withdrawal, confirming rapid achievement of opioid detoxification. In contrast to conventional detoxification achieved by gradual tapering of opioid doses, the unpleasant aspects of opioid withdrawal are passed through in a few hours, during which time a patient is anesthetized. This contributes to an increased success rate.

Profound increases in serum catecholamine concentrations during anesthesia-assisted opioid detoxification have been described manifesting as changes in systolic blood pressure or tachycardia. Previous administration of clonidine may blunt these changes. During anesthesia, manifestations of sympathetic nervous system hyperactivity may be treated with pharmacologic interventions such as administration of β-adrenergic antagonists. Deep general anesthesia with skeletal muscle paralysis and controlled ventilation are recommended. Although general anesthesia seems to be safely tolerated during rapid opioid detoxification, there is some concern regarding the occurrence of cardiac dysrhythmias (prolonged QT interval) and postoperative mortality. Naltrexone is often administered in the postanesthesia care unit, with adjunct medications, such as midazolam, ketorolac, and clonidine being administered as needed. The occurrence of mild to moderate withdrawal symptoms for 3 to 4 days after rapid opioid detoxification is expected.

Management of Anesthesia

Opioid addicts should have opioids or methadone maintained during the perioperative period. Preoperative medication may also include an opioid. Opioid agonist-antagonist drugs are not recommended because these drugs can precipitate acute withdrawal reactions. There is no advantage in trying to maintain anesthesia with opioids, as doses greatly in excess of normal are likely to be required. Furthermore, chronic opioid use leads to cross-tolerance to other central nervous system depressants. This may manifest as a decreased analgesic response to inhaled anesthetics such as nitrous oxide. Conversely, acute opioid administration decreases anesthetic requirements. Maintenance of anesthesia is most often with volatile anesthetics, remembering that these patients are likely to have underlying liver disease. There is a tendency for perioperative hypotension to occur, which may reflect inadequate intravascular fluid volume secondary to chronic infection, fever, malnutrition, adrenocortical insufficiency, or an inadequate opioid concentration in the brain.

Management of anesthesia for rehabilitated opioid addicts and patients on antagonist therapy often includes a volatile

TABLE 22-12	Time Course of Opioid Withdrawal Syndrome		
Drug	Onset	Peak Intensity	Duration
Meperidine	2–6 hours	8–12 hours	4–5 days
Dihydromorphine	6–18 hours	36–72 hours	7–10 days
Codeine	24–48 hours	3–21 days	6–7 weeks
Morphine			
Heroin			
Methadone			

anesthetic. Regional anesthesia may have a role in some patients, but it is important to remember the tendency for hypotension to occur, the increased incidence of positive serology, the occasional presence of peripheral neuritis, and the rare occurrence of transverse myelitis.

Opioid addicts often seem to experience exaggerated degrees of postoperative pain. For reasons that are not clear, satisfactory postoperative analgesia may be achieved when average doses of meperidine are administered in addition to the usual daily maintenance dose of methadone or other opioids. Methadone has minimal analgesic activity with respect to management of postoperative pain. Levomethadyl, like methadone, is a μ-opioid agonist that has a long half-life owing to its active metabolites. The advantage of levomethadyl over methadone is the option for less than daily dosing. Alternative methods of postoperative pain relief include continuous regional anesthesia with local anesthetics, neuraxial opioids, and transcutaneous electrical nerve stimulation.

Barbiturates

Long-term barbiturate abuse is not associated with major pathophysiologic changes. These drugs are most commonly abused orally for their euphoric effects to counter insomnia and to antagonize the stimulant effects of other drugs. There is tolerance to most of the actions of these drugs and cross-tolerance to other central nervous system depressants. Although the barbiturate doses required to produce sedative or euphoric effects increase rapidly, lethal doses do not increase at the same rate or to the same magnitude. Thus, a barbiturate abuser's margin of error, in contrast to that of opioid addicts, decreases as barbiturate doses are increased to achieve the desired effect.

Overdose

Central nervous system depression is the principal manifestation of barbiturate overdose. Barbiturate blood levels correspond with the degree of central nervous system depression (slurred speech, ataxia, irritability), with excessively high blood levels resulting in loss of pharyngeal and deep tendon reflexes and with the onset of coma. No specific pharmacologic antagonist exists to reverse barbiturate-induced central nervous system depression and the use of nonspecific stimulants is not encouraged. Depression of ventilation may be profound. As with opioid overdoses, maintenance of a patent airway, protection from aspiration, and support of ventilation using a cuffed endotracheal tube may be necessary. Barbiturate overdoses may be associated with hypotension due to central vasomotor depression, direct myocardial depression, and increased venous capacitance. This hypotension usually responds to fluid infusion, although occasionally vasopressors or inotropic drugs are required. Hypothermia is frequent and may necessitate aggressive attempts to restore normothermia. Acute renal failure due to hypotension and rhabdomyolysis may occur. Forced diuresis and alkalinization of the urine promote elimination of phenobarbital but are of lesser value with many of the other barbiturates.

TABLE 22-13 Time Course of Barbiturate Withdrawal Syndrome

Drug	Onset (hr)	Peak Intensity (days)	Duration (days)
Pentobarbital	12–24	2–3	7–10
Secobarbital	12–24	2–3	7–10
Phenobarbital	48–72	6–10	10+

Induced emesis or gastric lavage followed by administration of activated charcoal may be helpful in awake patients who ingested barbiturates less than 6 hours previously.

Withdrawal Syndrome

In contrast to opioid withdrawal, the abrupt cessation of excessive barbiturate ingestion is associated with potentially life-threatening responses. The time of onset, peak intensity, and duration of withdrawal symptoms for barbiturates are delayed compared to opioids (**Table 22-13**). Barbiturate withdrawal symptoms manifest initially as anxiety, skeletal muscle tremors, hyperreflexia, diaphoresis, tachycardia, and orthostatic hypotension. Cardiovascular collapse and hyperthermia may occur. The most serious problem associated with barbiturate withdrawal is the occurrence of grand mal seizures. Seizures are likely to be caused by an abrupt decrease in the circulating concentration of drug. Many of the manifestations of barbiturate withdrawal, particularly seizures, are difficult to abort once they develop.

Pentobarbital may be administered if evidence of barbiturate withdrawal manifests. Typically, the initial oral dose is 200 to 400 mg, with subsequent doses titrated to effect, since tolerance may disappear rapidly in these patients. Phenobarbital and diazepam may also be useful for suppressing evidence of barbiturate withdrawal.

Management of Anesthesia

Although there are few data concerning management of anesthesia in chronic barbiturate abusers, it is predictable that cross-tolerance to the depressant effects of anesthetic drugs occurs. For example, mice tolerant to thiopental awaken at higher barbiturate tissue concentrations than do control animals. Similarly, anecdotal reports describe the need for increased barbiturate doses for induction of anesthesia in chronic barbiturate abusers. Although acute administration of barbiturates has been shown to decrease anesthetic requirements, there are no reports of increased anesthetic requirements (MAC) in chronic barbiturate abusers. Long-term barbiturate abuse leads to induction of hepatic microsomal enzymes, introducing the potential for drug interactions with concomitantly administered medications (warfarin, digitalis, phenytoin, volatile anesthetics). Venous access is a likely problem in intravenous barbiturate abusers, as the alkalinity of the self-injected solutions is likely to sclerose veins.

Substance Abuse as an Occupational Hazard in Anesthesiology

Anesthesiologists represent 3.6% of all physicians in the United States. However, they are overrepresented in addictive treatment programs at a rate approximately three times higher than any other physician group. In addition, anesthesiologists are at highest risk of relapse of all physician specialties. At the present time, 12% to 15% of all physicians in treatment are anesthesiologists. The encouraging news is that, in a survey (1994–1995), it was revealed that the apparent incidence of substance abuse among anesthesiology residents was 0.40% with a faculty incidence of 0.1%. This represents a decline in incidence since 1986.

Why Anesthesiologists?

Numerous factors have been proposed to explain the high incidence of substance abuse among anesthesiologists. These include the following:

- Easy access to potent drugs, particularly opioids
- The highly addictive potential of accessible drugs, particularly fentanyl and sufentanil
- Diversion of these agents is relatively simple since only small doses will initially provide the effect desired by the abuser
- Curiosity about patients' experiences with these substances
- Control-oriented personality

Characteristics/Demographics of the Addicted Anesthesiologist

The curriculum on drug abuse and addiction compiled by the American Society of Anesthesiologists Committee on Occupational Health is a highly recommended in-depth source of information on this important topic. This curriculum revealed the following characteristics associated with addiction among anesthesiologists:

- Fifty percent are younger than 35 years old, but this may reflect the age distribution within the specialty.
- Residents are overrepresented. It may be that, due to the increased awareness of the high risk of substance abuse among anesthesiologists, training programs are looking more carefully for signs of addiction in this group. (Interestingly, a higher proportion of anesthesiology residents who are addicted are members of the Alpha Omega Alpha Honor Society.)
- Sixty-seven percent to 88% are male, and 75% to 96% are white.
- Seventy-six percent to 90% use opiates as the drug of choice.
- Thirty-three percent to 50% are polydrug users.
- Thirty-three percent have a family history of addictive disease, most frequently, alcohol.
- Sixty-five percent of anesthesiologists with a documented history of addiction are associated with academic departments.

Most Frequently Abused Drugs

Traditionally, opioids are the drugs selected for abuse by anesthesiologists. Fentanyl and sufentanil are the most commonly abused drugs, followed by meperidine and morphine. This choice is particularly evident in anesthesiologists younger than 35 years of age. Alcohol is seen as an abuse substance primarily in older anesthesiologists because the time to produce impairment is significantly longer than that observed with opiate addiction. The data also suggest that opiates are the substance of choice for abuse early in an anesthesiologist's career, while alcohol abuse is more frequently detected in anesthesia practitioners who have been out of residency for more than 5 years.

Other agents that have been abused include cocaine, benzodiazepines (midazolam), and, more recently, propofol. Over the past 5 years, there has been a major switch to "needleless" approaches for delivery of commonly abused agents. This approach provides a cleaner alternative to the more traditional intravenous or intramuscular routes. Every possible route of administration has been tried and reported including unusual intravenous sites (hidden veins in the feet, groin, thigh, and penis), oral/nasal administration (benzodiazepines), sublingual, and rectal routes. Volatile anesthetics are now entering the abuse arena as well. Sevoflurane has been reported as the drug of choice among inhalational agents. Regardless of the primary agent of abuse, after 6 months, there is an increasing incidence of polydrug abuse.

Methods of Obtaining Drugs for Abuse

Anesthesiologists have developed numerous and often creative methods for obtaining drugs for abuse. The most frequently employed methods are falsely recording drug administration, improper recording on the anesthesia record, and keeping rather than wasting leftover drugs. In addition, recent reports have highlighted a new practice involving secretly accessing multidose vials and then refilling and resealing them with other substances. It is important to be wary of the faculty member or resident who is too anxious to give breaks or volunteers to do late cases. One of the most frequently reported retrospective markers of addictive behavior was the desire to work overtime, particularly during periods when supervision may be reduced such as evenings and weekends.

Signs and Symptoms of Addictive Behavior

Regardless of which drugs are abused, any unusual and persistent changes in behavior should be cause for alarm. Classically, these behaviors include wide mood swings, such as periods of depression, anger, and irritability alternating with periods of euphoria. Key points to remember about addictive behavior include the following:

- Denial is universal.
- Symptoms at work are the last to appear (symptoms appear first in the community and then at home).
- The pathognomonic sign is self-administration of drugs.
- Detected addicts are often found comatose.

547

- Untreated addicts are often found dead!

The following is a list of the most frequently overlooked symptoms of addictive behavior.

- The desire to work alone
- Refusing lunch relief or breaks
- Frequently relieving others
- Volunteering for extra cases or call
- Patient pain needs in the postanesthetic care unit are out of proportion to the narcotics recorded as given
- Weight loss
- Frequent bathroom breaks

Associated Risks of Physician Drug Addiction

Although traditionally risk is primarily assigned to the individual physician, there are also significant risks to patients and potential risks for the hospital staff and administration when a physician becomes addicted.

Physician The principal risks to the anesthesia provider with addictive disease include increased risk of suicide by drug overdose and drug-related death. Unfortunately, the relapse rate for anesthesiologists is the highest of all physicians with a history of narcotic addiction. This risk of relapse is greatest in the first 5 years and decreases as time in recovery increases. The positive news is that 89% of anesthesiologists who complete treatment and commit to aftercare remain abstinent for more than 2 years. However, death is the primary presenting sign of relapse in opiate-addicted anesthesiologists!

Patient Patients can be affected by addictive behavior. The data show that impaired physicians (those who are actively abusing drugs) are at increased risk of malpractice suits. Data from both California and Oklahoma revealed a dramatic decrease in both the number and dollar value of claims filed following treatment for substance abuse.

Hospital/Institution Most states have laws requiring that hospital and medical staff report any suspected addictive behavior. Failure to report may have significant consequences depending on individual state statutes.

What to Do When Substance Abuse Is Suspected

This process will be significantly affected by the presence or absence of a physician assistance committee. If an institution does not have such a committee, one should be formed and policies developed so that the support needed for an impaired physician is in place when needed. The membership of this committee should include an anesthesiologist. In addition, this group should have a consulting agreement with local addiction specialists with experience in treating and referring physicians. Ideally, this treatment group would include a physician/counselor with experience and expertise in treating anesthesiologists. Finally, this committee should have a help line telephone number and a point of contact with at least one preselected addiction treatment program.

Reporting and Intervention

Admission to an alcohol or drug addiction treatment program is not a reportable event to state or national agencies.

This can be dealt with as a medical leave of absence. However, intervention must be initiated as soon as there is firm evidence that substances of abuse are being diverted. This evidence needs to be clear and convincing to the physician assistance committee.

The primary goal of intervention is to get the addicted individual into a multidisciplinary medical evaluation process composed of a team of experts at an experienced inpatient or residential treatment program. One-on-one intervention must be avoided. The expertise of the hospital physician assistance committee and county or state medical society can be used to help with the intervention. After an individual has been confronted and is awaiting final disposition, it is important not to leave him/her alone because newly identified addictive physicians are at increased risk of suicide following the initial confrontation.

Treatment

The specifics of substance abuse treatment for physicians are beyond the scope of this chapter. However, it is important that a member of the faculty, group, or impairment committee keep in contact with the addictive physician and his/her treatment team. There is no cure for addiction and recovery is a lifelong process. The most effective treatment programs are multidisciplinary in composition and can provide long-term follow-up for the impaired physician.

Benzodiazepines

Benzodiazepine addiction requires ingestion of *large* doses of drug. As with barbiturates, tolerance and physical dependence occur with chronic benzodiazepine abuse. Benzodiazepines do not significantly induce microsomal enzymes. Symptoms of withdrawal generally occur later than with barbiturates and are less severe owing to the prolonged elimination half-lives of most benzodiazepines and the fact that many of these drugs are metabolized to pharmacologically active metabolites that also have prolonged elimination half-lives. Anesthetic considerations in chronic benzodiazepine abusers are similar to those described for chronic barbiturate abusers.

Acute benzodiazepine overdose is much less likely to produce ventilatory depression than barbiturate overdose. It must be recognized, however, that the combination of benzodiazepines and other central nervous system depressants, such as alcohol, have proved to be life threatening. Supportive treatment usually suffices for treatment of a benzodiazepine overdose. Flumazenil, a specific benzodiazepine antagonist, is useful for managing severe or life-threatening overdose. Seizure activity suppressed by benzodiazepines could be unmasked after administration of flumazenil.

Amphetamines

Amphetamines stimulate the release of catecholamines, resulting in increased cortical alertness, appetite suppression, and decreased need for sleep. Approved medical uses of amphetamines are treatment of narcolepsy, attention-deficit disorders, and hyperactivity associated with minimal brain dysfunction in children. Tolerance to the appetite suppressant effects of amphetamines develops within a few weeks, making these drugs poor substitutes for proper dieting techniques. Physiologic dependence on amphetamines is profound, and daily doses may be increased to several hundred times the therapeutic dose. Chronic abuse of amphetamines results in depletion of body stores of catecholamines. Such depletion may manifest as somnolence and anxiety or a psychotic state. Other physiologic abnormalities reported with long-term amphetamine abuse include hypertension, cardiac dysrhythmias, and malnutrition. Amphetamines are most often abused orally but, in the case of methamphetamine, abuse is via the intravenous route.

Overdose

Amphetamine overdose causes anxiety, a psychotic state, and progressive central nervous system irritability manifesting as hyperactivity, hyperreflexia, and, occasionally, seizures. Other physiologic effects include increased blood pressure and heart rate, cardiac dysrhythmias, decreased gastrointestinal motility, mydriasis, diaphoresis, and hyperthermia. Metabolic imbalances such as dehydration, lactic acidosis, and ketosis may occur.

Treatment of oral amphetamine overdose includes induced emesis or gastric lavage followed by administration of activated charcoal and a cathartic. Phenothiazines may antagonize many of the acute central nervous system effects of amphetamines. Similarly, diazepam may be useful for controlling amphetamine-induced seizures. Acidification of the urine promotes elimination of amphetamines.

Withdrawal Syndrome

Abrupt cessation of excess amphetamine use is accompanied by extreme lethargy, depression that may be suicidal, increased appetite, and weight gain. Benzodiazepines are useful in the management of withdrawal if sedation is needed, and β-adrenergic antagonists may be administered to control sympathetic nervous system hyperactivity. Postamphetamine depression may last for months and require treatment with antidepressant drugs.

Management of Anesthesia

Chronic pharmacologic doses of amphetamine administered for medically indicated uses (narcolepsy, attention-deficit disorder) need not be discontinued before elective surgery. Patients requiring emergency surgery and who are acutely intoxicated from ingestion of amphetamines may exhibit hypertension, tachycardia, hyperthermia, and increased requirements for volatile anesthetics. Even intraoperative intracranial hypertension and cardiac arrest have been attributed to amphetamine abuse. In animals, *acute* intravenous administration of dextroamphetamine produces dose-related increases in body temperature and anesthetic requirements. For these reasons, it is prudent to monitor body temperature during the perioperative period. *Chronic* amphetamine abuse may be associated with markedly decreased anesthetic requirements, presumably as a result of catecholamine depletion in

the central nervous system. Refractory hypotension can reflect depletion of catecholamine stores. Direct-acting vasopressors, including phenylephrine and epinephrine, should be available to treat hypotension because the response to indirect-acting vasopressors such as ephedrine may be attenuated by the amphetamine-induced catecholamine depletion. Intraoperative monitoring of blood pressure using an intra-arterial catheter is a consideration. Postoperatively, there is the potential for orthostatic hypotension once patients begin to ambulate.

Hallucinogens

Hallucinogens, as represented by lysergic acid diethylamine (LSD) and phencyclidine, are usually ingested orally. Although there is a high degree of psychological dependence, there is no evidence of physical dependence or withdrawal symptoms when LSD is acutely discontinued. Long-term use of hallucinogens is unlikely. The effects of these drugs develop within 1 to 2 hours and last 8 to 12 hours. They consist of visual, auditory, and tactile hallucinations and distortions of the surroundings and body image. The ability of the brain to suppress relatively unimportant stimuli is impaired by LSD. Evidence of sympathetic nervous system stimulation includes mydriasis, increased body temperature, hypertension, and tachycardia. Tolerance to the behavioral effects of LSD occurs rapidly, whereas tolerance to the cardiovascular effects is less pronounced.

Overdose

Overdose of LSD has not been associated with death, although patients may suffer unrecognized injuries, reflecting the intrinsic analgesic effects of the drug. On rare occasions, LSD produces seizures and apnea. It can produce an acute panic reaction characterized by hyperactivity, mood lability, and, in extreme cases, overt psychosis. Patients should be placed in a calm, quiet environment with minimal external stimuli. No specific antidote exists, although benzodiazepines may be useful for controlling agitation and anxiety reactions. Supportive care in the form of airway management, mechanical ventilation, treatment of seizures, and control of the manifestations of sympathetic nervous system hyperactivity is warranted. Forced diuresis and acidification of the urine promotes elimination of phencyclidine but also introduces the risk of fluid overload and electrolyte abnormalities, especially hypokalemia.

Management of Anesthesia

Anesthesia and surgery have been reported to precipitate panic responses in these patients. If such an event occurs, diazepam is likely to be a useful treatment. Exaggerated responses to sympathomimetic drugs are likely. The analgesia and ventilatory depressant effects of opioids are prolonged by LSD.

Marijuana

Marijuana is usually abused via smoking, which increases the bioavailability of the primary psychoactive component, tetrahydrocannabinol (THC) compared to oral ingestion. Inhalation of marijuana smoke produces euphoria, with signs of increased sympathetic nervous system activity and decreased parasympathetic nervous system activity. The most consistent cardiac change is an increased resting heart rate. Orthostatic hypotension may occur. Chronic marijuana abuse leads to increased tar deposits in the lungs, impaired pulmonary defense mechanisms, and decreased pulmonary function. An increased incidence of sinusitis and bronchitis is likely. In predisposed persons, marijuana may evoke seizures. Conjunctival reddening is evidence of vasodilation. Drowsiness is a common side effect. Tolerance to most of the psychoactive effects of THC has been observed. Although physical dependence on marijuana is not believed to occur, abrupt cessation after chronic use is characterized by mild withdrawal symptoms, such as irritability, insomnia, diaphoresis, nausea, vomiting, and diarrhea. The one medical indication for marijuana use is as an antiemetic in patients receiving cancer chemotherapy.

Pharmacologic effects of inhaled THC occur within minutes but rarely persist more than 2 to 3 hours, decreasing the likelihood that acutely intoxicated patients will be seen in the operating room. Management of anesthesia includes consideration of the known effects of THC on the heart, lungs, and central nervous system. Animal studies have demonstrated drug-induced drowsiness and decreased dose requirements for volatile anesthetics following *intravenous* administration of THC. Barbiturate and ketamine sleep times are prolonged in THC-treated animals, and opioid-induced respiratory depression may be potentiated.

Cyclic Antidepressant Overdose

Deliberate overdose of antidepressant medication is a common cause of death due to drug ingestion. The cyclic antidepressant drugs account for most of this mortality. Potentially lethal doses of these drugs may only be five to 10 times the daily therapeutic doses. Overdose principally affects the central nervous system, parasympathetic nervous system, and cardiovascular system. Inhibition of neuronal uptake of norepinephrine and/or serotonin, anticholinergic effects, peripheral α-adrenergic blockade, and membrane depressant effects account for the toxicity. Evidence of intense anticholinergic effects include delirium, fever, tachycardia, mydriasis, flushed dry skin, ileus, and urinary retention (see Table 22-4). Cardiovascular toxicity consists of sinus tachycardia with prolongation of the PR interval, QRS and QTc, ventricular dysrhythmias, and myocardial depression and may be lethal. Seizures are not uncommon. The likelihood of seizures and cardiac dysrhythmias is rare when the maximal limb lead QRS duration is less than 100 milliseconds. Plasma concentrations of cyclic antidepressants are not usually measured because of the reliability of the limb lead QRS duration in predicting the risk of neurologic and cardiac complications. The obtundation/coma/seizure phase of cyclic antidepressant overdose lasts 24 hours or longer. Even after this phase passes, the risk of life-threatening cardiac dysrhythmias may persist for several days, necessitating prolonged electrocardiographic monitoring.

Initial treatment of cyclic antidepressant overdose in the presence of preserved upper airway reflexes includes gastric lavage and activated charcoal. Emesis should not be induced because progression from being alert with mild symptoms to being obtunded with life-threatening changes (seizures, hypoventilation, hypotension, coma) may be very rapid, and pulmonary aspiration may result. Depressed ventilation or coma may require tracheal intubation and mechanical ventilation. Serum alkalinization is the principal treatment and results in an increase of protein-bound drug, less free drug, and thereby less toxicity. Intravenous administration of sodium bicarbonate or hyperventilation to a pH between 7.45 and 7.55 should be accomplished to a clinical end point such as narrowing of the QRS or cessation of dysrhythmias. Lidocaine may be an additional treatment for cardiac dysrhythmias. If torsade de pointes is present, magnesium should be administered. Patients who remain hypotensive after volume expansion and alkalinization may benefit from vasopressor or inotropic support. Diazepam is useful for seizure control. Hemodialysis and hemoperfusion are ineffective in removing cyclic antidepressants because of the high lipid solubility and high degree of protein binding of these drugs.

Salicylic Acid Overdose

Once ingested, aspirin is converted to its active metabolite, salicylic acid. At toxic levels, salicylates are metabolic poisons that affect many organs by uncoupling oxidative phosphorylation and interfering with the Krebs cycle. This uncoupling of oxidative phosphorylation leads to accumulation of lactic and ketoacids.

Manifestations of salicylic acid overdose include tinnitus, nausea and vomiting, fever, seizures, obtundation, hypoglycemia, low cerebrospinal fluid glucose concentrations, coagulopathy, hepatic dysfunction, and direct stimulation of the respiratory center. The respiratory alkalosis resulting from this respiratory center stimulation assists in renal elimination of the drug by increasing the water-soluble ionized fraction of salicylic acid. Metabolic acidosis, on the other hand, favors the lipid-soluble nonionized fraction of the drug, which enhances the passage of drug into tissues and brain where toxic effects are produced. Noncardiogenic pulmonary edema often occurs during the first 24 hours after aspirin overdose.

Initial treatment of acute salicylic acid overdose includes gastric lavage and activated charcoal. A serum salicylate concentration should be measured initially and reassessed at a later time for evidence of continued absorption of drug such as might be seen with enteric-coated or sustained-release formulations. Empirical administration of dextrose will help prevent low cerebrospinal fluid glucose concentrations. Administration of sodium bicarbonate to increase arterial pH to 7.45 to 7.55 alkalinizes the urine, which dramatically increases renal clearance of salicylate. In addition, alkalemia promotes the movement of salicylate away from brain and other tissues into blood. Potential complications of this therapy include fluid overload and hypokalemia. Hemodialysis is indicated for potentially lethal concentrations of salicylic acid (>100 mg/dL) and for refractory acidosis, coma, seizures, volume overload, or renal failure.

Acetaminophen Overdose

Acetaminophen overdose is the most common medicinal overdose reported to poison control centers in the United States. Patients typically present with nausea and/or vomiting and abdominal pain. Acetaminophen toxicity is due to centrilobular hepatic necrosis caused by N-acetylbenzoquinonimine, which reacts with and destroys hepatocytes. Normally, this metabolite constitutes only 5% of acetaminophen metabolism and is inactivated by conjugation with endogenous glutathione. In overdose, the supply of glutathione becomes depleted and by N-acetylbenzoquinonimine is not detoxified.

Treatment of acetaminophen overdose begins with determination of the time of drug ingestion and with administration of activated charcoal to impede drug absorption. At 4 hours postdrug ingestion, a plasma acetaminophen concentration is measured and plotted on the Rumack-Matthew nomogram, which stratifies patients into no, possible, or probable risk of hepatotoxicity. All patients with possible or probable risk and anyone in whom the time of ingestion is not known are treated with N-acetylcysteine, which repletes glutathione, combines directly with by N-acetylbenzoquinonimine, and enhances sulfate conjugation of acetaminophen. Administration of N-acetylcysteine is virtually 100% effective in preventing hepatotoxicity when administered within 8 hours of drug ingestion.

POISONING

Methyl Alcohol Ingestion

Methyl alcohol (methanol) is found in paint remover, gas-line antifreeze, windshield washing fluid, and camper fuel. Methanol is a weak toxin, but it has very toxic metabolites. It is metabolized by alcohol dehydrogenase to formaldehyde and formic acid, resulting in an anion-gap metabolic acidosis. The target organs for its toxic effects are the retina, the optic nerve, and the central nervous system. Blurred vision, optic disk hyperemia, and blindness are hallmarks of methanol intoxication. Severe abdominal pain, possibly due to pancreatitis, that mimics a surgical emergency may occur.

Treatment of methyl alcohol poisoning includes supportive care and a secure airway. Activated charcoal does not adsorb alcohols. Intravenous administration of ethyl alcohol, which is preferentially metabolized by the enzyme alcohol dehydrogenase, will decrease the metabolism of methanol. Alternatively, the activity of alcohol dehydrogenase may be specifically inhibited by administration of fomepizole. Folinic acid will provide the cofactor for formic acid elimination. Hemodialysis may be indicated for refractory acidosis or visual impairment.

Ethylene Glycol Ingestion

Ethylene glycol (found in antifreeze, de-icers, and industrial solvents) is metabolized by alcohol dehydrogenase to glycolic acid resulting in a metabolic acidosis. Glycolic acid is then metabolized to oxalate. Accumulation and precipitation of calcium oxalate crystals in the renal tubules can produce acute tubular necrosis. Hypocalcemia due to oxalate chelation of calcium, myocardial dysfunction, pulmonary edema, and cerebral edema are additional features of ethylene glycol poisoning. Treatment of ethylene glycol ingestion is similar to that described for methyl alcohol ingestion. Inhibition of formation of toxic metabolites can be accomplished by administration of ethyl alcohol or fomepizole. Thiamine, pyridoxine, and sufficient calcium to reverse the hypocalcemia are also given. Urgent hemodialysis may be necessary.

Organophosphate Overdose

Organophosphate pesticides, carbamate pesticides, and organophosphorous compounds ("nerve agents") developed for chemical warfare (that have been used in terrorist attacks) all inhibit acetylcholinesterase, resulting in cholinergic overstimulation. These chemicals are absorbed by inhalation, by ingestion, and through the skin. There are several important differences between the nerve agents and the insecticides. The insecticides are oily, less volatile liquids with a slower onset to toxicity but longer-lasting effects. Nerve agents are typically watery and volatile, acting rapidly and severely but for a shorter period of time. Carbamate insecticides have a more limited penetration of the central nervous system, bind acetylcholinesterase reversibly, and result in a shorter, milder course than organophosphates. All can be aerosolized and vaporized. The manifestations of pesticide and nerve agent poisoning are influenced by the route of absorption, with the most severe effects occurring after inhalation (**Table 22-14**). Muscarinic signs and symptoms of organophosphate exposure include profuse exocrine secretions (tearing, rhinorrhea, bronchorrhea, salivation), gastrointestinal signs, and ophthalmic signs such as miosis. Exposure to larger doses results in stimulation of nicotinic receptors, producing skeletal muscle weakness, fasciculations, and paralysis. Cardiovascular findings may be mixed; tachycardia or bradycardia, hypertension or hypotension may be present. Central nervous system effects include cognitive impairment, convulsions, and coma. Acute respiratory failure is the primary cause of death and is mediated by bronchorrhea, bronchospasm, respiratory muscle/diaphragmatic weakness/paralysis, and inhibition of the medullary respiratory center.

Treatment of organophosphate overdose involves three strategies: an anticholinergic drug to counteract the acute cholinergic crisis, an oxime drug to reactivate inhibited acetylcholinesterase, and an anticonvulsant drug to prevent or treat seizures (**Table 22-15**). Atropine in 2-mg doses repeated every 5 to 10 minutes as needed is the main antidote for this poisoning. The clinical end point of atropine therapy is ease of breathing without significant airway secretions. Pralidoxime is an oxime that complexes with the organophosphate, resulting

TABLE 22-14 Signs of Organophosphate Poisoning

Muscarinic Effects
Copious secretions
  Salivation
  Tearing
  Diaphoresis
  Bronchorrhea
  Rhinorrhea
Bronchospasm
Miosis
Hyperperistalsis
Bradycardia
Nicotinic Effects
Skeletal muscle fasciculations
Skeletal muscle weakness
Skeletal muscle paralysis
Central Nervous System Effects
Seizures
Coma
Central apnea

TABLE 22-15 Goals of Treatment in Organophosphate Poisoning

Reverse the acute cholinergic crisis created by the poison
  Atropine 2 mg IV every 5–10 minutes as needed until ventilation improves
Reactivate the function of acetylcholinesterase
  Pralidoxime 600 mg IV
Prevent/treat seizures
  Diazepam or midazolam as needed
Supportive care

in its removal from the acetylcholinesterase enzyme and splitting of the organophosphate into rapidly metabolizable fragments. The removal of the organophosphate from acetylcholinesterase reactivates the enzyme, and its normal functions can be resumed. Benzodiazepines are the only effective anticonvulsants for the treatment of patients with organophosphate exposure. All patients with severe intoxication by these compounds should be administered diazepam or midazolam. Respiratory muscle weakness may require mechanical ventilation.

Carbon Monoxide Poisoning

Carbon monoxide (CO) poisoning is a common cause of morbidity and the leading cause of poisoning mortality in the United States. Exposure may be accidental (fire-related smoke inhalation, motor vehicle exhaust, poorly functioning heating systems, tobacco smoke) or intentional.

Pathophysiology

CO is a colorless, odorless, nonirritating gas that is easily absorbed through the lungs. The amount of CO absorbed is dependent on minute ventilation, duration of exposure, and ambient CO and oxygen concentrations. CO toxicity appears to result from a combination of tissue hypoxia and direct CO-mediated cellular damage. CO competes with oxygen for binding to hemoglobin. The affinity of hemoglobin for CO is more than 200 times greater than its affinity for oxygen. The consequence of this competitive binding is a shift of the oxygen-hemoglobin dissociation curve to the left, resulting in impaired release of oxygen to tissues (**Fig. 22-2**). However, the binding of CO to hemoglobin does not account for all the pathophysiologic consequences related to CO poisoning. CO also disrupts oxidative metabolism, increases nitric oxide concentrations, causes brain lipid peroxidation, generates oxygen free radicals, and produces other metabolic changes that may result in neurologic and cardiac toxicity. CO binds more tightly to fetal hemoglobin than adult hemoglobin, making infants particularly vulnerable to its effects. Children, because of their higher metabolic rate and oxygen consumption, are also very susceptible to CO toxicity. CO exposure has uniquely deleterious effects in pregnant women because CO readily crosses the placenta and fetal carboxyhemoglobin concentration may exceed the maternal carboxyhemoglobin concentration and fetal elimination of CO is slower than that of the mother.

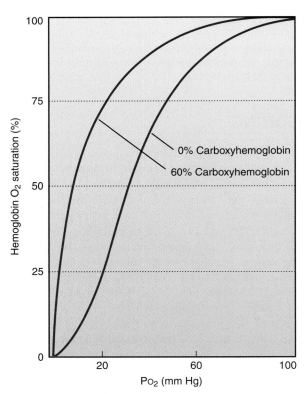

Figure 22-2 • Carboxyhemoglobin shifts the oxyhemoglobin dissociation curve to the left and changes it to a more hyperbolic shape. This results in decreased oxygen-carrying capacity and impaired release of oxygen at the tissue level. (*Adapted from Ernst A, Zibrak JD: Carbon monoxide poisoning. N Engl J Med 1998;339:1603–1608. Copyright 1998 Massachusetts Medical Society. All rights reserved.*)

Signs and Symptoms

The initial signs and symptoms of CO exposure are nonspecific. Headache, nausea, vomiting, weakness, difficulty concentrating, and confusion are common. The highly oxygen-dependent organs—the brain and the heart—show the major signs of injury. Tachycardia and tachypnea reflect cellular hypoxia. Angina pectoris, cardiac dysrhythmias, and pulmonary edema may result from the increased cardiac output necessitated by the hypoxia. Syncope and seizures may result from cerebral hypoxia and cerebral vasodilation, Of note, the presence of systemic hypotension in CO poisoning is correlated with the severity of central nervous system structural damage. The classic finding of cherry-red lips is not commonly seen.

The effects of CO are not confined to the period immediately following exposure. Persistent or delayed neurologic effects may be seen. Delayed neuropsychiatric syndrome, which may include cognitive dysfunction, memory loss, seizures, personality changes, parkinsonism, dementia, mutism, blindness, and psychosis, may occur following apparent recovery from the acute phase of CO intoxication. No clinical findings or laboratory tests reliably predict which patients are at risk of delayed neuropsychiatric syndrome, but patients who present comatose, older patients, and those with prolonged exposure seem to be at greater risk.

Diagnosis

Serum carboxyhemoglobin concentrations should be obtained from patients suspected of CO exposure. Arterial blood sampling is not necessary since arterial and venous carboxyhemoglobin levels correlate well. Measurement requires a co-oximeter, which, by spectrophotometry, can detect and quantify all normal and abnormal hemoglobins. Routine blood gas analysis does not recognize the presence of abnormal hemoglobins, and pulse oximetry cannot distinguish carboxyhemoglobin from oxyhemoglobin. SpO_2 values may, therefore, be quite misleading.

Treatment

Treatment consists of removing the individual from the source of the CO production, immediate administration of supplemental oxygen, and aggressive supportive care: airway management, blood pressure support, and cardiovascular stabilization. Oxygen therapy shortens the elimination half-time of CO by competing at the binding sites for hemoglobin and improves tissue oxygenation. Oxygen administration is continued until the carboxyhemoglobin concentrations have returned to normal. The half-life of carboxyhemoglobin is 4 to 6 hours when victims are breathing room air, 40 to 80 minutes when breathing 100% oxygen, and approximately 15 to 30 minutes when breathing hyperbaric oxygen. Hyperbaric oxygen therapy consists of delivery of 100% oxygen within a pressurized chamber resulting in huge increases in the amount of oxygen dissolved in blood. Hyperbaric oxygen therapy accelerates the elimination of CO and may decrease the frequency of the neurologic sequelae that can result from severe CO exposure. Hyperbaric oxygen therapy is controversial and not universally available and has some risks. However, it may be indicated in selected patients: those who are comatose or neurologically abnormal at presentation, those who have carboxyhemoglobin concentrations in excess of 40%, and those who are pregnant and have carboxyhemoglobin concentrations above 15%.

KEY POINTS

- Serotonin syndrome is a potentially life-threatening adverse drug reaction caused by overstimulation of central serotonin receptors. It can be caused by an excess of precursors, increased release, reduced reuptake, or reduced metabolism of serotonin. Many drugs are serotoninergic, i.e., involved in these processes, and include SSRIs, atypical and cyclic antidepressants, MAOIs, lithium, drugs of abuse, and narcotic analgesics.

- In addition to the seizure and its neuropsychiatric effects, ECT produces significant cardiovascular effects. The typical cardiovascular response to the electrically induced seizure consists of 10 to 15 seconds of parasympathetic stimulation producing bradycardia and a reduction in blood pressure. This is followed by sympathetic nervous system activation resulting in tachycardia and hypertension lasting several minutes.

- Neuroleptic malignant syndrome is a life-threatening adverse drug reaction caused by antipsychotic medication and presumed to be due to dopamine depletion in the central nervous system. It is characterized by fever and severe muscle rigidity, which may respond to dantrolene administration, but is not related to malignant hyperthermia.

- Substance abuse may be defined as self-administration of drugs that deviates from accepted medical or social use, which, if sustained, can lead to physical and psychological dependence. Physical dependence has developed when the presence of a drug in the body is necessary for normal physiologic function and prevention of withdrawal symptoms. Tolerance is the state in which tissues become accustomed to the presence of a drug such that increased doses of that drug become necessary to produce effects similar to those observed initially with smaller doses.

- Although alcohol appears to produce widespread nonspecific effects on cell membranes, there is evidence that many of its neurologic effects are mediated by actions at receptors for the inhibitory neurotransmitter GABA. Alcohol appears to increase GABA-mediated chloride ion conductance. A shared site of action for

Continued

KEY POINTS—cont'd

alcohol, benzodiazepines and barbiturates would be consistent with the ability of these different classes of drugs to produce cross-tolerance and cross-dependence.

- Acute cocaine administration is known to cause coronary vasospasm, myocardial ischemia, myocardial infarction, and ventricular cardiac dysrhythmias, including ventricular fibrillation. Associated systemic hypertension and tachycardia further increase myocardial oxygen requirements at a time when coronary oxygen delivery is decreased by the effects of cocaine on coronary blood flow. Cocaine use can cause myocardial ischemia and hypotension for as long as 6 weeks after discontinuing cocaine use. Excessive sensitivity of the coronary vasculature to catecholamines after chronic exposure to cocaine may be due in part to cocaine-induced depletion of dopamine stores.

- Anesthesiologists represent 3.6% of all physicians in the United States. However, they are overrepresented in addictive treatment programs at a rate approximately three times higher than any other physician group. In addition, anesthesiologists are at highest risk of relapse of all physician specialties. At the present time, 12% to 15% of all physicians in treatment for substance abuse are anesthesiologists.

- Traditionally opioids are the drugs selected for abuse by anesthesiologists. Fentanyl and sufentanil are the most commonly abused drugs, followed by meperidine and morphine. This choice is particularly evident in anesthesiologists younger than 35 years of age. Alcohol is seen as an abuse substance primarily in older anesthesiologists because the time to produce impairment is significantly longer than that observed with opiate addiction. It appears that opiates are the substance of choice for abuse early in an anesthesiologist's career, while alcohol abuse is more frequently detected in anesthesia practitioners who have been out of residency for more than 5 years.

- The primary goal of intervention is to get the addicted physician into a multidisciplinary medical evaluation process composed of a team of experts at an experienced inpatient or residential treatment program. One-on-one intervention must be avoided. The expertise of the hospital's physician assistance committee and county or state medical society can be used to help with the intervention. After an individual has been confronted and is awaiting final disposition, it is important not to leave him/her alone because newly identified addictive physicians are at increased risk of suicide following the initial confrontation.

- Acetaminophen overdose is the most common medicinal overdose reported to poison control centers in the United States. Patients typically present with nausea and/or vomiting and abdominal pain. Acetaminophen toxicity is due to centrilobular hepatic necrosis caused by a metabolite of acetaminophen that reacts with and destroys hepatocytes. Normally, this metabolite constitutes only 5% of acetaminophen metabolism and is inactivated by conjugation with endogenous glutathione. In overdose, the supply of glutathione becomes depleted and the destructive metabolite is not detoxified.

- Nerve agents are organophosphate poisons that have been used in warfare and in terrorist attacks. They inactivate acetylcholinesterase and create an acute, severe cholinergic crisis. Repeated large doses of atropine are an essential part of the emergency management of this poisoning.

- Routine blood gas analysis does not recognize the presence of abnormal hemoglobins, and pulse oximetry cannot distinguish carboxyhemoglobin from oxyhemoglobin. Therefore, in the presence of carbon monoxide poisoning, these monitors provide faulty data.

- The effects of CO are not confined to the period immediately following exposure. Persistent or delayed neurologic effects may be seen. Delayed neuropsychiatric syndrome, which may include cognitive dysfunction, memory loss, seizures, personality changes, parkinsonism, dementia, mutism, blindness, and psychosis, may occur following apparent recovery from the acute phase of CO intoxication. No clinical findings or laboratory tests reliably predict which patients are at risk of delayed neuropsychiatric syndrome, but patients who present comatose, older patients, and those with prolonged exposure seem to be at greater risk.

REFERENCES

Adnet P, Lestavel P, Krivosic-Horber R: Neuroleptic malignant syndrome. Br J Anaesth 2000;85:129–135.

American Society of Anesthesiologists' Committee on Occupational Health: Model curriculum on drug abuse and addiction for residents in anesthesiology. Available at: www.asahq.org/curriculum.pdf.

Boyer EW, Shannon M: The serotonin syndrome. N Engl J Med 2005;352:1112–1118.

Ding Z, White PF: Anesthesia for electroconvulsive therapy. Anesth Analg 2002;94:1351–1364.

Folk JW, Kellner CH, Beale MD, et al: Anesthesia for electroconvulsive therapy: A review. J ECT 2000;16:157–170.

Gold CG, Cullen DJ, Gonzales S, et al: Rapid opioid detoxification during general anesthesia: A review of 20 patients. Anesthesiology 1999;91:1639–1647.

Gold MS, Byars JA, Frost-Pineda K: Occupational exposure and addiction for physicians: Case studies and theoretical implications. Psychiatr Clin North Am 2004;27:745–753.

Kao LW, Nanagas KA: Carbon monoxide poisoning. Med Clin N Am 2005;89:1161–1194.

May JA, White HC, Leonard-White A, Warltier DC, Pagel PS: The patient recovering from alcohol and drug addiction: Special issues for the anesthesiologist. Anesth Analg 2001;92:1608–1610.

Mokhlesi B, Leikin JB, Murray P, Corbridge TC: Adult toxicology in critical care. Part II: Specific poisonings. Chest 2003;123:897–922.

Rumack BH, Matthew H: Acetaminophen poisoning and toxicity. Pediatrics 1975;55:871–876.

Sadock BJ, Sadock VA: Kaplan and Sadock's Pocket Handbook of Psychiatric Drug Treatment, 4th ed. Philadelphia, Lippincott Williams & Wilkins, 2005.

Zimmerman JL: Poisonings and overdoses in the intensive care unit: General and specific management issues. Crit Care Med 2003;31:2794–2801.

CHAPTER 23

Pregnancy-Associated Diseases

Ferne R. Braveman

Physiologic Changes Associated with Pregnancy
- Cardiovascular System
- Respiratory System
- Gastrointestinal
- Other Changes

Anesthetic Considerations
- Nonobstetric Surgery
- Obstetric Anesthesia Care

Pregnancy-Induced Hypertension
- Etiology
- Gestational Hypertension
- Preeclampsia
- Prognosis
- Management of Anesthesia
- HELLP Syndrome
- Eclampsia

Obstetric Complications
- Obstetric Hemorrhage
- Amniotic Fluid Embolism
- Uterine Rupture

- Vaginal Birth after Cesarean Delivery
- Abnormal Presentations and Multiple Births

Co-existing Medical Diseases
- Heart Disease
- Diabetes Mellitus
- Myasthenia Gravis
- Obesity
- Advanced Maternal Age
- Substance Abuse

Fetal Assessment/Neonatal Problems
- Electronic Fetal Monitoring
- Evaluation of the Neonate
- Hypovolemia
- Hypoglycemia
- Meconium Aspiration
- Choanal Stenosis and Atresia
- Diaphragmatic Hernia
- Tracheoesophageal Fistula
- Laryngeal Anomalies

Pregnancy and subsequent labor and delivery are accompanied by physiologic changes in multiple organ systems that may influence maternal responses to anesthesia and the choice of anesthetic techniques. Furthermore, the normal physiology of pregnancy may negatively interact with preexisting maternal conditions. In addition, medical diseases unique to parturients may influence management of anesthesia, especially during labor and delivery.

PHYSIOLOGIC CHANGES ASSOCIATED WITH PREGNANCY

Cardiovascular System

By 5 weeks of gestation, there is a significant increase in cardiac output. Cardiac output increases by 40% of nonpregnant values by the end of the first trimester, and 50% by the end of the second trimester. In labor, cardiac output increases by an additional 40% in the second stage. An additional 20% increase in cardiac output is seen during uterine contractions. Immediately postpartum, cardiac output can be as high as 75% above prelabor values. These changes can be significant for the patient with preexisting cardiovascular disease.

The increased cardiac output is due to an increase in heart rate early in pregnancy. By the end of the second trimester, stroke volume increases by approximately 30% and remains level until delivery. Stroke volume in labor increases due to auto-transfusion as blood is displaced from the uterus.

Supine hypotension syndrome occurs in more than 10% of parturients as they approach term. The incidence of supine hypotensive syndrome, which results from obstruction of the inferior vena cava by the gravid uterus when the pregnant woman is in the supine position, can be minimized by positioning the patient in the lateral position or mechanically displacing the uterus to the left (left uterine displacement) in the supine parturient.

Respiratory System

The combination of increased minute ventilation beginning during the first trimester and decreased functional residual capacity as the pregnancy progresses, speeds the rate at which changes in alveolar concentrations of inhaled anesthetics can be achieved. As a result, induction of anesthesia, emergence from anesthesia, and changes in the depth of anesthesia are notably faster in parturients than their nonpregnant counterparts. In addition, dose requirements for volatile anesthetic drugs (minimum alveolar concentration) may be decreased during surgery. The combination of accelerated onset of anesthesia and decreased anesthetic requirements makes pregnant patients susceptible to anesthetic overdose. Induction of anesthesia in parturients may be associated with marked decreases in arterial oxygenation if apnea is prolonged, as during tracheal intubation. This phenomenon reflects decreased oxygen reserves secondary to decreases in the functional residual capacity.

Capillary engorgement of the respiratory mucosa results in swelling of the nasal and oral pharynx, larynx, and trachea. Parturients thus may have symptoms consistent with an upper respiratory tract infection and laryngitis. These symptoms can be greatly exacerbated by fluid overload or the edema associated with preeclampsia. Of note, manipulation of the airway may cause bleeding and further edema.

Gastrointestinal System

Lower esophageal sphincter tone is decreased as a result of two factors: the displacement of the stomach upward and muscle relaxation due to the effects of progestins. In addition, heartburn is a frequent occurrence among parturients. Gastric emptying is not altered in pregnancy, although it is slowed during labor.

Pregnancy is characterized by insulin resistance, caused by placental lactogen secretion. This resistance resolves rapidly after delivery. Fasting glucose levels are lower in pregnancy than in the nonpregnant patient due to high glucose use by the fetus.

Other Changes

Pregnancy is a state of both increased platelet turnover and clotting. Platelet count can be decreased, but bleeding time remains normal. Clotting factors increase in pregnancy, resulting in shortened prothrombin time, and partial thromboplastin time. The changes observed in the thromboelastogram combined with the above are all suggestive of a hypercoagulable state.

Renal blood flow is increased in pregnancy. Glomerular filtration rate increases by 50%, resulting in a decrease in blood urea nitrogen and creatinine. Normal blood urea nitrogen and creatinine values at term are abnormal and indicate renal dysfunction (**Table 23-1**).

ANESTHETIC CONSIDERATIONS

Nonobstetric Surgery

One percent to 2% of all pregnant women in the United States will undergo surgical procedures unrelated to their pregnancy. The most frequent nonobstetric procedures are excision of ovarian cysts, appendectomy, breast biopsy, and surgery required because of trauma. In addition, treatment of an incompetent cervix (cervical cerclage) typically occurs early in pregnancy.

The objective of anesthetic management in patients undergoing nonobstetric operative procedures is maternal safety, safe care of the fetus, and prevention of premature labor related to the surgical procedure or drugs administered during anesthesia. To achieve these goals, the effects of the patient's altered physiology must be recognized and incorporated with this anesthetic plan. Induction and emergence from anesthesia are more rapid than in the nonpregnant state due to increased minute ventilation, decreased functional residual capacity, and the decreased minimum alveolar concentrate of volatile agents, which may be seen as early as 8 to 10 weeks of gestation. Supine hypotensive syndrome can occur as early as the second trimester.

It is important to remember that the effects of pregnant physiology are not limited to general anesthesia. There is an increased effect of local anesthetics during pregnancy; thus, the amount of local anesthetic administered should be reduced by 25% to 30% during any stage of pregnancy.

Teratogenicity may be induced at any stage of gestation. However, most of the critical organogenesis occurs in the first trimester. Although many commonly used anesthetics are

TABLE 23-1 Physiologic Changes Accompanying Pregnancy

Parameter	Average Change from Nonpregnant Value (%)
Intravascular fluid volume	+35
Plasma volume	+45
Erythrocyte volume	+20
Cardiac output	+40
Stroke volume	+30
Heart rate	+15
Peripheral circulation	
Systolic blood pressure	No change
Systemic vascular resistance	−15
Diastolic blood pressure	−15
Central venous pressure	No change
Femoral venous pressure	+15
Minute ventilation	+50
Tidal volume	+40
Breathing rate	+10
Pao_2	+10 mm Hg
$Paco_2$	−10 mm Hg
pHa	No change
Total lung capacity	No change
Vital capacity	No change
Functional residual capacity	−20
Expiratory reserve volume	−20
Residual volume	−20
Airway resistance	−35
Oxygen consumption	+20
Renal blood flow and glomerular filtration rate	−50
Serum cholinesterase activity	−25

oxyhemoglobin dissociation curve, resulting in the release of less oxygen to the fetus at the placenta. Maternal hypotension leads to a reduction in uterine blood flow and thus fetal hypoxia. Uterine hypertension, as occurs with increased uterine irritability, will also decrease uterine blood flow.

Anesthesia and surgery may also result in preterm labor during the intra- and postoperative periods. Abdominal and pelvic procedures are associated with the greatest incidence of preterm labor. Generally, elective surgery should be delayed until the patient is no longer pregnant and has returned to her nonpregnant physiologic state (approximately 2–6 weeks postpartum). Procedures that can be scheduled with some flexibility but that cannot be delayed until postpartum are best scheduled in the midtrimester. This lessens the risk of teratogenicity (first-trimester medication administration) or preterm labor (greater risk in the third trimester) (**Fig. 23-1**).

If emergency surgery is required, there are no data to support that any anesthetic technique is preferred over another, provided oxygenation and blood pressure are maintained and hyperventilation is avoided. Despite this statement, regional anesthesia should be considered as it minimizes fetal exposure to medications. If general anesthesia is needed, as emphasized previously, one must maintain normal oxygenation and blood pressure and avoid hyperventilation. Left uterine displacement should be used during the second and third trimesters and aspiration prophylaxis administered to all pregnant patients. For monitoring, pre- and postoperative fetal heart rate and uterine activity must be assessed at a minimum.

Obstetric Anesthesia Care
Regional Analgesic Techniques

The use of regional techniques in parturients requires an understanding of the neural pathways responsible for the transmission of pain during labor and delivery. The pain of labor arises primarily from receptors in uterine and perineal structures. Afferent pain impulses from the cervix and uterus travel in nerves that accompany sympathetic nervous system fibers and enter the spinal cord at T10-L1. Pain pathways from the perineum travel to S2-4 via the pudendal nerves. Pain during the first stage of labor (onset of regular contractions) results from dilation of the cervix, contraction of the uterus, and traction on the round ligament. The pain is visceral and is referred to dermatomes supplied by spinal cord segments T10-L1. During the second stage of labor (complete dilation of the cervix), pain is somatic and produced by distention of the perineum and stretching of fascia, skin, and subcutaneous tissues.

Lumbar Epidural Analgesia

When placing an epidural catheter for the provision of analgesia during labor and delivery or anesthesia for cesarean section, it is important to confirm the absence of intravascular or subarachnoid placement of the epidural catheter. In this regard, it is common to administer a test dose of a solution containing the local anesthetic and epinephrine (15 µg). An epinephrine-induced increase in the maternal heart rate alerts

teratogenic at high doses in animals, few, if any, studies support teratogenic effects of anesthetic or sedative medications in the doses used for anesthesia care in humans. There is some evidence of a link between maternal high-dose diazepam injection in the first trimester and cleft palate; however, medicinal doses of benzodiazepine are safe when needed to treat perioperative anxiety.

Nitrous oxide has also been suggested to be teratogenic in animals when administered for prolonged periods (1–2 days). Of concern for its use in humans is its effect on DNA synthesis. Although teratogenesis has been seen only in animals under extreme conditions, not likely to be reproduced in clinical care, some believe nitrous oxide use is contraindicated in the first two trimesters of pregnancy.

Intrauterine fetal asphyxia is avoided by maintaining maternal Pao_2, $Paco_2$, and uterine blood flow. $Paco_2$ can affect uterine blood flow as maternal alkalosis may cause a direct vasoconstriction. Alkalosis also shifts the

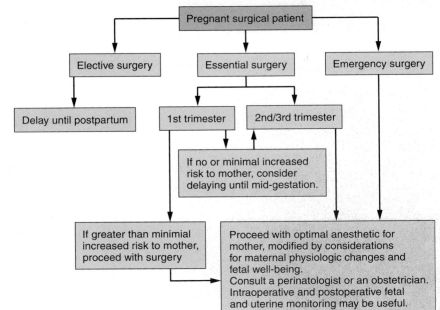

Figure 23-1 • Recommendations for management of parturients and surgical procedures. *(Adapted from Rosen MA: Management of anesthesia for the pregnant surgical patient. Anesthesiology 1999;91:1159–1163.* © *1999, Lippincott Williams & Wilkins.)*

the anesthesiologist to the possibility of an intravascular catheter. A rapid onset of analgesic suggests subarachnoid placement. Hypotension may require administration of small doses of ephedrine (5–10 mg IV) or phenylephrine (20–100 μg IV). Neuraxial analgesia in early labor does not increase the incidence of cesarean delivery and may shorten labor when compared to systemic analgesia. See **Table 23-2** for analgesic choices.

Combined Spinal-Epidural Analgesia

Combined spinal-epidural (CSE) analgesia in labor has been advocated as an alternative to epidural(CSE) analgesia. Advantages cited for the combined technique include more rapid onset of analgesia, increased reliability, effectiveness when instituted in a rapidly progressing labor, and minimal motor block. Subarachnoid administration of low doses of opioids such as fentanyl (12.5–25 μg) or sufentanil (5–10 μg) results in rapid (5 minutes), nearly complete pain relief during the first stage of labor. Low doses of local anesthetics such as 2.5 mg of bupivacaine may also be added to the opioid solution. Disadvantages of the combined technique include increased technical complexity and the possible risk

of postdural puncture headache. This technique should be considered when neuraxial analgesia is requested in very early labor or in a rapidly progressing multiparous labor.

Anesthesia for Cesarean Delivery

In 2007, more than 30% of parturients delivered by cesarean section. If epidural analgesia is used for labor, this technique can then be converted for use as a surgical anesthetic by changing the drug dose and concentration administered. Most elective cesarean deliveries and many urgent cesarean sections are done under spinal anesthesia. Hyperbaric bupivacaine solution provides reliable anesthesia, often with the addition of morphine or meperidine for postoperative analgesia. General anesthesia is reserved for the most emergent cases or when maternal condition contraindicates regional anesthesia. In patients undergoing unscheduled cesarean deliveries, the American College of Obstetrician and Gynecologists/American Society of Anesthesiologists consensus is that hospitals should have the capability to begin a cesarean delivery within 30 minutes of the decision to operate. However, not all indications for cesarean delivery require that 30-minute response time. Ironically, a time interval of greater than

TABLE 23-2	Epidural Labor Analgesia		
		INFUSION	
Bolus (10 mL)	**Local Anesthetic**	**Opioid**	
Bupivacaine 0.125% with hydromorphine 10 μg/mL	Bupivacaine 0.0625%–0.125%	Hydromorphine 3 μg/mL	
Bupivacaine 0.125% with fentanyl 5 μg/mL	Bupivacaine 0.0625%–0.125%	Fentanyl 2 μg/mL	
Bupivacaine 0.125% with sufentanil 1 μg/mL	Bupivacaine 0.0625%–0.125%	Sufentanil 2 μg/mL	
(Ropivacaine 0.075% may be used with opioid as above)	(Ropivacaine 0.075%–0.125% may be used)	(Any of the above)	

TABLE 23-3	Factors That Include Increasing Anesthesia Risk

Obesity
Facial and neck edema
Extreme short stature
Difficulty opening mouth
Arthritis of neck/short neck/small mandible
Abnormalities of face, mouth, or teeth
Large thyroid
Pulmonary disease
Cardiac disease

18, not 30, minutes from the onset of *severe* fetal heart rate decelerations to delivery is associated with poor neonatal outcome. One must consider the indication for unscheduled cesarean deliveries (e.g., arrest of labor, nonreassuring fetal heart rate, or maternal illness) versus the maternal risk/benefit when choosing the anesthetic. Maternal safety and well-being are paramount in determining the choice of anesthetic for nonscheduled cesarean delivery.

Ideally, all patients should be assessed by the anesthesiology team on admission for labor and delivery. At a minimum, the anesthesiology staff should be informed in advance and the patient evaluated when a complicated delivery is anticipated, when a patient has risk factors for increased anesthetic risk (**Table 23-3**), or at the first indication of a nonreassuring fetal heart rate trace. Obviously, preanesthetic assessment must include assessment for co-existing diseases as well as a thorough airway examination. Pulmonary aspiration and failed intubation account for three fourths of all maternal deaths related to anesthesia care. The incidence of aspiration of gastric contents is 1 in 661 patients undergoing cesarean section under general anesthesia compared to 1 in 2131 in the general surgical population. Fifteen percent to 20% of patients who experience aspiration pneumonitis may require mechanical ventilation or prolonged hospitalization. Prevention of aspiration pneumonitis should be with the use of appropriate premedication with H_2-blockers, the use of a nonparticulate antacid, and/or metoclopramide and/or famotidine to decrease the risk of significant aspiration pneumonitis. General anesthesia should be avoided whenever possible; cricoid pressure and an endotracheal tube should be used if general anesthesia is required. During labor, oral intake should be restricted to small amounts of clear fluids as one cannot predict which patients in labor will progress to cesarean section. The incidence of failed intubation in the obstetric population is 1 in 250, which is 10 times that in the general surgical population. Urgent cesarean delivery for a nonreassuring fetal heart rate pattern does not necessarily preclude the use of regional anesthesia. Rapid induction of spinal anesthesia is appropriate in many situations in which there is fetal compromise. Parturients at high risk of airway complications should have early induction of labor analgesia to preclude the need for general anesthesia should the emergent cesarean delivery

become necessary as labor analgesia can rapidly be converted to surgical anesthesia when cesarean section is necessary.

PREGNANCY-INDUCED HYPERTENSION

Etiology

Pregnancy-induced hypertension (PIH) encompasses a range of disorders collectively and formerly known as toxemia of pregnancy, which includes gestational hypertension (nonproteinuric hypertension), preeclampsia (proteinuric hypertension), and eclampsia. Occurring in 6% to 8% of all pregnancies, PIH is a major cause of obstetric and perinatal morbidity and mortality. The three principal mechanisms proposed as the etiology of PIH are vasospasm caused by abnormal sensitivity of vascular smooth muscles to catecholamines, antigen-antibody reactions between fetal and maternal tissues during the first trimester that initiates placental vasculitis, and an imbalance in the production of vasoactive prostaglandins (thromboxane A and prostacyclin), leading to vasoconstriction of small arteries and aggregation of platelets. The most common pathologic features seen in the placenta, kidneys, and brain are vascular endothelial damage and dysfunction (**Fig. 23-2**).

Gestational Hypertension

Diagnosis

Gestational hypertension is characterized by the onset of systemic hypertension, without proteinuria or edema, during the last few weeks of gestation or during the immediate postpartum period.

Treatment

Systemic hypertension is usually mild, and the outcome of pregnancy is not affected. Systemic blood pressure normalizes

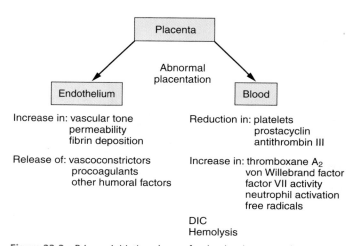

Figure 23-2 • Primary initiating change for the development of pregnancy-induced hypertension (preeclampsia) may be placental ischemia. DIC, disseminated intravascular coagulation *(Adapted from Mushambi MC, Halligan AW, Williamson K: Recent developments in the pathophysiology of preeclampsia. Br J Anaesth 1996;76:133–148. © The Board of Management and Trustees of the British Journal of Anaesthesia.)*

during the first few weeks postpartum, but often recurs during subsequent pregnancies.

Prognosis

It is believed that the risk of developing essential hypertension later in life is increased in these women.

Preeclampsia

Signs and Symptoms

Preeclampsia, a syndrome exhibited after 20 weeks of gestation, manifests as systemic hypertension, proteinuria, and generalized edema (**Table 23-4**). Generalized edema is not essential for the diagnosis, as edema is present in most normotensive parturients. Generalized edema associated with preeclampsia typically appears abruptly and is associated with accelerated weight gain. Signs and symptoms of preeclampsia usually resolve within 48 hours following delivery. Systemic blood pressures higher than 140/90 mm Hg with daily urine protein losses of more than 2 g are sufficient for the diagnosis of preeclampsia. Severe preeclampsia is present when systemic blood pressures exceed 160/110 mm Hg with daily urine protein losses of more than 5 g. These patients are likely to complain of headaches, visual disturbances, and epigastric pain, and they may exhibit altered consciousness.

Risk factors for the development of preeclampsia include nulliparity, advanced maternal age, hypertension, and obesity (**Table 23-5**).

TABLE 23-4	Manifestations and Complications of Preeclampsia
Systemic hypertension	
Congestive heart failure	
Decreased colloid osmotic pressure	
Pulmonary edema	
Arterial hypoxemia	
Laryngeal edema	
Cerebral edema (headaches, visual disturbances, changes in levels of consciousness)	
Grand mal seizures	
Cerebral hemorrhage	
Hypovolemia	
HELLP Syndrome (*Hemolysis, Elevated Liver Enzymes, Low Platelets*)	
Disseminated intravascular coagulation	
Proteinuria	
Oliguria	
Acute tubular necrosis	
Epigastric pain	
Decreased uterine blood flow	
Intrauterine growth retardation	
Premature labor and delivery	
Abruptio placentae	

TABLE 23-5 Risk Factors for Preeclampsia
Obesity
Nulliparity
Maternal age > 40 yr
Previous preeclampsia
Chronic hypertension
Diabetes
Renal disease
Multiple gestation

Diagnosis and Etiology

Preeclampsia is a syndrome that effects virtually all organ systems. It is associated with placental ischemia resulting from abnormal placenta. The abnormal placenta then may release factors that produce generalized vascular endothelial cell damage and lead to multiple organ system dysfunction (see Fig. 23-2).

Systemic hypertension is an early sign of preeclampsia and may result partly from severe vasospasm and generalized arterial vasoconstriction. Increased afterload can lead to left ventricular failure and pulmonary edema. Responses to circulating catecholamines and angiotensin II are exaggerated. Decreased intravascular fluid volume is common, especially in parturients with severe preeclampsia. Hypovolemia may result in an increased hematocrit and thus may obscure the presence of anemia.

Pulmonary edema may occur in severe preeclampsia. Low colloid osmotic pressure due to urinary losses of albumin and increased capillary permeability lead to interstitial accumulation of fluid in the lungs. Clinically, decreases in Pao_2 are suspicious for interstitial pulmonary edema. These parturients may be at increased risk of the development of pulmonary edema in response to intravenous fluid administration. Edema of the upper airway and larynx, which may accompany normal gestation, is exaggerated in preeclamptic patients. This change may influence the size of the endotracheal tube selected for tracheal intubation.

Visual disturbances (photophobia, diplopia, blurred vision) may accompany preeclampsia. Ischemia caused by vasospasm of the posterior cerebral arteries or cerebral edema in the occipital regions may be the cause of these visual disturbances. Headache and hyperreflexia are early warning signs of increased cerebral irritation. Grand mal seizures may occur and most likely reflect the effects of cerebral ischemia due to vasospasm, cerebral edema, and microinfarcts. The effectiveness of magnesium sulfate, a cerebral vasodilator, for controlling seizures lends support to the occurrence of cerebral vasospasm. A relationship between seizures and the severity of maternal systemic hypertension is questionable. Coma, in association with increased intracranial pressure, may follow seizures. Cerebral hemorrhage may occur and is fatal in these patients.

Preeclampsia is associated with decreased renal blood flow and glomerular filtration rate, with corresponding increases in serum creatinine concentration. Although oliguria is common, progression to acute renal failure is rare. Acute tubular necrosis is often the cause of reversible renal failure. Abruptio placentae, disseminated intravascular coagulation (DIC), and hypovolemia usually precede acute renal failure.

Impaired hepatic function in patients with severe preeclampsia may impair clearance of drugs metabolized by the liver. Spontaneous hepatic rupture is a rare but will likely be a fatal event. Abnormal liver function tests are seen alone and in conjunction with HELLP syndrome (see "HELLP Syndrome").

Thrombocytopenia may occur in preeclamptic patients reflecting low-grade DIC. Increased circulating concentrations of fibrin degradation products are also consistent with DIC. Thrombocytopenia may also involve autoimmune mechanisms as evidenced by increased immunoglobulin G levels. The effect of thrombocytopenia on bleeding is not clear, as prolonged bleeding times do not always parallel the platelet count. Nevertheless, bleeding times and platelet count usually correlate when the platelet count is less than 100,000/mm^3.

Maternal vascular prostacyclin concentrations are decreased with preeclampsia, and platelet thromboxane A_2 production is increased. The resulting imbalance between prostacyclin and thromboxane likely contributes to enhanced platelet activity and vascular damage.

Impaired placental circulation is the most likely explanation for the high incidence of intrauterine fetal death, intrauterine growth retardation, and perinatal mortality associated with preeclampsia. Placental abruption is also more common in patients with preeclampsia. Decreased uterine blood flow predisposes to a hyperactive uterus, and premature labor is common. Of note, clinically small and premature infants are more vulnerable to drug-induced depression from maternal drugs administered for labor analgesia or for seizure prophylaxis. In addition, meconium aspiration is a common problem in these neonates (see Table 23-3).

Treatment

The definitive treatment of preeclampsia is delivery. At term, a patient diagnosed with preeclampsia should be delivered. Remote from term, the risk of neonatal prematurity must be balanced against the risk to the mother and fetus of continuing the pregnancy.

If the preeclampsia is mild, and the patient remote from term, conservative management, with bed rest and monitoring until 37 weeks of gestation or until the status of the mother or fetus deteriorates are recommended. Women with severe preeclampsia (**Table 23-6**) should be delivered regardless of gestational age. Expectant management for 48 hours to allow corticosteroid administration to hasten fetal lung maturity is acceptable prior to delivery.

TABLE 23-6	Diagnostic Features of Severe Preeclampsia

≥5 g proteinuria over 24 hr
Oliguria
Pulmonary edema
Abnormal liver function
Right upper quadrant pain
Cerebral disturbances
Thrombocytopenia

Magnesium sulfate is administered for seizure prophylaxis. The anticonvulsant effect is at the N-methyl-M$_D$-aspartate receptors centrally. Other beneficial effects include a decrease in systemic vascular resistance and an increase in cardiac index.

Preeclamptic patients with blood pressures greater than 160 to 170 mm Hg systolic or greater than 105 to 110 mm Hg diastolic will require antihypertensive therapy. The goal of therapy is to achieve a blood pressure between 140 and 155 mm Hg systolic and 90 and 105 mm Hg diastolic. Lower blood pressures could compromise uteroplacental perfusion. Hydralazine, labetalol, and nifedipine are all effective antihypertensives in these patients. Refractory hypertension may necessitate a continuous infusion of an antihypertensive. Nitroglycerin, sodium nitroprusside, and fenoldopam all are useful as short-term therapy (**Table 23-7**). An intra-arterial catheter for blood pressure monitoring should be placed if a continuous infusion of any antihypertensive is used.

TABLE 23-7	Treatment of Systemic Hypertension Associated with Preeclampsia

Maintain diastolic blood pressure < 110 mm Hg
  Hydralazine 5–10 mg IV every 20–30 min
  Hydralazine 5–20 mg/hr IV as a continuous infusion following administration of 5 mg IV
  Labetalol 50 mg IV or 100 mg PO
  Labetalol 20–160 mg/hr IV as a continuous infusion
  Nitroglycerin 10 μg/min IV, titrated to response
  Nitroprusside 0.25 μg/kg/min IV, titrated to response
  Fenoldopam 0.1 μg/kg/min IV, increase by 0.05-0.2 μg/kg/min until reach desired response; average dose 0.25-0.5 μg/kg/min
Seizure prophylaxis
  Magnesium 4–6 g IV followed by 1–2 g/hr IV as a continuous infusion (goal is to maintain serum concentrations of 2.0–3.5 mEq/L)
  Toxicity
    4.0–6.5 mEq/L associated with nausea, vomiting, diplopia, somnolence, loss of patellar reflex
    6.5–7.5 mEq/L associated with skeletal muscle paralysis, apnea
    ≥10 mEq/L associated with cardiac arrest

Patients with preeclampsia are intravascularly volume depleted, and this deficit may need to be corrected prior to or in conjunction with antihypertensive therapy. If the patient develops oliguria, a fluid challenge of 500 to 1000 mL of crystalloid is indicated. Central cardiovascular monitoring may be useful if the oliguria is unresponsive to therapy or if pulmonary edema develops.

Prognosis

Maternal

Cerebral hemorrhage is a major cause of maternal death due to preeclampsia and eclampsia. When the mean arterial pressure exceeds 140 mm Hg, there is a significant risk of maternal cerebral hemorrhage. For these reasons, it is recommended that maternal systemic blood pressures higher than 170/110 mm Hg be aggressively treated with the goal of maintaining systemic blood pressures less than 170/110 mm Hg and greater than 130/90 mm Hg. This goal should decrease the risk of cerebral hemorrhage and preserve placental perfusion.

The preeclamptic patient may develop seizures or pulmonary edema within 24 to 48 hours of delivery; thus, anticonvulsant therapy and antihypertensive therapy should continue at least 48 hours postpartum.

Neonatal

Babies born to mothers with PIH are at greater risk of prematurity, of being small for gestational age, and of drug-related respiratory depression at the time of delivery.

Management of Anesthesia

Preanesthetic Assessment

Particular attention should be paid to airway assessment. Facial edema or stridor may indicate airway edema and thus a difficult intubation.

Preeclamptic patients are hypovolemic and prone to hypotension with the institution of neuraxial anesthesia. They are also at risk of pulmonary edema; thus, judicious hydration is indicated. A 500- to 1000-mL crystalloid preload is appropriate before neuroaxial abnormality. Invasive central monitoring may be indicated if the patient develops either pulmonary edema or oliguria unresponsive to a fluid challenge. Intra-arterial blood pressure monitoring is indicated for refractory hypertension, especially if an antihypertensive infusion is needed.

Laboratory assessment should include a complete blood count. An elevated hematocrit suggests hypovolemia. Thrombocytopenia occurs in approximately 15% of preeclamptic patients. A platelet count of less than 70,000/mm³ indicates an increased risk of epidural hematoma. A test of platelet function is useful in evaluating the patient's eligibility for regional anesthesia if the platelet count is in the range of 70,000 to 100,000/mm³.

Liver function tests, blood urea nitrogen, and creatinine are essential in determining the severity of the preeclampsia or in identifying the presence of HELLP syndrome. An arterial blood gas and a chest radiograph are indicated if there are signs or symptoms of pulmonary edema.

Labor Analgesia

Vaginal delivery in the presence of PIH and in the absence of fetal distress is an acceptable anesthetic plan. Cesarean section is necessary in the presence of fetal distress, which may reflect progressive deterioration of the uteroplacental circulation. Regardless of the choice of anesthetic technique, it is important to continue fetal heart rate monitoring until the start of surgery, especially if fetal distress is present.

Epidural analgesia is the preferred technique for labor analgesia, if not contraindicated. Epidural analgesia reduces maternal catecholamine levels and can facilitate blood pressure control in labor. Preeclampsia compromises uteroplacental perfusion because of the vasospastic component of the disease. Epidural analgesia may improve intervillous blood flow in preeclampsia, thus improving uteroplacental performance and, as a result, fetal well-being.

As these patients are at risk of cesarean delivery, early epidural placement can facilitate the use of epidural anesthesia for cesarean delivery, thus avoiding the risks of general anesthesia. Epidural analgesia is accomplished with continuous infusions of local anesthetic solutions containing ropivacaine or bupivacaine combined with an opioid (see Table 23-2) while maintaining left uterine displacement and fetal heart rate monitoring. Because of the hypersensitivity of the maternal vasculature to catecholamines, one might consider using local anesthetic solutions without the addition of epinephrine.

Anesthetic for Cesarean Delivery

General Anesthesia General anesthesia is indicated for preeclamptic patients undergoing cesarean section who refuse regional anesthesia or who are coagulopathic. Historically, parturients requiring emergency cesarean section for fetal distress have been managed most often with general anesthesia based on the notion that the time spent instituting regional anesthesia would be detrimental to the well-being of the fetus. Nevertheless, spinal anesthesia can be established in a timely manner, thereby avoiding the possible depressant effects of drugs on the fetus and the risk of failed or difficult tracheal intubation. General anesthesia is selected when hemorrhage or sepsis is the reason for an emergency cesarean section. In the presence of fetal distress, one should monitor the fetal heart rate continuously while placing the block or preparing for induction of anesthesia.

The risks of general anesthesia in parturients with preeclampsia include potentially difficult tracheal intubation owing to laryngeal edema, potential aspiration of gastric contents, increased sensitivity to nondepolarizing muscle relaxants, exaggerated pressor responses to direct laryngoscopy and tracheal intubation, and impaired placental blood flow. Mortality from general anesthesia in parturients is almost exclusively due to difficult airway management or failed tracheal intubation.

Before induction of anesthesia, it is essential to restore intravascular fluid volume and control blood pressure. Induction of anesthesia is usually accomplished using thiopental plus succinylcholine to facilitate tracheal intubation. Use of defasciculating doses of nondepolarizing muscle relaxants before the administration of succinylcholine is not necessary, as magnesium therapy (frequently given as adjuvant therapy in these patients) attenuates the fasciculations produced by succinylcholine.

Exaggerated edema of the upper airway structures may interfere with visualization of the glottic opening, and laryngeal swelling may result in the need to insert a smaller tracheal tube than anticipated. Laryngeal edema often occurs as part of the generalized edema and facial swelling that accompanies preeclampsia, but it may also occur with few warning signs. It is important to avoid repeated attempts at direct laryngoscopy, as this may worsen the existing edema. In preeclamptic parturients with impaired coagulation, any trauma associated with direct laryngoscopy could result in bleeding.

Systemic blood pressure responses to direct laryngoscopy and tracheal intubation are likely to be exaggerated in preeclamptic parturients, thereby increasing the risk of cerebral hemorrhage or pulmonary edema. Ideally, short-duration laryngoscopy is the most predictable method for minimizing the magnitude and duration of blood pressure and heart rate responses evoked by tracheal intubation. Hydralazine (5–10 mg IV administered 10–15 minutes before induction of anesthesia) labetalol (10–20 mg IV 5–10 minutes before induction of anesthesia), or nitroglycerin (1–2 µg/kg IV just before initiating direct laryngoscopy) may be administered to attenuate systemic blood pressure responses.

Low doses of volatile anesthetics (0.5–1.0 minimum alveolar concentrate) with or without 50% nitrous oxide can be used for maintenance of anesthesia. In this patient population, the major determinant of neonatal depression is a prolonged interval between the uterine incision and delivery, with the duration of anesthesia being important only with prolonged duration of administration (>20 minutes) prior to delivery. After delivery, the anesthetic is typically supplemented with opioids. Potentiation of muscle relaxants by magnesium may occur, and thus a peripheral nerve stimulator is essential for monitoring neuromuscular function.

Spinal Anesthesia Spinal anesthesia has traditionally been discouraged in parturients with preeclampsia because of the risk of severe hypotension. However, in patients with severe preeclampsia, the magnitude of maternal blood pressure decreases are similar following the administration of either spinal or epidural anesthesia for cesarean section. As with epidural anesthesia, institution of intravenous hydration before performing spinal anesthesia is essential. Should systolic blood pressure decrease more than 30% from the preblock value, treatment should consist of left uterine displacement and an increased rate of fluid infusion combined with a small dose of either ephedrine (5 mg IV) or phenylephrine (100 µg IV). A T4 sensory level is needed for cesarean section, keeping in mind that anesthetic requirements are decreased in parturients. In most instance, bupivacaine (12–15 mg) is adequate to achieve the desired T4 sensory level and 120 minutes of anesthesia. An opioid, meperidine (10 mg) or morphine (0.1–0.2 mg) should be added for postoperative analgesia.

HELLP Syndrome
Signs and Symptoms

Hemolysis, elevated liver transaminase enzymes, and low platelet counts are the characteristic features of HELLP syndrome, a severe form of preeclampsia. It is estimated that the HELLP syndrome occurs in up to 20% of parturients who develop severe preeclampsia. Clinical signs and symptoms include epigastric pain, upper abdominal tenderness, systemic hypertension, proteinuria, nausea and vomiting, and jaundice. The disease may progress to include such processes as pulmonary edema, pleural effusions, cerebral edema, hematuria, oliguria, acute tubular necrosis, and panhypopituitarism. DIC is a risk. Maternal and perinatal mortality is increased.

Treatment

The definitive treatment of HELLP syndrome is the delivery of the fetus, often by cesarean section. Vaginal delivery is acceptable if it can be achieved expeditiously. Platelet transfusion may be necessary before delivery. Packed red blood cell transfusion may be needed if anemia resulting from hemolysis is severe. In addition, monitoring urine output (via a bladder catheter) and central venous pressure monitoring may be helpful.

Management of Anesthesia

Management of anesthesia and the choice of a regional technique versus general anesthesia are influenced by the condition of the parturient and the fetus. Regional techniques may often be avoided because of coagulation defects. The precise selection of drugs will be influenced by the presence of renal and hepatic dysfunction that could alter drug clearance, metabolism, and elimination.

Eclampsia
Signs and Symptoms

Eclampsia is present when seizures are superimposed on preeclampsia.

Prognosis

Although signs and symptoms of preeclampsia usually precede the onset of eclampsia, it is possible for eclampsia to develop without warning. Eclampsia is associated with a maternal mortality of approximately 10%. Causes of maternal mortality due to eclampsia include congestive heart failure and cerebral hemorrhage. Eclampsia without generalized edema can occur.

Management of Anesthesia

The obstetric and anesthetic management of the eclamptic patient is directed at controlling the seizures and protecting the patient from aspiration pneumonitis should she have a prolonged period of semiconsciousness following the seizure. In addition, the patient should be observed for lateralizing neurologic signs following her seizure as this may be the first sign that she has had an intercranial hemorrhage.

A witnessed seizure should be treated with airway support, oxygenation, and immediate treatment to stop the seizure activity. A short-acting barbiturate such as thiopental, a benzodiazepine (diazepam), or a bolus of magnesium sulfate, if readily available, would all be appropriate therapy. Management of the seizure should be followed by institution of magnesium therapy for prophylaxis against subsequent seizures. If the patient is already on a magnesium infusion, levels should be checked immediately to determine whether the plasma levels are therapeutic and the dose adjusted accordingly.

If the parturient and fetus are stable following the eclamptic seizure, then management of the patient will proceed as it would for the management of a patient with preeclampsia.

OBSTETRIC COMPLICATIONS

Complications associated with delivery include hemorrhagic complications, amniotic fluid embolism, uterine rupture, vaginal birth after cesarean (VBAC), abnormal presentations, and multiple births.

Obstetric Hemorrhage

Obstetric hemorrhage remains a serious complication, contributing to maternal and perinatal morbidity and mortality. Although bleeding can occur at any time during pregnancy, third-trimester hemorrhage is the most threatening to maternal and fetal well-being (**Table 23-8**). Obstetric hemorrhage is the second leading cause of all pregnancy-related deaths and accounts for a significant portion of perinatal morbidity and mortality. Placenta previa and abruptio placentae are the major causes of bleeding during the third trimester. Uterine rupture can be responsible for uncontrolled hemorrhage that

manifests during active labor. Postpartum hemorrhage occurs after 3% to 5% of all vaginal deliveries. It is often due to uterine atony, but also to retained placenta or cervical or vaginal laceration.

Because of the increased blood volume and relative good health of the average pregnant patient, parturients tolerate mild to moderate hemorrhage with few clinical signs or symptoms. This can lead to an underestimation of blood loss.

Placenta Previa

Signs and Symptoms The cardinal symptom of placenta previa is painless vaginal bleeding. The first episode usually stops spontaneously. Bleeding typically manifests at approximately week 32 of gestation, when the lower uterine segment begins to form. When this diagnosis is suspected, the position of the placenta needs to be confirmed via ultrasonography or radioisotope scan.

Diagnosis Placenta previa occurs in up to 1% of full-term pregnancies. The cause of placenta previa is not known, although there may be an association with advanced maternal age and with high parity. The greatest risk factor is previous cesarean section. Placenta previa is classified as complete when the entire cervical os is covered by placental tissue, partial when the internal cervical os is covered by placental tissue when closed but not when fully dilated, and marginal when placental tissue encroaches on or extends to the margin of the internal cervical os. Approximately 50% of parturients with placenta previa have marginal implantations. The availability of more sophisticated obstetric ultrasonography has eliminated the need for a double set-up cervical examination to diagnose placenta previa. Magnetic resonance imaging and

TABLE 23-8	Differential Diagnosis of Third Trimester Bleeding		
Parameter	**Placenta Previa**	**Abruptio Placentae**	**Uterine Rupture**

Signs and symptoms	Painless vaginal bleeding	Abdominal pain
		Bleeding partially or wholly
		  concealed
		Uterine irritability
		Shock
		Coagulopathy
		Acute renal failure
		Fetal distress
			Abdominal pain
			Vaginal pain
			Recession of presenting part
			Disappearance of fetal heart
			  tones/fetal bradycardia
			Hemodynamic instability

Predisposing conditions	Advanced age	Advanced parity Advanced age Cigarette smoker Cocaine abuse Trauma	Previous uterine incision
	Multiple parity	Uterine anomalies Compression of the inferior vena cava Chronic systemic hypertension	Rapid spontaneous delivery Excessive uterine stimulation Cephalopelvic disproportion Multiple parity Polyhydramnios

color flow mapping during an ultrasound examination may identify, or at least raise suspicion of, placenta accreta.

Treatment Once the diagnosis is made, the obstetrician will determine timing and mode of delivery. Expectant management will be chosen if the bleeding stops and the fetus is immature. When fetal lung maturity is achieved, or at 37 weeks, delivery should proceed. Obviously, delivery will occur at any time that the mother exhibits cardiovascular instability. Except for a patient with a marginal previa who might elect vaginal delivery, the patient will be delivered by cesarean section.

Prognosis Maternal mortality is rare. Perinatal mortality is 12 per 1000 births. Maternal risk of cesarean hysterectomy increases with the number of previous cesarean sections.

Anesthetic Management Anesthetic management is dependent on the obstetric plan and the condition of the parturient.

Preoperative Mild to moderate blood loss is well tolerated by the patient and thus may be underestimated by the anesthesiologist. Adequate volume resuscitation is thus paramount to the patient's care. All patients should be typed and cross-matched to ensure continuous availability of packed red blood cells and, if needed, blood products.

Intraoperative Parturients with a total or partial previa will deliver by cesarean section. Anesthetic management will depend on maternal and fetal status and the urgency of the surgery. If the patient has not had recent bleeding and is scheduled electively, regional anesthesia is preferred, as it is for all patients undergoing cesarean delivery. Large-bore intravenous access should be established as the patient is at greater risk of intraoperative bleeding. Cross-matched blood should be immediately available.

If hemorrhage necessitates emergency delivery, general anesthesia is the anesthetic technique of choice. Ketamine and etomidate are the preferred induction agents in the hypovolemic patient. Maintenance of anesthesia will be determined by the hemodynamic status of the mother.

Placenta Accreta

Placenta accreta is when the placenta is abnormally adherent to the myometrium. Placenta accreta is an adherent placenta that has not invaded the myometrium. In placenta increta, the placenta has invaded the myometrium, and placenta percreta is invasion through the serosa. Massive hemorrhage may occur when removal of the placenta is attempted after delivery.

Signs and Symptoms Retained placenta and postpartum hemorrhage occur in patients with placenta accreta.

Diagnosis Risk factors include placenta previa and/or previous cesarean delivery, with the risk increasing with placenta previa in patients with multiple cesarean deliveries. Placenta implantation anteriorly in patients with previous cesarean deliveries also increases the risk. Magnetic resonance imaging and ultrasonography with Doppler flow mapping have identified placenta accreta antenatally. However, because the predictive value of these tests is poor, this diagnosis is often made at the time of surgery.

Treatment The majority of cases require cesarean hysterectomy.

Prognosis Maternal prognosis is good if she does not suffer from significant hemorrhage. If attempt is made to manually extract the placenta, profound hemorrhage may occur.

Anesthetic Management

Preoperative Significant hemorrhage should be anticipated and thus at least two large-bore intravenous catheters placed. An arterial catheter should be considered. Packed red blood cells should be immediately available and blood products readily available. The use of a cell saver should be considered after delivery. A preoperative interventional radiography consultation should be obtained as arterial embolization may reduce intraoperative blood loss.

Intraoperative Intraoperative management of a patient at risk of hemorrhage and/or cesarean hysterectomy is controversial. Many believe all patients should received general anesthesia (as discussed for patients with a placenta previa). Others argue that if needed, a cesarean hysterectomy can be performed under epidural anesthesia. There is a general agreement that if a patient is deemed a potential "difficult" airway, it is prudent to use general anesthesia.

Abruptio Placentae

Signs and Symptoms Signs and symptoms of abruptio placentae depend on the site and extent of the placental separation, but abdominal pain is always present. When the separation involves only placental margins, the escaping blood can appear as vaginal bleeding. Conversely, large volumes of blood loss can remain concealed within the uterus. Severe blood loss from abruptio placentae presents as maternal hypotension, uterine irritability and hypertonus, and fetal distress or demise. Clotting abnormalities can occur. The classic hemorrhagic picture includes thrombocytopenia, depletion of fibrinogen, and prolonged plasma thromboplastin times. Acute renal failure may accompany DIC, reflecting fibrin deposition in renal arterioles. Fetal distress reflects the loss of functional placenta and decreased uteroplacental perfusion because of maternal hypotension.

Diagnosis Abruptio placentae is defined as premature separation of a normally implanted placenta after 20 weeks of gestation. The precise causes are unknown, but the incidence is increased with high parity, uterine anomalies, compression of the inferior vena cava, PIH, and cocaine abuse. Abruptio placentae accounts for approximately one third of third trimester hemorrhages and occurs in 0.5% to 1% of all pregnancies. Diagnosis is made prior to delivery using ultrasonography and at delivery by examination of the placenta.

Treatment Definitive treatment of abruptio placentae is delivery of the fetus and placenta. Delivery may be vaginal if the abruption is not jeopardizing maternal or fetal well-being. Otherwise, delivery is by cesarean section.

Prognosis Maternal complications associated with abruptio placentae include DIC, acute renal failure, and uterine atony, which may lead to postpartum hemorrhage. DIC occurs in approximately 10% of patients with abruptio placentae.

Neonatal complications are significant. Perinatal mortality is 25-fold higher if a term pregnancy is complicated by abruption. Fetal distress is also common due to the disruption of placental blood flow.

Anesthetic Management If maternal hypotension is absent, clotting studies are acceptable, and there is no evidence of fetal distress due to uteroplacental insufficiency, epidural analgesia is useful for providing analgesia for labor and vaginal delivery. When the magnitude of placental separation and resulting hemorrhage are severe, emergency cesarean section is necessary; most often, general anesthesia is used, as regional anesthesia in a hemodynamically unstable patient may be unwise. Anesthetic management is similar to that employed with placenta previa. Blood and blood products should be readily available due to the risk of bleeding and DIC.

It is not uncommon for blood to dissect between layers of the myometrium after premature separation of the placenta. As a result, the uterus is unable to contract adequately after delivery, and postpartum hemorrhage occurs. Uncontrolled hemorrhage may require an emergency hysterectomy. Bleeding may be exaggerated by coagulopathy, in which case infusion of fresh frozen plasma and platelets may be indicated to replace deficient clotting factors. Clotting parameters usually revert to normal within a few hours after delivery of the neonate.

Postpartum Hemorrhage

Uterine Atony Uterine atony after vaginal delivery is a common cause of postpartum bleeding and a potential cause of maternal mortality. A completely atonic uterus may result in a 2000-mL blood loss in 5 minutes. Conditions associated with uterine atony include multiple parity, multiple births, polyhydramnios, a large fetus, and a retained placenta. Uterine atony may occur immediately after delivery or may manifest itself several hours later. Treatment is with intravenous oxytocin resulting in contraction of the uterus. Methylergonovine, administered intravenously or intramuscularly or intramuscular or intrauterine carboprost tromethamine (misoprostal) may also be used to control hemorrhage. In rare instances, it may be necessary to perform an emergency hysterectomy.

Retained Placenta Retained placenta occurs in approximately 1% of all vaginal deliveries and usually necessitates a manual exploration of the uterus. If an epidural has been used for vaginal delivery, manual removal of the retained placenta may be attempted under epidural anesthesia. Spinal anesthesia (saddleblock) or low-dose intravenous ketamine may provide adequate analgesia if an epidural is not in place. In rare cases, a general anesthetic may be needed. Low doses (40-μg boluses, as needed) of intravenous nitroglycerin are used to relax the uterus for placental removal when indicated.

Amniotic Fluid Embolism

Amniotic fluid embolism is a rare catastrophic and life-threatening complication of pregnancy that occurs in the setting of a disruption in barrier between the amniotic fluid and maternal circulation. The three most common sites for entry of amniotic fluid into the maternal circulation are the endocervical veins, the placenta, and a uterine trauma site. Multiparous parturients experiencing tumultuous labors are at increased risk of amniotic fluid embolism.

Signs and Symptoms

The onset of the signs and symptoms of amniotic fluid embolism are dramatic and abrupt, classically manifesting as dyspnea, arterial hypoxemia, cyanosis, seizures, loss of consciousness, and hypotension that is disproportionate to the blood loss. Fetal distress is present at the same time. More than 80% of these parturients experience cardiopulmonary arrest. Coagulopathy resembling DIC with associated bleeding is common and may be the only presenting symptom.

Pathophysiology

The principal defect created by amniotic fluid embolism is a mechanical blockage of part of the pulmonary circulation resulting in vasoconstriction of the remaining vessels, due to release of undefined chemicals such as prostaglandins, leukotrienes, serotonin, and histamine. As a result, pulmonary artery pressures increase, arterial hypoxemia occurs owing to ventilation-to-perfusion mismatching, and hypotension reflects decreased cardiac output and congestive heart failure due to right ventricular outflow obstruction and acute cor pulmonale.

Diagnosis

The diagnosis of amniotic fluid embolism is based on clinical signs and symptoms. These include increased pulmonary artery pressures and decreased cardiac output as determined by measurements from invasive monitors, and ultimately confirmation of amniotic fluid material in the parturient's blood aspirated from a central venous or pulmonary artery catheter. The presence of fetal squamous cells, fat, and mucin in samples of the parturient's blood are indicative of amniotic fluid embolism.

Conditions that can mimic amniotic fluid embolism include inhalation of gastric contents, pulmonary embolism, venous air embolism, and local anesthetic toxicity. Pulmonary aspiration is more likely when bronchoconstriction accompanies the clinical signs and symptoms. Indeed, bronchospasm is rare in parturients who experience amniotic fluid embolism. Pulmonary embolism is usually accompanied by chest pain. High sensory levels produced by spinal or epidural anesthesia may be confused with amniotic fluid embolism.

Treatment

Treatment of amniotic fluid embolism includes tracheal intubation and mechanical ventilation lungs with 100% oxygen, inotropic support as guided by central venous or pulmonary artery catheter monitoring, and correction of coagulopathy. Positive end-expiratory pressure is often helpful for improving oxygenation. Dopamine, dobutamine, and norepinephrine have been recommended as inotropes to treat acute left ventricular dysfunction and associated hypotension. Fluid therapy is guided by central venous pressure monitoring, keeping in mind that these patients are vulnerable to developing pulmonary edema. Treatment of DIC may include administration of fresh frozen plasma, cryoprecipitate, and platelets. Even with immediate and aggressive treatment, mortality due to amniotic fluid embolism remains higher than 80%.

Uterine Rupture

Uterine rupture occurs in up to 0.1% of full-term pregnancies and may be associated with separation of previous uterine surgical scars, rapid spontaneous delivery, excessive oxytocin stimulation, or multiple parity with cephalopelvic disproportion or unrecognized transverse presentations. Uterine rupture and dehiscence represent a spectrum ranging from incomplete rupture or gradual dehiscence of surgical scars to explosive rupture with intraperitoneal extrusion of uterine contents.

Signs and Symptoms

Uterine rupture may present with severe abdominal pain, often referred to the shoulder due to subdiaphragmatic irritation by intra-abdominal blood, maternal hypotension, and disappearance of fetal heart tones.

Diagnosis

An ultrasound examination is useful in making the diagnosis of uterine rupture. Visual examination of the uterus at cesarean delivery will detect rupture or dehiscence. Manual examination with vaginal delivery will detect dehiscence as well.

Treatment

Uterine rupture with maternal and/or fetal distress mandates immediate laparotomy, delivery, and surgical repair or hysterectomy.

Prognosis

Maternal mortality is rare. Fetal mortality is approximately 35%.

Anesthetic Management

Anesthetic management is similar to that for the unstable patient with placenta previa.

Vaginal Birth after Cesarean Section

Women who have undergone one low transfer cesarean delivery and have no other contraindications to a vaginal delivery are considered candidates for a vaginal birth after cesarean section (VBAC). Women with two previous cesarean deliveries may also be offered a VBAC. The risk of uterine rupture, however, increases with the number of previous uterine incisions. Women who have had more than two cesarean deliveries should not be offered VBAC. The American College of Obstetricians and Gynecologists Practice Bulletin for VBAC recommends that the potential complications of VBAC must be thoroughly discussed with the patient and that they be documented prior to offering the patient the option for VBAC. Both the American College of Obstetricians and Gynecologists and the American Society of Anesthesiologists recommend that personnel, including the obstetrician, anesthetist, and operating personnel be immediately available at all times to perform an emergency cesarean delivery when VBAC is being attempted. Despite the concern for uterine rupture in this patient population, the risk of uterine rupture in patients undergoing VBAC following one cesarean delivery is approximately 2%. Women who undergo VBAC rather than elective repeat cesarean delivery had a reduced morbidity associated with their delivery. However, there may be a higher incidence of perinatal death in the VBAC group.

Anesthetic Management

Epidural analgesia is an ideal technique for pain control in parturients attempting a VBAC. Because 60% to 80% of patients undergoing a trial for VBAC will ultimately have a cesarean delivery, the epidural analgesia can be quickly converted to surgical anesthesia in these patients. For this same reason, combined spinal epidural (CSE) is not recommended in this patient group as adequate functioning of the epidural catheter may not be determined prior to the need for its use for surgical anesthesia. Like other patients in labor, the patient attempting a VBAC should receive a dilute local anesthetic/opioid solution for her labor analgesia. It is recommended that one not use more dense anesthetics as this may delay recognition of the pain associated with uterine rupture.

Abnormal Presentations and Multiple Births

The presentation of the fetus is determined by the presenting part and the anatomic portion of the fetus felt through the cervix by manual examination. The description of the fetal position is based on the relationship of the fetal occiput, chin, or sacrum to the left or right side of the parturient. Approximately 90% of deliveries are cephalic presentations in either the occiput transverse or occiput anterior position. All other presentations and positions are considered abnormal.

Breech Presentation

Diagnosis Breech, rather than cephalic, presentations characterize approximately 3.5% of all pregnancies. The cause of breech presentation is unknown, but factors that seem to predispose to this presentation include prematurity, placenta previa, multiple gestations, and uterine anomalies. Fetal abnormalities, including hydrocephalus and polyhydramnios, are also associated with breech presentations.

Prognosis Breech vaginal deliveries result in increased maternal morbidity. Compared to cephalic presentations, there is a greater likelihood of cervical lacerations, perineal injury, retained placenta, and shock due to hemorrhage. Neonatal morbidity and mortality are also increased. These infants are more likely to experience arterial hypoxemia and acidosis during delivery because of umbilical cord compression. Prolapse of the umbilical cord occurs with increased frequency in breech presentations and is presumed to reflect failure of the presenting part to fill the lower uterine segment.

Treatment Fetuses in breech presentations are delivered by elective cesarean section. Vaginal breech delivery is rare and necessitates the immediate availability of anesthetic care as serious complications can occur.

Anesthetic Management Anesthetic care for patients undergoing elective cesarean delivery for breech presentation is usually performed under spinal anesthesia, as is routine for elective cesarean delivery.

Vaginal delivery may be complicated by umbilical cord prolapse or fetal head entrapment, necessitating emergency anesthesia for cesarean or instrumented vaginal delivery. Dense perineal anesthesia is needed for vaginal instrumentation and must be administered rapidly, either using 3% 2-chloroprocaine, if an epidural is in place, or by the induction of general anesthesia.

Multiple Gestations

The increasing use of assisted reproductive technologies has resulted in a markedly greater frequency of multiple gestations. Twin pregnancies are approximately 3% of all pregnancies. Triplet and higher order gestations have increased 500% from 1980 to 2001.

Treatment All triplet and higher order gestations are delivered by cesarean section. For twin gestations, presentation of the twins is considered when determining mode of delivery. If both are vertex, vaginal delivery is appropriate. If twin A is breech, cesarean delivery is recommended. The route of delivery for vertex/nonvertex twins is controversial, but often cesarean delivery is recommended.

Prognosis Maternal morbidity and mortality are increased because many obstetric complications are more common with multiple gestations. Perinatal mortality and morbidity are also increased, with preterm delivery the most common cause.

Anesthetic Management

Preoperative One must recognize that physiologic changes associated with pregnancy may be exaggerated with multiple gestations. The larger uterus causes a greater decrease in functional residual capacity. Maternal blood volume is 500 mL greater with twins, and cardiac output is greater. Supine hypotension syndrome is also more significant due to the larger uterus.

Intraoperative Epidural analgesia is preferred for labor analgesia as it will facilitate instrumented vaginal delivery or allow rapid induction of surgical anesthesia, if needed. Particular attention must be paid to left uterine displacement. Postpartum/intrapartum hemorrhage risk is increased; thus, large-bore IV access and a current type and screen should be available. The anesthesiologist must be prepared for vaginal (forceps) or abdominal operative delivery of twin B if a nonvertex presentation occurs.

For planned cesarean delivery, maternal and fetal status will dictate anesthetic choice. Severe aortocompression, despite left uterine displacement, may lead to profound hypotension, which should be treated aggressively.

CO-EXISTING MEDICAL DISEASES

Co-existing medical diseases may accompany pregnancy and thus assume importance out of proportion to the implications of the disease in the absence of pregnancy.

Heart Disease

Maternal heart disease is estimated to be present in approximately 1.6% of all parturients. Common causes are congenital malformations and acquired valvular heart disease. Many of the signs and symptoms of normal pregnancy can mimic those of cardiac disease. For example, dyspnea associated with interstitial pulmonary edema due to left ventricular failure may be difficult to distinguish from the labored breathing typical of normal pregnancy. Leg edema resulting from congestive heart failure can be mistaken for venous stasis from aortocaval compression. The presence of congestive heart failure is suggested by hepatomegaly and jugular venous distention, as these changes do not accompany normal pregnancy. It may be difficult to differentiate heart murmurs due to organic lesions from those due to increased blood flow. Rotation of the maternal heart, which occurs because of elevation of the diaphragm as pregnancy progresses, can be mistaken for cardiac hypertrophy.

Circulatory Changes and Co-Existing Heart Disease

Pregnancy and labor may lead to cardiovascular decompensation of the already diseased cardiovascular system. Cardiac output is increased approximately 40% during gestation and can be increased an additional 30% to 45% above prelabor values during labor and delivery. After delivery, relief of aortocaval obstruction contributes to even further increases in cardiac output above prelabor values. These increases, well tolerated by parturients with normal hearts, may result in congestive heart failure in the presence of co-existing heart disease. Fifty percent of patients with symptoms of heart disease during minimal activity or at rest when not pregnant develop congestive heart failure during pregnancy. Drugs administered to the patient with heart disease readily cross the placenta and may affect the fetus; for example, maternal blood lidocaine concentrations in excess of 5 µg/mL may be associated with neonatal depression. β-Blockers may produce fetal bradycardia and hypoglycemia. The elimination half-life of digoxin is significantly longer in the fetus. Were electrical cardioversion indicated, there is no adverse effects on the fetus.

Evaluation of preexisting heart disease is crucial when planning management of anesthesia during labor and delivery. Analgesia produced by epidural analgesia can minimize the adverse effects of increased cardiac output due to pain or anxiety.

Invasive monitoring during labor and delivery is usually not necessary in the absence of cardiac symptoms. Exceptions are parturients with pulmonary hypertension, right-to-left intracardiac shunts, or coarctation of the aorta. In these patients, the ability to measure cardiac output and cardiac filling pressures, as well as to calculate systemic and pulmonary vascular resistance, is helpful. Because the hemodynamic changes seen during labor and delivery can persist into the postpartum period, invasive cardiac monitoring should be continued for 48 hours after delivery in these patients.

Mitral Stenosis

Mitral stenosis is the most common type of cardiac valvular defect seen in pregnant patients. Parturients with mitral stenosis have an increased incidence of pulmonary edema, atrial fibrillation, and paroxysmal atrial tachycardia. Epidural analgesia producing segmental analgesia is useful for labor and vaginal delivery to minimize the undesirable effects of pain on the maternal heart rate and cardiac output. Perineal analgesia prevents the parturient's urge to push and eliminates the deleterious effects of the Valsalva maneuver on venous return. General or regional anesthesia can be used for cesarean section. If general anesthesia is selected, drugs that produce tachycardia and events that increase pulmonary vascular resistance (arterial hypoxemia, hypoventilation) must be avoided.

Mitral Regurgitation

Mitral regurgitation is the second most common cardiac valvular defect seen in pregnancy. In contrast to parturients with mitral stenosis, these patients usually tolerate pregnancy well. Clinical symptoms related to mitral regurgitation do not usually develop until later in life, usually after child-bearing age.

Epidural analgesia is recommended for labor and vaginal delivery, as it decreases the peripheral vasoconstriction associated with pain and thus helps to maintain forward left ventricular stroke volume, increase venous capacitance when venodilation results, such that intravenous fluids are required to maintain the filling volume of the left ventricle. General anesthesia is acceptable when cesarean section is planned.

Aortic Regurgitation

Complications of aortic regurgitation, like those of mitral regurgitation, usually develop after the child-bearing years. Therefore, these patients usually have an uneventful pregnancy, although congestive heart failure may develop in severe cases. Decreased systemic vascular resistance and a increased heart rate during pregnancy may decrease the regurgitant flow and the intensity of cardiac murmurs associated with aortic regurgitation. Conversely, increased systemic vascular resistance associated with pain during labor and vaginal delivery can lead to decreased forward left ventricular stroke volume. As with mitral regurgitation, epidural analgesia is recommended for analgesia during labor and vaginal delivery. General anesthesia is acceptable when cesarean section is planned.

Aortic Stenosis

The rarity of aortic stenosis seen during pregnancy reflects the typical 35- to 40-year latent period between acute rheumatic fever and symptoms of aortic stenosis. Asymptomatic parturients are not at increased risk during labor and delivery. Because of the fixed orifice valve lesion, however, these parturients are vulnerable to decreased stroke volume and hypotension if systemic vascular resistance is abruptly decreased. If regional anesthesia is used, a gradual onset of analgesia/anesthesia with epidural anesthesia is preferred. General anesthesia is acceptable when cesarean section is planned.

Tetralogy of Fallot

Pregnancy increases the morbidity and mortality associated with tetralogy of Fallot. Pain during labor and vaginal delivery may increase pulmonary vascular resistance, leading to an increase in the right-to-left intracardiac shunt, with decreased pulmonary blood flow and accentuation of arterial hypoxemia. In addition, normal decreases in systemic vascular resistance that accompany pregnancy can also increase right-to-left shunts and accentuate arterial hypoxemia. Indeed, most cardiac complications develop immediately postpartum, when systemic vascular resistance is lowest.

Regional anesthesia must be used with caution because of the hazards of decreased systemic blood pressure related to peripheral sympathetic nervous system blockade. General anesthesia is the preferred anesthetic technique for cesarean section. Invasive monitoring, including continuous measurement of arterial and cardiac filling pressures is helpful. Determination of the PaO_2 intraoperatively allows early detection of increased arterial hypoxemia, which can occur if the magnitude of right-to-left shunting is accentuated by decreased systemic blood pressure. Pulse oximetry may also reflect changes in arterial oxygenation.

Eisenmenger Syndrome

Eisenmenger syndrome consists of obliterative pulmonary vascular disease with resultant pulmonary hypertension, right-to-left intracardiac shunts, and arterial hypoxemia. Traditionally, if these anomalies are not well or completely corrected, then pregnancy is not well tolerated. Maternal mortality can approach 30%. The major hazards facing parturients with Eisenmenger syndrome are decreased systemic vascular resistance, which can lead to an increase in the magnitude of the right-to-left intracardiac shunt and thromboembolism, which may interfere with an already decreased pulmonary blood flow. The greatest risk to these patients is during delivery and immediately postpartum when cardiovascular perturbations are the greatest.

The major concern with any analgesia or anesthesia technique used in patients with Eisenmenger syndrome is avoiding decreases in systemic vascular resistance or cardiac output. Likewise, events that could further increase pulmonary vascular resistance (hypercarbia, increased arterial hypoxemia) must be avoided. Meticulous attention is required to prevent infusion of air through tubing used to deliver intravenous fluids, as the possibility of paradoxical air embolism is great.

Vaginal delivery is an acceptable goal. Analgesia provided with a continuous lumbar epidural minimizes the stress of labor. If epidural analgesia is selected, it is crucial that decreases in systemic vascular resistance be minimized. Epinephrine probably should not be added to local anesthetic solutions, as decreased systemic vascular resistance can be accentuated by the peripheral β-adrenergic effects of epinephrine absorbed from the epidural space. Alternatively, intrathecal opioid to provide analgesia for the first stage of labor followed by pudendal nerve block or activation of the epidural with CSE to provide anesthesia for the second stage of labor can be used.

Delivery by cesarean section is most often accomplished under general anesthesia. Epidural anesthesia has been used successfully for elective cesarean section in these patients; however, sympathetic blockade may lead to decompensation. Regardless of the anesthetic technique selected, antibiotics should be given preoperatively as protection against infective endocarditis. It should be recognized that arm-to-brain circulation times are rapid owing to right-to-left intracardiac shunts. Therefore, drugs given intravenously have a rapid onset of action. In contrast to parenteral drugs, the rate of increase of arterial concentrations of inhaled drugs is slow due to decreased pulmonary blood flow. Despite the slow onset, the myocardial depressant and vasodilating actions of volatile drugs may be hazardous in patients with Eisenmenger syndrome. Nitrous oxide may increase pulmonary vascular resistance and should be avoided. Positive-pressure ventilation of the lungs can decrease pulmonary blood flow. Invasive monitoring of arterial and cardiac filling pressures is indicated as the right ventricle is at greater risk of dysfunction than the left ventricle; thus, measuring the right atrial pressure is uniquely useful.

Coarctation of the Aorta

Coarctation of the aorta, like aortic stenosis, represents a fixed obstruction to the forward ejection of left ventricular stroke volume. Increases in cardiac output can be achieved primarily by increasing the heart rate. During periods of high demand, as during labor or acute increases in intravascular fluid volume produced by uterine contractions, the heart rate may not be able to increase to the extent necessary to maintain adequate cardiac output. This sequence of events may result in acute left ventricular failure. Another hazard during labor and vaginal delivery is damage to the vascular wall of the aorta. Specifically, with the increased heart rate and myocardial contractility that accompany the pain of labor, the rate of ejection of blood from the left ventricle increases and may lead to dissection of the aorta.

Maintenance of heart rate, myocardial contractility, and systemic vascular resistance are important considerations in the management of anesthesia. As with aortic stenosis, analgesia for labor and vaginal delivery is often provided using systemic medications or inhalation analgesia and pudendal block. Likewise, general anesthesia is recommended for cesarean section. In all cases, invasive monitoring of arterial and cardiac filling pressures is helpful.

Primary Pulmonary Hypertension

Primary pulmonary hypertension is seen predominantly in young women. Pain during labor and vaginal delivery is especially detrimental because it may further increase pulmonary vascular resistance and decrease venous return. Epidural analgesia is useful for preventing pain-induced increases in pulmonary vascular resistance. Dilute local anesthetic solutions with the addition of opioids will minimize the decrease in

systemic vascular resistance. General anesthesia is often recommended for cesarean section, although epidural anesthesia has also been used successfully. Spinal anesthesia is not recommended for cesarean section because of the potential for sudden decreases in systemic vascular resistance. The potential risks of general anesthesia in these patients include increased pulmonary artery pressures during laryngoscopy and tracheal intubation, the adverse effects of positive-pressure ventilation on venous return, and the negative inotropic effects of volatile anesthetics. Nitrous oxide may further increase pulmonary vascular resistance. Predelivery assessment of the effects of vasodilators, inotropes, oxytocin, and fluid administration may be of value during subsequent anesthetic management. In addition to oxygen, the administration of isoproterenol may be useful for decreasing pulmonary vascular resistance. Hemodynamic monitoring, including systemic and pulmonary arterial pressures, is indicated in these patients. Pulmonary artery rupture and thrombosis are risks with the use of pulmonary artery catheters in the presence of pulmonary hypertension, but the benefits in these critically ill patients appear to offset these potential hazards. Maternal mortality is more than 50%, with most deaths due to congestive heart failure occurring during labor and the early postpartum period.

Cardiomyopathy of Pregnancy

Diagnosis Left ventricular failure late in the course of pregnancy or during the first 6 weeks postpartum has been termed the cardiomyopathy of pregnancy. The precise etiology remains unknown. Suggested etiologies include myocarditis or an autoimmune response. Patients present with signs and symptoms of left ventricular failure, frequently after delivery or in the postpartum period.

Prognosis In approximately one half of these parturients, heart failure is transient, resolving within 6 months of delivery. In the remaining parturients, idiopathic congestive cardiomyopathy persists, and the mortality rate is as high as 25% to 50%.

Management Medical treatment of peripartum cardiomyopathy is similar to that for other dilated cardiomyopathies. This includes preload optimization afterload reduction and improvement of myocardial contractility. In addition, these patients may require anticoagulation because of the increased risk of thromboembolism. It is important to remember that angiotensin-converting enzyme inhibitors, which are routinely used for afterload reduction in the nonpregnant patients, are contraindicated during pregnancy. However, nitroglycerin or nitroprusside can be used for afterload reduction in the pregnant patient.

Collaboration among the obstetrician, cardiologist, and anesthesiologist is essential to optimize care of these patients. Induction of labor is usually recommended if the patient's cardiac status can be stabilized with medical therapy. However, if acute cardiac decompensation occurs, cesarean delivery may be required because of the inability of the mother to tolerate the stresses of labor.

Anesthetic Management Parturients with peripartum cardiomyopathy will likely require invasive monitoring including intra-arterial catheterization and pulmonary artery catheter to assess the patient's hemodynamic status and guide the intrapartum management. Acute cardiac decompensation during labor may require the administration of intravenous nitroglycerin or nitroprusside for preload and afterload reduction and dopamine or dobutamine for inotropic support. Early administration of epidural labor analgesia is essential to minimize the cardiac stress associated with the pain of labor. The invasive monitoring will guide fluid manage-ment, the titration of vasoactive drugs, and the induction of epidural analgesia.

If cesarean delivery is required, epidural or spinal anesthetic may be used with fluid management guided by the use of the invasive monitors. If spinal anesthesia is selected, a continuous technique should be used, as the use of a single-shot technique, with its concomitant rapid hemodynamic changes, will not be well tolerated. If general anesthesia is required, a high-dose opioid technique is often preferred using remifentanil; neonatal depression from the opioid is expected, and thus personnel for neonatal resuscitation must be available.

Diabetes Mellitus

Diabetes mellitus is one of the most common medical conditions in pregnancy, occurring in approximately 2% of parturients. The incidence is increasing because of the epidemic of obesity and the greater number of mothers at advanced maternal age. Ninety percent of patients are gestational diabetics, while the other 10% have preexisting diabetes. Pregnancy is a state of progressive insulin resistance, as discussed earlier in the chapter. Women who cannot produce enough insulin to compensate for this develop gestational diabetes. Patients with diabetes prior to pregnancy have increased insulin requirements in pregnancy. Patients with type 1 diabetes are at greater risk of diabetic ketoacidosis as pregnancy is associated with enhanced lipolysis and ketogenesis. Diabetic ketoacidosis occurs at lower glucose levels in pregnancy, as low as 200 mg/dL. β-Adrenergic drugs and glucosteroid administration may precipitate diabetic ketoacidosis.

Diagnosis

Patients with gestational diabetes are diagnosed if the routine 1-hour glucose tolerance test is abnormal, necessitating a 3-hour glucose tolerance test. If this is abnormal, the diagnosis of gestational diabetes is made. Patients with prepregnancy diabetes are classified by comorbidities (**Table 23-9**).

Treatment

Glycemic control is the major focus of the care of the pregnant diabetic. A blood sugar of 60 to 120 mg/dL is desirable, requiring frequent changes in insulin dose during pregnancy. Management of diabetic ketoacidosis is similar to that for nonpregnant patients. In patients with gestational diabetes, diet control is used initially. If glycemic control cannot be achieved, insulin therapy is initiated.

During the third trimester, antenatal surveillance is accomplished using twice-weekly nonstress tests, beginning at

TABLE 23–9	White's Classification of Diabetes During Pregnancy
Class	**Definition**
A₁	Diet-controlled gestational DM
A₂	Gestational DM requiring insulin
B	Preexisting DM, without complications (duration < 10 yr or onset > 20 yr)
C	Preexisting DM without complications (duration 10–19 yr or onset < 10–19 yr)
D	Preexisting DM (duration > 20yr or onset < 10yr)
F	Preexisting DM with nephropathy
R	Preexisting DM with retinopathy
T	Preexisting DM S/P renal transplant
H	Preexisting DM with heart disease

DM, diabetes mellitus; S/P, postoperative status.

28 weeks. A nonreactive nonstress test leads to a biophysical profile to determine timing and route of delivery. At 38 to 40 weeks, elective induction is commonly chosen to avoid neonatal risks associated with maternal diabetes.

Prognosis

Patients with gestational diabetes are at increased risk of type 2 diabetes later in life. In addition, the incidence of preeclampsia is increased, as is polyhydramnios.

Fetal effects of diabetes include a greater risk of anomalies in fetuses of women with preexisting diabetes mellitus. Intrauterine fetal death, including late-trimester stillbirth, occurs more frequently in diabetic mothers, probably secondary to poor uteroplacental blood flow. Macrosomia leads to a greater incidence of cesarean delivery, shoulder dystocia, and birth trauma. Neonates are at risk for hypoglycemia and may be at greater risk of respiratory distress.

Anesthetic Management

Preoperative Patients with pregestational diabetes should be assessed for diabetes-related complications. Appropriate assessment for gastroparesis, autonomic dysfunction, and cardiac, vascular, and renal involvement should be made.

Intraoperative Epidural labor analgesia decreases pain, resulting in decreased maternal plasma catecholamine levels; induced catecholamines increase and thus may improve uteroplacental blood flow. Patients with autonomic dysfunction are especially prone to hypotension with epidural analgesia, and thus hypervigilance and rapid treatment are indicated.

Because diabetic parturients are at increased risk of emergent cesarean sections, epidural analgesia is preferred to CSE as the catheter should be known to be functioning to minimize the need for general anesthesia in the event of a cesarean section.

The choice for anesthesia for cesarean delivery is, as in other patients, dependent on the status of the mother and fetus. Like all diabetics, blood sugar should be checked intraoperatively.

Myasthenia Gravis

Signs and Symptoms

The course of myasthenia gravis during gestation is highly variable and unpredictable. Exacerbations are most likely to take place during the first trimester or within the first 10 days of the postpartum period. Anticholinesterase drugs should be continued during pregnancy and labor. Theoretically, these drugs increase uterine contractility but without increasing the incidence of spontaneous abortion or premature labor.

Prognosis

Myasthenia gravis does not affect the course of labor. The use of sedatives should be avoided in view of the limited margin of reserve in these patients. Epidural analgesia is acceptable for labor and vaginal delivery. Outlet forceps may be used to shorten the second stage of labor, thereby minimizing skeletal muscle fatigue associated with expulsive efforts. Regional anesthesia can be used safely for cesarean section, but it is important to recognize that co-existing skeletal muscle weakness may lead to hypoventilation during anesthesia.

Neonatal myasthenia gravis occurs transiently in 20% to 30% of babies born to mothers with this disorder. Manifestations usually occur within 24 hours of birth and are characterized by generalized skeletal muscle weakness and expressionless faces. When breathing efforts are inadequate, tracheal intubation and mechanical ventilation of the infant's lungs should be initiated. Anticholinesterase therapy in neonates is usually necessary for approximately 21 days after birth.

Obesity

Obesity in the United States has become a national epidemic with more than 60% of the adult population being classified as overweight or obese. The pathophysiology associated with obesity results in a greater incidence of pregnancy-related complications when compared to nonobese patients. The pulmonary cardiovascular and gastrointestinal changes of pregnancy are often exaggerated in the obese parturient.

Prognosis

The presence of obesity during pregnancy has significant implications for both mother and fetus. Hypertensive disorders including chronic hypertension and preeclampsia are increased in these patients. Obese patients are more likely to develop gestational diabetes and are at increased risk of thromboembolic disease. Obese patients are more likely to have an abnormal labor, and failed induction is more likely to occur. The overall cesarean delivery rate and emergency cesarean delivery rate are increased in these patients. Factors that lead to these increased rates include preeclampsia and diabetes as well as an increased incidence of fetal macrosomia. Soft-tissue dystocia may also be a contributing factor. Prolonged surgical duration can be expected in these patients.

Obesity has been found to increase the risk of maternal death, related to the increased incidence of preeclampsia, diabetes, pulmonary embolism, and infection. Anesthesia-related maternal mortality is also increased in the obese parturient with airway difficulties being a major cause.

Perinatal outcome is adversely affected by obesity. The increased incidence of macrosomia leads to a greater risk of birth trauma and shoulder dystocia. Meconium aspiration occurs more frequently in infants of obese women, and these infants are at greater risk of neural tube defects and other congenital abnormalities.

Obstetric Management

Obesity presents specific technical problems with management of labor and delivery in that external fetal and contraction monitoring is difficult, necessitating internal monitoring of these parameters. As noted above, obesity leads to a greater incidence of cesarean delivery and the obesity itself creates greater technical problems related to the surgery. Thus, the duration of surgeries in these patients is greater than in the nonobese patient.

Anesthetic Management

Preanesthetic Evaluation The high incidence of medical disease associated with obesity as well as the difficulties encountered because of the patient's body habitus present a significant challenge in the management of the obese parturient. Preanesthetic evaluation and preparation should include a thorough airway examination and assessment of the patient's pulmonary and cardiac status. An arterial blood gas to assess for CO_2 retention, an electrocardiogram, and echocardiogram may be indicated. The availability of an appropriate size blood pressure cuff designed to fit the patient's arm is necessary for management.

Labor Analgesia Epidural analgesia is a reasonable choice for labor analgesia. It provides excellent pain relief, reduces oxygen consumption and may attenuate the cardiac responses to labor and delivery. Because obese women are at greater risk of cesarean delivery and the risk of general anesthesia in this patient population is substantial, the advantage of early epidural analgesia is the ability to extend the block for surgical anesthesia.

The technical challenge of performing epidural analgesia in the obese parturient cannot be underestimated. Long needles may be required to reach the epidural space and should be readily available in the labor and delivery unit. The sitting, rather than the lateral position, should facilitate successful identification of the epidural space. Because the failure rate for epidural analgesia is increased in obese patients, frequent monitoring of these patients and prompt replacement of epidural catheter if inadequate analgesia occurs must be provided.

Continuous spinal analgesia is an option for labor analgesia and may provide advantages over epidural analgesia in morbidly obese patients. Correct placement of the catheter is confirmed by aspiration of cerebrospinal fluid, and thus initial failure rates will be less than with epidural analgesia. A dislodged catheter will be more readily identified than with epidural analgesia. Continuous spinal anesthesia is associated with a small but significant risk of postural puncture headache, which may require treatment in the postpartum period.

Cesarean Delivery The incidence of cesarean delivery is increased in obese women compared to nonobese women. Longer surgical duration and increased blood loss must be anticipated by the anesthesiologist and because the obstetrician frequently requires cephalad retraction of the patient's panniculus. The anesthesiologist must be vigilant for signs and symptoms of maternal respiratory compromise due to increased chest wall compliance related to this retraction. These patients are at high risk of aspiration and thus should receive aspiration prophylaxis with sodium citrate and metoclopramide in combination with a H_2-receptor antagonist. Finally, the anesthesiologist must realize that technical difficulties are more likely to occur in the obese parturient regardless of the type of anesthetic chosen. Regional anesthesia is preferred whenever possible for the obese parturient. This is primarily due to the even greater risk of general anesthesia and airway difficulty in the obese parturient. Of significance with regional anesthesia is that the exaggerated spread of a local anesthetic in the obese parturient may result in a high spinal when a single-shot spinal anesthetic is used. For this reason, a continuous technique, spinal or epidural, may be a consideration in the morbidly obese patient. The continuous technique also has the advantage of maintaining anesthesia for what may be an extended surgical duration.

If general anesthesia is unavoidable, emergency airway equipment must be immediately available. If difficult intubation is anticipated, awake fiberoptic intubation should be elected.

Advanced Maternal Age

In 2002, approximately 14% of all births in the United States were to women 35 years or older. In Canada in 2002, 30% of all births were to women 30 to 34 years of age, 14% to women 35 to 39 years of age, 2% to women 40 years or older. Patients and health care professionals believe that advanced maternal age results in poor outcomes. This view is rationalized by the higher incidence of chronic medical conditions in older patients. Indeed, advanced maternal age is independently associated with maternal morbidities including gestational diabetes, preeclampsia, placental abruption, and cesarean delivery. In addition, older parturients are more likely to weigh greater than 70 kg and have preexisting hypertension or diabetes. Thus, these medical problems will complicate the pregnancy and its management.

Prognosis

The prognosis for outcome in the patient of advanced maternal age is related to the comorbidities, not to the patient's age. A healthy woman of advanced maternal age would be expected to have uneventful pregnancies and deliveries. However, almost half of patients of advanced maternal age have preexisting medical conditions or develop pregnancy-related illness. Their pregnancy outcomes are related to these illnesses.

Perinatal complications are significant in patients of advanced maternal age. Multiple gestations are more common in older gravida, as is miscarriage, congenital anomalies, preterm delivery, low birth weight, and intrauterine and neonatal death.

Obstetric Management

The focus of obstetric management is on the patient's comorbidities. Prenatal care should be focused on early diagnosis of pregnancy-related illnesses to allow early and aggressive management of these problems.

Cesarean delivery is performed more frequently in women of advanced maternal age. In some, the cesarean delivery is related to confounding problems. However, advanced maternal age is also independently associated with an increased likelihood of cesarean delivery and "request" cesarean delivery rates are much higher in women older than 34 years of age than in women 25 years of age or younger.

Anesthetic Management

As with obstetric management, anesthetic care of the parturient of advanced maternal age is related to her comorbidities, which have been discussed in other sections of this chapter.

Substance Abuse
Diagnosis

Diagnosis of substance abuse is often by history. Many commonly abused substances are mind altering or affect the cardiovascular system when the patient is acutely toxic. Diagnosis of the patient who is not under the effect of a substance at admission may be made when she, or her infant, develops withdrawal symptoms or the newborn is diagnosed with a syndrome related to in utero exposure.

Substances abused in pregnancy parallel those seen in society: alcohol, tobacco, opioids, and cocaine are frequently abused.

Alcohol Abuse

Signs and Symptoms Approximately 4% of pregnant women are heavy alcohol users. Maternal signs and symptoms may include abnormal liver function tests, but often diagnosis is not made until delivery when a diagnosis of fetal alcohol syndrome is made. Fetal alcohol syndrome occurs in approximately one third of infants born to mothers who drink more than 3 ounces of alcohol per day during pregnancy. However, studies have reported neurobehavioral deficit, intrauterine growth retardation, and other congenital abnormalities in infants of moderate alcohol consumers. Current recommendations support that there is no safe level of alcohol consumption during pregnancy. There has been no safe level of alcohol consumption defined during pregnancy.

Anesthetic Considerations Anesthetic care of the pregnant alcohol abuser are the same as those considerations in the nonpregnant patient (please see Chapter 19).

Tobacco Abuse

Signs and Symptoms Cigarettes are the most commonly abused drug during pregnancy. Because the pregnant smoker is relatively young, oftentimes there are minimal signs and symptoms associated with the tobacco abuse in this population. There is a strong association between cigarette smoking and low birth rate, abruptio placentae, and impaired respiratory function in newborns. In smokers of more than 20 cigarettes per day, the incidence of prematurity doubles. Sudden infant death syndrome occurs much more frequently in infants of mothers who smoke.

Anesthetic Considerations As with alcohol abuse, the anesthetic considerations for care of the tobacco abusing parturient are similar to those considerations in the nonpregnant patient.

Opioid Abuse

There are numerous medical complications of injected drug use. These include infectious complications such as human immunodeficiency virus and hepatitis. Patients may develop local abscesses, or, more significantly, they have endocarditis or thrombophlebitis. A pregnant patient admitted on chronic opioid therapy should be maintained on that therapy during her pregnancy and into the postpartum period. It is not recommended that these patients undergo detoxification during their pregnancy. In fact, withdrawal from opioids during the third trimester can result in perinatal asphyxia or neonatal death. Neonatal withdrawal from opioids can present as respiratory distress, seizures, hyperthermia, and sudden infant death syndrome. Neonates should be observed and treated for withdrawal symptoms as necessary.

Anesthetic Considerations Consideration for the care of the opioid-dependent parturient are similar to those in the nonpregnant patient.

Cocaine Abuse

Signs and Symptoms Cocaine abuse among parturients is associated with multiple organ involvement, including the cardiovascular, respiratory, neurologic, and hematologic systems. Cocaine is associated with maternal cardiovascular complications including systemic hypertension, myocardial ischemia and infarction, cardiac dysrhythmias, and sudden death. Sudden increases in systemic blood pressure may be the primary cause of cerebral hemorrhage. Alternatively, cerebrovascular spasm can produce local ischemia and infarction. Subarachnoid hemorrhage, intercerebral bleeding, aneurysmal rupture, and seizures have been associated with cocaine use during pregnancy. Thrombocytopenia may occur following cocaine use, resulting in prolonged bleeding times. The maternal use of cocaine may lead to metabolic and endocrine changes in both the fetus and mother, presumably reflecting cocaine-induced release of catecholamines. Pulmonary complications (asthma, chronic cough, dyspnea, pulmonary edema) occur most often in parturients who smoke free-base cocaine.

An increased incidence of significant obstetric complications occur in parturients who abuse cocaine during

TABLE 23-10 Obstetric Complications Associated with Cocaine Abuse During Pregnancy
Spontaneous abortion
Preterm labor
Premature rupture of membranes
Abruptio placentae
Precipitous delivery
Stillbirth
Maternal hypertension
Meconium aspiration
Low Apgar scores at birth

pregnancy (**Table 23-10**). The incidence of spontaneous abortion, stillbirth, and preterm labor is increased. High spontaneous abortion rates may be related to cocaine-induced vasoconstriction, enhanced uterine contractions, and abrupt changes in systemic blood pressure.

Diagnosis Identification of parturients abusing cocaine is difficult, as urine checks detect metabolites of cocaine for only 14 to 60 hours after use. One of the single most important predictors of cocaine abuse is the absence of perinatal care.

Prognosis Cocaine use during the third trimester may result in immediate uterine contractions, increased fetal activity, abruptio placentae, and preterm labor. Uteroplacental insufficiency results in decreased birth weight, intrauterine growth retardation, microcephaly, and prematurity. Cocaine administered during organogenesis is associated with fetal anomalies. Maternal systemic hypertension and vasoconstriction may be the cause of the increased incidence of abruptio placentae in cocaine-abusing parturients. Cocaine effects on the fetus may manifest as an increased incidence of meconium staining and low Apgar scores at birth.

Anesthetic Management

Preoperative Evaluation of parturients suspected of cocaine abuse includes an electrocardiogram and possibly echocardiography to check for the presence of valvular heart disease. In parturients presenting with severe cocaine-induced cardiovascular toxicity, hemodynamic stabilization must be established before induction of anesthesia.

Intraoperative Cocaine-induced thrombocytopenia must be excluded if regional anesthesia is planned. Epidural anesthesia is instituted gradually, with attention to hydration and left uterine displacement to prevent hypotension. Hypotension due to rapid sequence induction of general anesthesia or institution of regional anesthesia usually responds to ephedrine, although long-term cocaine abuse could deplete catecholamines and theoretically blunt responses to indirect-acting vasopressors. Thus, phenylephrine may be the better choice for treatment of hypotension in these patients. Ester-based local anesthetics, which undergo metabolism by plasma cholinesterase, may compete with cocaine, resulting in decreased metabolism for both drugs. Body temperature increases and sympathomimetic effects associated with cocaine may mimic malignant hyperthermia.

FETAL ASSESSMENT/NEONATAL PROBLEMS

Electronic Fetal Monitoring

Electronic fetal monitoring permits evaluation of fetal well-being by following changes in fetal heart rate, as recorded using an external monitor (Doppler) or fetal scalp electrode. The basic principle of electronic fetal monitoring is to correlate changes in fetal heart rate with fetal well-being and uterine contractions. For example, fetal well-being is evaluated by determining the beat-to-beat variability of the fetal heart rate, as computed from the R-R intervals on the fetal electrocardiogram. Another method is to evaluate the fetal heart rate decelerations associated with uterine contractions. The three major fetal heart rate decelerations are classified as early, late, and variable.

Beat-to-Beat Variability

The fetal heart rate varies 5 to 20 bpm, with a normal heart rate ranging between 120 and 160 bpm. This normal heart rate variability is thought to reflect the integrity of neural pathways from the fetal cerebral cortex through the medulla, vagus nerve, and cardiac conduction system. Fetal well-being is ensured when beat-to-beat variability is present. Conversely, fetal distress due to arterial hypoxemia, acidosis, or central nervous system damage is associated with minimal to absent beat-to-beat variability.

Drugs administered to parturients may blunt or eliminate fetal heart rate variability, even in the absence of fetal distress. Drugs most frequently associated with loss of beat-to-beat variability are benzodiazepines, opioids, barbiturates, anticholinergics, and local anesthetics, as used for continuous lumbar epidural analgesia. These drug-induced effects do not appear to be deleterious but may cause difficulty when interpreting the fetal heart rate monitoring results. In addition, the absence of heart rate variability may be normally present in the premature fetus and during fetal sleep cycles.

Early Decelerations

Early decelerations are characterized by the slowing of the fetal heart rate that begins with the onset of uterine contractions (**Fig. 23-3**). Slowing is maximum at the peak of the contraction, returning to near baseline at its termination. Decreases in heart rate are usually not more than 20 bpm or below an absolute rate of 100 bpm. This deceleration pattern is thought to be caused by vagal stimulation secondary to compression of the fetal head. Early decelerations are not prevented by increasing the fetal oxygenation but are blunted by the administration of atropine. Most important, this fetal heart rate pattern is not associated with fetal distress.

Treatment Early decelerations are caused by fetal head compressions and are generally mild and rarely result in

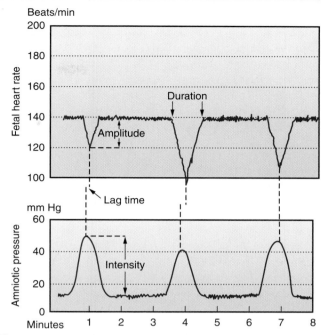

Figure 23-3 • Early decelerations of the fetal heart rate are characterized by a short lag time between the onset of uterine contractions and the beginning of fetal heart rate slowing. Maximum heart rate slowing is usually less than 20 bpm and occurs at the peak intensity of the contraction. Heart rate returns to normal by the time the contraction has ceased. The most likely explanation for this early deceleration is a vagal reflex response to compression of the fetal head. *(Adapted from Shnider SM: Diagnosis of fetal distress: Fetal heart rate. In Shnider SM [ed]: Obstetrical Anesthesia: Current Concepts and Practice. Baltimore, Williams & Wilkins, 1970;197–203.)*

poor fetal outcome. Change in maternal position may benefit the fetus. Fetal scalp stimulation may result in fetal heart rate acceleration in the presence of meconium or severe early decelerations. Fetal scalp sampling for further evaluation may be necessary.

Late Decelerations

Late decelerations are characterized by the slowing of the fetal heart rate that begins 10 to 30 seconds after the onset of uterine contractions. Maximum slowing occurs after the peak intensity of the contractions (**Fig. 23-4**). A mild late deceleration is classified as a decrease in heart rate of less than 20 bpm; profound slowing is present when the decrease is more than 40 bpm. Late decelerations are associated with fetal distress, most likely reflecting myocardial hypoxia secondary to uteroplacental insufficiency. Primary factors contributing to the appearance of late decelerations include maternal hypotension, uterine hyperactivity, and chronic uteroplacental insufficiency, such as may be seen with diabetes mellitus or hypertension. When this pattern persists, there is a predictable correlation with the development of fetal acidosis. Late decelerations can be corrected by improving fetal oxygenation. When beat-to-beat variability persists despite late decelerations, the fetus is still likely to be born vigorous.

Treatment Late decelerations are caused by uteroplacental insufficiency. Treatment involves left uterine displacement,

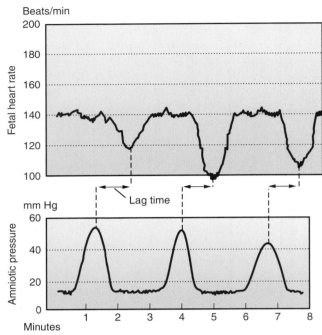

Figure 23-4 • Late decelerations of the fetal heart rate are characterized by a delay (lag time) between the onset of the uterine contraction and the beginning of fetal heart rate slowing. The fetal heart rate does not return to normal until after the contraction has ceased. A mild late deceleration pattern is present when slowing is less than 20 bpm; profound slowing is present when the fetal heart rate slows more than 40 bpm. Late fetal heart rate decelerations indicate fetal distress owing to uteroplacental insufficiency. *(Adapted from Shnider SM: Diagnosis of fetal distress: Fetal heart rate. In Shnider SM [ed]: Obstetrical Anesthesia: Current Concepts and Practice. Baltimore, Williams & Wilkins, 1970;197–203.)*

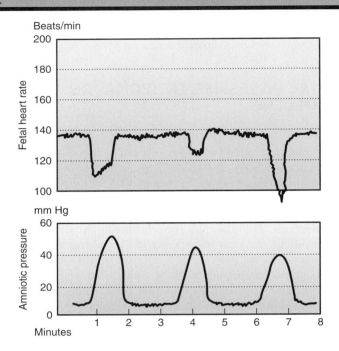

Figure 23-5 • Variable decelerations of the fetal heart rate are characterized by decreases in the heart rate of varying magnitude and duration that do not show a consistent relation to uterine contractions. This pattern of fetal heart rate slowing is associated with umbilical cord compression. *(Adapted from Shnider SM: Diagnosis of fetal distress: Fetal heart rate. In Shnider SM [ed]: Obstetrical Anesthesia: Current Concepts and Practice. Baltimore, Williams & Wilkins, 1970:197–203.)*

intravenous fluids, and, if maternal hypotension is present, ephedrine administration.

Variable Decelerations

Variable decelerations are the most common pattern of fetal heart changes observed during the intrapartum period. As the term indicates, these decelerations are variable in magnitude, duration, and time of onset relative to uterine contractions (**Fig. 23-5**). For example, this pattern may begin before, with, or after the onset of uterine contractions. Characteristically, deceleration patterns are abrupt in onset and cessation. The fetal heart rate almost invariably decreases to less than 100 bpm. Variable decelerations are thought to be caused by umbilical cord compression. Atropine diminishes the severity of variable decelerations, but administration of oxygen to the mother is without effect. If deceleration patterns are not severe and repetitive, there are usually only minimal alterations in the fetal acid-base status. Severe variable deceleration patterns that persist for 15 to 30 minutes are associated with fetal acidosis.

Treatment Variable decelerations are caused by umbilical cord compression and are also well tolerated by the healthy fetus. If severe, fetal compromise may occur and delivery may become necessary if variable decelerations persist or worsen.

Fetal Scalp Sampling

Fetal scalp sampling may be indicated to evaluate a fetus with an abnormal fetal heart rate tracing. Based on the results, suspected fetal hypoxia may be confirmed, establishing a need for urgent delivery. Good neonatal outcomes are associated with a pH of greater than 7.20, while a pH of less than 7.20 suggests fetal compromise necessitating immediate delivery.

Fetal Pulse Oximetry

Fetal pulse oximetry is a newer technique evaluating intrapartum fetal oxygenation. It is currently an adjunct to electronic fetal heart rate monitoring and currently may be used when the fetal heart rate monitor shows a nonreassuring trace. The fetal pulse oximeter provides continuous fetal arterial oxygen saturation readings when placed through the cervix to lie alongside the fetal cheek or temple. Normal fetal oxygen saturations range between 30% and 70%. Saturations less than 30% are suggestive of fetal academia.

Ultrasonography

Ultrasound examination of the fetus when the mother is in labor may be useful to determine the fetal presenting part. Also, if fetal heart tones are undetectable using Doppler scanning, ultrasonography may confirm intrauterine fetal health or demise. Ultrasonography may also determine the quantity of amniotic fluid present in the uterus and is used to diagnose placental abruption and placenta previa.

TABLE 23-11 Evaluation of Neonates Using the Apgar Score

Parameter	0	1	2
Heart rate (bpm)	Absent	<100	>100
Respiratory effort	Absent	Slow	Crying
		Irregular	
Reflex irritability	No response	Grimace	Crying
Muscle tone	Limp	Flexion of extremities	Active
Color	Pale	Body pink	Pink
	Cyanotic	Extremities cyanotic	

Evaluation of the Neonate

The importance of assessment immediately after birth is that depressed neonates who require active resuscitation are identified promptly. As a guide to identifying and treating depressed neonates, the Apgar score has not been surpassed.

The Apgar score assigns a numerical value to five vital signs measured or observed in neonates 1 minute and 5 minutes after delivery (**Table 23-11**). Of the five criteria, the heart rate and the quality of the respiratory effort are the most important factors; color is the least informative for identifying distressed neonates. A heart rate of less than 100 bpm generally signifies arterial hypoxemia. Disappearance of cyanosis is often rapid when ventilation and circulation are normal. Nevertheless, many healthy neonates still have cyanosis at 1 minute owing to peripheral vasoconstriction in response to cold ambient temperatures in the delivery room. Acidosis and pulmonary vasoconstriction are the most likely causes of persistent cyanosis.

Apgar scores correlate well with acid-base measurements performed immediately after birth. When scores are greater than 7, neonates have either normal blood gases or mild respiratory acidosis. Infants with scores of 4 to 6 are moderately depressed; those with scores of 3 or below have combined metabolic and respiratory acidosis. Mildly to moderately depressed infants (Apgar scores of 3–7) frequently improve in response to oxygen administered by face mask, with or without positive-pressure ventilation of the lungs. Tracheal intubation and perhaps external cardiac massage are indicated when Apgar scores are less than 3. Apgar scores are not sufficiently sensitive to detect drug-related changes reliably or to provide data necessary to evaluate the subtle effects of obstetric anesthetic techniques on neonates.

Immediate Neonatal Period

Major changes in the neonatal cardiovascular system and respiratory system occur immediately following delivery. For example, with clamping of the umbilical cord at birth, systemic vascular resistance increases, left atrial pressure increases, and flow through the foramen ovale ceases. Expansion of the lungs decreases pulmonary vascular resistance, and

the entire right ventricular output is diverted to the lungs. In normal newborns, increase in Pa_{O_2} to more than 60 mm Hg causes vasoconstriction and functional closure of the ductus arteriosus. When adequate oxygenation and ventilation are not established after delivery, a fetal circulation pattern persists characterized by increased pulmonary vascular resistance and decreased pulmonary blood flow. Furthermore, the ductus arteriosus and foramen ovale remain open, resulting in large right-to-left intracardiac shunts with associated arterial hypoxemia and acidosis.

A high index of suspicion must be maintained for serious abnormalities that can be present at birth or manifest shortly after delivery. They include meconium aspiration, choanal stenosis and atresia, diaphragmatic hernia, hypovolemia, hypoglycemia, tracheoesophageal fistula, and laryngeal anomalies.

Hypovolemia

Newborns with mean arterial pressures less than 50 mm Hg at birth are likely to be hypovolemic. Poor capillary refill, tachycardia, and tachypnea are present. Hypovolemia frequently follows intrauterine fetal distress, during which larger than normal portions of fetal blood are shunted to the placenta and remain there after delivery and clamping of the umbilical cord. Umbilical cord compression is also frequently associated with hypovolemia.

Hypoglycemia

Hypoglycemia can manifest as hypotension, tremors, and seizures. Infants with intrauterine growth retardation and those born to diabetic mothers or after severe intrauterine fetal distress are vulnerable to hypoglycemia.

Meconium Aspiration

Meconium is the breakdown product of swallowed amniotic fluid, gastrointestinal cells, and secretions. It is seldom present before 34 weeks of gestation. After approximately 34 weeks, intrauterine arterial hypoxemia can result in increased gut motility and defecation. Gasping associated with arterial hypoxemia causes the fetus to inhale amniotic fluid and debris into the lungs. If delivery is delayed, meconium is broken down and excreted from the lungs. If birth occurs within 24 hours of aspiration, the meconium is still present in the major airways and is distributed to the lung periphery with the onset of spontaneous breathing. Obstruction of small airways causes ventilation-to-perfusion mismatching. The breathing rate may be more than 100 breaths per minutes, and lung compliance decreases to levels seen in infants with respiratory distress syndrome. In severe cases, pulmonary hypertension and right-to-left shunting through the patent foramen ovale and ductus arteriosus (persistent fetal circulation) lead to severe arterial hypoxemia. Pneumothorax is also a common problem in the presence of meconium aspiration.

In the past, treatment of meconium aspiration consisted of placing a tracheal tube immediately after delivery and attempting to suction meconium from the newborn's airways.

Currently, a more conservative approach is recommended because routine tracheal intubation of all infants with meconium staining (approximately 10% of all newborns) may cause unnecessary airway complications. Routine oropharyngeal suctioning is recommended at the time of delivery, but tracheal intubation and suctioning is performed selectively, depending on the infant's condition (those with Apgar scores of more than 7 are managed conservatively). Infants with low Apgar scores or who are clinically obstructed with meconium require active resuscitation, including tracheal intubation and attempts to remove meconium via suctioning.

Choanal Stenosis and Atresia

Nasal obstruction should be suspected in neonates who have good breathing efforts but in whom air entry is absent. Cyanosis develops if these infants are forced to breathe with their mouths closed. Unilateral or bilateral choanal stenosis is diagnosed based on the failure to pass a small catheter through each naris; such failure may reflect congenital (anatomic) obstruction or more commonly functional atresia due to blood, mucus, or meconium. The congenital form of choanal atresia must be treated surgically during the neonatal period. An oral airway may be necessary until surgical correction can be accomplished. Functional choanal atresia is treated by nasal suctioning. Opioids often cause congestion of the nasal mucosa and obstruction. Such congestion can be treated with phenylephrine nose drops.

Diaphragmatic Hernia

Severe respiratory distress at birth, associated with cyanosis and a scaphoid abdomen, suggests a diaphragmatic hernia. Chest radiographs demonstrate abdominal contents in the thorax. Initial treatment in the delivery room includes tracheal intubation and ventilation of the lungs with oxygen. A pneumothorax on the side opposite the hernia is likely if attempts are made to expand the ipsilateral lung.

Tracheoesophageal Fistula

A tracheoesophageal fistula should be suspected when polyhydramnios is present (see Chapter 24). An initial diagnosis in the delivery room is suggested when a catheter is inserted into the esophagus but cannot be passed into the stomach. Copious amounts of oropharyngeal secretions are usually present. Chest radiographs with the catheter in place confirm the diagnosis.

Laryngeal Anomalies

Stridor is present at birth as a manifestation of laryngeal anomalies and subglottic stenosis. Insertion of a tube into the trachea beyond the obstruction alleviates the symptoms. Vascular rings are anomalies of the aorta that may compress the trachea, producing both inspiratory and expiratory obstruction. It may be difficult to advance a tracheal tube beyond the obstruction produced by vascular rings.

KEY POINTS

- Physiologic changes of pregnancy affect all organ systems. They influence maternal compensation for comorbidities and maternal responses to anesthesia.

- There is less fetal drug exposure with regional anesthesia. Any well-conducted anesthetic is safe.

- Maintain blood pressure, oxygenation, and normocarbia.

- PIH delivery is the definitive treatment. Temporize only if the risk of neonatal immaturity outweighs maternal risk.

- Co-existing medical diseases may result in maternal decompensation related to physiologic changes of pregnancy.

- Fetal assessment permits evaluation of fetal well-being and guides neonatal management.

REFERENCES

Bridges EJ, Womble S, Wallace M, McCartney J: Hemodynamic monitoring in high-risk obstetrics patients. II. Pregnancy-induced hypertension and preeclampsia. Crit Care Nurse 2003;23:53–57.

Casey BM, McIntire DD, Leveno KJ: The continuing value of the Apgar score for the assessment of newborn infants. N Engl J Med 2001;344:467–471.

Davies S: Amniotic fluid embolus: A review of the literature. Can J Anaesth 2001;48:88–98.

Eisenach JC: Combined spinal-epidural analgesia in obstetrics. Anesthesiology 1999;91:299–302.

Koren G, Pastusak A, Ito S: Drugs in pregnancy (review). N Engl J Med 1998;338:1128–1137.

Mushambi MC, Halligan AW, Williamson K: Recent developments in the pathophysiology and management of pre-eclampsia. Br J Anaesth 1996;76:133–148.

Roberts JM, Lain KY: Recent insights into the pathogenesis of preeclampsia. Placenta 2002;23:359–372.

Rosen MA: Management of anesthesia for the pregnant surgical patient. Anesthesiology 1999;91:1159–1163.

Visalyaputra S, Rodanant O, Somboonviboon W, et al: Spinal versus epidural anesthesia for cesarean delivery in severe preeclampsia: A prospective randomized, multicenter study. Anesth Analg 2005;101:862–868.

Wong CA, Scavone BM, Peaceman AM, et al: The risk of cesarean delivery with neuraxial analgesia given early versus late in labor. N Engl J Med 2005;352:655–665.

CHAPTER 24

Pediatric Diseases

Charles Lee
Igor Luginbuehl
Bruno Bissonnette
Linda J. Mason

- Postintubation Laryngeal Edema
- Foreign Body Aspiration
- Laryngeal Papillomatosis
- Lung Abscess

Malignant Hyperthermia
- Signs and Symptoms
- Diagnosis
- Treatment
- Prognosis
- Identification of Susceptible Patients
- Management of Anesthesia

Familial Dysautonomia
- Signs and Symptoms
- Diagnosis

- Treatment
- Prognosis
- Management of Anesthesia

Solid Tumors
- Neuroblastoma
- Nephroblastoma

Oncologic Emergencies
- Mediastinal Tumors

Burn (Thermal) Injuries
- Signs and Symptoms
- Cardiac Output
- Systemic Hypertension
- Airway

UNIQUE CONSIDERATIONS IN PEDIATRIC PATIENTS

The needs of infants and young children differ greatly from those of adults. Pediatric patients, especially neonates and infants younger than 6 months of age, have anatomic and physiologic differences that place them at higher risk of anesthetic complications than adults. Differences in responses to pharmacologic agents in this population further add to the complexity of administering anesthesia to these patients. Many diseases present exclusively or with greater frequency in this age group.

Airway Anatomy

The large head and tongue, mobile epiglottis, and anterior position of the larynx characteristic of neonates makes tracheal intubation easier with the neonate's head at a neutral or slightly flexed position than with the head hyperextended. Because the infant's larynx is higher in the neck than in adults, the infant's tongue obstructs the airway more easily. The cricoid cartilage (as opposed to the vocal cords in adults) is the narrowest portion of the larynx in pediatric patients and necessitates the use of tracheal tubes that minimize risks of trauma to the airway and subsequent development of subglottic edema. As in adults, angulation of the right mainstem bronchus favors right endobronchial intubation if the tracheal tube is inserted beyond the carina.

Physiology

Physiologic differences between children and adults are important determinants when planning management of anesthesia in pediatric patients. Monitoring vital signs and organ function during the perioperative period is especially important, as neonates and infants have decreased physiologic reserves.

Respiratory System

The single most important difference that physiologically distinguishes pediatric patients from adult patients is oxygen consumption. Oxygen consumption of neonates is more than 6 mL/kg, which is approximately twice that of adults on a weight basis (**Table 24-1**). To satisfy this high demand, alveolar ventilation is doubled compared with that in adults. Because the tidal volume on a weight basis is similar for infants and adults, the increased alveolar ventilation is accomplished by an increased breathing rate. PaO_2 increases rapidly after birth, but several days are needed to achieve the levels present in older children.

Cardiovascular System

Birth and the initiation of spontaneous ventilation initiate circulatory changes, permitting neonates to survive in an extrauterine environment. Fetal circulation is characterized by high pulmonary vascular resistance, low systemic vascular resistance (placenta), and right-to-left shunting of blood through the foramen ovale and ductus arteriosus. The onset of spontaneous ventilation at birth is associated with decreased pulmonary vascular resistance and increased pulmonary blood flow. As the left atrial pressure increases, the foramen ovale functionally closes. Anatomic closure of the foramen ovale occurs between 3 months and 1 year of age, although 20% to 30% of adults have probe-patent foramen ovales. Functional closure of the ductus arteriosus normally occurs 10 to 15 hours after birth, with anatomic closure taking place in 4 to 6 weeks. Constriction of the ductus arteriosus occurs in response to increased arterial oxygenation that develops after birth. Nevertheless, the ductus arteriosus may reopen during periods of arterial hypoxemia. A diagnosis of persistent fetal circulation can be confirmed by measuring the PaO_2 in blood samples obtained simultaneously from preductal (right radial) and postductal (umbilical, posterior tibial,

TABLE 24-1 Mean Pulmonary Function Values

Parameter	Neonates (3 kg)	Adults (70 kg)
Oxygen consumption (mL/kg/min)	6.4	3.5
Alveolar ventilation (mL/kg/min)	130	60
Carbon dioxide production (mL/kg/min)	6	3
Tidal volume (mL/kg)	6	6
Breathing frequency (min)	35	15
Vital capacity (mL/kg)	35	70
Functional residual capacity (mL/kg)	30	35
Tracheal length (cm)	5.5	12
Pao_2 (room air, mm Hg)	65–85	85–95
$Paco_2$ (room air, mm Hg)	30–36	36–44
pH	7.34–7.40	7.36–7.44

TABLE 24-2 Intraoperative Fluid Therapy for Pediatric Patients

Procedure	NORMAL SALINE OR/LACTATED RINGER'S SOLUTION (mL/kg/hr)		
	Maintenance	Replacement	Total
Minor surgery (herniorrhaphy)	4	2	6
Moderate surgery (pyloromyotomy)	4	4	8
Extensive surgery (bowel resection)	4	6	10

dorsalis pedis) arteries. The presence of Pao_2 differences of more than 20 mm Hg in these simultaneously obtained blood samples confirms the diagnosis.

Neonates are highly dependent on heart rate to maintain cardiac output and systemic blood pressure. Vasoconstrictive responses to hemorrhage are less in neonates than in adults. For example, a 10% decrease in intravascular fluid volume is likely to cause a 15% to 30% decrease in mean arterial pressure in neonates. The hypotension that accompanies administration of volatile anesthetics to premature neonates is most likely due to decreased intravascular fluid volume and/or anesthetic overdose.

Distribution of Body Water

Total body water content and extracellular fluid (ECF) volume are increased proportionately in neonates. The ECF volume is equivalent to approximately 40% of body weight in neonates compared with approximately 20% in adults. By 18 to 24 months of age, the proportion of ECF volume relative to body weight is similar to that in adults. The increased metabolic rate characteristic of neonates results in accelerated turnover of ECF and dictates meticulous attention to intraoperative fluid replacement. Intraoperative fluid replacement often includes glucose, although the clinical impression that pediatric patients are more susceptible than adults to hypoglycemia during fasting periods has been challenged (**Table 24-2**).

Renal Function

The glomerular filtration rate is greatly decreased in term neonates but increases nearly fourfold by 3 to 5 weeks. Preterm neonates may show delayed increases in the glomerular filtration rate. Neonates are obligate sodium losers and cannot concentrate urine as effectively as adults. Therefore, adequate exogenous sodium and water must be provided during the perioperative period. Conversely, neonates are likely to excrete volume loads more slowly than adults and are therefore more susceptible to fluid overload. Decreased renal function can also delay excretion of drugs dependent on renal clearance for elimination.

Hematology

Characteristics of fetal hemoglobin influence oxygen transport. For example, fetal hemoglobin has a P_{50} (the partial pressure of oxygen at which hemoglobin is 50% saturated) of 19 mm Hg compared with 26 mm Hg for adults, which results in a leftward shift of the fetal oxyhemoglobin dissociation curve. Subsequent increased affinity of hemoglobin for oxygen manifests as decreased oxygen release to peripheral tissues. This decreased release is offset by increased oxygen delivery provided by the increased hemoglobin concentrations characteristic of neonates (**Table 24-3**). By 2 to 3 months of age, however, physiologic anemia results. After 3 months, there are progressive increases in erythrocyte mass and hematocrit. By 4 to 6 months, the oxyhemoglobin dissociation curve approximates that of adults. In view of the decreased cardiovascular reserve of neonates and the leftward shift of the oxyhemoglobin dissociation curve, it may be useful to maintain the neonate's hematocrit closer to 40% than 30%, as is often accepted for older children. Calculation of the estimated erythrocyte mass and the acceptable erythrocyte loss provides a useful guide for intraoperative blood replacement (**Table 24-4**).

The need for routine preoperative hemoglobin determinations is controversial. Routine preoperative hemoglobin determinations in children younger than 1 year of age results in the detection of only a small number of patients with hemoglobin concentrations less than 10 g/dL, and this rarely influences management of anesthesia or delays planned surgery. Because of the potential benefit of identifying anemia during infancy, routine preoperative hemoglobin testing may be justifiable only in this age group.

TABLE 24-3 Normal Hemogram Values in Neonates, Infants, and Children

Age	Hemoglobin (g/dL)	Hematocrit (%)	Leukocytes (cells/mm^3)
1 day	19.0	61	18,000
2 wk	17.3	54	12,000
1 mo	14.2	43	
2 mo	10.7	31	
6 mo	12.3	36	10,000
1 yr	11.6	35	
6 yr	12.7	38	
10–12 yr	13.0	39	8000

Thermoregulation

Neonates and infants are vulnerable to the development of hypothermia during the perioperative period. Body heat is lost more rapidly in this age group than in older children or adults because of the large body surface area relative to body weight, the thin layer of insulating subcutaneous fat, and a decreased ability to produce heat. Shivering is of little significance during heat production in neonates, whose primary mechanism is nonshivering thermogenesis mediated by brown fat. Brown fat is a specialized adipose tissue located in the neonate's posterior neck, in the interscapular and vertebral areas, and surrounding the kidneys and adrenal glands. Metabolism of brown fat is stimulated by norepinephrine and results in triglyceride hydrolysis and thermogenesis.

An important mechanism for loss of body heat in operating rooms is radiation. To minimize oxygen consumption, the neonate must be in a neutral thermal environment. Neutral temperature is defined as the ambient temperature that results in the least oxygen consumption (**Table 24-5**). The critical temperature is that ambient temperature below which an unclothed, unanesthetized person cannot maintain a normal core body temperature (see Table 24-5). Most operating rooms are below the critical temperature of even a term neonate, and it is imperative that heat loss be minimized. Steps aimed at decreasing loss of body heat include transporting neonates in heated modules, increasing the ambient temperature of operating rooms, using a heating mattress, radiant warmer, corrective forced-air warming devices, and humidifying and warming inspired gases.

Pharmacology

Pharmacologic responses to drugs may differ in pediatric patients and adults. They manifest as differences in anesthetic requirements, responses to muscle relaxants, and pharmacokinetics.

Anesthetic Requirements

Full-term neonates require *lower* concentrations of volatile anesthetics than do infants 1 to 6 months of age. For example, the minimum alveolar concentration (MAC) is approximately 25% less in neonates than in infants. Furthermore, MAC in preterm neonates less than 32 weeks' gestational age is less than MAC in preterm neonates 32 to 37 weeks' gestational age, and MAC for both of these age groups is less than that in full-term neonates. Decreased anesthetic requirements in neonates may be related to immaturity of the central nervous system and to increased circulating concentrations of progesterone and β-endorphins. MAC steadily increases until 2 to 3 months of age, but after 3 months, the MAC steadily declines with age, although there are slight increases at puberty.

In contrast, sevoflurane, which has essentially replaced halothane for use in pediatric anesthesia, is unique among the currently used volatile anesthetics. The MAC of sevoflurane in neonates and infants younger than 6 months (3.2%) and in infants older than 6 months and children up to 12 years (2.5%) remains constant. The reason that the MAC of sevoflurane does not decline with advancing age in childhood, as is seen with the other volatile anesthetics, is unclear.

TABLE 24-4 Estimation of Acceptable Blood Loss*

A 3.2-kg term neonate is scheduled for intra-abdominal surgery. The preoperative hematocrit is 50%. What is the acceptable intraoperative blood loss to maintain the hematocrit at 40%?

Parameter	Calculation
Estimated blood volume	85 mL/kg × 3.2 kg = 272 mL
Estimated erythrocyte mass	272 mL × 0.5 = 136 mL
Estimated erythrocyte mass to maintain hematocrit at 40%	272 mL × 0.4 = 109 mL
Acceptable intraoperative erythrocyte loss	136 mL − 109 mL = 27 mL
Acceptable intraoperative blood loss to maintain hematocrit at 40%	27 × 2[†] = 54 mL

*These calculations are only guidelines and do not consider the potential impact of intravenous infusion of crystalloid or colloid solutions on the hematocrit.
[†]Factor to correct the original hematocrit to 50%.

TABLE 24-5	Neutral and Critical Temperatures	
Patient Age	Neutral Temperature (°C)	Critical Temperature (°C)
Preterm neonate	34	28
Term neonate	32	23
Adult	28	1

Muscle Relaxants

Morphologic and functional maturation of the neuromuscular junctions are not complete until approximately 2 months of age, but the implications of this initial immaturity on the pharmacodynamics of muscle relaxants are not clear. Due to immature muscle composition, the infant's diaphragm is paralyzed at the same time as the peripheral muscles (as opposed to later in adults). This has led to the suggestion that infants may be more sensitive to the effects of nondepolarizing muscle relaxants, but the relatively large volume of distribution results in initial doses that are similar on a weight basis to those for adults. Immaturity of hepatic or renal function could prolong the duration of action of muscle relaxants that are highly dependent on these mechanisms for their clearance. Antagonism of neuromuscular blockade seems to be reliable in infants, and requirements for anticholinesterase drugs may be decreased due to longer clearance times than in adults.

Neonates and infants require more succinylcholine on a body weight basis than do older children to produce comparable degrees of neuromuscular blockade. Presumably, this response reflects increased ECF volumes characteristic of this age group, resulting in larger volumes of distribution of succinylcholine. The incidence of adverse side effects of succinylcholine (myoglobinuria, malignant hyperthermia [MH], hyperkalemia) limits the use of this drug in children (especially younger than age 5) to rapid securing of the airway and treatment of laryngospasm.

Pharmacokinetics

Pharmacokinetics differ in neonates and infants compared with adults. For example, uptake of inhaled anesthetics is more rapid in infants than in older children or adults. This accelerated uptake most likely reflects the infant's high alveolar ventilation relative to functional residual capacity. More rapid uptake may unmask negative inotropic effects of volatile anesthetics, resulting in an increased incidence of hypotension in neonates and infants during administration of volatile anesthetics. Considering these factors, a decreased margin of safety when volatile anesthetics are administered to infants is predictable.

An immature blood-brain barrier and decreased ability to metabolize drugs could increase the sensitivity of neonates to the effects of barbiturates and opioids. As a result, neonates might require lower doses of barbiturates for induction of anesthesia. Nevertheless, children between the ages of 5 and 15 years require somewhat higher doses of thiopental than do adults for induction of anesthesia. Similarly, the non-barbiturate hypnotic, propofol demonstrates a higher dose requirement in infants (ED_{50} of 3.0 mg/kg in infants ages 1–6 months) than in older children (ED_{50} of 2.4 mg/kg in children aged 10–16 years) for induction of anesthesia.

Decreased hepatic and renal clearance of drugs, which is characteristic of neonates, can produce prolonged drug effects. Clearance rates increase to adult levels by 5 to 6 months of age and during early childhood may even exceed adult rates. Protein binding of many drugs is decreased in infants, which could result in high circulating concentrations of unbound and pharmacologically active drugs.

Monitoring

Oscillometric methods for noninvasive measurements of systemic blood pressure are reliable for pediatric patients. Selecting the proper cuff size is critical, as a cuff that is too large for the patient's arm results in falsely low readings. A catheter placed in a peripheral artery may be the method selected to monitor systemic blood pressure and to obtain blood samples for analysis of blood gases and pH. The peripheral artery selected in neonates is uniquely important, as blood sampled from an artery that arises distal to the ductus arteriosus (left radial artery, umbilical artery, posterior tibial artery) may not accurately reflect the PaO_2 being delivered to the retina or brain in the presence of a patent ductus arteriosus. If retinopathy of prematurity (ROP) is a consideration, a preductal artery, such as the right radial artery should be cannulated.

Monitoring body temperature is useful during the perioperative period to detect the development of hypothermia as well as the rare patient manifesting malignant hyperthermia (MH). Hypothermia, as is likely to occur in neonates or infants during anesthesia, results in increased total body oxygen consumption, depression of ventilation, bradycardia, metabolic acidosis, and hypoglycemia. Monitoring end-tidal carbon dioxide concentrations is reliable in children, although there are some limitations in neonates and infants. For example, because of small tidal volumes and high inspired gas flows, exhaled carbon dioxide concentrations may be diluted, producing falsely low values when measuring end-tidal carbon dioxide concentrations.

DISEASES OF THE NEONATE

In the past, infants weighing less than 2500 g at birth were considered premature. However, term infants can weigh less than 2500 g depending on in utero exposure to certain drugs, infections, toxemia, placental insufficiency, and maternal malnutrition. Infants are considered premature if they are born before 37 weeks of gestation. In general, preterm infants can be divided into three groups (**Table 24-6**).

Respiratory Distress Syndrome

Respiratory distress syndrome (RDS), or hyaline membrane disease, is responsible for 50% to 75% of deaths

TABLE 24-6	Classification of Prematurity
Degree of Prematurity	Gestational Age (wk)
Borderline	36–37 wk
Moderate	31–36 wk
Severe	24–30 wk

in preterm neonates. Incidence is inversely proportional to the gestational age and birth weight. This syndrome manifests as progressive impairment of gas exchange at the alveolar level due to deficient production and secretion of surface-active phospholipids known as surfactant. Surfactant, produced by type II pneumocytes, helps maintain alveolar stability by reducing alveolar surface tension. Without surfactant, alveoli collapse and there is failure to develop a functional residual capacity, leading to right-to-left shunting, arterial hypoxemia, and metabolic acidosis. Mature levels of pulmonary surfactant are not present until 35 weeks of gestation.

Signs and Symptoms

Signs of RDS usually become apparent within minutes of birth. Tachypnea, prominent grunting, intercostal and subcostal retractions, nasal flaring, and duskiness are typically noted. Cyanosis, which may not improve despite oxygen administration, and dyspnea progressively worsen. Apnea and irregular respirations are ominous signs of fatigue requiring immediate intervention. Without adequate treatment, hypotension, hypothermia, a mixed respiratory-metabolic acidosis, edema, ileus, and oliguria may ensue.

Diagnosis

The clinical course, chest radiograph, and blood gas analysis help to establish the diagnosis of RDS. The typical radiographic appearance of the lungs is a fine reticular granularity of the parenchyma and air bronchograms. Blood gas findings are characterized by progressive hypoxemia, hypercarbia, and variable metabolic acidosis. Group B streptococcal sepsis may be indistinguishable from RDS, but maternal colonization, gram-positive cocci in the gastric or tracheal aspirates, and buffy coat smear may help distinguish this diagnosis. Congenital alveolar proteinosis is a rare familial disease that often presents as a severe and lethal form of RDS.

Treatment

Because most cases of RDS are self-limiting, care is primarily supportive. The primary defect requiring treatment is progressive impairment in pulmonary exchange of oxygen and carbon dioxide. Until adequate surfactant can be produced, arterial oxygenation must be maintained using supplemental oxygen, with or without mechanical ventilation of the lungs. Infants with severe RDS or those who develop persistent apnea or who cannot maintain an arterial oxygen tension greater than 50 mm Hg while breathing 70% to 100% oxygen require assisted mechanical ventilation. Acceptable ranges of blood gas values during mechanical ventilation are Pao_2 of 55 to 70 mm Hg, Pco_2 of 45 to 55 mm Hg, and pH of 7.25 to 7.45. During mechanical ventilation, oxygenation is improved by increasing the Fio_2 or the mean airway pressure (by increasing the peak inspiratory pressure (PIP), gas flow, inspiratory to expiratory ratio, or positive end-expiratory pressure) and carbon dioxide elimination is achieved by increasing the PIP (tidal volume) or the rate of ventilation. High-frequency oscillatory ventilation may improve carbon dioxide elimination, lower mean airway pressure, and improve oxygenation in infants who do not respond to conventional ventilators.

Prognosis

In most cases, gradual improvement occurs after several days, heralded by spontaneous diuresis and reduced oxygen requirements. Death is usually associated with alveolar air leaks from interstitial emphysema or pneumothorax and pulmonary or intraventricular hemorrhage. Antenatal corticosteroid administration, postnatal surfactant use, improved modes of ventilation, and skilled supportive care have resulted in steadily declining mortality from RDS.

Management of Anesthesia

During anesthesia, the Pao_2 in patients with RDS is maintained near its preoperative levels. Volatile anesthetics can alter arterial oxygenation by decreasing cardiac output. An intra-arterial catheter is useful during surgery to assess oxygenation, avoid hyperoxia, and prevent respiratory and metabolic acidosis. Ideally, the Pao_2 is monitored from blood obtained from a preductal artery. However, the patient may already have an umbilical artery catheter or arterial cannulation may not be feasible, in which case the umbilical artery catheter or pulse oximetry (for short procedures) may be acceptable for monitoring oxygenation. Pneumothorax secondary to barotrauma is an ever-present danger and should be considered if oxygenation deteriorates abruptly during mechanical ventilation. Hypotension is a frequently encountered problem during anesthesia. Administration of albumin (1 g/kg IV) to premature neonates with RDS will likely increase the blood volume and glomerular filtration rate. Maintaining the neonate's hematocrit near 40% may optimize oxygen delivery to tissues. Excessive hydration is to be avoided as this may reopen the ductus arteriosus. Patients who tolerate early extubation should be monitored postoperatively for apnea and bradycardia.

Bronchopulmonary Dysplasia

Bronchopulmonary dysplasia (BPD) is a chronic disease of lung parenchyma and small airways that most commonly results from lung injury in small premature infants requiring prolonged mechanical ventilation. Although prematurity, mechanical pulmonary trauma, and oxygen toxicity are crucial factors in the pathogenesis of BPD, other risk factors also play a role (**Table 24-7**).

TABLE 24-7 Factors That Contribute to the Pathogenesis of Bronchopulmonary Dysplasia

Factors Associated with Prematurity
Positive pressure ventilation
High inspired oxygen concentration
Inflammation (alone or associated with infection)
Pulmonary edema (due to patent ductus arteriosus or excess fluid administration)
Pulmonary air leak
Nutritional deficiencies
Airway hyperreactivity
Early adrenal insufficiency

Other Factors
Meconium aspiration pneumonia
Neonatal pneumonia
Congestive heart failure
Wilson-Mikity syndrome

Signs and Symptoms

BPD results when some neonates with RDS develop persistent respiratory distress characterized by increased airway reactivity and resistance, decreased pulmonary compliance, ventilation-to-perfusion mismatch, hypoxemia, hypercarbia, tachypnea, and, in severe cases, right heart failure. Oxygen consumption is increased by as much as 25%. Failure to thrive is a sign of chronic hypoxia. Auscultation of the lungs may not reveal wheezing because the site of airway hyperreactivity is primarily in the small airways in the periphery of the lungs.

Diagnosis

BPD is a clinical diagnosis defined as oxygen dependence at 36 weeks' postconceptual age with oxygen requirements (to maintain Pa_{O_2} >50 mm Hg) beyond 28 days of life in infants with birth weights less than 1500 g. The radiographic appearance of the lungs gradually changes from a picture of almost complete opacification with air bronchograms and interstitial emphysema to one of small, round, radiolucent areas alternating with areas of irregular density resembling a sponge.

Treatment

Most infants with moderate to severe BPD remain oxygen dependent, with or without ventilator dependence, beyond 4 weeks of age. Maintenance of adequate oxygenation (with Pa_{O_2} >55 mm Hg and Sp_{O_2} >94%) is necessary to prevent or treat cor pulmonale and to promote growth of lung tissue and remodeling of the pulmonary vascular bed. Reactive airway bronchoconstriction is treated with bronchodilating agents. Cor pulmonale and severe chest retractions that draw fluid into the interstitial space cause fluid retention, necessitating fluid restriction and diuretic administration in order to decrease pulmonary edema and improve gas exchange.

Prognosis

Pulmonary dysfunction in patients with BPD is most marked during the first year of life. Infants with mild BPD may eventually become asymptomatic, but airway hyperreactivity may persist.

Management of Anesthesia

Before anesthetizing a child with a history of BPD, a baseline oxygen saturation measurement should be obtained with a pulse oximeter. Desaturation may be rapid when apnea occurs. The choice of drugs for anesthesia in patients with BPD is not as important as management of the airway. In children with a history of mechanical ventilation, an endotracheal tube one size smaller than the appropriate size for the patient's age should be available as subglottic stenosis may be present. Tracheomalacia and bronchomalacia may also present as sequelae of prolonged intubation in patients with BPD. The possible presence of airway hyperreactivity and increased risk of bronchospasm warrants establishing a surgical level of anesthesia before instrumenting the airway. Children who have or have had BPD can be assumed to have reactive airway disease (RAD) and should be treated similarly to those with asthma. Some patients with BPD may require increased peak airway pressures and oxygen concentrations intraoperatively. High airway pressures may cause pneumothorax. Adequate oxygen should be delivered to maintain a Pa_{O_2} of 50 to 70 mm Hg. Patients with metabolic alkalosis from furosemide therapy may exhibit a compensatory retention of CO_2. Hyperventilation of patients with compensated metabolic alkalosis may cause hypotension from severe alkalosis. Fluid administration should be monitored and minimized to avoid pulmonary edema.

Intracranial Hemorrhage

The four types of intracranial hemorrhage that occur during the neonatal period are subdural, primary subarachnoid, intercellular, and periventricular-intraventricular (intraventricular hemorrhage [IVH]). The most frequent and important type of intracranial hemorrhage is IVH. Its incidence is inversely related to gestational age or birth weight and is a major complication in premature neonates. Incomplete autoregulation of cerebral blood flow and immaturity of neonatal cerebral capillary beds predispose the vessels in the germinal matrix to rupture as a result of abrupt or severe changes in blood flow, with resultant hemorrhage. Although newborn prematurity is the single most important risk factor for intracranial hemorrhage, both perinatal and postnatal events have been identified in the etiology of IVH.

Signs and Symptoms

Clinical features can range from subtle and not easily elicited neurologic aberrations to catastrophic deterioration with rapid onset of coma.

Diagnosis

The diagnosis of IVH can be made by maintaining a high index of suspicion in susceptible neonates, by clinical signs of encephalopathy, and neuroimaging. Cranial ultrasonography, or echoencephalography, is the method of choice for diagnosis of IVH.

Treatment

The administration of antenatal corticosteroids and prevention or delay of preterm delivery with tocolytic therapy has been associated with a reduced incidence of intracranial hemorrhage as a result of decreasing the risk of RDS. Important supportive measures in the prevention of IVH include expanding volume slowly, maintaining blood pressure stability, and avoiding blood pressure fluctuations that may adversely affect cerebral blood flow velocity.

Prognosis

Intraventricular hemorrhage occurs in 40% to 60% of neonates of less than 34 weeks of gestation or very low birth weight ($\leq$1250 g). Those patients with the lowest gestational ages and extremely low birth weights are more likely to experience the highest grades of hemorrhage. Clinical events such as pneumothoraces and seizures, which are known to increase cerebral blood flow, can extend acute IVH. Hydrocephalus and death are more common in infants with the highest grades of hemorrhage.

Management of Anesthesia

There is no evidence to suggest that the stress of general anesthesia worsens preexisting intraventricular hemorrhage. Metabolic derangements (e.g., acidosis, hypoglycemia, hypercarbia, hypocarbia, hypoxia, hyponatremia, hypernatremia, hypocalcemia) can cause hemodynamic instability and must be corrected. Incomplete autoregulation of cerebral blood flow places the premature neonate's normal blood pressure at the lower range of the autoregulatory limit. In view of the impaired autoregulation of cerebral blood flow, systolic blood pressures should be maintained within normal ranges to decrease the risk of cerebral hyperperfusion. Hypotension, hypertensive spikes, and rapid volume expansion can all cause alterations in cerebral circulation, and attempts should be made to minimize these occurrences.

Retinopathy of Prematurity

Retinopathy of prematurity (ROP), formerly known as retrolental fibroplasia, is a vasoproliferative retinopathy of multifactorial etiology that occurs almost exclusively in preterm infants in whom retinal vasculogenesis is incomplete. The risk of retinopathy is inversely related to birth weight and gestational age.

The immature retina responds to injury to the developing retinal capillaries by arrest of normal vasculogenesis followed later by disorganized reactive neovascularization and fibrous tissue formation in the retina and vitreous humor. Retinal vasculogenesis is complete by 44 weeks postconception, after which time the risk of ROP is negligible.

The risk factors associated with ROP are not fully known. Hyperoxia is a major risk factor, but oxygen alone is not sufficient to produce ROP, which has been documented even in the absence of oxygen therapy. Concentration, duration, timing, and fluctuation of oxygen may all play a role in the development of ROP. Nevertheless, prematurity with associated retinal immaturity is unquestionably the strongest risk factor. Other identified risk factors for ROP include sepsis, congenital infections, congenital heart disease, mechanical ventilation, RDS, blood transfusions, IVH, hypoxia, hyper- and hypocapnia, asphyxia, and vitamin E deficiency.

Signs and Symptoms

Clinical manifestations range from mild, transient changes of the peripheral retina to severe progressive extraretinal vasoproliferation (over the surface of the retina as well as into the vitreous humor), cicatrization, and subsequent retinal detachment. Retinal detachment is the primary cause of visual impairment and blindness in ROP.

Diagnosis

Ophthalmologic examination at 6 weeks of chronologic age or at 32 weeks' postconceptual age is recommended in premature infants weighing less than 1500 g at birth and in those born before 28 weeks of gestation. In the normal developing retina, there is a gradual transition from vascularized to avascular retina. In patients with ROP, there is an abrupt termination of the vessels, marked by a linear demarcation in the retina.

Treatment

Transscleral cryotherapy or laser photocoagulation is used to destroy the peripheral avascular areas of the retina, resulting in slowing or reversing the abnormal growth of blood vessels, which may reduce the risk of retinal detachment. Central vision is preserved at the expense of some peripheral vision. Surgical options aimed at relieving cicatrix-induced traction on the retina allow the retina to relax and reattach and may be considered in infants who do not respond to laser or cryotherapy. Scleral buckle may be performed on infants if a shallow retinal detachment develops due to traction from fibrovascular scar tissue.

Prognosis

Fortunately, approximately 80% to 90% of acute cases of ROP undergo spontaneous regression with little or no residual effects or visual disability. Infants who develop ROP are at higher risk of developing ophthalmologic problems later in life including retinal tears, retinal detachment, myopia, strabismus, amblyopia, and glaucoma.

Management of Anesthesia

Management of anesthesia in patients with ROP introduces the dilemma of trying to minimize oxygen administration to a group of patients who are also susceptible to arterial hypoxemia. The STOP-ROP multicenter controlled trial revealed that the use of supplemental oxygen at pulse oximetry saturations of 96% to 99% did not worsen preexisting prethreshold ROP. Because the optimal intraoperative oxygen saturation for these infants is yet to be determined, it would seem prudent to limit oxygen supplementation, especially to those infants without a diagnosis of ROP, during the period of retinal vascularization. Efforts should be made to maintain Pa_{O_2} between 50 and 80 mm Hg and Pa_{CO_2} between 35 and 45 mm Hg, maintaining oxygen saturation at a pulse oximetry target of 89% to 94%. While it is desirable to avoid hyperoxia, arterial hypoxemia can be life threatening and more deleterious. Oxygen should not be withheld from patients who require high inspired oxygen concentrations to maintain cardiovascular stability and neurologic function. Infants undergoing peripheral retinal ablation have an increased incidence of apnea and bradycardia both during the procedure and in the following 1 to 3 days.

Apnea

Apnea is defined as a cessation of breathing that lasts longer than 20 seconds or of any duration if accompanied by cyanosis and bradycardia. Periodic breathing and apnea are common in preterm infants and are usually due to idiopathic apnea of prematurity. However, it may also be the presenting sign of other neonatal diseases. Idiopathic apnea of prematurity is a disorder of respiratory control and may be obstructive, central, or mixed. Obstructive apnea can result from pharyngeal instability, neck flexion, and nasal occlusion. Central apnea is attributed to an immature respiratory control mechanism.

Signs and Symptoms

In central apnea, there is a complete cessation of airflow and respiratory efforts with no chest wall movement. In obstructive apnea, on the other hand, airflow is absent despite chest wall movements. The majority (50%–75%) of apnea episodes in preterm neonates are of mixed etiology. Apnea episodes of short duration tend to be central, whereas those of long duration are often mixed.

Diagnosis

Idiopathic apnea of prematurity varies inversely with gestational age. Onset of idiopathic apnea typically occurs on the second to seventh days of life. Onset of apnea after the second week of life in a previously asymptomatic premature neonate or at any time in a term infant may be a worrisome occurrence that warrants investigation. Apnea must be differentiated from periodic breathing, which is characterized by regular breathing that is interrupted by short pauses or apnea lasting 5 to 10 seconds without cyanosis or changes in heart rate. The apneic pauses are followed by a burst of rapid respirations. Periodic breathing may be exhibited in normal full-term infants as well as in premature infants and is considered a normal characteristic of neonatal respiration without long-term significance.

Treatment

Apnea monitors should be used on infants at risk of apnea. Infants with mild episodes may require only gentle cutaneous stimulation, while infants with recurrent and prolonged episodes require immediate bag and mask ventilation. Oxygen should be administered to treat hypoxia, which increases minute ventilation. Oxygen improves carbon dioxide sensitivity, decreases hypoxic respiratory depression, decreases periodic breathing, and enhances diaphragmatic strength and activity. Theophylline (orally) or aminophylline (intravenously) is given as a loading dose of 5 mg/kg followed by a maintenance regimen of 1 to 2 mg/kg given every 6 to 8 hours. Caffeine is administered as a loading dose of 10 mg/kg followed by maintenance doses of 2.5 mg/kg per day orally. Obstructive or mixed apneas may be effectively treated with high-flow nasal cannula therapy (1–2.5 L/min) and nasal continuous positive airway pressure of 3 to 6 cm H_2O. Continuous positive airway pressure splints the upper airway and may increase functional residual capacity, improving oxygenation. Transfusions of packed red blood cells may be helpful in severely anemic infants.

Prognosis

Apnea of prematurity usually resolves by 36 weeks' postconceptual age. In the absence of significant life-threatening events, monitoring can often be discontinued at 44 to 45 weeks' postconceptual age.

Management of Anesthesia

Life-threatening apnea has been reported postoperatively in former preterm infants following even minor surgeries such as inguinal hernia repair. The risk of apnea in prematurely born infants correlates inversely to both gestational age as well as postconceptual age. In addition to a history of apnea, anemia (hematocrit < 30) is also a risk factor for postoperative apnea, independent of gestational or postconceptual age.

Inhaled and injected anesthetics affect the control of breathing and contribute to upper airway obstruction, thus increasing the likelihood of apneic episodes for up to 12 hours postoperatively, especially in preterm infants less than 60 weeks' postconceptual age. The use of pure regional anesthetic techniques unsupplemented by sedative agents is associated with greatly reduced, but not eliminated, risk of postoperative apnea in ex-premature infants. Consequently, ex-premature infants with a history of apnea spells are probably not suitable candidates for outpatient surgery. It is recommended that these patients be admitted and monitored with pulse oximetry and apnea monitors for at least 12 hours after surgery. The risk of postoperative apnea appears to be significantly decreased beyond 50 to 52 weeks' gestational age, leading some authorities to still recommend postponement of nonessential and ambulatory surgery in preterm infants until after this age.

Kernicterus

Hyperbilirubinemia is a common and usually benign problem in neonates. Jaundice may be observed during the first week of life in up to 60% of term infants and 80% of premature infants. Physiologic jaundice results because newborns have higher rates of bilirubin production than adults due to a shorter life span and turnover of red blood cells combined with a diminished ability of an immature liver to conjugate bilirubin into an excretable form.

Kernicterus is a neurologic syndrome caused by the toxic effects of deposition of unconjugated bilirubin in the basal ganglia and brainstem nuclei. The blood-brain barrier of neonates, especially premature neonates, is immature, which may explain the ability of bilirubin to enter the brain and produce cell damage.

Signs and Symptoms

Signs and symptoms of kernicterus typically become apparent 2 to 5 days after birth in term infants and as late as the day 7 in premature infants. The initial signs are nonspecific, being indistinguishable from those of sepsis, asphyxia, hypoglycemia, intracranial hemorrhage, and other acute systemic illnesses in neonates. In neonates with acute kernicterus, lethargy, poor feeding, and loss of the Moro reflex may progress to diminished tendon reflexes and respiratory distress, followed by hypo- and hypertonia, opisthotonus, twitching of the face or limbs, and a shrill high-pitched cry. In advanced cases, convulsions and spasm occur. The classic sequelae of kernicterus is a tetrad of athetoid cerebral palsy, hearing loss, impairment of upward gaze, and enamel dysplasia of the primary teeth.

Diagnosis

Kernicterus is currently diagnosed clinically by a combination of history, physical examination, and laboratory tests. The diagnosis is suggested by a history of jaundice, characteristic neurologic symptoms, and laboratory confirmation of hyperbilirubinemia.

Treatment

Treatment includes phototherapy, exchange blood transfusions, and drugs that induce or enhance activity of the hepatic conjugation system. Modern high-intensity phototherapeutic techniques have greatly decreased the need for more invasive treatment modalities.

Prognosis

Neonates with overt neurologic signs have a grave prognosis. Greater than 75% of infants with neurologic symptoms die. Eighty percent of affected survivors develop bilateral choreoathetosis with involuntary muscle spasms. Mental retardation, deafness, and spastic quadriplegia are common sequelae.

Management of Anesthesia

There are no data concerning effects of anesthesia on the serum concentrations of bilirubin in premature infants. Benzyl alcohol, a preservative agent that was added to normal saline flush solutions in the 1970s, has been implicated in causing kernicterus possibly by displacing bilirubin from albumin and therefore facilitating its entry into the brain. Normal saline diluents and flush solutions preserved with benzyl alcohol can still be found in some operating rooms and should be avoided in neonates. Acidosis, hyperoxia, and hyperosmolarity should also be avoided or corrected in neonates with hyperbilirubinemia.

Hypoglycemia

Hypoglycemia is the most common metabolic problem occurring in newborn infants. Inadequate glycogen stores and deficient gluconeogenesis are important factors in the newborn's susceptibility to hypoglycemia. The incidence of symptomatic hypoglycemia is highest in small-for-gestational age infants. Infants may be at risk of hypoglycemia due to alterations in maternal metabolism, intrinsic neonatal problems, and endocrine or metabolic disorders (**Table 24-8**).

Signs and Symptoms

Many neonates with low serum glucose levels are asymptomatic. The onset of symptoms varies from a few hours to a week after birth. Hypoglycemia that persists beyond the first week of life is uncommon and most often is due to congenital hyperinsulinism. Signs of hypoglycemia in neonates include irritability, apnea, cyanotic spells, seizures, hypotonia,

---

TABLE 24-8 Causes of Neonatal Hypoglycemia

A. Maternal factors
  1. Intrapartum administration of glucose
  2. Drug treatment
    a. β-adrenergic blocking agents (terbutaline, ritodrine, propranolol)
    b. Oral hypoglycemic agents
    c. Salicylates
  3. Maternal diabetes/gestational diabetes
B. Neonatal factors
  1. Depleted glycogen stores
    a. Asphyxia
    b. Perinatal stress
  2. Increased glucose utilization (metabolic demands)
    a. Sepsis
    b. Polycythemia
    c. Hypothermia
    d. Respiratory distress syndrome
    e. Congestive heart failure (cyanotic congenital heart disease)
  3. Limited glycogen stores
    a. Intrauterine growth retardation
    b. Prematurity
  4. Hyperinsulinism/endocrine disorders
    a. Infants of diabetic mothers
    b. Erythroblastosis fetalis, fetal hydrops
    c. Insulinomas
    d. Beckwith-Wiedemann syndrome
    e. Panhypopituitarism
  5. Decreased glycogenolysis, gluconeogenesis, or utilization of alternate fuels
    a. Inborn errors of metabolism
    b. Adrenal insufficiency

lethargy, and difficulty feeding. Many of the clinical manifestations are subtle or nonspecific, and a high index of suspicion must be maintained in high-risk neonates.

Diagnosis

No studies to date have established an absolute serum glucose concentration or duration of hypoglycemia that causes CNS injury in neonates. However, it is known that serum glucose levels are rarely less than 35 to 40 mg/dL in the first 24 hours of life or less than 45 mg/dL thereafter. Central nervous system or systemic signs of hypoglycemia will usually be observed when serum glucose concentrations decrease to less than 20 mg/dL in the premature, 30 mg/dL in term infants during the first 72 hours, and 40 mg/dL thereafter. It may be prudent to keep serum glucose concentrations at greater than 40 mg/dL in all newborns.

Treatment

Infants with symptoms other than seizures should receive an intravenous bolus of 200 mg/kg (2 mL/kg) of 10% dextrose. If the infant is experiencing convulsions, an intravenous bolus of 4 mL/kg of 10% dextrose is indicated. Following bolus administration, a 10% dextrose infusion should be given at 8 mg/kg per minute and titrated to maintain the serum glucose at more than 40 mg/dL. Causes of recurrent and persistent neonatal hypoglycemia include hyperinsulinism, endocrine deficiency, and disorders of carbohydrate, amino acid, or fatty acid metabolism.

Prognosis

The prognosis for normal outcome is good in asymptomatic neonates with transient hypoglycemia. The prognosis for subsequent normal intellectual development is more guarded in symptomatic infants, particularly low birth weight infants, those with persistent hyperinsulinemic hypoglycemia, and infants of diabetic mothers.

Management of Anesthesia

In neonates less than 48 hours old, premature or small-for-gestational age infants, and those born to diabetic mothers, the risk of intraoperative hypoglycemia is significant. As in adults, hypoglycemia is not always symptomatic and manifestations of hypoglycemia may be further attenuated by anesthetic drugs, suggesting the potential value of intraoperative monitoring of blood glucose concentrations and supplemental glucose administration in at-risk neonates. Maintenance fluid requirements may be replaced with a glucose-containing solution 5% dextrose and 0.2 normal saline ([D5 0.2 NS] 4 mL/kg per hour or 10% dextrose in water [D10W] at 2–3 mL/kg per hour) to safeguard against intraoperative hypoglycemia. Hyperglycemia (plasma glucose $\geq$150 mg/dL) may occur in stressed neonates receiving infusions of glucose-containing solutions intraoperatively. Thus, fluid deficits and blood and "third space" losses should be replaced with dextrose-free solutions. Serum glucose concentrations in excess of 125 mg/dL can result in osmotic diuresis from glucosuria, with subsequent dehydration, and

further release of insulin, leading to rebound hypoglycemia. Additionally, a hyperosmolar state in neonates, especially premature very low birth weight neonates, is associated with intraventricular hemorrhage.

Hypocalcemia

Neonates at particular risk of hypocalcemia are low birth weight and premature infants, particularly infants with intrauterine growth retardation, infants of insulin-dependent diabetics, and infants with birth asphyxia associated with prolonged, difficult deliveries. Late neonatal hypocalcemia occurring 5 to 10 days after birth is usually due to ingestion of cow's milk, which contains high levels of phosphorous. It is not seen in breast-fed infants because human breast milk has a lower phosphate content. The high phosphate content of cow's milk, in conjunction with decreased phosphate excretion associated with renal immaturity, can cause hyperphosphatemia and secondary hypocalcemia in the neonate. Other notable causes of hypocalcemia in the newborn include maternal hypercalcemia and DiGeorge syndrome.

Signs and Symptoms

Early neonatal hypocalcemia is one of the most common causes of neonatal seizures, which may be the first manifestation in infants. Along with seizures, signs of hypocalcemia in newborns may include irritability, increased skeletal muscle tone, twitching, tremors, and hypotension. Additional nonspecific symptoms of neonatal hypocalcemia such as poor feeding, vomiting, and lethargy often prompt investigation for sepsis, intracranial hemorrhages, and meningitis.

Diagnosis

Hypocalcemia is defined as serum calcium concentration less than 8 mg/dL in term neonates and less than 7 mg/dL in preterm neonates, or serum ionized calcium concentration less than 4.4 mg/dL (or 1.1 mmol/L). The serum calcium concentration should be corrected for albumin concentration as each 1 g/dL of albumin binds approximately 0.8 mg/dL of calcium. Hypoalbuminemia may falsely suggest a diagnosis of hypocalcemia because the total serum calcium is low even though the ionized calcium concentration remains normal. The ionized calcium concentration, rather than the total calcium, is low in true hypocalcemia.

Treatment

Symptomatic hypocalcemia requires immediate treatment with intravenous administration of calcium. Acute correction of hypocalcemia can be achieved with either the chloride or gluconate forms of calcium. Calcium gluconate 10% (100 mg/mL calcium gluconate and 9 mg/mL of elemental calcium) is commonly used in neonates. It is given at a dose of 100 to 200 mg/kg (1–2 mL/kg) and repeated every 6 to 8 hours until the calcium level stabilizes. Too rapid an infusion rate can cause bradycardia and even asystole due to inhibition of the sinus node. Cardiac monitoring is mandatory, and atropine should be available during replacement therapy. Other potential complications of treatment include soft-tissue necrosis due to extravasation, precipitation in intravenous tubing and small veins when administered concomitantly with bicarbonate, and digitalis toxicity in patients on digoxin.

Prognosis

Early neonatal hypocalcemia usually resolves within a few days without treatment in asymptomatic newborns. Serum calcium levels typically normalize within 1 to 3 days with treatment in symptomatic early neonatal hypocalcemia.

Management of Anesthesia

Hypocalcemia should be corrected preoperatively when possible, and efforts should be made to prevent further decreases in the ionized calcium concentration intraoperatively. Intraoperative metabolic derangements such as alkalosis resulting from hyperventilation and sodium bicarbonate administration can precipitate hypocalcemia by causing calcium to bind to albumin, thereby lowering the ionized calcium concentration. Hypocalcemia can also occur during infusions of albumin and citrated blood products. Rapid intraoperative infusions of citrate, as may occur during exchange transfusions or infusions of citrated blood or fresh frozen plasma, may result in hypocalcemia due to calcium chelation by sodium citrate ions. Hypotensive effects of citrate-induced hypocalcemia can be minimized by administering calcium gluconate (1–2 mg IV) for each milliliter of blood transfused.

Sepsis

As many as 10% of infants experience infections in the first month of life due to immaturity of the immune system. This may be particularly true of premature or low birth weight infants who have a three- to 10-fold higher incidence of infection than full-term, normal birth weight infants. Other circumstances that place this patient population at increased risk are the frequent requirements for prolonged intravenous access, endotracheal intubation, and other invasive procedures that provide a portal of entry for microorganisms. Most nosocomial infections in hospitalized newborns are bloodstream infections related to intravascular catheters.

Signs and Symptoms

Sepsis in neonates may present as acute catastrophic multi-organ dysfunction, but the clinical manifestations are often nonspecific. Consequently, evaluation of sepsis has become an integral part of the evaluation of critically ill neonates. A high level of suspicion must be maintained whenever suggestive signs of sepsis are observed in neonates (**Table 24-9**).

Diagnosis

In contrast to adults, increased body temperature or leukocytosis may be absent in neonates. Fever or temperatures higher than 37.8°C (axillary) may be observed in only approximately 50% of newborns with infection. Neutropenia is more common than neutrophilia in severe neonatal sepsis, but it lacks specificity as it is also associated with preeclampsia and intrauterine growth retardation.

TABLE 24-9	Signs and Symptoms of Infection in Neonates
Fever	
Temperature instability	
Hypoglycemia	
Feeding intolerance	
Apnea	
Respiratory distress	
Cyanosis	
Tachycardia	
Hypotension	
Bradycardia	
Poor perfusion with pallor and mottled skin	
Metabolic acidosis	
Lethargy	
Seizures	

Positive blood cultures are important for confirming the diagnosis of sepsis. When clinical findings suggest an acute infection in the absence of a clear etiology, additional studies including lumbar puncture, urine studies, and a chest radiograph are indicated.

Treatment

Once appropriate cultures have been obtained, antibiotic therapy should be instituted immediately. Initial empirical treatment of bacterial infections in neonates should consist of ampicillin and gentamicin (or another aminoglycoside).

Supportive care includes providing adequate oxygenation of tissues. Due to low functional residual capacity, ventilatory support is frequently necessary for respiratory failure in neonates and young infants with severe sepsis. Shock and metabolic acidosis are treated with fluid resuscitation and inotropic agents as needed. Hyperbilirubinemia should be treated aggressively because the risk of kernicterus increases in the presence of sepsis

Prognosis

Sepsis in neonates is associated with mortality approaching 50%. Complications of sepsis include respiratory failure, pulmonary hypertension, endocarditis, cardiac failure, shock, renal failure, liver dysfunction, cerebral edema or thrombosis, adrenal hemorrhage and/or insufficiency, bone marrow dysfunction (neutropenia, thrombocytopenia, anemia), meningitis, and DIC. The case fatality rate for neonatal sepsis is highest for gram-negative and fungal infections.

Management of Anesthesia

Patients may present for emergency surgical procedures in the presence of fulminant sepsis. Supportive therapy initiated prior to arrival in the operating room should be continued intraoperatively. Care should be taken not to disrupt inotrope and/or vasopressor support in the presence of hemodynamic instability, but the importance of adequate volume resuscitation should not be overlooked. Fluids, electrolytes, and glucose levels should be monitored carefully and deficits corrected as indicated. Arterial cannulation and central vascular access may be necessary to obtain accurate blood pressure measurements and to facilitate aggressive fluid resuscitation in the face of shock and cardiac dysfunction. Corticosteroids should be administered only for adrenal insufficiency that is proven or suggested by profound hypotension refractory to both volume expansion and inotrope therapy.

NEONATAL SURGICAL DISEASES

Neonatal surgical diseases during the first days of life may require immediate life-saving surgery or be best managed by medical stabilization of the neonate followed by corrective surgery (**Table 24-10**). In addition to physiologic aberrations produced by the disease process, incomplete adaptation to the extrauterine environment may further complicate perioperative management.

Congenital Diaphragmatic Hernia

The reported incidence of congenital diaphragmatic hernia (CDH) is approximately 1 in 5000 live births with a male-to-female ratio of 1:1.8. This defect is usually characterized by pulmonary hypoplasia due to in utero compression of the developing lungs by the herniated viscera. In addition to the effects of lung compression, there may be an underlying primary abnormality in airway branching that results in pulmonary hypoplasia. There is incomplete embryologic closure of the diaphragm. The most common and largest diaphragmatic defect occurs through the left posterolateral pleuroperitoneal canal (foramen of Bochdalek), accounting for 75% of cases. The remainder of defects occurs at the right posterolateral foramen of Bochdalek, the anterior foramen of Morgagni, and paraesophageal.

Signs and Symptoms

Signs and symptoms of a CDH evident soon after birth include scaphoid abdomen, barrel-shaped chest, detection of bowel sounds during auscultation of the chest, and profound arterial hypoxemia. Chest radiographs show loops of intestine

TABLE 24-10 Neonatal Surgical Diseases
Congenital diaphragmatic hernia
Esophageal atresia
Abdominal wall defects
Omphalocele
Gastroschisis
Hirschsprung's disease
Imperforate anus
Pyloric stenosis
Necrotizing enterocolitis
Congenital hyperinsulinism
Lobar emphysema

in the thorax and a shift of the mediastinum to the opposite side. Arterial hypoxemia reflects the presence of right-to-left shunting through the ductus arteriosus as manifestations of persistent fetal circulation. Increased pulmonary vascular resistance is further aggravated by arterial hypoxemia, hypercarbia, and acidosis, ensuring that the ductus arteriosus remains patent and fetal circulation patterns persist. There is a high incidence of congenital heart disease and intestinal malrotation in neonates with CDH.

Diagnosis

The diagnosis of CDH is now commonly made prenatally due to the use of routine ultrasonography. Prenatal findings that correlate with poor prognosis include polyhydramnios, displacement of the stomach above the diaphragm, and diagnosis made prior to 20 weeks of gestation.

A chest radiograph showing loops of bowel in the chest along with mediastinal shift confirms the diagnosis. Occasionally, congenital cystic adenomatoid malformations of the lung can mimic CDH by producing a similar radiographic appearance. Ultrasonography or injection of contrast material into the stomach may be necessary to distinguish cystic lesions from dilated intestine.

Treatment

Immediate treatment of neonates with suspected CDH includes decompression of the stomach with an orogastric or nasogastric tube and administration of supplemental oxygen. Positive-pressure ventilation by mask should be avoided, as the passage of gas into the esophagus may increase stomach volume and further compromise pulmonary function. Indeed, awake tracheal intubation should be performed if the need for mechanical ventilation of the neonate's lungs is anticipated for any sustained period of time. After tracheal intubation, positive airway pressures during mechanical ventilation of the lungs should not exceed 25 to 30 cm H_2O, as excessive airway pressures can result in damage to the neonate's normal lung, manifesting as pneumothorax.

Congenital diaphragmatic hernias do not require immediate surgery, as the primary problem after birth is not herniation of abdominal viscera into the chest but rather severe uncorrectable pulmonary hypoplasia and potentially reversible pulmonary hypertension. Preoperative stabilization (sedation, skeletal muscle paralysis, mechanical ventilation of the lungs, extracorporeal membrane oxygenation [ECMO]) for a period of hours or days may decrease the mortality rate among unstable patients. Extracorporeal membrane oxygenation may improve survival in selected neonates. Although initial resuscitation has traditionally relied on modest hyperventilation (Pa_{CO_2} of 25–30 mm Hg), equal or improved survival and decreased need for ECMO has been reported with permissive hypercapnia ($P_{CO_2} < 60$ mm Hg) with gentle ventilation to minimize airway inflation pressures and barotrauma. Although pulmonary hypertension associated with CDH results from a combination of reversible (constriction of relatively normal arteries) and fixed (hypoplastic, dysplastic arteries) vasoconstriction of the pulmonary arteries, inhaled nitric oxide has not proven to be effective in improving survival or decreasing the requirement for ECMO in infants with CDH.

Prognosis

Reported survival in live-born infants with CDH ranges from 42% to 75% despite improvements in diagnosis and supportive modalities including ECMO. Prognosis is related to the degree of pulmonary hypoplasia and associated anomalies. Factors associated with a poor prognosis include severe pulmonary hypoplasia and herniation to the contralateral hemithorax, onset of symptoms in the first 24 hours of life, severe right-to-left shunting that requires ECMO, associated major developmental anomalies, and delivery in a nontertiary center.

Survivors exhibit evidence of restrictive lung disease and reactive airways that may improve with time. In fact, survivors of CDH who require only conventional management may lead healthy, normal lives free of significant respiratory problems. On the other hand, the incidence of neurologic abnormalities is nearly threefold higher in those infants requiring ECMO.

Management of Anesthesia

Management of anesthesia for neonates with a congenital diaphragmatic hernia begins with awake tracheal intubation following preoxygenation. In addition to routine monitors, preductal arterial cannulation (right radial) is useful for monitoring systemic blood pressure, blood gases, and pH. The infant may arrive in the operating room with umbilical arterial and venous access already in place, in which case a pulse oximeter applied to the right hand may provide additional information about preductal arterial oxygen saturation. Venous access should be avoided in the lower extremities because venous return may be limited due to compression of the inferior vena cava following reduction of the hernia.

Anesthesia can be induced and maintained with low concentrations of inhaled anesthetics. Nitrous oxide should be avoided, as its diffusion into loops of intestine present in the chest may result in distention of these loops with subsequent compression of functional lung tissue. If the level of arterial oxygenation permits, the delivered concentration of oxygen can be diluted by adding air to the oxygen until the desired concentration of oxygen is attained, as reflected by an oxygen analyzer. Because prolonged postoperative ventilation of the lungs is required by almost all neonates with congenital diaphragmatic hernia, an alternative approach to inhaled drugs for anesthesia is the use of opioids such as fentanyl plus muscle relaxants.

During intraoperative mechanical ventilation of the lungs, airway pressures should be monitored and maintained at less than 25 to 30 cm H_2O to minimize the risk of pneumothorax. A sudden decrease in lung compliance or deterioration of oxygenation or blood pressure suggests a pneumothorax. Hypothermia must be avoided. Complications associated with hypothermia include increased pulmonary vascular resistance with resultant right-to-left shunting. Hypothermia also causes increased oxygen consumption, which may result in inadequate oxygen delivery and acidosis, which then further increases pulmonary vasoconstriction and worsens arterial desaturation.

Reduction of the diaphragmatic hernia is usually accomplished through a left subcostal abdominal incision, although the repair can be accomplished through a thoracotomy incision as well. The abdominal approach facilitates the correction of intestinal malrotation. After reduction, an attempt to inflate the hypoplastic lung is not recommended, as it is unlikely to expand and the contralateral lung may be damaged by excessive positive airway pressures. In addition to a hypoplastic lung, these neonates are likely to have an underdeveloped abdominal cavity, such that a tight surgical abdominal closure causes increased intra-abdominal pressure, with cephalad displacement of the diaphragm, decreased functional residual capacity, and compression of the inferior vena cava. To prevent excessively tight abdominal surgical closures in infants with large defects, it is often necessary to create a ventral hernia (which can be surgically repaired later) and close the skin or to place a Silastic pouch. A pulse oximeter applied to the lower extremity at the time of anesthetic induction may forewarn of abdominal compartment syndrome and circulatory compromise.

In some institutions, surgery for CDH may be performed in the neonatal intensive care unit to avoid the stresses of transport and sudden changes in ventilation parameters. If surgery is performed in the neonatal intensive care unit without a conventional anesthesia machine and/or while the patient is on unconventional modes of ventilation or ECMO, a high-dose intravenous opioid and muscle relaxant technique is chosen. Drugs can be given directly into the circuit for those on ECMO.

Postoperative Management

Postoperative management of neonates with congenital diaphragmatic hernias presents significant challenges. The prognosis of these neonates is ultimately determined by the degree of pulmonary hypoplasia. There is no effective treatment for pulmonary hypoplasia, other than keeping these neonates alive with the hope that lung maturation will occur.

The postoperative course, after surgical reduction of congenital diaphragmatic hernias, is often characterized by rapid improvement, followed by sudden deterioration with profound arterial hypoxemia, hypercapnia, and acidosis, resulting in death. The mechanism for this deterioration is the reappearance of fetal circulation patterns, with right-to-left shunting through the foramen ovale and ductus arteriosus. If shunting occurs through the ductus arteriosus, there is a 20-mm Hg or more difference in the Pao_2 measured in samples obtained simultaneously from preductal and postductal arteries. If the shunting is predominantly through the foramen ovale, no such gradient exists. Proper sedation is necessary as any stressful stimulus can further exacerbate already elevated pulmonary pressures with resultant increases in shunt flow and further desaturation.

Esophageal Atresia and Tracheoesophageal Fistula

Esophageal atresia (EA) is the most frequent congenital anomaly of the esophagus, with an approximate incidence of 1 in 4000 neonates. Greater than 90% of affected individuals have an associated tracheoesophageal fistula (TEF). The most common form of EA manifests as a blind upper esophageal pouch and a distal esophagus that forms a TEF (**Fig. 24-1**). Survival of neonates with EA and no associated defects approaches 100%. Nevertheless, 50% of infants with EA have associated anomalies, most often associated with the VATER (*v*ertebral defects, imperforate *a*nus, *t*racheoesophageal fistula, *c*ardiac, *r*adial and renal dysplasia)/VACTERL (VATER but including *c*ardiac and *l*imb anomalies) association. Approximately 20% of neonates with EA have major coexisting cardiovascular anomalies (ventricular septal defect, tetralogy of Fallot, coarctation of the aorta, atrial septal defect), and 30% to 40% are born before term.

Signs and Symptoms

The neonate with EA typically presents with respiratory distress associated with episodes of coughing, cyanosis, and frothing at the mouth and nose. Feeding exacerbates these symptoms and causes regurgitation. Pulmonary aspiration is likely to occur. Infants with an isolated TEF in the absence of EA may elude diagnosis until later in life when the patients come to medical attention for recurrent pneumonias and refractory bronchospasm.

Diagnosis

Prenatally, EA should be suspected if maternal polyhydramnios is present. However, EA is usually diagnosed soon after birth when an oral catheter cannot be passed into the stomach or when the neonate exhibits cyanosis, coughing, and choking during oral feedings. Plain radiographs of the chest and abdomen will reveal coiling of a nasogastric tube in the esophageal pouch and possibly an air-filled stomach in the presence of a co-existing TEF. In contrast, pure EA may present as an airless, scaphoid abdomen.

Treatment

Initial therapeutic measures include maintaining a patent airway and preventing aspiration of secretions. Feedings are obviously stopped. The neonate is placed in a head-up position to minimize regurgitation of gastric secretions through the fistula. Continuous suctioning of the proximal esophageal segment prevents aspiration of pharyngeal secretions. Endotracheal intubation is avoided, if possible, because of the potential to worsen distention of the stomach, which can lead to gastric rupture. Gastric distention can be of sufficient magnitude to impair ventilation and venous return, resulting in cardiopulmonary arrest. Should life-threatening gastric distention occur, one-lung ventilation may be necessary until the stomach can be decompressed.

Primary repair without gastrostomy is routine. Repair of a TEF is urgent. However, neonates with EA, particularly those who are premature, may exhibit significant associated anomalies or have severe lung disease, and in these neonates, a staged surgical approach with an initial gastrostomy created under local anesthesia may be selected. Definitive repair of the TEF can then be delayed until the neonate's condition has improved.

Prognosis

A consistent pathologic finding in neonates with EA is decreased tracheal cartilage. This decreased support can

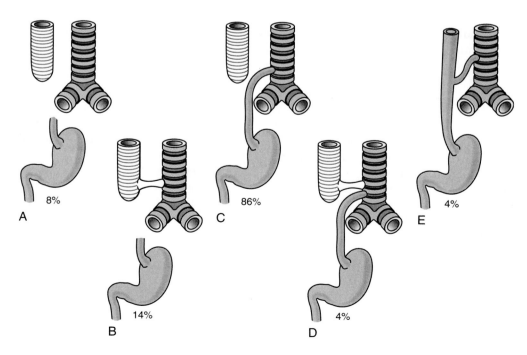

Figure 24-1 • Types of esophageal atresia (EA). Pure EA (**A**); proximal fistula (**B**); EA, distal fistula (**C**); proximal and distal fistula (**D**); pure tracheoesophageal fistula (**E**). (*Adapted from Ravitch MM, et al. [eds]: Pediatric Surgery, Volume 1, 3rd ed. Chicago, Year Book Medical Publishers, 1979 and Smith BM, Matthes-Kofidis C, Golianu B, Hammer GB: Pediatric general surgery. In Jaffe RA, Samuels SI [eds]: Anesthesiologists Manual of Surgical Procedures, 3rd ed. Philadelphia, Lippincott Williams & Wilkins, 2004, p 1019.*)

8%

14%

86%

4%

4%

A

B

C

D

E

result in tracheal collapse after tracheal extubation, requiring immediate reintubation of the trachea. Some degree of esophageal stricture, which may require dilatation, is likely to occur within the first year after repair. Strictures become less severe with age, and most patients are either asymptomatic or have only mild dysphagia by adulthood. Chronic gastroesophageal reflux and dysphagia can predispose children to recurrent aspiration pneumonitis following corrective surgery, necessitating antireflux surgical procedures at a later time in life. The highest risk of death is in those neonates weighing less than 1500 g at birth and in those with associated cardiac or chromosomal anomalies. Early deaths are the result of cardiac or chromosomal abnormalities, whereas later deaths are usually the result of respiratory complications. Survival among infants with other anomalies is also decreased.

Management of Anesthesia

Ideally, awake intubation with spontaneous ventilation allows the appropriate positioning of the endotracheal tube while minimizing the risk of ventilatory impairment associated with gastric distention due to positive-pressure ventilation and passage of gases through the fistula. However, awake intubation may be difficult and traumatic in a vigorous infant. If inhalation induction is chosen, the trachea can be intubated without the use of muscle relaxants and the neonate allowed to ventilate spontaneously. If induction by the intravenous route is chosen, care must be exercised during ventilation to minimize PIP and potential inflation of the stomach. Proper placement of the tracheal tube is critical; it should be above the carina but below the TEF. It is important that the tracheal tube be above the carina, as the right lung is compressed during thoracotomy. Accidental right main stem bronchus placement of the tracheal tube results in a precipitous decrease in arterial oxygenation, especially during surgical retraction of the lung. The endotracheal tube can be gently advanced into the right mainstem bronchus and then withdrawn until bilateral breath sounds are present. If the neonate does not have a gastrostomy, care must be exercised to avoid excessive airway pressures and further gastric distention. After tracheal intubation, the use of a pediatric fiberoptic bronchoscope is valuable for confirming the proper position of the tracheal tube.

Selection of anesthetic technique during surgical correction of EA depends on the physiologic status of the neonate. Low-dose volatile anesthetics in conjunction with air/O$_2$/opiate is usually well tolerated if the neonate is adequately hydrated. A nondepolarizing muscle relaxant can be administered after the airway is secured and ventilation is deemed satisfactory. The use of low PIP will minimize gastric distention by gases passing through the fistula. In addition to routine monitors, a catheter placed in a peripheral artery permits continuous monitoring of systemic blood pressure and measurement of arterial blood gases and pH. Pulse oximetry is useful for detecting acute changes in arterial oxygenation.

Intraoperative insensible and third-space fluid losses should be replaced with crystalloid at a rate of 6 to 8 mL/kg per hour. Blood loss may be replaced with 5% albumin and blood to maintain a hematocrit greater than 35%. Heart rate, blood pressure, urine output, and serial arterial blood gases and hematocrits are useful in monitoring the adequacy of fluid and blood replacement. The use of a warming mattress and corrective forced-air warming devices and warming all fluids and gases will decrease the risk of hypothermia.

Ligation of the TEF and primary esophageal anastomosis is usually performed via a right thoracotomy. During surgery, lung retraction may impair ventilation and surgical manipulation of the trachea may cause airway obstruction. Close communication between the surgeon and anesthesiologist is mandatory. Intermittent release of traction on the lung and trachea may be necessary to improve oxygenation and ventilation. Intraoperatively, accumulation of secretions and blood may also cause airway obstruction. Frequent tracheal suctioning may be required. Rarely, the endotracheal tube may become completely occluded by a clot that cannot be removed by suctioning, necessitating immediate replacement of the tube.

Extubation of term infants in the operating room at the end of surgery is preferable, but usually not feasible. Continued intubation and ventilation are necessary if cardiac or pulmonary complications arise intraoperatively, or if the adequacy of ventilation is in question. Infants at risk of developing respiratory failure should remain intubated postoperatively and be weaned from ventilatory support when adequate gas exchange and respiratory effort are demonstrated. Excessive neck extension and reintubation can compromise the new anastomosis.

Abdominal Wall Defects

Omphalocele and gastroschisis are congenital defects of the anterior abdominal wall that permit external herniation of abdominal viscera.

Omphalocele

Omphalocele manifests as external herniation of abdominal viscera through the base of the umbilical cord. The abdominal contents are contained within a sac formed by the peritoneal membrane internally and the amniotic membrane externally, without overlying skin. The incidence of herniation of intestines into the cord is approximately 1 in 5000 live births, while herniation of liver and intestines occurs in 1 in 10,000 live births, with a male predominance. Omphalocele is associated with a 75% incidence of other congenital defects, including cardiac anomalies, trisomy 21, and Beckwith-Wiedemann syndrome (omphalocele, organomegaly, macrosomia, macroglossia, hypoglycemia). Approximately 33% of neonates with omphaloceles are preterm. Cardiac defects and prematurity are the major causes of the 30% mortality among newborns with an omphalocele.

Gastroschisis

Gastroschisis manifests as external herniation of abdominal viscera through a small (usually < 5 cm) defect in the anterior abdominal wall. In most cases, the defect occurs laterally, just to the right of the normally inserted umbilical cord. Unlike the omphalocele, a hernial sac does not cover the herniated abdominal viscera. Gastroschisis is rarely associated with other congenital anomalies. The incidence of pre-term birth, however, is higher than in neonates with ompha-loceles. As with omphalocele, there appears to be a male preponderance.

Diagnosis

Omphalocele and gastroschisis can be diagnosed prenatally by fetal ultrasonography. The differences between omphalo-cele and gastroschisis are summarized in **Table 24-11**.

Treatment

Gastroschisis requires urgent repair. The sooner the bowel is reduced, the more likely primary closure can be achieved and the less severe the degree of bowel wall edema and accu-mulation of fibrinous coating. Placing the infant's lower body and exposed intestine immediately after delivery into a plastic drawstring bowel bag reduces evaporative fluid and heat loss from the large surface area of exposed bowel. While ompha-locele also requires urgent corrective surgery, the frequency of associated cardiac anomalies warrants preoperative cardiology evaluation and echocardiography.

Primary closure is not always possible. Staged closure is very successful and avoids potential complications of increased abdominal pressure following reduction of herniated viscera. Primary closure may cause respiratory compromise, decreased venous return, and circulatory dysfunction if the abdomen is too tense. A profound decrease in cardiac output and organ perfusion can result in acidosis, anuria, and bowel necrosis. Lower extremity congestion and cyanosis may also be seen if venous return from the lower body is impaired.

Blood pressure and pulse oximetry measurements from a lower extremity will help identify circulatory problems. If inspiratory pressures are greater than 25 to 30 cm H_2O or intravesical or intragastric pressures are greater than 20 cm H_2O, primary closure is not recommended. The viscera should be covered with a prosthetic silo and the abdominal viscera allowed to slowly reduce over a period of several days to 1 week.

Prognosis

The survival rate for gastroschisis is 90% or better. Infants who required a silo or had associated intestinal atresia typi-cally have a longer time to feeding and longer hospital stays but no increase in mortality. Survival rates for omphalocele range from 70% to 95%. Mortality is primarily related to associated cardiac and chromosomal abnormalities.

Preoperative Management

The primary concerns during preoperative preparation of the neonate with an omphalocele or gastroschisis are pre-vention of infections and minimization of fluid and heat loss from exposed abdominal viscera. Covering exposed viscera with moist dressings and a plastic bowel bag and maintaining a neutral thermal environment are effective methods of decreasing fluid and heat loss. The stomach should be decompressed with an orogastric tube to decrease the risk of regurgitation and pulmonary aspiration. The initial fluid requirement in these neonates is increased and should be admi-nistered at a rate two to four times the daily maintenance requirements (≥8–16 mL/kg per hour). These neonates expe-rience considerable protein loss and third-space translocation. To maintain normal oncotic pressures, protein-containing solutions (5% albumin) should constitute approximately 25% of the replacement fluids. Hypovolemia is indicated by

TABLE 24-11	Comparison of Omphalocele and Gastroschisis	
	Omphalocele	**Gastroschisis**
Etiology	Failure of midgut migration from yolk sac into abdomen	Abnormal development of right omphalomesenteric artery or umbilical vein with ischemia to right paraumbilical area
Location	Within umbilical cord	Periumbilical (usually to right of cord)
Covering	Membranous sac	None (exposed viscera)
Associated conditions	Beckwith-Wiedemann syndrome Congenital heart disease Trisomies 13, 18, 21 Malrotation of gastrointestinal tract Pentalogy of Cantrell Exstrophy of bladder	Malrotation of gastrointestinal tract, prematurity Intestinal atresia

Adapted from Roberts JD Jr, Cronin JH, Todres ID: Neonatal emergencies. In Cote CJ, Todres ID, Goudsouzian NG, Ryan JF (eds): A Practice of Anesthesia for Infants and Children, 3rd ed. Philadelphia, Saunders, 2001, p 309.

hemoconcentration and metabolic acidosis. Sodium bicarbonate administration to correct metabolic acidosis that does not respond to fluid therapy should be guided by arterial pH measurements.

Management of Anesthesia

Important aspects of the management of anesthesia for surgical treatment of omphalocele and gastroschisis include preservation of body temperature and continuation of fluid replacement. After decompression of the stomach and preoxygenation, anesthesia may be induced with either inhalation or intravenous agents. Following administration of a nondepolarizing muscle relaxant, the trachea is intubated with an endotracheal tube suitable for ventilation with PIPs greater than 20 cm H_2O. Primary closure may require the ability to ventilate the patient with high PIPs into the postoperative period. Repair of a large defect will require maximal relaxation intraoperatively and during the initial postoperative period. Anesthesia is maintained with opioids such as fentanyl or sufentanil or volatile anesthetics titrated to avoid hypotension. Nitrous oxide is avoided because of its potential to diffuse into the intestinal tract and interfere with the reduction of eviscerated bowel back into the abdomen. It must be remembered that these neonates have an underdeveloped abdominal cavity; tight surgical abdominal closure can result in compression of the inferior vena cava and decreased diaphragmatic excursion, resulting in impaired abdominal organ perfusion and decreased pulmonary compliance. Monitoring airway pressures is helpful for detecting changes in pulmonary compliance due to abdominal closure. Evidence of unacceptable intra-abdominal pressure requires removal of fascial sutures and closure of only the skin or addition of a prosthesis.

Intensive intraoperative and postoperative monitoring is recommended. Direct monitoring of arterial blood gases and pH is helpful for guiding fluid therapy. Intraoperative fluid requirements of at least 25% of estimated blood volume is to be expected during surgical repair of large abdominal defects. Mechanical ventilation of the neonate's lungs is often necessary for 24 to 48 hours following omphalocele or gastroschisis repair.

Hirschsprung's Disease

Hirschsprung's disease, or congenital aganglionic megacolon, is the most common cause of lower intestinal obstruction in full-term neonates. The incidence is approximately 1 in 5000 live births, with a pronounced male predominance. It is a disease characterized by the absence of parasympathetic ganglion cells in the large bowel. This disorder extends a variable distance proximally from the anus but is usually limited to the rectum and sigmoid colon. In rare cases, aganglionosis extends the entire length of the gastrointestinal tract, a condition that is often fatal. There may be deficiencies of nitric oxide synthase activity in the affected intestinal walls. The lack of nitric oxide–producing nerve fibers in the aganglionic bowel probably contributes to the inability of intestinal smooth muscle to relax appropriately, thereby impairing peristalsis. Tonic contraction of involved bowel produces a functional obstruction.

Signs and Symptoms

Constipation leads to dilatation of the proximal bowel and abdominal distention. Progressive bowel distention results in increasing intraluminal pressure, which may result in decreased blood flow and deterioration of the mucosal barrier. A persistent state of small intestinal and colonic stasis promotes bacterial proliferation, which may lead to enterocolitis with associated signs of bowel obstruction and sepsis. Enterocolitis of Hirschsprung's disease manifests as abdominal distention, fever, and explosive diarrhea following a rectal examination.

Diagnosis

Hirschsprung's disease should be suspected in any full-term neonate with delayed passage of stool. The diagnosis should also be entertained in any young child with a history of chronic constipation dating back to the newborn period. In these children, the rectum may be empty on examination while a large fecal mass may be palpable in the left lower quadrant. Rectal examination of patients with Hirschsprung's disease reveals normal anal tone or a tight anus that may be incorrectly diagnosed as anal stenosis.

A classic radiographic finding, following a contrast enema, is the presence of a transition zone between normal dilated proximal colon and a narrow, spastic distal colon segment caused by nonrelaxation of the aganglionic bowel. Anorectal manometry measures internal anal sphincter pressure during rectal distention with a balloon. The normal response to rectal distention is a reflex decrease in internal sphincter tone. In patients with Hirschsprung's disease, the internal sphincter pressure fails to decrease or paradoxically increases with rectal distention. Rectal biopsy is the diagnostic gold standard. The diagnosis is confirmed by the absence of ganglion cells and the presence of hypertrophied nerve bundles that stain positively for acetylcholinesterase.

Treatment

Surgical treatment aimed at bringing ganglionated bowel down to the anus usually provides satisfactory long-term results. A primary endorectal pull-through procedure is the preferred approach to infants with Hirschsprung's disease. However, a decompressive colostomy is indicated in infants presenting with severe enterocolitis or who have a markedly dilated proximal colon that might preclude the feasibility of a primary pull-through procedure.

Prognosis

The outcomes for patients with surgically treated Hirschsprung's disease are reasonably good. Most patients attain fecal continence. However, patients with retained or acquired aganglionosis, severe strictures, dysfunctional bowel, and intestinal neuronal dysplasia may require reoperation.

Management of Anesthesia

Anesthesia may be induced by either inhalation or intravenous routes. Anesthesia can be maintained with a mixture of air, oxygen, volatile agent, and a muscle relaxant. Intravenous catheters should be placed in the upper extremities because the lower extremities may be included in the surgical field. Intraoperative blood loss is usually mild, but third-space fluid losses can be significant. Patients may require an initial bolus of 10 to 20 mL/kg IV of crystalloid to offset the volume deficit resulting from bowel preparation and fasting. Epidural anesthesia provides excellent intraoperative as well as postoperative analgesia in patients undergoing open abdominal procedures. Extubation at the end of surgery is routine.

Anorectal Malformations

Anorectal anomalies include a spectrum of defects, most of which involve a fistula between the lower intestinal tract and the genitourinary structures. Imperforate anus without fistula occurs in a small number of patients, especially in association with Down syndrome. Imperforate anus is often also associated with the VACTERL association.

Spinal and vertebral anomalies also occur in up to 50% of patients with anorectal malformations. Tethered cord is the most frequent spinal abnormality seen. Cardiovascular anomalies are present in approximately one third of patients with imperforate anus. The most common cardiac lesions are atrial septal defect and patent ductus arteriosus, followed by tetralogy of Fallot and ventricular septal defect.

Signs and Symptoms

Inspection of the perineum will reveal an anorectal malformation. The neonate may fail to pass meconium in the first 24 to 48 hours of life.

Diagnosis

Meconium seen on the neonate's perineum is evidence of a rectoperineal fistula. Meconium in the urine indicates a rectourinary fistula. Rectovestibular fistula in females and rectourethral fistula in males are the most common presentations.

Treatment

Preliminary treatment for high lesions is a diverting colostomy followed at a later date by a posterior sagittal surgical approach that facilitates placing the rectum within the pelvic muscles and allows division and closure of rectourinary or rectovestibular fistulae. Low lesions such as perineal fistulas, on the other hand, may be repaired during the neonatal period without a protective colostomy.

Prognosis

The degree of sacral development correlates well with final functional prognosis. The greater the degree of sacral malformation, the greater is the likelihood of fecal and urinary incontinence. The majority of patients with perineal fistula and rectal atresia are expected to be fully continent following repair of their defects.

Management of Anesthesia

Anesthetic induction of patients presenting for decompressive colostomy or primary repair should be treated as for any infant with bowel obstruction. Definitive anorectal reconstruction is usually performed 1 to 12 months later. All defects can be repaired through a posterior sagittal approach, although some patients may also require an abdominal approach to mobilize a high rectum or vagina. Electrical muscle stimulation is used throughout the procedure to identify muscle structures and to define the anterior and posterior limits of the new anus. Blood loss and third-space fluid losses are usually moderate. Intravenous catheters should be placed in upper extremities because surgical positioning of the legs may impede venous flow or limit access to the intravenous site. Patients are usually extubated at the end of surgery.

Pyloric Stenosis

Pyloric stenosis is a common cause of gastric outlet obstruction in infants. Idiopathic hypertrophy of the circular muscle of the pylorus results in compression and narrowing of the pyloric channel. Pyloric stenosis occurs in approximately 1 in every 300 live births. It occurs in males, especially first borns, approximately four times more often than in females.

Signs and Symptoms

Pyloric stenosis generally manifests as nonbilious projectile vomiting at 2 to 5 weeks of age. However, symptoms may develop as early as the first week and as late as the fifth month of life. Vomiting may not be frequent or projectile in nature initially, but emesis progressively becomes forceful and usually occurs within 30 to 60 minutes after feeding. Jaundice may occur in some infants and is thought to be due to hepatic glucuronyl transferase deficiency associated with starvation, as occurs in proximal gastrointestinal obstruction. The indirect hyperbilirubinemia typically resolves rapidly following relief of the obstruction.

Persistent vomiting results in the progressive loss of gastric fluid, which contains sodium, potassium, chloride, and hydrogen. As chloride and hydrogen ions are lost, the kidneys initially attempt to maintain serum pH by excreting potassium in exchange for hydrogen ions and excreting HCO_3^- and sodium to compensate for chloride losses. With persistent vomiting, volume contraction ensues and the kidneys respond by defending extracellular volume in preference to serum pH by conserving sodium and excreting hydrogen ions. The initially alkaline urine thereby becomes acidic, and this paradoxic aciduria worsens the existing metabolic alkalosis. Hyponatremia, although present, may not be evident in serum electrolyte studies because of hypovolemia. Although the total body potassium deficit typically results in hypokalemia, hyperkalemia is not infrequently observed. Hypocalcemia may also be present in association with hyponatremia.

Compensatory respiratory acidosis is frequently seen, resulting from hypoventilation and periodic apnea. In contrast, severe dehydration and hypovolemic shock may manifest as metabolic acidosis with hyperventilation and respiratory alkalosis. However, the most frequent presentation is hypokalemic, hypochloremic primary metabolic alkalosis with a secondary respiratory acidosis.

Diagnosis

A thorough history and physical examination will lead to a clinical diagnosis in the majority of cases. An olive-like mass can usually be palpated in the epigastrium. Feeding an infant with pyloric stenosis may also aid in the diagnosis. After feeding, a gastric peristaltic wave may be observed progressing across the abdomen from left to right. However, patients in whom the pyloric mass is not identified require further diagnostic studies. Confirmation of the diagnosis by upper gastrointestinal contrast studies (barium swallow) has largely, but not completely, been replaced by abdominal ultrasonography. Ultrasonography has been demonstrated to have a diagnostic sensitivity of approximately 95% and a specificity of 100%. Ultrasonography is clearly becoming the diagnostic study of choice for pyloric stenosis.

Treatment

Pyloromyotomy, either open or laparoscopic, is the definitive treatment for pyloric stenosis. Pyloric stenosis, however, is not a surgical emergency. Severe, protracted vomiting results in significant fluid, electrolyte, and acid-base disturbances that require urgent resuscitation prior to surgical intervention. Severely dehydrated infants should receive an initial 20-mL/kg bolus of isotonic sodium chloride to re-expand the intravascular volume. Further resuscitation is given as 5% dextrose in 0.45% NaCl at 1.5 times the maintenance rate to prevent rapid changes in volume and electrolyte concentrations, which can lead to seizures and other complications. Potassium chloride 10 to 40 mEq/L can be added to the fluids if necessary when adequate urine output is demonstrated. Fluid resuscitation should be guided by measurement of serum electrolyte concentrations, which is essential for estimating the degree of dehydration, alkalosis, and metabolic derangements in patients with pyloric stenosis.

Surgery is performed nonemergently after correction of fluid and electrolyte deficits, which usually can be achieved within 12 to 48 hours of resuscitation. Metabolic alkalosis must be corrected prior to surgery to prevent postoperative apnea, which may be associated with anesthesia. Laboratory indices that indicate readiness for surgery are a serum chloride greater than 100 mEq/dL and serum bicarbonate less than 28 mEq/dL.

Prognosis

Surgical treatment of pyloric stenosis is curative. Feedings can usually be initiated within 4 to 6 hours following surgery.

Management of Anesthesia

Patients with pyloric stenosis should be regarded as having full stomachs. Pulmonary aspiration of gastric fluid is a definite risk in infants with gastric outlet obstruction. This risk of aspiration is further increased in infants who have undergone radiographic examination of the upper gastrointestinal tract using barium. Therefore, the stomach should be emptied as completely as possible with a large-bore orogastric catheter after premedication with atropine and before induction of anesthesia. Awake tracheal intubation is indicated when a difficult intubation is anticipated. Otherwise, rapid-sequence induction with sodium pentothal or propofol and succinylcholine or rocuronium is recommended. Maintenance of anesthesia with volatile agents is acceptable. Skeletal muscle relaxation, as provided by muscle relaxants, is usually not needed during maintenance of anesthesia. However, the need for additional muscle relaxant administration will depend on the speed of the surgeon. After intubation of the trachea, an orogastric tube is reinserted and left in place during surgery so that air can be insufflated in the stomach, to test for mucosal perforation after the hypertrophied muscle is split. Opioids are usually unnecessary intraoperatively and should be avoided to reduce the risk of delayed emergence and postoperative apnea. Infiltration of the incision sites with local anesthetics generally provides sufficient postoperative analgesia.

Postoperative Management

Postoperative depression of ventilation often occurs in infants with pyloric stenosis. The cause is unknown but may be related to cerebrospinal fluid (CSF) alkalosis and intraoperative hyperventilation of the infant's lungs. For this reason, infants should be fully awake, vigorous, and demonstrating a stable and regular breathing pattern before tracheal extubation. Apnea monitoring for the first 12 hours after surgery is indicated. Glucose levels should be monitored because occasionally hypoglycemia may occur 2 to 3 hours after surgical correction of pyloric stenosis, most likely due to inadequate liver glycogen stores and cessation of intravenous dextrose infusions.

Necrotizing Enterocolitis

Necrotizing enterocolitis (NEC) is characterized by various degrees of mucosal or transmural necrosis of the intestine, most frequently involving the terminal ileum and proximal colon. It is the most common neonatal surgical emergency, resulting in substantial perinatal morbidity and mortality. Incidence and case fatality rates are inversely related to gestational age and birth weight. Neonates at greatest risk are those born at less than 32 weeks of gestation and weighing less than 1500 g.

Although the greatest risk factor for NEC is prematurity, the etiology of NEC appears to be multifactorial. Perinatal asphyxia, systemic infections, umbilical artery catheterization, exchange blood transfusions, hypotension, RDS, patent ductus arteriosus, cyanotic congenital heart disease, and aggressive hyperosmolar formula feedings have all been implicated as causes.

Signs and Symptoms

Early clinical findings, which tend to be nonspecific, include recurrent apnea, lethargy, temperature instability, glucose instability, and shock. More specific signs of NEC are abdominal distention, high gastric residuals after feeding, and bloody or mucoid diarrhea. Metabolic acidosis is very common secondary to generalized peritonitis and hypovolemia. Neutropenia and thrombocytopenia are usually present and appear to be associated with gram-negative sepsis and platelet binding by endotoxin.

Diagnosis

The diagnosis of NEC is made with clinical correlation of plain abdominal radiographic findings. Pneumatosis intestinalis, air in the intestinal wall, is diagnostic of NEC in newborns. Air in the intestinal wall represents gas produced by bacterial fermentation that penetrates the damaged mucosa and enters the submucosal region. Pneumoperitoneum indicates intestinal perforation. However, perforation is frequently present without evidence of free air in the peritoneal cavity.

Treatment

Medical treatment, consisting of cessation of feeding, gastric decompression, intravenous fluids, and antibiotics, is often successful in the management of neonates with NEC. Mechanical ventilation is indicated if abdominal distention is contributing to hypoxia and hypercapnia. Hypotension is treated with crystalloid and blood products. Dopamine may be required to improve cardiac output and bowel perfusion. Umbilical artery catheters should be removed, if present, to avoid compromising mesenteric blood flow.

Surgery is reserved for neonates in whom medical management fails, as evidenced by bowel perforation, sepsis (peritonitis), and progressive metabolic acidosis indicating bowel necrosis. As many as 50% of infants with NEC require surgical intervention.

Prognosis

Medical management fails in approximately 20% of patients with pneumatosis intestinalis at diagnosis, and as many as 25% of these patients may die. Those who undergo extensive intestinal resection may suffer from short-bowel syndrome, complications related to central venous catheters for total parenteral alimentation, and cholestatic jaundice.

Management of Anesthesia

Neonates with NEC are usually hypovolemic and require vigorous fluid resuscitation with crystalloid and colloid solutions before induction of anesthesia. Blood and platelet transfusions are often necessary. Adequate monitoring of fluid resuscitation is critical. A catheter placed in a peripheral artery provides the ability to measure systemic blood pressure continuously and to monitor arterial blood gases, pH,

hematocrit, and electrolytes. It must be appreciated that rapid fluid administration to preterm neonates may cause intracranial hemorrhage or reopening of the ductus arteriosus.

These infants are usually on mechanical ventilation prior to surgery. If not already intubated on arrival in the operating room, full stomach precautions are in order. Preoxygenation and premedication with atropine should be given prior to induction and laryngoscopy. An endotracheal tube should be chosen to allow ventilation with PIPs greater than 20 cm H_2O, as high intra-abdominal pressures and decreased pulmonary compliance are likely to be encountered. Volatile anesthetics can produce significant hypotension in these neonates, particularly in the presence of sepsis and hypovolemia. Therefore, decreased doses of ketamine, fentanyl, or sufentanil plus nondepolarizing muscle relaxants are preferred for the maintenance of anesthesia.

Inotropes such as dopamine may be required to maintain adequate cardiac output and bowel perfusion. Massive third-space losses necessitate aggressive volume resuscitation. Fluids and the operating room should be appropriately warmed to maintain normothermia. Postoperative mechanical ventilation of the neonate's lungs is usually required because of abdominal distention and co-existing RDS.

Congenital Hyperinsulinism

Congenital hyperinsulinism in infancy or persistent hyperinsulinemic hypoglycemia of infancy, formerly known as nesidioblastosis, is characterized by inappropriately elevated plasma insulin levels in relation to blood glucose levels. It is the most common cause of persistent hypoglycemia in early infancy and is a major risk factor for the development of mental retardation and epilepsy. Onset is usually from birth to 18 months of age.

Signs and Symptoms

Some hyperinsulinemic newborns may be macrosomic due to the anabolic effects of insulin in utero. Macrosomic infants may experience hypoglycemia within hours or days of birth. Those infants with lesser degrees of hyperinsulinemia may not manifest hypoglycemic symptoms until after the first few weeks to months of life when the frequency of feedings is decreased to allow the infant to sleep through the night and hyperinsulinemia prevents the mobilization of glucose.

Diagnosis

In patients with congenital hyperinsulinism in infancy, insulin levels are elevated relative to a concurrent state of hypoglycemia. Clinical diagnosis of congenital hyperinsulinism in infancy is based on evidence of excess insulin activity during a state of hypoglycemia. The diagnostic criteria include (1) serum insulin level in excess of 10 μU/mL in the presence of a blood glucose concentration less than 50 mg/dL, (2) inappropriate suppression of lipolysis and ketogenesis, (3) requirement of a glucose infusion rate greater than 10 mg/kg per minute to maintain a blood glucose concentration of more than 35 mg/dL, and (4) a positive glycemic response to glucagon despite hypoglycemia.

Treatment

Prevention of hypoglycemia and its resultant effects on CNS development is imperative in the neonatal period. Immediate attention must be given to administering sufficient glucose to maintain blood glucose concentrations in a normal range. Blood glucose levels less than 50 mg/dL should be vigorously treated. Pancreatectomy is performed in an attempt to prevent recurrent episodes of neuroglycopenia and long-term neurologic sequelae. Diffuse disease often requires near-total pancreatectomy, which is associated with a long-term risk of diabetes mellitus. Conversely, focal disease may be cured with a partial pancreatectomy, with little risk of the subsequent development of diabetes mellitus.

Prognosis

Because pancreatectomy is an inexact procedure, the results are not entirely predictable and hypoglycemia may persist postoperatively, especially following subtotal resection. Reoperation may occasionally be required at the risk of permanent diabetes mellitus and exocrine pancreatic insufficiency.

Management of Anesthesia

Supplemental glucose should be continued into the intraoperative period as hypoglycemia must be avoided. The glucose requirements in infants with hyperinsulinism may be as high as 10 mg/kg per minute or more preoperatively, but the hyperglycemic response to surgery may reduce the requirement intraoperatively. Frequent monitoring of blood glucose concentrations is essential. Release of pancreatic lipase may result in omental fat saponification and hypocalcemia. Extensive third spacing of fluids and the potential for major hemorrhage during pancreatic dissection should be anticipated. Placement of an arterial catheter will facilitate monitoring of blood gases and serum glucose. Blood glucose concentrations must be monitored closely in the postoperative period, as near total pancreatectomy may result in hyperglycemia requiring insulin administration, whereas subtotal pancreatectomy may result in persistent hypoglycemia.

Congenital Lobar Emphysema

Congenital lobar emphysema is a rare cause of respiratory distress in neonates that results from localized bronchial obstruction. The affected bronchus allows passage of air on inspiration but limits expulsion of air on expiration, leading to air trapping and lobar overexpansion. Pathologic causes of congenital lobar emphysema include collapse of bronchi due to hypoplasia of supporting cartilage, bronchial stenosis, mucous plugs, obstructing cysts, and vascular compression of bronchi. The most frequent site of involvement is the left upper lobe (40%–50%), followed by the right middle lobe (30%–40%), and then the right upper lobe (20%). Acquired lobar emphysema may result from barotrauma associated with

the treatment of bronchopulmonary dysplasia. Right lower lobe involvement is common in these cases due to endotracheal tube positioning. There is an increased incidence of congenital heart disease, particularly ventricular septal defect and patent ductus arteriosus, in patients with congenital lobar emphysema.

Signs and Symptoms

The clinical manifestations of congenital lobar emphysema usually become apparent in the neonatal period, with 25% of cases diagnosed at birth and 50% of cases diagnosed by 1 month of age. The clinical presentation may range from mild tachypnea and wheezing to severe dyspnea and cyanosis.

Diagnosis

Diagnostic studies include chest radiography, computed tomography (CT), and ventilation/perfusion scan. As lobar emphysema progresses, atelectasis of the ipsilateral normal lung may be followed by mediastinal shift and impaired function of the contralateral lung. Chest radiograph often reveals a radiolucent lobe and a mediastinal shift but at the time of birth, the affected lobe may appear radiopaque due to delayed clearance of fetal lung fluid.

Treatment

Resection of the diseased lobe is the treatment of choice for symptomatic, progressive lobar emphysema. Some infants with only very mild symptoms and without evidence of progression of lobar emphysema may not require surgery.

Prognosis

Long-term pulmonary growth and function are excellent following lobectomy. Infants who undergo lobectomy compensate with new alveolar development and demonstrate minimal respiratory function differences from normal individuals.

Management of Anesthesia

Infants may be at greatest risk during induction of anesthesia, as positive-pressure ventilation of the lungs before the chest is opened may cause abrupt, exaggerated expansion of emphysematous lobes (gas enters but cannot leave due to a ball-valve effect), with sudden mediastinal shift and cardiac arrest. For this reason, tracheal intubation without muscle relaxants and maintenance of spontaneous breathing with minimal positive airway pressures is recommended. Intubation of the contralateral bronchus, facilitated by the use of muscle relaxants, and the use of positive-pressure ventilation have been suggested as an alternative means of airway management by some. The surgeon should be present at induction in the event that sudden cardiopulmonary decompensation necessitates urgent thoracotomy. Placement of an arterial catheter allows serial blood gas monitoring and earlier detection of hemodynamic changes. General anesthesia may be supplemented with local anesthesia until the chest is opened and the emphysematous lobe is delivered through the incision.

Thereafter, these infants may be paralyzed and their lungs mechanically ventilated. Nitrous oxide should not be used, as its diffusion into the diseased lobes can cause further distention. Severely decompensated infants may require emergency needle aspiration or thoracotomy for decompression of the affected lobe or lobes.

NERVOUS SYSTEM

Cerebral Palsy

Cerebral palsy is a symptom complex rather than a specific disease. It comprises a group of nonprogressive, but often changing, motor impairment syndromes secondary to lesions or anomalies of the brain that arise during the early stages of development. Cerebral palsy is classified according to the extremity involved (monoplegia, hemiplegia, diplegia, quadriplegia) and the characteristics of the neurologic dysfunction (spastic, hypotonic, dystonic, athetotic). The high frequency of epilepsy (approximately one third of children with cerebral palsy) and cognitive disorders among individuals with this disease suggests that these disorders have common or related origins.

The prevalence of moderately severe or severe cerebral palsy is 1.5 to 2.5 per 1000 live births. It has been assumed, but unproven, that problems during the birth process (midforceps delivery) and signs and symptoms that were present in newborn infants (low Apgar scores) are related to the subsequent development of cerebral palsy. Babies whose birth weight is less than 2500 g account for approximately one third of all those who later develop signs and symptoms of cerebral palsy. Despite the perceived association between a multitude of factors and cerebral palsy, the cause of most cases of cerebral palsy is unknown.

Signs and Symptoms

The most common manifestation of cerebral palsy is skeletal muscle spasticity. Extrapyramidal cerebral palsy is associated with choreoathetosis and dystonia, and cerebellar ataxia is characteristic of atonic cerebral palsy. Varying degrees of mental retardation and speech defects can accompany cerebral palsy. Seizure disorders co-exist in approximately one third of individuals afflicted with cerebral palsy.

Children with cerebral palsy may have varying degrees of spasticity of different skeletal muscle groups, resulting in contractures and fixed deformities of several joints of both upper and lower extremities. They include fixed flexion and internal rotation deformities of the hip joint due to involved adductor and flexor muscles and plantar flexion of the ankles due to involvement of the Achilles tendon.

Treatment

These children often undergo elective orthopedic corrective procedures, such as Achilles tendon lengthening, hip adductor and iliopsoas release, derotational osteotomy of the femur, and correction of scoliosis. Stereotactic surgery may be performed in attempts to decrease skeletal muscle rigidity, spasticity, and dyskinesia. Dental restorations requiring general anesthesia are frequently necessary in children with cerebral palsy. Gastroesophageal reflux is common in children with central nervous system disorders, and antireflux operations may be required.

Children with cerebral palsy frequently receive medications to treat seizures and to relieve skeletal muscle spasticity. Medications used to relieve muscle spasm includes dantrolene, botulinum neurotoxin (Botox) injections, and baclofen. Baclofen may be administered orally or intrathecally and should not be discontinued abruptly in the perioperative period due to the potential for withdrawal symptoms, including seizures, hallucinations, delirium, and pruritus, which may persist up to 72 hours. Phenytoin may lead to gingival hyperplasia and megaloblastic anemia. Phenobarbital stimulates hepatic microsomal enzymatic activity and may lead to altered responses to drugs that undergo metabolism in the liver. Valproic acid is also associated with hepatotoxicity, bone marrow suppression, and platelet dysfunction.

Management of Anesthesia

Management of anesthesia in children with cerebral palsy includes tracheal intubation because of the propensity for gastroesophageal reflux and poor function of laryngeal and pharyngeal reflexes. The use of volatile anesthetic agents is safe in these patients as there is no increased risk of MH. Although children with cerebral palsy have skeletal muscle spasticity, succinylcholine does not produce abnormal potassium release. Children on anticonvulsants may be more resistant to nondepolarizing muscle relaxants due to hepatic enzyme induction. Body temperature should be monitored, as these children may be susceptible to the development of hypothermia during the intraoperative period. Emergence from anesthesia may be quite slow due to cerebral abnormalities or hypothermia. Tracheal extubation should be delayed until these children are fully awake and body temperature has returned to near normal. Postoperatively, these children have a high incidence of pulmonary complications.

Hydrocephalus

Hydrocephalus is a congenital or acquired increase in the amount of CSF resulting in enlarged cerebral ventricles. Hydrocephalus can be caused by obstruction to the flow of CSF (e.g., tumor), as well as overproduction or decreased absorption of CSF (**Table 24-12**). Patients with hydrocephalus usually present with an increase in intracranial pressure (ICP). Hydrocephalus can occur at any age depending on the cause.

Signs and Symptoms

The clinical presentation depends on the age of the child and the presence of increased ICP. Congenital hydrocephalus typically presents at birth or soon after birth with an enlarged head featuring separation of cranial sutures, inferiorly deviated eyes ("sunsetting eyes") dilated scalp veins, and thin shiny skin. Late-onset hydrocephalus may not result in an enlarged

TABLE 24-12 Classification of Hydrocephalus

I. Excessive production of cerebrospinal fluid
   i. Chorioid plexus papilloma
II. Obstruction of CSF pathways
   A. Obstruction within the ventricular system
     i. Lateral ventricular (atrium, body, foramen of Monro)
     ii. Third ventricular
     iii. Aqueductal (congenital stenosis, mass lesions)
     iv. Fourth ventricular (Dandy-Walker)
   B. Obstruction within the subarachnoid space
     i. Basal cisterns (Chiari I malformation, postinfectious)
     ii. Convexity
III. Decreased absorption of cerebrospinal fluid
   A. Obstruction at the arachnoid villi (plugging by tumor cells, protein, blood, bacteria, etc.)
   B. Obstruction at the major dural venous sinuses (thrombus, hematologic malignancies, infection)
   C. Obstruction at extracranial venous sinuses (achondroplasia)

head but may lead to significantly increased ICP. Normal pressure hydrocephalus is a condition, often considered a syndrome, with distinct clinical and neuroimaging characteristics. The association of an abnormal gait combined with dementia and urinary incontinence is often described as the clinical triad of normal pressure hydrocephalus.

Diagnosis

Serial head circumference measurements, skull radiographs, and CT confirm the diagnosis. Patients presenting for CSF shunting procedures may present with a broad spectrum of symptoms and clinical signs, varying from an apparently healthy child with minimal disability to a seriously ill comatose patient for whom surgery is urgent. Common causes leading to the blockade of the CSF flow are reported in **Table 24-13**. In patients with an existing shunt, a shunt scan is useful in determining the site of malfunction.

Treatment

Treatment depends on the mechanisms responsible for hydrocephalus. When surgical excision of obstructive lesions is not feasible or is unsuccessful, a shunting procedure is necessary. The most common neurosurgical operation for hydrocephalus is the ventriculoperitoneal shunt.

TABLE 24-13 Common Causes of Cerebrospinal Fluid Blockage

1. Infectious: abscess, meningitis, encephalitis
2. Neoplastic: astrocytoma, ependymoma, choroid plexus papilloma, oligodendroglioma, medulloblastoma, meningioma
3. Vascular: arteriovenous malformations, aneurysm
4. Congenital: arachnoid cysts, colloid cysts, Chiari malformation, encephalocele

Ventriculoperitoneal shunts frequently require revisions or replacement due to infections involving the shunt or malfunction due to malposition of the distal end of the catheter, reflecting normal patient growth. Malfunctions may occur proximally (80%), distally, and in the form of peritoneal catheter obstruction (10%), and, rarely, both ventricular and peritoneal catheters will need to be replaced. Patients presenting with increased ICP secondary to shunt malfunction may have their ICP lowered acutely by tapping the proximal reservoir. Three types of ventricular shunts are used: ventriculoperitoneal, ventriculoatrial, and ventriculopleural shunts.

Management of Anesthesia

Preoperative Delayed gastric emptying and vomiting are indications for a rapid-sequence induction technique. Children with severe neurologic compromise may present with a gastrostomy tube, which should be aspirated prior to induction of anesthesia and left open during induction to prevent gastric distention and regurgitation.

Intraoperative Arterial catheterization is usually reserved for the patient with uncontrolled ICP and hemodynamic instability. The technique for induction of anesthesia depends on the presence of raised ICP. Inhalation or intravenous induction is acceptable in the child without clinical evidence of elevated ICP. On the other hand, the child with increased ICP and/or delayed gastric emptying should be induced intravenously following preoxygenation. Atropine premedication is recommended in infants, especially in the presence of increased ICP, due to the immaturity of the sympathetic autonomic system. Although laryngoscopy is a potent stimulus that may cause significant increase in ICP, the benefit of lidocaine administration prior to laryngoscopy has not been demonstrated to prevent sudden increases in ICP in infants and small children. However, sudden cardiac arrest in infants receiving 1.0 to 1.5 mg/kg of lidocaine intravenously at time of induction of anesthesia has been reported. Mild hypocapnia (32–35 mm Hg) following tracheal intubation may prevent further elevation of the ICP; however, aggressively decreasing the Pa_{CO_2} increases the risk of brain ischemia. Normocapnia should be maintained in patients with normal ICP. Intraoperative spontaneous ventilation is not recommended due to the risk of air embolism during craniotomy and ventriculoatrial shunt placement, and due to the risk of pneumothorax during ventriculopleural shunt placement.

In neuroanesthesia, the use of nitrous oxide is not recommended for two reasons: (1) it significantly increases cerebral blood flow and volume, which can contribute to elevating the ICP, and (2) it is associated with a strong emetic effect that may confuse the evaluation of the patient postoperatively. Ventricular shunt procedures usually do not result in significant blood or third-space losses. Preservation of body temperature is important during shunt procedures despite their relatively short duration because a large body surface area is exposed and surgically prepped, causing infants to cool rapidly.

Prior to extubation of the trachea, the patient should be awake and demonstrate an appropriate gag reflex in order to protect the airway against aspiration on emergence. However, patients undergoing shunt procedures may have poor airway control due to the presence of severe neurologic deficits.

Postoperative Patients with severe neurologic deficits may be more prone to postoperative respiratory problems. Analgesics should be used judiciously and under close supervision in neurologically impaired patients. The infiltration of the skin with local anesthetic at time of surgery can substantially reduce the requirement for opioid analgesics.

Intracranial Tumors

Neoplasms of the central nervous system account for a major proportion of all solid tumors in children younger than 15 years of age. It is the second most common cancer in childhood after leukemia. The survival of children affected with brain tumors has improved significantly in recent years; however, patients diagnosed at less than 3 years of age have a poor prognosis.

Supratentorial Tumors

Supratentorial lesions account for 50% of all pediatric brain neoplasms. Most of these tumors originate from midline structures and tend to impinge on the ventricular system, leading to obstructive hydrocephalus. During the first year of life, the frequency of all intracranial neoplasms is approximately twice as high in infants compared with the overall incidence in older children (37% compared with 16%–24%).

Signs and Symptoms Patients affected with intracranial tumors may show evidence of increased ICP. The clinical presentation will vary according to the location and size of the tumor. Brain tumors usually present with one of three syndromes: (1) a subacute progression of a focal neurologic deficit, (2) seizures, and (3) a nonfocal disorder such as headache, dementia, personality change, and gait disorder.

Diagnosis Computed tomography and magnetic resonance imaging are the most reliable tests to confirm the presence of an intracranial mass effect, resulting from expansion of the neoplastic tissue and focal edema. Brain tumors routinely produce a vasogenic pattern of edema, most often in the area around the tumor (penumbra). Positron emission tomography and single-photon emission tomography are used to distinguish tumor recurrence from tissue necrosis, especially after brain radiation. Lumbar puncture for CSF analysis should not be performed in patients with primary brain tumors because of the risk of brain herniation in the presence of elevated ICP.

Treatment Corticosteroids are the cornerstone of therapy in patients affected with brain tumors. Glucocorticoids improve neurologic function by reducing the volume of edema surrounding the tumor, which then increases brain perfusion and oxygenation of the cells located in the penumbra regions. Dexamethasone (0.1 mg/kg up to 10 mg; 12–20 mg/day)

represents the best choice because of its limited mineralocorticoid effect. Anticonvulsants are used in patients presenting with seizures. Patients with gliomas have an increased incidence of deep vein thrombosis and pulmonary embolism associated with release of procoagulant factors into the systemic circulation.

Management of Anesthesia

Preoperative. It is essential to determine the presence and degree of ICP elevation. Patients with large mass lesions, significant tumor edema, or obstruction to CSF outflow will require an anesthetic approach aimed at reducing ICP and improving cerebral perfusion. Preoperative neurologic deficits should be assessed and documented. Intracranial pathology can present with syndrome of inappropriate secretion of antidiuretic hormone. Laboratory tests, especially electrolytes, serum osmolality, and urine osmolality should be performed, and information about urine output should be obtained.

Intraoperative. It is recommended that all patients undergoing subdural surgical procedures receive an arterial catheter for beat-to-beat hemodynamic monitoring and blood chemistry sampling. The placement of a central venous catheter is indicated when there is a potential for significant blood loss, leading to hemodynamic instability or an increased risk of air embolism. A urinary catheter is essential because of the duration of the surgical procedure, the use of diuretic therapy, and detecting development of diabetes insipidus.

Stimulation during laryngoscopy should be minimized and the airway rapidly secured. Although nasotracheal intubation is often recommended for patients in whom postoperative ventilation is expected or in small infants in whom the tube may be better stabilized, the risk of bacterial contamination via the cribriform plate to the meninges should be weighed against the benefit of this technique.

Patients with increased ICP are generally hyperventilated. Although hyperventilation is of paramount importance in the patient with significantly elevated ICP, the degree of hypocapnia must never be less than 30 mm Hg unless a jugular bulb catheter is used to monitor the presence of brain cell ischemia caused by a more profound vasoconstriction induced by the decrease in Pa_{CO_2}. Once the dura is opened, the Pa_{CO_2} should progressively be returned to its normal range, thus preserving the benefit of sudden hyperventilation and CO_2 vasoconstrictive effect when needed. In patients with impaired oxygenation, the use of a minimal amount of positive end-expiratory pressure (5 cm H_2O) does not affect cerebral venous drainage and ICP, but should be implemented gradually to prevent impairment of venous return. Fluid management will be affected by pre- and intraoperative diuretic therapy (furosemide and mannitol) aimed at decreasing brain tissue volume and allowing better intracranial compliance. The use of isotonic solutions is mandatory to maintain normotonicity across the blood-brain barrier and to avoid the development of vasogenic edema.

The decision to extubate the trachea at the end of the surgical procedure is guided by the intraoperative course and expected level of consciousness following surgery. The trachea should be extubated once the child is awake and demonstrating an appropriate gag reflex. Neonates with poor pulmonary compliance or an immature respiratory drive may require ventilating support postoperatively.

Postoperative. Patients requiring postoperative ventilation will require sedation and possibly muscle relaxation to avoid agitation and increased ICP. Children who fail to awaken or who exhibit hyperventilation in the postoperative period should be suspected of having a sudden increase in ICP (e.g., bleeding) and should have a CT scan performed immediately under anesthesia supervision. To reduce the use of systemic opioids, pain management can be supplemented with local anesthetic infiltration of the wound and/or blockade of the superficial cervical plexus. Special attention must be given to the systemic blood pressure because the most common contributor to postoperative increased ICP is uncontrolled hypertension. Persistent hypertension despite appropriate analgesic administration should be treated with vasodilators or a β-blocker, particularly labetalol, which has both β- and α-blocking properties and does not cross the blood-brain barrier. Seizures frequently occur in the immediate postoperative period, especially in infants and young children, and the prophylactic administration of anticonvulsants is recommended.

Craniopharyngioma

Craniopharyngiomas are the most common intracranial tumors of nonglial origin in the pediatric population. It is a benign encapsulated tumor of the hypophysis cerebri. However, craniopharyngiomas commonly cause progressive neurologic deterioration and can cause death because of their close relation to important structures such as the hypothalamus, optic nerves, and pituitary stalk. Three main types have been described: sellar, prechiasmatic, and retrochiasmatic.

Signs and Symptoms Headaches and endocrine dysfunction are pathognomonic of a sellar craniopharyngioma. Patients with prechiasmatic tumors have reduced visual acuity, field cuts, and optic atrophy. Obstructive hydrocephalus and increased ICP with papilledema is frequently observed with the retrochiasmatic tumors.

Diagnosis CT is superior to magnetic resonance imaging in demonstrating intratumoral calcification. Prior to surgery, all patients should undergo formal neuro ophthalmologic, neuroendocrinologic, and, if possible, neuropsychological assessments.

Treatment This tumor can be treated either surgically, via radiation therapy, or with a combination of both modalities. The first approach to all craniopharyngiomas is attempted total removal. Total resection can be achieved in more than 65% of patients.

Management of Anesthesia

Preoperative Preoperative evaluation of the child with a craniopharyngioma is focused on determining the presence of hydrocephalus and endocrine dysfunction that could affect anesthetic management. Hypothyroidism, growth hormone deficiency, corticotropin deficiency, and diabetes insipidus have been reported. Diabetes insipidus can develop intraoperatively but most often occurs 4 to 6 hours postoperatively. Characteristically, patients produce a copious quantity of dilute urine in association with an increasing serum osmolality and low urine osmolality (usually < 200 mOsm $\bullet$ L^{-1}). In the presence of diabetes insipidus, the urine specific gravity will be lower than 1.002. Hypernatremia and hypovolemia complete the clinical presentation.

Intraoperative If diabetes insipidus is diagnosed intraoperatively, fluid therapy must be started and hourly urine output must be measured. Maintenance fluids should be administered along with three fourths of the previous hour's urine output. Although it has been suggested that the fluid therapy should always consist of an hypotonic solution such as half-normal saline with D5W, the choice of solution should be dictated by the serum electrolyte levels. Vasopressin should be administered early when the diagnosis is confirmed. DDAVP (1-deamino-8-D-arginine vasopressin [desmopressin]) should be administered intravenously in its aqueous solution or intranasally. Postoperatively intranasal DDAVP 5 to 30 μg/day is given in two divided doses. The intravenous solution must be administered with caution because it may occasionally produce transient hypertension. The dose should be one tenth of the intranasal dose, also divided into two doses daily. Vasopressin can also be administered as an infusion at a rate of 0.5 mU $\bullet$ kg^{-1} per hour, titrated to antidiuretic effect.

Postoperative An endocrinologist should be consulted in the postoperative period for the appropriate management of steroid, thyroid, and sex hormone replacement. Insulin-dependent diabetics may experience a reduction in insulin requirements after surgery. Seizures have been reported in the postoperative period due to intraoperative surgical trauma to the frontal lobes. Anticonvulsant prophylaxis should be instituted intraoperatively and be continued into the postsurgical period. Injury to the hypothalamic thermoregulatory mechanisms may result in hyperthermia. Efforts should be made to maintain normothermia and reduce the risk of hypermetabolic cell injury.

Posterior Fossa Tumors

The incidence of posterior fossa tumors is greater in children than in adults. More than half of all pediatric brain tumors are located in the infratentorial compartment. The four common types include medulloblastoma (30%), cerebellar astrocytoma (30%), brainstem glioma (30%), and ependymoma (7%). The remaining 3% include acoustic neuroma, meningioma, ganglioglioma, chordomas, and others. Cerebellar astrocytomas have no gender predilection, whereas medulloblastoma occurs more frequently in males.

Signs and Symptoms Because the posterior fossa compartment is a very limited space, even small tumors will lead to an increase in ICP, rapid obstruction of CSF flow, and hydrocephalus with negative effects on the brainstem respiratory and cardiovascular regulatory centers. The typical clinical history is one of worsening headaches, most often in the morning, accompanied by nausea and vomiting. The association of an abnormal gait or unsteadiness of arm movements may be the initial symptoms of a cerebellar hemispheric tumor. Rapid obtundation, stupor, and/or coma may develop if intratumoral hemorrhage occurs, requiring urgent decompression.

Diagnosis The common symptoms of a posterior fossa tumor in children are due to hydrocephalus, which is present in 90% of patients affected with medulloblastoma and in virtually all children with cerebellar astrocytoma. Ideally, a CT or magnetic resonance imaging scan should be obtained with or without contrast enhancement. Typically, medulloblastomas are mildly hyperdense masses on CT scans, filling the fourth ventricle, presenting calcification in 15% and demonstrating increased vascularization. Astrocytomas are more likely to have calcifications (50%) and large cysts (>2 cm in diameter). The use of lumbar punctures is contraindicated in patients with posterior fossa tumors and obstructive hydrocephalus because of the risk of tonsillar herniation.

Treatment Most posterior fossa tumors will require surgical decompression and tumor debulking. The severity of hydrocephalus determines the urgency of the surgical procedure.

Management of Anesthesia

Preoperative Children with posterior fossa tumors should be monitored closely if preoperative sedation is to be given. The anesthesiologist must pay particular attention to the neurologic symptoms such as cerebellar dysfunction, evidence of upper airway obstruction (inspiratory stridor), cardiovascular instability, and increased ICP. Patients presenting with decreased level of consciousness, usually secondary to increased ICP from obstructive hydrocephalus, will require respiratory support and airway protection from gastric aspiration.

Intraoperative The induction of anesthesia must be aimed at preserving cerebral perfusion pressure and providing an appropriate depth of anesthesia during laryngoscopy to prevent sudden changes in ICP. A major challenge of infratentorial surgery is to prevent further neurologic injury from surgical position, exploration, and mechanical retraction on tissue. Monitoring should include an arterial catheter and possibly a central venous line. The use of electrophysiologic somatosensory evoked potential monitoring helps detect the development of intraoperative ischemia and/or compromised perfusion of the brainstem or cranial nerves. Surgical positioning is most often prone; therefore, the risk of intraoperative venous air embolism is reduced but not completely eliminated and should always be kept in mind. To minimize the possibility that the tracheal tube may be kinked and/or obstructed in the prone position, a reinforced armored orotracheal tube may be used.

The choice of anesthetic is not as crucial as the manner in which the medications are administered. As with induction of anesthesia, no single anesthetic technique is superior and the maintenance regimen must be tailored to the needs of the patient and the requirement of the surgical procedure. Sevoflurane and isoflurane are the most commonly used inhalational anesthetic agents in neuroanesthesia. Their ability to preserve the cerebrovascular reactivity to carbon dioxide is very useful. The goal of anesthesia is to provide a "slack brain" that will reduce the amount of retractor pressure and maintain adequate cerebral perfusion and oxygenation in the nonautoregulated brain. The use of a nondepolarizing muscle relaxant can facilitate ventilation in the prone position, facilitate venous return, and reduce cerebral venous stasis. During the initial surgical approach, intermittent positive pressure ventilation is adjusted to maintain the Pa_{CO_2} in the range of 28 to 30 mm Hg. However, once the dura mater is opened, the Pa_{CO_2} should be increased to 32 mm Hg for the duration of the procedure. Patients are typically awakened immediately at the end of the procedure to allow a neurologic evaluation.

Postoperative An understanding of the pathologic process will dictate the correct airway management postoperatively (e.g., tracheal intubation is essential postoperatively following resection of intramedullary tumors). Postoperative pain medications should be chosen to minimize effects on the patient's sensorium and the pupillary reactivity.

Cerebral Vascular Anomalies

Arteriovenous malformations (AVMs) are congenital vascular malformations characterized by direct arterial-to-venous communications without intervening capillary circulation. Specific structures involved in vascular anomalies in the pediatric population include the posterior cerebral artery and the great vein of Galen. AVMs may present clinically in the newborn period with congestive heart failure. Hydrocephalus due to the obstruction of the aqueduct of Sylvius is often associated with a dilatation of the great vein of Galen. Although moyamoya disease is not neurologically classified as an AVM, this chronic occlusive cerebrovascular disease of the basal cerebral arteries leads to severe dilatation of perforating arteries at the base of the brain and requires similar anesthetic management. It is important to note that moyamoya has been reported to be associated with progressive myopathy.

Signs and Symptoms

AVMs are congenital anomalies that usually are not detected until the fourth or fifth decade of life. However, 18% may manifest before the age of 15 years, usually with severe intracranial hemorrhage. An AVM can manifest itself in several ways: (1) intraparenchymal hemorrhage, thrombosis, and cerebral infarction; (2) compression of adjacent neural structures; (3) parenchymal ischemia as a result of circulatory "steal" from the low resistance vascular network; (4) congestive heart failure and tissue hypoperfusion; and (5) surgical disruption or diversion of the blood flow. Symptomatology varies with the age at which the disease presents. Older children most commonly present with subarachnoid hemorrhage and headache or IVH. Seventy percent of pediatric patients presenting with spontaneous subarachnoid hemorrhage have AVMs as the cause. Seizure is the presenting symptom in approximately 25% of patients. The neonatal presentation of cerebral AVM is the most challenging because it is associated with congestive heart failure.

Diagnosis

Fifty percent of AVMs become symptomatic due to a small amount of bleeding within the parenchyma and within the CSF pathways (hallmark of a ruptured AVM). It is also detectable within 72 hours on high-quality CT, especially with the presence of blood in the basal cisterns. The presence of yellowish CSF (due to lysis of red cell and production of bilirubin) can be detected after 6 hours in a lumbar puncture. CT is the test of choice for the detection of ruptured AVMs. A four-vessel angiography is generally performed to localize and define the anatomic details of the lesion involved. Lesions can often be treated using endovascular techniques at the time of the initial angiogram. The use of a transcranial Doppler sonography is recommended to detect the onset of cerebral vasospasm and follow its course and response to therapy.

Treatment

Patients with AVMs may undergo surgical excision, radiographic embolization of the arterial blood supply, or stereotactic radiosurgery as definitive or adjunctive therapy. Stereotactic localization may be required to safely excise deep-seated AVMs. Surgical clipping of feeding vessels may be performed as a single or staged procedure.

Management of Anesthesia

Preoperative Patients without evidence of congestive heart failure can be premedicated to reduce agitation and systemic pressure changes at the time of induction of anesthesia.

Intraoperative Central to induction of anesthesia in children with an AVM without congestive heart failure is prevention of hypertension during laryngoscopy and tracheal intubation. Inhalation or intravenous induction may be performed in the child without evidence of increased ICP. A nondepolarizing muscle relaxant is recommended to facilitate tracheal intubation and/or reduce the doses of hypnotic agents that could cause hemodynamic instability. The anesthetic management for neonates and infants presenting with congestive heart failure will be dictated by the severity of this problem and the need to maintain proper cardiac output and brain tissue perfusion. Hyperventilation might be required in patients with hydrocephalus to reduce the ICP. However, once the dura mater is opened, normocarbia must be maintained to avoid shunting additional blood flow to the low-resistance malformed vessels, increasing the risk of rupture and worsening the congestive heart failure.

In the absence of congestive heart failure, a hypotensive anesthesia technique may be indicated at the time of ligation of the arteriovenous malformation to facilitate surgical manipulation. Neonates and infants presenting with congestive heart failure are usually on inotropic support and will not tolerate hypotensive anesthesia. Fluid management requires special attention in neonates who do not tolerate excessive fluid loads. In addition, preoperative attempts to decrease brain water can lead to rapid circulatory collapse in the event of brisk intraoperative bleeding and is therefore not recommended. While cerebral protection might be achieved with mild hypothermia (35°C), it is essential to aggressively treat hyperthermia until the patient is no longer at risk of ischemic neurologic injury. Hyperthermia has been shown to exacerbate cerebral ischemic injury in animal models. Two large bore intravenous catheters, an indwelling arterial catheter and a central venous catheter allow rapid control of blood pressure, infusion of vasoactive drugs, assessment of adequacy of fluid therapy, and monitoring of cerebral perfusion pressure. Urinary catheter placement is mandatory following induction of anesthesia.

Postoperative It is paramount to the management of these patients to avoid sudden changes in blood pressure. Vasospasm is not a common postoperative complication in children but must be considered in the face of neurologic deterioration. Transcranial Doppler sonography has become useful in the diagnosis of this complication.

Myelomeningocele

Neural tube defects, or myelodysplasia, refers to an abnormality in the fusion of the embryologic neural groove that normally closes in the first month of gestation. Failure of the canal end of the neural tube to close can result in spina bifida (characterized by defects of the vertebral arches) or formation of a saclike herniation of the meninges (meningocele) or herniation containing neural elements (myelomeningocele). In both cases, CSF is contained in the defect. However, children affected with myelomeningomyelocele often present an Arnold-Chiari type II malformation. The spinal cord is often tethered caudally by the sacral roots, resulting in orthopedic or urologic symptoms later during childhood if not surgically corrected.

Signs and Symptoms

The clinical presentation will vary significantly according to the anatomic defect involved. Children with meningoceles are usually born without neurologic deficits; those with myelomeningoceles are likely to have varying degrees of motor and sensory deficits. For example, children with lumbosacral myelomeningoceles exhibit flaccid paraplegia, loss of sensation to pinprick, and loss of anal, urethral, and bladder-sphincter tone. Associated congenital conditions include clubfoot, hydrocephalus, dislocation of the hips, exstrophy of the bladder, prolapsed uterus, Klippel-Feil syndrome, and congenital cardiac defects. Severe dilation of the upper urinary tract may develop in these children, necessitating urinary diversion procedures such as vesicostomy, cutaneous ureterostomy, and ileal or colon conduit construction. They are likely to experience recurrent urinary tract infections, which may be complicated by gram-negative sepsis. The need for corrective orthopedic procedures on the lower extremities is predictable. As these patients mature, they have a tendency to develop varying degrees of scoliosis, often requiring posterior spinal fusion.

Diagnosis

The Chiari II malformation is usually found at birth in combination with hydrocephalus and myelomeningocele. CT will confirm the presence of this anomaly. In the older child, the diagnosis of spina bifida is often made incidentally when plain films are obtained for other reasons, such as lower back pain. Less severe conditions, such as dermal sinus tracts, diastematomyelia, lipomyelomeningocele, and tethered cord manifestation, will most often result in back pain, progressive lower extremity weakness, spasticity, and bladder and bowel dysfunction. These lesions can be found at any age. Magnetic resonance imaging is the most useful radiographic test to confirm the presence of neural tube defects and/or spinal cord anomalies.

Treatment

Early neurosurgical repair of a myelomeningocele will lead to the restoration of a more normal configuration of the spine, which will facilitate the care and future handling of the back of the child. Open neural tube defects will often require subcutaneous skin flaps to close the defect, which may lead to significant bleeding. The more severe anomalies will be detected at birth and will require a surgical intervention within the first 24 hours of life to reduce the risk of infection of exposed central nervous system tissue. However, the incidence of ventriculitis is directly proportional to the time with which the myelomeningocele is surgically repaired.

Management of Anesthesia

Preoperative Infants presenting for repair of a meningomyelocele defect rarely present with increased ICP. The association of Arnold-Chiari malformation and hydrocephalus does not always require placement of a ventriculoperitoneal shunt. Neonates with a myelomeningocele, however, may have an abnormal ventilatory response to hypoxia and hypercarbia. These neonates often have gastroesophageal reflux and abnormal vocal cord motility, emphasizing the need to take precautions against aspiration. The surgical closure of a myelomeningocele sac must be tight enough to prevent leakage of CSF, as confirmed by increasing the pressure in the sac with positive airway pressure. Blood loss can be insidious, especially if the sac is large and significant undermining of the subcutaneous space must be performed to ensure closure of the defect. Invasive monitoring should be used for patients presenting with large defects, such as a multilevel myelomeningocele where significant cutaneous undermining will be needed. Myelomeningoceles may present with significant vascular volume contraction because of large third-space losses.

Hypothermia is a frequent complication of these procedures considering the surface area of tissue exposed and the age of the patient. However, care must be taken to prevent drying or causing thermal injury to the exposed neural tissue by the use of radiant heat lamps.

Intraoperative If general anesthesia is selected, awake tracheal intubation may be performed with these children in the lateral decubitus position to avoid pressure on the meningocele sac. Anesthesia may also be induced with neonates in the supine position with the meningocele sac protected by elevating it on a doughnut-shaped support. Maintenance of anesthesia is with inhaled anesthetics delivered using mechanical ventilation of the lungs. The operative procedures are performed with these neonates in the prone position. Although succinylcholine may be used to facilitate tracheal intubation, long-acting nondepolarizing muscle relaxants are avoided, as the surgeon may need to use a nerve stimulator to identify functional neural elements.

Postoperative Postoperatively, neonates should be maintained in the prone position, with a high index of suspicion maintained for the development of increased ICP. Older children with a myelomeningocele require numerous corrective procedures, primarily involving the urologic and musculoskeletal systems. Although the myelomeningoceles produce both upper and lower motor neuron dysfunction, succinylcholine does not elicit a hyperkalemic response.

Children with a myelomeningocele may have an increased incidence of sensitivity to latex (natural rubber), which manifests as intraoperative cardiovascular collapse and bronchospasm. It is possible that chronic exposure to indwelling catheters results in sensitization to latex. A preoperative history of itching, rashes, or wheezing after wearing latex gloves or inflating toy balloons is suggestive of latex allergy.

Craniosynostosis
Signs and Symptoms

Craniosynostosis (or craniostenosis) refers to a condition where one or more cranial sutures fuse prematurely leading to focal or global growth delay of the skull. With the developing brain inducing the growth of the cranial vault, this may result not only in aesthetic abnormalities (i.e., abnormal shape of the head), but also severe functional abnormalities (i.e., increased ICP, hydrocephalus, developmental delay, amblyopia). The premature fusion of a suture leads to compensatory increase in growth of the bone plates parallel (instead of perpendicular) to the affected suture.

Craniosynostosis affects approximately 1 in 2000 to 3000 live births. Sagittal and coronal craniosynostoses are the most common types and are approximately four times more frequent in males than in females. However, unicoronal craniosynostosis is more common in females. For the other forms, the distribution is approximately equal between the two genders.

Craniosynostosis may occur as an isolated deformity or as part of a genetic malformation syndrome. A positive family history is present in up to 40% of cases, with genetic syndromes accounting for at least 50% of those cases.

Nonsyndromic forms account for as many as 80% of all craniosynostoses and are commonly limited to a single suture (sagittal, coronal, or metopic suture) and not associated with increased ICP. Syndromic craniosynostosis (approximately

20% of all craniosynostoses) most commonly refers to patients with acrocephalosyndactyly syndromes (i.e., Apert, Pfeiffer, Saethre-Chotzen, and Crouzon syndromes), where premature fusion of more than one suture (total craniosynostosis, bicoronal [isolated], or in combination with sagittal craniosynostosis) is typical and may result in hydrocephalus with increased ICP and developmental delay.

Craniosynostoses are differentiated according to the affected suture(s) (**Table 24-14**).

Diagnosis

Diagnosis should be suspected in presence of abnormal head circumference and shape, fontanelle size, and palpable bony ridges along affected sutures. The diagnosis is confirmed with plain radiographs, ultrasonography, CT, and/or magnetic resonance imaging.

Treatment

Surgical intervention should be performed early in infancy to prevent the further progression of the deformity and potential complications associated with increased ICP. Also, the cranial vault of children younger than the age of 9 months is still very malleable, and deformations therefore are easier to correct.

Current surgical technique for craniosynostosis carries a high risk of major blood loss (often significantly more than one circulating blood volume) and consists of either total cranial vault reconstruction or (endoscopic) strip craniectomy followed by molding helmet therapy for 6 to 8 months postoperatively.

Prognosis

More than half of the patients suffering from increased ICP preoperatively show some signs of mental retardation. Intraoperative death is primarily a consequence of massive blood loss.

Anesthetic Management

Intracranial pressure may be elevated in syndromic children and their airway management may be challenging (upper airway obstruction) because of other concomitant craniofacial anomalies. In the presence of increased ICP, high-dose sedative premedication, ketamine, and succinylcholine should be avoided. In patients with a difficult airway, spontaneous ventilation should be maintained until the airway is secured. Alternative airway management techniques (e.g., laryngeal mask airway, fiberoptic bronchoscope) should be available.

In the presence of increased ICP, specific anesthetic measures must be considered (avoiding hypercapnia, hypoxemia, arterial hypotension).

Large-bore intravenous access is required for major craniosynostosis repair and an arterial indwelling catheter is recommended to allow for real-time blood pressure measurements and repeated blood sampling. Requirements of blood transfusions should be based on hemodynamic parameters rather than simply on hematocrit values. For craniosynostosis

TABLE 24-14 Classification of Craniosynostosis Based on Involved Cranial Sutures

Affected Suture	Morphology	Increased Intracranial Pressure	Mental Retardation
Sagittal (40%)	Scaphocephaly or dolichocephaly (decreased biparietal and increased anteroposterior diameter, i.e., long, narrow head)	Uncommon	Uncommon
Unicoronal (15%)	Anterior plagiocephaly (marked craniofacial asymmetry, "lopsided" appearance)	Uncommon	Uncommon
Bicoronal (20%)	Brachycephaly (short anteroposterior diameter of the skull with a broad, flat, recessed forehead)	Common	Common
Metopic (4%)	Trigonocephaly (pointed forehead and narrow triangular skull)	Uncommon	Uncommon
Lambdoid (5%) Bilateral Unilateral	 Brachycephaly Posterior plagiocephaly	 Common Uncommon	 Common Uncommon
Multisuture (most frequently the sagittal and coronal sutures)	Oxycephaly (high conical or pointed skull)	Common	Common
Kleeblattschadel (all sutures except the metopic)	Cloverleaf skull	Common	Common
Total (10%)	Microcephaly	Common	Common

repair, packed red blood cells should be available in the operating room upon skin incision.

Techniques to reduce allogenic blood transfusions include cell saver, preoperative acute normovolemic hemodilution, and controlled arterial hypotension. Hypotensive anesthesia is most often achieved by using volatile anesthetics, opioids, and/or sympathoadrenergic receptor–blocking drugs. However, to maintain sufficient cerebral perfusion pressure, arterial hypotension should not be used in patients with increased ICP.

Depending on the positioning of the patient, a precordial Doppler ultrasound probe may be indicated to detect intraoperative venous air embolism. Some anesthesiologists insert a long central venous catheter to evacuate air from the right side of the heart in case of significant air embolism. Because intraoperative venous air embolism may occur in more than 80% of cases, although often not hemodynamically relevant, nitrous oxide should be avoided.

Positive-pressure ventilation should be initiated once the airway has been secured and the ventilation parameters adjusted to yield normocapnia. Some anesthesiologists prefer to have the endotracheal tube sutured in place to avoid accidental extubation intraoperatively, which could potentially result in a "cannot ventilate/cannot intubate" situation (due to blood and facial swelling).

Facial swelling related to surgery can be quite pronounced (particularly when the surgery extends below the orbital ridge) and require postoperative mechanical ventilation.

Some surgeons prefer to suture the eyelids together rather than simply keep them closed by self-adhesive tape, which often comes loose during surgical manipulation.

Normothermia should be maintained. Infusion of significant amounts of cold fluids (e.g., blood products) may contribute to a rapid drop in body temperature. The use of warmed infusions and convective forced-air warming devices is therefore recommended.

DOWN SYNDROME (TRISOMY 21)

Trisomy 21 or Down syndrome is the most common human chromosomal syndrome. Overall, the prevalence is approximately 1 in 700 live births; however, with increasing maternal age older than 40 years, the prevalence can be as high as 1 in 350 live births. This disease is most often caused by maternal nondisjunction during meiosis I, resulting in three separate copies of chromosome 21. Translocation of the third chromosome onto chromosome 14 or 21 accounts for a minority of cases.

Signs and Symptoms

The clinical features are quite variable. Common features affect the head (brachycephaly, a flat occiput, dysplastic ears, epicanthal folds with typical up-slanting of the palpebral folds [mongoloid slanting] and strabismus, and Brushfield spots on the iris). The tongue is normal at birth, but later becomes enlarged due to hypertrophy of the papillae. Midface hypoplasia, a high-arched palate, and micrognathia complicate this problem. To compensate for their restricted airways, these children

habitually hold their mouths open with their tongues slightly protruding. Skeletal anomalies may include short stature and a short, broad neck with occipito-atlantoaxial instability (approximately 20% of patients). The hands are usually short and broad with a simian crease, and the middle phalanx of the fifth finger is often hypoplastic. The muscle tonus is reduced and the joints are hypermobile.

Respiratory problems can be caused by a floppy soft palate, enlarged tonsils, laryngotracheal or subglottic stenosis, obstructive sleep apnea, and recurrent pulmonary infections. As many as 40% of these patients have a congenital cardiac defect (e.g., atrial septal defect, ventricular septal defect [25%], endocardial cushion defect [50%], patent ductus arteriosus, or tetralogy of Fallot). Pulmonary hypertension should be suspected in the presence of uncorrected cardiac defects and may even lead to Eisenmenger complex. Visceral anomalies may include gastroesophageal reflux, duodenal atresia (300 times more frequent in Down syndrome), imperforate anus, and Hirschsprung's disease.

Diagnosis

Diagnoses can be established antenatally by chorionic villous sampling or by amniocentesis. Postnatally, the diagnosis is based on the typical clinical features and confirmed by karyotyping.

Prognosis

There is a 10- to 20-fold increased risk of developing leukemia (acute myelocytic leukemia or acute lymphocytic leukemia), which on average occurs approximately 3 years earlier than in otherwise healthy children. Hypothyroidism, precocious Alzheimer's disease, and conductive hearing loss are other common problems associated with Down syndrome.

Management of Anesthesia

The preoperative assessment should start with a thorough clinical review of the current respiratory and cardiac status. Airway management can be difficult (due to relative macroglossia, micrognathia, narrow hypopharynx, and muscular hypotonia), and careful airway assessment is therefore mandatory. The risk of spinal cord compression due to occipitoatlantoaxial instability should be kept in mind during intubation or positioning for surgical procedures. Since lateral radiographs of the neck in flexion and extension do not reliably detect occipito-atlantoaxial instability, it is controversial whether they should be obtained prior to anesthesia. Thus, it is important to elicit a history of gait anomalies, a preference for the sitting position, hyperreflexia, and signs of clonus, which could all be suggestive of spinal canal stenosis/cord compression. Symptomatic children may require posterior cervical spine fusion and possible fiberoptic bronchoscope intubation.

The anesthetic risk is increased in the presence of cardiac disease, particularly when associated with pulmonary hypertension, which may dictate the selection of anesthetic technique and a need for subacute bacterial endocarditis prophylaxis. Bradycardia during induction of anesthesia is more common in patients with trisomy 21. Vascular access is often challenging secondary to xerodermia, atopic dermatitis, and obesity. Choanal atresia, or narrowing of the nasal passage (due to midface hypoplasia) and the trachea (subglottic stenosis), is common and may require a smaller endotracheal tube than expected. Postintubation stridor occurs in almost 2% of these patients. The teeth are often smaller than normal with conical roots increasing the risk of dental damage during direct laryngoscopy. Reduced immune competence predisposes these patients to recurrent infections and requires strict asepsis with all invasive procedures. Airway abnormalities increase the risk of obstructive sleep apnea and mandate close monitoring in the early postoperative period. Although the intellectual capacity of these patients varies significantly, it may be advantageous to administer premedication (oral midazolam) and/or have the primary caregiver present for the induction of anesthesia as well as for the recovery period. Occasionally, a small dose of intramuscular ketamine facilitates preparation for induction of anesthesia in an uncooperative patient. Increased sensitivity to atropine has been reported in some patients manifesting mydriasis and profound tachycardia.

CRANIOFACIAL ABNORMALITIES

Cleft Lip and Palate

Cleft lip and/or cleft palate are among the most common congenital anomalies and comprise a heterogeneous group of facial malformations, although the cause of orofacial clefts is not well known. Beside chromosomal abnormalities, drugs (e.g., steroids, antiepileptics [benzodiazepines]), chemotherapy, excessive maternal vitamin A intake), folic acid deficiency, maternal tobacco or alcohol abuse (fetal alcohol syndrome), maternal diabetes mellitus, and, although controversial, maternal age (younger than 20 years or older than 39 years of age) and increased paternal age, have all been associated with orofacial clefting. Overall, a form of orofacial clefting is estimated to affect 1 in 500 to 600 newborns. The cleft may occur as an isolated anomaly or a familial trait anomaly or be part of a syndrome, e.g., Pierre Robin syndrome, trisomy 21, Treacher Collins syndrome, Stickler syndrome). The primary palatal development begins in the fifth week of gestation, with weeks 6 to 9 being the most critical ones. It is estimated that approximately one in six newborns with a cleft has other congenital defects (often affecting heart or kidney).

Signs and Symptoms

Newborns with a cleft lip usually do not have problems maintaining airway patency. However, in infants with a cleft palate or cleft lip/palate, the tongue may fall into the cleft and obstruct the airway (nose breathing). Feeding problems may be present secondary to weak or uncoordinated sucking and difficulties swallowing, which may potentially result in recurrent pulmonary aspirations and failure to thrive. Due to insufficient ventilation of the eustachian tubes in children with cleft palate, recurrent or chronic otitis media is common and often requires myringotomy and tube insertions.

Diagnosis

The diagnosis is most commonly made postnatally; however, in utero diagnosis with ultrasonography is possible as early as at the beginning of the second trimester of pregnancy. While cleft lip and cleft lip/palate should easily be detectable, an isolated cleft palate may be more discrete, sometimes requiring meticulous inspection, and palpation of the hard and soft palate.

Treatment

There is a wide variety in treatment options in terms of timing and the preferred surgical technique. In cleft lip, surgery to close the defect and reconstruct the normal anatomy is commonly performed at the age of approximately 3 months. However, the variation in age range at which the cleft palate is repaired varies significantly (most often neonatal period to approximately 18 months of age), before the development of speech.

Prognosis

In children with isolated orofacial clefting, the prognosis is excellent, although in some cases (mainly in cleft palate patients), further corrective surgeries (e.g., pharyngo- and palatoplasty) may be required.

Management of Anesthesia

In infants with nonsyndromic clefting, an inhalational induction is usually preferred and after establishing venous access, a small dose of neuromuscular blocker and opioid (fentanyl or morphine) are administered followed by securing the airway with an oral Ring-Adair-Elwyn (RAE) endotracheal tube. In infants with syndromic clefting, spontaneous ventilation should be maintained until the airway has been secured. Local anesthetics should be used to minimize pain intra- and postoperatively. Either local infiltration by the surgeon and/or an infraorbital nerve block by the anesthesiologist can serve this purpose.

The patient may be extubated once fully awake. Gentle, but thorough suctioning of the mouth and pharynx prior to extubation is recommended, as well as confirming that any throat pack inserted during surgery has been removed.

Cool mist in the postoperative period has been used successfully to keep these children comfortable and prevent airway complications. The nose may be stented initially. The arms are often splinted to prevent the infant or young child from removing nasal stents or disrupting the repair.

Mandibular Hypoplasia

Mandibular hypoplasia is a prominent feature of several syndromes that affect pediatric patients. The small mandible leaves little room for the tongue and makes the larynx appear to be anterior. Therefore, upper airway obstruction and difficult tracheal intubation are likely.

Pierre Robin Syndrome

Pierre Robin syndrome consists of micrognathia usually accompanied by glossoptosis (posterior displacement of the tongue) and cleft palate. Mandibular hypoplasia may be responsible for displacement of the tongue into the pharynx, which subsequently prevents fusion of the palate. Acute upper airway obstruction can occur in neonates or infants with Pierre Robin syndrome. Feeding problems, failure to thrive, and cyanotic episodes are other early complications of this syndrome. Associated congenital heart disease is frequent. Fortunately, sufficient mandibular growth during early childhood markedly reduces the degree of airway problems in later years.

Treacher Collins Syndrome

Treacher Collins syndrome is the most common of the mandibulofacial dysostoses. Inheritance of this syndrome is as an autosomal dominant trait with variable expression. A lethal prenatal defect occurs frequently, as fetal wastage is common in affected families. Miller syndrome has facial features similar to those associated with Treacher Collins syndrome as well as severe deformities of the extremities.

Micrognathia results in early airway problems similar to those experienced by infants with Pierre Robin syndrome. Approximately 30% of children with Treacher Collins syndrome have an associated cleft palate. Congenital heart disease, particularly a ventricular septal defect, frequently accompanies this syndrome. Other features include malar hypoplasia, colobomas (notching of the lower eyelids), and an antimongoloid slant of the palpebral fissures. Ear tags and gross deformities of the external ear canals and ossicular chain are common. Mental retardation is not a primary feature of Treacher Collins syndrome but may result from hearing loss. Tracheal intubation, as in infants with Pierre Robin syndrome, is difficult and sometimes impossible, especially once full dentition has been achieved. Patients with Treacher Collins syndrome may present for upper airway management, palatoplasty, treatment of chronic otitis media, and correction of congenital heart defects. In addition, some patients with Treacher Collins syndrome undergo extensive craniofacial osteotomies to correct cosmetic deformities (see "Hypertelorism").

Goldenhar Syndrome

Goldenhar syndrome is characterized by unilateral mandibular hypoplasia. Associated anomalies include eye, ear, and vertebral abnormalities on the affected side. Ease of tracheal intubation is highly variable. Some patients present little difficulty for tracheal intubation, whereas for others, intubation is extremely difficult.

Nager Syndrome

Nager syndrome is a rare form of acrofacial dysostosis that includes characteristic craniofacial abnormalities (malar hypoplasia, severe micrognathia). These children are likely to require multiple surgical interventions early in life to correct orthopedic and craniofacial abnormalities.

Management of Anesthesia

Preoperative Evaluation Preoperative evaluation of children with severe mandibular hypoplasia begins with evaluation of the upper airway and formulation of plans for tracheal intubation. In addition, preoperative assessment should focus on the cardiovascular system and the hemoglobin concentration. Some patients with chronic airway obstruction experience chronic arterial hypoxemia and develop pulmonary hypertension. Inclusion of anticholinergic drugs in the preoperative medication is recommended to decrease upper airway secretions. Opioids and other ventilatory depressants are often avoided in the preoperative medication.

Intraoperative Several approaches to tracheal intubation may be considered, but alternative methods must be immediately available, including facilities for emergency bronchoscopy, cricothyrotomy, or tracheostomy. Attempts at direct laryngoscopy may be preceded by intravenous administration of atropine to minimize the likelihood of vagal stimulation and resultant bradycardia. Preoxygenation before initiation of direct laryngoscopy is recommended. Administration of muscle relaxants to these patients is not recommended until the airway is secured by successful tracheal intubation. Awake tracheal intubation with the aid of fiberoptic intubation can sometimes be accomplished by the oral or nasal route after adequate topical anesthesia has been established. Awake tracheal intubation may produce undue trauma to the child's upper airway and does not eliminate the risk of pulmonary aspiration. More often, fiberoptic tracheal intubation is accomplished after inhalation induction of anesthesia with volatile anesthetics, such as sevoflurane, provided a patent upper airway can be maintained until an adequate depth of anesthesia is attained. Spontaneous ventilation is desirable during induction of anesthesia to ensure continuous airway control and to avoid inflating the child's stomach with air. Jaw thrust may facilitate maintenance of a patent upper airway until a sufficient depth of anesthesia can be achieved. Fiberoptic intubation should not be attempted until a sufficient depth of anesthesia has been established. Forward traction of the tongue along with jaw thrust may facilitate fiberoptic laryngoscopy and intubation. Use of laryngeal mask airways may be an alternative to tracheal intubation in selected patients or when tracheal intubation proves impossible. The laryngeal mask airway is also useful as a conduit for fiberoptic tracheal intubation. Tracheostomy under local anesthesia may be required when all other attempts to maintain the airway have failed. Tracheostomy in these children may be technically difficult, however, and associated with immediate and delayed complications such as bleeding and poor positioning of the tracheostomy site.

Tracheal extubation following surgery is delayed until these patients are fully awake and alert. Equipment for urgent tracheal reintubation must be immediately available.

Hypertelorism

Hypertelorism is an increased distance between the eyes and is associated with many craniofacial anomalies, such as Crouzon and Apert syndromes. Crouzon syndrome consists of hypertelorism, craniosynostosis, shallow orbits with marked proptosis, and midface hypoplasia. Apert's syndrome is characterized by essentially the same features, with the addition of syndactyly of all extremities. Other anomalies associated with hypertelorism are cleft palate, synostosis of the cervical spine, hearing loss, and mental retardation. Hypertelorism is representative of many craniofacial disorders amenable to facial reconstructive surgery.

Treatment

Correction of major craniofacial deformities may involve mandibular osteotomies, craniotomy with wide exposure of the frontal lobes, maxillary osteotomies with forward displacement of the maxilla, medial displacement of the orbits, and multiple rib grafts. Such complex operations may require several hours for completion and involve more than 100 separate surgical steps. Surgical correction is often performed during infancy, before ossification of the facial bones occurs.

Management of Anesthesia

Management of anesthesia for craniofacial surgery in children with hypertelorism is a complex undertaking that begins with meticulous preoperative assessment and preparation and extends into the postoperative period for several days. Craniofacial surgery should be attempted only by qualified teams of physicians under ideal circumstances, recognizing the possibility of multiple potential anesthetic problems.

Management of the patient's airway must not interfere with the exposure required to perform the corrective surgery. Predictably, tracheal intubation may be difficult. Intraoperatively, the tracheal tube may become dislodged or kinked during maxillary advancement, mandibular osteotomy, or repositioning of the head and neck. In addition, the tracheal tube may be displaced into a main stem bronchus when the child's neck is flexed, or the tube may be accidentally cut by the osteotome. Dry or inadequately humidified inspired gases are likely to lead to mucous plugs in the tracheal tube during these long operations, especially if small-diameter tubes are required.

Blood loss generally occurs in a steady ooze from multiple osteotomies and bone graft donor sites, averaging approximately one to two blood volumes. Quantitation of blood loss is difficult because of the diffuse oozing. Measurement of serial hematocrits, central venous pressure, and urine output are helpful for estimating blood loss and guiding intravenous fluid replacement. The availability of appropriate amounts of packed red blood cells, platelets, and fresh frozen plasma should be confirmed before surgery. Intravenous catheters must be of sufficient number and diameter to permit rapid transfusions of blood.

Blood loss may be decreased by positioning the patient in a 15- to 20-degree head-up position. In addition, controlled hypotension, using nitroprusside during phases of surgery when major hemorrhage is anticipated, may be useful. The mean arterial pressure, as measured at the level of the circle of Willis, should probably not be decreased to less than approximately 50 mm Hg during controlled hypotension. Blood must be filtered, warmed, and, if given rapidly to small children, accompanied by calcium gluconate (1–2 mg IV for every milliliter of blood infused) to decrease the possibility of citrate intoxication.

Complex craniofacial reconstruction surgeries are predictably prolonged. Hypothermia during these lengthy operations can be minimized by placing children on warming blankets, warming intravenous fluids and blood, and using warmed, humidified inspired gases. Pressure necrosis and nerve injuries can be minimized by careful positioning and padding, with an emphasis on avoiding traction on the patient's brachial plexus. Despite these precautions, peripheral nerve injury may still occur (especially ulnar neuropathy) in the absence of an obvious explanation.

Hyperventilation of the lungs to maintain the $PaCO_2$ between 30 and 35 mm Hg, maintenance of the head-up position, and administration of furosemide, mannitol, and corticosteroids are used to minimize brain swelling. Free water is limited by administering an isotonic solution. An anesthetic technique that minimizes brain edema is useful. Intraoperative brain swelling can be minimized by continuous drainage of lumbar CSF. Many reconstructive procedures are extracranial, and cerebral edema is not a significant issue.

Corneal abrasions are likely in children when ocular proptosis is pronounced. Therefore, eye ointment should be used and the eyelids sutured closed. In addition, ocular or orbital manipulations can evoke the oculocardiac reflex. Release of pressure on the orbits or administration of small doses of atropine rapidly blocks the reflex.

In addition to routine monitors, a catheter placed in a peripheral artery for continuous measurement of systemic blood pressure is mandatory. Blood from the arterial catheter also permits determination of arterial blood gases, pH, hematocrit, electrolytes, and plasma osmolarity. A central venous catheter and a Foley catheter are helpful for evaluating the adequacy of intravenous fluid replacement. Capnography is useful for following the adequacy of ventilation and prompt recognition of dislodgement of the tube from the trachea.

Postoperatively, the entire head may be wrapped in a pressure dressing through which only the endotracheal tube protrudes. The child's mouth may be wired shut. Pharyngeal bleeding, laryngeal edema, and increased ICP may be present. Therefore, no attempt is made to reverse opioid or muscle relaxant effects at the end of the operation, as mechanical ventilation of the lungs may be required for several days postoperatively.

DISORDERS OF THE UPPER AIRWAY

Acute Epiglottitis (Supraglottitis)

Acute epiglottitis is a short-lived disease that presents most often in children 2 to 7 years of age, although infants and adults may also be affected. The most common pathogen is *Haemophilus influenzae* type B, but, fortunately, the incidence of epiglottitis has decreased markedly since routine immunization for *H. influenzae* type B was instituted in the late 1980s. Nevertheless, acute epiglottitis remains a formidable challenge as its onset may be abrupt, progressing to respiratory obstruction in a matter of hours, and may be fatal if upper airway obstruction is not treated promptly. At times, however, classic signs and symptoms are not present, and it may be difficult to differentiate acute epiglottitis from laryngotracheobronchitis (croup) (**Table 24-15**). Edema of supraglottic tissues and the epiglottis is the reason some prefer to designate this disease acute supraglottitis rather than acute epiglottitis.

Signs and Symptoms

Classically, children with acute epiglottitis present with a history of acute difficulty swallowing, high fever, and inspiratory stridor. Characteristic signs and symptoms (see Table 24-15) usually develop over a period of less than 24 hours. Children naturally assume the characteristic posture of sitting upright and leaning forward with the chin up and mouth open in an attempt to maintain the airway. In fact, changes in posture may cause increased degrees of upper airway obstruction. Pulmonary edema, pericarditis, meningitis, and septic arthritis may accompany acute epiglottitis. However, *Neisseria meningitidis*, group A streptococcus, and *Candida albicans* are now the primary causes of meningitis and epiglottitis.

Diagnosis

Acute epiglottitis is a medical emergency. It is mandatory that children with suspected acute epiglottitis be admitted to the hospital. The diagnosis of acute epiglottitis is based principally on clinical signs. The history can be quickly obtained and the child examined for signs of upper airway obstruction. A lateral radiograph of the neck is obtained only in stable patients. Evidence of a large, swollen epiglottis ("thumb sign") is diagnostic. If the diagnosis of epiglottitis is strongly suspected or the child is in severe distress, radiographic examination is unnecessary and should not be pursued. Attempts to directly visualize the epiglottis should be deferred as any instrumentation, even a tongue blade, may provoke laryngospasm. Arterial blood gas sampling, venipuncture, and intravenous catheter placement are also avoided to prevent agitating the child.

Treatment

Management of acute epiglottitis should involve a team composed of a pediatric intensivist, an anesthesiologist, and an otolaryngologist. When airway obstruction is impending, it is common to bring the child to the operating room, where preparations are completed for tracheal intubation and possible emergency tracheostomy. It should be remembered that total upper airway obstruction can occur at any time, especially with instrumentation of the upper airway, perhaps reflecting glottic obstruction by the edematous epiglottis, laryngospasm from aspirated saliva, and respiratory muscle fatigue. Physicians skilled in airway management must accompany these children at all times.

Definitive treatment of acute epiglottitis includes prompt establishment of a secure airway and administration of antibiotics effective against *H. influenzae*, after blood and throat cultures are obtained. Corticosteroids are of unproven efficacy for decreasing epiglottic edema. Translaryngeal tracheal intubation during general anesthesia is the recommended approach for securing the child's airway.

Prognosis

As many as 6% of children with epiglottitis without an artificial airway (endotracheal tube or tracheostomy) may die as compared with less than 1% of those with an artificial airway. The duration of intubation depends on the clinical course of

TABLE 24-15	Clinical Features of Acute Epiglottitis and Laryngotracheobronchitis	
Parameter	**Acute Epiglottitis**	**Laryngotracheobronchitis**
Age group affected	2–7 yr	<2 yr
Incidence	Accounts for 5% of children with stridor	Accounts for about 80% of children with stridor
Etiologic agent	Bacterial (*Haemophilus influenzae*)	Viral
Onset	Rapid over 24 hr	Gradual over 24–72 hr
Signs and symptoms	Inspiratory stridor, pharyngitis, drooling, fever (often > 39°C), lethargic to restless, insists upon sitting up and leaning forward, tachypnea, cyanosis	Inspiratory stridor, "barking" cough, rhinorrhea, fever (rarely > 39°C)
Laboratory	Neutrophilia	Lymphocytosis
Lateral radiographs of the neck	Swollen epiglottis	Narrowing of the subglottic area
Treatment	Oxygen, urgent tracheal intubation tracheostomy during general anesthesia, fluids, antibiotics, corticosteroids (?)	Oxygen, aerosolized racemic epinephrine, humidity, fluids, corticosteroids, tracheal intubation for severe airway obstruction

the patient. Because the response to antibiotics is rapid, extubation may be achieved within 2 to 3 days in most cases.

Management of Anesthesia

An otolaryngologist should be present at the time of induction. Induction and maintenance of anesthesia for tracheal intubation are accomplished with the volatile anesthetic sevoflurane (halothane historically) in oxygen. High inspired concentrations of oxygen permitted by the use of volatile anesthetics facilitate optimal oxygenation in these patients. Before induction of anesthesia, preparations are made for an emergency cricothyrotomy or tracheostomy, which may be required if airway obstruction suddenly occurs and translaryngeal tracheal intubation is not possible.

Inhalation induction of anesthesia is initiated with the child in the sitting position. After the onset of drowsiness, the child is placed supine, and assisted mask ventilation is provided if necessary to overcome upper airway obstruction. Once an adequate depth of anesthesia has been established, an intravenous catheter is placed and direct laryngoscopy and intubation (with a styletted endotracheal tube that is one half size smaller than would ordinarily be selected) are performed. After successful tracheal intubation, a thorough direct laryngoscopy is performed to confirm the diagnosis of acute epiglottitis. Some anesthesiologists prefer to replace the orotracheal tube with a nasotracheal tube under direct vision if the switch can be made confidently without losing the airway. A nasotracheal tube is more comfortable for awake children, decreases salivation, and prevents biting of the tube. After intubation is accomplished and the endotracheal tube is well secured, the child is allowed to awaken from the anesthetic and transferred to the intensive care unit

Tracheal extubation may be considered when the child's fever and other signs of infection such as neutrophilia have waned. A clinical sign of resolution of the epiglottic swelling is the development of an air leak around the tracheal tube. Regardless of the clinical impression, the airway is examined by direct laryngoscopy or flexible fiberoptic laryngoscopy while under sedation or general anesthesia to confirm that inflammation of the epiglottis and other supraglottic tissues has resolved before the trachea is extubated.

Laryngotracheobronchitis (Croup)

Laryngotracheobronchitis (croup) is a viral infection of the upper respiratory tract that typically afflicts children between 6 months and 6 years of age, particularly those younger than 2 years of age (see Table 24-15). Parainfluenza, adenovirus, myxovirus, and influenza A virus have been implicated as causative agents. Laryngotracheobronchitis and acute epiglottitis share certain clinical features and at times are difficult to differentiate (see Table 24-15).

Signs and Symptoms

Laryngotracheobronchitis, in contrast to acute epiglottitis, has a gradual onset over 24 to 72 hours. There are signs of upper respiratory tract infection, such as rhinorrhea, pharyngitis, and low-grade fever. Leukocyte counts are normal or only slightly increased with lymphocytosis. Patients present with a characteristic "barking" cough, hoarse voice, and inspiratory stridor. Symptoms worsen with agitation and crying and at night. The child with croup may prefer to sit up or be held upright.

Diagnosis

Croup is a clinical diagnosis. However, if a radiograph of the neck is obtained, a characteristic subglottic narrowing or "steeple sign" frequently may be evident on the anteroposterior view. Unfortunately, the steeple sign is not pathognomonic of croup and does not correlate well with disease severity. Infants with mild subglottic stenosis may present with a history of recurrent respiratory infections and symptoms confused with croup.

Treatment

Croup occasionally presents with life-threatening airway obstruction. Treatment of mild to moderate laryngotracheobronchitis includes administration of supplemental oxygen and cool mist. It should be noted that in children presenting with wheezing and croup concomitantly, cool mist may exacerbate bronchospasm. In cases of severe respiratory distress with cyanosis and retractions, nebulized racemic epinephrine (0.05 mL/kg up to 0.5 mL of 2.25% epinephrine solution in 3 mL normal saline) in addition to oxygen may help relieve airway obstruction. Treatment with nebulized racemic epinephrine presumably reduces laryngeal mucosal edema due to its vasoconstrictive effect and has been shown to decrease the need for tracheal intubation. Patients receiving nebulized racemic epinephrine therapy should be admitted for observation because they often require repeated treatments 1 to 4 hours apart and may experience a rebound effect manifested as increased obstruction following an initial state of improvement. Administration of corticosteroids, such as dexamethasone (0.5–1.0 mg/kg IV) or inhalation of budesonide are effective in relieving symptoms of croup by decreasing edema in the laryngeal mucosa.

Tracheal intubation is required if physical exhaustion occurs, as evidenced by increased Pa_{CO_2}. When airway obstruction is compounded by accumulation of thick, inspissated secretions, intubation and aggressive pulmonary toilet are indicated. The trachea should be intubated with a smaller than normal tube to minimize the edema associated with intubation. In the event that a smaller than normal tracheal tube fits too tightly in the subglottic area, a tracheostomy may be required.

Prognosis

Most patients, especially older children, with croup experience only stridor and mild dyspnea before recovering. In more severe cases, the use of nebulized epinephrine has significantly decreased the need for tracheostomies. Although laryngotracheobronchitis is generally a short-lived illness, airway hyperreactivity may persist. The duration of intubation is longer than that for epiglottitis and depends on the development of an air leak around the endotracheal tube, generally 3 to 5 days.

Management of Anesthesia

When intubation is necessary, the procedure should be performed in the operating room as for a child with epiglottitis. A surgeon should be present in case a tracheostomy becomes necessary.

Postintubation Laryngeal Edema

Postintubation laryngeal edema or postintubation croup is a potential complication of tracheal intubation in all children, although the incidence is highest in children between the ages of 1 and 4 years. Symptoms are typically caused by mucosal edema in the subglottic region, but edema may also occur at the glottic level. Studies to delineate the cause of postintubation laryngeal edema are lacking, but certain predisposing factors seem predictable (**Table 24-16**).

Signs and Symptoms

Postintubation laryngeal edema may manifest as stridor, a "barking" or "brassy" cough, hoarseness, retractions, flaring of the alae nasi, hypoxemia, and mental status changes. The severity of the symptoms correlates to the severity of airway obstruction. Symptoms generally occur within 1 hour of extubation, with peak intensity within 4 hours and resolution of stridor within 24 hours.

Diagnosis

Inspiratory stridor suggests airway obstruction at or above the level of the vocal cords, whereas expiratory stridor suggests airway obstruction below the level of the vocal cords.

Treatment

Treatment of postintubation laryngeal edema is aimed at reducing airway edema. Hourly administration of aerosolized racemic epinephrine may be required until symptoms subside. The aerosolized dose of racemic epinephrine is 0.05 mL/kg (maximum 0.5 mL) in 3.0 mL of saline. The clinical effect of racemic epinephrine dissipates within 2 hours. Because of the potential for the rebound phenomenon associated with nebulized racemic epinephrine therapy, day surgery patients should be observed for up to 4 hours after the last treatment. In severe cases of postintubation laryngeal edema, helium and oxygen mixtures have proven to be useful.

Although the administration of dexamethasone to treat postintubation laryngeal edema is widespread, the therapeutic efficacy remains controversial. Steroids also do not reliably prevent postintubation laryngeal edema when given prophylactically, although the progression of airway edema may be prevented. While dexamethasone has been shown to be of use in treating laryngotracheobronchitis, 4 to 6 hours are required to achieve maximum effect.

Prognosis

In most cases, postintubation laryngeal edema is self-limited. Mild cases may improve with cool mist therapy alone. For those requiring racemic epinephrine, one or two treatments usually produce significant improvement. Reintubation of the trachea or a tracheostomy is rarely needed.

Management of Anesthesia

The use of uncuffed endotracheal tubes has traditionally been recommended in children younger than the age of 8 years because of concerns that cuffed endotracheal tubes might contribute to the risk of subglottic edema. The replacement of high-pressure, low-volume cuffs with low-pressure, high-volume cuffs on modern endotracheal tubes appears to make cuffed endotracheal tubes of no greater risk of postintubation stridor than uncuffed tubes. In fact, the use of a cuffed endotracheal tube one half to one size smaller than the uncuffed tube that would normally be selected, theoretically could decrease the number of reintubation attempts due to a tube that is either too tight or too small (having an excessive leak). Extubation can be contemplated when a leak around the endotracheal tube is demonstrated, indicating adequate improvement in the laryngeal edema.

Foreign Body Aspiration

Foreign body aspiration into the airways, with its resultant airway obstruction, can produce a wide range of responses. For example, complete obstruction at the level of the larynx or trachea can result in death from asphyxiation. At the opposite end of the spectrum, passage of a foreign body into distal airways may elicit only mild symptoms that may go unnoticed.

Signs and Symptoms

Common clinical features of foreign body aspiration are cough, wheezing, and decreased air entry into the affected lung. The most frequent site of aspiration is the right mainstem bronchus, followed by the trachea to a much lesser extent. Severity of symptoms varies with the site of the foreign body and the degree of obstruction it produces. Chronically retained airway foreign bodies often present with the misdiagnosis of upper respiratory tract infections, asthma, or

TABLE 24-16 Factors Associated with Postintubation Laryngeal Edema
Age younger than 4 years
Tight-fitting endotracheal tube, no audible leak at 15–25 cm H_2O
Traumatic or repeated intubation
Prolonged intubation
High-pressure, low-volume cuff
Patient "bucking" or coughing while intubated
Head repositioning while intubated
History of infectious or postintubation croup
Neck/airway surgery
Upper respiratory infection
Trisomy 21

pneumonia. The type of foreign body aspirated can influence the clinical course. For example, nuts and certain vegetable materials are highly irritating to the bronchial mucosa.

Diagnosis

In a previously healthy child with no other signs of upper respiratory infection or airway abnormalities, choking or coughing episodes accompanied by wheezing are highly suggestive of an airway foreign body. Bronchial foreign bodies manifest as coughing, wheezing, dyspnea, and decreased air entry in the affected side. Chest radiography provides direct evidence if the aspirated object is radiopaque. If the aspirated foreign body is radiolucent, indirect evidence can be obtained by demonstrating hyperinflation of the affected lung (due to air trapping) and shifting of the mediastinum toward the opposite side on expiratory chest radiograph. Atelectasis occurs as a late finding, distal to the obstruction. Laryngeal foreign bodies present with complete obstruction and asphyxiation unless promptly relieved or with partial obstruction and croup, hoarseness, cough, stridor, and dyspnea. Tracheal foreign bodies most frequently present with choking, stridor, and wheezing.

Treatment

Treatment for aspirated foreign bodies requires endoscopic removal using direct laryngoscopy and rigid bronchoscopy. The goal is to remove the foreign body within 24 hours after aspiration. Risks of leaving the foreign body in the airways for longer than 24 hours include migration of the aspirated material, pneumonia, and residual pulmonary disease.

Prognosis

Aspirated peanuts and beans soften and are subject to fragmentation when grasped by forceps. Fragmentation during the course of removal is an extremely dangerous situation that can result in death if the pieces occlude both main-stem bronchi and prevent ventilation. Laryngeal or tracheal occlusion usually is associated with a grave outcome, but, fortunately, most objects small enough to pass through the vocal cords rarely occlude the trachea.

Management of Anesthesia

Few cases demand as much flexibility on the part of the anesthesiologist as do children with aspirated foreign bodies. Each child mandates individualization of the anesthetic technique to fit the clinical situation. Techniques for induction of anesthesia depend on the severity and location of the airway obstruction. When a laryngeal foreign body or airway obstruction is present, induction of anesthesia using only volatile anesthetics such as sevoflurane in oxygen is useful. Induction of anesthesia with intravenous drugs followed by inhalation of volatile anesthetics is acceptable if the airway is less tenuous. Allowing spontaneous ventilation requires that an adequate depth of anesthesia be attained to prevent coughing during laryngoscopy and bronchoscopy. Spraying the larynx with a lidocaine solution is effective in preventing laryngospasm when endoscopic manipulation is performed. Administration

of atropine (10–20 µg/kg IV) or glycopyrrolate (3–5 µg/kg IV) is useful to decrease the likelihood of bradycardia from vagal stimulation during endoscopy.

Muscle relaxants are often avoided during bronchoscopy because positive airway pressures could contribute to distal migration of foreign bodies, complicating their extraction. In addition, if foreign bodies produce a ball-valve phenomenon, the use of positive-pressure ventilation of the lungs could contribute to hyperinflation and possibly pneumothorax. Spontaneous ventilation is desirable until the nature and location of the foreign body have been identified by bronchoscopy. Muscle relaxants may be useful during removal of a foreign body distal to the carina because the duration of these procedures tends to be long.

Total intravenous anesthesia using propofol can have advantages over inhalational anesthesia, particularly in long cases involving bronchial foreign bodies. A propofol infusion will ensure a steady level of anesthesia regardless of intermittent ventilation or ventilation-perfusion mismatches. After the rigid bronchoscope is placed in the trachea, the anesthesia circuit can be attached to the breathing sidearm of the bronchoscope. Spontaneous ventilation or manual ventilation, if the patient is paralyzed, can then be resumed. When endoscopic instruments are placed through the bronchoscope, ventilation through the breathing sidearm becomes ineffective due to high resistance. An apneic oxygenation technique may need to be applied in which ventilation is held during endoscopy. When the oxygen saturation begins to decrease, the endoscopic instruments are removed, the bronchoscope is withdrawn above the level of the carina, and the proximal open end is occluded so that the patient can be hyperventilated before instrumentation resumes. A large air leak around the bronchoscope is frequently present. High fresh gas flows are often required to overcome a substantial air leak.

Occasionally, the endoscopist must intermittently remove the bronchoscope and place an endotracheal tube to allow adequate ventilation if the air leak is so large as to prohibit adequate ventilation. If during retrieval, a foreign body becomes dislodged in the trachea or larynx causing airway occlusion and prompt retrieval is not possible, the foreign body should be pushed back into one of the main bronchi so that ventilation can be accomplished with at least one lung. The patient can be mask ventilated, or an endotracheal tube can be placed in the trachea until another attempt at retrieval is made. Skeletal muscle paralysis produced with succinylcholine or short-acting nondepolarizing muscle relaxants may be required to remove the bronchoscope and foreign body if the object is too large to pass through the moving vocal cords. After completion of bronchoscopy, the patient is intubated with an endotracheal tube and extubated when the appropriate criteria are met.

Despite the concerns that adverse effects of aspirated foreign bodies may be influenced by the method of ventilation selected during anesthesia (spontaneous versus controlled ventilation), there is no evidence that outcomes during and following bronchial or tracheal foreign body removal are influenced by the ventilatory management strategy employed. Fortunately, most patients are relatively stable at presentation, allowing preoperative studies to be obtained and adequate emptying of the stomach. Dexamethasone is frequently given prophylactically to decrease subglottic edema. Nebulized racemic epinephrine is useful in treating postintubation croup. Chest radiographs should be obtained after bronchoscopy to detect atelectasis or pneumothorax. Postural drainage and chest percussion enhance clearance of secretions and decrease the subsequent risk of infections.

Laryngeal Papillomatosis

Laryngeal papillomatosis is the most common benign laryngeal neoplasm in children. The most likely cause is a tissue response to human papillomavirus. The mechanism of human papillomavirus infection in the larynx is unclear. In many cases, it is suspected, but unproven, that transmission of the virus to the child from a mother with genital warts occurs during vaginal delivery.

Signs and Symptoms

A change in the character of the child's voice is the most common initial symptom of laryngeal papillomatosis. Children present with hoarseness, whereas infants may present with an altered cry and sometimes stridor. Progressive dyspnea and airway obstruction may ensue if left untreated. Most children with papillomatosis present with symptoms before the age of 7 years. Some degree of airway obstruction is present in more than 40% of patients.

Diagnosis

Diagnosis is confirmed by microlaryngoscopy and biopsy of lesions.

Treatment

Various forms of treatment for laryngeal papillomatosis have been used, including surgical excision, cryosurgery, topical 5-fluorouracil, exogenous interferon, and laser ablation. Because the disease is ultimately self-limiting, the complications of therapy must be avoided. For example, seeding of the distal airways can occur after tracheostomy (although the spread of lesions is usually limited to the tracheostomy site). Tracheostomy can be life saving and is usually reserved for cases with rapid recurrence and accompanying airway obstruction. Surgical therapy with laser coagulation has been the mainstay of treatment. Because papillomas recur, frequent laser ablation is required until the patient experiences spontaneous remission. More recently, excision of papillomas with the laryngeal microdébrider has gained popularity in some centers.

Prognosis

Distal involvement of the lower tracheobronchial tree represents an aggressive variant that may be fatal. Malignant degeneration of juvenile papillomas is rare but can occur in older children. Papillomas usually regress spontaneously at puberty.

Management of Anesthesia

Management of anesthesia for removal of laryngeal papillomas depends on the severity of the airway obstruction. Maintaining spontaneous ventilation is recommended until the extent and nature of airway obstruction is determined. Awake tracheal intubation is recommended for severe airway obstruction but is not always feasible in children. Intubating the trachea after inducing anesthesia with sevoflurane in oxygen while the otolaryngologist stands by is usually a safe approach. Children with severe airway obstruction should not be given muscle relaxants in an attempt to facilitate tracheal intubation. Indeed, in some children, the glottic opening can be identified only with the child breathing spontaneously. A partially obstructed airway may become completely obstructed with the onset of anesthesia or with positive-pressure ventilation, as in the case of a pedunculated vocal cord or supraglottic papilloma. A rigid bronchoscope must be readily available, and it may be the only means to secure an airway in some children. Difficulty ventilating the lungs can be encountered after intubation if a papilloma is dislodged into the trachea or obstructs the endotracheal tube. It should be appreciated that the degree of airway obstruction can vary greatly in the same patient presenting for subsequent papilloma excisions.

Surgical therapy for papillomatosis by laser ablation or forceps excision is usually done as a microlaryngoscopic procedure. During microlaryngoscopy, the vocal cords must be quiescent. Skeletal muscle paralysis or deep anesthesia therefore is required to produce acceptable operating conditions. Short-acting nondepolarizing muscle relaxants are useful for this purpose. Muscle relaxants should be administered only after the ability to provide positive-pressure ventilation by mask is demonstrated. Cuffed tracheal tubes of smaller-than-predicted diameters should be used for tracheal intubation and should improve visualization of the glottis by the endoscopist. In some instances, apneic oxygenation techniques with temporary removal of the tracheal tube are useful. The usual safety precautions concerning laser use should be observed for laser ablation of papillomas. After resection of papillomas, the tracheal tube should be removed only when the child is fully awake and laryngeal bleeding has ceased. After tracheal extubation, inhalation of aerosolized racemic epinephrine and intravenous administration of dexamethasone may decrease subglottic edema.

Lung Abscess

A lung abscess develops when localized infection in the lung parenchyma becomes necrotic and cavitates. A number of conditions predispose children to the development of pulmonary abscesses. The most common cause of lung abscess in a child is aspiration of gastric secretions containing disease-producing bacteria. Pneumonitis impairs drainage of the aspirated material and leads to localized inflammation and parenchymal ischemia, resulting in tissue necrosis and liquefaction. In addition, bronchial obstruction by tumor or a foreign body may result in lung abscesses distal to sites of airway obstruction. The use of endotracheal intubation and pharyngeal packing has reduced the incidence of lung abscesses resulting from aspiration of blood and tissue during oropharyngeal procedures.

Signs and Symptoms

The most common symptoms caused by lung abscess in the pediatric population include fever, cough, pleuritic chest pain, productive sputum, anorexia, weight loss, hemoptysis, dyspnea, and tachypnea.

Diagnosis

Lung abscess is usually diagnosed from a chest radiograph classically demonstrating a cavity containing an air-fluid level. Infected congenital bronchogenic or pulmonary cysts may be indistinguishable from lung abscess on chest radiographs. A chest CT can be a useful adjunct in obtaining additional information about the anatomic character and the location and size of the diseased lung region. If a satisfactory sputum sample is unobtainable, percutaneous needle aspiration of the abscess cavity under CT guidance or diagnostic bronchoscopy with direct transbronchial aspiration of purulent fluid may help isolate the causative organism.

Treatment

The initial treatment consists of parenteral antibiotic therapy that covers both aerobic and anaerobic organisms until a specific bacteriologic diagnosis is established. Chest physiotherapy and postural drainage of the abscess in conjunction with antibiotic therapy are often effective, but therapeutic bronchoscopy and transbronchial drainage of the abscess may be necessary. Surgical intervention is indicated for the cases that do not respond to antibiotic therapy.

Prognosis

Medical therapy is frequently unsuccessful in neonates and immunocompromised children. However, the prognosis for previously healthy patients with no underlying medical disorders is quite good, with most symptoms resolving within 7 to 10 days, although fever may persist for several weeks.

Management of Anesthesia

Placing a double-lumen endobronchial tube is often used to minimize the risk of contamination of the lungs and airways with purulent material from the lung abscess. In infants and small children, endobronchial intubation may be required for lung isolation (as double-lumen tubes are too large). High inspired concentrations of oxygen are necessary, as one-lung anesthesia may result in increased right-to-left intrapulmonary shunting, resulting in decreased Pa_{O_2}

MALIGNANT HYPERTHERMIA

Malignant hyperthermia (MH) is an example of a pharmacogenetic clinical syndrome. Susceptible patients have a genetic predisposition for the development of this disorder, which does not manifest until they are exposed to triggering agents or stressful environmental factors. All volatile inhalation anesthetic agents are the most commonly implicated pharmacologic triggers of MH.

The overall incidence of MH during general anesthesia has been reported as 1 in 3000 to 15,000 children and 1 in 50,000 to 100,000 adults. The incidence is higher when succinylcholine is used with other triggering agents. The incidence has an apparent geographic variation, as it is more prevalent in certain areas of North America. MH usually occurs in children and young adults (the incidence of acute MH is highest in the first three decades of life) but has been reported at the extremes of age, ranging from infants in the delivery room to 70 years.

The recognized modes of inheritance for MH susceptibility are autosomal dominant with reduced penetrance and variable expression, autosomal recessive, or multifactorial and unclassified. Reduced penetrance means that fewer offspring are affected than would be predicted by a perfectly dominant pattern. Variable expression is a difference of susceptibility between families with little variation within the same family.

In pigs, the porcine stress syndrome or pale soft exudative pork syndrome, is an animal model for MH. Certain breeds of pig show a classic presentation of MH on induction of anesthesia with potent inhalation agents and succinylcholine. A single-point mutation occurs at the *RYR1* gene locus and is then transmitted as an autosomal recessive genetic disorder. This syndrome can be triggered by stressors other than anesthesia (e.g., shipping, preparation for slaughter). The gene for MH is located on human chromosome 19, which is also the genetic coding site for the calcium release channels of skeletal muscle sarcoplasmic reticulum (ryanodine receptors RYR1 locus). It is presumed that a defect in the calcium release channels results in MH susceptibility. Although 25% of MH families in North America who have been studied have a genetic mutation of the *RYR1* gene, these mutations do not always relate to a positive in vitro contracture test to halothane. MH in humans is not a single disease as in the pig but a syndrome with multiple sites of causation and multiple mutations at these sites.

Even the presentation of MH is not the same in all patients. Some 30% of MH patients have had up to three uneventful anesthetics. A spectrum can occur from minor reactions to rapid temperature increase, muscle rigidity, acidosis, arrhythmias, and death. Some reactions have greater latency to onset and may not manifest until the postoperative period. MH may not always occur in response to triggering agents. Thus, there may be different genes causing MH in different families or other predisposing factors being expressed differently in patients or families. MH may be described as a heterogeneous genetic disorder with a highly variable clinical presentation.

Signs and Symptoms

There are no clinical features that are specific for MH, and the diagnosis depends on knowledge of features that can occur during an episode (**Table 24-17**). MH is characterized by signs and symptoms of hypermetabolism (up to 10 times normal). The clinical manifestations of this disorder are nonspecific and include tachycardia, tachypnea, arterial

TABLE 24-17 Clinical Feature of Malignant Hyperthermia

Timing	Clinical Signs	Changes in Monitored Variables	Biochemical Changes
Early	Masseter spasm		
	Tachypnea	Increased minute ventilation	
	Rapid exhaustion of soda lime	Increasing end-tidal carbon dioxide concentrations	Increased Paco$_2$
	Warm soda lime canister		
	Tachycardia		Acidosis
	Irregular heart rate	Cardiac dysrhythmias Peaked T waves on the ECG	Hyperkalemia
Intermediate	Patient warm to touch	Increasing core body temperature	
	Cyanosis	Decreasing hemoglobin oxygen saturation	
	Dark blood in surgical site		
	Irregular heart rate	Cardiac dysrhythmias Peaked T waves on the ECG	Hyperkalemia
Late	Generalized skeletal muscle rigidity		Increased creature kinase concentrations
	Prolonged bleeding		
	Dark urine		Myoglobinuria
	Irregular heart rate	Cardiac dysrhythmias Peaked T waves on the ECG	Hyperkalemia

Adapted from Hopkns PM: Malignant hyperthermia: Advances in clinical management and diagnosis. Br J Anaesth 2000:118–128.

hypoxemia, hypercarbia, metabolic and respiratory acidosis, hyperkalemia, cardiac dysrhythmias, hypotension, skeletal muscle rigidity, trismus or masseter spasm after administration of succinylcholine, and increased body temperature.

The earliest signs of MH are those related to enormous increases in the patient's metabolic rate reflecting the ability of triggering drugs to cause an imbalance in calcium homeostasis in skeletal muscle cells. In some patients, metabolic stimulation is evident clinically within 10 minutes of administration of volatile anesthetics, whereas in others, several hours may elapse. Increased intracellular calcium concentrations stimulate metabolism both directly through activation of phosphorylase to increase glycolysis and indirectly because of increased demands for adenosine triphosphate production. Hypermetabolism leads to increased carbon dioxide production with associated tachypnea. In addition, lactic acidosis develops, and the presence of mixed respiratory and metabolic acidosis stimulates sympathetic nervous system activity with associated tachycardia. Increased carbon dioxide production occurs early, emphasizing the value of continuous capnography. Temperature rise may be a late sign, but core temperature may increase as early as 15 minutes after exposure to a triggering agent. Cardiac dysrhythmias, such as ventricular bigeminy, multifocal ventricular premature beats, and ventricular tachycardia, may also occur, especially when hyperkalemia resulting from rhabdomyolysis and sympathetic nervous system stimulation accompany this syndrome. Cutaneous changes may vary from flushing, caused by vasodilation, to blanching secondary to intense vasoconstriction. Other complications are hemolysis, myoglobinemia, and renal failure.

Diagnosis

MH is a disorder of increased metabolism with increased oxygen consumption and CO_2 production. The cardiovascular and respiratory systems respond to this by increasing cardiac output and respiratory rate. In a spontaneously breathing patient, the first clinically evident signs of MH are an increase in end-tidal CO_2, tachycardia, and tachypnea (see Table 23-17). The CO_2 absorber in a semiclosed system may become hot, and the canister absorber will be exhausted. Without hypercapnia and acidosis, the diagnosis of MH is questionable.

Tachycardia may be attributed to "light" anesthesia and cause a delay in the diagnosis. The first indication that an individual may be susceptible to MH is the development of exaggerated initial responses to succinylcholine manifesting as increased tension of the masseter muscles. If sufficiently sensitive measuring equipment is used, jaw stiffness after administration of succinylcholine can be detected in most patients but is often more pronounced in children (**Fig. 24-2**). Conversely, in others, drug-induced masseter spasm is mild and transient or even absent. It is recommended that signs of hypermetabolism (metabolic and respiratory acidosis, increased body temperature) should be sought after masseter spasm is noted before a diagnosis of MH is contemplated. It has been suggested, however, that children in whom masseter spasm develops have a 50% incidence of susceptibility to MH.

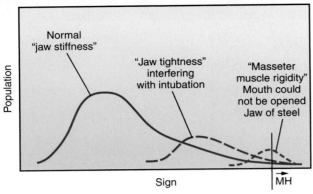

Figure 24-2 • The spectrum of masseter muscle responses to succinylcholine varies from a slight jaw stiffness that does not interfere with endotracheal intubation to the extreme "jaws of steel," which is masseter muscle tetany, not allowing the mouth to be opened. It is likely that the latter response is more highly associated with malignant hyperthermia. It should be noted that, even with the inability to open the mouth, the patient should still be able to be ventilated by bag and mask since all other muscles are relaxed. (*Adapted from Kaplan RF. Malignant Hyperthermia. Annual Refresher Course Lectures. Washington, DC, American Society of Anesthesiologists, 1993.*)

Whether one proceeds with the anesthetic after masseter muscle rigidity (MMR) is a source of controversy. If the decision is made to continue with the procedure, it is recommended that the halogenated agent be discontinued and that maintenance of anesthesia continue with a nitrous oxide/narcotic-intravenous hypnotic/nondepolarizing muscle relaxant technique (i.e., nontriggering technique) as indicated. Skeletal muscle biopsies are positive for MH susceptibility in all patients in whom plasma creatine kinase concentrations exceed 20,000 IU/L after succinylcholine-induced masseter spasm.

Monitoring must include continuous capnography and temperature monitoring. The urine must be examined for myoglobinuria. If myoglobin is present, hydration, diuresis, and possibly alkalinization should be maintained to prevent rhabdomyolytic renal failure. Patients should remain hospitalized until the urine is free of myoglobin. Postanesthesia serum creatine kinase levels should be checked every 6 to 8 hours for 24 hours. At least 12 hours of observation after MMR is recommended, even when signs of hypermetabolism or myoglobinuria are initially absent. Patients with evidence of hypermetabolism should be admitted and treated for acute MH.

Body temperature increases are often late manifestations of MH. Indeed, the diagnosis of MH should not depend on increased body temperature. Nevertheless, increased body temperature may be precipitous, increasing at a rate of 0.5°C every 15 minutes and reaching levels as high as 46°C.

Analysis of arterial and central venous blood reveals arterial hypoxemia, hypercarbia ($Paco_2$ 100–200 mm Hg), respiratory and metabolic acidosis (pH 7.15–6.80), and marked central venous oxygen desaturation. Hyperkalemia may occur early in the course of MH, but after normothermia returns, the serum potassium concentrations decrease rapidly. Serum concentrations of transaminase enzymes and creatine kinase are markedly increased, although peak levels may not occur for 12 to 24 hours after acute episodes. Plasma and urine myoglobin concentrations (give urine a color similar to that caused by hemoglobin) are also increased, reflecting massive rhabdomyolysis. Late complications of untreated MH include disseminated intravascular coagulation, pulmonary edema, and acute renal failure. Central nervous system damage may manifest as blindness, seizures, coma, or paralysis.

Differential Diagnosis

A differential diagnosis of MH can be seen in **Table 24-18**. Also hyperglycemic, hyperosmolar nonketotic syndrome may give a similar presentation to MH rhabdomyolysis. Dantrolene therapy is also used to treat this condition.

Treatment

Successful treatment of MH depends on early recognition of the diagnosis and institution of a preplanned therapeutic regimen. Treatment of MH can be categorized as causal or symptomatic. Causal treatment is directed at correcting the underlying causative mechanisms. Symptomatic treatment is directed toward maintaining renal function and correcting hyperthermia, acidosis, and arterial hypoxemia.

Dantrolene, administered intravenously, is the only drug that is reliably effective for the treatment of MH (**Table 24-19**). Treatment of acute episodes of MH is with dantrolene (2–3 mg/kg IV). This dose is repeated every 5 to 10 minutes to maximum doses of 10 mg/kg, depending on the patient's temperature and metabolic responses. Typically, dantrolene (2–5 mg/kg IV) is required for treatment of acute episodes of MH. Occasionally, doses higher than 10 mg/kg IV may be needed. Diluting dantrolene with 40°C water rather than operating room temperature water (20°C or below) will speed dantrolene reconstitution.

Symptomatic treatment for MH includes immediate termination of the administration of the inhaled anesthetics and prompt conclusion of the surgical procedure (see Table 24-19). Under no circumstances should the administration of volatile anesthetics be continued with the false hope that anesthetic-induced vasodilation will aid in cooling or that high concentrations of these drugs will decrease the metabolic rate. The patient's lungs are hyperventilated with 100% oxygen, and active cooling is initiated. Active cooling may be done with surface cooling and intracavitary lavage of the stomach and bladder using cold saline solutions. Intravenous saline solutions infused through peripheral intravenous catheters should also be cooled. Cooling is discontinued when body temperature decreases to 38°C. Other symptomatic therapy includes intravenous administration of sodium bicarbonate to correct metabolic acidosis and hyperkalemia, hydration with saline, and maintenance of urine output at 2 mL/kg per hour with the administration of osmotic or tubular diuretics. Intravenous administration of glucose combined with regular insulin helps drive potassium intracellularly and provides an exogenous energy source with which to replace depleted cerebral metabolic substrates. Failure to maintain diuresis may result

TABLE 24-18 Differential Diagnosis of Malignant Hyperthermia

Diagnosis	Distinguishing Traits
Hyperthyroidism	Symptoms and physical findings often present, blood gas abnormalities increase gradually
Sepsis	Usually normal blood gases
Pheochromocytoma	Similar to MH except marked blood pressure swings
Metastatic carcinoid	Same as pheochromocytoma
Cocaine intoxication	Fever, rigidity, rhabdomyolysis similar to malignant neuroleptic syndrome
Heat stroke	Similar to MH except that the patient is outside the operating room
Masseter spasm (MMR)	May progress to MH, total body spasm more likely than isolated MMR
Malignant neurolept	Similar to MH, usually associated with the use of syndrome antidepressants
Serotogenic syndrome	Similar to MH and malignant neuroleptic syndrome, associated with the administration of mood-elevating drugs

MH, malignant hyperthermia; MMR, masseter muscle rigidity.
Adapted from Bissonnette B, Ryan JF: Temperature regulation: Normal and abnormal [malignant hyperthermia]. In Cote CJ, Todres ID, Goudsouzian NG, Ryan JF, (eds): A Practice of Anesthesia for Infants and Children, 3rd ed. Philadelphia, Saunders, 2001, p 621.

TABLE-24-19 Treatrment of Malignant Hyperthermia

Etiologic Treatment
Dantrolene (2-3 mg/kg IV) as an initial bolus, followed with repeat doses every 5–10 minutes until symptoms are controlled (rarely need total dose > 10 mg/kg)
Prevent recrudescence (dantrolene 1 mg/kg IV every 6 hours for 72 hours)

Symptomatic Treatment
Immediately discontinue inhaled anesthetics and conclude surgery as soon as possible
Hyperventilate the lungs with 100% oxygen
Initiate active cooling (iced saline 15 mL/kg IV every 10 minutes, gastric and bladder lavage with iced saline, surface cooling)
Correct metabolic acidosis (sodium bicarbonate 1–2 mEq/kg IV based on arterial pH)
Maintain urine output (hydration, mannitol 0.25 g/kg IV, furosemide 1 mg/kg IV)
Treat cardiac dysrhythmias (procainamide 15 mg/kg IV)
Monitor in an intensive care unit (urine output, arterial blood gases, pH, electrolytes)

in acute renal failure due to deposition of myoglobin in the renal tubules.

The important fact is that within 45 minutes, the patient should be responding to treatment; if not, intensive therapy should be pursued. Recrudescence may occur in 25% of patients, usually within 4 to 8 hours after the initial episode but recrudescence as late as 36 hours has been reported. Patients may smolder, with symptoms such as continued hyperkalemia, residual muscle rigidity, massive fluid requirements, and oliguria progressing to anuria. Dantrolene should probably be repeated even if the initial episode is under control at a dose 1 to 2 mg/kg intravenously every 6 hours for a 24-hour period. If there are no signs of recurrence,

dantrolene can be discontinued after 24 hours; however, some recommend continuing oral dantrolene 1 mg/kg every 4 to 8 hours for 48 hours. More recent findings suggest that a continuous infusion started 5 hours after emergency treatment with an individualized infusion rate dependent on the number of initial bolus(es) may be preferable.

Creatine kinase elevations (which may not manifest for 6–12 hours) may be followed as a rough guide for therapy and how long to continue the dantrolene. Furosemide (0.5–1.0 mg/kg IV) can also be given to enhance renal output.

Disseminated intravascular coagulation may occur, likely resulting from release of thromboplastins secondary to shock and/or release of cellular contents or membrane destruction. The usual regimen for treating disseminated intravascular coagulation should be followed.

Prognosis

After recovery from acute episodes of MH, patients should be closely monitored in an intensive care unit for up to 72 hours. Urine output, arterial blood gases, pH, and serum electrolyte concentrations should be determined frequently. It must be appreciated that MH may recur in the intensive care unit in the absence of obvious triggering events. Therapy with dantrolene has reduced mortality from 70% to less than 5%.

Identification of Susceptible Patients

The advantages of detecting patients susceptible to MH before anesthesia are obvious. Detailed medical and family histories, with particular reference to previous anesthetic experiences, should be obtained.

Linkage of MH with other diseases has been problematic: only central core disease appears to be truly linked, and most families with central core disease have been a mutation at the RYR1 locus. Other syndromes associated with multicore myopathy are Evan's myopathy and the King-Denborough syndrome/phenotype. An exceptionally rare phenomenon of stress-induced MH affects a small number of MH-susceptible patients. These patients do not require exposure to anesthetic-triggering agents to develop MH. Stress-related triggers may include trauma, anxiety, vigorous exercise, and high environmental temperature. It must be emphasized that most MH episodes are associated only with exposure to anesthetic-triggering agents.

In Duchenne's muscular dystrophy, the balance of opinion has shifted from an association with MH to an anesthesia-induced rhabdomyolysis. The two processes share common clinical and biochemical characteristics, such as hyperkalemia, metabolic acidosis, myoglobinuria, and elevated creatine kinase. However, the underlying mechanism of rhabdomyolysis is different, in that the anesthetic agents stress a muscle cell membrane that is fragile or unstable because of the progressive X-linked myopathy (short arm of the X chromosome), not the autosomal dominant MH (long arm of chromosome 19). This further increases membrane permeability, resulting in a compensatory hypermetabolic response in an attempt to reestablish membrane stability and prevent calcium ion fluxes.

A negative caffeine halothane contracture test has been documented in patients with confirmed Duchenne's muscular dystrophy. A caffeine halothane contracture test on dystrophin-deficient mdx mouse muscle demonstrates that the absence of dystrophin does not predispose to MH susceptibility. A recent large retrospective review of 444 anesthetics in Duchenne's muscular dystrophy and Becker's muscular dystrophy patients found 15 complications, only one of which was thought to be MH. This was based on "beer-colored" urine and an elevated creatine kinase level, which could equally have been attributable to rhabdomyolysis. The more common complication associated with succinylcholine administration in Duchenne's muscular dystrophy patients is the occurrence of acute hyperkalemic cardiac arrest.

It may seem trivial to dismiss this association, especially when the triggering agents are the same for both MH and anesthesia-induced rhabdomyolysis. It is, however, important to be alert to the diagnostic differential. So great is the concern over the association with MH that some have advocated pretreatment with dantrolene. Dantrolene, although life saving

when used appropriately, is not without side effects including muscular weakness (particularly undesirable in a patient with Duchenne's muscular dystrophy). More importantly, dantrolene does not treat anesthesia-induced rhabdomyolysis and may detract from the more appropriate management course.

Approximately 70% of susceptible patients have increased resting plasma concentrations of creatine kinase. By contrast, persons in some families with susceptibility to MH have normal creatine kinase levels. Other conditions, such as muscular dystrophy and skeletal muscle trauma, also produce increased creatine kinase concentrations. Although the creatine kinase level should be measured in patients being evaluated for susceptibility to MH, the measurement of creatine kinase levels is not a definitive screening test for MH. Electromyographic changes are present in 50% of patients susceptible to MH. These findings include an increased incidence of polyphasic action potentials and fibrillation potentials. Patients with exercise-induced rhabdomyolysis may be considered for skeletal muscle biopsies and in vitro contracture tests to determine MH susceptibility. The complexity of the molecular genetics of MH precludes a total DNA-based diagnosis of MH susceptibility.

In vitro contracture testing allows one to predict whether a patient with a history of MMR may safely receive potent inhalational agents for future general anesthetics. Contracture testing is not appropriate in children younger than 6 years or who weigh less than 20 kg due to the amount of muscle needed to perform the test. Because of the controversy surrounding the association of MMR with MH, it is preferable to take a biopsy sample from the patient with MMR before testing other family members. Follow-up of patients who have had MMR should include the following (**Table 24-20**).

Skeletal muscle biopsies with in vitro contracture testing provide definitive confirmation of susceptibility to MH. Biopsy specimens are typically obtained from the vastus muscles of the thighs using local or regional anesthesia. A nontriggering general anesthetic may be required in younger children. These muscle biopsies post-incision can be clamped under tension and stored in Krebs buffer maintained at room temperature for 22 to 26 hours with accurate caffeine and halothane-induced contractures. This has implications for

---

TABLE 24-20	Follow-up of Patients with Masseter Muscle Rigidity

1. Medic-Alert bracelet or other conspicuous form of identification; the patient and first-degree relatives must be assumed to have malignant hyperthermia susceptibility (MHS) unless the patient is subsequently proved to have caffeine halothane contracture test.
2. Referral of the patient to malignant hyperthermia nonsusceptible states (MHS), Malignant Hyperthermia Association of the United States (MHAUS) (800-98MHAUS; www.mhaus.org). MHAUS can refer the patient to an MH diagnostic center.
3. Review of the family history for adverse anesthetic events or suggestion of heritable myopathy.
4. Consider evaluation for temporomandibular joint disorder.
5. Consider neurologic consultation to evaluate for a potential myotonic disorder; if rhabdomyolysis is severe, consider evaluation for a dystrophinopathy (eg., Duchenne's or Becker's muscular dystrophy) or a heritable metabolic disorder (eg., carnitine palmitoyltransferase II deficiency or McArdle's disease).

remote testing of MH-susceptible patients. Histologic changes in skeletal muscles from MH-susceptible patients are not diagnostic. The two most widely used protocols for the diagnosis of MH susceptibility using in vitro skeletal muscle contracture tests both use separate exposures to halothane and caffeine.

There are differences in the North American Malignant Hyperthermia Group and European Malignant Hyperthermia Group protocols. With the North American protocol, abnormal contracture to either halothane or caffeine results in the patient being labeled as MH susceptible. Whereas in the European group protocol, MH-susceptible assignment requires abnormal contracture test to both halothane and caffeine; however, abnormal contracture with either caffeine or halothane results in MH-equivocal status, and these patients are treated as MH-susceptible patients when they require anesthetic care. Both have 97% to 99% sensitivity (frequency of positive results in patients with clinically established MH) and acceptable 78% to 94% specificity (frequency of negative results in low-risk controls). The false-negative result is less than 1% for the European and less than 3% for the North American protocol. To improve the specificity of caffeine halothane contracture test and potentially reclassify MH-equivocal patients as having either MH-susceptible or MH-negative, biopsy centers have evaluated the use of the ryanodine contracture test or 4-chloro-m-cresol (a ryanodine agonist test). There are other tests being developed with greater specificity, but currently the caffeine halothane contracture test is the most reliable one in clinical use.

Management of Anesthesia

Dantrolene Prophylaxis

Prophylaxis with dantrolene is usually unnecessary if one adheres to a nontriggering technique. If a severe MH reaction has previously occurred, dantrolene, 2 to 4 mg/kg IV, may be administered over 10 to 30 minutes as prophylaxis just prior to induction of anesthesia; for continued protection, one half the dose is repeated in 6 hours. Diuresis may accompany intravenous administration of dantrolene, reflecting the addition of mannitol to the dantrolene powder in an effort to make the solution isotonic. For this reason, it is recommended that patients receiving intravenous dantrolene also have a urinary catheter in place. Large doses of dantrolene administered acutely for prophylaxis against MH may cause nausea, diarrhea, blurred vision, and skeletal muscle weakness, which may be of sufficient magnitude to interfere with adequate ventilation or protection of the lungs from aspiration of gastric fluid. In the absence of signs of MH intraoperatively, it is probably not necessary to continue administration of dantrolene into the postoperative period.

Drug Selections

Patients susceptible to MH should be well sedated before induction of anesthesia. All preparations for the treatment of MH must be made before induction of anesthesia (see "Treatment"). Drugs that can trigger MH include volatile anesthetics and succinylcholine. Administration of calcium entry–blocking drugs in the presence of dantrolene has been associated with the development of hyperkalemia and myocardial depression. Drugs considered safe for administration to MH-susceptible patients include barbiturates, propofol, opioids, benzodiazepines, dexmedetomidine, ketamine, droperidol, and nondepolarizing muscle relaxants (**Table 24-21**). Prolonged neuromuscular blockade in response to nondepolarizing muscle relaxants may occur in patients susceptible to MH who have been pretreated with dantrolene. Conceivably, nitrous oxide could influence the course of MH indirectly through its capacity to stimulate the sympathetic nervous system but is generally considered safe. Antagonism of nondepolarizing muscle relaxants has not been shown to trigger MH in susceptible patients.

Anesthesia Machine

No studies have confirmed that MH can be triggered by residual concentrations of volatile anesthetics delivered from previously used anesthesia machines. Nevertheless, some have advocated use of a "dedicated" anesthesia machine that has never been used to deliver volatile anesthetics for administration of anesthesia to patients susceptible to MH. A more practical, acceptable alternative is to use a conventional anesthesia machine with a disposable anesthesia breathing circuit and fresh gas outlet hoses, fresh carbon dioxide absorbent, no vaporizers (removed or taped), and a continuous flow of oxygen at 10 L/min for 10 to 60 minutes (see manufacturer's recommendations) before using the machine to deliver anesthesia to patients susceptible to MH.

Regional Anesthesia

Regional anesthesia is an acceptable choice for anesthesia in MH susceptible patients. In the past, avoidance of amide-based local anesthetics was recommended, as it was believed that these drugs could trigger MH in susceptible patients.

TABLE 24-21 Nontriggering Drugs for Malignant Hyperthermia

Barbiturates
Propofol
Etomidate
Benzodiazepines
Opioids
Droperidol
Nitrous oxide
Nondepolarizing muscle relaxants
Anticholinesterases
Anticholinergics
Sympathomimetics
Local anesthetics (esters and amides)
α_2-Agonists
  Clonidine
  Dexmedetomidine

This opinion, however, is probably not valid, and ester- and amide-based local anesthetics are considered acceptable for regional or local anesthesia, as may be needed to perform skeletal muscle biopsies.

Postoperative Discharge Home

It is acceptable to perform surgery in ambulatory centers on patients susceptible to MH as long as they are monitored for at least 1 hour after a nontriggering anesthetic. Dantrolene and appropriate monitoring devices should be available at all anesthetizing locations.

FAMILIAL DYSAUTONOMIA

Familial dysautonomia (FD) or Riley-Day syndrome is an autosomal recessive inherited neurodegenerative disorder with complete penetrance and has mainly been reported in the Ashkenazi Jewish population. This progressive disorder mainly results in a loss of unmyelinated nerve fibers, which, among other functions, are involved in central autonomic nervous system control and the perception of pain and temperature.

Signs and Symptoms

Children affected with FD present in early infancy with feeding difficulties due to poor sucking and swallowing (dysphagia) from pharyngeal dyscoordination, which eventually leads to failure to thrive. Other symptoms include generalized hypotonia, gastroesophageal reflux, recurrent vomiting and aspirations with pulmonary problems, absence of overflowing tears on emotion, a reduction or absence of lingual fungiform papillae, pallor, delayed developmental milestones, and diminished response to nociceptive stimuli. Body temperature regulation is labile. Muscle biopsies show a loss of Golgi tendon organs explaining decreased or absent deep tendon reflexes, delayed walking, and ataxia. Generalized seizures may occur in up to 40% of patients and may be associated with decerebrate posturing following a breath-holding episode.

The lack of autonomic nerve terminals on peripheral blood vessels seems to be at least in part responsible for the often profound postural hypotension and extreme response to adrenergic and cholinergic drugs, suggestive of functional autonomic denervation. With increasing age, autonomic blood pressure dysregulation (profound orthostatic hypotension, supine hypertension), peripheral sensory dysfunction, and ataxia become worse. After the age of approximately 3 to 6 years, about 40% of all FD patients suffer from recurrent episodes of dysautonomic crises, a state characterized by nausea and cyclic vomiting, profuse sweating, mottled skin, agitation, and a rapidly changing pattern of arterial hyper- and hypotension with brady- and tachycardia. These crises can be triggered by already mild emotional or physical stress (e.g., visceral pain) and may result in serious complications (e.g., pulmonary aspiration).

Baseline norepinephrine serum concentrations are reduced in FD patients. Hemodynamic lability may present in a variety of ways, including orthostatic hypotension without reflex tachycardia, tachycardia, bradycardia and atrioventricular block, or severe supine hypertension. Almost 40% of FD patients have also been diagnosed with long QT syndrome.

Diagnosis

In the past, the diagnosis of FD was based on the five clinical features: (1) Ashkenazi Jewish origin and a reduction in or absence of (2) lacrimation, (3) deep tendon reflexes, (4) lingual fungiform papillae, and (5) axon flare after intradermal histamine injection. The diagnosis is now confirmed by DNA analysis by genetic linkage testing. Prenatal diagnosis and carrier genetic testing (in the case of a positive family history) are available.

Treatment

Due to failure to thrive, these patients often present for placement of a gastrostomy tube for supplemental food and fluid replacement. Nissen fundoplication is another frequent procedure on these patients to reduce gastroesophageal reflux and the risk of aspiration with its sequelae.

Almost all FD patients have some degree of scoliosis, which is at least in part due to osteoporosis. In severe cases, this combined with chronic aspiration may lead to atelectasis, consolidation, recurrent pneumonia, and finally restrictive lung disease with potential cor pulmonale.

Prognosis

The decreased mortality of FD patients over the past decades has mainly been attributed to early access to centralized and more advanced treatment, supplemental feeding (gastrostomy), and strict efforts to reduce pulmonary aspiration and its sequelae. Although before 1960, half of these patients died before the age of 5 years, current statistics show a 50% chance for a newborn to reach the age of 40 years. Sudden death (with approximately two thirds occurring during sleep) and pulmonary and renal complications represent the main causes of death.

Management of Anesthesia

Dysfunctional chemoreceptors seem to be responsible for the decreased ventilatory response to hypoxia and hypercarbia and the increased incidence of central sleep apnea in these patients. Several reports of respiratory arrest exist, emphasizing the importance of careful and continuous perioperative monitoring.

Even moderate hypoxia results in central ventilatory depression with hypoventilation, arterial (systolic and diastolic) hypotension, bradycardia, and potentially respiratory arrest. Minor stress or events such as crying or laughing may change the depth of ventilation enough to trigger breath holding and decerebrate posturing. On emergence from anesthesia, respiratory efforts may be weak and arterial hypertension may result from hypoxia and hypercapnia.

A preoperative electrocardiogram is warranted in these patients due to the prevalence of long QT syndrome.

Preoperative blood work should include serum concentrations of electrolytes, creatinine, and blood urea nitrogen. During a dysautonomic crisis, which can be triggered by stress or pain, profuse sweating and vomiting may result in severe and life-threatening electrolyte imbalances (e.g., hyponatremia-induced seizures, arrhythmias). Appropriate premedication and pain control are therefore essential.

These patients have an increased risk of hypovolemia (excessive losses secondary to sweating and vomiting and decreased fluid intake due to dysphagia), which requires pre-operative correction to reduce the risk of hemodynamic instability. Treatment of arterial hypotension should begin with intravenous volume replacement therapy, especially given the fact that these patients may be highly sensitive to adrenergic and cholinergic agents.

Benzodiazepines (e.g., midazolam) for premedication have been used successfully and are recommended to prevent stress and dysautonomic crises. Thiopental, propofol, and ketamine have all been safely used for induction of anesthesia. A smaller dose than normal is advised to avoid hypotension and bradycardia, and the administration of a preoperative fluid bolus may help to blunt the hemodynamic instability.

Due to the high incidence of gastroesophageal reflux, a rapid sequence induction is recommended. Succinylcholine, vecuronium, and rocuronium have been used without problems. Mask induction can be necessary in the absence of a peripheral intravenous catheter, but care should be taken to avoid hypo- or hyperventilation during spontaneous breathing. Opioids are not contraindicated; however, short-acting drugs are often preferred to allow titration to control pain and respiratory depression. Regional anesthesia alone or in combination with general anesthesia has been used safely and may be beneficial for postoperative pain control. There should be a low threshold for invasive monitoring, given the frequency of hemodynamic instability (arterial catheter) and preoperative hypovolemia (central venous catheter).

Alacrima requires intraoperative lubrication and protection of the eyes to prevent corneal ulcerations. Thermoregulation is poor, and monitoring of core temperature is recommended to avoid hypothermia. Nonsteroidal anti-inflammatory drugs are useful in this population; however, they should be used with caution if renal function is impaired.

The postoperative management in the intensive care unit may be warranted due to the fact that intraoperative challenges and problems may extend well into the postoperative period. Appropriate pain control is important in the prevention of not only a dysautonomic crisis but also pulmonary complications. Generalized muscle weakness and preexisting lung problems may require postoperative ventilatory support. The potential for hemodynamic instability and/or electrolyte imbalances requires continuous and careful monitoring.

Diazepam is the drug of choice to control dysautonomic crises. Persistent arterial hypertension responds well to oral clonidine. More potent antihypertensive drugs (e.g., labetalol, hydralazine) may be required, but should be used cautiously since hemodynamic instability can manifest as hypotension.

SOLID TUMORS

Cancer is second only to accidental trauma as a cause of death in children ages 1 to 14 years. Nearly 60% of intra-abdominal tumors in children reflect leukemia involving the liver and spleen. Conversely, most intra-abdominal tumors in infants are benign and of renal origin. Retroperitoneal solid tumors are also likely to be of renal origin. Two thirds of these renal masses are cystic lesions, such as hydronephrosis, and the remainder are nephroblastomas (Wilms' tumors). Neuroblastoma is another example of a solid tumor that tends to occur in the retroperitoneal space.

Neuroblastoma

Neuroblastoma is the most common extracranial solid tumor in infants and children, resulting from malignant proliferation of sympathetic ganglion cell precursors. Neuroblastomas account for 8% to 10% of all childhood malignancies. These tumors may arise anywhere along the sympathetic ganglion chain from the neck to the pelvis, but 75% occur in the retroperitoneum, in either the adrenal medulla (50%) or the paraspinal ganglia (25%). Neuroblastoma may metastasize by direct invasion into surrounding structures, lymphatic infiltration, or hematogenous spread.

Signs and Symptoms

Children with neuroblastomas typically present with protuberant abdomens, often discovered by the parents. On clinical examination, neuroblastomas are large, firm, nodular, sometimes painful flank masses that are usually fixed to surrounding structures. Some children present with pulmonary metastases, although the most common sites of metastasis are the long bones, skull, bone marrow, liver, lymph nodes, and skin. Paraspinal neuroblastomas may extend through the neural foramina into the epidural space, producing paraplegia. Tumor located in the upper posterior mediastinum or neck may involve the stellate ganglion and cause Horner syndrome. Neuroblastomas may secrete a vasoactive intestinal peptide, which is responsible for persistent watery diarrhea with loss of fluid and electrolytes. These tumors also synthesize catecholamines, but the incidence of hypertension is relatively low.

Diagnosis

The median age at diagnosis is 2 years, while 90% of cases are diagnosed by 5 years of age. Ultrasonography, CT, and magnetic resonance imaging are the primary diagnostic procedures for evaluating abdominal masses in children. Calcification and hemorrhage within the tumor are often seen on CT, distinguishing neuroblastoma from Wilms tumor, which usually does not calcify. Helical CT or magnetic resonance angiography is helpful for delineating the extent of involvement of the great vessels by the tumors and their resectability. Urinary excretion of vanillylmandelic acid is increased in most children with neuroblastomas, reflecting the metabolism of catecholamines produced by these tumors.

Treatment

Treatment of neuroblastoma consists of surgical removal, including local metastases and involved lymph nodes. If the tumor cannot be resected completely, a biopsy is performed. Complete resection is delayed until after completion of chemotherapy and/or radiation therapy. Radiation therapy can be given as a palliative or a therapeutic measure. Drugs used for chemotherapy in varied combinations include cyclophosphamide, doxorubicin, cisplatin, and vincristine. Possible adverse effects of chemotherapy must be considered during the preoperative evaluation of these patients.

Prognosis

Prognosis depends on multiple factors such as molecular markers and degree of tumor differentiation, but patient age and tumor stage are the two most important independent prognostic factors. Infants younger than 1 year at diagnosis have a significantly improved outcome across all tumor stages. Surgical excision of the tumor is usually curative in patients with a favorable stage.

Management of Anesthesia

Management of anesthesia for resection of neuroblastoma is as described for children with nephroblastoma. Adequate intravenous access is particularly essential because neuroblastomas are quite vascular and often adhere to or surround the great vessels, creating the potential for significant blood loss. A peripheral arterial catheter may be helpful in detecting sudden hypertension caused by excessive catecholamine release from the tumor. Despite the high incidence of catecholamine production associated with neuroblastoma, adrenergic blockade (as required for a pheochromocytoma) is generally unnecessary. Because of the extensive upper abdominal incisions frequently required for retroperitoneal tumor resection, epidural analgesia is a beneficial adjunct so long as tumor does not involve the spine.

Nephroblastoma

Nephroblastoma (Wilms' tumor) is the most common malignant renal tumor and the second most common malignant abdominal tumor in children, accounting for 6% of all pediatric malignancies. Three fourths of patients are diagnosed by 4 years of age; one third of these tumors occur in children younger than 1 year of age, while the median age at onset is 3 years. It is a congenital tumor thought to arise from anomalous differentiation of embryonal renal elements. The most common site of metastasis is the lungs. Nephroblastoma is associated with certain congenital anomalies including WAGR syndrome (*W*ilms' tumor, *a*niridia, *g*enitourinary malformations, and mental *r*etardation), Beckwith-Wiedemann syndrome (hemihypertrophy, visceromegaly, macroglossia, and hyperinsulinemic hypoglycemia), and Denys-Drash syndrome (pseudohermaphroditism, progressive glomerulopathy, and Wilms' tumor). A minor familial predisposition (1%–2% of cases) is also reported.

Signs and Symptoms

Nephroblastomas typically present as asymptomatic flank masses in otherwise healthy children. The mass is usually accidentally discovered by the parents or by a physician during a routine physical examination. Nephroblastomas vary in size and are usually firm, nontender, and free from surrounding structures. Pain, fever, and hematuria are usually late manifestations. These children may exhibit malaise, weight loss, anemia, disturbed micturition, and symptoms such as vomiting or constipation due to compression of adjacent portions of the gastrointestinal tract by tumor. Systemic hypertension may be a manifestation of nephroblastoma, particularly if the tumor involves both kidneys. Increases in systemic blood pressure are usually mild, but on rare occasions, hypertension is so severe that encephalopathy and congestive heart failure develop. Systemic hypertension may reflect renin production by the tumor or indirect stimulation of renin release due to compression of the renal vasculature. Secondary hyperaldosteronism and hypokalemia may be present. Hypertension usually disappears after nephrectomy but may recur if metastases develop.

Diagnosis

Radiography of the abdomen demonstrates a renal mass and occasional calcification. Intravenous pyelography shows distortion of the renal collecting system and occasionally absence of excretion by the involved kidney. This diagnostic test also assesses the function of the contralateral kidney. An inferior vena cavagram may indicate tumor invasion of this blood vessel. An arteriogram shows the extent of the tumor and involvement of the contralateral kidney. Chest radiographs or liver scans may demonstrate metastatic disease.

Treatment

Treatment of nephroblastomas consists of nephrectomy, with or without subsequent radiation and chemotherapy, depending on the stage of involvement. Preoperative chemotherapy is generally administered to patients with bilateral tumors who will undergo parenchyma-sparing procedures, patients with extensive intravascular (inferior vena caval) tumor extension, or those with inoperable tumors. Extensive tumor may necessitate radical en bloc resection, including portions of the inferior vena cava, pancreas, spleen, and diaphragm. The presence of metastases may require multiple surgical procedures. If the tumor is inoperable at the initial exploration or if the child is in poor clinical condition, radiation therapy is given initially to shrink the tumor, and the child is then surgically re-explored. In other patients, renal-sparing procedures (partial nephrectomy, enucleation of tumor nodules) before or after chemotherapy are acceptable.

Bilateral nephroblastomas occur in up to 7% of children. Two thirds of these tumors occur at the same time; in the remainder, involvement of the contralateral kidney occurs at a later date. Depending on the magnitude of the tumor involvement, surgical treatment can consist of bilateral partial nephrectomy or bilateral total nephrectomy followed by dialysis and eventually renal transplantation.

Prognosis

Two broad histologic categories, favorable and unfavorable, are recognized. The favorable histologic type is devoid of ectopia or anaplasia and carries a good prognosis. The unfavorable histologic type is characterized by focal or diffuse anaplasia and is associated with high rates of tumor relapse and death. Tumor size, stage, and histology are major prognostic factors. Multimodal treatment of nephroblastomas is associated with a survival rate approaching 90% in patients with favorable histology and stage and a survival rate greater than 60% across all stages.

Management of Anesthesia

Infants or children scheduled for exploration and resection of neuroblastomas or nephroblastomas are in varying degrees of general health. For example, if the tumor is diagnosed at a late stage, it is likely that anemia is severe. In addition, adverse effects related to chemotherapy must be considered. Anemia is corrected to a hemoglobin concentration of approximately 10 g/dL. Adequate amounts of blood should be cross-matched preoperatively, as resection of neuroblastomas or nephroblastomas may be associated with excessive surgical blood loss. These children must be well hydrated preoperatively, and their electrolyte and acid-base imbalances must be corrected, especially in the presence of excessive fluid and electrolyte losses due to diarrhea. Maintenance of anesthesia is acceptably provided with volatile anesthetics in air and oxygen plus opioids. Muscle relaxants are necessary to optimize surgical exposure.

In addition to routine monitoring, placing a catheter in a peripheral artery is indicated to permit constant monitoring of systemic blood pressure and frequent determination of arterial blood gases and pH. Intraoperative hypotension is not uncommon owing to sudden surgical blood loss, which is most likely to occur during dissection of the tumor from around major blood vessels. Catheters for infusion of intravenous fluids should be placed in the upper extremities or the external jugular veins. Lower extremity veins should be avoided, as it may be necessary to ligate or partially resect the inferior vena cava. Measurement of central venous pressure is helpful for evaluating intravascular fluid volume and the adequacy of fluid replacement. Likewise, a Foley catheter to facilitate monitoring urine output aids in maintaining an optimal intravascular fluid volume. Tumor extension into the suprahepatic vena cava and right atrium requires intraoperative cardiopulmonary bypass. Epidural analgesia should be avoided in these patients due to potential complications associated with full heparinization.

Precautions should be taken during induction of anesthesia to prevent pulmonary aspiration, particularly if tumors are causing compression of the gastrointestinal tract. In children in poor general condition, sudden hypotension may develop during the induction of anesthesia, particularly if intravascular fluid volume has not been restored by preoperative infusion of crystalloid or colloid solutions. Systemic hypertension, as is present in some of these children, must be considered and measures taken to prevent excessive increases in systemic blood pressure during tracheal intubation. Manipulation of the inferior vena cava containing metastatic tumor can result in a tumor embolism to the heart or pulmonary artery.

ONCOLOGIC EMERGENCIES

Mediastinal Tumors

Mediastinal tumors may initially present as an anterior mediastinal mass in 1 in 25,000 children. In infants and children 0 to 2 years old, neurologic tumors (benign and malignant) are most common; in children 2 to 10 years old, neurologic and lymphatic tumors are equally common; and in children older than 10 years of age, lymphoma and Hodgkin's disease are most prevalent.

Signs and Symptoms

Cardiovascular and respiratory symptoms are particularly pronounced. The severity of symptoms depends on the size and location of the tumor within the mediastinum. Important respiratory findings in the history and physical examination include tachypnea, orthopnea, and nocturnal dyspnea, suggesting an airway compression. Patients may preferentially lie or sleep in a particular position.

Tumors may compress or weaken long segments of the tracheobronchial tree. The severity of this mass effect is associated with the weight of the tumor, duration of the pressure, and position of the patient. The patient's respiratory status may appear normal in the sitting, prone, or decubitus position, but in the supine position, decreased lung volume and gravitational exertion on the tumor will compress the airway, particularly during expiration when the pleural pressure is close to 0.

Cardiovascular structures can also be compressed or constricted by an enlarging mediastinal tumor. Pericardial encasement may produce constriction or effusion. Compression of atrium or pulmonary artery may be asymptomatic. However, a Valsalva effect (which decreases venous return) may be associated with syncopal events. Aortic involvement may be asymptomatic because the thicker muscular wall and the intra-abdominal pressure can withstand greater extrinsic pressure. Superior vena cava syndrome presents with facial and periorbital edema, shortness of breath, engorgement of jugular veins, and mild central nervous system symptoms (headache and visual disturbances) that worsen in the supine position.

Diagnosis

Chest radiograph, computed axial tomography, and magnetic resonance imaging are static pictures of airway compression and may not accurately quantitate the degree of compression. Airway obstruction with general anesthesia is likely to occur if the diameter of the trachea is decreased by 50%. Flow volume loops sitting and supine may give a more dynamic assessment of the airway as well as flexible fiberoptic bronchoscopy done under local anesthesia or sedation. This may not be possible in younger patients. Cardiovascular evaluation must focus on restrictions in cardiac output and venous return. Orthopnea, pulsus paradoxus, and superior vena cava syndrome are concerning. If any of these are present, a two-dimensional echocardiogram and CT scan of the chest are indicated.

Treatment

When superior vena cava syndrome is present, radiation therapy may be the treatment of choice in this emergency. When superior vena cava syndrome is associated with lymphoma, chemotherapy may be as effective as radiation in alleviating the effects of superior vena cava syndrome.

Procedures that may need general anesthesia or sedation include computed axial tomography scan, biopsy of cervical nodes, and central venous line catheter placement. In addition, thoracotomy with removal of the tumor may be indicated if the tumor is not responsive to radiation or chemotherapy. Prior to surgery, the indications for preoperative chemotherapy, radiation therapy, and steroid therapy to shrink symptomatic tumors must be considered. Treating and decreasing the size of the tumor prior to surgery are often beneficial. One viable therapy option that can shrink the tumor without obscuring the tissue diagnosis is 4 to 24 hours of steroids, which is worth trying.

Management of Anesthesia

Preoperative In order to safely anesthetize these children, limitations in respiratory and cardiovascular reserves must be evaluated and further deterioration anticipated. A strategy to prevent cardiorespiratory collapse under anesthesia must also be established.

Intraoperative Premedication should be avoided and intravenous access should be established prior to induction, preferably in a lower extremity if superior vena cava obstruction is present. Inhalation or intravenous induction with maintenance of spontaneous ventilation at all times and avoidance of all muscle relaxants are recommended. Some patients without apparent symptoms in the supine position when awake may deteriorate when anesthesia is induced. Placing the patient in the left lateral decubitus or sitting positions may relieve the obstruction. Anesthesia may be induced in the sitting position, but it is difficult to intubate and hypotension may occur precipitously. The left lateral decubitus or semidecubitus position may be preferable.

Intravenous agents commonly used are ketamine and/or midazolam. If indicated, the trachea may be intubated under deep sevoflurane anesthesia. In older children, the airway may be secured under sedation and topical anesthesia via fiberoptic bronchoscopy. An arterial line or a reliable noninvasive blood pressure monitor must be present. If the child deteriorates during induction, turning him or her in the left lateral decubitus position may improve cardiorespiratory function. Other options if collapse of the airway occurs is rigid bronchoscopy, pushing the endotracheal tube past the obstruction, and upward traction on the sternum to stent open the vessels. Cardiopulmonary bypass (femorofemoral bypass) or venovenous bypass may be necessary if either complete airway obstruction or vessel occlusion is anticipated. This must be planned and organized with the appropriate surgical specialities well in advance of the procedure. In addition, extra long endotracheal tubes in small sizes should be available to pass through fixed narrowed airways.

A helium (70%) and oxygen (30%) (Heliox) mixture may be used to improve oxygenation in patients with airway compression due to mediastinal tumors. Heliox has one third the density of oxygen, permitting more laminar gas flow and decreasing resistance in the conducting airways. It can be attached to the anesthesia machines air inlet, but the rotameter will read inaccurately so one must read the F_{IO_2} with an oxygen analyzer. The lowest oxygen and the highest concentration of helium will give the best clinical effect because the decreased density is directly related to the amount of helium delivered. Patient's oxygen saturations are the key to the optimum mixture. Extubation is best accomplished with the child awake, ensuring adequate return of airway reflexes and prevention of laryngospasm.

Postoperative Recovery room personnel must be notified of the effect of position on the patient's cardiorespiratory status. Children with significant tracheomalacia may manifest tracheal obstruction and respiratory difficulties in recovery. Often these may be corrected by repositioning the child in the decubitus or prone positions, but may necessitate reintubation. Unilateral re-expansion pulmonary edema may be associated with lung re-expansion after mediastinal tumor removal. This complication may manifest itself immediately after tumor removal or as a delayed response in the recovery period.

BURN (THERMAL) INJURIES

As many as one third of burn-related injuries and deaths occur in children. Survival after burn injuries depends on the patient's age and the percentage of body area burned, with younger patients having higher morbidities and mortalities due to higher surface area–to–body weight ratio, thinner skin, and decreased physiologic reserves. Burns are classified according to the total body surface area involved (**Table 24-22**), the depth of the burn (**Table 24-23**), and the presence or absence of inhalation injury. The total body surface area burned is calculated using the rule of nines, which accurately predicts the body surface area involved in adults. Even modified versions of the rule of nines, however, appear to underestimate the extent of burn injury in children (**Figs. 24-3 and 24-4**).

Signs and Symptoms

Burn injuries produce predictable pathophysiologic responses (**Table 24-24**). Mediators released from the burn wound contribute to local inflammation and burn wound edema. With minor burns, the inflammatory process is limited to the burned area. With major burns, local injury triggers the release of circulating mediators, resulting in systemic responses characterized by hypermetabolism, immunosuppression, and the systemic inflammatory response syndrome (**Fig. 24-5**). Cytokines appear to be the primary mediators of systemic inflammation after burn injuries. These responses must be considered when formulating plans for management of anesthesia for burned patients.

TABLE 24-22 Definition of Major Burns

Third-degree (full-thickness) burn injuries involving more than 10% of the total body surface area

Second-degree (partial-thickness) burn injuries involving more than 25% of the total body surface area in adults (at extremes of age 20% of total body surface area)

Burn injuries involving the face, hands, feet, or perineum

Inhalation burn injuries

Chemical burn injuries

Electrical burn injuries

Burn injuries in patients with series co-existing medical diseases

Adapted from MacLennan N, Heimbach DM, Cullen BF: Anesthesia for major thermal injury. Anesthesiology 1998;89:749–770.

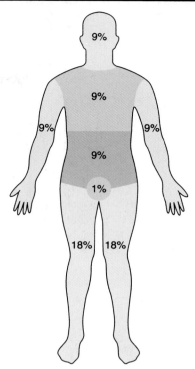

Figure 24-3 • Rule of nines for determining the percentage of body surface area burned in adults. (*Adapted from MacLennan N, Heimbach DM, Cullen BF: Anesthesia for major thermal injury. Anesthesiology 1998;89:749–770.*)

Cardiac Output

Cardiac output decreases dramatically during the immediate postburn period. The initial decrease precedes any measurable loss of intravascular fluid volume and may reflect the presence of circulating low molecular weight myocardial depressant factors. Of note, cardiac output remains decreased until the beginning of the second postburn day. After the initial 24 hours of fluid resuscitation, the circulatory system enters a hyperdynamic state that persists well into the postburn period. The systemic blood pressure and heart rate are increased, and cardiac output stabilizes at approximately twice normal.

Systemic Hypertension

Approximately 30% of children with extensive thermal injury become hypertensive during the postburn period. The onset of systemic hypertension is usually within the first 2 weeks. Males younger than 10 years of age are at greatest risk of the development of systemic hypertension. Systemic hypertension is usually transient but on occasion persists for several weeks. Left untreated, hypertensive encephalopathy manifesting as irritability and headache, with or without seizures, develops in approximately 10% of these children. The cause of systemic hypertension is unknown but may be related to increased serum concentrations of catecholamines and/or activation of the renin-angiotensin system. Treatment with antihypertensive drugs is needed in some children.

Airway

Direct burn injuries to the airway, with the exception of steam inhalation, do not occur below the level of the vocal cords, reflecting the low thermal capacity of air and the efficient cooling ability of the upper air passages. Burn or chemical injuries of the upper airway, however, can cause severe edema. Laryngeal edema manifesting as hoarseness, stridor, and tachypnea demand prompt airway evaluation, as swelling of supraglottic tissues can result in sudden, complete upper airway obstruction within hours after the original thermal injury.

TABLE 24-23 Classification of Burn Injuries

Classification	Depth of Burn Injury	Outcome and Treatment
First degree (superficial)	Epidermis	Heals spontaneously
Second degree (partial thickness)		
Superficial dermal burn	Epidermis and upper dermis	Heals spontaneously
Deep dermal burn	Epidermis and deep dermis	Requires excision and grafting for rapid return of function
Third-degree (full thickness)	Destruction of epidermis and dermis	Wound excision and grafting required
		Some limitation of function and scar formation
Fourth degree	Skeletal muscles	Complete excision
	Fascia	Limited function
	Bone	

Adapted from MacLennan N, Heimbach DM, Cullen BF: Anesthesia for Major thermal injury. Anesthesiology 1998;89:749–770.

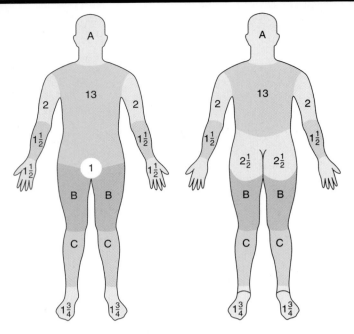

RELATIVE PERCENTAGES OF AREAS AFFECTED BY GROWTH
(Age in years)

Area	0	1	5	10	15	Adult
A: Half of head	$9\frac{1}{2}$	$8\frac{1}{2}$	$6\frac{1}{2}$	$5\frac{1}{2}$	$4\frac{1}{2}$	$3\frac{1}{2}$
B: Half of thigh	$2\frac{3}{4}$	$3\frac{1}{4}$	4	$4\frac{1}{4}$	$4\frac{1}{2}$	$4\frac{3}{4}$
C: Half of leg	$2\frac{1}{2}$	$2\frac{1}{2}$	$2\frac{3}{4}$	3	$3\frac{1}{4}$	$3\frac{1}{2}$

Figure 24-4 • Methods to determine the percentage of body surface area burned in children. (*Adapted from MacLennan N, Heimbach DM, Cullen BF: Anesthesia for major thermal injury. Anesthesiology 1998;89:749–770.*)

Smoke Inhalation

Inhalation of suspended particles (smoke) and toxic products of incomplete combustion results in chemical pneumonitis similar to that resulting from aspiration of acidic gastric fluid. Most individuals with smoke inhalation have associated face and neck burns or a history of being trapped in a closed space. Smoke inhalation victims often experience asymptomatic periods lasting as long as 48 hours before respiratory distress becomes overt. Initial chest radiographs may be clear, but the Pao_2 is consistently decreased while these individuals are breathing room air. Production of carbonaceous sputum and detection of wheezes and rales during auscultation of the chest herald impending ventilatory failure.

Carbon monoxide poisoning often complicates burns that occur in closed spaces and is the most common immediate cause of death from fires. Measurement of carboxyhemoglobin concentrations can serve as a useful diagnostic marker of smoke inhalation.

Gastrointestinal Tract

Adynamic ileus is virtually universal after burn injuries of more than 20% of the body surface area. Therefore, early

decompression of the stomach through a nasogastric tube is indicated. Acute ulceration of the stomach or duodenum, known as Curling's ulcer, is the most frequent life-threatening gastrointestinal complication. Duodenal ulcers occur twice as frequently in children with burn injuries as in adults (14% versus 7%). Most patients with Curling's ulcer can be managed conservatively with antacids or H_2-antagonist drugs, but occasional patients require vagotomy with or without partial gastrectomy.

Renal Function

Immediately after burn injury, cardiac output and intravascular fluid volume decrease and plasma catecholamine concentrations increase, resulting in decreased renal blood flow and glomerular filtration rates. Diminished renal blood flow activates the renin-angiotensin-aldosterone system and stimulates the release of antidiuretic hormone. The net effect on renal function is retention of sodium and water and exaggerated losses of potassium, calcium, and magnesium. Following adequate fluid resuscitation, renal blood flow and glomerular filtration may increase dramatically.

Endocrine Responses

Endocrine responses to burn injuries are characterized by massive outpourings of corticotropin, antidiuretic hormone, renin, angiotensin, aldosterone, glucagon, and catecholamines. Serum concentrations of insulin may be increased or decreased. Nevertheless, serum glucose concentrations are increased owing to increased concentrations of glucagon and catecholamine-induced glycogenolysis in the liver and skeletal muscles. Indeed, glycosuria occurs frequently in nondiabetic burn patients. Burn patients may be particularly susceptible to the development of nonketotic hyperosmolar coma, especially if total parenteral nutrition is being used.

Rheology

Liver Function Liver function tests are frequently abnormal in burn patients, even when the areas of burn injury are small. Overt liver failure is uncommon, however, unless the postburn course is complicated by hypotension, sepsis, or multiple blood transfusions.

Treatment

Intravascular Fluid Volume Intravascular fluid volume deficits after thermal injury are roughly proportional to the extent and depth of the burn injury. After burn injuries, fluid accumulates rapidly in the injured area and to a lesser extent in unburned tissues. If burn injuries involve at least 10% to 15% of the total body surface area, hypovolemic shock develops unless there is effective, rapid intervention.

On the first postburn day, the vascular compartment becomes permeable to plasma proteins, including fibrinogen. This increased permeability exists throughout the vascular system but is most pronounced in the area of the burn injury. Extravasated plasma proteins exert an osmotic pressure that can hold large volumes of fluid in an extravascular third space.

TABLE 24-24 Pathophysiologic Responses Evoked by Burn Injuries

Cardiovascular Responses
Early
  Hypovolemia (burn shock)
  Impaired myocardial contractility
Late
  Systemic hypertension
  Tachycardia
  Increased cardiac output

Pulmonary Responses
Early direct effects
  Upper airway obstruction (burns)
  Effects of smoke inhalation (chemical pneumonitis, carbon
    monoxide)
  Asphyxia
Early indirect effects
  Effects of inflammatory mediators
  Pulmonary edema (complication of resuscitation)
Late direct effects
  Chest wall restriction (thoracic burn injuries)
Late indirect effects (complications of ventilation and airway
    management)
  Oxygen toxicity
  Barotrauma
  Infections
  Laryngeal damage
  Tracheal stenosis

Metabolism and Thermoregulation
Increased metabolic rate
Increased carbon dioxide production
Increased oxygen utilization
Impaired thermoregulation

Renal and Electrolyte Responses
Early
  Decreased renal blood flow
  Myoglobinuria
  Hyperkalemia (tissue necrosis)
Late
  Increased renal blood flow
  Variable drug clearance
  Hypokalemia (diuresis)

Endocrine Responses
Increased serum norepinephrine concentrations
Hyperglycemia (susceptible to development of nonketotic
    hyperosmolar coma)

Gastrointestinal Responses
Stress ulcers
Impaired gastrointestinal barrier to bacteria
Endotoxemia

Coagulation and Theology
Early
  Activation of thrombotic and fibrinolytic systems
  Hemoconcentration
  Hemolysis
Late
  Anemia

Immune Responses
Impaired immune function (sepsis, pneumonia)
Endotoxemia
Multiple organ system failure

Adapted from MacLennan N, Heimbach DM, Cullen BF: Anesthesia for major thermal injury. Anesthesiology 1998;89:749–770.

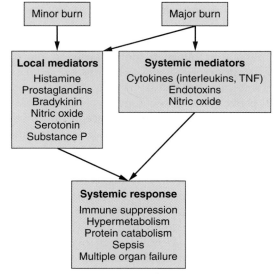

Figure 24-5 • Mediators released with thermal injuries and responses to their release. (*Adapted from MacLennan N, Heimbach DM, Cullen BF: Anesthesia for major thermal injury. Anesthesiology 1998;89:749–770.*)

Severe hypoproteinemia is the primary cause of tissue edema. Pulmonary capillary permeability does not increase unless smoke inhalation occurs. Consequently, colloids do not need to be withheld during the early phases of resuscitation. The loss of fluid from the vascular compartment on the first postburn day is approximately 4 mL/kg for each percent of body surface burned. For example, in a 40-kg child with a 50% burn, fluid needed for the first 24 hours would be 8000 mL of Ringer's lactated solution or isotonic crystalloid. The most effective restoration of intravascular fluid volume occurs when one half of this fluid is given within the first 8 hours after the burn and the remainder over the next 16 hours.

On the second postburn day, capillary integrity is largely restored, and fluid and plasma protein losses are markedly decreased. Decreasing amounts of fluid are required to maintain the intravascular fluid volume. Further rapid administration of electrolyte solutions at this time may result in edema in excess of any gain in circulatory dynamics. Therefore, infusion of crystalloid solutions is decreased after the first postburn day, but replacement volume must be individually adjusted based on clinical response.

Airway Management Fiberoptic laryngoscopy is indicated if the diagnosis of upper airway edema is in doubt. The airway should be secured before respiratory decompensation occurs, as translaryngeal tracheal intubation after progression of edema of the airway is likely to be difficult. Tracheal intubation may be required for several days until edema subsides. The small caliber of the child's airway accentuates the impact of airway edema on resistance to breathing. If tracheal intubation is required for a child, a nasotracheal tube may be preferred, as this route is more comfortable and easily secured than an oral tube.

Tracheostomy is reserved for patients with late pulmonary complications requiring prolonged ventilatory support. Performing a tracheotomy in a burned child with swelling of the face and neck is a formidable surgical challenge. Early complications of tracheostomy in burn patients include hemorrhage, pneumothorax, and malposition of the tracheostomy tube; late complications are related to mechanical factors (displacement of the cannula) and to cannula erosion into blood vessels with massive hemorrhage.

Smoke Inhalation Treatment of respiratory distress related to smoke inhalation is symptomatic. Administration of warm humidified oxygen and bronchodilators is indicated. Early institution of positive-pressure ventilation of the lungs with positive end-expiratory pressure should be considered if the Pa_{O_2} is less than 60 mm Hg while breathing room air. Prophylactic antibiotic administration is not beneficial, and the value of corticosteroids is controversial. The best treatment for carbon monoxide poisoning is ventilation of the victim's lungs with 100% oxygen, which decreases the half-life of carboxyhemoglobin from 4 to 6 hours to 40 to 80 minutes.

Metabolism and Thermoregulation The metabolic rate increases in proportion to the extent of burn injury. The metabolic rate can be more than doubled in individuals with burn injury involving 50% of the body surface area. Total parenteral nutrition may be required to meet these increased metabolic requirements. Accompanying these hypermetabolic responses, the metabolic thermostat is reset upward so burn patients tend to increase skin and core temperatures somewhat above normal, regardless of the environmental temperatures. Early enteral alimentation of burn patients has several benefits, including attenuation of the hypermetabolic responses to burn injury.

Thermoregulatory functions of the skin, including vasoactivity, sweating, piloerection, and insulation, are abolished or diminished by thermal injury. In addition, skin no longer functions as an effective water vapor barrier, resulting in the loss of ion-free water. In children, intense vasoconstriction in the non-burned areas of skin can result in an increased body temperature sufficient to cause febrile seizures. Conversely, when metabolism and peripheral vasoconstriction are depressed, as during general anesthesia, children with burn injuries may experience a rapid decrease in body temperature.

Fluid, Electrolytes, and Blood Products Hourly urine output remains the most readily available guide to the adequacy of fluid resuscitation. For example, urine output should be approximately 1.0 mL/kg per hour in adequately hydrated children. Increased serum potassium concentrations due to tissue necrosis and hemolysis are common during the first two postburn days. This is followed over the next several days by marked hypokalemia due to accentuated renal loss of potassium. Diarrhea and gastric suction further exaggerate the potassium loss.

Hemolysis of erythrocytes in response to burn injuries is not extensive. Therefore, early transfusions of whole blood or packed erythrocytes, in the absence of other indications, is rarely necessary. Nevertheless, generalized suppression of erythrocyte production and decreased erythrocyte survival time follow burn injuries and may persist well into the postburn period. Therefore, transfusions of erythrocytes is often needed by approximately the fifth postburn day to maintain the hemoglobin concentration at more than 10 g/dL.

Serum concentrations of ionized calcium may be decreased during postburn periods. Because children are more sensitive than adults to the effects of citrate and potassium in stored blood, children with extensive burn injuries who are receiving large volumes of rapidly infused whole blood should receive 1 to 2 mg of calcium gluconate for every milliliter of infused blood.

Prognosis

Survival after severe (nonairway-related) burns in the pediatric population has improved dramatically in the past two decades. Children with more than 80% total body surface area burn treated between 1982 and 1996 had a mortality rate of 33%, improved from earlier reported rates exceeding 80%. The most frequent cause of death remains severe multiple organ dysfunction due to overwhelming late sepsis (typically after a period of weeks).

Management of Anesthesia

Preoperative Historic information regarding the time and type of burn injury is pertinent for the management of anesthesia in acutely burned children (**Table 24-25**). For example, the time of burn injury is important, as initial fluid requirements are based on the time elapsed since the burn occurred.

The physical examination should focus on the status of the patient's airway. Head and neck burns, burned nasal hairs, and hoarseness are signs that supraglottic edema may develop or is already present. Carbonaceous sputum, wheezing, and diminished breath sounds suggest the presence of smoke inhalation injury. Abdominal distention may indicate ileus, warranting special precautions during the induction of anesthesia to decrease the risk of pulmonary aspiration. A careful search should be made during the preoperative evaluation for sites suitable for placing intravenous catheters and monitoring devices.

Children who were trapped in closed spaces are likely to have experienced smoke inhalation injury. Measurement of arterial blood gases and pH and evaluation of chest radiographs are indicated in patients suspected of having experienced smoke inhalation. Serum carboxyhemoglobin concentrations are helpful only for the first few hours after burn injuries. In the

TABLE 24-25 Anesthetic Considerations for Excision and Grafting of Major Burn Injuries

Preoperative Medication
Provide adequate analgesia
Limit period of fluid fasting

Vascular Access
Establish appropriate intravenous access
Consider invasive monitoring

Airway Management
Consider alternative to direct laryngoscopy
Consider awake fiberoptic intubation (neck or facial contractures)

Ventilation
Minute ventilation requirements increased (increased metabolic rate, parenteral hyperalimentation)
Mechanical ventilation (smoke inhalation, acute respiratory failure)

Fluids and Blood
Anticipate possibility of rapid and large blood loss
Evaluate coagulation status

Temperature Regulation
Increase ambient temperatures of the operating rooms
Warm intravenous fluids

Anesthetic Drugs
Include opioids
Consider effects of increased circulating catecholamine concentrations
Muscle Relaxants
Avoid succinylcholine
Anticipate resistance to neuromuscular blocking effects of nondepolarizing muscle relaxants

Postoperative Period
Anticipate increased analgesic (opioids) requirements

Adapted from MacLennan N, Heimbach DM, Cullen BF: Anesthesia for major thermal injury. Anesthesiology 1998;89:749–770.

presence of carboxyhemoglobin, the pulse oximeter may overestimate saturation of hemoglobin with oxygen, emphasizing the need for caution in relying solely on this monitor in patients who have recently experienced carbon monoxide exposure. Serum glucose concentrations and osmolarity are determined, particularly if burn patients are receiving total parenteral nutrition. Measures of renal function are indicated after extensive electrical burns. Coagulation profiles should be obtained in patients in whom extensive intraoperative blood loss is anticipated. It has been shown that severe burn injury does not affect the kinetics of gastric emptying and that clear liquids given 2 hours before anesthesia is safe. This may have special implications in patients who come for repeated surgeries.

Intraoperative Establishing intravenous infusion lines may be difficult in severely burned individuals. In some instances, it is necessary to use veins in areas that have escaped burn injury, such as the axilla, scalp, or web spaces between the digits. Reliable intravenous catheters of sufficient caliber are essential for patients undergoing excision of burn eschars, as large amounts of blood can be lost in brief periods of time. Even split-thickness skin grafts are associated with approximately 80 mL of blood loss for each 100 cm^2 of skin that is harvested for grafting.

Airway management in pediatric burn patients can be challenging. Mask ventilation may be a problem with facial burns. Depending on the age of the burns, edema, scarring, or contractures may narrow the mouth opening and limit the neck movements. Fixing the endotracheal tube for prone positioning in the presence of facial burns is best achieved by suturing it to the teeth or the nares. In children requiring high inspiratory pressures during mechanical ventilation, a cuffed endotracheal tube may be necessary.

Children with extensive burn injuries may require intensive monitoring, yet not have an unburned limb available for placing a blood pressure cuff. Pulse oximeters may need to be placed on the tongue to obtain adequate monitoring. Catheters placed in peripheral arteries occasionally must be inserted through burn eschars. Septic complications are likely, such that catheters placed through eschars should be removed as soon as possible. Venous cannulation sites are likewise vulnerable to septic complications. Decreases in body temperature are exaggerated during the intraoperative period, reflecting the loss of the insulating properties of the skin, evaporative loss of water from eschars, and depression of the metabolic rate by general anesthesia. Routine measures for decreasing heat loss include the use of warming blankets, forced air warmers, and radiant overhead warmers. Inspired gases may be warmed and humidified, and intravenous fluids are administered through a warmer. Ambient temperatures of the operating room should be maintained near 25°C. A number of pathophysiologic alterations produced by burn injuries affect drug responses. Immediately after burn injury, organ and tissue blood flow is decreased as a result of hypovolemia, depressed myocardial function, and release of vasoactive substances. Absorption of drugs administered by any route other than intravenously is predictably delayed. Intravenous and inhaled drugs may have increased effects on the brain and heart because of relative increases in blood flow to these organs. After adequate fluid resuscitation, the hypermetabolic phase begins approximately 48 hours after burn injury. During this time, oxygen and glucose consumption is markedly increased. Serum albumin concentrations are decreased after burn injuries; thus, albumin-bound drugs (benzodiazepines, anticonvulsants) have increased circulating free and pharmacologically active fractions. Conversely, serum concentrations of α_1-acid glycoprotein are increased, so drugs bound to this protein (muscle relaxants, tricyclic antidepressant drugs) have decreased free fractions. Pharmacologic alterations may persist after recovery from burn injuries. It has been shown that thiopental requirements are increased in children for more than 1 year after burn injuries. Opioid requirements may also be decreased in burn patients.

Of all the classes of drugs, the effects of burn injury on muscle relaxants have been studied most extensively. Hyperkalemic responses to succinylcholine are well known. The risk of hyperkalemia is probably related to the severity of the burn injury and the time elapsed from the burn injury to succinylcholine administration. The greatest risk appears to be 10 to 50 days after the burn injury. Nevertheless, these zones are poorly defined, and the safest recommendation may be to avoid succinylcholine. Several studies have shown that burn patients develop marked resistance (up to threefold increases in dose requirements) to nondepolarizing muscle relaxants. Approximately 30% or more of the body must be burned to produce resistance to nondepolarizing muscle relaxants, manifesting approximately 10 days after burn injury, peaking at 40 days, and declining after approximately 60 days. Despite this typical time sequence, one report described prolonged resistance to the effects of nondepolarizing muscle relaxants that was still present after 463 days. Pharmacodynamic explanations as the principal mechanisms for resistance to effects of nondepolarizing muscle relaxants are documented by the need to achieve higher serum drug concentrations to produce given degrees of twitch suppression in burn-injured patients compared with nonburn-injured patients. It is speculated that proliferation of extrajunctional cholinergic receptors is responsible for this resistance to the effects produced by nondepolarizing muscle relaxants. This increased number of extrajunctional cholinergic receptors would also increase the available sites for potassium exchange to occur after administration of succinylcholine to burn-injured patients, leading to the possibility of hyperkalemia. Despite these theories, there is evidence that burn injuries are not associated with an increased number of extrajunctional cholinergic receptors. Instead, altered affinity of cholinergic receptors for acetylcholine or nondepolarizing muscle relaxants may be the basis for burn injury–induced resistance to these drugs. With both vecuronium and rocuronium use in patients with major burns, the onset time was found to be slower in burned patients as compared with nonburned patients, but the recovery profiles were significantly shorter in burned patients. Resistance to the neuromuscular effects of rocuronium is partially overcome by increasing the dose, with 1 to 2 mg/kg providing good tracheal intubating conditions after major burns.

Ketamine has been used for years for anesthesia in burn-injury patients, especially for dressing changes and escharotomy. The drug can be administered intravenously or intramuscularly with good effect. Administration of ketamine is often preceded by anticholinergic drugs, as excessive salivation is likely. Ketamine (1–2 mg/kg IV) provides excellent somatic analgesia for skin grafting procedures. Recovery of consciousness from single intravenous doses of ketamine is usually rapid, allowing early return to oral nutritional support. Nitrous oxide can be administered to decrease random motion of the patient's limbs, which often accompanies ketamine anesthesia. Ketamine in combination with benzodiazepine or propofol to reduce the adverse psychodynamic effects may be used in analgesia and anesthetic doses depending on the desired effect. Excessive movement during emergence from anesthesia may dislodge skin grafts or promote hemorrhage, resulting in early graft loss. Sevoflurane is the most likely inhaled drug to be used for anesthesia in children with burn injuries. In addition, injection of tumescent local anesthesia (a maximum dose of 2 mg/kg lidocaine) prior to burn incision and grafting can give excellent postoperative analgesia and decrease the amount of inhalational anesthetic agent needed.

Postoperative A combination of prolonged prone positioning and relatively high fluid volume administration may cause significant airway swelling. It is best to wait until an air leak is present around the endotracheal tube before tracheal extubation because this indicates resolution of edema. If there is still no air leak and the patient is deemed ready for tracheal extubation, direct or fiberoptic laryngoscopy may be necessary to determine the extent of residual edema. Once extubated, the patient should be closely monitored for progressive airway obstruction during the subsequent 24 to 48 hours.

Postoperative pain from the skin graft site can be managed with regional nerve blocks (e.g., continuous fascia iliaca compartment block for thigh donor sites), reducing the need for opioid analgesics that may cause respiratory depression and postoperative nausea and vomiting.

For background analgesia, analgesics such as acetaminophen can be used for their opioid-sparing effect and are combined with generous administration of oral opioids. Nonsteroidal anti-inflammatory drugs have antiplatelet effects and may not be appropriate for patients who require extensive excision and grafting procedures. In addition, burn patients can also manifest the nephrotoxic effects of nonsteroidal anti-inflammatory drugs.

KEY POINTS

- One of the most important physiologic differences between pediatric and adult patients is oxygen consumption, which in neonates is approximately twice that of adults on a weight basis. The alveolar ventilation is doubled in neonates, manifested as increased respiratory rate, to meet this increased oxygen demand.

- Because cardiac stroke volume is relatively fixed by a noncompliant and immaturely developed left ventricle in infants, cardiac output is highly dependent on heart rate.

- MAC of volatile anesthetics steadily increases until approximately 3 months of age after which MAC steadily decreases with age, except for sevoflurane, which has a relatively constant MAC in children between 6 months and 12 years of age.

KEY POINTS—cont'd

- Pyloric stenosis is a medical, not a surgical, emergency that requires adequate fluid and electrolyte replacement therapy prior to surgery.

- MH and anesthesia-induced rhabdomyolysis are distinct entities that may mimic each other in clinical presentation.

- Airway emergencies in pediatric patients require a coordinated management effort that should include the anesthesiologist, otolaryngologist, and pediatric intensivist. A physician skilled in airway management should accompany the child during transport to and from the operating room.

- Neurosurgical emergencies in the pediatric population frequently are associated with congenital anomalies in addition to trauma. Increased ICP frequently accompanies congenital intracranial anomalies, necessitating minimal stimulation during laryngoscopy and expedient securing of the airway by a skilled practitioner.

- Extensive burn injuries produce long-lasting physical and physiologic derangements in multiple organ systems. These changes such as upregulation of neuromuscular receptors and injury to the face and airway affect the choice of anesthetic drugs and techniques.

- Symptomatic anterior mediastinal masses in children represent one of the greatest anesthetic challenges. There is significant potential for an airway disaster during induction of anesthesia. The anesthetic plan must be discussed with the perioperative team well in advance and may even require preparations for partial cardiopulmonary bypass.

- Craniofacial surgery in pediatric patients, especially infants, requires meticulous attention to temperature preservation, airway, and fluid management. Intraoperative cardiac arrest is most frequently associated with inadequate volume resuscitation.

REFERENCES

Axelrod FB: Familial dysautonomia. Muscle Nerve 2004;29:352–363.

Borland LM, Colligan J, Brandom BW: Frequency of anesthesia-related complications in children with Down syndrome under general anesthesia for noncardiac procedures. Paediatr Anaesth 2004;14:733–738.

Chadd GD, Crane DL, Phillips RM, et al: Extubation and reintubation guided by the laryngeal mask airway in a child with the Pierre-Robin syndrome. Anesthesiology 1992;76:640–641.

Cote CJ, Zaslavsky A, Downes JJ, et al: Postoperative apnea in former preterm infants after inguinal herniorrhaphy. A combined analysis. Anesthesiology 1995;82:809–822.

Dunne MJ, Cosgrove KE, Shepherd RM, et al: Hyperinsulinism in infancy: From basic science to clinical disease. Physiol Rev 2004;84:239–275.

Faberowski LW, Black S, Mickle JP: Incidence of venous air embolism during craniectomy for craniosynostosis repair. Anesthesiology 2000;92:20–23.

Garner L, Stirt JA, Finholt DA: Heart block after intravenous lidocaine in an infant. Can Anaesth Soc J 1985;32:425–428.

Glickstein JS, Schwartzman D, Friedman D, et al: Abnormalities of the corrected QT interval in familial dysautonomia: An indicator of autonomic dysfunction. J Pediatr 1993;122:925–928.

Islander G, Twetman ER: Comparison between the European and North American protocols for diagnosis of malignant hyperthermia susceptibility in humans. Anesth Analg 1999;88:1155–1160.

Lerman J, Sikich N, Kleinman S, et al: The pharmacology of sevoflurane in infants and children. Anesthesiology 1994;80:814–824.

Prinzhausen H, Crawford MW, O'Rourke J, Petroz GC: Preparation of the Drager Primus anesthetic machine for malignant hyperthermia-susceptible patients. Can J Anaesth 2006;53:885–890.

The STOP-ROP Multicenter Study Group: Supplemental Therapeutic Oxygen for Prethreshold Retinopathy of Prematurity (STOP-ROP), a randomized, controlled trial. I: Primary outcomes. Pediatrics 2000;105:295–310.

Uyar M, Hepaguslar H, Ugur G, Balcioglu T: Resistance to vecuronium in burned children. Paediatr Anaesth 1999;9:115–118.

Wass CT, Lanier WL, Hofer RE, et al: Temperature changes of > or = 1 degree C alter functional neurologic outcome and histopathology in a canine model of complete cerebral ischemia. Anesthesiology 1995;83:325–335.

Westrin P: The induction dose of propofol in infants 1-6 months of age and in children 16 years of age. Anesthesiology 1991;74:455.

CHAPTER 25

Geriatric Disorders

Zoltan G. Hevesi

Public Health and Aging Trends

Physiology of Aging
- Nervous System
- Cardiovascular Changes
- Respiratory Alterations
- Hepatic, Gastrointestinal, and Renal Aging
- Endocrine Function in the Elderly
- Hematology, Oncology, and Immune Function Changes

Geriatric Syndromes
- Osteoporosis
- Osteoarthritis

- Emphysema
- Parkinson's Disease
- Dementia
- Delirium

Geriatric Anesthesia Strategies

Ethical Challenges in Geriatric Anesthesia and Palliative Care

Summary

PUBLIC HEALTH AND AGING TRENDS

The elderly population, persons 65 years or older, numbered 36.3 million in the United States in 2004. This represented 12.4% of the U.S. population. By 2030, there will be approximately 71.5 million elderly individuals, and the number of persons aged older than 80 years is expected to increase from 9.3 million in 2000 to 19.5 million. The number of people 65 years and older is expected to grow to be 20% of the population by 2030 (**Fig. 25-1**).

The median age of the world's population is increasing because of a decline in fertility and an increase in the average life span during the 20th century. Worldwide, the average life span is expected to extend another 10 years by 2050.

The growing number of older adults increases demands on the public health systems and on social services. In the United States and other developed countries, the health care cost per capita for the elderly is three to five times greater than the cost

for younger persons. Chronic diseases, which affect older adults disproportionately, contribute to disability and diminish quality of life. Increased life expectancy reflects, in part, the success of public health interventions. Now public health programs must respond to the future challenges created by this achievement, including the growing concerns about future health care costs of chronic illnesses, injuries, and disabilities (**Fig. 25-2**).

The overall health of older Americans is improving. Still, many are disabled and suffer from chronic conditions. The proportion of this population with a disability decreased significantly in recent decades; however, 14 million people age 65 and older reported some level of disability in the Census of 2000 (**Fig. 25-3**). Currently individuals older than 65 years of age comprise only 12% of the United States population and undergo almost one third of the 25 million surgical procedures performed annually. In addition, they consume approximately one half of the $140 billion annual U.S. federal health

PERCENT AGED 65 AND OVER OF THE TOTAL POPULATION:
2000 TO 2050

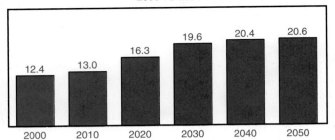

Figure 25-1 • Aging of the U.S. population. The reference population for these data is the resident population. (*Adapted from 2000 U.S. Census Bureau, 2001, Table PCT12; 2010 to 2050, U.S. Census Bureau, 2004.*)

care budget. The aging of the U.S. population will result in significant growth in the demand for surgical services. Based on the assumption that age-specific per capita use of surgical services will remain constant, the amount of work in all surgical fields is predicted to increase 14% to 47%. These increases will vary widely by specialty.

For anesthesiologists, it is a great responsibility to develop strategies to address this increased demand while maintaining quality of care for our senior patients. Elderly individuals are obviously prone to develop more or less the same illnesses as the rest of the population. However, the diminished baseline physiologic reserve, the chronic persistence of disease, and the cumulative effect of morbidities warrant separate and focused discussion of this age group. This chapter focuses on the age-related biologic alterations first and then provides a description of a few prevalent age-specific conditions affecting the elderly.

A sound understanding of the age-related physiologic changes is an essential first step in providing the high-quality care elderly citizens deserve. Emphasis should be placed on cautious preanesthesia screening and evaluation, so that comorbidities are thoughtfully considered in relationship to the planned anesthetic when caring for the patient.

PHYSIOLOGY OF AGING

Nervous System

There is a continual loss of neuronal substance with advancing age that is accompanied by a similarly reduced cerebral blood

flow and diminished production of neurotransmitters (i.e., norepinephrine and dopamine). However, this reduction in neuronal density that occurs with age is not directly proportional with the general level of mental functioning. This can be explained by the considerable redundancy of the neuronal network in younger individuals. Gray matter is more affected by atrophy than white matter, and there is a compensatory increase of cerebrospinal fluid volume. There is a great individual variability to the degree these changes manifest in the elderly. In general, nervous system function tends to decline with age, leading to impairments in cognition, motor, sensory, and other behaviors. Much needs to be learned regarding the cellular and molecular mechanisms responsible for the selective vulnerability of brain cells and regions to age-dependent dysfunction and neurodegeneration, such as occurs in Parkinson's and Alzheimer's diseases. Most central nervous system pathologies are progressively more prevalent with increasing age; examples include cerebral atherosclerosis, Parkinson's disease, depression, dementia, Alzheimer's disease, and delirium.

The autonomic nervous system is no exception to the overall decline of function as we age. With advancing age, parasympathetic outflow declines, while sympathetic autonomic activity increases. However, elderly patients generally manifest a reduced responsiveness to β-adrenergic stimulation. Changes of sympathetic and parasympathetic responsiveness are reflected as compromised thermoregulation, decreased baroreceptor sensitivity, and common dehydration. Hypothermia, heat stroke, orthostatic hypotension, and syncope are common problems in the elderly and are frequently worsened by the presence of diabetic autonomic dysfunction.

It is most important to note clinically that most geriatric patients have a reduced requirement for various anesthetic agents. A prime example of this alteration is the reduced minimum alveolar concentration necessary in elderly patients to produce anesthesia. Moreover, clearance of various pharmaceutical compounds is often compromised by reduced renal and hepatic capacity. The incidence of postoperative cognitive dysfunction is much increased by advanced age, independent of the type of anesthetic techniques employed.

Cardiovascular Changes

"Seventy is the new fifty" is a frequently expressed phrase today. In fact, a large number of elderly individuals report

PARENT SUPPORT RATIOS: 1960 TO 2050
(Number of people aged 85 and over per 100 people aged 50 to 64)

Figure 25-2 • Aging population presents increasing challenge for health care. The reference population for these data is the resident population. (*Adapted from 1960, U.S. Bureau of Census, 1964, Table 155; 1970 and 1980, U.S. Bureau of the Census, 1983, Table 42; 1990, U.S. Bureau of the Census, 1991, Table QT-PI; 2000, U.S. Census Bureau, 2001, Table PCT12; 2010 to 2050, U.S. Census Bureau, 2004.*)

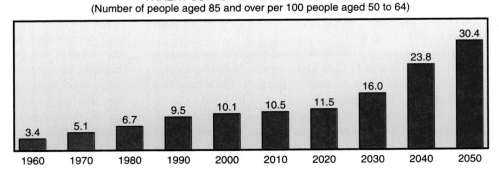

NURSING HOME RESIDENTS AMONG PEOPLE
AGED 65 AND OVER BY AGE AND SEX: 1999

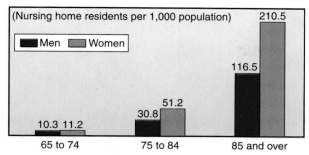

Figure 25-3 • Care use increases with advanced age. The reference population for these data is nursing home residents, excluding residents in personal care or domiciliary care homes. (*Adapted from National Center for Health Statistics, 2003a, Table 97*).

strenuous and frequent athletic activity and look much younger than their stated age. As a result, a broad spectrum of individual differences exists. Therefore, the need for individualized cardiac functional assessment cannot be overstated.

It is controversial as to whether aging is associated with decreases in cardiac output and stroke volume to a significant degree at rest. However, exercise tolerance (maximal attainable heart rate, stroke volume, and cardiac output) is typically reduced in older adults. Progressive loss of vascular elasticity tends to lead to compensatory left ventricular hypertrophy and hypertension as we age. Chronically elevated blood pressure results in decreased baroreceptor sensitivity. The incidence of coronary arteriosclerosis and valvular heart disease is also higher with advancing age. In more severe cases of cardiac pathophysiology, various forms of arrhythmias and congestive heart failure may compound the problem of prescribing an age-appropriate anesthetic regimen.

In the assessment of cardiac risk, patient self-report of daily physical activities and exercise tolerance is the most valuable source of insight for the clinician. Chemical cardiac stress tests are frequently used to differentiate cardiac and noncardiac etiologies of limited exercise tolerance. When multiple risk factors are identified, stress echocardiography or cardiac catheterization may also be indicated to provide a more specific and precise quantitative description of the cardiac compromise.

Respiratory Alterations

Gradual tissue degeneration is the main cause for respiratory system aging. Protective reflexes, especially coughing and swallowing, are diminished with increasing age. The result is chronic pulmonary inflammation and loss of alveolar surface area from repeated "microaspirations" and contamination of the lower airway with enteral organisms. Moreover, chronic noxious environmental exposure may be a major contributing factor in smokers and various subgroups of agricultural and industrial workers.

In general, physiologic responsiveness to hypercapnia and hypoxemia is also diminished in the elderly. In addition to the reduced respiratory drive, the work of breathing is increased due to a reduced chest wall elasticity and increasingly

turbulent flow that are seen in narrowing airway passages. Progressive mismatch between increasing respiratory work and weakening respiratory muscles results in an increased incidence of shortness of breath during regular daily activities and, in severe cases, during rest. As a result of these changes, forced vital capacity and forced expiratory volume in 1 second (FEV_1) decline progressively in the elderly. Intraparenchymal elastic forces in some pulmonary segments may become insufficient to maintain patent distal airways. Consequently, air trapping occurs, and closing capacity and residual volume increase. The residual volume to total lung capacity ratio is 20% at 20 years of age and 40% by age 70.

Maldistribution of ventilation and, less often, pulmonary perfusion lead to a decreased efficiency of oxygenation and carbon dioxide removal. The two most frequently seen forms of ventilation-perfusion mismatch are dead space (regional excess of ventilation compared to perfusion) and pulmonary venous admixture (pulmonary perfusion in excess of ventilation). Dead space manifests primarily in a reduced ventilatory efficiency, as increased minute ventilation is necessary to achieve equal alveolar ventilation and maintain the same arterial carbon dioxide level. In contrast, pulmonary venous admixture affects arterial oxygen tension, as deoxygenated blood from the pulmonary artery passes through insufficiently ventilated areas of the lungs and lowers pulmonary venous, and ultimately systemic, oxygen tension. Mean arterial oxygen tension decreases from 95 mm Hg at age 20 to less than 70 mm Hg at age 80.

Hepatic, Gastrointestinal, and Renal Aging

Parenchymal atrophy, sclerotic vascular decline, and diminished function are often described when age-related changes of various viscera are discussed. Hepatic synthetic and metabolic capacity, renal blood flow and clearance, gastrointestinal motility, and sphincter function are frequently compromised in the elderly. These gradual changes persist at a subclinical level in most cases for a long period of time before the subtle laboratory alterations and reduced functional reserve progress to clinically observable pathology. Hepatic tissue mass is typically significantly reduced in later years in life, but baseline function is often relatively well preserved. Renal tissue atrophy results in an approximate 50% reduction in the number of functioning glomeruli by age 80, with a corresponding 1% to 1.5% decline per year in glomerular filtration rate when compared to terms seen in young adulthood. Creatinine clearance also declines with age. However, serum creatinine level remains frequently within normal limits due to less skeletal muscle mass and less creatinine production. Maintenance of adequate urine output (>0.5 mL/kg per hour) is crucial in preventing postoperative renal dysfunction because postsurgical acute renal failure carries a high mortality in the critically ill elderly. It is a great professional challenge for the anesthesiologist to entertain and investigate the possibility of reduced organ function that may be inconsequential preoperatively but will pose a significant and relevant risk during the stressful preoperative period.

TABLE 25-1	T β, Elimination Half-life Difference by Age	
Drug	**Young Adults**	**Elderly Adults**
Fentanyl	250 min	925 min
Midazolam	2.8 hr	4.3 hr
Vecuronium	16 min	45 min

Various pharmacodynamic and pharmacokinetic alterations, such as increased volume of distribution for lipid-soluble drugs, reduced plasma volume, less plasma protein binding, slower hepatic conjugation, and diminished renal elimination will also influence the clinical planning and decision-making process in the elderly (**Table 25-1**).

Endocrine Function in the Elderly

Just like all other parenchymal organs, the endocrine glands tend to atrophy in the elderly and reduction hormone production frequently leads to impaired function (i.e., serum glucose homeostasis). Compounds like insulin, thyroxin, growth hormone, renin, aldosterone, and testosterone are often deficient. Diabetes, hypothyroidism, impotence, and osteoporosis are also common, along with chronic electrolyte abnormalities. Of note, basal metabolic rate declines approximately 1% per year after age 30.

Hematology, Oncology, and Immune Function Changes

In the bone marrow and lymph nodes of elderly individuals, various cellular elements are produced at a reduced rate compared to healthy young adults. Anemia is especially concerning when diminished oxygen-carrying capacity is present in combination with coronary artery disease.

Compromised cellular immunity (leukocytopenia, lymphocytopenia) results in increased vulnerability to a variety of infectious diseases, ranging from simple community-acquired infections to less common entities such as tuberculosis and shingles. Age is the most significant risk factor for cancer. The incidence of cancer is less than 2% before age 20 and more than 25% after age 65. The prevalence of autoantibodies and autoimmune disorders is also higher with advanced age.

GERIATRIC SYNDROMES

Correlation between biologic and chronologic age is not always strong, but it is important to recognize that the unavoidable physiologic decline seen with advancing age always leads to similar pathologies. In the geriatric population, the increased prevalence of these syndromes makes it essential for the anesthesiologist to be familiar with them.

Osteoporosis

Aging of the musculoskeletal system is frequently an easily observable change at the first preoperative encounter with

Normal bone   Osteoporosis

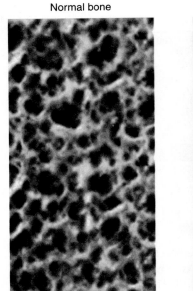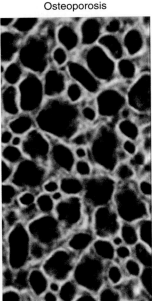

Figure 25-4 • Comparison of normal (*left*) and osteoporotic (*right*) bone. With aging, bone becomes fragile with loss of normal structure.

the patient. Loss of skeletal muscle (lean body mass) and increased percentage of body fat are typical changes associated with aging. Osteoporosis is characterized by microarchitectural deterioration and decreased bone density, with consequent increased bone fragility and susceptibility to fracture. Osteoporosis is often largely asymptomatic until a fracture occurs, although patients may note a loss of height and gradually increasing kyphosis secondary to vertebral compression fractures. Prevention is a key aspect of management (**Fig. 25-4.**)

In the United States, approximately 10 million people have osteoporosis. Another 14 to 18 million have osteopenia. Approximately 1.5 million fractures per year are attributed to osteoporosis, and more than 37,000 people die of subsequent fracture-related complications. Among women who sustain a hip fracture, 50% spend time in a nursing home while recovering, and 14% of all patients with hip fractures remain in nursing homes 1 year later. Whites, especially of northern European descent, and Asians are at increased risk of osteoporosis. The peak incidence is in people aged 70 years or older. Besides demographics, estrogen deficiency, male hypogonadism, smoking, increased alcohol consumption, calcium deficiency, cancer, immobilization, and chronic corticosteroid administration are well-documented risk factors.

For screening purposes, plain radiography is not as accurate as bone mineral density testing. In symptomatic patients, however, radiographs are useful to identify osteopenia and fractures.

Regular weight-bearing exercises and adequate calcium and vitamin D intake are key elements of prevention. Hormone replacement therapy is considered an effective treatment option for postmenopausal women. Parenteral or intranasal calcitonin is typically reserved for the treatment of cancer-related bone absorption.

Osteoarthritis

Osteoarthritis is the most common joint disease, affecting more than 20 million individuals in the United States alone. More than half of the population older than 65 years displays radiographic signs of osteoarthritis, although most are asymptomatic. Prevalence increases with age. Middle-aged men and women are affected equally, but prevalence is greater in women in the elderly. Other risk factors include obesity, joint trauma, infection, and metabolic and neuromuscular disorders.

Pathologic findings suggest that articular cartilage is the site of the primary abnormality, but the reactive changes also affect the periarticular tissues and surrounding bones. Predominantly, the weight-bearing joints are affected, such as the knees, hips, cervical and lumbosacral spine, and feet. Pain and dysfunction of the affected joints are major causes of chronic inactivity, disability, and morbidity. There are no specific laboratory abnormalities are associated with osteoarthritis. The diagnosis is based on clinical assessment and positive radiographic findings on the affected joints (**Fig. 25-5**).

Nonpharmacologic interventions are the cornerstones of osteoarthritis therapy and include patient education, weight loss, physical therapy, occupational therapy, and reduction of joint stress. In addition, acetaminophen and nonsteroidal anti-inflammatory drugs are administered to improve patient mobility. Muscle relaxants are considered selectively for patients with evidence of muscle spasm. Intra-articular glucocorticoid injections, narcotics, and arthroplasty are reserved for patients with the most severe pain.

Decreased mobility and discomfort are obvious concerns for all caregivers, but cervical spinal mobility and stability carry special implications for the anesthesiologist when laryngoscopy and tracheal intubation is planned. Cervical osteoarthritis may interfere with visualizing the glottic opening. Flexion and extension cervical radiographs can be instrumental in deciding which technique offers the safest approach for

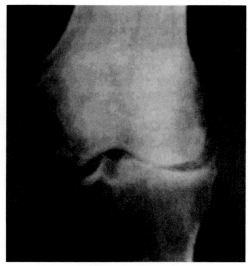

Figure 25-5 • Classic osteoarthritis of the knee with associated changes in the articular cartilage.

tracheal intubation without causing neck injury or compromising the spinal cord.

Emphysema

Typically, patients present in their fifth decade of life with a history of productive cough or an acute chest illness. The cough usually is worse in the morning and produces a colorless sputum from a concomitant chronic bronchitis. Breathlessness, the most significant symptom, rarely occurs until the sixth decade of life. In the United States, 4% to 6% of male adults and 1% to 3% of female adults are estimated to have emphysema. Cigarette smoking is by far the single most clearly established environmental risk factor for emphysema. Most patients with emphysema have a smoking history of greater than 20 pack-years before the common symptoms develop. The incidence of emphysema has increased 2.8 times by smoking. Intravenous drugs, α_1-antitrypsin deficiency, immunodeficiency, and connective tissue disorders are also potential risk factors.

The pathologic changes manifest as emphysematous destruction distal to the respiratory bronchioles and small airway inflammation. In these affected areas, occlusion of the lumen occurs by mucous plugging, and airflow limitation develops. Clinically, the severity of airflow obstruction is more prevalent in patients with chronic cough and sputum production and is associated with an accelerated decline in lung function.

The cellular composition of the airway inflammation seen in chronic obstructive pulmonary disease is predominantly mediated by the neutrophils. Cigarette smoking induces macrophages to release neutrophil chemotactic factors and elastases, leading to tissue destruction. By the time FEV_1 has decreased to 30% of predicted, the patient is breathless on minimal exertion. With disease progression, the intervals between acute exacerbations become shorter; as a result, cyanosis and right heart failure may develop.

The respiratory rate increases in proportion to disease severity. On physical examination, the use of accessory respiratory muscles and paradoxical chest wall movement are evident. In advanced disease, cyanosis, elevated central venous pressure, and anasarca can be observed. Changes in the FEV_1 component of the pulmonary function tests is the most commonly used index of airflow obstruction. On chest radiographs, hyperinflation, flattening of diaphragms, increased retrosternal air space, and hyperlucency of the lungs are characteristic for this disease. (**Fig. 25-6**).

Smoking cessation, bronchodilators, and supplemental oxygen therapy are the most frequently prescribed maintenance treatments for emphysema. Approximately 30% of patients demonstrated an increase in FEV_1 of 15% or more following bronchodilator therapy. In smokers, the laboratory finding of polycythemia is frequently observed. With exacerbations of the disease, the sputum becomes purulent with an excessive number of neutrophils and a mixture of organisms on Gram stain. When this occurs, antibiotics and anti-inflammatory agents are indicated. In addition, mucolytics and phosphodiesterase inhibitors can also be considered.

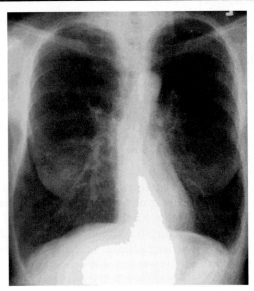

Figure 25-6 • Chest radiograph and associated radiographic changes in emphysema. Note the classic changes of flattening of the diaphragms and hyperlucency of the lungs.

In α_1-antitrypsin deficiency, available augmentation strategies include pharmacologic attempts to increase endogenous production of α_1-antitrypsin by the liver (e.g., tamoxifen). Administration of purified α_1-antitrypsin by repeated intravenous infusion or inhalation is also an option.

Individuals with cigarette smoking–related emphysema have a variable prognosis. One long-term study demonstrated a 40% 12-year survival rate in those with an initial FEV_1 of 1.25 L and approximately 5% for those with an initial FEV_1 of 0.75 L. Surgical treatment is reserved for the most severe forms of emphysema when other alternatives are exhausted without acceptable symptomatic relief. Bullectomy and lung volume reduction surgery are offered to patients when the presence of giant bullae can be confirmed with computed tomography, and significant improvement of postoperative exercise tolerance is expected. In end-stage lung disease where all traditional therapeutic modalities have failed, lung transplantation may be the only option.

Parkinson's Disease

This disease deserves separate mention as there are multiple perioperative concerns pertaining to its optimal management. Parkinson's disease is a disorder of the extrapyramidal system and is one of the most common neurodegenerative disease. Although the cause of Parkinson's disease is largely unknown, it has long been hypothesized that neurodegeneration is induced by genetic, environmental, or infectious disorders. Age is the single most consistent risk factor, and it has been estimated that Parkinson's disease affects approximately 3% of the population older than 66 years of age. In addition, more than 50% of individuals older than 85 years of age have some related symptoms of Parkinson's disease.

Parkinson's disease is characterized by the progressive depletion of selected neuronal populations, including those dopaminergic neurons of the substantia nigra of the basal ganglia (**Fig. 25-7**). Patients present with clinical signs when approximately 80% of dopaminergic activity is lost. Imbalance between the inhibitory actions of dopamine and the excitatory actions of acetylcholine lead to excessive thalamic inhibition with the classic triad of rigidity, resting tremor, and bradykinesis. These classic clinical features are not exclusive to Parkinson's disease and may be exhibited in other parkinsonian syndromes.

There is no one specific test to confirm the diagnosis Parkinson's disease; the diagnosis is made mainly on clinical grounds. The goal of treatment of Parkinson's disease is directed at allowing the patient to pursue normal daily activities. The mainstay of treatment is drug therapy using L-DOPA or dopamine receptor agonists. Surgical treatment of Parkinson's disease has been advocated with promising developments in recent years; namely, subthalamic deep brain stimulation and fetal mesencephalic tissue implantation have been shown to improve outcome in this condition in certain patient populations.

When anesthesia care is needed for these patients, aspiration prophylaxis and close monitoring for adequate perioperative respiratory function are paramount. The patient's usual drug regimen (i.e., drugs used to treat the Parkinson's symptoms) should be administered as close to the regular schedule as possible. Drugs that precipitate or exacerbate Parkinson's disease should be avoided, including phenothiazines, butyrophenones, and metoclopramide. If drug-induced extrapyramidal symptoms develop or sedation is required, diphenhydramine has been described as effective.

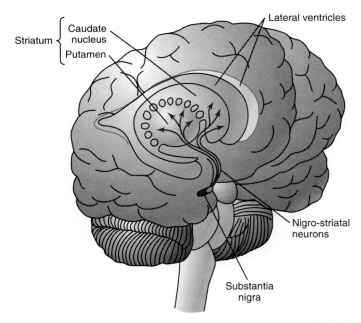

Figure 25-7 • Dopaminergic neurons of the basal ganglia become depleted in Parkinson's disease.

Concomitant autonomic nervous system dysfunction is common; thus, continuous intraoperative monitoring of hemodynamic parameters may be required, including both non-invasive and invasive techniques.

Dementia

Intellectual decline is one of the early hallmarks of dementia. There are major differences in the elderly regarding the level of intellectual functioning compared to their own baseline in early adulthood. In any patient with a known slowly progressive degenerative dementia, sudden changes in cognitive, behavioral, or health status may occur. Mental status is often a barometer of health in the patient with dementia, and abrupt changes necessitate a search for additional superimposed problems that may be occurring (**Table 25-2**). Perhaps the most important challenge in treating dementia is identifying the uncommon cases of reversible dementia such as chronic drug intoxication, vitamin deficiencies, subdural hematoma, major depression, normal pressure hydrocephalus, and hypothyroidism. Obviously, the management of such cases is aimed at diagnosing the underlying disease process.

Unfortunately, most cases of dementia, including degenerative brain diseases (i.e., Alzheimer's disease) and other common multi-infarct states, are incurable. This, however, does not mean that symptoms cannot be treated and ameliorated. The pharmacotherapy of dementia is tailored to the specific problems confronted such as behavioral and sleep disorders and prevention of further intellectual decline and neurodegeneration. Those treatments include vitamin E, nonsteroidal anti-inflammatory drugs, estrogen replacement, and centrally acting acetylcholinesterase inhibitors.

For the anesthesiologist, the challenges when taking care of the elderly patient with declining mental capacity are many. Perioperative interaction with patient and family should consider compromised ability to process general and medical information, and especially obtaining a true informed consent. Establishing and documenting baseline may become significant when encountering postoperative alteration of mental functioning. If acute deterioration is suspected, a neurology consultation with input from the patient's primary physician is advised.

A common problem in this age group is postoperative cognitive dysfunction. Cognition is defined as the mental processes of perception, memory, and information processing that allow the individual to acquire knowledge, solve problems, and plan for the future. It comprises the mental processes required for everyday living and should not be confused with intelligence.

Postoperative cognitive dysfunction is strongly associated with increasing age, and as many as one in every four elderly surgical patients may be affected. It is not related to perioperative hypotension or hypoxia and typically resolves by 3 months after surgery. It is usually expressed as a failure to perform simple cognitive tasks or to complete mental tasks. In the absence of cognitive testing, it may manifest as decreased activity during this period. Patients may be helped by recognition that the problem is genuine and reassured that it is likely to be transient.

Delirium

Characterized by an acute change in cognition and disturbances of consciousness, delirium usually results from an underlying medical condition, from medication, and, at times, drug withdrawal. Delirium affects 10% to 30% of hospitalized patients with medical illness. Following general anesthesia, the prevalence of delirium in the elderly has been reported to be between 10% and 15%. The associated morbidity and mortality make early and precise diagnosis of this condition extremely important (**Table 25-3**). It has been suggested that postoperative delirium and cognitive dysfunction are more likely to occur in patients with preoperative cognitive dysfunction. On this basis, one may consider that a Mini-Mental State Examination should be a part of preoperative assessment in the elderly. A low score and what it might represent may serve as an early warning to both hospital staff and family and possibly even decrease its likelihood by strict attention to the several possible causative factors in the perioperative period.

Patients with delirium can present with a variety of symptoms including agitation, somnolence, withdrawal, and

TABLE 25-2 Comparison of Different Central Nervous System Disorders			
Diagnosis	**Distinguishing Feature**	**Symptoms**	**Course**
Dementia	Memory impairment	Disorientation, agitation	Slow onset, progressive, chronic
Delirium	Fluctuating levels of consciousness, decreased attention	Disorientation, visual hallucination, agitation, apathy, withdrawal, memory and attention impairment	Acute; most cases remit with correction of underlying medical condition
Psychotic disorders	Deficit in reality testing	Social withdrawal, apathy	Slow onset with prodromal syndrome; chronic with exacerbations
Depression	Sadness, loss of interest and pleasure in usual activities	Disturbances of sleep, appetite, concentration; low energy; feelings of hopelessness and worthlessness; suicidal ideation	Single episode or recurrent episodes; may be chronic

TABLE 25-3 Components of Delirium

For delirium, a patient must show each of the features listed
- Disturbance of consciousness (i.e., reduced clarity of awareness about the environment) with reduced ability to focus, sustain, or shift attention
- A change in cognition (e.g., memory deficit, disorientation, language disturbance) or development of a perceptual disturbance that is not better accounted for by a preexisting, established, or evolving dementia
- The disturbance develops over a short period of time (usually hours to days) and tends to fluctuate during the course of a day
- Evidence from the history, physical examination, or laboratory findings indicates that the disturbance is caused by direct physiologic consequences of a general medical condition

psychosis. This variation in presentation can lead to diagnostic confusion and, in some cases, incorrect attribution of symptoms to a primary psychiatric disorder. To make the distinction, it is important to obtain the history of the onset and course of the condition from family members or caregivers. Without careful assessment, delirium can easily be confused with a number of primary psychiatric disorders because many of the signs and symptoms of delirium are also present in conditions such as dementia, depression, and psychosis.

Risk factors for delirium include advanced age (i.e., older than 70), underlying dementia, various comorbidities drugs, and electrolyte abnormalities.

Almost any acute illness, or an exacerbation of any chronic illness, may precipitate delirium (**Table 25-4**). Hospitalized patients with delirium demonstrated up to a 10-fold higher risk of developing other medical complications (including mortality), longer hospitalization, higher hospital costs, and increased need for long-term care after discharge.

Once identified, the organic disorder causing delirium must be treated. At every opportunity, staff and family members should help orient a person with delirium to time

TABLE 25-4 Factors That Can Precipitate Delirium

Drug use (especially when the drug is introduced or the dose is adjusted)
Electrolyte and physiologic abnormalities (e.g., hyponatremia, hypoxemia)
Lack of drugs (withdrawal)
Infection (especially urinary or respiratory infection)
Reduced sensory input (blindness, deafness, darkness, change in surroundings)
Intracranial problems (stroke, bleeding, meningitis, postictal state)
Urinary retention and fecal impaction
Myocardial problems (myocardial infarction, arrhythmia, heart failure)

and place. They should explain what is going on around the patient, including tests or treatments the person is about to receive. Behavioral control may be necessary to ensure patient comfort and safety. For acute control of delirium, 0.25 to 2 mg of oral haloperidol is the preferred treatment but diazepam, droperidol, and chlorpromazine are also often used with good results. Prompt correction of the underlying disorder causing delirium is essential to prevent permanent brain damage and may result in a complete recovery.

GERIATRIC ANESTHESIA STRATEGIES

One hundred years ago, the age of 50 (and certainly older) was considered a contraindication to surgical procedures. With advances in health care, pharmacology, and technology, a chronologic age contraindication for most surgical procedures no longer exists. However, normal age-related changes do increase the risks of perioperative complications and death due to an increased prevalence of age-related, concomitant disease.

Comprehensive preoperative evaluation of an elderly individual's health status can be very challenging. In the elderly, several factors make taking history more difficult and time-consuming than usual. For example, impaired hearing and vision can interfere with effective communication. Furthermore, it is important to separate the effects of aging per se from the consequences of age-related disease. Many elderly patients underreport potentially important symptoms because they consider these illnesses to be a normal consequence of aging. Baseline function in most elderly patients is sufficient to meet daily needs, but under conditions of physiologic stress, impairment in functional reserve may become evident.

It is evident that older surgical patients have significant comorbidities. Aging produces progressive fibrosis, loss of elasticity, and atrophy in virtually all tissues and organs. Anesthesiologists' knowledge of the physiology of aging affords early identification of any potential problems as well as effective prevention and treatment of complications during the perioperative period. Seemingly minor concerns can make a big difference when taking care of someone with multiple compromised organ systems and diminished reserves. Attention to detail is important for all anesthesiologists but rarely as important as it is when taking care of the extremes of age. The incidence of adverse drug effects is increased by age-related alterations in the pharmacokinetics and pharmacodynamics. Moreover, older patients are likely to be taking numerous drugs, and polypharmacy can result in undesirable drug interactions.

In the elderly, decreased skin elasticity increases the risk of injury from the use of various adhesive tapes. Adding a thin layer of cotton batting wrap before applying the noninvasive blood pressure cuff may be a simple but effective maneuver for the prevention of neurovascular complication. Another concern is a thinner layer of subcutaneous fat, which predisposes elderly patients to the potential for pressure sores. Protecting elderly patients' bony prominences, padding with pillows and arm-support devices is best achieved if it is a part of a systemic, uniform protocol.

Elderly patients are often dehydrated, reflecting a diminished sensation of thirst, reduced renal capacity to conserve water and sodium, and frequent use of diuretics. Because of decreased left ventricular compliance and limited β-adrenergic receptor responsiveness, these patients are predictably more prone to develop hypotension when volume depleted and congestive heart failure when hypervolemic. Prior to the induction of general anesthesia, a thorough assessment of intravascular volume status is essential. Elderly patients respond to hypothermia by shivering during the perioperative period, which results in increased oxygen demands. It is an especially pronounced concern in the presence of coronary disease or those with compromised cardiovascular reserve.

Appropriate thermoregulatory measures must be followed in order to conserve the patients' body heat and decrease their risks for hypothermia. Prolonged elimination of anesthetic agents and slower postoperative awakening also can occur as a result of poorly controlled intraoperative heat loss. Interventions available for protecting from hypothermia include increasing operating room temperature, using warm blankets or other warming devices to cover patients, administering heated anesthetic gas mixtures, and infusing warmed intravenous fluids.

Most general anesthetic agents depress cardiovascular function, which is why it is often advocated that regional anesthesia be employed in geriatric patients whenever possible. One further perceived advantage emphasizes that maintenance of consciousness during surgery permits prompt recognition of acute changes in cerebral function or the onset of cardiovascular derangement such as angina. The respective benefits of regional and general anesthesia were addressed by several meta-analyses. These studies failed to identify any meaningful difference in mortality and morbidity except for a clearly reduced incidence of deep venous thrombosis associated with regional anesthesia. There is some additional evidence that regional anesthesia may decrease intraoperative blood loss in certain subsets of surgical patients.

When administering an anesthetic, one must keep in mind the age-related circulatory, hepatic, and renal alterations as described earlier in this chapter. Decreased cardiac output may contribute to a slow onset of drug effects followed by prolonged action secondary to delayed clearance (i.e., barbiturates, benzodiazepines). There is no evidence that any specific inhaled or injected anesthetic drugs are preferable for induction and maintenance of anesthesia in elderly patients. However, some agents, because of their pharmacokinetic and pharmacodynamic properties, lend themselves better to the geriatric anesthesia population. One must keep in mind that minimal alveolar concentration of inhalation anesthetics decreases with age (4% for each decade after age 40), which parallels loss of neurons and decreased cerebral metabolism. Short-acting intravenous drugs and volatile anesthetics with lower partition coefficients provide the advantage of more rapid elimination, brisk emergence, and reorientation to the

patient's surroundings, and potentially lower incidence of confusion and delirium during recovery. However, the recovery of cognitive function, measured by the Mini-Mental State Examination, has not been shown to be different between various agents.

Most surgical morbidity and mortality, including myocardial ischemia, cerebrovascular events, renal insufficiency, pneumonia, and delirium, occur in the postoperative period. The most common morbidity following noncardiac surgery is respiratory complications. The incidence of postoperative hypoxia is 20% to 60% in the elderly. Diminished laryngeal protective reflexes, declining hypoxic and hypercarbic drive, reduced respiratory muscle strength, and an increased ventilation-perfusion mismatch are all potential contributors to this increase in morbidity. Additionally, apnea and hypoventilation following administration of narcotics and sedatives are more common in the aging population. Poor respiratory effort secondary to pain may further increase the likelihood of respiratory complications. As a result of these respiratory changes, increased use of supplemental oxygen therapy, pulse oximetry, and capnography are essential components in anesthesia for the elderly.

The same basic principles that guide acute pain management in the general population apply to the geriatric group. However, optimal analgesia for elderly individuals is more pressing because they might receive the most potential harm as well as the greatest potential benefit from improved control of postoperative pain. Because of common ischemic heart disease and diminished pulmonary capacity, the elderly patient is more vulnerable to the physiologic consequences of inadequate analgesia and to the side effects of various analgesics.

The postoperative catabolic state is more detrimental for elderly patients as they have decreased nutritional reserve; this process is exaggerated when pain control is suboptimal. Finally, acute pain management in the elderly may have a major effect on rehabilitation and subsequent functional status. Early ambulation is encouraged in an effort to decrease the incidence of thromboembolic complications.

ETHICAL CHALLENGES IN GERIATRIC ANESTHESIA AND PALLIATIVE CARE

Essential ethical principles are identical in all adult patient populations. Common challenges include patient autonomy, surrogate decision making, and do-not-resuscitate status in the hospital and in the operating room. The ultimate decision of what medical therapy is to be employed rests with the patient. The legal doctrine embodying this principle is the informed consent. Essential criteria for informed consent include providing sufficient information, patient competence, and voluntary decision making (**Table 25-5**). Patients with possible dementia should be referred for competency evaluations to assess mental functioning and decision-making capacity. When the patient is mentally too compromised, a surrogate is identified based on a living will or a durable power of attorney. Each state has a legal hierarchy to appoint

TABLE 25-5 Essential Elements of Informed Consent
Sufficient information for patient
Competence of consenter
Voluntary decision making without pressure

TABLE 25-6 Definition of Palliative Care by the World Health Organization
Affirms life and regards dying as a normal process
Neither hastens nor postpones death
Provides relief from pain and other distressing symptoms
Integrates the psychological and spiritual aspects of patient care
Offers a support system to help the family cope during the patient's illness and their own bereavement

a proxy decision maker if these documents are not available to guide the process.

Cause and prognosis of cardiac arrest and the success rate of resuscitation is markedly different if it happens in the operating room. However, informed consent (or informed refusal) of medical intervention is guided by the same moral principles during end-of-life care, regardless of location. However, to ensure that institutional legal guidelines are followed, please refer to your institution's protocols and policies regarding do-not-resuscitate status in the operating room and postanesthetic care unit. For high-risk surgical procedures, comprehensive discussions of patient's preferences are well advised.

It is established in the medical literature that a significant portion of the elderly, cancer patients in particular, experience pain and discomfort of various origins during the last years of their life. Palliative care is gaining more recognition, especially in the industrially developed aging societies. Palliative medicine is defined as the all-inclusive care of patients whose disease is not responsive to curative treatment (**Table 25-6**). This requires a multidisciplinary approach to treat symptoms, control pain, and address the psychological, social, and spiritual needs of the patient and his or her family. By training, anesthesiologists are invaluable experts of pharmacologic and procedural pain management. These modalities are key pieces of successful palliative care.

SUMMARY

Aging is a multifactorial, all-encompassing process. It produces a gradual decline in the functional reserve of most of the body's major organ systems, thereby resulting in a decreased capacity for adaptation. Aging is not a disease but carries an increased potential for development of various age-related pathologies. Therefore, there is no one "ideal anesthetic" for the elderly patient. A sound understanding of the aging-related physiologic changes and the altered pharmacokinetic and pharmacodynamic responses of these patients helps to design and implement the optimal anesthetic for these elderly patients. Since this patient subset is not only physiologically but also physically fragile, they require special attention throughout the perioperative process to prolong their life span and maintain good function and quality of living including the incorporation of their wishes regarding end-of-life issues.

KEY POINTS

- As the age of the population increases, a thorough appreciation of age-appropriate anesthetic concerns will allow the provision of optimal perioperative care.

- Aging is not a disease, but the incidence of various morbidities increases in the elderly.

- The correlation of calendar age and physiologic age is variable and can be significantly different in some individuals.

- A thorough exploration of medical history, combined with a detailed examination and sound understanding of age-related physiologic alterations, allows the foundation providing for optimal medical care in this population.

REFERENCES

Alagiakrishnan K, Wiens CA: An approach to drug induced delirium in the elderly. Postgrad Med J 2004;80:388–393.

Altman RD, Lozada CJ: Clinical features of osteoarthritis. In Hochberg MC, Silman AJ, Smolen JS, et al (eds): Practical Rheumatology. Philadelphia, Mosby, 2004, pp 503–510.

Bodis-Wollner I: Visualizing the next steps in Parkinson disease. Arch Neurol 2002;59:1233–1234.

Desai AK, Grossberg GT: Diagnosis and treatment of Alzheimer's disease. Neurology 2005;64:S34–S39.

Fabbri LM, Luppi F, Beghe B: Update in chronic obstructive pulmonary disease 2005. Am J Respir Crit Care Med 2006;173:1056–1065.

Hanning CD: Postoperative cognitive dysfunction. Br J Anaesth 2005;95:82–87.

Hogenmiller MS, Lozada CJ: An update on osteoarthritis therapeutics. Curr Opin Rheumatol 2006;18:256–260.

Kaduszkiewicz H, Zimmermann T, Beck-Bornholdt HP: Cholinesterase inhibitors for patients with Alzheimer's disease: Systematic review of randomised clinical trials. BMJ 2005;331:321–327.

Kenny AM, Prestwood KM: Osteoporosis. Pathogenesis, diagnosis, and treatment in older adults. Rheum Dis Clin North Am 2000;26:569–591.

Mannino DM, Watt G, Hole D: The natural history of chronic obstructive pulmonary disease. Eur Respir J 2006;27:627–643.

Pahwa R, Wilkinson SB, Overman J, Lyons KE: Bilateral subthalamic stimulation in patients with Parkinson disease: Long-term follow up. J Neurosurg 2003;99:71–77.

Papi A, Luppi F, Franco F: Pathophysiology of exacerbations of chronic obstructive pulmonary disease. Proc Am Thorac Soc 2006;3:245–251.

Price CC, Garvan CW, Monk TG: Neurocognitive performance in older adults with postoperative cognitive dysfunction. Anesthesiology 2003;99:A50.

Rasmussen LS, Johnson T, Kuipers HM, et al: Does anaesthesia cause postoperative cognitive dysfunction? A randomised study of regional versus general anaesthesia in 438 elderly patients. Acta Anaesthesiol Scand 2003;47:260–266.

Sethi KD: Clinical aspects of Parkinson disease. Curr Opin Neurol 2002;15:457–460.

Vestbo J: Clinical assessment, staging, and epidemiology of chronic obstructive pulmonary disease exacerbations. Proc Am Thorac Soc 2006;3:252–256.

Watts NB: Treatment of osteoporosis with bisphosphonates. Rheum Dis Clin North Am 2001;27:197–214.

Weldon C, Mahla ME, Van der Aa MT, Monk TG: Advancing age and deeper intraoperative anesthetic levels are associated with higher first year death rates. Anesthesiology 2002; 97(Suppl):A1097.

INDEX

Note: Page numbers followed by *b* indicate boxes; *f*, figures; *t*, tables.

A

AAI pacing, 83
Abdominal aortic aneurysm, 143–145
Abdominal wall defects, in neonates, 594–596, 595*t*
Aberrant left pulmonary artery, 59–60
Abnormal presentations in delivery, 567–568
Abruptio placentae, 564*t*, 565–566
Absent pulmonic valve, 60
Acanthocytosis, 409–410
ACE inhibitors. *See* Angiotensin-converting enzyme inhibitors.
Acetaminophen, in porphyria patients, 316*t*
Acetaminophen overdose, 262, 549
Acetylcholine receptors, in myasthenia gravis, 450, 451*f*, 453
N-acetylcysteine, for renal failure, 328
Achondroplasia, 460–461
Acid-base balance, 359
Acid-base disorders, 359–363
Acidosis
    metabolic, 346, 361–362
    respiratory, 360–361, 361*t*
    systemic, 359–360, 360*t*
Acoustic neuroma, 207
Acquired cardiomyopathy, 115*t*
Acquired immunodeficiency syndrome (AIDS)
    anesthesia management in, 491–492
    overview of, 488–489
    pneumonia in, 483, 489
    pregnancy and, 492
    renal insufficiency in, 341
    tuberculosis in, 490
Acromegaly, 402–403
ACTH. *See* Corticotropin (ACTH).
Activated partial thromboplastin, 418
Acute arterial occlusion, 147–148
Acute back pain, 462
Acute cholecystitis, 274–275
Acute coronary syndrome, 5–7
Acute epiglottitis, 612–614, 613*t*
Acute fatty liver of pregnancy, 272–273

Acute heart failure, 105, 112–114. *See also* Heart failure.
Acute hemorrhagic stroke, 217–220
Acute HIV infection, 489
Acute idiopathic polyneuritis, 254–255, 255*t*
Acute intermittent porphyria, 315
Acute intrinsic restrictive lung disease, 177
Acute liver failure, 272–273, 272*t*
Acute pancreatitis, 291–292
Acute pericarditis, 125–126
Acute porphyria, 314–315
Acute renal failure (ARF)
    in cancer patients, 505
    cardiovascular complications of, 327
    complications of, 327
    definition of, 325
    diagnosis of, 327
    drug dosing and, 328–329, 329*t*
    gastrointestinal complications of, 327
    incidence of, 325–326, 326*t*
    in nephrotic syndrome, 341
    neurologic complications, 327
    risk factors, 327
    signs and symptoms, 327
    treatment of, 327–328
Acute respiratory distress syndrome (ARDS)
    alveolar overdistention in, 189–190
    barotrauma and, 189
    complications of, 188–189
    corticosteroids for, 187
    diagnosis of, 185, 185*f*
    epidemiology of, 184–185, 185*t*
    fluid intake and, 187
    infection in, 189
    monitoring in, 189–191, 190*t*
    pathogenesis of, 184–185, 185*t*
    signs and symptoms, 185
    treatment of, 186–188
Acute stroke, 216–217
Acute-colonic pseudo-obstruction, 295–296
Acyanotic congenital heart disease, 44–50, 45*f*
    See also Congenital heart disease.
Addiction, in anesthesiologists, 545

Adenocarcinoma, overview of, 508–509
Adenosine
    in angina pectoris, 2
    in antidromic AV nodal reentrant tachycardia, 72
    for dysrhythmia, 79
    in heart disease imaging, 3
    in supraventricular tachycardia, 66
Adenosine deaminase deficiency, 525
ADH. *See* Vasopressin.
Adhesive capsulitis, 462
Adrenal cortex, 393–394
Adrenal gland, 393–394
Adrenal gland dysfunction, 393–398
Adrenal insufficiency
    in cancer, 505
    overview of, 396–398, 397*t*
Age
    aortic stenosis and, 36
    breast cancer and, 511
    heart disease and, 1, 2*t*
    pregnancy and advanced maternal, 573
Aging
    cardiovascular system in, 638–639
    immune system in, 640
    nervous system in, 638
    physiology of, 638–640, 639*f*
    public health and, 637–638, 638*f*
    respiratory system in, 639
AIDS. *See* Acquired immunodeficiency syndrome (AIDS).
Airway secretion clearance, 176
ALA synthetase. *See* Aminolevulinic acid (ALA) synthetase.
Albumin, in malnutrition, 311
Alcohol. *See also* Cirrhosis.
    abuse, 539–541
    γ-aminobutyric acid receptors and, 540
    delirium tremens and, 541
    intoxicated patients, 271
    overdose, 540
    pregnancy and, 541, 573
    Wernicke-Korsakoff syndrome and, 541
    withdrawal, 540–541